Complete Review of

Pathology

& Hematology for NBE

Covering 2500+ Qs with Explanations, 100+ IBQs & 1000+ Colored Illustrations/Images

Fully Updated from Robbin's 10/e (Basic Edition), Robbin's 9/e,
Wintrobe's 13/e, Sternberg's 6/e, Ackerman's 11/e, WHO 2015 Lung,
WHO 2016 Male Genital System and WHO 2017 CNS/Hematopoietic Classifications

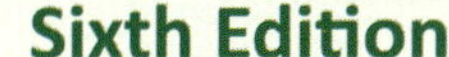

Sixth Edition

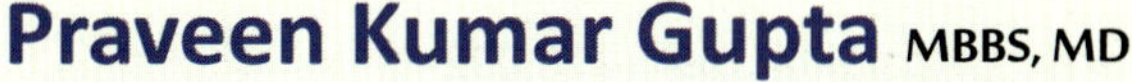

Praveen Kumar Gupta MBBS, MD

MBBS (Honours), Medical College and Hospital, Kolkata, West Bangal
MD, Ex Senior Resident (Laboratory Medicine), AIIMS, New Delhi

Consultant Pathologist & Lab Head
Primus Super Speciality Hospital, New Delhi

Vandana Puri MBBS, MD (Pathology), DNB (Pathology), MNAMS

MBBS, CMC, Coimbatore, Tamil Nadu
MD & Ex SR Lady Hardinge Medical College, New Delhi
Ex SRA, Hematology, AIIMS, New Delhi
Ex Assistant Professor, UCMS, New Delhi

Associate Professor
Department of Pathology
Lady Hardinge Medical College, New Delhi

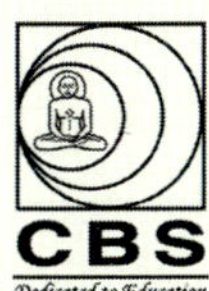

CBS Publishers & Distributors Pvt Ltd

• New Delhi • Bengaluru • Chennai • Kochi • Kolkata • Mumbai
• Hyderabad • Nagpur • Patna • Pune • Vijayawada

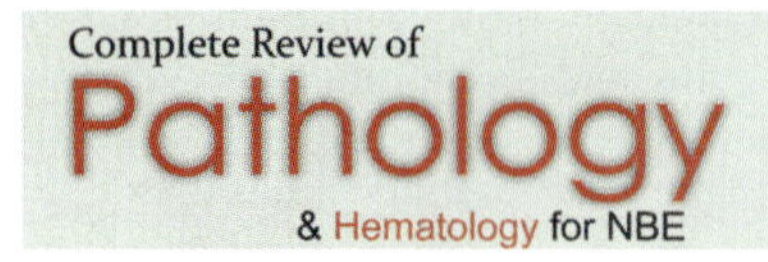

ISBN: 978-81-945783-3-8

Sixth Edition: 2020
Fifth Edition: 2019-20
Fourth Edition: 2018

Published by **Satish Kumar Jain** and produced by **Varun Jain** for

CBS Publishers and Distributors Pvt Ltd

4819/XI Prahlad Street, 24 Ansari Road, Daryaganj, New Delhi 110 002, India.

Ph: 23289259, 23266861, 23266867   Website: www.cbspd.com

Fax: 011-23243014

e-mail: delhi@cbspd.com; cbspubs@airtelmail.in.

Corporate Office: 204 FIE, Industrial Area, Patparganj, Delhi 110 092

Ph: +91-11-4934 4934 Fax: 4934 4935

e-mail: feedback@cbspd.com; bhupesharora@cbspd.com

Branches

- ***Bengaluru:*** Seema House 2975, 17th Cross, K.R. Road, Banasankari 2nd Stage, Bengaluru 560 070, Karnataka
  Ph: +91-80-26771678/79   Fax: +91-80-26771680   e-mail: bangalore@cbspd.com
- ***Chennai:*** No. 7, Subbaraya Street, Shenoy Nagar, Chennai 600 030, Tamil Nadu
  Ph: +91-44-26680620, 26681266   Fax: +91-44-42032115   e-mail: chennai@cbspd.com
- ***Kochi:*** 68/1534, 35, 36-Power House Road, Opp. KSEB, Cochin-682018, Kochi, Kerala
  Ph: +91-484-4059061-65   Fax: +91-484-4059065   e-mail: kochi@cbspd.com
- ***Kolkata:*** 6/B, Ground Floor, Rameswar Shaw Road, Kolkata-700014 (West Bengal)
  Ph: +91-33-22891126, 22891127, 22891128   e-mail: kolkata@cbspd.com
- ***Mumbai:*** 83-C, Dr E Moses Road, Worli, Mumbai-400018, Maharashtra
  Ph: +91-22-24902340/41   Fax: +91-22-24902342   e-mail: mumbai@cbspd.com

Representatives

- **Hyderabad**   +91-9885175004
- **Pune**   +91-9623451994
- **Patna**   +91-9334159340
- **Vijayawada** +91-9000660880

Printed At : Goyal Offset Works (P) Limited

Dedicated to

My parents for their love and support, my loving wife Dr Meenakshi and cute little angel Myra, it is a privilege to share my life and love with you.

Dr Praveen Kumar Gupta

My soulmate Dr Shakti Tiwari, my kids Arsh and Amaira, my parents for their unconditional support and my teachers and students for their inspiration, love and guidance.

Dr Vandana Puri

Dr Praveen Kr Gupta, *MBBS, MD,* is presently working as Consultant Pathologist and Lab Head at Primus Super Speciality Hospital, New Delhi. He did his MBBS from Medical College and Hospital, Kolkata, West Bengal and MD as well as Senior Residency from the prestigious All India Institute of Medical Sciences, New Delhi. He has an excellent academic record and has been the recipient of many awards in various states and national level competitions in Clinical Pathology and Hematology. He has authored several books, including the popular AIIMS PGMEE series and has many National and International publications to his name. Teaching is his passion and he is well known for his emphasis on concept building and focused learning. He is the co-founder of "AIM4AIIMS-PG" group, which has been mentoring and guiding over 50,000 PG aspirants all over the country. It gives us immense pleasure to announce the release of Pathology App by Dr Praveen Kr Gupta, which will aid many students all over the country to understand the basic concepts of pathology. This is available on Android and IOS and can be bought for a nominal cost.

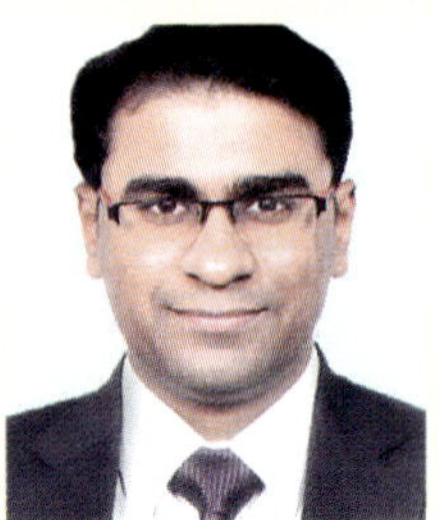

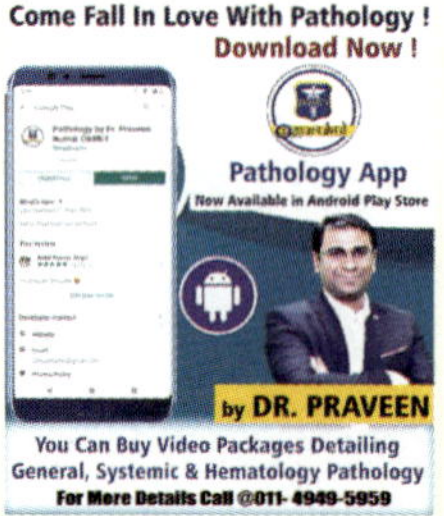

Join Author's **Facebook Discussion Group** – www.facebook.com/Pathology by Dr Praveen or
https://www.facebook.com/groups/390769121404969/ or

Dr Vandana Puri, *MBBS, MD (Pathology), DNB (Pathology), MNAMS,* is presently working as Associate Professor Pathology at Lady Hardinge Medical College and Associated Hospitals, New Delhi. She did her MBBS from Coimbatore Medical College, Coimbatore, Tamil Nadu, India. Following this, she pursued her MD and Senior Residency in Pathology from Lady Hardinge Medical College, New Delhi. She did her Senior Research Associateship in Hematology from AIIMS, New Delhi. Before joining Lady Hardinge Medical College, she had worked as Assistant Professor in Department of Pathology, University College of Medical Sciences and GTB Hospital, Delhi. She has more than 40 International and National Publications to her name. Besides, she has been co-author of important chapters in many National and International books. She has vast teaching experience and she orients the students in concept building in advanced pathology by making them understand the basics of pathology. She has more than 54,000 student followers at her Facebook group "Dr Vandana Pathology Study Circle" who are regularly benefitted and updated by discussions. She is also author of book-PICS (*coming soon*) and has both android and iOS apps with DocTutorials where in you can subscribe for pathology. You can sign up both on apps and website too (www.doctutorials.com)

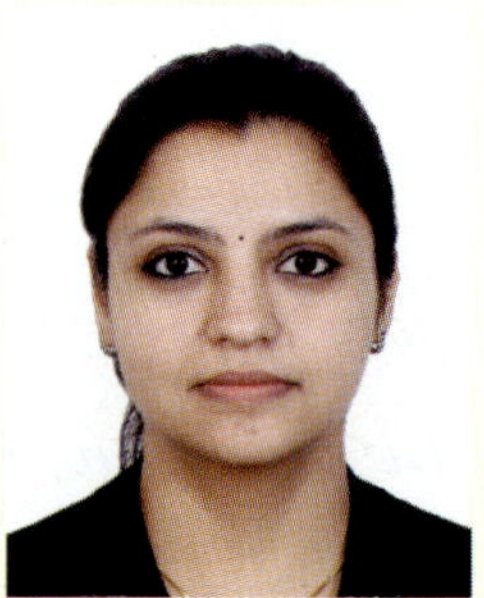

Follow authors you tube channel and Facebook group
https://www.youtube.com/channel/UCrYYtBBSscRAhAaUyMJTKpA or

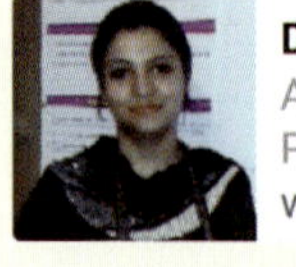

&

https://www.Facebook.com/groups/1444287919221567/ or

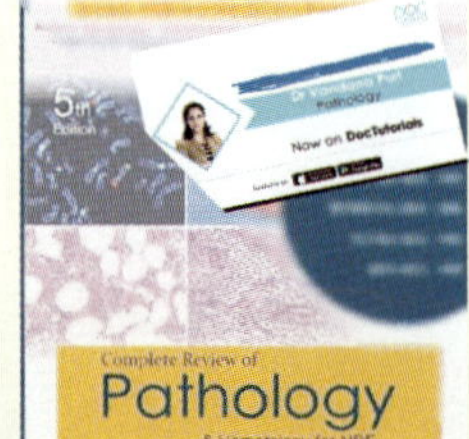

Join Author's **Facebook Discussion Group** – www.facebook.com/Dr Vandana Pathology study circle

Preface

"The best way to predict your future is to create it."

Abraham Lincoln

Achieving **success in Postgraduate Medical Entrance Exams (PGMEE)** and to be able to pursue a specialty of choice in the premier medical institutes of the country has been the ultimate dream of every medical student. To make this dream a reality—**a belief in self, setting realistic goals, 'intelligent hard work', 'smart and productive studying'** and **selection of the right study material** are some of the very important factors.

To cover more than 15 subjects of medical curriculum in a limited time span is definitely not an easy task, however it's not impossible.

As, **impossible itself says I'm possible!**

It is very important to **strengthen your fundamentals and get your basics right! Pathology is the backbone of medical science.** One cannot understand clinical subjects, like **Medicine, Surgery, Pediatrics** and **Gynecology** without being well-versed with the basic pathology of diseases. By the time a student appears for any PGMEE, usually during or after internship, preclinical subjects, like **Pathology tend to fade away from the memory** as the clinical subjects largely dominate the mind.

In the recent NBE pattern examinations, **25–30 MCQs out of 300** are being asked from core pathology. Most of the MCQs asked from Medicine and Surgery also have one or two options related to Pathology, which makes contribution of **50–60 MCQs from pathology; which is almost 15–20% of any examination. In AIIMS Nov 2015 exam, there were over 60 Image-based Questions** which re-emphasized the importance of conceptual learning with figures rather than nearly solving repeats.

Solving recent NBE based, AIIMS, PGI and other state entrance exam questions not only requires **mastery over the repeated MCQs** but also **thorough knowledge** of topics with **special emphasis on concepts and high-yielding facts**.

For the first time AIIMS New Pattern 2019 Model Questions have been added to ace your preparation practice before upcoming AIIMS examination. Chapter-wise NEXT Pattern Qs have been added as per the changing scenario of upcoming examination.

With so many MCQ-based guidebooks flooding the market, there was a felt need for a book on Pathology which is *student friendly, lucid, interesting, not full of big paragraphs loaded with heavy information, but which covers all topics and relevant information that can be revised in limited time and is updated with all recent facts and advances.*

This book is useful **not only** for the students preparing for various PGME exams, but also for the **undergraduate students and pathology students pursuing postgraduation**, it will also help in concept building as well as **quick revision**.

Praveen Kumar Gupta

Vandana Puri

Highlights of 6th edition

The overwhelming response by the students and 100% Pathology (including many Medicines, Pediatrics) MCQs from AIIMS, PGI, JIPMER and NEET entrance exams from this book made it a roaring sensation in the market. It gives us immense pleasure to bring to you the sixth edition of Complete Review of Pathology & Hematology with fully revised content, most recent updates, recent questions, high-yield points and annexures.

- **Pretexts:** Detailed yet concise, pointwise overview of the entire topic. High-yielding MCQs and repeated MCQs have been highlighted.

- **Flow charts:** Flow diagrams have been added wherever necessary for easy understanding including most updated points from recent editions of books. New chapters on "Diseases of Muscle and Tumors of Bones and Joints" have been added. Over 80 new labelled and explained images have been added for proper explanation of texts and better understanding of Image-Based Questions.

- **Recent updates:** All additions and changes are according to latest Robbin's 10th edition and are highlighted separately, so that students are updated with recent advances in relevant topics. These are potential MCQs in upcoming PGMEEs.

- **MCQs:** All MCQs of NBE pattern up to January 2020, AIIMS up to November 2019, PGI up to December 2019 and JIPMER up to November 2019 have been included, and the recent Qs have been highlighted separately. MCQs have been arranged chronologically with recent ones coming earlier, so that more stress is put on recent pattern questions. Repeated MCQs have been clubbed together to avoid unnecessary duplication and time wastage.

- **AIIMS new pattern 2019 model questions:** Since you all must be aware that AIIMS PG exam has announced new patterns of MCQs from this session onwards, we have added many new pattern Qs including "match the following, arrange in sequence, reason and assertion and concept-based multiple answers" in the current edition to benefit the aspiring students.

- **Image-based MCQs:** As PGMEEs have shifted to online CBT exams, there has been an increase in image-based questions. We have included potential image-based MCQs at the end of every topic to familiarize the students with the same. Students can learn identification points of images from the pretext and then quickly answer Image-based Questions for strong hold in subject.

- **Video-based questions have been added to cater recent AIIMS pattern.**

- **Authentic explanations:** Explanations from standard and recent edition textbooks have been provided for each answer. Difficult and controversial MCQs have been explained in detail discussing each option and excluding the incorrect ones. This will help a student to develop his/her analytical skills.

- **Annexures:** A new Annexure on Autoantibodies in Autoimmune Disease has been added for quick revision.

- **NEXT pattern questions** have been added.

Although utmost care has been taken to avoid all possible errors, some minor errors might have crept in inadvertently. We request the readers to kindly point out the same and give their valuable suggestions or feedback on the address provided in About the Authors page.

We wish you all the very best for your upcoming exams and for your bright future!

Acknowledgements

Firstly, we would like to express our eternal gratitude to the blessings of Almighty GOD. We thank our parents for their blessings, everlasting love and support.

We wish to sincerely thank our teachers and faculty for being the source of our inspiration and knowledge, and who helped us to achieve a lot in our personal and professional lines:

- Prof Manjula Jain-ex. Director Professor, Department of Pathology, LHMC
- Prof AK Mukhopadhyay-Professor & Head, Department of Laboratory Medicine, AIIMS
- Prof Sunita Sharma-Director Professor and Head, Department of Pathology, LHMC
- Prof Renu Saxena-Head of Department, Department of Hematology, AIIMS
- Prof Usha Rusia-Previous Head of Department, Department of Pathology, UCMS
- Prof Meera Sikka -Head of Department, Department of Pathology, UCMS
- Prof Sarman Singh-Professor, Department of Laboratory Medicine, AIIMS
- Prof M Irshad-Professor, Department of Laboratory Medicine, AIIMS
- Prof Kiran Agarwal-Director Professor, Department of Pathology, LHMC
- Prof Shilpi Agarwal-Director Professor, Department of Pathology, LHMC
- Prof Anita Nangia-Director Professor, Department of Pathology, LHMC
- Prof Shailja Shukla-Director Professor, Department of Pathology, LHMC
- Dr Sonal Sharma & Dr Mrinalini Kotru-Professor, Department of Pathology, UCMS
- Dr Subhadra Sharma, Purva Mathur & Dr Arulselvi S-Associate Professor, Department of Laboratory Medicine, AIIMS
- Dr Sangeeta Pahuja & Dr Smita Singh-Associate Professor, Department of Pathology, LHMC
- Dr Mukta Pujani-Associate Professor, Department of Pathology, ESI Medical College, Faridabad
- Dr Venkateswaran Iyer (Associate Professor), Dr Prasenjit Das, Dr Sudip Arava, Dr Soumya (Assistant Professor) Department of Pathology, AIIMS, Prateek Bhatia (Asst Professor, PGI, Chandigarh), Dr Manupriya Nain (Assistant Professor, Hindu Rao Hospital)
- Dr Gaurav Chabbra, Dr Sudip Datta, Dr Raghavendra L, Dr Shyam Prakash-Assistant Professor, Lab Medicine, AIIMS

A special thanks to *Dr Meenakshi (Dr Praveen's wife) for her immense motivation and support. She has been instrumental in conceptualization, formatting and designing of our book.*

We thank our friends/students/well-wishers, for their invaluable contribution & support in writing this book

- Dr Shakti Tiwari-Consultant Anesthetist, Sant Parmanand Hospital (Dr Vandana's husband)
- Dr Sawan Kumar-Consultant Pathologist, Primus Hospital, New Delhi, Dr Apoorv Singh (MBBS, AIIMS)
- Dr Zainab Vora, Dr Ravi Sharma, Dr Amit Gupta, Dr Anil Shekhwat (AIIMS, New Delhi)
- Dr Param Prakash, Postgraduate Resident, LHMC for helping in framing of NEXT Pattern Questions

We are also grateful to our following well-wishers, whose ideas and suggestions have helped us immensely

- Dr Akhilesh Raj Jhamad, Dr Rajat Jain, Dr Vivek Jain, Dr Thameem Saif, Dr Mukesh Bhatia, Dr Vineet, Dr Nachiketa Bhatia, Dr Apurv Mehra, Dr Sourav Bhatia, Dr Shashwat Ray, Dr Manish Soni, Dr Ashish, Dr Sonu Panwar, Dr Surendra Nath Reddy, Dr Rajeswar Gudadhe, Dr Ashwini, Dr Saurabh Bhatia, Dr Sidharth Sekhar Mishra, Mr Dhruv, Mr Amit Bhatia, Mr Rajiv, Mr Roshan, Dr T Piyush, Dr Kumar Sarvottam, Dr Pritesh Singh, Dr Manjunatha A.

We are extending our special thanks to **Mr Satish Kumar Jain** (Chairman) and **Mr Varun Jain** (Managing Director), M/s CBS Publishers and Distributors Pvt Ltd for their wholehearted support in publication of this book. We have no words to describe the role, efforts, inputs and initiatives undertaken by **Mr Bhupesh Arora** (Vice President - Publishing & Marketing, PGMEE and Nursing Division) for helping and motivating us.

We sincerely thank the entire CBS team for bringing out the book with utmost care and attractive presentation. We would like to thank Dr Mrinalini Bakshi (Editorial Head & Content Strategist) for her editorial support and Ms Nitasha Arora (Production Head & Content Strategist), Dr Anju Dhir (Project Manager & Senior Scientific Coordinator), Mr Shivendu Bhushan Pandey (Senior Editor), Mr Ashutosh Pathak (Senior Proof Reader) and all the production team members Mr Chaman Lal, Mr Prakash Gaur, Mr Phool Kumar, Mr Bunty Kashyap, Ms Tahira Parveen, Ms Manorama Gupta, Ms Babita Verma, Mr Chander Mani, Mr Raju Sharma, Mr Manoj Chaudhary, Mr Vikram Chaudhary, Mr Manoj Malakar, Mr Arun Kumar and Mr Rahul Negi for devoting laborious hours in designing and typesetting of the book.

Contents

ANNEXURES

1. CELL AS A UNIT OF HEALTH AND DISEASE

2. CELL ADAPTATION, INJURY AND DEATH

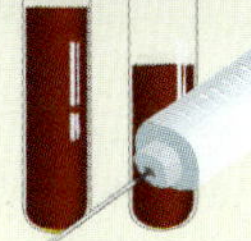

21. CENTRAL NERVOUS SYSTEM AND ITS DISORDERS

22. BLOOD BANKING AND TRANSFUSION MEDICINE

23. TUMORS OF SOFT TISSUE & HEAD & NECK

24. DISEASES OF MUSCLES

25. TUMORS OF BONE AND JOINTS

26. RECENT TECHNIQUES IN PATHOLOGY

27. STAINS AND FIXATIVES

Recent Pattern Questions 2020 at a Glance

1. Histological picture of a lesion excised from the right cervical region is shown below. What is your diagnosis?

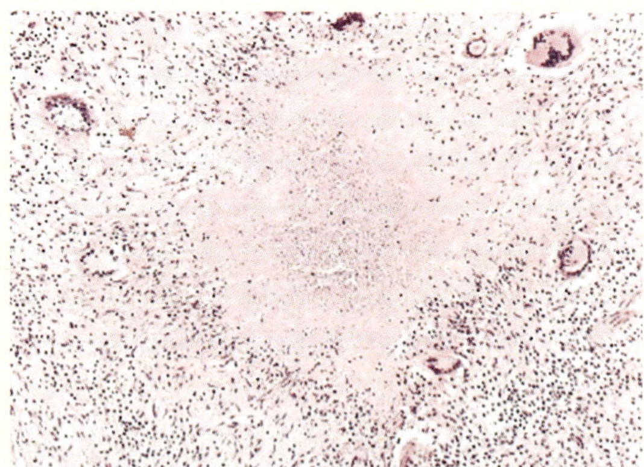

   a. Necrotizing granulomatous inflammation
   b. Neurofibroma
   c. Schwannoma
   d. Hodgkin lymphoma

2. Which of the following has a major role in thrombus formation?
   a. Endothelial injury
   b. Vasoconstriction
   c. Platelet activation
   d. Coagulation cascade

3. Mutation in DNA Helicase causes
   a. Wermer syndrome
   b. Werner syndrome
   c. Sipple syndrome
   d. Autoimmune lymphoproliferative syndrome

4. Which of the following mode of inheritance is shown below?

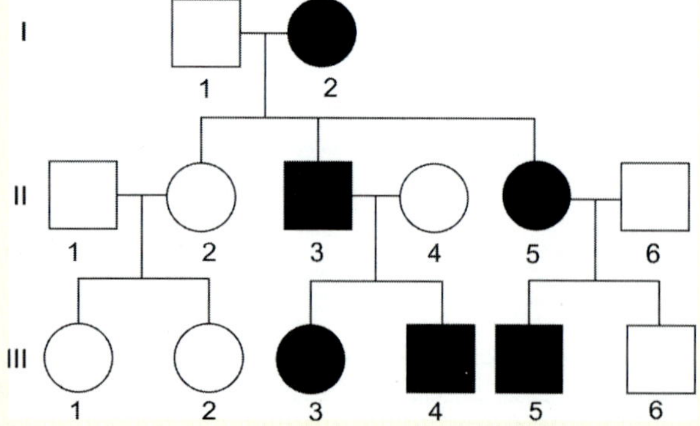

   a. AD
   b. AR
   c. X linked dominant
   d. X linked recessive

5. An 8-year-old child presented with history of recurrent infections. The child had rashes. Investigations revealed low platelets. What could be the probable cause?
   a. Job syndrome
   b. Wiskott-Aldrich syndrome
   c. Henoch-Schonlein purpura
   d. Hyper IgM syndrome

6. B cells are induced to produce IgE by which of the following?
   a. IL 2   b. IL 4
   c. IL 1   d. IL 6

7. Graft between Identical twins is:
   a. Allograft   b. Xenograft
   c. Isograft   d. Autograft

8. Identify the parasite in the intestinal biopsy of a HIV positive patient.

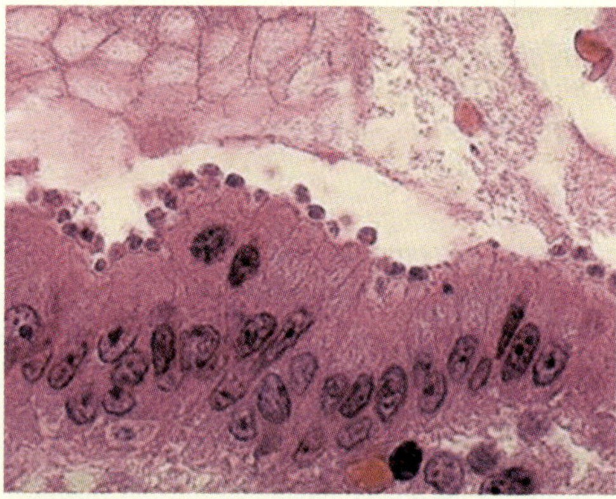

   a. Giardia   b. CMV
   c. Amoebic colitis   d. Cryptosporidium

9. A 75-year-old male, known smoker presented to pulmonology department with history of cough. Biopsy was taken which showed the following. What is the change shown?

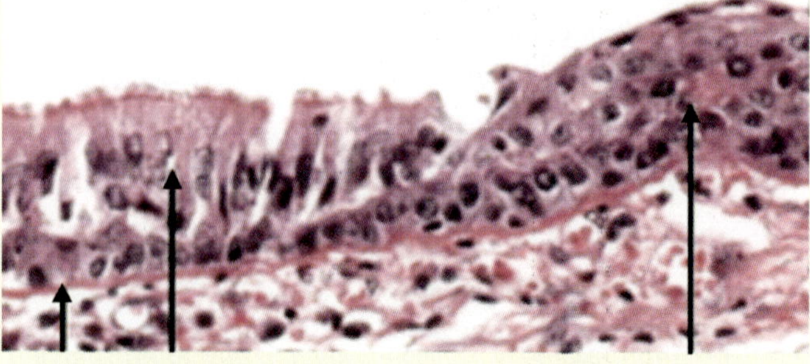

   a. Dysplasia   b. Metaplasia
   c. Hyperplasia   d. Atrophy

Ans.

1. a
2. a
3. b
4. a
5. b
6. b
7. c
8. d
9. b

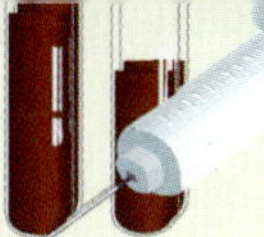

10. **Cardiac biopsy of a patient who died following myocardial infarction is shown below. What is the finding is a feature of reperfusion injury?**

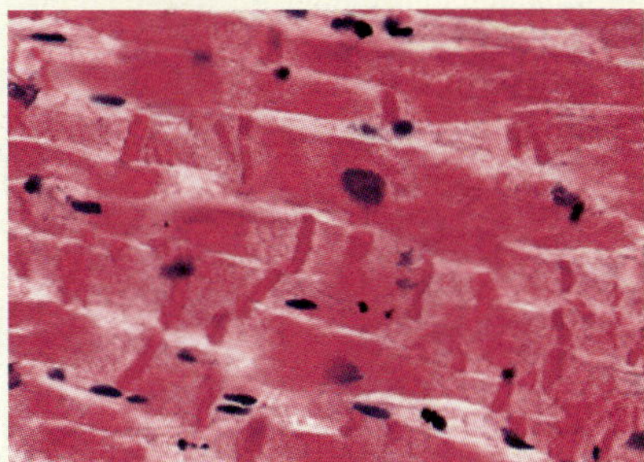

   a. Waviness of fibers
   b. Neutrophils in cardiac muscle
   c. Eosinophilic contraction bands
   d. Swelling of cells

11. **Bulky friable vegetations are seen in:**
   a. Rheumatic carditis
   b. Infective endocarditis
   c. Libman sack's endocarditis
   d. Non-bacterial thrombotic endocarditis

12. **Histological picture of a lesion excised from the right cervical region is shown below. What is your diagnosis?**

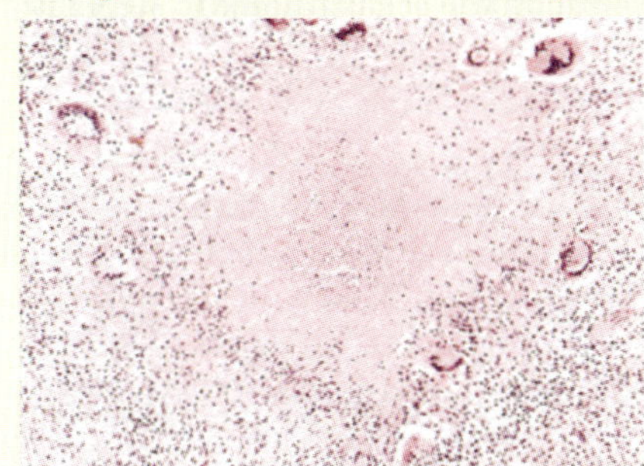

   a. Necrotizing granulomatous inflammation
   b. Neurofibroma
   c. Schwannoma
   d. Hodgkin lymphoma

13. **A 30-year old male presented with history of dyspnoea, cough and sputum production. The patient died of respiratory failure. Gross image of lung is shown below. What is the likely etiology?**

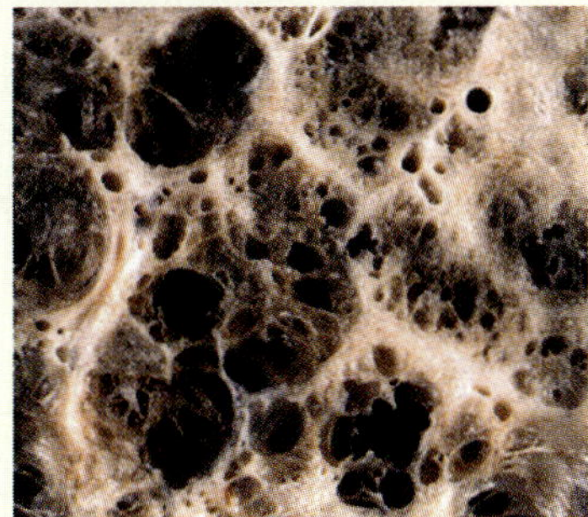

   a. Cystic fibrosis
   b. Mutation in dynein arms
   c. Alpha 1 antitrypsin deficiency
   d. Antibodies against type IV collagen

14. **A 75-year-old male, known smoker presented to pulmonology department with history of cough. Biopsy was taken which showed the following. What is the change shown?**

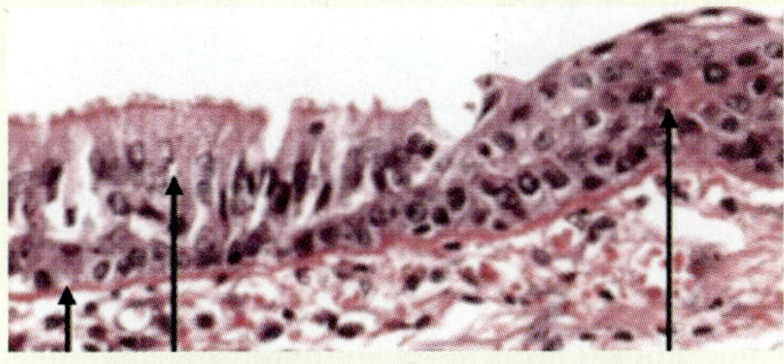

   a. Dysplasia   b. Metaplasia
   c. Hyperplasia   d. Atrophy

15. **A 23-year-old lady presented with diarrhea, vomiting and poor appetite. Biopsy showed crypt hyperplasia, villous atrophy and CD8+ cells in the lamina propria. Skin manifeatations have been shown. What could be the diagnosis?**

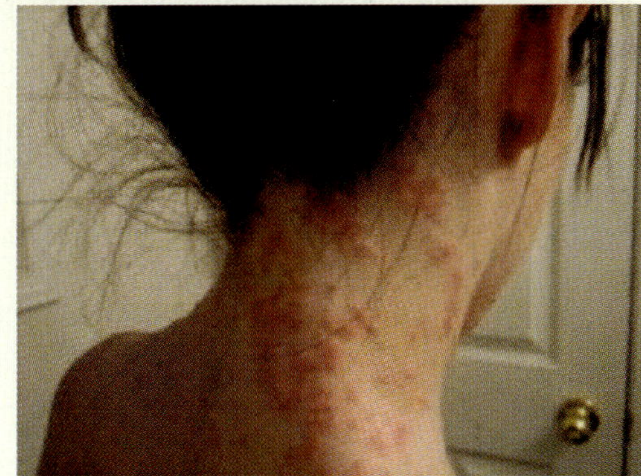

   a. Whipple's disease
   b. Chronic pancreatitis
   c. Environmental enteropathy
   d. Celiac disease

16. **Identify the parasite in the intestinal biopsy of a HIV positive patient.**

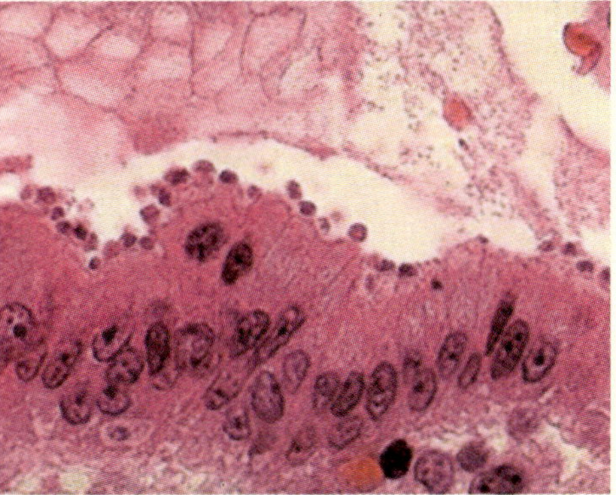

   a. Giardia
   b. CMV
   c. Amoebic colitis
   d. Cryptosporidium

Ans.

10.	c
11.	b
12.	a
13.	c
14.	b
15.	d
16.	d

17. A 5 year-old boy presented with bleeding per rectum. PR showed rectal polyp, biopsy showed the following. What is your diagnosis?

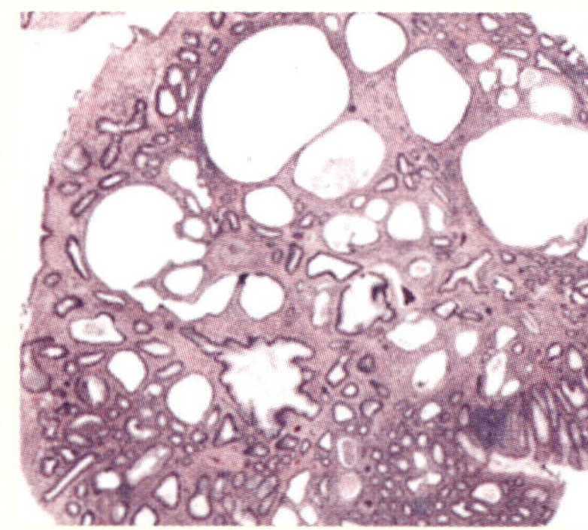

a. Villous adenoma
b. Peutz-Jeghers polyp
c. Juvenile polyp
d. Serrated adenoma

18. A 50-year-old male presented with hematuria. Investigations revealed normal glucose levels, proteinuria and creatinine of 9 mg%. Electron microscopic image is shown below. What other investigations could help in the diagnosis?

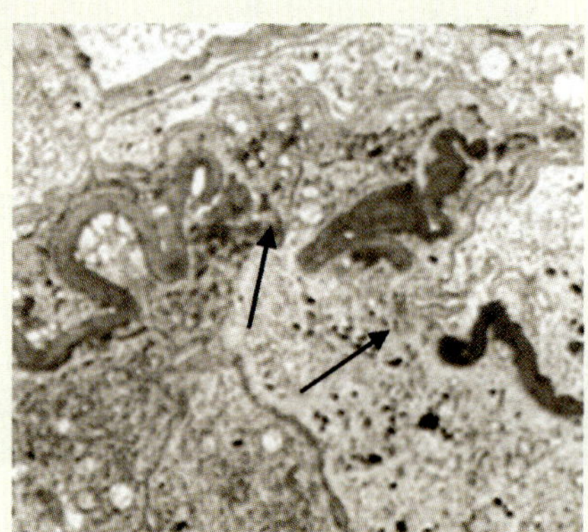

a. ANA
b. HIV serology
c. Electrophoresis
d. Anti GBM antibodies

19. A 30-year-old female presented with 4 cm mass in the right breast. Biopsy showed densely packed cells with bland nuclei and mucin infiltrating the stroma. What is your diagnosis?

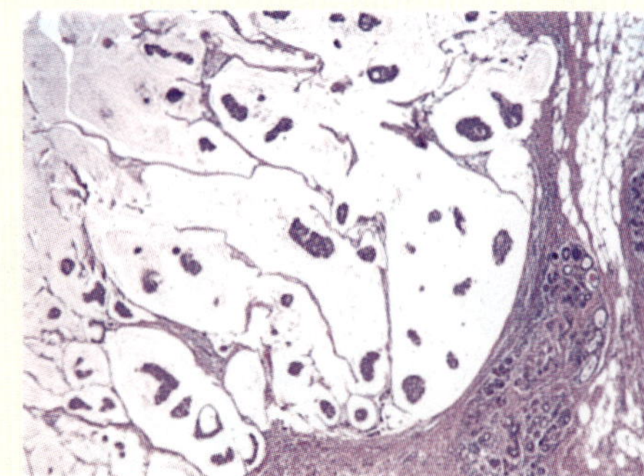

a. Invasive papillary carcinoma
b. Medullary carcinoma
c. Apocrine carcinoma
d. Colloid carcinoma

20. 25-year-old female presented with swelling in front of neck. TSH levels were elevated. Biopsy showed lymphocytic infiltration and Hurthle cells. Which of the following is the possible diagnosis?

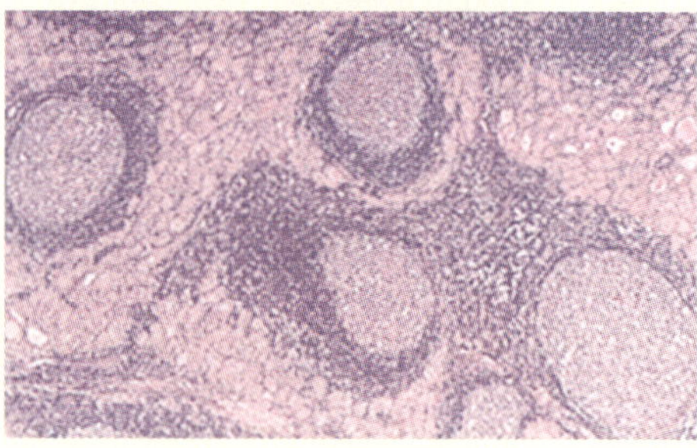

a. Graves' disease
b. Hashimoto's thyroiditis
c. Medullary carcinoma thyroid
d. Papillary carcinoma thyroid

21. Patient came with swelling in midline of neck measuring 2 cm in size. Histopathological examination showed Orphan Annie eye nuclei. What is the most likely diagnosis?

a. Medullary carcinoma
b. Papillary carcinoma thyroid
c. Toxic nodular goitre
d. Follicular thyroid carcinoma

22. Most common site of gastrinoma in MEN 1 is:

a. Stomach
b. Jejenum
c. Duodenum
d. Appendix

23. A 25-year-old male presented with swelling in the wrist joint. Histopathological examination showed spindle cells and Verocay bodies. What is the most likely diagnosis?

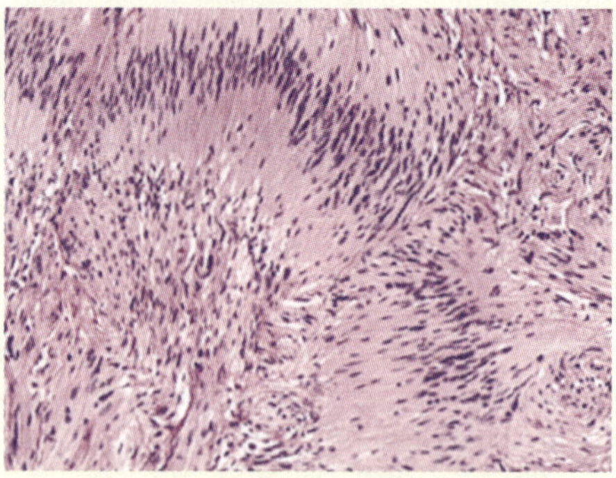

a. Neurofibroma
b. Schwannoma
c. Lipoma
d. Squamous cell carcinoma

24. Why is CPDA better than ACD for storage of blood?
a. Improves oxygen transport
b. More citrate ions
c. It is less acidic
d. Hypertonicity of blood

25. Which of the following translocation is seen in Myxoid liposarcoma?
a. t (11:22)
b. t (14:18)
c. t (x:18)
d. t (12:16)

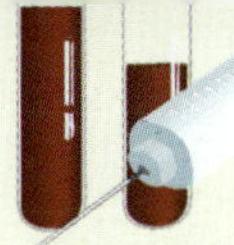

AIIMS New Pattern 2019 Model Questions

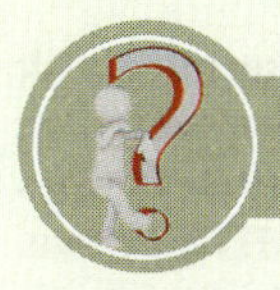

GENERAL PATHOLOGY

PATTERN 1: MULTIPLE TRUE /FALSE TYPE

1. In an experiment, a cell line derived from a human malignant neoplasm is grown in culture. A human IgG antibody is added to the culture, and the tumor cells become coated by the antibody, but they do not undergo lysis. Next, human cells are added that are negative for CD3, CD19, and surface immunoglobulin, but are positive for CD16 and CD56. The tumor cells are observed to undergo lysis. Which of the following statement denotes correctly about the cell types most likely to have killed the tumor cells?
   1. B cells have surface immunoglobulin and can lyse the tumor cells
   2. CD8+ cell are positive for CD16 and can lyse the tumor cells
   3. Dendritic cells can lyse the tumor cells
   4. Macrophage express MHC II and can lyse the tumor cells
   5. Natural killer cells show ADCC and can lyse the tumor cells
   a. Option 1, 3, 4 are true
   b. Option 2 and 5 are true
   c. Option 5 is true, all others are false
   d. All options are false

Ans. (c) Option 5 is true, all others are false

CD8 + CELL is not positive for CD16 ans c

2. Which of the following are true about deficiencies in complement pathway
   1. Deficiency of decay-accelerating factor → paroxysmal nocturnal hemoglobinuria
   2. Deficiency of C6 and C7 → recurrent pyogenic bacterial infections
   3. Deficiency of C1 esterase inhibitor → hereditary angioedema
   4. Deficiency of C3 and C5 → recurrent pyogenic bacterial infections
   5. Deficiency of C6, C7, and C8 →recurrent infections with Neisseria species
   a. Option 1, 3, 4 are true
   b. Option 2 and 5 are true
   c. Option 5 is true, all others are false
   d. All options are false

Ans. (a) Option 1, 3, 4 are true

PATTERN 2 : MATCH THE FOLLOWING

3.

A. Mast cells	1. Granulomatous response
B. Langhans giant cells	2. Cytotoxic lymphocytes
C. CD8 + cells	3. Humoral immunity
D. Dendritic cells	4. Elaborate type I interferons
	5. Surface-bound IgE
	6. Express MHC 1

a. A-5, B-1, C-2, D-4   b. A-5, B-1, C-2, D-6
c. A-5, B-1, C-6, D-4   d. A-5, B-6, C-2, D-4

Ans. (a) A-5, B-1, C-2, D-4

4.

A. c-abl	1. Small cell carcinoma of the lung
B. L-myc	2. Neuroblastoma
C. N-myc	3. Breast cancer
D. c-myc	4. Burkitt's lymphoma
	5. Chronic myelocytic leukemia (CML)
	6. Squamous cell carcinoma of the lung

a. A-5,B-1,C-2,D-4   b. A-5,B-1,C-2,D-6
c. A-5,B-1,C-6,D-4   d. A-5,B-6,C-2,D-4

Ans. (a) A-5,B-1,C-2,D-4

5.

A. CD8	1. Helper T cells,
B. CD4	2. Pan T cell marker
C. CD3	3. T cell receptor
D. CD2	4. Receptor for sheep erythrocyte (E rosette)
	5. Cytotoxic T cells
	6. Receptor for Fc portion of IgG

a. A-5,B-1,C-2,D-4   b. A-5,B-1,C-2,D-6
c. A-5,B-1,C-6,D-4   d. A-5,B-6,C-2,D-4

Ans. (a) A-5,B-1,C-2,D-4

6.

A. Centromere	1. Smith (SLE),
B. Speckled (non-DNA extractable nuclear proteins)	2. Double-stranded DNA (SLE)
C. Rim (peripheral)	3. T cell receptor
D. Nucleolar (RNA)	4. Progressive systemic sclerosis
	5. CREST syndrome
	6. Histones

a. A-5,B-1,C-2,D-4
b. A-5,B-1,C-2,D-6
c. A-5,B-1,C-6,D-4
d. A-5,B-6,C-2,D-4

Ans. (a) A-5,B-1,C-2,D-4

Contd...

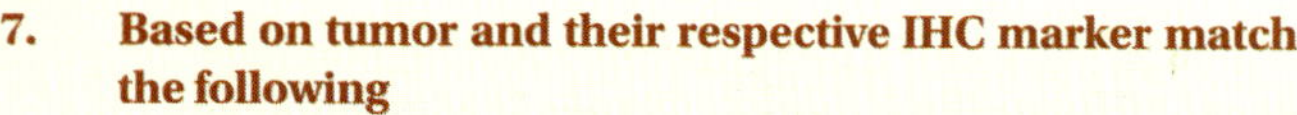

7. Based on tumor and their respective IHC marker match the following

A. Carcinoma	1. CD 45
B. Lymphoma	2. NSE
C. Sarcoma	3. Vimentin
D. Melanoma	4. CK
E. Neuroendocrine Tumor	5. HMB45

a. A-5, B-1,C-2, D-3, E-4 b. A-4, B-1,C-3, D-5, E-2
c. A-3, B-2,C-4, D-1, E-5 d. A-1, B-2,C-3, D-4, E-5

Ans. (b) A-4, B-1,C-3, D-5, E-2

PATTERN 3: SEQUENCE Q

8. A 63-year-old man has increasing malaise and back pain for the past 4 months. A radiograph of his spine shows rounded lucent lesions. The microscopic appearance of his liver with Congo red stain and with polarized light is shown in the figure. What is the correct sequence to diagnose this condition

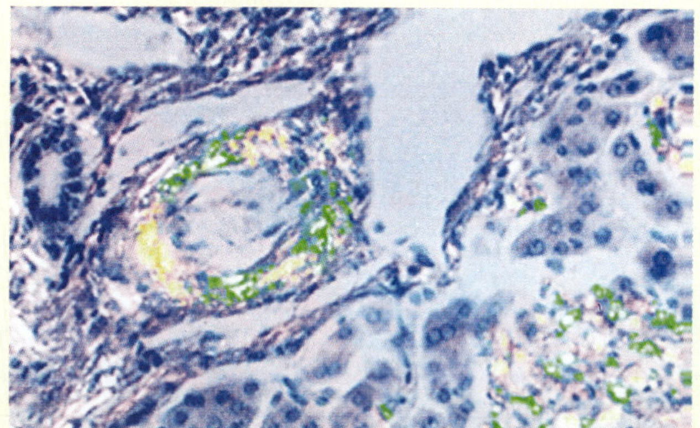

a. Biopsy –h & e –congo red –polarising light under congo red
b. Biopsy - polarising light under congo red – mahagony brown on gross
c. Biopsy-masson trichrome-electron microscopy
d. Biopsy –congo red –h & e -polarising light under congo red

Ans. (a) Biopsy –H & E -congo red –polarising light under congo red

Now this is sequence biopsy fb h and e which shows pink colour deposits and then we do special stain like congo red fb seeing it under polarizing mic so ans is A.

9. A 48-year-old woman has fingers that are tapered and claw-like, with decreased motion at the small joints. There are no wrinkle lines on her facial skin. The microscopic appearance of the skin is shown in the figure. The patient also has diffuse interstitial fibrosis of the lungs, with pulmonary hypertension and cor pulmonale. Which of the following dermal inflammatory cells is the most likely initiator of the process that is the cause of her skin disease?

10. An epidemiologic study is conducted to determine risk factors for HIV infection. The study documents that individuals with coexisting sexually transmitted diseases such as chancroid are more likely to become HIV-positive. It is postulated that an inflamed mucosal surface is an ideal location for the transmission of HIV during sexual intercourse. Which of the following cells in these mucosal surfaces is most instrumental in transmitting HIV to CD4+ T lymphocytes?

a. CD8+ cells b. Dendritic cells
c. Natural killer cells d. Neutrophils
e. Plasma cells f. CD4+ lymphocyte
g. Mast cell

Ans. (b) Dendritic cells; (f) CD4+ lymphocyte

11. Which of the following are the characteristics of Exudative pleural effusion?

1. Pleural fluid protein/serum protein > 0.5
2. Pleural fluid protein/serum protein < 0.5
3. Pleural fluid LDH/serum LDH > 0.6
4. Pleural fluid LDH/serum LDH < 0.6

Select the correct answer using the code given below:

a. 1 and 3 b. 1 and 4
c. 2 and 3 d. 2 and 4

Ans. (a) 1 and 3

Light's criteria (Sensitivity 99%, Specificity 98%)

Criteria	Transudate	Exudate
Pleural fluid protein: Serum: protein ratio	<0.5	>0.5
Pleural fluid LDH: Serum LDH	<0.6	>0.6
Pleural fluid LDH	<200	>200

PATTERN 4: MULTIPLE CORRECT OPTIONS

12. A 37-year-old man who is HIV-positive has noticed an increasing number and size of skin lesions on his face, trunk, and extremities, as shown in the figure, over the past 18 months. Some of the larger lesions appear to be nodular. Which among the following is/ are correct options?

A. HIV is not detected in the spindle cells that proliferate in Kaposi sarcoma.
B. Cytomegalovirus is implicated cause of above lesion
C. Epstein-Barr virus is usually not associated with skin lesions
D. Kaposi sarcoma is associated with Kaposi sarcoma herpes virus.
E. Human herpesvirus-8 is the implicated cause
a. Option A, C, D, E are true
b. Option A, C, D are true, B and E are false
c. Option E is true, all others are false
d. All options are false

Ans. (a) Option A,C,D,E are true

This is kaposi sarcoma. Kaposi sarcoma is associated with Kaposi sarcoma herpes virus (kshv). KSHV is also called HHV8. Human herpesvirus-8 is the implicated cause OF KS –true. HIV is not detected in the spindle cells that proliferate in Kaposi sarcoma. Remember Epstein-Barr virus is usually not associated with skin lesions. So ans is A.

13. **A 23-year-old girl is infected with HPV. Which among below are correct lesions that can be associated with above lesion**
    A. Verruca vulgaris
    B. Condyloma
    C. Cervical neoplasia
    D. Carcinoma of the nasopharynx
    E. African Burkitt's lymphoma
    a. Option A,B,C are true
    b. Option A,C,D are true, B and E are false
    c. Option E is true, all others are false
    d. All options are false

Ans. (a) Option a,b,c are true

PATTERN 5: BEST ONE ANSWER

14. **Lymphocyte phenotype test is done for?**
    a. Agammaglobulinemia   b. SCID
    c. Sepsis   d. Acute leukemia

Ans. (c) Sepsis

Clinical signs and symptoms of sepsis are nonspecific and often indistinguishable from those of nonseptic critical illness

This ambiguity frequently delays the diagnosis of sepsis until culture results can confirm the presence or absence of an infectious organism. Lymphocyte phenotyping can be conducted rapidly and may provide information on the presence of infection before culture results are available. Hence answer is sepsis c.

15. **True about repeats in Fragile X syndrome?**
    a. CGG repeats   b. CAG repeats
    c. CTG repeats   d. GCT repeats

Ans. (c) CTG repeats

Carcinoid heart disease: PV stenosis, TV regurgitation

PATTERN 6: ASSERTION REASONING

16. **Assertion: majority of people with HIV have a symptomatic disease.**
    Reason: HIV causes progressive destruction of CD4 cells.
    a. If both **Assertion** and **Reason** are true and the **Reason** is the correct explanation of the **Assertion**.
    b. If both **Assertion** and **Reason** are true but the **Reason** is not the correct explanation of the **Assertion**.
    c. If **Assertion** is true but **Reason** is false.
    d. If **Assertion** is false and **Reason** is true.

Ans. (d) If Assertion is false and Reason is true.

17. **Assertion: Natural Killer Cells are a part of innate immunity.**
    Reason: Natural Killer Cells do not need previous sensitization
    a. If both **Assertion** and **Reason** are true and the **Reason** is the correct explanation of the **Assertion**.
    b. If both **Assertion** and Reason are true but the **Reason** is not the correct explanation of the Assertion.
    c. If **Assertion** is true but **Reason** is false.
    d. If **Assertion** is false and **Reason** is true .

Ans. (a) If both Assertion and Reason are true and the Reason is the correct explanation of the Assertion.

PATTERN 6: SCENERIO TYPE Q

18. **A 45-year-old female patient presented with vaginal discharge. Her pap smear revealed HSV infection. What inclusions do u suspect in this case**
    a. Cowdry A bodies
    b. koilocytosis
    c. Guarnieri bodies
    d. Warthin-Finkeldey giant cells
    e. Ground-Glass Change
    f. Atypical lymphocytes

Ans. (a) Cowdry A bodies

19. **A 4-year-old child presented with measles. He showed many giant cells in his lymph node biopsy. Which of the following is the correct about inclusions seen in this entity**
    a. Cowdry A bodies
    b. koilocytosis
    c. Guarnieri bodies
    d. Warthin-Finkeldey giant cells
    e. Ground-Glass Change
    f. Atypical lymphocytes

Ans. (d) Warthin-Finkeldey giant cells

20. **Deficiency of which immune function results in tubercular infections?**
    1. Defective phagocytic function
    2. Defect in T cell function
    3. Defect in B cell function
    4. Defect in antibody productivity
    a. Only 1   b. Only 1 and 3
    c. Only 2   d. None of above

Ans. (c) Only 2

T-lymphocytes play a major role in conferring immunity against M. tuberculosis.

21. **Syndrome X includes:**
    a. Hyperlipidemia, Obesity, Type 2 DM
    b. Obesity, CAD, COPD
    c. Hyponatremia, Hyperlipidemia with type 2 DM
    d. Hyponatremia, Hyperlipidemia with type 2 DM

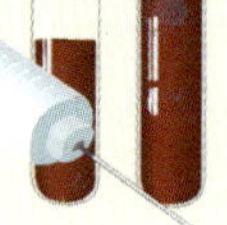

Ans. (a) Hyperlipidemia, Obesity, Type 2 DM

Metabolic syndrome, sometimes known as Syndrome X, is a clustering of at least three of the five following medical conditions: central obesity, high blood pressure, high blood sugar (type 2 diabetes mellitus), high serum triglycerides, and low serum high density lipoprotein (HDL).

22. Cutaneous manifestations of tuberculosis include:
   a. Erythema nodosum and lupus vulgaris
   b. Erythema marginatum and lupus vulgaris
   c. Phlyctenular conjunctivitis and erythema multiform
   d. Pyoderma gangrenosum and Dactylitis

Ans. (a) Erythema nodosum and lupus vulgaris

Lesion associated with TB

- Erythema nodosum (EN), also known as subacute migratory panniculitis of Villanova an inflammatory condition characterized by inflammation of the fat cells under the skin resulting in render red nodules or lumps that are usually seen on both shins.
- Lupus vulgaris (also known as tuberculosis luposa) are painful cutaneous tuberculosis skin lesion with nodular appearance, most often on the face around the nose, eyelids, lips, cheeks, ear and neck. It is the most common Mycobacterium tuberculosis skin infection.

23. Killer T cells which are responsible for defence against intracellular pathogen are expressed by which of the following CD phenotypes?

   1. CD 2   2. CD 8
   3. CD 5   4. CD 10
   5. CD 4   6. CD 16
   a. 2, 5, 6   b. 3, 4, 5
   c. 1, 5, 6   d. None

Ans. (a) 2, 5, 6

Natural killer T-cells/NKT cells include both NK 1.1* and NK 1.1 as well as CD4, CD4, CD8 cells, CD 16, CD 16

HEMATOLOGY

PATTERN 1: MULTIPLE TRUE FALSE TYPE

24. Identify the correct statements regarding Polycythemia
   1. Most cases of Polycythemia vera are due to mutation of the JAK2 gene on the short arm of chromosome 9.
   2. Increase in bone marrow production of RBCs is seen in relative polycythemia
   3. Ectopic release of EPO may occur in renal cell carcinoma
   4. Hypoxic stimulus for EPO release can cause increase in bone marrow production of RBCs
   5. Plasma volume is increased in relative polycythemia
   a. Option 1, 3, 4 are true
   b. Option 2 and 5 are true
   c. Option 5 is true, all others are false
   d. All options are false

Ans. (a) Option 1, 3, 4 are true

Option 2 and 5 is false. No increase in bone marrow production of RBCs in relative polycythemia. plasma volume is decreased.

25. Safe transfusion practices regarding Patient cross match for a blood transfusion
   1. Before blood is transfused into newborns or patients with T-cell deficiencies, it must be irradiated to kill donor lymphocytes
   2. Blood group AB patients have natural antibodies.
   3. Major cross match is Patient serum is mixed with a sample of RBCs from a donor unit.
   4. Blood group O individuals are considered universal donors.
   5. Direct Coombs test to identify atypical antigens on the persons RBCs
   a. Option 1, 3, 4 are true
   b. Option 2 and 5 are true
   c. Option 5 is true, all others are false
   d. All options are false

Ans. (a) Option 1, 3, 4 are true

Option 2 and 5 is false-Direct Coombs test to identify atypical IgG antibodies on the persons RBCs and Blood group AB patients lack natural antibodies.

PATTERN 2 : MATCH THE FOLLOWING

26.

A. Spleen in portal hypertension (PH)	1. Macrophages with a soap bubble appearance
B. Niemann-Pick disease	2. Macrophages with a fibrillary appearance
C. Gaucher disease	3. Humoral immunity
D. Red pulp of spleen	4. Fixed macrophages and sinusoids
	5. Thickened ("sugar-coated") capsule
	6. B and T cells

   a. A-5, B-1, C-2, D-4   b. A-5, B-1, C-2, D-6
   c. A-5, B-1, C-6, D-4   d. A-5, B-6, C-2, D-4

Ans. (a) A-5, B-1, C-2, D-4

Spleen in portal hypertension (PH)

- Gross findings
  - Spleen is covered by a thickened ("sugar-coated") capsule from perisplenitis
- Microscopic findings
  - Calcium and iron concretions called Gamna-Gandy bodies are deposited in collagen

PATTERN 3: SEQUENCE Q

27. **Identify the correct sequence in primary hemostasis. What is the correct sequence to diagnose this condition**
   a. Vessel injury-Platelet adhesion to Vwf-Platelet release of aggregating agents-platelet gp2b3a binding to fibrinogen
   b. Vessel injury-platelet gp2b3a binding to fibrinogen -Platelet adhesion to Vwf-Platelet release of aggregating agents
   c. Vessel injury-Platelet adhesion to Vwf-platelet gp2b3a binding to fibrinogen -Platelet release of aggregating agents
   d. Platelet adhesion to Vwf-Platelet release of aggregating agents-platelet gp2b3a binding to fibrinogen –injury

Ans. (a) Vessel injury-Platelet adhesion to Vwf-Platelet release of aggregating agents-platelet gp2b3a binding to fibrinogen

PATTERN 4: MULTIPLE CORRECT OPTIONS

28. **A 37-year-old man presents with Thrombocytopenia. What of the following can be causes of decreased platelet count**
   A. Thrombotic thrombocytopenic purpura
   B. Hypersplenism
   C. Idiopathic thrombocytopenic purpura
   D. Thrombotic thrombocytopenic purpura.
   E. Decreased production of platelets
   a. Option A,B,C,D,E are true
   b. Option A,C,D are true, Band E are false
   c. Option E is true, all others are false
   d. All options are false

Ans. (a) Option A,B,C,D,E are true

PATTERN 5: BEST ONE ANSWER

29. **Lymphocytic and histiocytic (L&H) cells are seen in?**
   a. Nodular sclerosis
   b. Mixed cellularity classical HL
   c. Nodular lymphocyte predominant HL
   d. Lymphocyte depleted classical HL

Ans. (c) Nodular lymphocyte predominant HL

PATTERN 6: ASSERTION REASONING

30. **Assertion: antiphospholipid antibodies produces strokes**
   Reason: antiphospholipid antibodies are associated with arterial thrombosis specially cerebral vessels
   a. If both **Assertion** and **Reason** are true and the **Reason** is the correct explanation of the **Assertion**.
   b. If both **Assertion** and **Reason** are true but the **Reason** is not the correct explanation of the **Assertion**.
   c. If **Assertion** is true but **Reason** is false.
   d. If **Assertion** is false and **Reason** is true.

Ans. (a) If both Assertion and Reason are true and the Reason is the correct explanation of the Assertion.

Cerebral vessels thrombosis (most common site of APLA; produces strokes)

31. **Assertion: Allergic transfusion reactions are most common transfusion reaction**
   Reason: It is due to type I IgE-mediated hypersensitivity reaction (HSR) against proteins (allergens) that are present in the donor blood
   a. If both **Assertion** and **Reason** are true and the **Reason** is the correct explanation of the **Assertion**.
   b. If both **Assertion** and **Reason** are true but the **Reason** is not the correct explanation of the **Assertion**.
   c. If **Assertion** is true but **Reason** is false.
   d. If **Assertion** is false and **Reason** is true .

Ans. (a) If both Assertion and Reason are true and the Reason is the correct explanation of the Assertion.

A –understand Allergic transfusion reactions

- Since the patient has been previously sensitized to an allergen that is present in donor blood, IgE antibodies are already present on the patient's mast cells
- Exposure to the allergen from the donor blood leads to cross-linking of IgE antibodies specific for the allergen on the mast cell membranes.
- IgE triggering causes an early phase reaction that is characterized by mast cell release of preformed mediators.
  - Preformed chemicals include histamine, eosinophil chemotactic factor, and serotonin.

PATTERN 7: SCENERIO TYPE Q

32. **A febrile child presented with Lytic lesions are present in the skull, Central diabetes insipidus (CDI) and Exophthalmos**

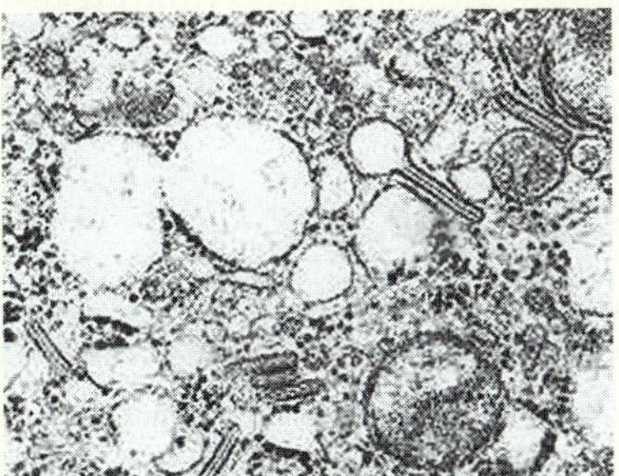

Diagnosis
The electron microscopy shown above is typically seen in this child. What is the electron microscopy showing
   a. Letterer-Siwe disease
   b. Hand-Schüller-Christian (HSC) disease
   c. Urticaria pigmentosa
   d. Lymphocyte depleted classical HL
   e. Eosinophilic granuloma
   f. Birbeck granules

Ans. (b) Hand-Schüller-Christian (HSC)

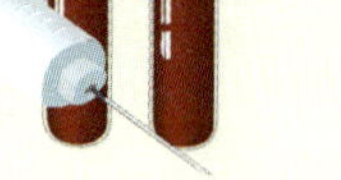

Hand-Schüller-Christian (HSC) disease shows Classic triad due to infiltrative disease
- Lytic lesions are present in the skull.
- Central diabetes insipidus (CDI), due to invasion of the posterior pituitary stalk
- Exophthalmos from infiltration of the orbit 2nd– f-Electron micrograph showing racket-shaped Birbeck granules in a histiocyte

33. **Which of the following conditions are associated with prolonged prothrombin time?**
1. Factor VIII deficiency
2. Factor VII deficiency
3. Heparin anticoagulation
4. Warfarin anticoagulation

Select the correct answer using the code given below:

a. 1 and 4
b. 1 and 3
c. 2 and 3
d. 2 and 4

Ans. (d) 2 and 4

The prothrombin time can be prolonged as a result of deficiencies in vitamin K, warfarin therapy, malabsorption, or lack of intestinal colonization by bacteria (such as in newborn). In addition, poor factor VII synthesis (due to liver disease) or increased consumption (in disseminated intravascular coagulation) may prolong the PT.

34. **Match the following vials in column (A) with the color coding in column (B)?**

Column A-Vials	Column B-color coding
A. EDTA vial	a. Light blue
B. Plain vial	b. Purple
C. Coagulation profile vial	c. Yellow
D Heparin vial	d. Red
	e. Gray
	f. Green

Ans. A-b, B-d, C-a, D-f

SYSTEMIC PATHOLOGY

PATTERN 1 : MULTIPLE TRUE FALSE TYPE

35. **A patient presents with biventricular failure and narrow pulse pressure. His CXR was suggestive of Dilated cardiomyopathy. Which of the following statements tell correctly about etiology**
1. Idiopathic (most common)
2. Genetic (most common)
3. Postpartum state can be a causative
4. Alcohol can cause direct toxicity to cause DCM
5. Most common cause of sudden death in young athletes

a. Option 1, 3, 4 are true
b. Option 2 and 5 are true
c. Option 5 is true, all others are false
d. All options are false

Ans. (a) Option 1, 3, 4 are true

A-Hypertrophic cardiomyopathy (HCM) is most common cause of sudden death in young athletes and is mostly genetic

36. **A 30-year-old man has sudden onset of hematemesis after a weekend in which he consumed large amounts of alcohol. The bleeding stops, but he has another episode under similar circumstances 1 month later. Upper gastroesophageal endoscopy shows longitudinal tears at the gastroesophageal junction. What is the most likely mechanism to cause his hematemesis?**
1. Most cases occur in the context of alcohol abuse
2. This is a case of cirrhosis from alcohol abuse.
3. Mallory-Weiss syndrome with esophageal tears results from severe vomiting.
4. The bleeding due to this condition is usually not very life-threatening
5. This is case of Herpes simplex virus infection

a. Option 1, 3, 4 are true
b. Option 2 and 5 are true
c. Option 5 is true, all others are false
d. All options are false

Ans. (a) Option 1, 3, 4 are true

Portal hypertension leads to dilation of esophageal submucosal veins, which can bleed profusely; in this case, the patient's age argues against the presence of cirrhosis from alcohol abuse

37. **Bronchiolitis obliterans with organizing pneumonia (BOOP) is characterized histologically in the lung by**
1. Loose fibrous tissue within bronchioles and alveoli
2. Asteroid bodies in giant cells within bronchioles
3. It occurs due to smoking
4. Steroid responsive
5. Multiple rheumatoid nodules within the interstitial tissue

a. Option 1,3,4 are true
b. Option 2 and 5 are true
c. Option 5 is true, all others are false
d. All options are false

Ans. (a) Option 1, 3 ,4 are true

The lungs respond to these agents, causing bronchiolar injury by forming loose, fibrous tissue within the bronchioles (bronchiolitis obliterans) and alveoli (organizing pneumonia).

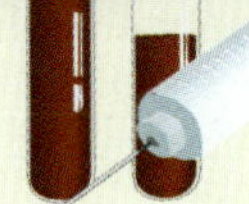

PATTERN 2 : MATCH THE FOLLOWING

38.

A. MC site for Cardiac metastasis	1. Rhabdomyoma
B. Tuberous sclerosis	2. Cardiac myxoma
C. Ball-valve effect	3. Hypertrophic cardiomyopathy (HCM)
D. Endocardial fibroelastosis	4. Restrictive cardiomyopathy
	5. Pericardium
	6. β-Blockers

a. A-5, B-1, C-2, D-4   b. A-5, B-1, C-2, D-6
c. A-5, B-1, C-6, D-4   d. A-5, B-6, C-2, D-4

Ans. (a) A-5, B-1, C-2, D-4

39.

A. Turcot syndrome	1. SMAD4
B. Juvenile polyposis	2. STK11
C. Peutz-Jeghers syndrome	3. TSC
D. Cowden syndrome	4. PTEN
	5. APC
	6. MYH

a. A-5,B-1,C-2,D-4   b. A-5,B-1,C-2,D-6
c. A-5,B-1,C-6,D-4   d. A-5,B-6,C-2,D-4

Ans. (a) A-5,B-1,C-2,D-4

40.

A. MEN 2B	1. Wermer's Syndrome
B. Type 1 MEN	2. Medullary carcinoma of thyroid
C. Sipple's Syndrome	3. Membranous glomerulonephropathy (MGN)
D. MEN4	4. Heterozygous inactivating mutations in the CDKN1B gene
	5. Mucosal neuromas
	6. Minimal change disease (lipoid nephrosis)

a. A-5,B-1,C-2,D-4   b. A-5,B-1,C-2,D-6
c. A-5,B-1,C-6,D-4   d. A-5,B-6,C-2,D-4

Ans. (a) A-5,B-1,C-2,D-4

A MEN4 is caused by heterozygous inactivating mutations in the CDKN1B gene (12p13.1-p12) encoding p27, a cyclin-dependent kinase inhibitor that acts as a negative regulator of cell cycle progression

Type 1 (Wermer's Syndrome)
- Parathyroid
- Pituitary
- Pancreas

Type 2 (Sipple's Syndrome)
- Parathyroid
- Medullary carcinoma of thyroid
- Pheochromocytoma

Type 3 (MEN 2B)
- Medullary carcinoma of thyroid
- Pheochromocytoma
- Mucosal neuromas

41.

A. Fats	1. PAS-positive, diastase-sensitive
B. Glycogen	2. Prussian blue
C. Hemosiderin	3. Von Kossa
D. α1 antitrypsin	4. PAS-positive, diastase-resistant
	5. Oil red O
	6. Congo red

a. A-5,B-1,C-2,D-4   b. A-5,B-1,C-2,D-6
c. A-5,B-1,C-6,D-4   d. A-5,B-6,C-2,D-4

Ans. (a) A-5,B-1,C-2,D-4

42.

A. Minimal change disease (lipoid nephrosis)	1. Thickening of basement membrane ("spikes and domes")
B. Membranous glomerulonephropathy (MGN)	2. Mesangial deposits
C. IgA nephropathy	3. Subendothelial deposits
D. FSGS	4. Apol1 mutation
	5. EM reveals fusion of foot processes of podocytes
	6. K w lesions

a. A-5,B-1,C-2,D-4   b. A-5,B-1,C-2,D-6
c. A-5,B-1,C-6,D-4   d. A-5,B-6,C-2,D-4

Ans. (a) A-5,B-1,C-2,D-4

The risk variants G1 (S342G:I384M) and G2 (del.N388/Y389) are two coding variants in the APOL1 gene on chromosome 22q13. The mutant alleles confer protection against trypanosomal infections. Its mutations are associated with FSGS

PATTERN 3: SEQUENCE Q

43.   A 63-year-old man died de to mi. Correct sequence of events

a. Coagulation necrosis-Neutrophils-Macrophages-Granulation tissue and collagen formation

b. Granulation TISSUE -Coagulation necrosis-Neutrophils-Macrophages-collagen formation

c. Neutrophils-Coagulation necrosis--Macrophages-Granulation tissue and collagen formation

d. Coagulationnecrosis-Neutrophils-Macrophages-collagen formation-Granulation TISSUE

Ans. (a) Coagulation necrosis- Neutrophils- Macrophages- Granulation tissue and collagen formation

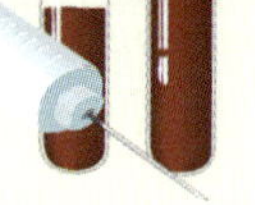

44. **A child presented with VSD, PV stenosis, RVH and cyanosis after 1 year of age. Diagnosis**
    a. Tetralogy of Fallot
    b. Coarctation of the aorta
    c. TV atresia
    d. Truncus arteriosus
    e. Complete transposition of the great arteries
    f. VSD

Ans. (a) Tetralogy of Fallot

Tetralogy of Fallot presents with A-VSD, Infundibular (most common) or PV stenosis, RVH, Dextrorotated aorta with a right-sided aortic arch

45. **A 48-year-old woman has leg claudication and hypertension. On examination, increase in the upper extremity blood pressure is observed. Disparity between upper/lower extremity blood pressure >10 mm Hg is seen. Which of the following is the correct diagnosis of this entity?**
    a. Tetralogy of Fallot
    b. Coarctation of the aorta
    c. TV atresia
    d. Truncus arteriosus
    e. Complete transposition of the great arteries
    f. VSD

Ans. (b) Coarctation of the aorta

46. **Identify the correct the classic adenoma-carcinoma sequence**
    a. APC –b-catenin -K-RAS –TP53-LOH at 18q21-Telomerase activation
    b. APC –TP53 -K-RAS –LOH at 18q21-Telomerase activation
    c. APC – K-RAS –TP53-LOH at 18q21-Telomerase activation
    d. APC –b-catenin -K-RAS –Telomerase activation -LOH at 18q21

Ans. (a) APC –b-catenin -K-RAS –TP53-LOH at 18q21-Telomerase activation

---

PATTERN 4: MULTIPLE CORRECT OPTIONS

47. **Many complications are associated with ST ELEVATION MYOCARDIAL INFARCTION (STEMI). WHICH among below are correct options about the above lesion**
    A. Congestive heart failure: Usually occurs within the first 24 hours
    B. Mural thrombus: has high danger of embolization
    C. Ventricular fibrillation: MCC death in STEMI
    D. Fibrinous pericarditis occurs between day 1 to 7 of a STEMI.
    E. Myocardial rupture: MC at 3–7 days
    a. Option A,B,C,D,E are true
    b. Option A,C,D are true, B and e are false
    c. Option E is true, all others are false
    d. All options are false

Ans. (a) Option A,B,C,D,E are true

48. **A 65-year-old woman is being treated in the hospital for pneumonia complicated by septicemia. She has required multiple antibiotics and was intubated and mechanically ventilated earlier in the course. On day 20 of hospitalization, she has abdominal distention. At laparotomy, a portion of distal ileum and cecum is resected. The gross appearance of the mucosal surface is shown in the figure.**
    A. The opened colon shows pseudomembranes that are patches of fibrinopurulent debris attached to the mucosa.
    B. It's a complication of broadspectrum antibiotic therapy
    C. It results from overgrowth of Clostridium difficile or other organisms that are capable of inflicting mucosal injury
    D. Clostridium septicum is most often associated with malignancy or immunosuppression
    E. Its image of toxic megacolon is an uncommon complication of ulcerative colitis.
    a. Option A,B,C,D are true
    b. Option A,C,D are true, B and e are false
    c. Option e is true, all others are false
    d. All options are false

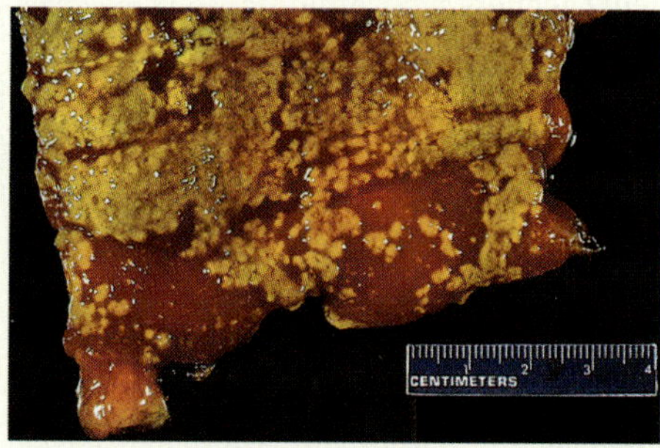

Ans. (a) Option a,b,c,d are true

The opened colon shows pseudomembranes that are patches of fibrinopurulent debris attached to the mucosa. Pseudomembranous enterocolitis is a complication of broad-spectrum antibiotic therapy, which alters gut flora to allow overgrowth of Clostridium difficile or other organisms that are capable of inflicting mucosal injury. Clostridium septicum infection can lead to myonecrosis that is most often associated with malignancy or immunosuppression. This gross pattern also can appear from ischemic injury that is vascular or mechanical, but this patient's history and the time course support an iatrogenic cause. An ischemic colitis resulting from mesenteric artery thrombosis could appear similar, but it is not associated with C. difficile. A dilated, thinned, toxic megacolon is an uncommon complication of ulcerative colitis

49. **A 57-year-old male presents with a lesion similar to that seen in this gross photograph of a sagittal section of the lung. Which one of the listed characteristics, if present in this lesion, would favor the diagnosis of mesothelioma?**
    A. Arises from the pleural surfaces
    B. Negative staining with CEA and Leu-M1.
    C. Long microvilli seen by electron microscopy
    D. Lamellar bodies seen by electron microscopy
    E. Its image of adenocarcinoma

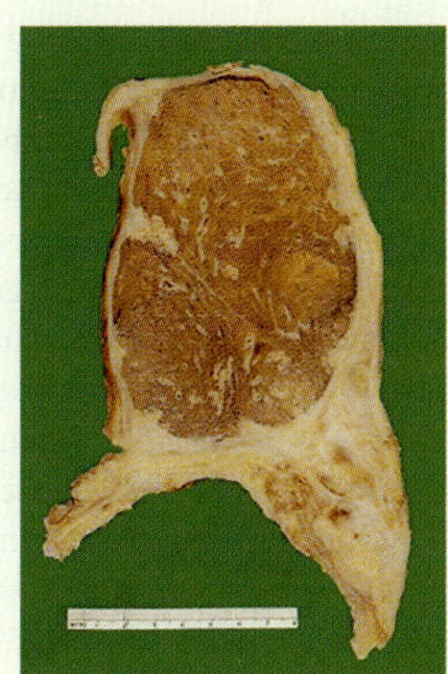

a. Option a,b,c are true
b. Option a,c,d are true, b and e are false
c. Option e is true, all others are false
d. All options are false

Ans. (a) Option a,b,c are true

PATTERN 5: BEST ONE ANSWER

50. **Sterile, nondestructive vegetations present on the MITRAL VALVE?**
    a. Libman-Sacks endocarditis
    b. Infective endocarditis (IE)
    c. Nonbacterial thrombotic endocarditis
    d. Carcinoid heart disease

Ans. (c) Nonbacterial thrombotic endocarditis

Carcinoid heart disease: PV stenosis, TV regurgitation

51. **A 53-year-old woman undergoes a routine checkup. The only abnormal finding is a stool specimen that contains Occult blood. Colonoscopy shows a 1.5-cm, solitary, rounded, erythematous polyp on a 0.5-cm stalk at the splenic flexure. Her colonic lesion is most likely associated with which of the following?**
    a. Low risk for development of carcinoma
    b. Inheritance of an abnormal tumor suppressor gene
    c. Presence of similar lesions in the small intestine
    d. Risk for development of endometrial carcinoma

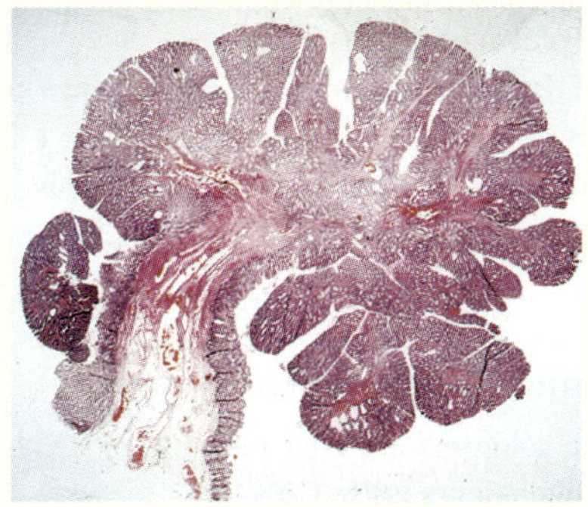

Ans. (a) Low risk for development of carcinoma

The figure shows a solitary pedunculated adenoma of the colon with no evidence of malignancy

52. **Histologic sections from a 3-cm mass found in the mandible of a 55-year-old female reveal a tumor consisting of nests of tumor cells that appear dark and crowded at the periphery of the nests and loose in the center (similar to the stellate reticulum of a developing tooth). Grossly, the lesions consist of multiple cysts filled with a thick, "motor oil"–like fluid. What is the correct diagnosis for this tumor?**
    a. Pleomorphic adenoma   b. Ameloblastoma
    c. Mucoepidermoid carcinoma
    d. Adenoid cystic carcinoma
    e. Acinic cell carcinoma

Ans. (b) Ameloblastoma

Rare tumor of the oral cavity (found most commonly in the mandible) that is similar to the enamel organ of the tooth is the ameloblastoma. This locally aggressive tumor consists of nests of cells that at their periphery are similar to ameloblasts and centrally are similar to the stellate reticulum of the developing tooth

PATTERN 6: ASSERTION REASONING

53. **Assertion: Pharynx is the only site for infection leading to Rheumatic fever (RF).**
    Reason: Nephrogenic strains of group A streptococcus that produce poststreptococcal glomerulonephritis, lack the types of matrix (M) proteins (virulence factors) in their cell wall that are present in pharyngeal strains; hence they never produce RF.
    a. If both **Assertion** and **Reason** are true and the **Reason** is the correct explanation of the **Assertion**.
    b. If both **Assertion** and **Reason** are true but the **Reason** is not the correct explanation of the **Assertion**.
    c. If **Assertion** is true but **Reason** is false.
    d. If **Assertion** is false and **Reason** is true.

Ans. (a) If both Assertion and Reason are true and the Reason is the correct explanation of the Assertion.

54. **Assertion: patient presents with secretory diarrhea syndrome.**
    Reason: The figure shows a large villous adenoma which can cause these manifestations

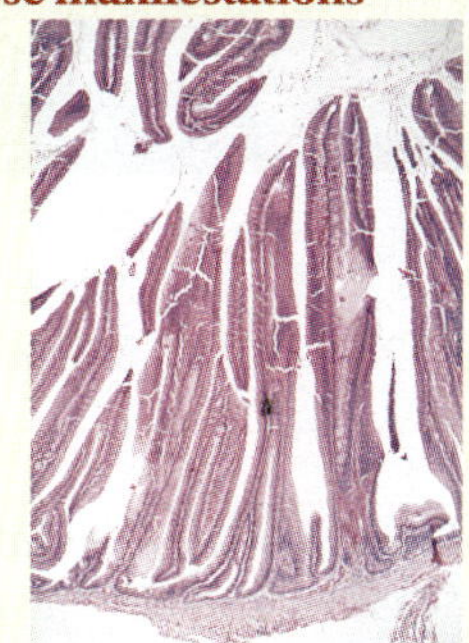

    a. If both **Assertion** and **Reason** are true and the **Reason** is the correct explanation of the **Assertion**.
    b. If both **Assertion** and **Reason** are true but the **Reason** is not the correct explanation of the **Assertion**.
    c. If **Assertion** is true but **Reason** is false.
    d. If **Assertion** is false and **Reason** is true.

Ans. (a) **If both Assertion and Reason are true and the Reason is the correct explanation of the Assertion.**

55. **Assertion: squamous cell carcinomas of the urinary bladder are quite rare except in Egypt and other areas of the Middle East.**

Reason: these areas predominantly have schistosomiasis

a. If both **Assertion** and **Reason** are true and the Reason is the correct explanation of the Assertion.

b. If both **Assertion** and **Reason** are true but the Reason is not the correct explanation of the **Assertion**.

c. If **Assertion** is true but **Reason** is false.

d. If **Assertion** is false and **Reason** is true.

Ans. (a) **If both Assertion and Reason are true and the Reason is the correct explanation of the Assertion.**

PATTERN 7: EMQ

56. **A 19-year-old man is advised to see his physician because genetic screening has detected a disease in other family members. On physical examination, a stool sample is positive for occult blood. A colonoscopy is performed, followed by a colectomy. The figure shows the gross appearance of the mucosal surface of the colectomy specimen**

1. Molecular analysis of this patient's normal fibroblasts is most likely to show a mutation in which of the following genes?

2. Patients of chron's disease are associated with which mutation?

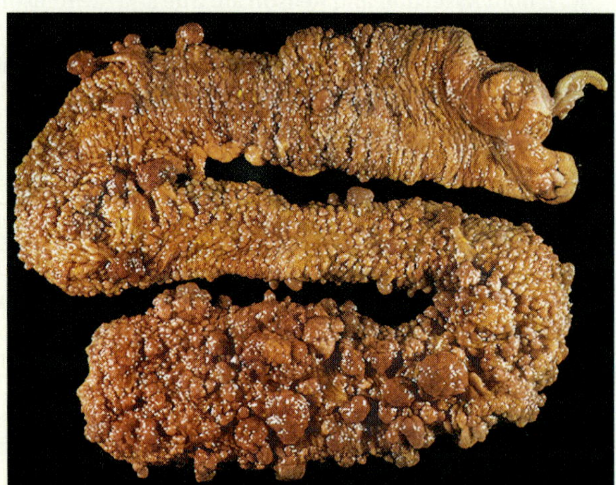

a. APC	b. MLH1
c. KRAS	d. NOD2
e. p53	f. MSH2

Ans. 1-a, 2 - d

This young patient's colon shows hundreds of polyps. This is most likely a case of familial adenomatous polyposis (FAP) syndrome, which results from inheritance of one mutant copy of the APC tumor-suppressor gene (a few FAP cases are associated with DNA mismatch repair genes). Every somatic cell of this patient most likely has one defective copy of the APC gene. Polyps are formed when the second copy of the APC gene is lost in many colon epithelial cells. Without treatment, colon cancers arise in 100% of these patients because of accumulation of additional mutations in one or more polyps, typically before 30 years of age. Patients with a gene for hereditary nonpolyposis colorectal carcinoma, such as MLH1 and MSH2, also have an inherited susceptibility to develop colon cancer, but in contrast to patients with FAP, they do not develop numerous polyps. Sporadic colon cancers may have CpG island hypermethylation along with KRAS mutations, whereas others have p53 mutations, but the somatic cells of patients with these cancers do not show abnormalities of these genes. NOD2 mutations are linked with Crohn's disease.

57. **A 66-year-old male presents to his family physician, complaining of bloating, which has developed over the course of several weeks. After evaluation, an exploratory laparotomy is performed. When the peritoneum is entered, the surgeon finds a large amount of gelatinous material. Of the following, what is the most likely anatomic site for the condition causing this change?**

a. Lung	b. Liver
c. Stomach	d. Appendix
e. Large intestine	f. Prostate

Ans. (d) Appendix

The description is that of pseudomyxoma peritonei. The gross features are associated with both benign and malignant neoplasms, and the classification and naming of the lesion is controversial; however, in a vast majority of cases, the neoplasm responsible for the changes in the peritoneal cavity is found in the appendix (D). Although a variety of neoplasms could give rise to the finding of pseudomyxoma peritonei, neoplasms in the appendix are by far the most common source, which indicates that the other answers (A-C, E-F) are not the best choice.

58. **Consider the following statements regarding changes in pregnancy:**

1. Plasma volume increases up to 30-50%
2. Pregnancy is a hypercoagulable state
3. Hematocrit is decreased
4. Total plasma proteins increases

Which of the statements given above is/are correct?

a. 1 only	b. 1, 2, 3 and 4
c. 1 and 2 only	d. 3 and 4 only

Ans. (b) 1, 2, 3 and 4

Hematological changes in pregnancy

- Plasma volume: Increase by 30-40%
- Fibrinogen: Increase by 50%
- Hematocrit: Decrease by 6%
- Total plasma proteins: Increase by 30%

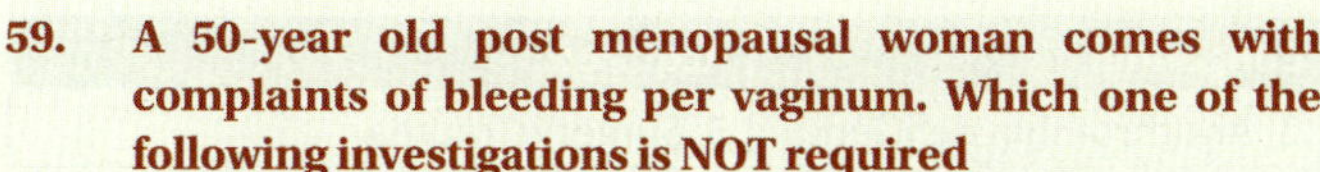

59. **A 50-year old post menopausal woman comes with complaints of bleeding per vaginum. Which one of the following investigations is NOT required**

a. Endometrial biopsy   b. Diagnostic laparoscopy

c. Hysteroscopy   d. Pap smear

Ans. (b) Diagnostic laparoscopy

Evaluation of postmenopausal bleeding

- Abnormal endometrium may have to be investigated by a hysteroscopy with a biopsy or a dilation and curettage.
- Pap smear is done to rule out carcinoma cervix

60. **Which of the following statements regarding β Human chorionic Gonadotropin are NOT correct**

1. It is a glycoprotein hormone.
2. Serum levels increase in pregnancy, germ cells tumor and gestational trophoblastic disease
3. Its levels are same in single and multiple pregnancy
4. It has common and Alpha subunit with other hormones FSH, LH and TSH.

Select the correct answer using the code given below:

a. 1, 2 and 4   b. 1, 2 and 3

c. 2, 3 and 4   d. 1, 3 and 4

Ans. (a) 1, 2 and 4

High levels of hCG could be detected in multiple pregnancy (levels are not same in single pregnancy and multiple pregnancy).

61. **Which of the following is/are the common infectious syndrome (s) associated with Klebsiella pneumonia?**

1. Pneumonia
2. Intra-abdominal infections
3. Hepatitis

Select the correct answer using the code given below:

a. 1 only   b. 1 and 2 only

c. 1, 2 and 3   d. 2 only

Ans. (c) 1, 2 and 3

The range of clinical disease caused by Klebsiella pneumonia includes pneumonia thrombophlebitis, urinary tract infection, cholecystitis, diarrhea, upper respiratory tract infection, wound infection, osteomyelitis, meningitis, and bacteremia and septicemia.

62. **Consider the following statements with regard to acute anterior poliomyelitis:**

1. It is caused by a virus belonging to picornavirus family
2. Muscle pain and cramps may be associated with diffuse transient fasciculations
3. Tonsillectomy reduces the risk of bulbar poliomyelitis
4. Cerebrospinal fluid may show mild pleocytosis with increase polymorphonuclear cells in early course of disease

Which of the above statements are correct?

a. 1, 2 and 3   b. 2, 3 and 4

c. 1, 2 and 4   d. 1, 3 and 4

Ans. (c) 1, 2 and 4

Polio

- Polivirus, the causative agent of poliomyelitis (commonly known as polio), is a human entervirus and member of the family of picomaviridae.
- Virus invasion cause inflammation of the nerve cells of anterior horn cells of spinal cord, leading to damage or destruction of motor neuron ganglia. With the destruction of nerve cells, the muscles no longer receive signals from the brain or spinal cord; without nerve stimulation, the muscles atrophy, becoming weak, floppy and poorly controlled, and finally completely paralyzed Maximum paralysis progresses rapidly (two or four days), and usually involves fever and muscle pain.
- Tonsillectomy increases the risk of bulbar poliomyelitis.
- Analysis of the patient's cerebrospinal fluid (CSF), which is collected by a lumber puncture ("spinal tap"), reveals an increased number of white blood cells and a mildly elevated protein level.

63. **Which of the following are the Indications for lung transplantation?**

1. Emphysema
2. Primary pulmonary hypertension
3. Obliterative bronchiolitis

Select the correct answer using the code given below:

a. 1 and 2 only   b. 2 and 3 only

c. 1 and 3 only   d. 1, 2 and 3

Ans. (a) 1 and 2 only

As of 2005, the most common reasons for lung transplantation in the United States were:

- 27% chronic obstructive pulmonary disease (COPD), including emphysema:
- 16% idiopathic pulmonary fibrosis:
- 14% cystic fibrosis:
- 12% idiopathic (formerly known as "primary") pulmonary hypertension:
- 5% alpha 1 antitrypsin deficiency:
- 2% replacing previously transplanted lungs that have since failed:
- 24% other causes, including bronchiectasis and sarcoidosis.

64. **Which of the following are common risk factors for contrast induced Nephrotoxicity?**

1. Use of high osmolality, ionic contrast media
2. Diabetes Mellitus
3. Myeloma

Select the correct answer using the code given below:

a. 1 and 2 only   b. 2 and 3 only

c. 1 and 3 only   d. 1, 2 and 3

Ans. (d) 1, 2 and 3

There are multiple risk factors of contrast induced nephropathy, whereof a review in 2016 emphasized chronic kidney disease, diabetes mellitus, high blood pressure, reduced intravascular volume, use of contrast agents with high osmolality (limited use today) and/or old age.

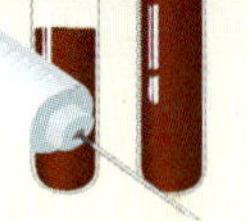

65. In a 40-year-old woman, pap smear shows atypical glandular cells, The next step of management should be:
 a. Repeat pap smear after three months
 b. Colposcopic directed cervical biopsy
 c. Colposcopy: cervical biopsy, endocervical curettage and endometrial biopsy
 d. Hysteroscopy and directed endometrial biopsy

Ans. (c) Colposcopy, cervical biopsy, endocervical curettage and endometrial biopsy.

The Papanicolaou test (abbreviated as Pap test, also known as Pap smear, cervical smear, or smear test) is a method of cervical screening used to detect potentially precancerous and cancerous processes in the cervix. Abnormal findings are often followed up by more sensitive diagnostic procedures, and if warranted, interventions that aim to prevent progression to cervical cancer. The test was invented by and named for doctor Aurel Babe' and doctor Georgios Papanikolaou.

66. A patient develops skin necrosis 3 days after being started on warfarin for deep vein thrombosis. What is the most likely cause?
 1. Antiphospholipid antibody syndrome
 2. Protein C deficiency
 3. Disseminated intravascular coagulation
 4. Thrombotic thrombocytopenic ....

a. Only 1	b. Only 3
c. 1 and 3	d. 1, 2, 3

Ans. (b) Only 3

Protein C is vitamin K dependent. Patients with Protein C deficiency are at an increased risk of developing skin necrosis while on warfarin. Protein C has a short half-life (8 hours) compared with other vitamin K dependent factors and therefore is rapidly depleted with warfarin initiation, resulting in a transient hypercoagulable state.

67. Which of the following is associated with hypercoagulable state?
 1. Protein C deficiency
 2. Antiphospholipid syndrome
 3. Homocysteinemia
 Select the correct answer using the code given below:

a. Only 1	b. Only 3
c. 1 and 3	d. 1, 2, 3

Ans. (d) 1, 2 and 3

Congenital & acquired hypercoagulable states

Congenital	Acquired
1. Protein C deficiency	1. Antiphospholipid antibody syndrome
2. Protein S deficiency	2. Malignancy

Contd...

Congenital	Acquired
3. Antithrombin deficiency	3. Surgery/Trauma
4. Factor V leiden	4. Pregnancy/Oral contraceptives
5. Prothrombin gene G20210A mutation	5. Prolonged immobilization
6. Hyper-horocysteinemia	6. Older age
7. Dysfibrinolysis	

68. Which of the following conditions is associated with cigarette smoking?
 1. Non-specific interstitial pneumonia
 2. Acute interstitial pneumonia
 3. Cryptogenic organizing pneumonia
 4. Desquamative interstitial pneumonia
 a. Only 1
 b. Only 3
 c. Only 4

Ans. (c) Only 4

Desquamative interstitial pneumonia is a form of idiopathic interstitial pneumonia featuring elevated levels of macrophages. Its name is derived from the former belief that these macrophages were pneumocytes that had desquamated. It is associated with patients with a history of smoking.

69. Consider the following statements about infective endocarditis:
 1. Modified Duke criteria are used for clinical diagnosis
 2. Echocardiographic findings form one of the major Duke criteria
 3. Presence of one major and two minor criteria is considered as diagnostic of endocarditis
 4. Presence of glomerulonephritis is a minor Duke criterion
 Which of the statements given above are correct?

a. 1, 2 and 3 only	b. 1, 2 and 4 only
c. 3 and 4 only	d. 1, 2, 3 and 4

Ans. (b) 1, 2 and 4 only

Infective endocarditis

- Established in 1994 by the Duke Endocarditis Service and revised in 2000, the Duke criteria are a collection of major and minor criteria used to establish a diagnosis of infective endocarditis. According to the Duke criteria, diagnosis of infective endocarditis can be definite, possible, or rejected.
- Evidence of endocardial involvement with positive echocardiogram is a major criteria
- Immunological problems is a minor criteria: glomerulonephritis, Osler's nodes, Roth's spots, Rheumatoid factor.

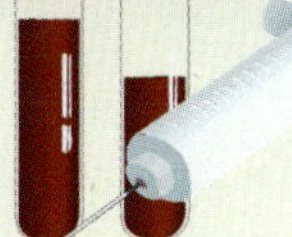

70. **A young female presented to medicine OPD with complaints of diarrhoea and fatigue. She had history of significant weight loss. Her physical examination is non significant and stool examination is normal. An endoscopy performed after microscopic examination and modified her diet. She is started on a special diet with no wheat or barely gains products. The dietary substitution causes marked improvement in her symptoms. Which of the following microscopic findings to be seen in the biopsy specimen?**

    a. Lymphatic obstructions

    b. Noncaseating granulomas

    c. Atrophy of villi with blunting and flattening

    d. Foamy macrophages within lamina propria

    e. Increased in intraepithelial lymphocytes.

    1. a, c are correct   2. a, d are correct

    3. c, b are correct   4. c, d are correct

    5. c, e are correct

Ans. (5) c, e are correct

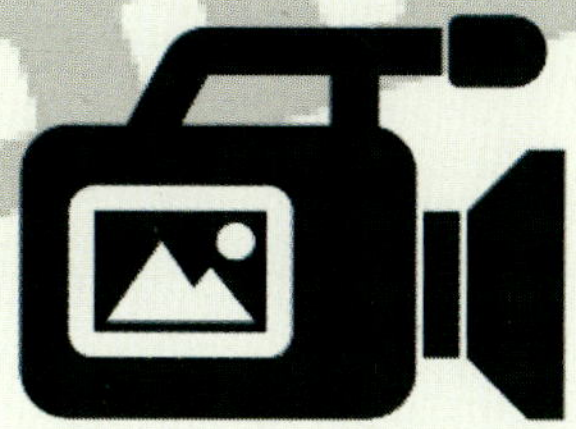

Sample Video Questions

1. Identify the technique?

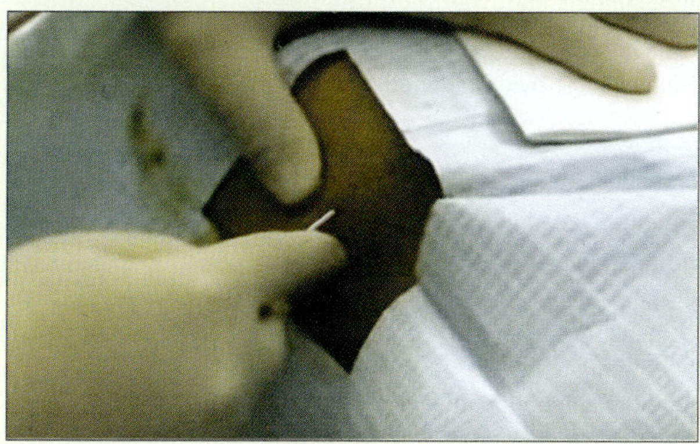

  a. Bone marrow aspiration b. CSF aspirate
  c. Blood culture d. Pleural tap

2. Identify the technique?

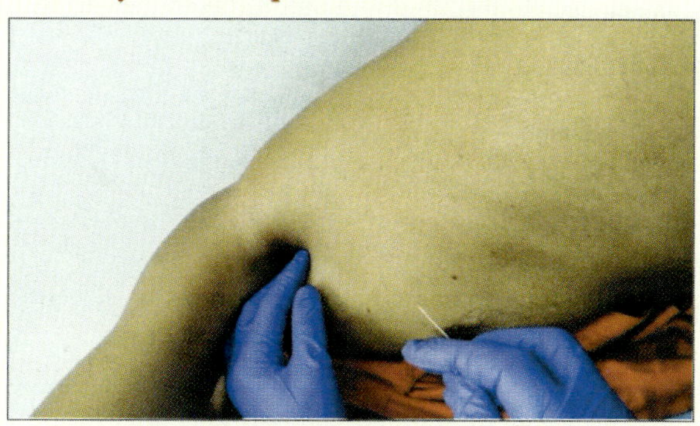

  a. Bone marrow aspirate b. FNAC
  c. Blood culture d. Pleural tap

3. What is this brush used for

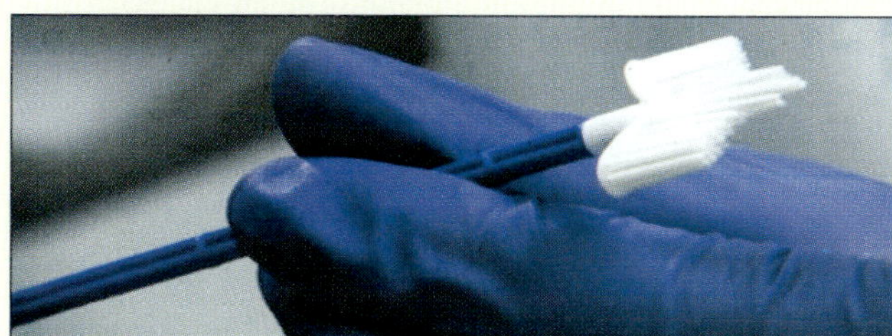

  a. Liquid based cytology b. Conventional cytology
  c. CSF needle d. Pleural tapping

4. What is this way of taking samples called:

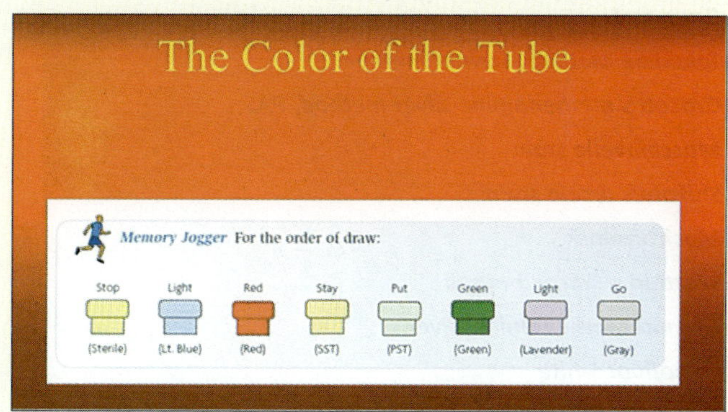

  a. Order of draw b. Collection sample order
  c. Universal protocol d. None

5. What is the solution used when there is blood spill

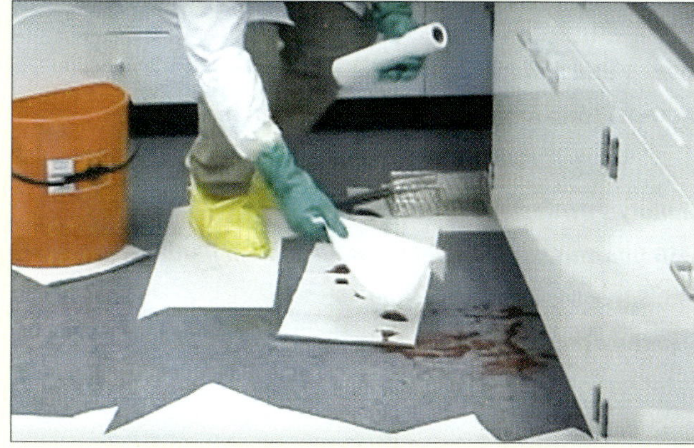

  a. Hypochlorite
  b. H_2SO_4
  c. HCl
  d. Formalin

For video, scan this QR Code

Ans.

1. a
2. b
3. a
4. a
5. a

Annexure 1

1. Important Special Stains and Fixatives

Name of stain	Elements stained
For Microorganisms	
Ziehl-Neelsen stain, Kinyoun stain	Acid-Fast Organism
May - Grünwald Giemsa Stain	Bacteria, blood elements
Gram stain	Bacteria
Toluidine Method, Steiner method	Helicobacter pylori (stained black)
Grocott's methenamine silver method, PAS	Fungi
Macchiavello stain	Rickettsia and viral inclusions
Shikata's orcein stain	Hepatitis B Antigen
Mucicarmine	Cryptococcus
Warthin – Starry method	Spirochetes
Gomori Methenamine silver	Fungus (stained black)
Calcofluor white	Acanthamoeba (stained white)
For Connective tissue and lipids	
Hematoxylin & Eosin stain (H&E)	All tissues (most commonly used stain)
Trichrome Stain	Collagen
Verhoeff - Van Gieson's stain (Best for Elastin)	Elastic fibers
Luna stain	Elastin & Mast cells
Silver Methenamine stain	Reticulin
Oil red O stain (on Fresh specimen/Frozen section)	Fat
Sudan black (on fixed specimen)	
Mallory's PTAH stain	Muscle striations
MSB (martius scarlet blue) (1st stain to stain fibrin in various stages)	Fibrin
PAS, Silver Methenamine stain	Basement membrane
Bielschowsky (silver stain)	Neurofibrillary tangles, Senile plaques
Luxol fast blue	Myelin
Papanicolau stain	Cervical Exfoliative cytology
For Carbohydrates	
PAS	Glycogen/neutral mucin or mucoprotein
Alcian blue	Differentiates Acid & neutral mucopolysaccharides
(at pH 2.5: positive for acid mucopolysaccharides)	
Mucicarmine stain (specific)	Acidic epithelial Mucin
Alcian blue at pH 1	Highly acidic mucins (sulphated mucins)

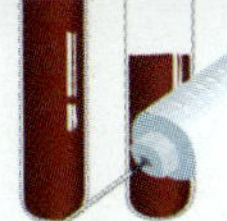

For Amyloid	
Congo Red stain	Amyloid (Gold standard is Congo red staining with apple green birefringence under polarized light)
Metachromatic stains like crystal violet	
For Minerals, pigments and miscellaneous	
Von Kossa stain *(most commonly used)*	Calcium
alizarin red S at pH 4.2 *(specific for Calcium)*	
Prussian blue	Iron
Fontana Masson Silver stain	Melanin
Modified fouchets	Bile pigments
Orcein	Copper
Modified rhodamine *(method of choice)*	
For Hematological cells	
Romanowsky stain (Giemsa, Leishman, Wright, Genner)	Routine blood & bone marrow
Myeloperoxidase	Myeloid cells
Sudan Black B	Myeloid cells
Non-specific Esterase	Monocytic cells
Acid Phosphatase	T-lymphocytes
PAS	Lymphoblasts (block positive), Dysplastic Erythroids, Megakaryocytes (granular positive)
TRAP (Tartrate-resistant Acid Phosphatase)	Hairy cell Leukemia
Toluidine blue	Mast cells & Basophils

2. Important Fixatives

HISTOPATHOLOGY	
Routine fixative	10% buffered normal Formalin (most commonly used)
Electron Microscopy	Glutaraldehyde (most commonly used), Osmium tetraoxide
Special Tissues	**Fixatives**
GI Biopsies & testicular Bx for infertility diagnosis	Bouin's fluid
Bone Marrow Biopsies	Zenker's fluid, B-5
Brain Tissues	Formalin ammonium Bromide
Adrenal Medulla	Orth's fluid
CYTOPATHOLOGY	
Nuclear fixatives	Carnoy's Fluid
Cytoplasmic Fixatives	Champy's Fluid
PAP smears	95% ethyl alcohol
Cell blocks	Bouin's fluid

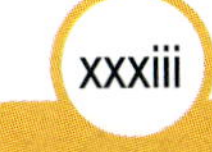

Annexure 2

3. Cytokines and Cytokine Receptors

Cytokine	Receptor	Cell Source	Cell Target	Biologic Activity
IL-1,		Monocytes/macrophages, B cells	All cells	• Explained in detail in text
IL-2		T cells[q]	T cells, B cells	• T cell activation and proliferation[q], • B cell growth[q]
IL-3		T cells	Bone marrow progenitors[q]	• Hematopoietic progenitor stimulation.[q]
IL-4		T cells		• T_H2 differentiation and proliferation.[q] • B cell Ig class switching[q]
IL-5		T cells, mast cells & eosinophils	Eosinophils,[q] basophils[q]	• Eosinophil activation.[q]
IL-6	Gp130	Monocytes/macrophages, B cells		• Myeloma cell[q] growth, • Osteoclast growth and activation.[q] • T and B cell differentiation and growth[q]
IL-7		Bone marrow, thymic epithelial cells[q]		• Important for T-cell development[q]
IL-8	CXCR1, CXCR2	Monocytes/macrophages	Neutrophils	• Neutrophil migration[q] (neutrophil chemotactic factor) • Stimulates angiogenesis.[q] • Suppresses hepatic precursor proliferation.[q]
IL-9		T cells	Bone marrow progenitors	• Induces mast cell proliferation and function[q]
IL-10		Monocytes/ macrophages, T cells, B cells		• Anti-inflammatory molecule[q]
IL-11	Gp130	Bone marrow stromal cells	Megakaryocytes,	• Induces megakaryocyte colony formation[q]
IL-12		Activated macrophages	T cells	• Induces T_H1 T helper cell formation & lymphokine-activated killer cell formation.[q]
IL-13		T cells (T_H2)		• Inhibits macrophage proinflammatory cytokine production.[q]
IL-14		T cells	B cells	• Induces B cell proliferation
IL-15		Monocytes/macrophages,	T cells	• T cell activation and proliferation. • Promotes angiogenesis[q]
IL-16	CD4	Mast cells,CD8+ T cells	CD4+ T cells,	• Chemoattraction of CD4+ T cells,[q] • Inhibits HIV replication.[q]
IL-17		CD4+ T cells		• Neutrophil recruitment[q]
IL-18		Keratinocytes, macrophages		• Upregulated IFN production[q]
IL-21		CD4 T cells	NK cells	• Down-regulates NK cell activating molecules, NKG2D/DAP10[q]
IL-23		Macrophages	T cells	• Opposite effects of IL-12 (IL-17, -IFN)[q]

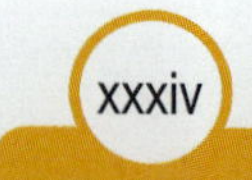

Annexure 3

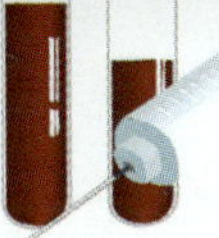

4. Type of Modified Macrophages

Modified Macrophages	Location
Adipose tissue macrophages	Adipose tissue
Monocyte	Bone Marrow/Blood
Kupffer cell	Liver
Sinus histiocytes	Lymph node
Alveolar macrophages (dust cell)	Pulmonary alveolus of lungs
Tissue macrophages (Histiocyte) leading to Giant cells	Connective tissues
Langerhans cell	Skin and mucosa
Microglia	Central Nervous System
Hofbauer cell	Placenta
Intraglomerular mesangial cell	Kidney
Osteoclasts	Bone
Epithelioid cells	Granulomas
Red Pulp Macrophage (Sinusoidal lining cells)	Red pulp of spleen
Peritoneal macrophages	Peritoneal cavity

5. Types of Giant Cells

Variety	Characteristics
Physiological giant cells	Osteoclasts, syncytiotrophoblasts and megakaryocytes.
Langhan giant cell	Nuclei present in the periphery, in a **horseshoe pattern,** seen in is **tuberculosis.**[Q]
Foreign body giant cell	<ul><li>Nuclei are arranged randomly or haphazardly here.</li><li>Seen in granuloma formed by **foreign bodies**, like sutures (intravenous drug abuse, talc)</li><li>Appears **refractile**[Q] when viewed with polarized light</li></ul>
Touton giant cells	<ul><li>Seen in **xanthomas, fat necrosis, xanthogranulomatous inflammation, dermatofibroma.**[Q]</li><li>Formed by fusion of epithelioid cells</li><li>Contain a ring of nuclei surrounded by foamy cytoplasm.</li></ul>
Warthin-Finkeldey giant cells	**Measles.**[Q]
Reed-Sternberg cells	**Hodgkin's lymphoma**[Q]
Tumor giant cells[Q]	Tumors, e.g. HCC

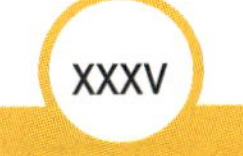

Annexure 4

6. Important Translocations

Translocation	Gene (Chromosome)	Malignancy
(9;22)(q34;q11)[Q]	**Bcr–Abl**	**Chronic myeloid leukemia**[Q]
(11;14)(q13;q32)	**Bcl1–IgH**	**Mantle cell lymphoma**[Q]
(8;21)[Q]	*RUNX1-RUNX1T1*	*Acute myeloid leukemia*[Q]
(15;17)[Q]	*PML-RARA*	
(16;16)[Q]	*CBFB-MYH11*	
(14;18)(q32;q21)	*BCL2–IgH*	*Follicular lymphoma*[Q]
(11;22)(q24;q12)	*FLI1–EWS*	*Ewing's sarcoma*[Q]
(1;7)(p34;q35)[Q]	LCK–TCRB	T cell acute lymphocytic leukemia
(8;14)(q24;q32)	**Myc–IgH**	**Burkitt's lymphoma**[Q] **B cell acute lymphocytic leukemia**[Q]
(2;13)(q35;q14)	PAX3 –FKHR/ALV	*Alveolar rhabdomyosarcoma*[Q]
(1;13)(p36;q14)	PAX7 –KHR/ALV	
Inv (2p13;p11.2-14)	REL–NRG	Non-Hodgkin's lymphoma
(10;17)(q11.2;q23)	RET–PKAR1A	Thyroid carcinoma
(1;3)(p34;p21)[Q]	**TAL1–TCTA**[Q]	*Acute T cell leukemia*[Q]
Inv1(q23;q31)	TRK–TPM3	Colon carcinoma
(12;22)(q13;q12)[Q]	ATF1–EWS	Malignant melanoma of soft parts
(11;22)(p13;q12)[Q]	WT1–EWS[Q]	*Desmoplastic small round cell tumor*[Q]

7. Important Genes & Chromosome

Gene	Chromosome No.
Rb	13q14.3
p53	17q13.1
APC	5q21
NF1 (Hamartin)	17q11
NF2	22p12
WT$_1$	11p13
BRCA1	17q21
BRCA2	13q12
VHL	3p25
p16	9p21
RET (MEN2 syndrome)	10q
ABO	9
Rh	1
PRSS1	7q
FXN (Friedrich ataxia)	9q21.1
DMPK (Myotonic dystrophy)	19q13.3
Menin (MEN1 syndrome)	11q

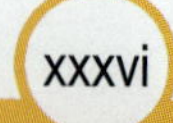

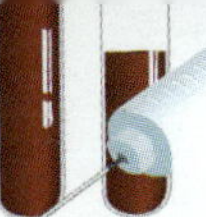

8. Chromosomal Abnormality

Chromosomes involved	Neoplasm
t(9;22)	CML[Q] (p210), ALL (p190, FAB types L1 and L2)
t(8;14)	Burkitt's[Q] lymphoma, ALL (type L3), Immunoblastic B cell lymphoma
t(15;17)	Acute Promyelocytic Leukemia[Q]
t(11;14)	Mantle zone Lymphoma, Multiple myeloma, CLL[Q]
t(11;22)	Ewing's sarcoma[Q]
t(14;18)	Follicular lymphomas, DLBCL (20%)[Q]
t(6;14)	Cystadenocarcinoma of ovary[Q]
t(3;8)	Renal adenocarcinoma, Mixed parotid tumor (benign)
Trisomy 12	Chronic lymphocytic leukemia
Chr 8 and 17	Blast crisis of CML[Q]
5q- and 7q-	MDS, AML
1p-	Neuroblastoma[Q]
13q-	Retinoblastoma[Q], Osteosarcoma[Q], Small- cell carcinoma of lung[Q]
Chr 22	Meningioma

Annexure 5

9. Cancer Predisposition Syndromes and Associated Gene

Syndrome	Gene	Chr.	Inherit.	Tumors
Ataxia telangiectasia	*ATM*	11q22	AR	Breast
Bloom syndrome	*BLM*	15q26	AR	Acute Leukemia
Cowden syndrome	PTEN	10q23	AD	Breast, thyroid
Familial adenomatous polyposis	APC	5q21	AD	Intestinal adenoma, colorectal
Familial melanoma	*p16INK4*	9p21	AD	Melanoma, pancreatic
Familial Wilms' tumor	*WT1*	11p13	AD	Kidney (pediatric)
Hereditary breast/ovarian cancer	*BRCA1 BRCA2*	17q21 13q12	AD	Breast, ovarian, colon, prostate
Her. diffuse gastric Ca	*CDH1*	16q22	AD	Stomach
Hereditary multiple exostoses	*EXT1 EXT2*	8q24	AD	Exostoses, chondrosarcoma
Hereditary retinoblastoma	*RB1*	13q14	AD	Retinoblastoma, osteosarcoma
Hereditary nonpolyposis colon cancer (HNPCC)	*MSH2/6*	2p16	AD	Colon, endometrial, ovarian, stomach, small bowel, ureter Ca
Hereditary papillary renal carcinoma	MET	7q31	AD	Papillary kidney
Juvenile polyposis	*SMAD4*	18q21	AD	Gastrointestinal, pancreatic
Li-Fraumeni Synd	*TP53*	17p13	AD	Sarcoma, breast
Multiple endocrine neoplasia type 1	*MEN1*	11q13	AD	Parathyroid, endocrine, pancreas, and pituitary
Multiple endocrine neoplasia type 2a	RET	10q11	AD	Medullary thyroid carcinoma, pheochromocytoma
Neurofibromatosis type 1	*NF1*	17q11	AD	Neurofibroma, neurofibrosarcoma, brain
Neurofibromatosis type 2	*NF2*	22q12	AD	Vestibular schwannoma, meningioma, spine
NBCCS (Gorlin syndrome)	PTCH	9q22	AD	Basal cell carcinoma, medulloblastoma, jaw cysts
Tuberous sclerosis	TSC	9q34 16p13	AD	Angiofibroma, renal angiomyolipoma
Von Hippel–Lindau	*VHL*	3p25	AD	Kidney, cerebellum, pheochromocytoma

Annexure 6

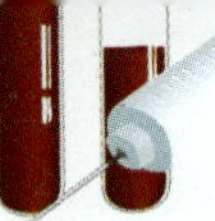

10. CD Markers used for Hematolymphoid Neoplasms, Location/Characteristics

Hematological cells	Immunophenotyping Markers (on Flow Cytometry)
Blasts	**CD34,**[Q] tdt (Lymphoblasts), HLADR
RBCs	Glycophorin A
Megakaryocytic marker	**CD41,**[Q] **CD61**
WBCs	**CD 45**[Q] **(Leukocyte Common Antigen)**[Q]
Myeloid cells	**Anti- MPO,**[Q] CD13, CD33, CD14, CD117
B –cells	**CD19,**[Q] CD20, CD22, FMC7, CD23, **CD79 a**, CD79 b, S lg, IgM
T-cells	**CD3,**[Q] CD2, CD5, CD7, CD8, TCR-α/β, **TCR-γ/δ**
NK cells	**CD16,**[Q] **CD56,**[Q] CD57
Plasma cells	**CD38,**[Q] **CD138,**[Q] kappa and Lambda light chains

CD Marker	Location/ Characteristics
CD1	**CD1a: Cortical thymocytes, dendritic cells (DCs), epidermal Langerhans cells**
	CD1b: Langerhans cells
	CD1c: **Thymocytes, B cells,** mantle zone, and umbilical cord
	CD1d: Intestinal epithelium, kidney tubular epithelia, hepatocytes, and thymus
CD2	Thymocytes, T cells
CD3	Signaling component of **T cell receptor** (TCR) complex
CD4	A co-receptor for MHC Class II; also a receptor **used by HIV** to enter T cells
CD5	T cells, **thymocytes, and B cells, Seen in CLL**, Mantle cell lymphoma and T-cell lymphoma
CD7	**Thymocytes**, some T cells
CD8	Co-receptor for **MHC Class I**
CD9	**Pre B cells**, eosinophils, basophils and platelets
CD10	**Pre-B cells, germinal-center B** cells, ALL, **follicular B- cell lymphomas**
CD11c	Dendritic cells and **hairy cell leukemia** cells
CD13	Myelomonocytic cells, AML, lymphoma and lymphocytic leukemia
CD14	**Macrophages** which binds to bacterial lipopolysaccharide
CD16	Fc receptor for IgG on NK cells
CD19	Component of the **B-cell co-receptor**
CD20	Transmembrane protein found on **B cells**
CD21	**CR2,** mature B cells, **Receptor for complement (C3d) and Epstein-Barr virus (EBV)**
CD22	Inhibitory receptor for **B cell receptor (BCR) signaling**
CD23	Mature B cells, monocytes, activated macrophages, Seen in **CLL**
CD24	**B lymphocytes**
CD25	High-affinity receptor for **IL-2; Hairy cell leukemias**
CD28	T-cells, **co-stimulatory effect on the T-cell**
CD30	Present on **activated T and B cell**; Hodgkin disease, **anaplastic large cell lymphomas**
CD31	**PECAM-1**, a cell adhesion molecule on platelets and endothelial cells

Contd....

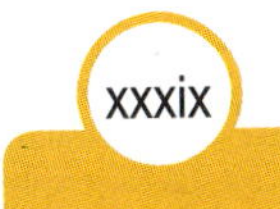

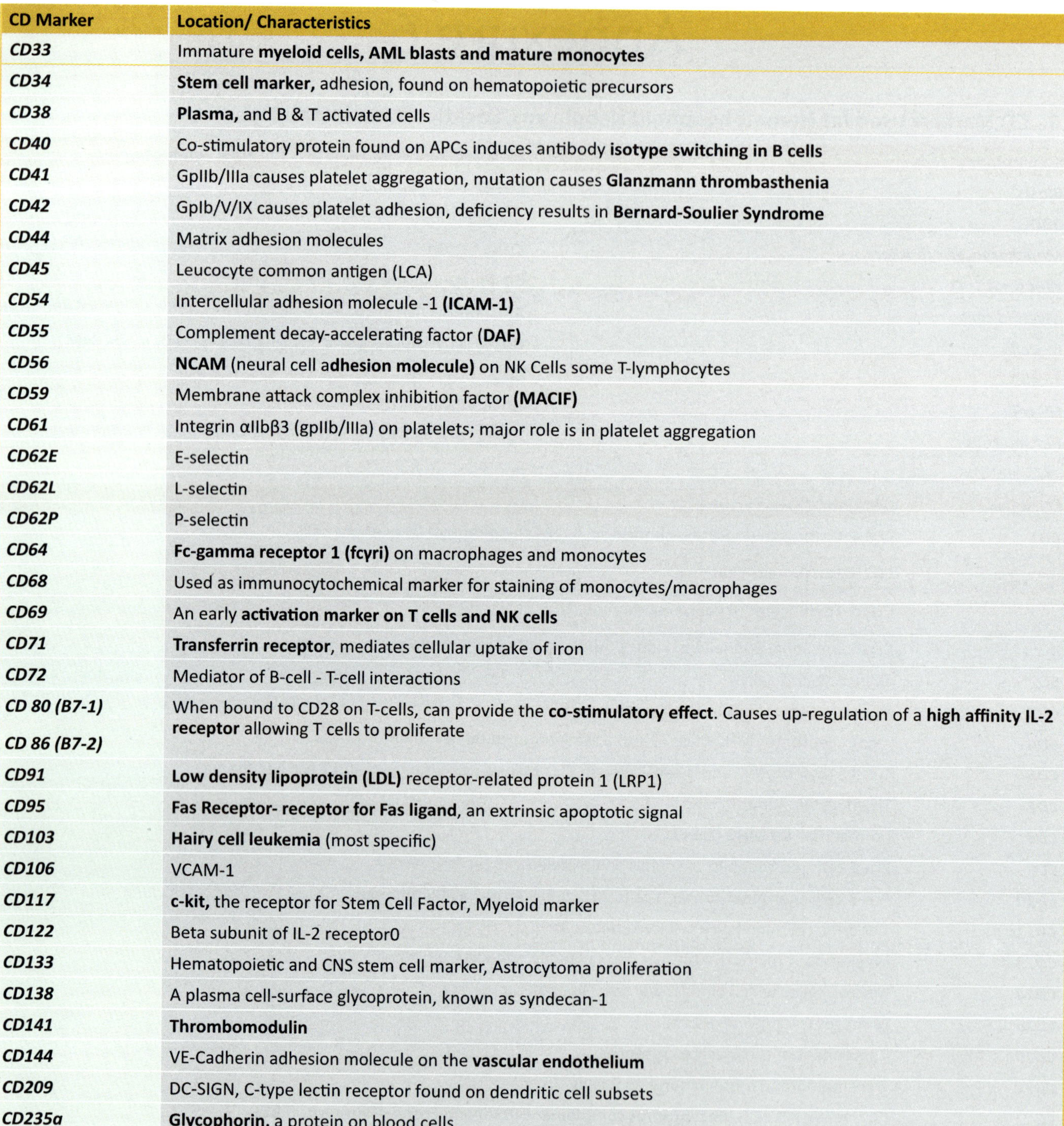

CD Marker	Location/ Characteristics
CD33	Immature **myeloid cells, AML blasts and mature monocytes**
CD34	**Stem cell marker,** adhesion, found on hematopoietic precursors
CD38	**Plasma,** and B & T activated cells
CD40	Co-stimulatory protein found on APCs induces antibody **isotype switching in B cells**
CD41	GpIIb/IIIa causes platelet aggregation, mutation causes **Glanzmann thrombasthenia**
CD42	GpIb/V/IX causes platelet adhesion, deficiency results in **Bernard-Soulier Syndrome**
CD44	Matrix adhesion molecules
CD45	Leucocyte common antigen (LCA)
CD54	Intercellular adhesion molecule -1 **(ICAM-1)**
CD55	Complement decay-accelerating factor **(DAF)**
CD56	**NCAM** (neural cell a**dhesion molecule)** on NK Cells some T-lymphocytes
CD59	Membrane attack complex inhibition factor **(MACIF)**
CD61	Integrin $\alpha IIb\beta 3$ (gpIIb/IIIa) on platelets; major role is in platelet aggregation
CD62E	E-selectin
CD62L	L-selectin
CD62P	P-selectin
CD64	**Fc-gamma receptor 1 (fcyri)** on macrophages and monocytes
CD68	Used as immunocytochemical marker for staining of monocytes/macrophages
CD69	An early **activation marker on T cells and NK cells**
CD71	**Transferrin receptor**, mediates cellular uptake of iron
CD72	Mediator of B-cell - T-cell interactions
CD 80 (B7-1) CD 86 (B7-2)	When bound to CD28 on T-cells, can provide the **co-stimulatory effect**. Causes up-regulation of a **high affinity IL-2 receptor** allowing T cells to proliferate
CD91	**Low density lipoprotein (LDL)** receptor-related protein 1 (LRP1)
CD95	**Fas Receptor- receptor for Fas ligand**, an extrinsic apoptotic signal
CD103	**Hairy cell leukemia** (most specific)
CD106	VCAM-1
CD117	**c-kit,** the receptor for Stem Cell Factor, Myeloid marker
CD122	Beta subunit of IL-2 receptor0
CD133	Hematopoietic and CNS stem cell marker, Astrocytoma proliferation
CD138	A plasma cell-surface glycoprotein, known as syndecan-1
CD141	**Thrombomodulin**
CD144	VE-Cadherin adhesion molecule on the **vascular endothelium**
CD209	DC-SIGN, C-type lectin receptor found on dendritic cell subsets
CD235a	**Glycophorin,** a protein on blood cells

Annexure 7

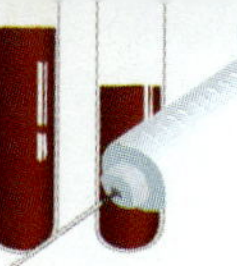

11. Features of the Peripheral Blood Smear

RBC Morphology	Images	Definition	Associated conditions
Normal RBC		**Central palor**	None
Polychromasia		**Large, bluish** (due to residual **RNA**) RBCs **lacking central pallor**	**Rapid production & release** of RBCs from BM; **Elevated retic % (hemolytic anemia)**
Basophilic stippling		**Small bluish dots** in RBCs (**clustered polyribosomes**)	**Hemolytic anemia & lead poisoning** (lead **inhibits pyrimidine 5' nucleotidase**, which normally digests the residual RNA)
Pappenheimer bodies		**Grayish, irregular inclusions** in RBCs composed of aggregates of **ribosomes, ferritin & mitochondria**	Hemoglobinopathies, splenic hypofunction; megaloblastic anemia
Target RBCs		**Central round staining in RBCs**	**Liver disease**, Dysbetalipoproteinemia, **Hemolytic anemia, Severe IDA**
Heinz bodies		Several grayish, round inclusions represent aggregates of denatured hemoglobin	Indicative of oxidative injury **G6PD deficiency**, or unstable hemoglobin
Howell-jolly bodies		**Few purplish inclusions** on RBC represent residual fragments of nuclei containing chromatin	**Splenic hypofunction, post-splenectomy, severe hemolytic anemia**
Schistocytes		**Fragmented RBCs** helmet-shaped cells; indicative of shearing of the erythrocyte within the circulation	Microangiopatic hemolytic anemias, including **DIC, TTP** or **HUS**, mechanical causes of hemolysis, such as prosthetic valves
Spherocytes		RBCs that have **lost their central pallor** and appear **spherical**.	**H.S, AIHA, Toxins, Burns**
Teardrop cells		**Pear-shaped RBCs** indicative of mechanical stress on the RBC during release from the BM or passage through the spleen	**Thalassemia, megaloblastic anemia; myelofibrosis**, myelophthisis (BM replacement)
Burr cells (echinocytes)		**Smooth undulations** present on RBC surface circumferentially	**Uremia**, drying artifact
Spur cells (acanthocytes)		**Spiny points** present on the surface circumferentially; reflective of normal lipid composition of RBC membrane	**Liver disease**, abetalipoproteinemia, RBCs lacking the Kell blood group antigen

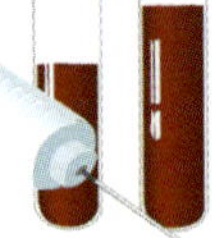

12. Blood-Clotting Factors

Factor	Names	Plasma Half-Life
I	**Fibrinogen**[Q]	**2–4 d**[Q]
II	**Prothrombin**[Q]	**3-4 d**[Q]
III	**Thromboplastin**[Q]	–
IV	**Calcium**[Q]	–
V	**Proaccelerin, labile factor**[Q], accelerator globulin	**36 hr**[Q]
VII	Proconvertin, SPCA, stable factor	**4-6 hr (min)**[Q]
VIII	**Antihemophilic factor A (AHF)**[Q]	**8-12 hr**[Q]
IX	**Christmas factor**[Q], **antihemophilic factor B**[Q]	18-24 hr
X	**Stuart–Prower factor**[Q]	**40-60 hr**[Q]
XI	Plasma thromboplastin antecedent (PTA), antihemophilic factor C	40-70 hr
XII	**Hageman factor**[Q], glass factor	60 hr
XIII	Fibrin-stabilizing factor, **Laki–Lorand factor**[Q]	**11-14 d (max)**[Q]
HMW-K	High-molecular-weight kininogen, **Fitzgerald factor**[Q]	150 hr
Pre-K$_a$	Prekallikrein, Fletcher factor	35 hr
PL	Platelet phospholipid	–

Annexure 8

13. Crystals in Urine

Triple Phosphate		• Seen in **alkaline urine** • Rectangular shape
Uric acid		• Seen in **acidic urine** • Brown lemon shaped or star shaped • Birefringent with polarized light
Calcium oxalate		• Envelope shaped • Seen in **acidic urine**

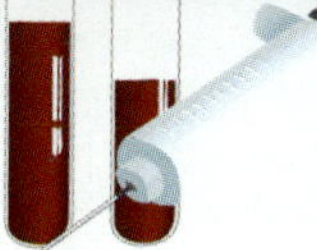

14. Different Types of Urinary Casts

Type	Images	Description	Significance
Plain casts (Cast Matrix)			
Hyaline		Consists of Tamm-Horsfall protein	Nonspecific; **0-2/lpf is normal**[Q] **Most frequently observed cast**[Q] Increased number in: **renal diseases, dehydration**[Q]**, fever**[Q]**, congestive heart failure, diuretic therapy**[Q]
Waxy		Easily visualized due to high refractive index	Observed most frequently in **Chronic Renal Failure;**[Q] Broad waxy casts are called **"Renal Failure Casts"**[Q] Also seen in **acute & chronic Renal Allograft Rejection**[Q]
Cellular casts			
RBC		Appears red-orange	**Pathognomonic of glomerulonephritis (RPGN)**[Q] Indicator of **bleeding within the nephron** Also seen in: **IgA Nephropathy**[Q]**, Lupus Nephritis, Bacterial endocarditis, Renal infarction**[Q]
WBC		Protein matrix with WBCs	**Pyelonephritis**[Q] **& tubulointerstitial disease**[Q]**,** Also seen in **glomerular diseases**[Q]**, Lupus Nephritis, Interstitial Nephritis**[Q]
Epithelial cell		Protein matrix with tubular cells	**Acute Tubular Necrosis**[Q]**, Viral infection (CMV), Heavy Metal**[Q]**, Salicylate poisoning**[Q]
Inclusion Casts			
Granular		Glycoprotein matrix with protein or cellular debris	Glomerular, **tubular, tubulointerstitial diseases, Renal graft rejection**, lead poisoning, after strenuous exercise Coarse: in **Renal Papillary Necrosis**[Q] Fine: May be **physiological**[Q]**, Hyperparathyroidism**[Q]
Fatty		**"Maltese cross pattern"** in polarized light	Commonly seen in heavy proteinuria, characteristic of **nephrotic syndrome**[Q]
Crystal	*(See Next page)*	Urates, **Ca oxalate**[Q]	Indicate deposition of **crystals** in tubules or **collecting ducts**
Other Casts			
Pigment		Granular casts with pigment stain	Usually occurs in acute kidney injury due to **hemolysis**[Q] **or rhabdomyolysis**[Q] or in acute tubular necrosis; **Bilirubin cast** in **obstructive jaundice**
Broad		Diameter 2 to 6 times of normal casts	Typically seen in Chronic Renal Failure[Q] Indicate poor prognosis[Q]

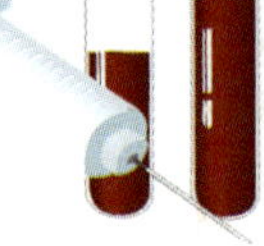

Annexure 9

15. Rosettes

Rosette Type	Schematic Diagram	Definition	Associated Tumors
Homer Wright rosette		• Ball-like arrangement of cells that enclose meshwork of fibers. • **Fibers represent primitive neuronal processes**[Q]	• **Neuroblastoma,**[Q] • **Medulloblastoma,**[Q] • PNET • Pineoblastoma
Flexner-Wintersteiner rosette		• Tumor cells circumscribe a **central lumen** • Lumen contains small **cytoplasmic extensions of the encircling cells.**[Q]	• **Retinoblastoma,**[Q] Pineoblastoma, Medulloepithelioma
True ependymal rosette		• Rosettes with an **empty** appearing lumen	• **Ependymoma**[Q]
Perivascular pseudorosette		• Spoke-wheel arrangement of cells • Tapered cellular processes **radiates around a wall of a centrally-placed vessel.**[Q]	• **Ependymoma,**[Q] • Medulloblastoma, • PNET • Central neurocytoma, • Glioblastoma, • Monomorphous pilomyxoid astrocytomas
Pineocytomatous & Neurocytic rosette		• **Neuropil-rich rosettes** similar to Homer-Wright rosettes • **Larger and more irregular in contour**	• **Pineocytoma**[Q] • **Central neurocytoma**

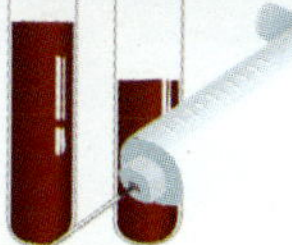

16. Familial Cancer Syndromes with Cutaneous Manifestations

Disease	Inheritance	Chromosomal Location	Gene/Protein
Ataxia-telangiectasia	**AR**[Q]	11q22.3	*ATM*/ATM[Q]
Nevoid basal cell carcinoma syndrome	AD	9q22.3	*PTCH*/PTCH[Q]
Cowden syndrome	AD	10q23	*PTEN*/PTEN[Q]
Familial melanoma syndrome	**AD**	**9p21**[Q]	*CDKN2*/p16/INK4;[Q] *CDKN2*/p14/ARF[Q]
Muir-Torre syndrome	AD	2p22	*MSH2*/MSH2;[Q] *MLH1*/MLH1
Tuberous sclerosis	AD	9q34, 16p13.3	*TSC1*/hamartin;[Q] *TSC2*/tuberin[Q]
Neurofibromatosis I	**AD**	**17q11.2**[Q]	*NF1*/neurofibromin[Q]
Neurofibromatosis II	AD	22q12.2	*NF2*/merlin[Q]
Xeroderma pigmentosum	**AR**[Q]	9q22 and others	*XPA*/XPA and others

17. Relationship between Proteins and Neurodegenerative Diseases

Protein	Diseases with Inclusions
Aβ	**Alzheimer disease**[Q]
Tau	**Alzheimer disease**[Q] **Frontotemporal lobar degeneration**[Q] **Parkinson disease (with LRRK2 mutations)**[Q] **Progressive supranuclear palsy** **Corticobasal degeneration**[Q]
TPD-43	Frontotemporal lobar degeneration **Amyotrophic lateral sclerosis**[Q]
FUS	**Frontotemporal lobar degeneration**[Q] Amyotrophic lateral sclerosis
α-synuclein	**Parkinson disease**[Q] **Multiple system atrophy**[Q]
Polyglutamine aggregates **(distinct proteins per disease)**	**Huntington's disease**[Q] Some forms of spinocerebellar ataxia Spinal bulbar muscular atrophy

Annexure 10

18. Pattern of Injury and Associated Agents

Pattern of Injury	Examples of Associated Agents
Budd-Chiari syndrome	Oral contraceptives
Peliosis hepatis (Dilated sinusoids)	**Anabolic steroids, Danazol, OCPs, tamoxifen**[Q]
Hepatic adenoma	Oral contraceptives, anabolic steroids
Hepatocellular carcinoma	**Thorotrast**[Q]
Cholangiocarcinoma	Thorotrast
Angiosarcoma	Thorotrast, **vinyl chloride, Arsenic, Thorium dioxide**[Q]
Cholestatis	**OCPs** and anabolic steroids[Q]
Cholestatic hepatitis	Chlorpromazine, Statins
Spotty hepatocyte necrosis	Methyldopa, phenytoin
Submassive necrosis, zone 3	Paracetamol, **halothane**[Q]
Massive necrosis	**Isoniazid, phenytoin**[Q]
Macrovesicular Steatosis	Ethanol, methotrexate, corticosteroids, TPN
Microvesicular Steatohepatitis with Mallory bodies	**Amiodarone, ethanol**[Q]
Fibrosis and cirrhosis	Methotrexate (Periportal fibrosis), isoniazid, enalapril
Noncaseating Granulomas	**Sulfonamides**[Q]

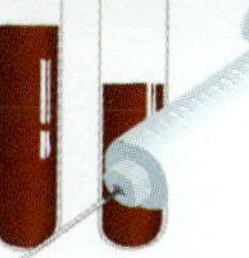

Annexure 11

19. Morphological Differentiation of Malaria Parasites

	P. falciparum	*P. vivax*	*P. ovale*	*P. malariae*
Infected red cells	Normal size,[a] Maurer's clefts[b]	Enlarged; Schuffner's dots[c]	Enlarged; oval and fimbriated; Schuffner's dots[c]	Normal or microcytic; stippling not usually seen
Ring forms (early trophozoites)	Delicate; frequently 2 or more; accole forms;[d] small chromatin dot	Large, thick; usually single (occasionally 2 in cell; large chromatin dot)	Thick compact rings	Very small, compact rings
Later trophozoites	Compact, vacuolated; sometimes 2 chromatin dots	Amoeboid; central vacuole; light blue cytoplasm	Smaller than *P. Vivax*, slightly amoeboid	Band across cell; deep blue cytoplasm
Schizonts	18-24 merozoites filling 2/3 of cell	12-24 merozoites, irregularly arranged	8-12 merozoites filling 3/4 of cell	6-12 merozoites in daisy-head around central mass of pigment
Pigment	Dark to black clumped mass	Fine granular; yellow brown	Coarse light brown	Dark, prominent at all stages
Gametocytes	Crescent of sausage-shaped; diffuse chromatin; single nucleus	Spherical compact, almost fills cell; single nucleus	Oval, fills 3/4 of cell; similar to but smaller than *P. vivax*	Round; fills 1/2 to 2/3 of cell; similar to *P. vivax* but smaller, with no Schuffner's dots

Falciparum Ring forms

Vivax Trophozoite

Falciparum gametocyte

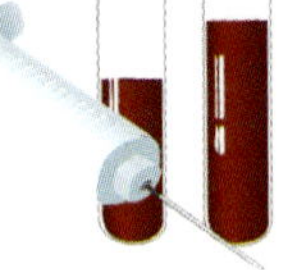

Annexure 12

20. Autoantibodies in Autoimmune Disease

Autoantibodies	Disease	Test sensitivity (%)
Anti-acetylcholine receptor	Myasthenia gravis	>85
Anti-basement membrane	Goodpasture syndrome	>90
Anticentromere	CREST syndrome Diffuse systemic sclerosis	40 <2
Antiendomysial IgA	Celiac disease	95
Antigliadin IgA	Celiac disease	80
Anti histone	Drug-induced lupus	90-95
Anti-insulin	Systemic lupus erythematosus, Type 1 diabetes	50-70 50
Anti-islet cell	Type 1 diabetes	75-80
Anti-intrinsic factor	Pernicious anemia	60
Anti-parietal cell	Pernicious anemia	90
Anti microsomal	Hashimoto thyroiditis	97
Anti-Smith (Sm)	Systemic lupus erythematosus	20-30
Anti-SS-A (Ro)	Sjögren syndrome Systemic lupus erythematosus	70-95 30-50
Anti-SS-B (La)	Sjögren syndrome	60-90
Antithyroglobulin	Systemic lupus erythematosus Hashimoto thyroiditis	10-15 85
Anti-tissue transglutaminase IgA	Celiac disease	98
Anti-DNA topoisomerase	Diffuse systemic sclerosis	30-70
Antimitochondrial	CREST syndrome Primary biliary cirrhosis	10-20 90-100
Anti myeloperoxidase	Microscopic polyangiitis	80 (p-ANCA)
Antinuclear	Systemic lupus erythematosus Systemic sclerosis Dermatomyositis	-100 70-90 <30
Antiproteinase 3	Polymyositis MCTD Primary biliary cirrhosis Wegener granulomatosis	30-60 95-99 50 >90 (c-ANCA)
Anti-ribonucleoprotein	MCTD Systemic lupus erythematosus	85 30-40
Anti-TSH receptor	Graves disease	85

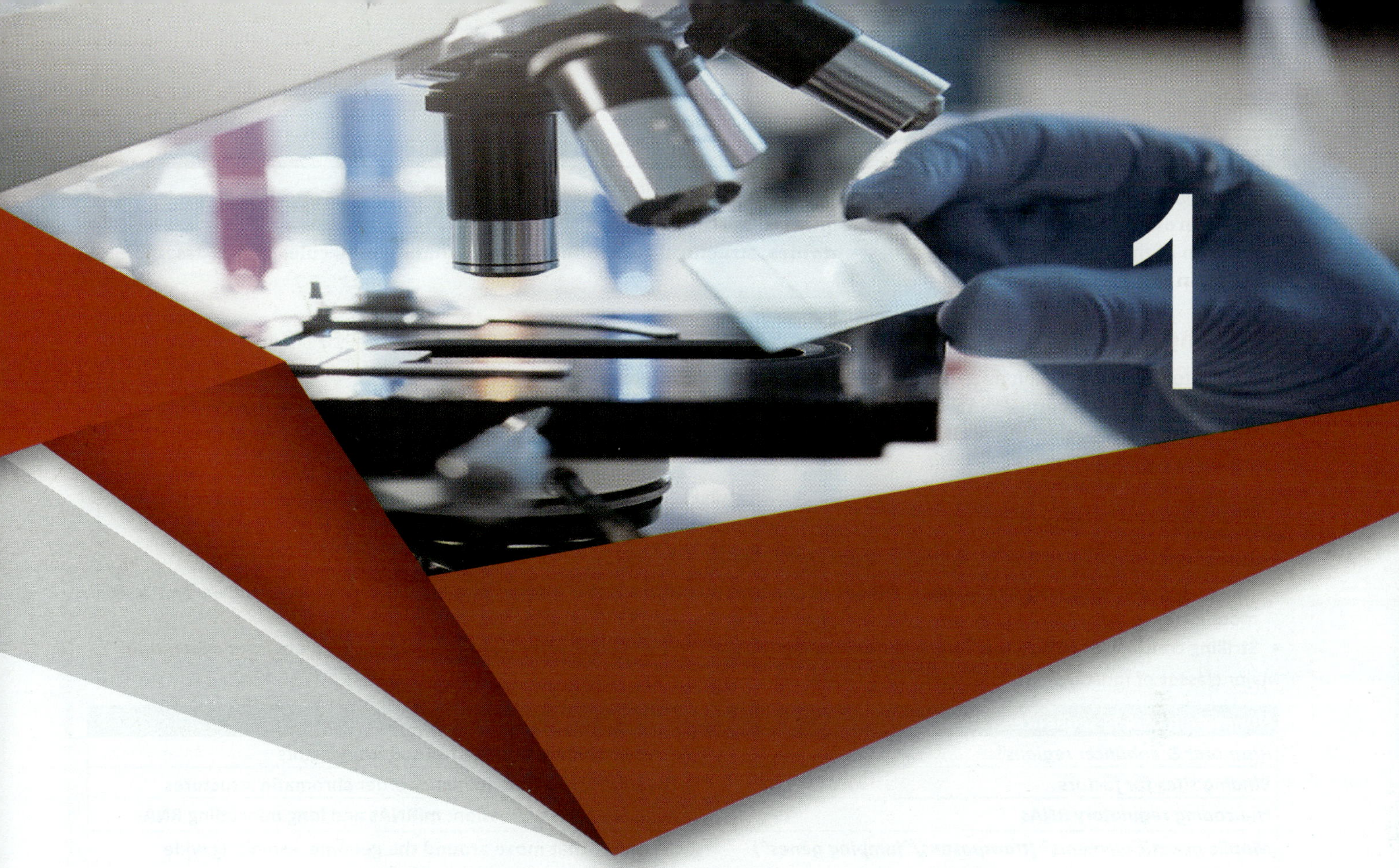

Cell as a Unit of Health and Disease

THE HUMAN GENOME

- Human genome contains **3.2 billion DNA base pairs.**[Q]
- **20,000 protein-encoding genes**[Q], comprising only **1.5% of the genome.**[Q]
- Function of these **protein encoding** genes: enzymes, structural components, and signaling molecules and to **assemble and maintain** all cells in the body.

Noncoding DNA

- It refers to the **98.5%** of human genome that does **not encode proteins.**
- **The amount of noncoding DNA varies greatly among species.** E.g., in bacteria, only 2% of genome is noncoding DNA.
- Noncoding DNA is **also transcribed into functional noncoding RNA molecules (e.g., transfer RNA, ribosomal RNA, and regulatory RNAs)**

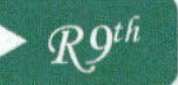

R9th Latest Update

ENCODE (ENCyclopedia of DNA Elements) project: 2007
- This project has systematically **mapped regions of transcription, transcription factor association, chromatin structure and histone modification.**
- Striking conclusion: 80% of the human genome, even the noncoding regions either **binds proteins** or **regulate gene expression.**

Major **classes** of functional **nonprotein-coding sequences:**

Nonprotein coding sequences	Characteristics
Promoter & enhancer regions[Q]	Provide **binding sites** for transcription factors
Binding sites for factors	**Organize and maintain** higher order **chromatin structures**
Noncoding regulatory RNAs	Regulate gene expression: **miRNAs** and **long noncoding RNAs**
Mobile genetic elements[Q] (transposons/"jumping genes")	Segments **that move around the genome**, exhibiting **wide variation** in number and positioning; Role in gene regulation and chromatin organization
Special structural regions of DNA	Chromosome ends (**Telomeres**) and "tethers" (**centromeres**)

POLYMORPHISM

Any two individuals share greater than 99.5% of their DNA sequences.[Q] *So what is the reason of genetic variations?*

The most common forms of DNA variation in the human genome is shown in Flowchart 1.

Flowchart 1: DNA variation in human genome

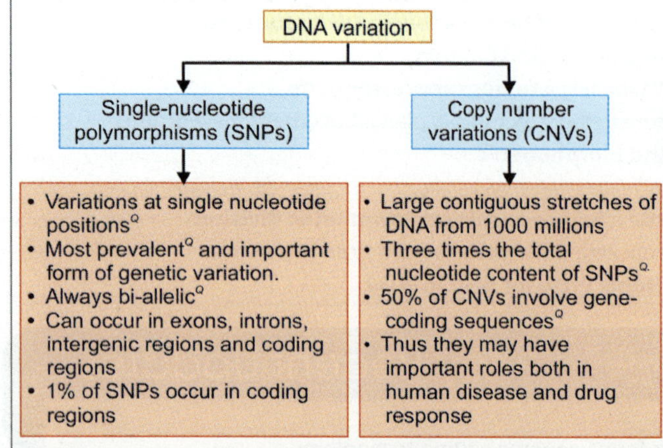

Role of SNPs

- SNPs located in **noncoding regions** are **regulatory elements**[Q] in the genome
- They **alter gene expression**[Q] and have **direct influence** on **disease susceptibility**
- Even if any SNP has no effect on gene function (**Neutral SNP**)[Q], it may be coinherited with the "actual disease causing gene," if located close to that gene → "**Linkage disequilibrium**"[Q]
- May act as **markers of multigenic complex diseases**, E.g. Diabetes, Hypertension.

Epigenetics

- **Definition**
  - **Heritable changes**[Q] in **gene expression, not caused by** alterations in **DNA sequence.**[Q]
- **Epigenetic factors**
  - Histones and histone-modifying factors
    - **Histone methylation, Histone acetylation, Histone phosphorylation, DNA methylation, Chromatin organizing factors**

- *Significance*
  - Epigenetic **Dysregulation** → **central role in malignancy**
  - Many other diseases are associated with **inherited or acquired epigenetic alterations. E.g. Genomic imprinting in Prader Willi syndrome**
  - Epigenetic alterations like histone acetylation and DNA methylation are **reversible** and are **responsive to drugs**; So, **HDAC inhibitors and DNA methylation inhibitors** are being tested in the treatment of cancer
- *Diagnosis*
  - **Sequencing**
  - Chip on chip (**Microarray technology**)
  - Using **Methylation specific primers** in Polymerase chain reaction (PCR)
  - **Bisulphite method**: Bisulphite **converts unmethylated cytosine to uracil**, which **acts like thymine** in downstream reactions. The unmethylated (modified) DNA is detected by sequence analysis.

High Yield Facts

- **SNP** is the most common type of **DNA polymorphism**[Q]
- **SNP** can be **detected by SNP Cytogenomic Array.**
- **Linkage analysis** can be used to detect **SNPs** with **profound effects and high penetrance.**[Q]
- **Linkage analysis** is used to **identify unknown genes**[Q] associated with a disease
- **GWAS** can be used **to identify unknown genes NOT** in 'Linkage disequilibrium'[Q]
- The 2 types of genetic polymorphisms most useful for linkage analysis are **SNPs and repeat length polymorphisms**[Q]
- Repeat length polymorphisms can be **mini-satellite (1-3 kb)**[Q] or **Micro-satellite repeats (<1 kb)**[Q]
- **Genome-wide association study (GWAS)** refers to 'Genome Wide Association Studies'[Q]
- In **GWAS, entire genome** of **large number of individuals** with and without a disease are examined for common **genetic variants or polymorphisms** that are over represented in patients with the disease.

NONCODING REGULATORY RNA

A. Micro-RNA (miRNA): Small **noncoding RNA molecule (22 nucleotides)** which causes **RNA silencing** and **post-transcriptional regulation** of gene expression.

- Generation and mode of action of miRNA is shown in Flowchart 2.

Flowchart 2: Generation of MicroRNA (miRNA) and their mode of action

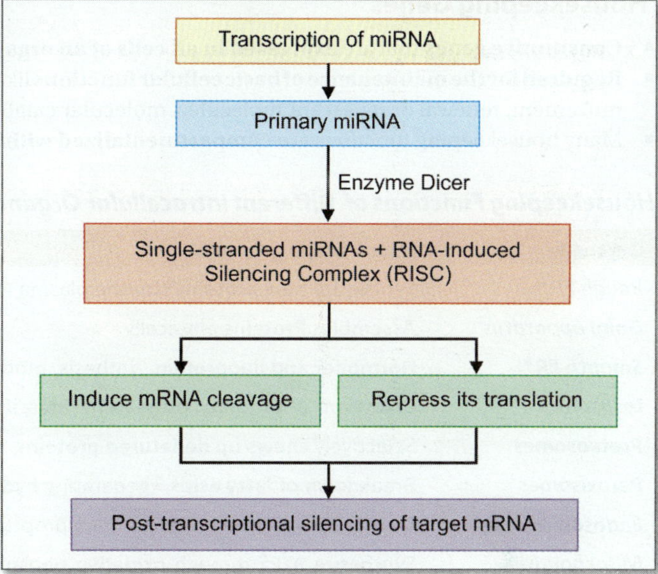

Small Interfering RNAs (siRNAs)

- miRNA **introduced experimentally** into cells and inhibit them
- So-called **"knockdown technology"**
- Possible **therapeutic agents** to **silence pathogenic genes**, such as **oncogenes** involved in neoplastic transformation.

B. Long Noncoding RNA (lncRNA or long ncRNAs): **Nonprotein coding** transcripts **longer than 200 nucleotides**[Q]

lncRNAs modulate gene expression in following ways:

Mechanism	Characteristics
Gene activation	Can **facilitate transcription factor binding** → promote gene activation
Gene suppression	Can preemptively **bind transcription factors** → prevent gene transcription.
Histone & DNA modification	Bind to and **direct acetylases/ methylases** (or deacetylases/ demethylases)
Assembly of protein complexes	Act as scaffolding to stabilize secondary/ tertiary structures and/or multi-subunit complexes influencing chromatin architecture or gene activity
Repressive function	Example: **XIST** → role in physiologic X chromosome inactivation

High Yield Facts

- **lncRNAs** have been found to have link with diseases like **atherosclerosis & cancer.**
- **XIST** refers to **'X-inactive specific transcript'**[Q]
- **XIST** is a RNA gene (17 kb) on the **X** chromosome that acts as **major effector of the X inactivation process.**
- **XIST is expressed on the inactive X chromosome** and not on the active one.

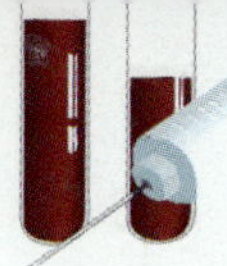

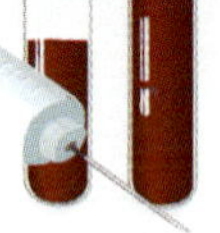

CELLULAR HOUSEKEEPING

'Housekeeping Genes'[Q]

- **Constitutive genes** that are **expressed in all cells of an organism**[Q]
- **Required for the maintenance of basic cellular functions** like protection from environment, nutrient acquisition, communication, movement, renewal of senescent molecules, molecular catabolism, and energy generation.
- Many housekeeping functions are **compartmentalized within intracellular organelles.**

Housekeeping Functions of Different Intracellular Organelles

Organelle	House-keeping function
Rough ER*	**Synthesize new proteins**[Q] for the plasma membrane
Golgi apparatus	**Assembles Proteins** physically
Smooth ER*	**Hormone**[Q] and **lipoprotein** synthesis, **modification** of hydrophobic[Q] compounds into water-soluble molecules
Lysosomes	**Digestion**[Q] of proteins, polysaccharides, lipids, nucleic acids
Proteosomes	Selectively **chews up denatured proteins, releasing peptides**[Q]
Peroxisomes	**Breakdown of fatty acids,**[Q] generating **hydrogen peroxide**
Endosomal vesicles	**Shuttle internalized material**[Q] to appropriate intracellular sites
Mitochondria	**Synthesize ATP**[Q] through **oxidative phosphorylation** & synthesize metabolic **intermediates** needed for anabolic metabolism

* ER → Endoplasmic Reticulum

PLASMA MEMBRANE

Fluid bilayer of amphipathic phospholipids with **hydrophilic head** and **hydrophobic lipid tails** that **forms a barrier to passive diffusion** of large or charged molecules.

Phospholipids in Plasma Membrane and their Functions

Phospholipid	Location	Function
Phosphatidylinositol	**Inner** leaflet of membrane	Acts as **electrostatic scaffold** for intracellular proteins **Hydrolyzed by phospholipase C** to generate 2nd messengers like diacylglycerol (**DAG**) and inositol trisphosphate (**IP3**).[Q]
Phosphatidylserine	**Inner** face	Confers a **−ve charge**[Q] involved in electrostatic protein interactions
	Extracellular face	Acts as **"eat me" signal**[Q] for phagocytes, in cells undergoing **apoptosis**[Q]
	Platelets	Serves as **a cofactor in the clotting**[Q] of blood
Glycolipids and sphingomyelin	**Extracellular** face	Important in cell-cell and cell-matrix interactions including **inflammatory cell recruitment** and **sperm-egg interaction**[Q]

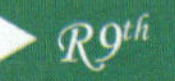 **Latest** Update

Mechanisms of movement across plasma membrane
1. Passive Membrane Diffusion:
- Transfers:
  - **Small, nonpolar**[Q] molecules (e.g. O_2 and CO_2)
  - **Hydrophobic**[Q] molecules (e.g., estradiol or vitamin D)
  - **Polar molecules <75 daltons**[Q] (e.g., water, ethanol, and urea).
- **Effective barrier to:** polar molecules >75 daltons e.g., Glucose & Ions, due to their charge and high degree of hydration.

Contd...

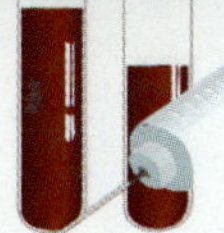

2. Channels and Carrier proteins:
- For low molecular weight molecules (<1000 daltons)
- Each transported molecule (e.g., ion, sugar, nucleotide) requires a specific transporter

Characteristics	Channel proteins	Carrier proteins
Mechanism	Create **hydrophilic**[Q] **pores**	Bind their specific solute → **undergo conformational changes** → transfer the ligand across the membrane
Speed of transport	**Rapid**[Q]	**Relatively slow**[Q]
Direction of movement	**Along** concentration gradient	**Against**[Q] concentration gradient
Active transport	**Cannot occur**[Q]	**Can mediate active transport**[Q]

Receptor-mediated and Fluid-phase Uptake

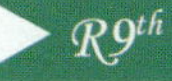 **Latest Update**

Endocytosis: Mechanism of uptake of **fluids or macromolecules** by the cell; Occurs by two major mechanisms:

Characteristics	Caveolae-mediated endocytosis	Receptor-mediated endocytosis
Includes	**Potocytosis (*"cellular sipping"*)**[Q]	**Pinocytosis (*"cellular drinking"*)**
Protein involved	Caveolin	Clathrin
Mechanism	**Caveolae ("little caves")** or **noncoated** plasma membrane invaginations are formed ↓ Internalization of caveolae with any bound molecules and associated extracellular fluid	Begin at **Clathrin-coated pit** in plasma membrane ↓ **Invaginates & pinches off** to form a **clathrin-coated vesicle** containing the macromolecules ↓ **Vesicles uncoat and fuse with** an acidic intracellular structure **(Early endosome)** ↓ **Discharge their contents** for digestion & passage to **lysosome** ↓ Endocytosed vesicles **may recycle** back to plasma membrane for another round of ingestion
Significance	Transports **vitamins like folate** & Regulate **transmembrane signaling** and/or **cellular adhesion** via **Integrins**	Major uptake mechanism for certain macromolecules like **transferrin and low-density lipoprotein (LDL)**

High Yield Facts

- Multi Drug Resistance **(MDR) protein** is a **Transporter ATPase**[Q] which pumps polar compounds (Chemotherapy drugs) out of cells & **may render cancer cells resistant** to treatment
- **Hypertonicity** (extracellular salt > in cytosol) causes a **net movement of water out**[Q] of cells.
- **Hypotonicity** causes a net movement of **water into cells.**[Q]
- Most cytosolic enzymes work at pH 7.4 whereas **lysosomal enzymes** function best at **pH ≤ 5.**[Q]
- **Exocytosis:** The process by which **membrane-bound vesicles**[Q] fuse with the plasma membrane and discharge their contents to the **extracellular space.**
- **Transcytosis** is the **movement of endocytosed vesicles** between the **apical and basolateral**[Q] compartments of cells, for transferring **intact proteins**[Q] across epithelial barriers.
- **Phagocytosis** involves **non-clathrin-mediated**[Q] **membrane invagination** of **large particles**, by specialized phagocytes.

CYTOSKELETON

Intracellular scaffolding of proteins that helps a cell to adopt a **particular shape,**[Q] maintain **polarity,**[Q] organize the relationship of intracellular organelles, and **move.**[Q]

Three Major Classes of Cytoskeletal Proteins

1. **Actin Microfilaments**
   - **5- to 9-nm diameter fibrils** formed from the **globular protein** actin (**G-actin**),
   - **Most abundant cytosolic protein in cells.**[Q]
   - G-actin monomers **noncovalently polymerize** into long **filaments (F-actin)** that intertwine to form **double-stranded helices** with a defined polarity; (positive and negative)
   - **In muscle:** Myosin binds to actin with ATP and **cause muscle contraction.**[Q]
   - In **nonmuscle cells:** F-actin assembles into well-organized **bundles and networks** that control **cell shape and movement.**[Q]

Theory

2. **Intermediate Filaments**
   ○ Impart **tensile strength**[Q] to tolerate **mechanical stress**.
   ○ Characteristic **tissue-specific patterns of expression**[Q]
   ○ Can be **useful for assigning a cell of origin**[Q] for **poorly differentiated tumors**.

Intermediate Filaments	Tissue
Lamin A, B, and C	**Nuclear lamina** of all cells
Vimentin	Mesenchymal cells (**fibroblasts, endothelium**)[Q]
Desmin	**Muscle cells,**[Q] forming the scaffold on which actin & myosin contract
Neurofilaments	**Axons of neurons**[Q], imparting **strength and rigidity**
Glial fibrillary acidic protein	**Glial cells** around neurons
Cytokeratins	**Acidic (type I)** and **neutral/basic (type II)**; different types present in different cells: used as cell markers

3. **Microtubules**
   ○ 25-nm thick fibrils composed of non-covalently polymerized dimers of α- and β-tubulin
   ○ **2 varieties** of these motor proteins:
     • Kinesins: for anterograde (– to +) transport
     • Dyneins: for retrograde (+ to –) transport
   ○ **Functions:**
     • Serve as connecting cables for **"molecular motor"** proteins that use **ATP to move vesicles, organelles, or other molecules** around the cells;
     • Participate in **sister chromatid separation during mitosis**.
     • Adapted to **form motile cilia** (bronchial epithelium) or **flagella (in sperm)**.[Q]

- The largest protein molecule in skeletal muscle is Titin.
- Communicating junctions (Gap junctions) consists of connexons[Q] formed by connexins[Q]

CELL-CELL INTERACTIONS

Cells **interact** and **communicate with one another** by forming **junctions** that provide **mechanical links** and enable surface receptors to **recognize ligands on other cells**.

Three Basic Types

1. **Occluding junctions (Tight junctions):**
   ○ Seal adjacent cells together to create a **continuous barrier** that **restricts**[Q] the **paracellular (between cells) movement of ions and other molecules**.
   ○ Proteins involved are **Occludin, Claudin, Zonulin and Catenin.**[Q]
2. **Anchoring junctions (Desmosomes)**[Q]
   ○ **Mechanically attach cell and their intracellular cytoskeletons—to other cells or to the extracellular matrix (ECM)**
   ○ **Types**

Spot desmosome or Macula adherens	When the adhesion focus is **small and rivet-like**; Proteins involved: **desmogleins** and **desmocollins**
Hemidesmosome	When such a focus attaches the **cell to the ECM integrins; E-cadherins**
Belt desmosomes	Similar adhesion domains occurring as **broad bands between cells**
Cell-cell desmosomal junctions	Formed by homotypic association of **transmembrane glycoproteins** called **Cadherins**

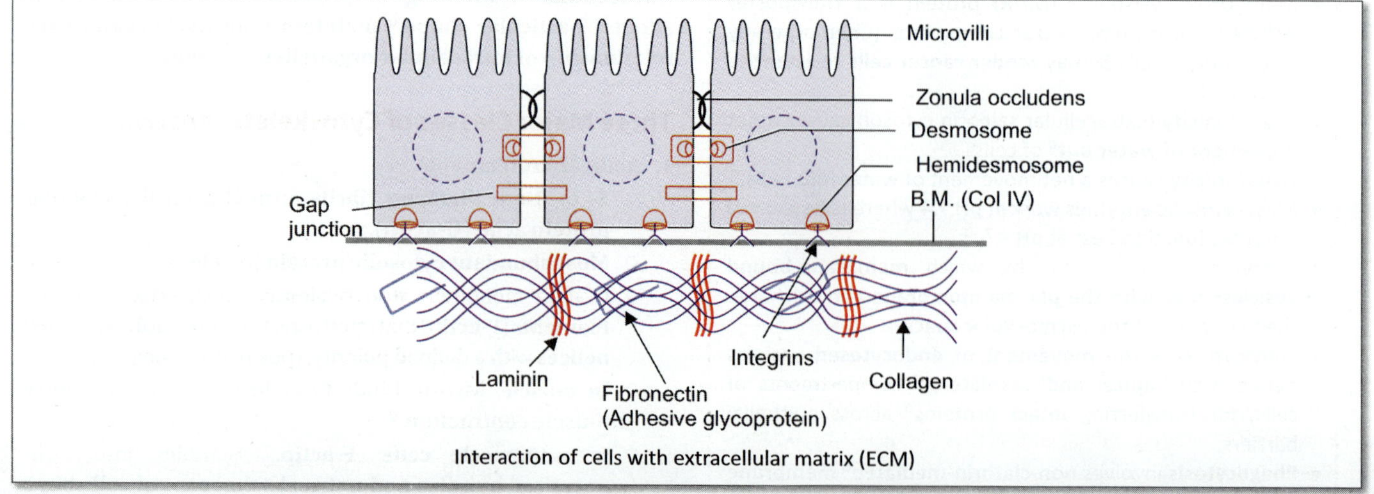

Interaction of cells with extracellular matrix (ECM)

3. **Communicating junctions (Gap junctions)**
   - Mediate the passage of **chemical or electrical signals** from **one cell to another**.
     - Consists of a dense planar array of 1.5–2-nm **pores** called **connexons**[Q]
     - Formed by hexamers of transmembrane **proteins** called **connexins**[Q]

SIGNAL TRANSDUCTION PATHWAYS

- **First messengers:** The extracellular ligands that bind to receptors
- **Second messengers**: The intracellular mediators of action, following binding of ligand to receptor

Newer receptors that are must to know

Receptors	Mechanism	Role in
Notch family receptors	**Proteolytic cleavage of the receptor** ↓ Nuclear translocation of the cytoplasmic piece ↓ Formation of a transcription complex	Development: • Neuronal development • Angiogenesis • T cell development Diseases: **T-ALL, Multiple Sclerosis**
Frizzled family receptors for Wnt protein ligands	APC-β-catenin degradration complex not formed ↓ β-catenin translocates to the nucleus ↓ Causes **transcriptional activation** & cell proliferation	• Action of **APC gene** • Disease: Adenomatosis Polyposis Coli & **Colorectal Carcinoma**[Q]

High Yield Facts

- Mutation in TTN gene on chromosome 2 causes dilated Cardiomyopathy
- TGF β family includes BMP[Q], Activins, Inhibins, Mullerian Inhibiting substance[Q]
- TGF β is an anti-inflammatory[Q] cytokine and causes fibrosis[Q]

GROWTH FACTORS

- Growth factor activity is mediated through binding to specific receptors, ultimately influencing the expression of genes that can:
  - **Promote entry** of cells **into the cell cycle**
  - **Relieve blocks** on cell cycle progression (thus promoting replication)
  - **Prevent apoptosis**
  - Enhance **biosynthesis of cellular components** (nucleic acids, proteins, lipids, carbohydrates) required for a mother cell to give rise to two daughter cells

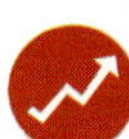

High Yield Facts

- All growth factors are proto-oncogenes, except TGF β,[Q] which is a tumor suppressor gene.
- Bone Morphogenic Protein (BMP) is both mitogenic & morphogenic[Q]
- Hypoxia[Q] is the most important inducer of **VEGF** production
- EGF receptor family includes ERB-B1(EGFR1) & ERB-B2 (HER2)[Q]
- Mutation of **ERB-B1** causes **Lung Adenocarcinoma**
- Mutation of **ERB-B2** causes **Breast Carcinoma**

EXTRACELLULAR MATRIX (ECM)

Cell interactions with ECM are critical for **development and healing**, as well as for maintaining **normal tissue architecture.**

Functions of ECM

- **Mechanical support**[Q] for cell **anchorage**, **migration** and cellular **polarity**
- **Control of cell proliferation**, Scaffolding for **tissue renewal**, Establishment of **tissue microenvironments**

Two Basic forms of ECM

Interstitial matrix & Basement membrane.

Characteristics	Interstitial matrix	Basement membrane
Location	**Present in the spaces between cells in** connective tissue, and **between parenchymal epithelium and supportive** vascular and smooth muscle structures	"Chicken wire" mesh (porous) **Present between epithelium & mesenchymal cells**
Synthesized by	**Mesenchymal cells (e.g., fibroblasts)**	Overlying epithelium & underlying mesenchymal cells
Major constituents	**Fibrillar & non-fibrillar** collagens, fibronectin, elastin, proteoglycans and hyaluronate	Amorphous **non-fibrillar type IV collagen** and **laminin**

Theory

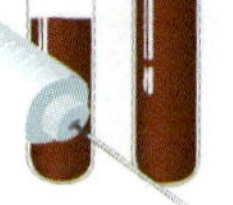

Components of the Extracellular Matrix

- **Fibrous structural proteins**
  - **Collagens:** confer tensile strength and recoil.
  - **Elastin**
    - Help tissues to **recoil and recover their shape** after physical deformation
    - Found in: **Cardiac valves**, large blood vessels, uterus, skin and ligaments.
    - Consist of a **central core of elastin** with an associated **mesh-like network** composed of **fibrillin.**
  - **Proteoglycans:**
    - **Hydrated compressible gels** that confer **resistance to compressive forces**
    - In joint cartilage: provides a layer of **lubrication between adjacent bony surfaces.**
    - **Structure:** Proteoglycans consists of **long polysaccharides** (glycosaminoglycans) eg: Keratin and chondroitin sulphate
    - Action of proteoglycan is shown in Flowchart 3

- **Fibrillin** synthetic defects lead to skeletal abnormalities and weakened aortic walls, as in individuals with **Marfan's syndrome**

Fibrillar Collagen
- **Types I, II, III, and V collagens** form **linear fibrils** stabilized by **interchain hydrogen bonding.**
- **Found in:** bone, tendon, cartilage, blood vessels, and skin, healing wounds and scars.

Non-Fibrillar Collagens
- **Type IV collagen:** contribute to the structures of planar **basement membranes**
- **Type IX collagen in cartilage:** help regulate **collagen fibril diameters** or collagen-collagen **interactions** via 'Fibril-Associated Collagen with Interrupted Triple helices' (**FACITs**)
- **Type VII collagen:** provide **anchoring fibrils** to basement membrane beneath stratified squamous epithelium

Flowchart 3: Action of proteoglycan

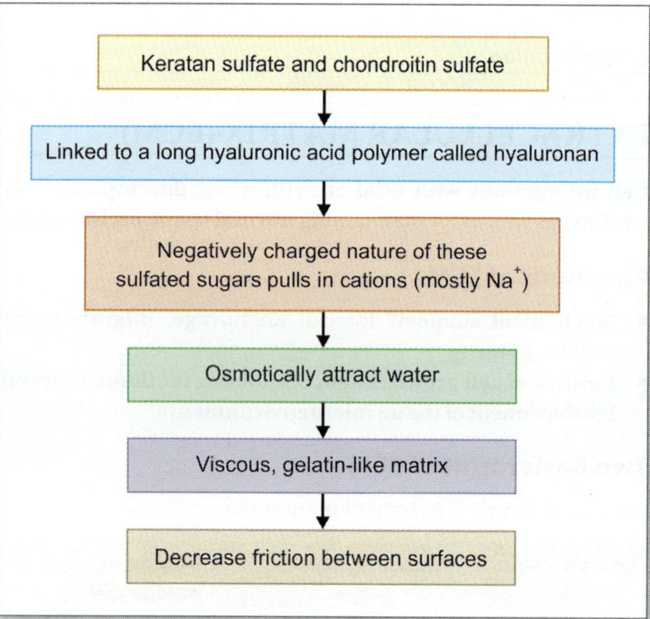

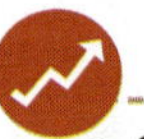

- **Cell Adhesion** molecules include **immunoglobulins, cadherins^Q and selectins**
- **E-Cadherin gene mutation is associated with Gastric Carcinoma^Q**
- **Germ-line loss of function mutation in E-Cadherin gene (CDH1) is associated with Autosomal Dominant familial Gastric Carcinoma**
- **E-Cadherin binds and sequesters β-catenin in the WNT pathway.^{Q}**
- **Laminin^Q is the most abundant glycoprotein in basement membrane**
- **Collagen I is most the most abundant collagen in the body.^{Q}**
- **Collagen I is the main component of the organic part of bone.^{Q}**
- **Collagen II is most abundant in Cartilage.^{Q}**

- **Adhesive Glycoproteins and Adhesion Receptors**
  - Involved in **cell-to-cell adhesion**, linking **cells to the ECM**, and the interactions **between ECM components.**
  - Prototypical adhesive glycoproteins include:
    - **Fibronectin:** A major component of the **interstitial ECM**
    - **Laminin:** A major constituent of **basement membrane** (most abundant glycoprotein in basement membrane)
    - **Integrins:** are representative of the **adhesion receptors,** also known as **cell adhesion molecules (CAMs)**

STEM CELLS

Definition

Undifferentiated cells^Q capable of giving rise to one or more different types of **specialized cells** and replace **damaged cells** and maintain tissue populations.

Stem Cells are Characterized by Two Important Properties

- **Self-renewal^Q:** Which permits stem cells to **maintain their numbers.**
- **Asymmetric division^Q:** In which **one daughter cell enters a differentiation** pathway and gives rise to mature cells, while the **other remains undifferentiated and retains its self-renewal capacity.**

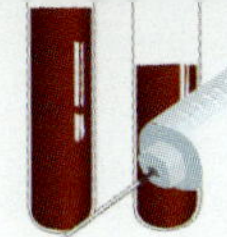

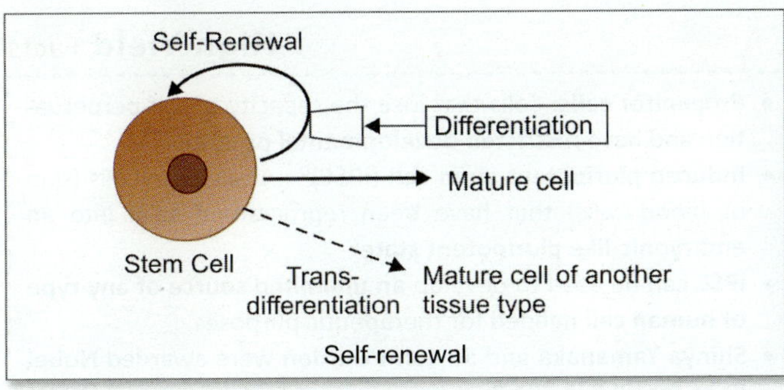

Types of Stem Cells

Embryonic Stem Cells (ES Cells)

Characteristics

- Most **undifferentiated**[Q]
- Present in the **inner cell mass**[Q] of the blastocyst
- **Limitless cell renewal capacity**[Q]
- **Totipotent**[Q]: Can give rise to every cell in the body

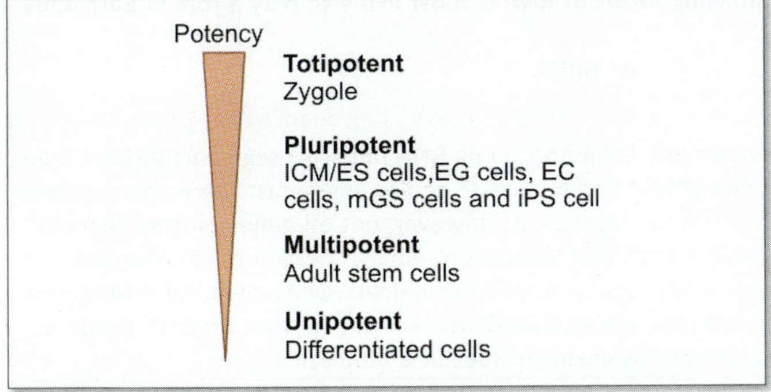

ES cells induced under appropriate culture conditions form specialized cells of **all three germ cell layers**[Q], including neurons, cardiac muscle, liver cells, and pancreatic islet cells.

Tissue Stem Cells (Also Called Adult Stem Cells)

Undifferentiated cells, found throughout the body after development that multiply to **replenish dying cells** and **regenerate damaged tissues**.

Important types of adult stem cells are:

A. Hematopoietic Stem Cells
- Found in **Bone Marrow**[Q]
- Replenish all **cellular elements of the blood**
- Isolated directly from **bone marrow** or from the **peripheral blood** after administration of colony stimulating factors **(CSF)**[Q]
- Stem cells **can be used to repopulate marrows** depleted after chemotherapy (e.g., for leukemia),
- Provide **normal precursors** to correct various blood cell defects[Q]

B. Mesenchymal Stem Cells
- Found in **Bone marrow**[Q]
- **Multipotent** cells that can differentiate into a variety of stromal cells including chondrocytes (cartilage), osteocytes (bone), adipocytes (fat), and myocytes (muscle)[Q]
- Manufactures **stromal cellular scaffolding** for **tissue regeneration**[Q]

C. Stem cell niches: **Microenvironment** where **tissue stem cells** are found, which **interacts with stem cells to regulate cell fate normally**

Stem Cell Niches	Location
Skin stem cells	Hair follicle bulge[Q], Sebaceous glands[Q], Interfollicular areas[Q] of the surface epidermis
Small intestine stem cells[Q]	Base of a crypt[Q], above Paneth cells
Liver stem cells (oval cells)[Q]	Canals of Hering[Q]
Corneal stem cells[Q]	Limbus region[Q]

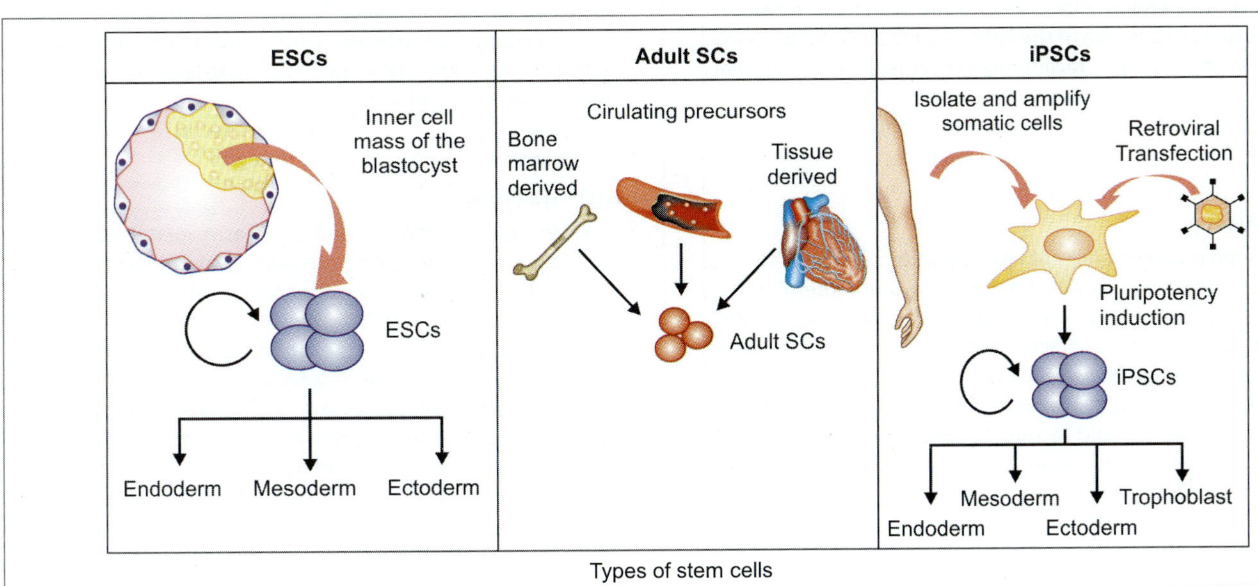

Types of stem cells

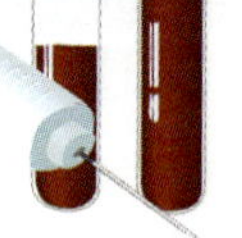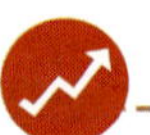

High Yield Facts

- **Transdifferentiation[Q]:** Irreversible conversion of cells from **one differentiated cell type to another[Q]**
- **Developmental plasticity[Q]:** capacity of a **cell to transdifferentiate** into diverse lineages[Q]
- **Dedifferentiation[Q]:** Reverse developmental process in which **differentiated** cells with specialized functions become **undifferentiated progenitor cells.[Q]**
- **Transit amplifying cells:** rapidly dividing cells[Q] generated by somatic stem cells

- **Progenitor cells:** Cells that lose the capacity of self-perpetuation and have **restricted developmental potential[Q]**
- **Induced pluripotent stem cell (iPSC)[Q]** : Adult stem cells (skin or blood cells) that have been reprogramed back into an **embryonic-like pluripotent state[Q]**
- **iPSC** can be used to develop **an unlimited source of any type of human cell** needed for therapeutic purposes.
- **Shinya Yamanaka** and **Sir John Gurdon** were awarded **Nobel Prize for iPSC in 2012[Q]**

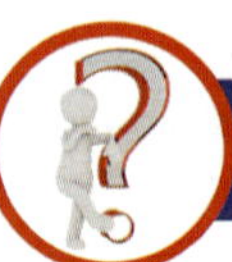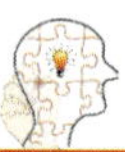

NEXT Pattern Questions

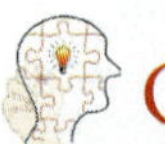

Q's

1. A study of peripheral blood smears shows that neutrophil nuclei of women have a Barr body, whereas those of men do not. The Barr body is an inactivated X chromosome. Which of the following forms of RNA is most likely to play a role in Barr body formation?

   a. lncRNA   b. mRNA   c. miRNA   d. siRNA

Ans. (a) lncRNA

- There are forms of noncoding RNA that play a role in gene expression. Long noncoding RNA (lncRNA) segments greater than 200 nucleotides in length can bind to chromatin to restrict access of RNA polymerase to coding segments. The X chromosome transcribes XIST, a lncRNA that binds to and represses X chromosome expression. However, not all genes on the "inactive" X chromosome are switched off. The RNA transcribed from nuclear DNA that directs protein synthesis through translation is mRNA. MicroRNAs (miRNAs) are noncoding RNA sequences that inhibit the translation of mRNAs. Gene-silencing RNAs (small interfering RNAs [siRNAs]) have the same function as miRNAs, but they are produced synthetically for experimental purposes. Transfer RNA (tRNA) participates in the translation of mRNA to proteins by linking to specific amino acids.

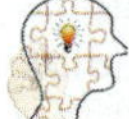

Q's

2. At the site of a surgical incision, endothelial cells elaborate vascular endothelial growth factor. There is sprouting with migration of endothelial cells into the wound to establish new capillaries. Which of the following intracellular proteins is most important in facilitating movement of endothelial cells?

   a. Actin   b. Cytokeratin
   c. Desmin   d. Lamin

Ans. (a) Actin

- Actin is a microfilament involved with cell movement.
- The other possibilities listed in B to D are intermediate filaments, which are larger than actin but smaller than myosin (a thick filament interdigitating with actin, required for muscle movement). Cytokeratins form cytoskeletal elements of epithelial cells. Desmin forms the scaffold in muscle cells on which actin and myosin contract. Lamin is associated with the nuclear membrane.

Q's

3. A 62-year-old man has increasing knee pain with movement for the past 10 years. The knee joint surfaces are eroded and the joint space narrowed. There is loss of compressibility and lubrication of articular cartilaginous surfaces. Loss of which of the following extracellular matrix components has most likely occurred in this man?

   a. Elastin   b. Fibronectin
   c. Hyaluronan   d. Integrin

Ans. (c) Hyaluronan

- He has osteoarthritis, or degenerative joint disease, with loss of articular hyaline cartilage. Hyaluronan (hyaluronic acid) is a large mucopolysaccharide, one form of proteoglycan, which forms a hydrated, compressible gel contributing to the shock-absorbing function of joint surfaces. Elastin is a fibrillar protein that provides recoil in tissues such as skin, arterial walls, and ligaments that need to stretch and return to their original shape. Fibronectin is a form of glycoprotein that serves an adhesive function. Integrins are glycoproteins that serve as cellular receptors for extracellular matrix components; they can link to intracellular actin so that cells can alter their shape and mobility

Multiple Choice Questions

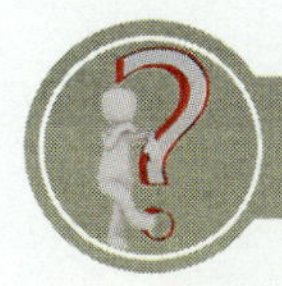

1. Which of the following tumor(s) is/are related to DICER1 Gene mutation: *(PGI May 2019)*
   a. Retinoblastoma
   b. Pleuropulmonary blastoma
   c. Cystic nephroma
   d. Thyroid carcinoma
   e. Sertoli-Leydig cell tumor

2. Integrin binds to: *(AIIMS Nov 18)*
   a. Fibronectin
   b. Vitronectin
   c. Collagen
   d. Laminin

3. The small inner circles in the given image of EM signifies which of the following? *(AIIMS May 18)*

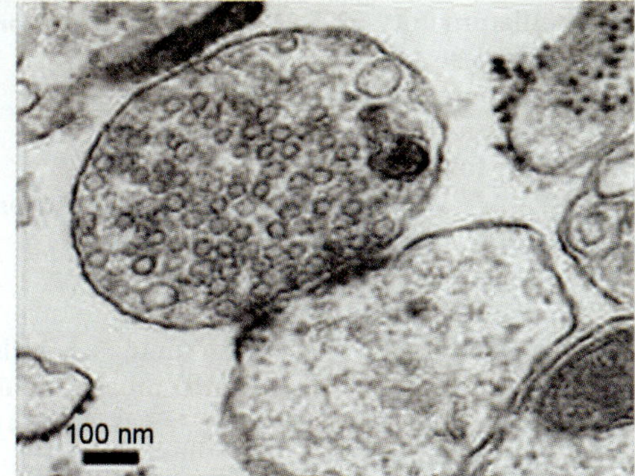

   a. Neuro transmitter
   b. Neurosecretory granules
   c. Collagen fibril
   d. Microtubules

4. False about micro satellites is? *(JIPMER 18)*
   a. Repeat size more than 10 to 15 nucleotides
   b. More prone to variation
   c. Found in colonic carcinoma
   d. DNA repeats present

5. Type 1 collagen is present in all except? *(AIIMS May 18)*
   a. Bone
   b. Cartilage
   c. Ligament
   d. Aponeurosis

6. Which among the following is not seen in disorder to deficiency in elastin production? *(AIIMS May 18)*
   a. Aortic dissection
   b. Lens subluxation
   c. Ligament hyperlaxity
   d. bone fracture

7. Which Vitamin increases iron Absorption? *(AIIMS May 18)*
   a. Vitamin C
   b. Biotin
   c. Vitamin B6
   d. Vitamin E

8. Which of the following plays a role in gene editing? *(AIIMS May 2017)*
   a. Gene Xper
   b. CRISPR
   c. Health care apps
   d. Big data

9. Cell to cell permeability occurs through: *(Recent Question 2016-17)*
   a. Occludin
   b. Zona adherens
   c. Connexins
   d. Zonulin

10. Tensile strength of tendon depends on *(Recent Question 2016-17)*
    a. Fibrillin
    b. Collagen
    c. Fibronectin
    d. Elastin

11. Which of the following mechanism is mainly involved in Genomic imprinting? *(AIIMS Nov 2015)*
    a. Methylation
    b. Acetylation
    c. Deamination
    d. Phosphorylation

12. The term pathology was coined by? *(APPGMEE 2015)*
    a. Robert Kochs
    b. Rudolf Virchow
    c. Lois Pasteur
    d. Gregor Mendal

13. Which Collagen is typical of basement membrane? *(AIIMS May 2015)*
    a. Type I
    b. Type V
    c. Type IV
    d. Type III

14. Which of the following function is done by RNAi in a gene? *(AIIMS May 2015)*
    a. Knock in
    b. Knock out
    c. Knock down
    d. Knock up

15. All of the following are Intermediate filament except? *(Recent Question 2016)*
    a. Lamin
    b. Cadherin
    c. Vimentin
    d. Desmin

16. Tight junction consists of all except? *(Recent Question 2016)*
    a. Occludin
    b. Claudin
    c. Zonulin
    d. Cadherin

17. Titin protein mutated in? *(Recent Question 2016)*
    a. DCM
    b. HOCM
    c. RCM
    d. Non functional cardiomyopathy

18. Peripheral protein in cell membrane are attached by? *(Recent Question 2016)*
    a. GpI
    b. Desmosome
    c. Catenins
    d. Cadherins

19. Bridging fibrosis in large wounds is due to *(Recent Question 2015)*
    a. Keratinocyte growth factor
    b. Epidermal growth factor
    c. Platelet derived growth factor
    d. Transforming growth factor-β

20. Major cytokine involved in fibrosis
    a. Transforming growth factor-α *(Recent Question 2015)*
    b. Transforming growth factor-β
    c. Fibroblast growth factor
    d. Epidermal growth factor

21. Types of collage playing important role in wound healing *(Recent Question 2015)*
    a. I and III
    b. II and V
    c. III and IV
    d. V and IX

22. Oval stem cells are located in *(Recent Question 2015)*
    a. Canal of schlemm
    b. Canal of herring
    c. Space of disse
    d. Basal lamina of myotubules

23. Stem cells are present in? *(Recent Question 2015)*
    a. Cornea
    b. Base of crypts
    c. Bile duct of liver
    d. Mesonephros

24. Human genome contains *(Recent Question 2015)*
    a. 3.2 billion DNA base pairs
    b. 2.3 billion DNA base pairs
    c. 3.2 million DNA base pairs
    d. 2.3 million DNA base pairs

25. **Protein-encoding genes comprises what percentage of genome** *(Recent Question 2015)*
    a. 98.5%
    b. 1.5%
    c. 5%
    d. 95%

26. **Jumping genes take part in:** *(Recent Question 2015)*
    a. Gene regulation
    b. Chromosomal aberrations
    c. Gene movement in a species
    d. Carry out gene amplification

27. **The most-commen form of DNA variation is?** *(Recent Question 2015)*
    a. Single nucleotide polymorphism
    b. Copy Number Variations (CNVs)
    c. Transposons
    d. Mutations

28. **Linkage disequilibrium refers to?** *(Recent Question 2015)*
    a. Never co-inherited gene
    b. Inherited but not with disease causing gene
    c. Genetic mutations
    d. Co-inherited with the disease causing gene

29. **Heritable changes in gene expression not caused by alterations in DNA sequence refers to?** *(Recent Question 2015)*
    a. Genetics
    b. Epigenetics
    c. Mutations
    d. Transposons

30. **Epigenetic factors refers to?** *(Recent Question 2015)*
    a. Histone methylation
    b. Histone phosphorylation
    c. DNA methylation
    d. All of the above

31. **Function of Peroxisomes is?** *(Recent Question 2014)*
    a. Protein synthesis
    b. Carbohydrate metabolism
    c. Generating H_2O_2
    d. DNA replication

32. **Collagen present in cornea?** *(Recent Question 2015)*
    a. Type 1
    b. Type 2
    c. Type 4
    d. Type 7

33. **Gene silencing RNA-** *(Recent Question 2014)*
    a. rRNA
    b. tRNA
    c. miRNA
    d. None

34. **Epigenetics deals with genetic modification that do not alter the sequence of DNA. All of the following can detect epigenetic modifications except?** *(AIIMS Nov 14)*
    a. Chip on chip
    b. Bisulphite method
    c. HPLC
    d. Methylation specific PCR

35. **Coding DNA constitutes what proportion of total DNA?** *(AIIMS May 2014)*
    a. 0.02
    b. 0.25
    c. 0.4
    d. 0.1

36. **GWAS stands for:** *(PGI Nov 2014)*
    a. Genome wide Association syndrome
    b. Genome wide Association studies
    c. Genetic wide array studies
    d. Genetic wide amplification studies
    e. Genomic way of association studies

37. **Genetic polymorphisms include -** *(PGI Nov 10)*
    a. SNP
    b. Microsatellites
    c. Mutations
    d. Translocation
    e. Mini satellites

38. **Function of miRNA is/are:** *(PGI May 12)*
    a. Gene silencing
    b. Gene activation
    c. Transcription inhibition
    d. Translation repression
    e. Breaking of messenger RNA

39. **Most abundant collagen in the body?** *(Recent Question 2015)*
    a. Type I
    b. Type II
    c. Type III
    d. Type IV

40. **FACIT collagen is?** *(Recent Question 2015)*
    a. Type I
    b. Type III
    c. Type IX
    d. Type XI

41. **Gap junctions comprise of?** *(Recent Question 2015)*
    a. Catenins
    b. Cadherins
    c. Connexins
    d. Claudin

42. **All of the following are true about TGF-β except:** *(Recent Question 2014)*
    a. Anti-inflammatory
    b. Causes fibrosis
    c. Tumor suppressor gene
    d. Anti-Angiogenic

43. **Which of the following statement is not true?** *(Recent Question 2013)*
    a. Cytokeratin is the marker of muscle cells
    b. Vimentin is used to stain fibroblasts
    c. Neurofilamentsare present in neurons
    d. Desmin can be used as a marker for muscle cells

44. **Which of the following is both morphogenic and mitogenic?** *(AIIMS May 2014)*
    a. Insulin growth factor
    b. Bone morphogenic factor
    c. Fibroblast growth factor
    d. Epidermal growth factor

45. **The function of Proteoglycans and Hyaluronanis ?**
    a. Lubrication and reduces resistance
    b. Cell growth
    c. Connect ECM components
    d. Provides tensile strength

46. **Mutation in COL4A5 chain leads to?** *(AIIMS May 2013)*
    a. Alport's syndrome
    b. Good pasture's syndrome
    c. Hereditary Non-polyposis Colon Cancer
    d. Xeroderma Pigmentosum

47. **Oncogene tyrosine kinase involves:** *(PGI May 2012)*
    a. PML-BRCA 1
    b. BCR-ABL
    c. HAAJ
    d. JUN
    e. NJKK

48. **Epidermal growth factor is/are formed by:** *(PGI May 12)*
    a. Platelet
    b. Fibroblast
    c. Mast cell
    d. Endothelial cell
    e. Keratinocyte

49. **Which of the following statements is not correct regarding stem cell?** *(DPG 11)*
    a. Developmental elasticity
    b. Transdifferentiation
    c. Can be harvested from embryo
    d. Knock out mice made possible because of it

50. **Which of the following is involved in stem cell self-renewal?** *(PGI May 2014)*
    a. Oct 3/4
    b. sox 2
    c. c-myc
    d. FLT3 ligand
    e. c-kit

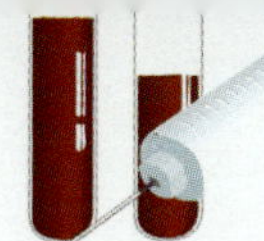

51. Which of the following statements about hematopoietic stem cell is false? *(AP PGMEE 2014)*
a. Stem cells have self-renewal property
b. Subset of stem cells normally circulate in peripheral blood
c. Marrow derived stem cells can seed other tissues and develop into non-hematopoietic cells as well
d. Stem cells resemble lymphoblasts morphologically

52. In an ablated animal, If Myeloid Stem Cells are injected, which type of cells are induced after the incubation period? *(AIIMS May 12)*
a. T-Lymphocyte
b. Erythroid
c. Fibroblast
d. Hematopoietic Stem Cells

53. Location of small intestine stem cells is? *(Recent Question 12)*
a. Jejunum epithelial cells
b. Terminal ileum mucosa
c. Crypt base
d. Mucosa throughout

54. True about stem cell *(PGI Nov 12)*
a. Undifferentiated
b. Pluripotent
c. Dedicated to one cell line
d. Used for cell repair and tissue regeneration
e. Can form any cell

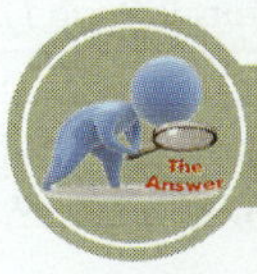

Answers with Explanations

1. Ans. (b) Pleuropulmonary blastoma; (c) Cystic nephroma; (d) Thyroid carcinoma; (e) Sertoli-Leydig cell tumor *(Ref: Robbins 9th/pg 5; pg 1033)*

Dicer is a type III cytoplasmic endoribonuclease that is involved in the maturation of several classes of small non-coding RNAs, such as microRNAs. Germline loss-of-function mutations in DICER1 are associated with pleuropulmonary blastoma (PPB), ovarian sex cord-stromal tumors, ciliary body medulloepitheliomas, nasal chondromesenchymal hamartomas, multinodular goiter and differentiated thyroid carcinomas, cystic nephroma and, more rarely, anaplastic sarcoma of kidney. DICER1 mutations have also been documented in pediatric tumors including Wilms' tumor and in pituitary blastoma (PitB).

2. Ans. (d) Laminin > Fibronectin

Integrins localised in the plasma membrane are the major adhesion receptors connecting cells with components of the extracellular matrix. Integrins interact directly with laminin, fibronectin present in the basal lamina and intracellularly contact actin through intermediate proteins, such as alpha-actinin, vinculin, and talin

3. Ans. (b) Neurosecretory granules

Neurosecretion is the storage, synthesis and release of hormones from neurons. These neurohormones, produced by neurosecretory cells, are normally secreted from nerve cells in the brain that then circulate into the blood.

4. Ans. (a) Repeat size more than 10 to 15 nucleotides

5. Ans. (b) Cartilage

Please Refer to Explanation of Q.21

6. Ans. (d) Bone fracture

7. Ans. (a) Vitamin C

8. Ans. (b) CRISPR *(Ref. R 9th/p 5-6)*

CRISPR-Cas9 is a genome editing tool essential in adaptive immunity in select bacteria enabling the organisms to respond to and eliminate invading genetic material

9. Ans. (c) Connexins *(Ref: Robbins 9th/ pg 11)*

- Communicating junctions (Gap junctions): mediate the passage of chemical or electrical signals from one cell to another.
- Consists of pores called connexions and formed by hexamers of transmembrane proteins called connexins

10. Ans. (b) Collagen *(Ref: Robbins 9th/ pg 12-13)*

Fibrous structural proteins like Collagens confer tensile strength and & elastins provide recoil to the tension

11. Ans. (a) Methylation *(Ref: Robbins 9th/pg 3-4)*

- Genomic imprinting selectively inactivates either the maternal or paternal allele.
- Occurs in the ovum or the sperm, before fertilization, and then is stably transmitted to all somatic cells through mitosis

Mechanisms

- **Histones and histone modifying factors**
- Histone methylation
  - Histone acetylation
  - Histone phosphorylation
- **DNA methylation**
- **Chromatin organizing factors**

12. Ans. (b) Rudolf Virchow *(Ref: Robbins 9th/pg 1)*

Pathology (from the Ancient Greek roots of pathos, meaning "experience" or "suffering", and -logia, "an account of") is a significant component of the causal study of disease and a major field in modern medicine and diagnosis. The term cellular pathology was coined by Rudolf Virchow.

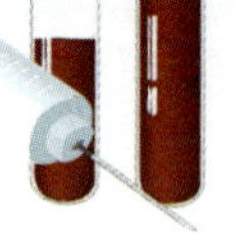

13. **Ans. (c) Type IV** (*Ref: Robbins 9th/pg 20-23*)

14. **Ans. (c) Knock down** (*Ref: Robbins 9th/pg 3-4*)

Small interfering RNAs (siRNAs)

- Short RNA sequences **introduced experimentally** into cells
- Their action is similar to **endogenous miRNAs**.
- Synthetic **siRNAs targeted against specific mRNA** have become useful laboratory tools to study gene function (so-called "**knockdown technology**")

15. **Ans. (b) Cadherin** (*Ref: Robbins 9th/pg 21-24*)

Intermediate filaments are 10-nm diameter fibrils which provide tensile strength to a cell.

Cadherins **are cell-cell desmosomal junctions are formed by homotypic association of transmembrane glycoproteins.**

16. **Ans. (d) Cadherin** (*Ref: Robbins 9th/pg 21-24*)

Occluding Junctions (Tight Junctions)

- Seal adjacent cells together to create a **continuous barrier** that **restricts[Q]** the **paracellular (between cells) movement of ions and other molecules**.
- Proteins involved are **Occludin, Claudin, Zonulin and Catenin**

17. **Ans. (a) DCM** (*Ref: Robbins 9th/pg 21-24*)

Mutations in TTN, a gene on chr 2q31 that encodes titin (so-called because it is the largest protein expressed in humans) causes 20% of all cases of Dilated Cardiomyopathy (DCM)

18. **Ans. (a) GpI** (*Ref: Robbins 9th/pg 21-24*)

Proteins are linked to cell via glycophosphatidylinositol (GPI) structures.

19. **Ans. (d) Transforming growth factor-β** (*Ref: R 9th/pg 20*)

Functions of TGFβ are:

- Anti-inflammatory, fibrosis, tumor suppressor gene, angiogenesis

20. **Ans. (b) Transforming growth factor-β** (*Ref: R 9th/pg 20*)

21. **Ans. (a) I and III** (*Ref: Robbins 9th/pg 20-23*)

Major types of Collagens & disorders associated with them:

Type	Present in	Disorders
I	Bone[Q], Cornea,[Q] Scar tissue, tendons, skin, artery walls, endomysium of myofibrils[Q], fibrocartilage, teeth	Osteogenesis-imperfecta[Q], Ehlers-Danlos Syndrome[Q], Caffey's disease[Q]
II	Hyaline cartilage[Q], Vitreous humor[Q] of the eye.	Collagenopathy

Contd...

Type	Present in	Disorders
III	Granulation tissue[Q], Reticular fiber, artery walls, skin, intestines and the uterus	Ehlers-Danlos Syndrome[Q]
IV	Basement membrane[Q], eye lens[Q], Glomerular Basement membrane	Alport syndrome[Q] (COL4α5) Goodpasture's syndrome[Q] (COL4α3)

22. **Ans. (b) Canal of herring** (*Ref: Robbins 9th/ pg 27-28*)

Liver stem cells (oval cells)[Q] are present in canals of Hering[Q]

23. **Ans. (b) Base of crypts** (*Ref: Robbins 9th/pg 27-28*)

24. **Ans. (a) 3.2 billion DNA base pairs** (*Ref: Robbins 9th/ pg 1*)

25. **Ans. (b) 1.5%** (*Ref: Robbins 9th/ pg 1*)

In humans, there are 20,000 protein-encoding genes[Q], comprising only 1.5% of the genome.[Q]

26. **Ans. (a) Gene regulation** (*Ref: Robbins 9th/ pg 2*)

Jumping genes

- They are **Mobile genetic elements,** also called '**transposons**'
- Segments **that move around the genome**, exhibiting **wide variation** in number and positioning;
- Role in **gene regulation** and **chromatin organization**

27. **Ans. (a) Single nucleotide polymorphism** (*Ref: R 9th/ pg 3*)

Single-Nucleotide Polymorphisms (SNPs)

- Variations at **single nucleotide positions[Q]**
- **Most prevalent[Q]** and **important form of genetic variation.**
- Always **bi-allelic[Q]**
- Can occur in **exons, introns, intergenic regions and coding regions**
- **1% of SNPs occur in coding regions**

28. **Ans. (d) Co-inherited with the disease causing gene**

(*Ref: Robbins 9th/ pg 3*)

Even if any SNP has no effect on gene function (Neutral SNP)[Q], it may be co-inherited with the "actual disease causing gene," if located close to that gene. This is called "Linkage disequilibrium"[Q]

29. **Ans. (b) Epigenetics** (*Ref: Robbins 9th/ pg 3-4*)

Epigenetics refers to heritable changes in gene expression, not caused by alterations in DNA sequence.

Epigenetic factors include:

- Histones and **histone modifying factors** like Histone methylation, acetylation and phosphorylation
- **DNA methylation**
- **Chromatin organizing** factors

30. **Ans. (d) All of the above** (*Ref: Robbins 9th/ pg 3-4*)

31. **Ans. (c)** **Generating H$_2$O$_2$** *(Ref: Robbins 9th/ pg 6-7)*

Functions of some important cell organelles:

- *Lysosomes:*
- **Digestion**[Q] of **proteins, polysaccharides, lipids, nucleic acids**
- *Proteasomes:*
  - Selectively **chews up denatured proteins, releasing peptides**[Q]
- *Peroxisomes:*
  - **Breakdown of fatty acids,**[Q] generating **hydrogen peroxide**

32. **Ans. (a)** **Type 1** *(Ref: Robbins 9th/ pg 20-23)*

33. **Ans. (c)** **miRNA** *(Ref: Robbins 9th/ pg 4-5)*

34. **Ans. (c)** **HPLC** *(Ref: Robbins 9th/ pg 3-4)*

35. **Ans. (a)** **0.02** *(Ref: Robbins 9th/ pg 1)*

Coding DNA constitutes 0.02 or 1.5-2% of total DNA; Refer Ans 3 above

36. **Ans. (b)** **Genome wide association studies**

(Ref: Robbins 9th/ pg 179)

GWAS refers to 'Genome Wide Association Studies'[Q]

In GWAS, entire genome of large number of individuals with and without a disease are examined for common genetic variants or polymorphisms that are overrepresented in patients with the disease.

37. **Ans. (a, b, e)** **a. SNP; b. Microsatellites; e. Mini satellites**

(Ref: Robbins 9th/ pg 3)

- The 2 types of genetic polymorphisms are **single nucleotide polymorphisms (SNPs) & repeat length polymorphisms**
- Repeat length polymorphisms can be **mini-satellite (1-3 kb)**[Q] or **Micro-satellite repeats (<1 kb)**[Q]

38. **Ans. (a, d, e)** **a. Gene silencing; d. Translation repression; e. Breaking of messenger RNA**

(Ref: Robbins 9th/ pg 4-5)

39. **Ans. (b)** **Type II** *(Ref: Robbins 9th/ pg 20-23)*

- **Collagen I is most the most abundant collagen in the body.**[Q]
- **Collagen I is the main component of the organic part of bone.**[Q]
- **Collagen II is most abundant in Cartilage.**[Q]

40. **Ans. (c)** **Type IX** *(Ref: Robbins 9th/ pg 20-23)*

Type IX collagen in cartilage: help regulate collagen fibril diameters or collagen-collagen interactions via 'Fibril-Associated Collagen with Interrupted Triple helices' (FACITs).

41. **Ans. (c)** **Connexins** *(Ref: Robbins 9th/ pg 11)*

Communicating junctions (Gap junctions)

- Mediate the passage of **chemical or electrical signals** from **one cell to another**.
- Consists of a dense planar array of 1.5–2-nm **pores** called **connexons**[Q]
- Formed by hexamers of transmembrane **proteins** called **connexins**[Q]

42. **Ans. (d)** **Anti-Angiogenic** *(Ref: Robbins 9th/ pg 20)*

43. **Ans. (a)** **Cytokeratin is the marker of muscle cells**

(Ref: Robbins 9th/pg 11)

44. **Ans. (b, a)** **b. Bone morphogenic factor > a. Insulin like Growth Factor**

(Ref: Robbins 9th/ pg 19-20; International journal of molecular medicine 2007;20: 53-57)

Discussing the options one by one:

A. Insulin growth factor (IGF)	• **IGF-1** is **mitogenic** for **growth plate chondrocytes** and stimulates chondrocyte synthesis of matrix macromolecules, including proteoglycan and collagen. • Causes **skeletal growth and development** by acting on epiphyseal growth plate
B. Bone morphogenic factor or protein (BMP)	• Act as **chemotactic, mitogenic** and help in **differentiating mechanisms** • During embryogenesis, BMPs **regulate dorsal-ventral patterning**, establishment of embryonic **body plan, cell apoptosis, differentiation of neural cells, patterning of the limb bud and epithelial-mesenchymal interactions** during organogenesis **(morphogenesis)**
C. Fibroblast growth factor (FGF)	• **Chemotactic and Mitogenic for** and **fibroblasts;** • Stimulates **angiogenesis** and ECM protein synthesis
D. Epidermal growth factor (EGF)	• **Mitogenic** for hepatocytes and fibroblasts; • Stimulates **granulation tissue formation**

45. **Ans. (a)** **Lubrication and reduces resistance**

(Ref: Robbins 9th/pg 20-24)

Function of proteoglycans and hyaluronan is to provide a layer of lubrication between adjacent bony surfaces and reduces friction & resistance.

46.   **Ans. (a)**   **Alport's syndrome** *(Ref: Robbins 9th/ pg 20-23)*

47.   **Ans. (b, d)**   **b. BCR-ABL; d. JUN** *(Ref: Robbins 9th/pg 16-17)*

48.   **Ans. (e)**   **Keratinocyte** *(Ref: Robbins 9th/pg 19)*

EGF and TGF–α are produced by macrophages and a variety of epithelial cells, including keratinocytes and are mitogenic for hepatocytes, fibroblasts, and a host of epithelial cells.

49.   **Ans. (a)**   **Developmental elasticity**

(Ref: Robbins 9th/pg 27-28)

Stem cells show developmental plasticity (transdifferenti-ation) and not developmental elasticity;
Transdifferentiation indicates a change in the lineage commitment of a stem cell.

50.   **Ans. (a, b, d, e)**   **a. Oct 3/4; b. sox 2; d. FLT3 ligand; e. c-kit**

(Ref: Robbins 9th/ pg 27-28, 580-581)

Discussing the options one by one:

A. Oct 3/ pg4 (octamer-binding transcription factor)	• Also known as **POU5F1**; • It is critically involved in the **self-renewal** of undifferentiated embryonic stem cells. • It is frequently **used as a marker for undifferentiated cells**.
B. Sox 2	SRY (sex determining region Y)-box 2, also known as SOX2, is a transcription factor that is essential for maintaining self-renewal or pluripotency of undifferentiated embryonic stem cells
C. C myc	Proto-oncogene involved in Burkitt lymphoma; Not involved in stem cell self-renewal;
D. FLT3 ligand	Flt3 ligand (FL) is a hematopoietic cytokine. It is structurally homologous to stem cell factor (SCF) and colony stimulating factor 1 (CSF-1). Flt3 ligand **stimulates proliferation & differentiation of various blood cell progenitors.**
E. C-kit	• Mast/stem cell growth factor receptor (SCFR), also known as CD117 • Signalling through CD117 plays a role in **cell survival, proliferation, and differentiation**. • It binds to a substance called stem cell factor (SCF), which causes **stem cell proliferation**

51.   **Ans. (b)**   **Subset of stem cells normally circulate in peripheral blood** *(Ref: Robbins 9th/ pg 27-28)*

Discussing the options one by one:

A.	True	**Self-renewal takes place by asymmetric division,** which permits stem cells to **maintain their numbers**
B.	False	Hematopoietic stem cells **can be found inperipheral bloodafter administration of colony stimulating factors (CSF)**[Q]
C.	True	**Mesenchymal stem cells** found in **Bone marrow** are **multipotent** cells that can differentiate into a variety of stromal cells including chondrocytes (cartilage), osteocytes (bone), adipocytes (fat), and myocytes (muscle).
D.	True	Stem cells resemble lymphocytes or lymphoblasts morphologically

52.   **Ans. (b)**   **Erythroid** *(Ref: Robbins 9th/ pg 27-28, 580-581)*

Neutrophils, Monocytes, Basophils, Erythroids and Mega-karyocytes are myeloid in origin while lymphocytes are Lymphoid in origin. Hematopoietic Stem Cells give rise to myeloid stem cells and not the reverse.

53.   **Ans. (c)**   **Crypts base** *(Ref: 9th/ pg 27-28)*

54.   **Ans. (a, b, d, e)**   **a. Undifferentiated; b. Pluripotent; d. Used for cell repair and tissue regeneration; e. Can form any cell** *(Ref: Robbins 9th/ pg 27-28)*

Discussing the options one by one:

• **Undifferentiated → True**
• **Pluripotent → True; embryonic stem cells or ES cells, are pluripotent, that is, they can generate all tissues of the body**
• Dedicated to one cell line False, stem cells are pluripotent or multipotent and can give rise to multiple cell lines
• **Used for cell repair and tissue regeneration True; Mesenchymal stem cells manufacture stromal cellular scaffolding for tissue regeneration**
• **Can form any cell → True; Embryonic (pluripotent) stem cells can generate all tissues of the body. Pluripotent stem cells give rise to multipotent stem cells, which have more restricted developmental potential, and eventually produce differentiated cells from the three embryonic layers.**

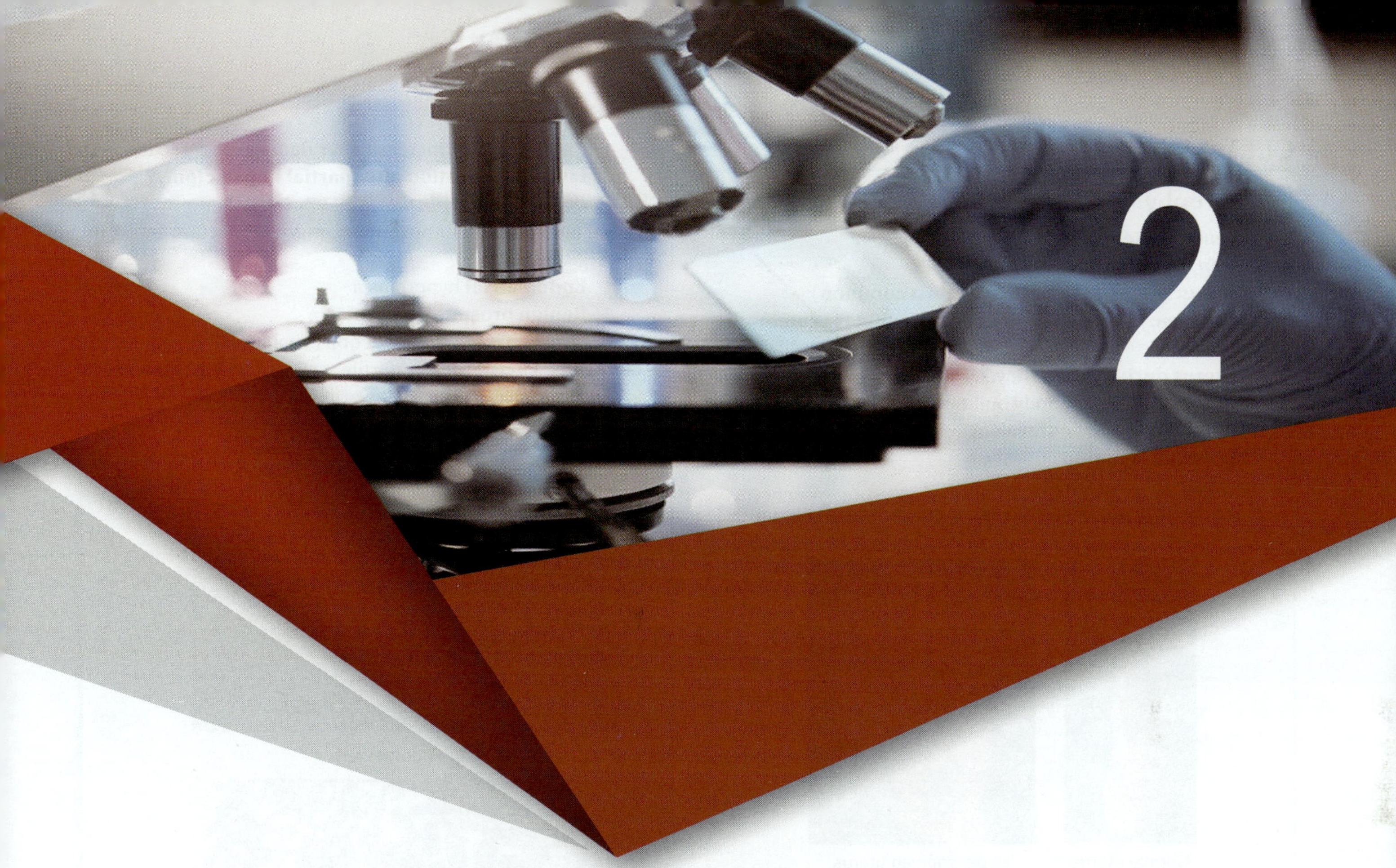

2

Cell Adaptation, Injury and Death

CELL ADAPTATIONS

Hypertrophy

- **Increase in the size of cells**[Q]
- *Seen in:* **Nondividing cells.**[Q]
- *Stimulus:* **Increased workload**[Q] **(Most common)**
- *Mechanism:* **Increased production of cellular proteins.**[Q]
- *Examples*
  - **Uterus during pregnancy.**[Q]
  - Bulging muscles of body builders.
  - Hypertension or faulty valves → heart hypertrophy
  - **Breast in lactation**[Q]
- *Outcome*
  - **Reversible** process; Does not predispose to malignancy[Q]

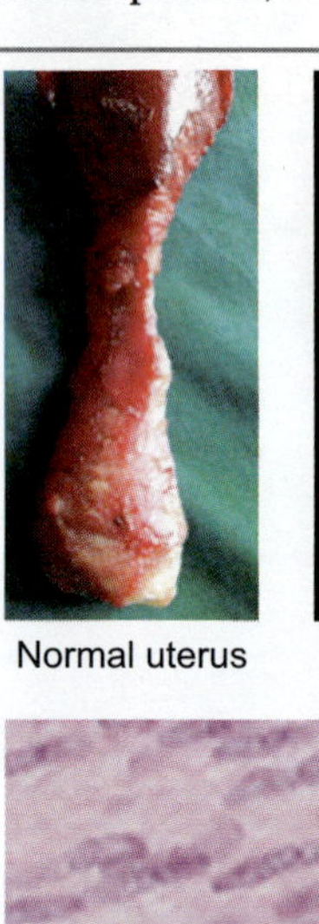
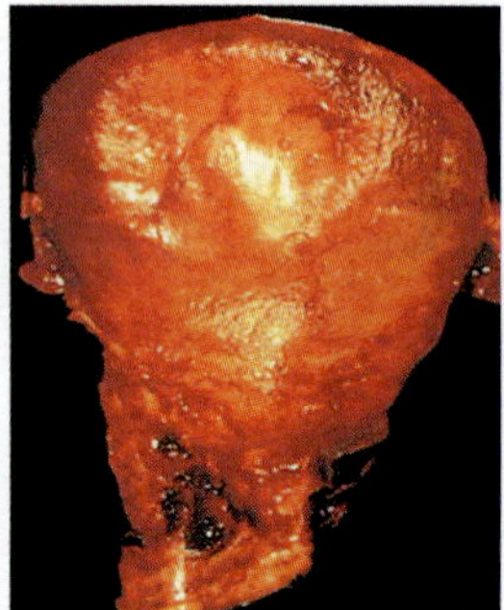

Normal uterus   Hypertrophied uterus

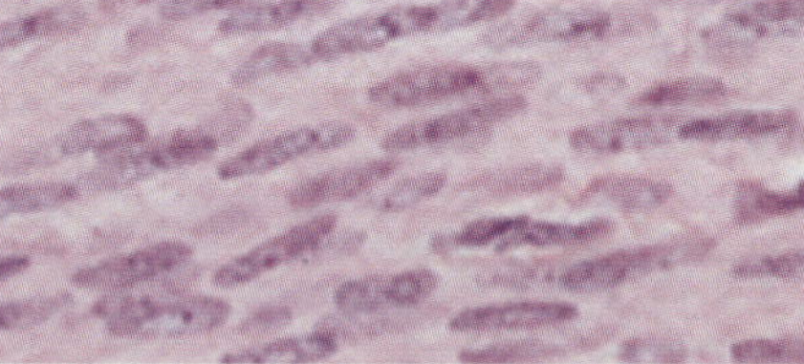

Normal muscle

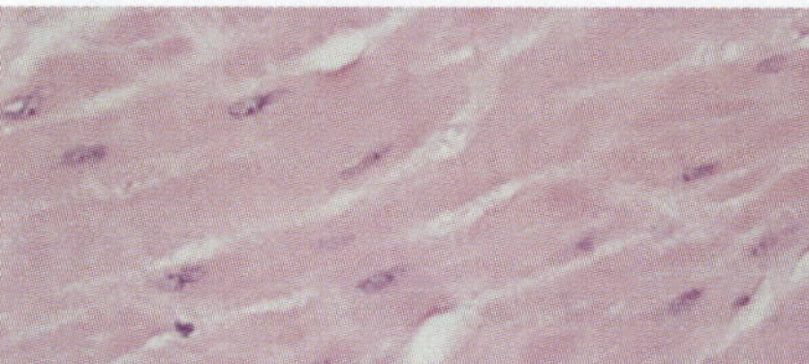

Hypertrophied smooth muscle

Hyperplasia

- Increase in **number of cells** in an organ or tissue in response to a stimulus.[Q]
- *Seen in:* **Dividing cells.**[Q]
- *Mechanism:*
- **Growth factor-driven proliferation**[Q] of mature cells
- Increased output of new cells from tissue stem cells (rare)
- *Types with examples*
  - *Physiologic hyperplasia:*
    - Action of **hormones or growth factors** in hormone responsive organs
  - Breast in pregnancy and during puberty
    - **Bone marrow**[Q] in response to deficiency of terminally differentiated blood cells.

- Compensatory increase after damage or resection, e.g. **Liver regeneration after partial hepatectomy**[Q]
  - *Pathologic hyperplasia*
  Excessive action of hormones or growth factors acting on target cells.
    - **Endometrial** hyperplasia
    - **Benign prostatic hyperplasia**
    - **Skin warts**-by viral infections such as HPV[Q]
- *Outcome*: Constitutes a fertile soil in which **cancerous proliferations** may eventually arise

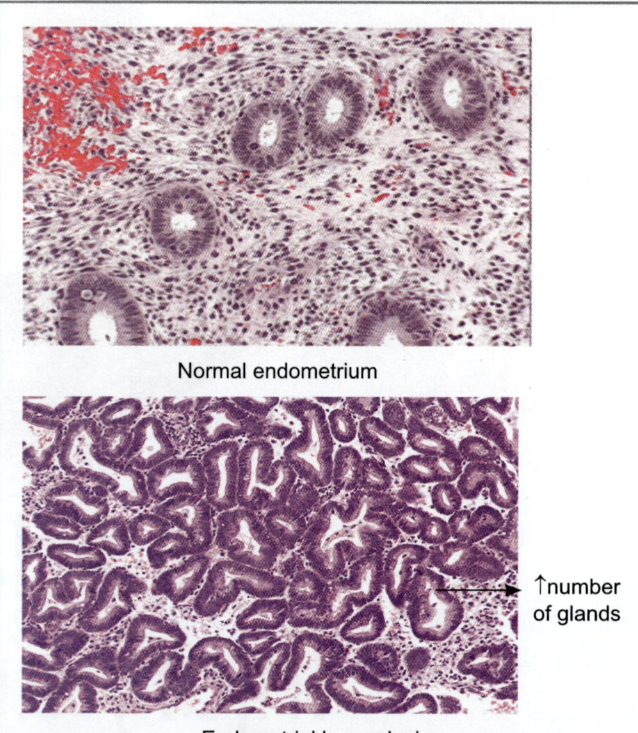

Normal endometrium

↑number of glands

Endometrial hyperplasia

> **R10th Latest Update**
> - **Combined hypertrophy + hyperplasia: uterus in pregnancy**[Q]
> - **Hypertrophy: Breast in lactation**[Q]
> - **Atrophy: Breast at menopause**[Q]

Atrophy

- Reduction in the size of an organ or tissue due to a **decrease in cell size and number**[Q]
- *Mechanism:* **Decreased protein synthesis**[Q] and increased protein degradation in cells.
- *Types with examples*
  - **Physiologic atrophy:**
    - During **normal development** e.g **notochord and thyroglossal duct**[Q]
    - Decrease in size of **uterus after parturition**[Q]
  - **Pathologic atrophy**
    - **Disuse** atrophy: Most common due to decreased workload

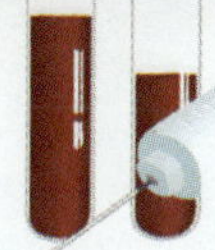

- **Denervation** atrophy: Due to loss of innervation
- **Senile** atrophy: Due to diminished **blood supply**; seen in **aging brain**[Q]
- **Pressure** atrophy: Atrophy of surrounding uninvolved tissues due to an enlarging benign tumor
- **Brown atrophy-lipofuscin granules** seen → **brown** discoloration of tissue
- **Inadequate nutrition**: protein-calorie malnutrition
- **Loss of endocrine stimulation: menopause** → physiologic **atrophy** of the **endometrium**, vaginal epithelium & **breast**

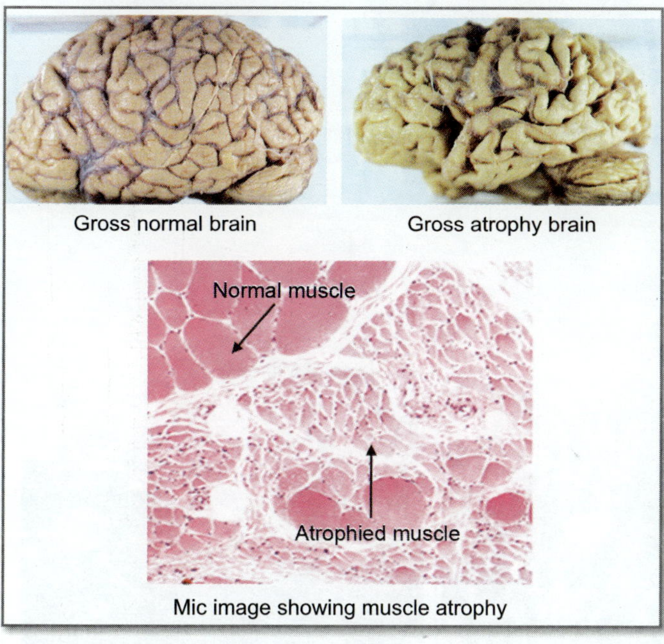

Gross normal brain

Gross atrophy brain

Mic image showing muscle atrophy

Metaplasia

- **One differentiated** cell type (epithelial or mesenchymal) is **replaced by another cell type; Reversible**

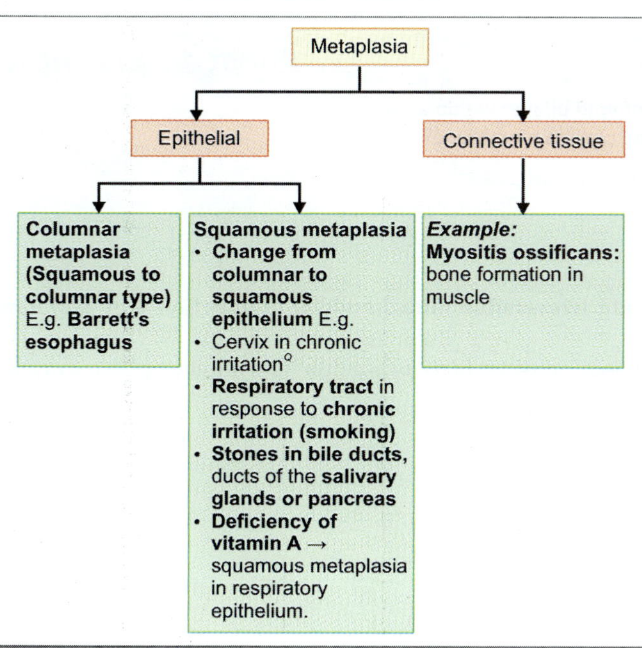

- ***Mechanism*: Reprograming of stem cells** or **undifferentiated** mesenchymal cells[Q] in normal tissues
- ***Outcome:*** If persistent, can initiate **malignant transformation** in metaplastic epithelium

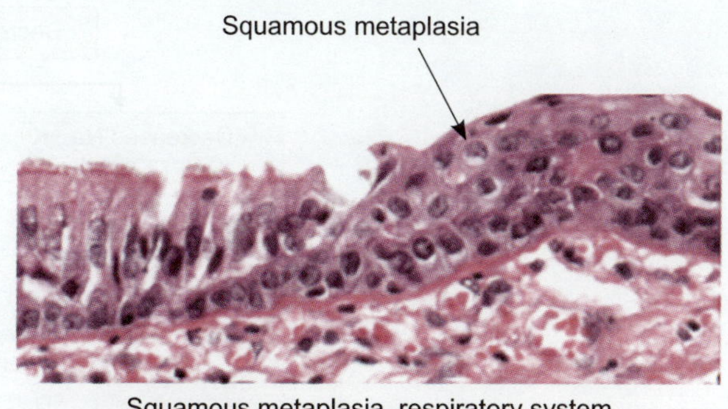

Squamous metaplasia, respiratory system

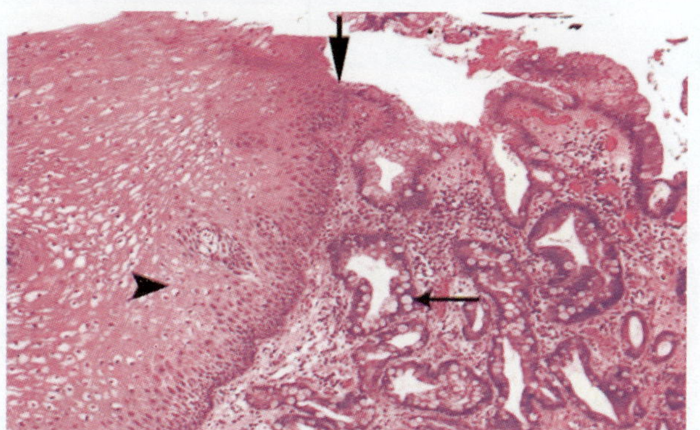

Barrett's metaplasia

Barrett's metaplasia of esophagus is defined as replacement of the normal squamous epithelium of distal esophagus by metaplastic glandular epithelium containing intestinal-type goblet cells. Note the squamous epithelium on the left (arrow head) is continuous with the metaplastic epithelium containing goblet cells (long thin arrow) on the right. The transition is shown by downward arrow on the top.

CELL INJURY

- **Hypoxia is** the most common cause of cell injury
- **Ischemia is** the most common cause of hypoxia

Reversible Injury

- **Cellular swelling (Hydropic Change/vacuolar degeneration):** Microscopic examination may show small, clear vacuoles within the cytoplasm; these represent distended and pinched-off **segments of the endoplasmic reticulum (ER)**
- Features of **reversible cell injury** seen in **light microscopy** are **cellular swelling and fatty change.**[Q]
- **The earliest change of reversible cell injury- cellular swelling**[Q]
- **The earliest morphological change** in reversible cell injury[Q] occur due to **accumulation of water intracellularly**[Q]
- Other features are demonstrated in the flow diagram below
- **Nuclear alterations** in reversible injury include **disaggregation of granular and fibrillar elements**

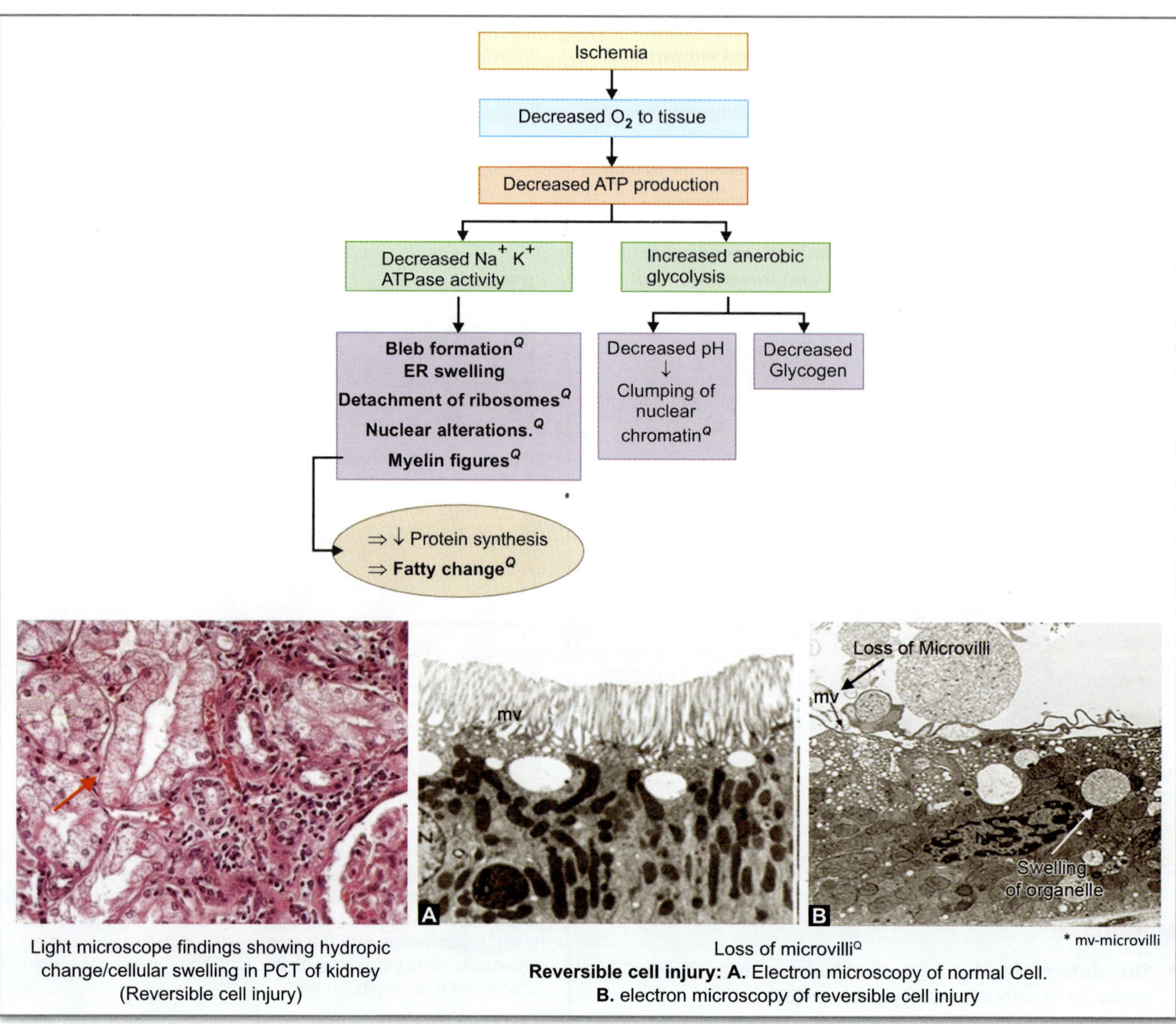

Light microscope findings showing hydropic change/cellular swelling in PCT of kidney (Reversible cell injury)

Loss of microvilli[Q]
Reversible cell injury: A. Electron microscopy of normal Cell. **B.** electron microscopy of reversible cell injury

* mv-microvilli

POINTS TO REMEMBER

- **Myelin figures** are rolled-up or are present in scroll-like arrangement of **lipid bilayer** within a cell
- Myelin figures are derived from damaged membranes of organelles and plasma membrane[Q]
- Myelin figures can be seen both in reversible and irreversible cell injury

Irreversible Cell Injury

- **Membrane damage is** the central factor for irreversible injury
- Two phenomena that **consistently characterize irreversibility** are **irreversible mitochondrial dysfunction** and **profound disturbances in membrane function**
- Electron microscopy features of irreversible injury are: large amorphous densities in mitochondria[Q] and intracytoplasmic myelin figures[Q]

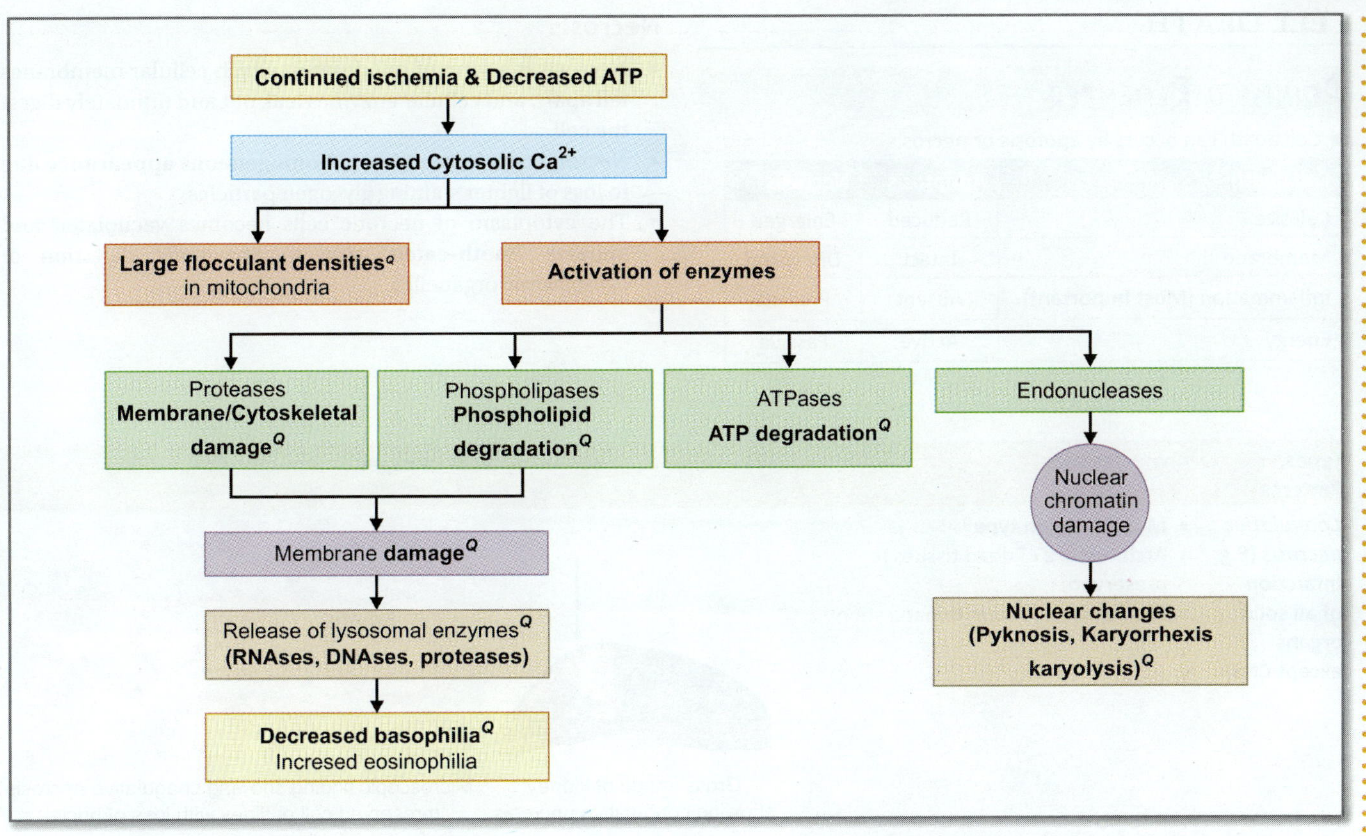

Features of Irreversible Injury

- **Severe swelling of mitochondria**[Q] and **large, flocculant, amorphous densities**[Q] due to **increased Ca²⁺ influx**[Q]
- **Severe swelling of lysosomes**[Q]: Injury to lysosomal membrane with release of enzymes leading to:
  - **Decreased basophilia, Increased eosinophilia**[Q]
  - **Nuclear changes (Pyknosis, karyolysis, Karyorrhexis)**[Q]
  - **Protein digestion**[Q]
  - **Severe damage to plasma membrane**[Q]

Stains

- Stain used in histopathology is **Hematoxylin and Eosin**.
- Hematoxylin stains—DNA & RNA of nucleus.
- **Eosin:** Stains cytoplasmic process.
- Necrotic/dying cells appear more pink as
  - Eosin binds strongly to denatured proteins
  - Loss of DNA & RNA causes loss of blue color

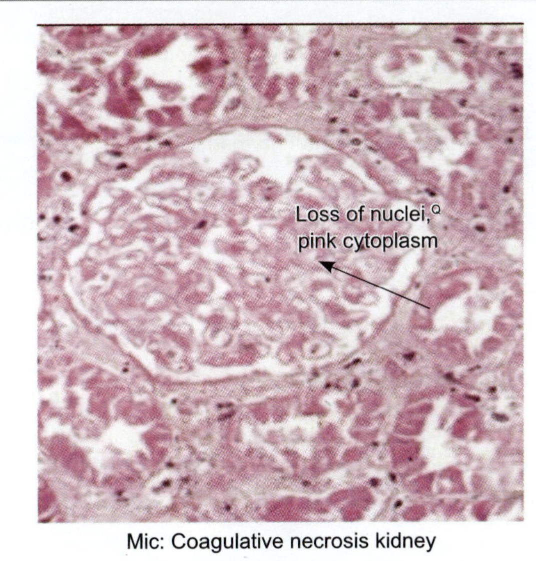

Mic: Coagulative necrosis kidney

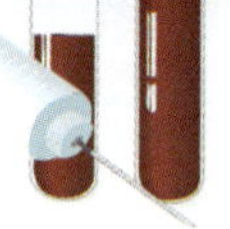

CELL DEATH

POINTS TO REMEMBER

- Cell death can occurs by apotosis or necrosis

Cell death	Apoptosis	Necrosis
Cell size	Reduced	Enlarged
Membrane	Intact	Disrupted
Inflammation (**Most Important**)	Absent	Present
Energy	Active	Passive

Necrosis

- Necrosis is a form of cell death in which cellular membranes fall apart, and cellular enzymes leak out and ultimately digest the cell
- Necrotic cells have a **glassy, homogeneous appearance** due to loss of lighter staining glycogen particles
- The cytoplasm of necrotic cells becomes vacuolated and appears "**moth-eaten**" due to enzymatic digestion of cytoplasmic organelles

Types/Patterns	Characteristics	Images
Coagulative necrosis (E.g. Infarction of all solid organs except CNS)	• **Most common type**[Q] • **Architecture** of dead tissues is **preserved** • **Mechanism:** Protein denaturation	Gross image of kidney showing coagulative necrosis. Microscopic finding showing coagulative necrosis (preserved cell outlines with loss of nuclei)
Liquefactive necrosis	• **Digestion** of the dead cells, resulting in **transformation of tissue into a liquid** viscous mass • Focal bacterial or, occasionally, fungal **infections** are seen; E.g. Necrosis in **CNS**[Q] • **Mechanism:** Enzymatic action.	Gross: Brain showing liquefactive necrosis. Mic: Image shows dissolution of tissue (Liquefactive necrosis in the brain)
Gangrenous necrosis	• Commonly used term in clinical practice, but **not a specific pattern of cell death**[Q] • **Wet** gangrene (type of Liquefactive necrosis) and **Dry** gangrene (type of Coagulative necrosis)	Dry gangrene. Wet gangrene
Caseous necrosis (CN)	• Characterised by **granuloma-**collection of fragmented or lysed cells & **amorphous granular debris**[Q] enclosed within a distinctive inflammatory border. • E.g. **Tuberculous infection**[Q] fungi-**histoplasma**[Q], **coccidiomycosis**[Q]	Gross-lung showing CN (red arrow). Microscopy-showing CN (green arrow) along with langhans giant cell (red arrow)

Gross image of kidney showing coagulative necrosis

Microscopic finding showing coagulative necrosis (preserved cell outlines with loss of nuclei)

Gross: Brain showing liquefactive necrosis

Mic: Image shows dissolution of tissue

Dry gangrene

Wet gangrene

Gross-lung showing CN (red arrow)

Microscopy-showing CN (green arrow) along with langhans giant cell (red arrow)

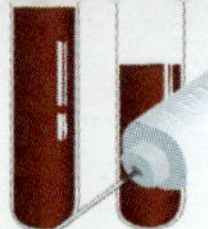

Types/ Patterns	Characteristics	Images
Fat necrosis	<ul><li>**Focal** areas of **fat destruction**; Not a specific pattern of necrosis.[Q]</li><li>**Lipases** → **split triglyceride esters** → **fatty acids** → combine with **calcium** to produce grossly visible **chalky-white areas (fat saponification)**[Q]</li><li>E.g. Acute pancreatitis, Injury to breast, Abdomen, Buttocks[Q]</li></ul>	Microscopy-showing chalky white deposits (arrow)
Fibrinoid necrosis	<ul><li>Due to **immune reactions** involving blood vessels</li><li>Deposits of "**antigen –antibody complexes**"[Q] and **fibrin** that has leaked out of vessels, result in a bright **pink and amorphous appearance in H & E stains.**[Q]</li><li>Seen **in PAN, malignant hypertension, acute rheumatic fever, Libman sacks endocarditis**[Q]</li></ul>	Microscopy-wall of artery showing fibrinoid necrosis (arrow)

High Yield Facts

- **Coagulative necrosis: The most common type of necrosis**[Q]: occurs due to degenerated cytoplasmic proteins[Q]
- **A localized area of coagulative necrosis is called an infarct.**[Q]
- **Caseous necrosis is most often** seen in **tuberculous infection**[Q]
- **Cause of caseous necrosis-mycolic acid**[Q]
- **Zenker's degeneration** is **a true necrosis**[Q] **(coagulative necrosis)**[Q] affecting muscles (**skeletal > cardiac**)[Q], during acute infections (especially typhoid[Q]).
- In Zenker's degeneration, Rectus and diaphragm are the most common muscles affected[Q]

- Cell loss in proliferating cell populations[Q]
- **Epithelial cells- in intestinal crypts**, as to maintain a constant number (homeostasis).
- Elimination of potentially harmful **self-reactive lymphocytes**[Q]
- Death of host cells that have served their useful purpose- **neutrophils in an acute inflammatory response**[Q]
- *Pathological situations*
  - DNA damage- **radiational injuries**[Q]
  - Accumulation of **misfolded proteins**[Q]
  - Cell death in certain viral infections- E.g. **councilman bodies in hepatitis B virus**[Q]
  - **Atrophy** in parenchymal organs after duct obstruction. E.g. **pancreas, parotids and kidneys**[Q]
- **Mechanisms:**
  - Two pathways: **Mitochondrial pathway (intrinsic) and the death receptor pathway (extrinsic)**
  - Activation of **caspases (cysteine protease enzymes that cleave proteins after aspartic residues)**[Q]

Apoptosis

- **Pathway of cell death** induced by a **tightly regulated suicide program**[Q] leading to activation of intrinsic enzymes **that degrade the cell's own DNA and proteins.**[Q]
- *Important characteristics*
  - **No loss of membrane integrity**[Q]
  - **No leakage of cellular contents**[Q]
  - **No host reaction**[Q]
- *Examples:*
  - *Physiologic Situations*
    - **Embryogenesis**[Q]
    - Hormone-dependent tissues upon **hormone withdrawal**

Intrinsic (Mitochondrial) Pathway of Apoptosis

- M**ajor mechanism**[Q] of apoptosis in all mammalian cells.
- Results from release of pro-apoptotic molecules from mitochondrial **intermembrane space** into the cytoplasm.[Q]

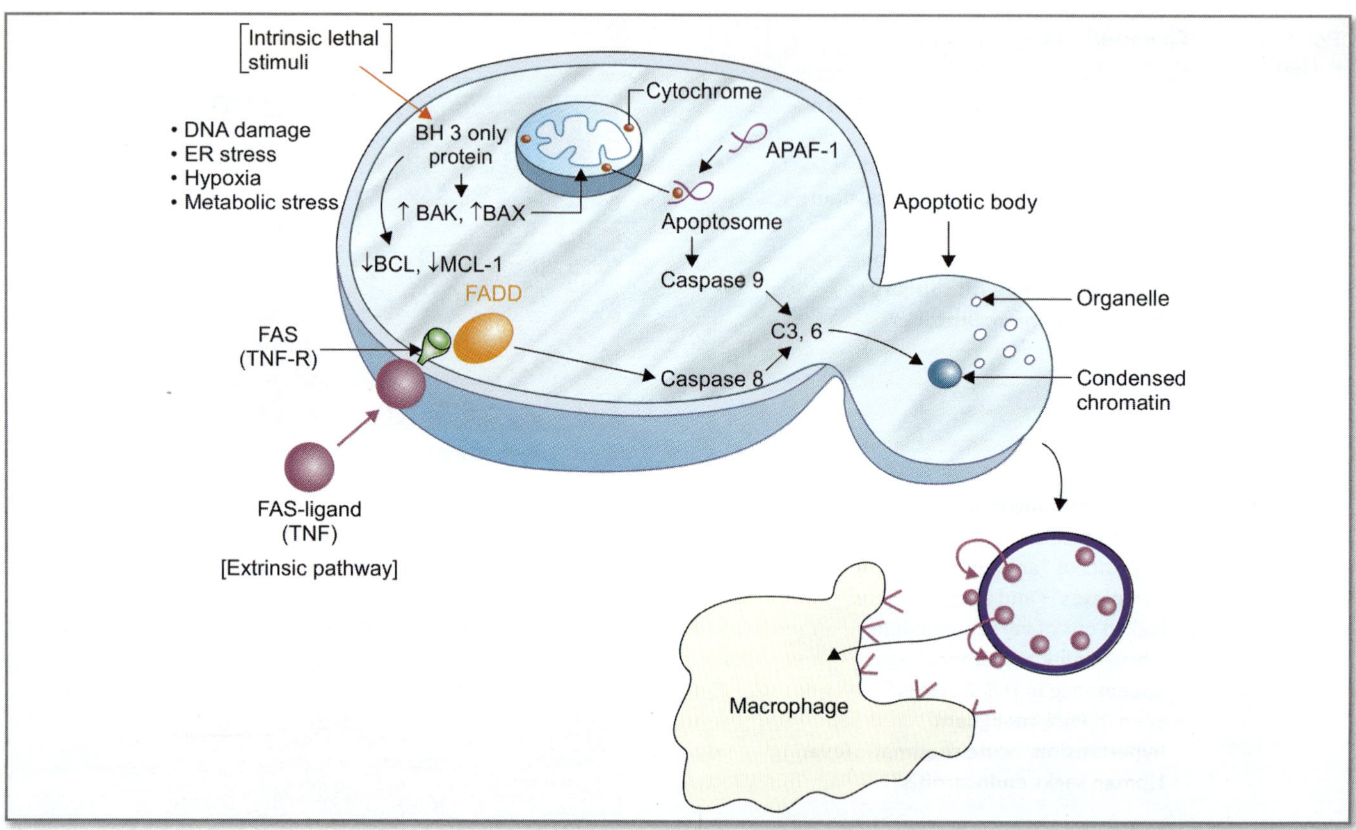

***Sensors:** Contain 3rd of 4 BH domains (BH3-only proteins)–BAD, BID, BIM, Puma, Noxa

Extrinsic (Death Receptor-Initiated) Pathway of Apoptosis

- Initiated by **engagement of plasma membrane death receptors**
- Death receptors are members of the **TNF receptor family[Q]** that contain a cytoplasmic domain involved in protein-protein interactions and is called the **death domain[Q]** because it is essential for delivering apoptotic signals.
- **Death receptors**: TNFR1 and FasR (**CD95**)

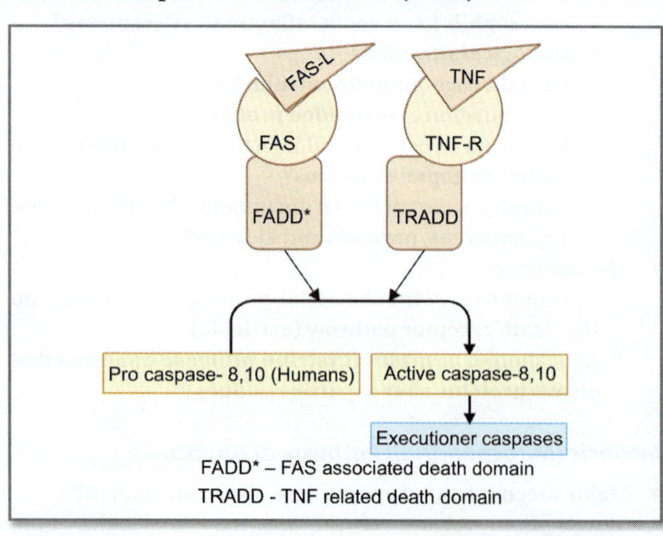

R9th **Latest** Update

Regulatory molecules in Apoptosis	
Anti-apoptotic	**Pro-apoptotic**
BCL2, BCL-XL, and MCL1	BAX and BAK
Possess four BH domains **(called BH 1-4)[Q]**	Possess four BH domains **(called BH 1-4)**
• Present in **outer mitochondrial & ER membranes & cytosol** • **Prevent leakage** of **cytochrome c** into the cytosol	• Form a **channel in outer mitochondrial membrane** • Allows **leakage** of **cyt c** from intermembranous space

- Biochemical Features of Apoptosis
  - *Protein cleavage*
    - **Active caspases[Q]** cleave many vital cellular proteins and break up nuclear scaffold and cytoskeleton
  - *DNA Breakdown[Q]*
    - Characteristic breakdown of DNA into large 50 to 300 kilobase piece
    - Subsequent **internucleosomal cleavage[Q]** of DNA into oligonucleosomes, in multiples of **180 to 200 base pairs[Q]**, by Ca^{2+} and Mg^{2+} dependent **endonucleases[Q]**
  - *Phagocytic recognition:* Expression of **phosphatidyl serine, thrombospondin[Q]** → early recognition of dead cells by macrophages → phagocytosis **without the release of proinflammatory cellular components[Q]**

Morphology of Apoptosis

- **Cell shrinkage**[Q]
- **Chromatin condensation: most characteristic feature**[Q] of apoptosis.
- **Formation of cytoplasmic blebs and apoptotic bodies**[Q]
- **Plasma membrane** remains **intact**[Q] during apoptosis
- Apoptosis in contrast to necrosis **doesn't elicit inflammation**[Q].

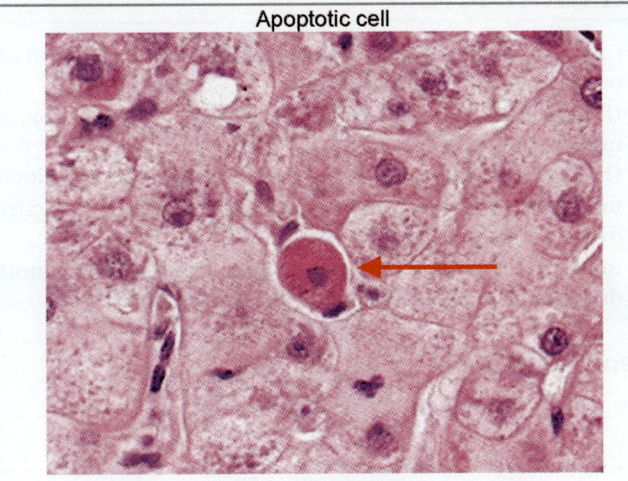

Reduced cell size with condensed chromatin

Diagnosis of Apoptosis

- Chromatin condensation is seen by hematoxylin, Feulgen and acridine orange staining.
- Estimation of **cytochrome 'c'**[Q]
- Estimation of activated caspases
- Estimation of **Annexin V** (apoptotic cells express **phosphatidylserine / thrombospondin**[Q] on the outer layer of plasma membrane because of which these cells are recognized by the dye **Annexin V**[Q].)
- DNA breakdown **(Internucleosome cleavage by endonuclease into 200bp oligonucleosomes is a characteristic)**[Q] at specific sites → fragments can be detected by **'step ladder pattern'** on agarose gel electrophoresis or TUNEL (TdT mediated d-UTP Nick End Labelling) technique[Q].

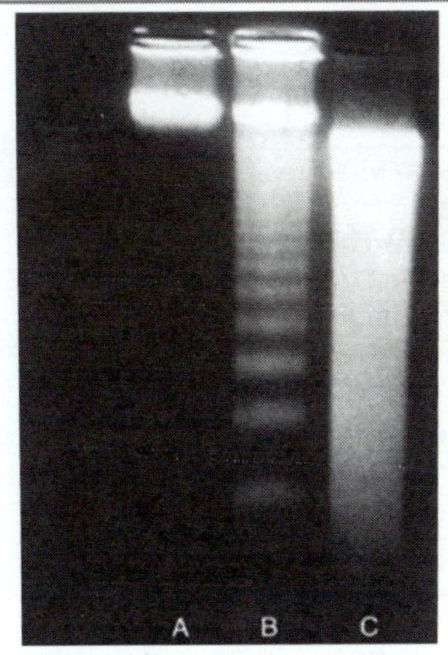

Electrophoresis showing step ladder pattern in (B) and Smudged pattern in (C)

Electron Microscopy of apoptosis

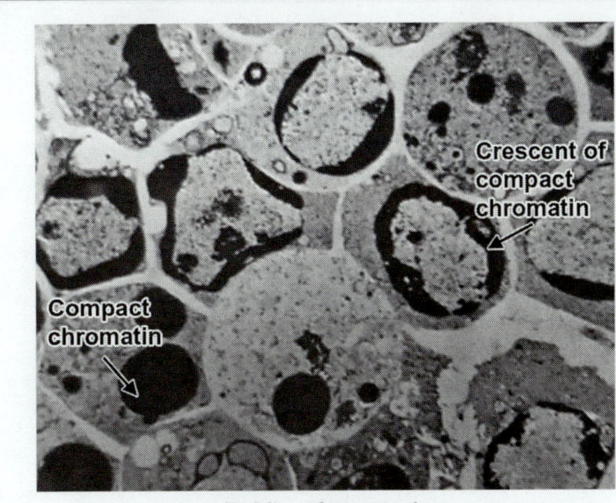

E. Mic. of apoptosis

- Initiator caspase:
  - Intrinsic pathway – caspase **9**[Q]
  - Extrinsic pathway – caspase **8, 10**[Q]
- Executionary pathway-caspase 3 (most important), **6**[Q]
- Necrosis and apoptosis together[Q]-Injurious stimuli like chemotherapy and radiation can induce apoptosis[Q] if the insult is mild but large doses of same stimuli can induce necrotic cell death[Q]

Necroptosis

Programed necrosis or "caspase-independent" programed cell death[Q]

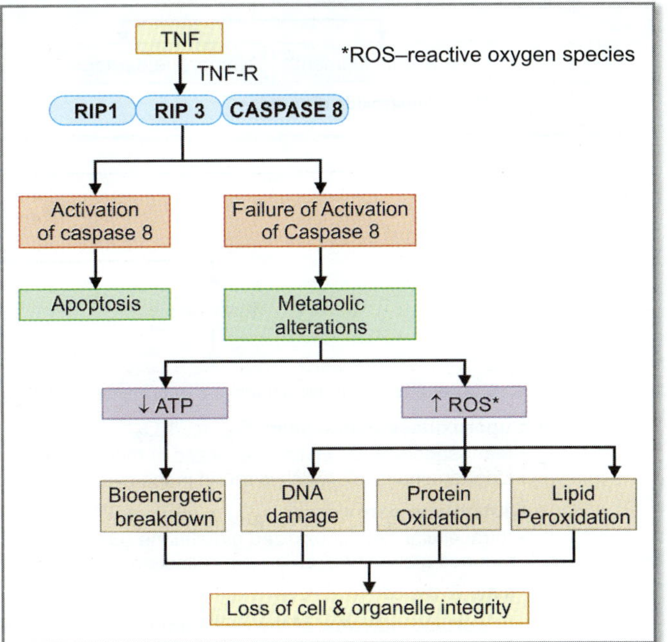

Pyroptosis

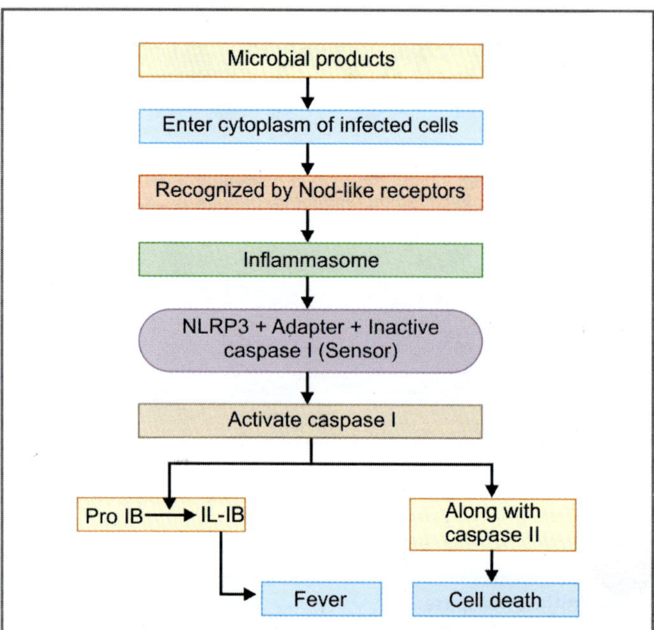

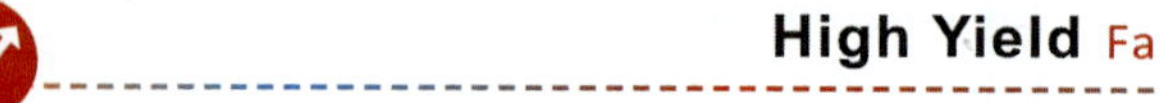

High Yield Facts

Examples of Necroptosis
- Formation of the mammalian bone growth plate[Q]
- Cell death in steatohepatitis and acute pancreatitis[Q]
- Reperfusion injury[Q]
- Neurodegenerative diseases such as Parkinson's disease[Q]

FREE RADICALS

- Chemical species that have a **single unpaired electron**[Q] in an outer orbit.
- Unpaired electrons are highly reactive and attack inorganic or organic chemicals
- **Oxidative stress**[Q] - excess of these free radicals due to either increased production or decreased scavenging of reactive oxygen species (ROS).
- Implicated in **cell injury, cancer, aging, and some degenerative diseases such as Alzheimer disease.**[Q]

Generation of Free Radicals[Q]

The generation and role of ROS in cell injury is given below.

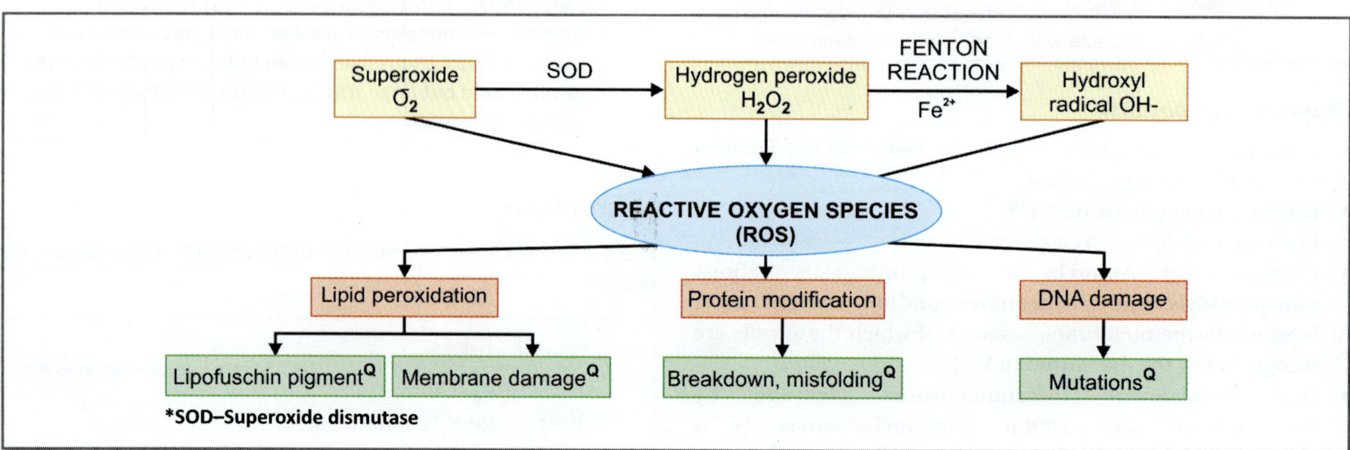

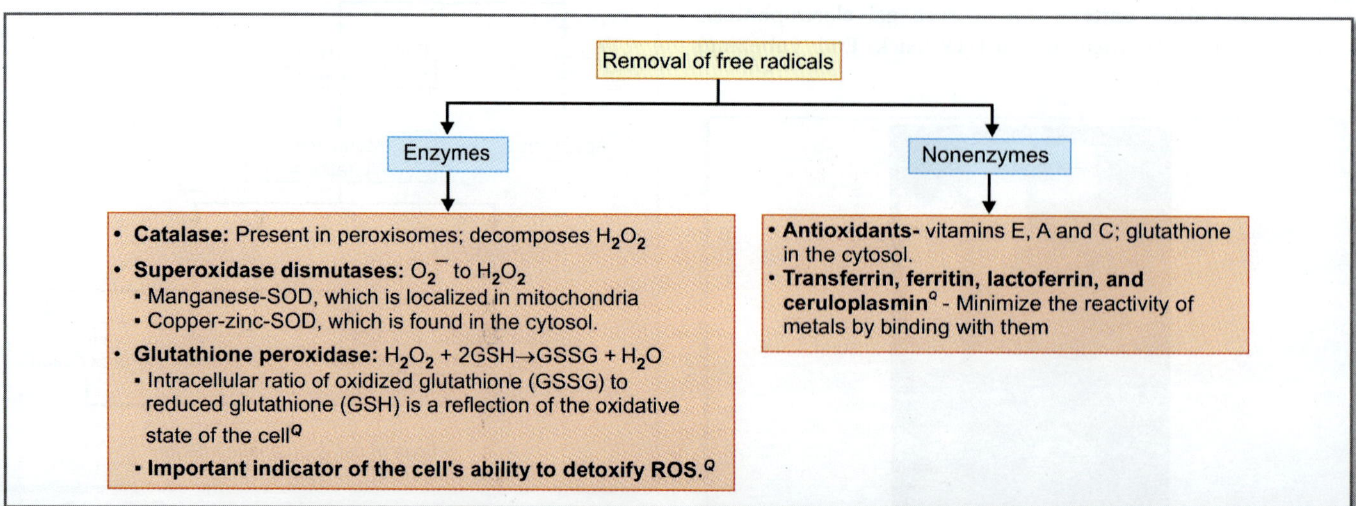

- **Superoxide dismutase**: **Enzyme** that protects the brain from free radical injury[Q]
- **Telltale sign** of free radical injury: **Lipofuscin pigment**[Q]

CELLULAR ACCUMULATIONS

Lipids

Triglycerides

- **Steatosis** (Fatty Change): accumulations of triglycerides within parenchymal cells
- **Organs** involved-liver, heart, muscle, and kidney
- **Tigered effect**: Fatty change in heart

Cholesterol and Cholesterol Esters

- **Foam cells**: Cholesterol-laden macrophages
- Accumulation of cholesterol and cholesterol esters occurs in following conditions:
  - **Xanthomas**
  - **Cholesterolosis**: In the lamina propria of **gall bladder**[Q]
  - **Niemann-Pick disease**, **type C:** Mutations affecting an enzyme involved in cholesterol trafficking, resulting in cholesterol accumulation in multiple organs

Phospholipids

Components of the **myelin figures**[Q] found in necrotic cells

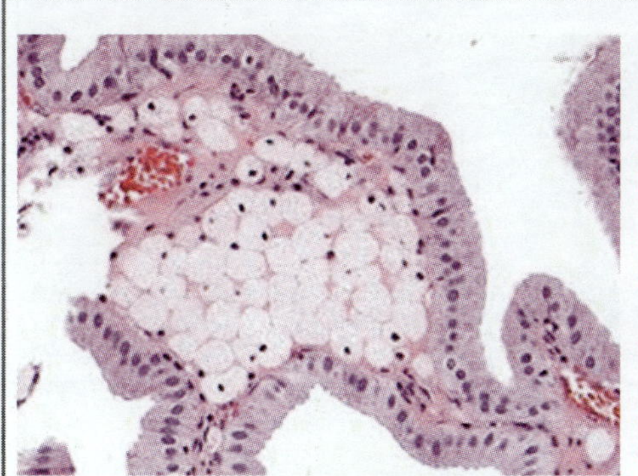

Image showing foam cells

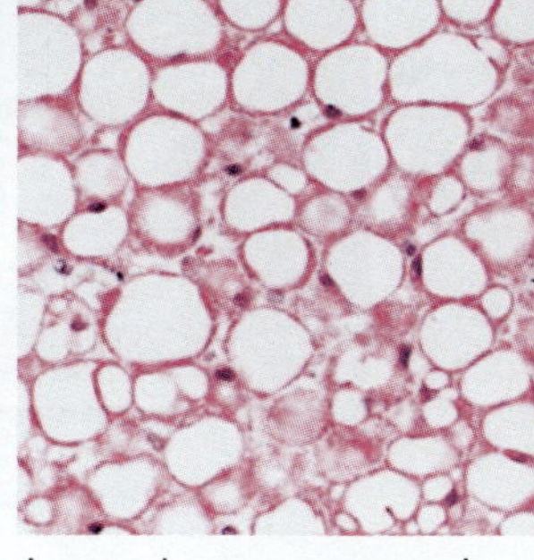

Image shows macrovascular steatosis

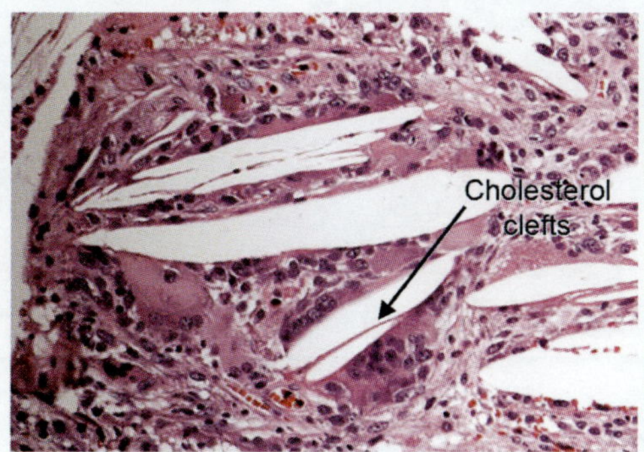

Image showing cholesterol clefts (arrow)

Proteins

Resorption Droplets

- **Appear as rounded, eosinophilic droplets, vacuoles, or aggregates in the cytoplasm.**[Q]
- Examples of Protein Accumulates are given below:

```
                        Proteins

  Resorption        Russell bodies°     Accumulation of
  droplets°                             cytoskeletal proteins

• In proximal renal   • Immunoglobulin   • Microtubules (20-25
  tubules in            accumulation in     mm in diameter)°
  disorders with        ER of cell - seen • Thin actin filaments
  heavy proteinuria     in multiple         (6-8 nm)°
• Appears as pink       myeloma°          • Thick myosin filaments
  hyaline droplets                          (15 nm)°
  within the                             • Intermediate filaments
  cytoplasm of the                          (10 nm)°
  tubular cell

                                         • CK
                                         • Vimentin
                                         • Desmin
                                         • GFAP
                                         • NF
```

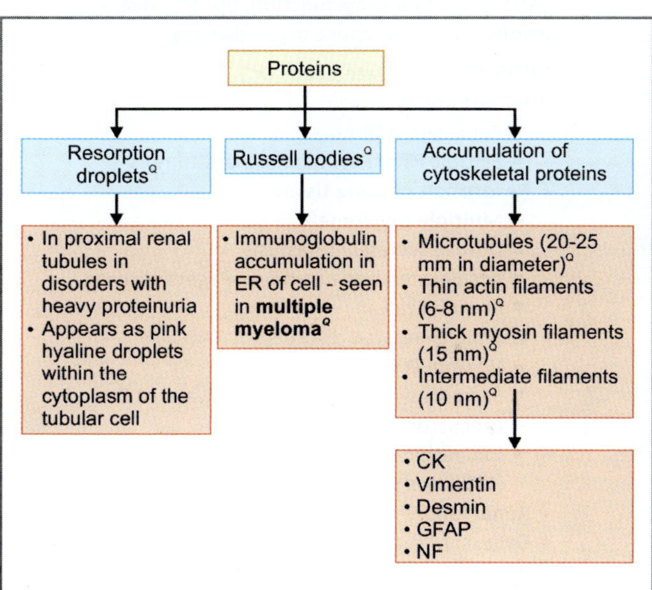

Image showing reabsorption droplets in PCT

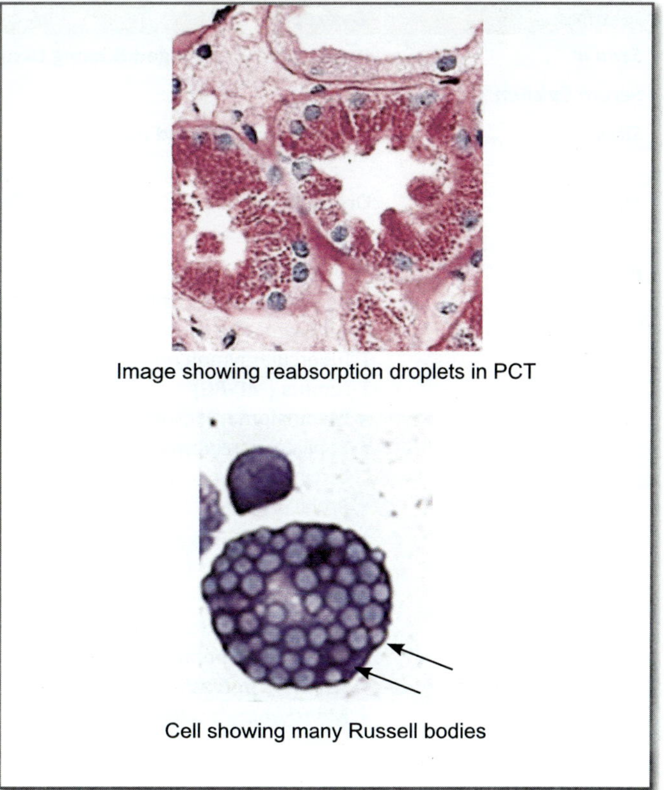

Cell showing many Russell bodies

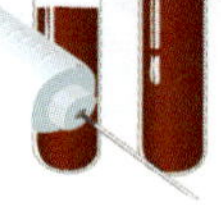

Hyaline Change

- Any intracellular or extracellular accumulation with pink homogenous appearance
- Descriptive histologic term rather than a specific marker for cell injury

Glycogen

- **Appears as clear vacuoles** within the cytoplasm

- Best fixed in absolute alcohol

Best stain:

- **Best carmine or PAS with diastase** (Diastase hydrolyzes glycogen)
- **Seen in:**
  1. **Diabetes mellitus:** Glycogen accumulates in renal tubular epithelial cells, liver cells, β cells of the islets of Langerhans, and heart muscle cells
  2. **Glycogen storage diseases[Q],** or glycogenoses

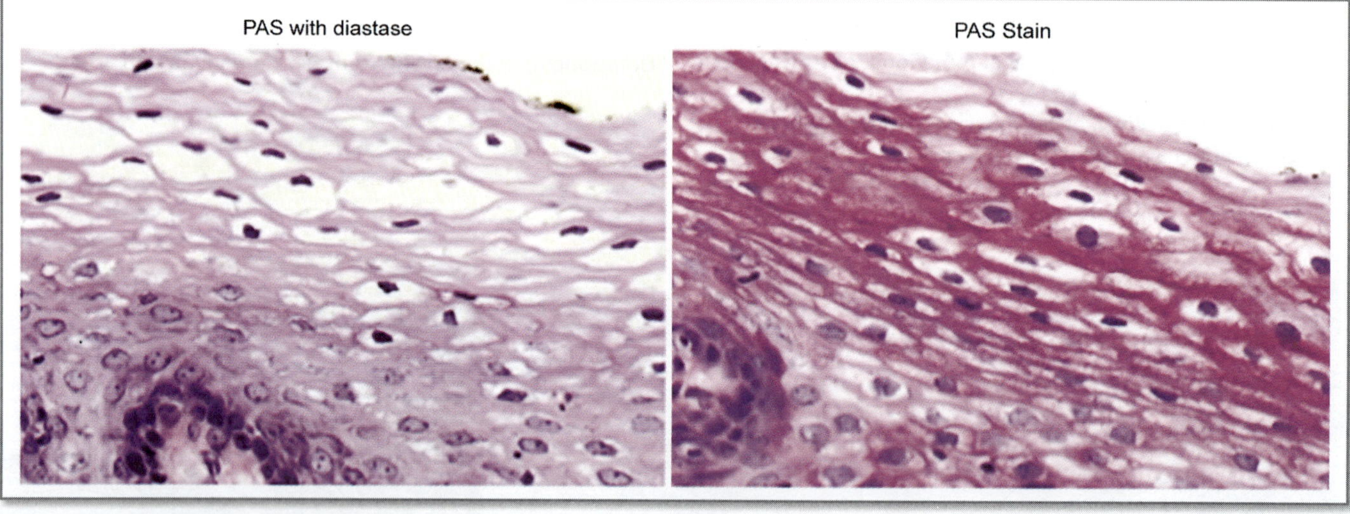

Calcification

- Abnormal tissue deposition of **calcium salts**, with small amounts of **iron, magnesium and other mineral salts.**[Q]
- It can be of the following two types:

Features	Dystrophic	Metastatic
Seen in	**Dead tissues[Q], damaged & aging tissues**	**Living tissues**
Serum Calcium	**Normal[Q]**	**Elevated**
Sites	Seen in **cell injury and necrosis[Q]**	Mainly affects **gastric mucosa[Q], kidneys[Q], lungs[Q], systemic arteries[Q] & pulmonary veins.[Q]**
Effect	**Organ dysfunction**	Usually **no clinical dysfunction, but massive involvement may cause organ damage**
Etiology	"R-A-T-T" **R**-Rheumatic heart ds (Cardiac valves) **A**-Atheromatous plaque **T**-Tubercular lymph node **T-Tumors (MP-PG)** • Meningioma, Mesothelioma • Papillary carcinoma of thyroid, Ovary (serous carcinoma) • Prolactinoma • Glucagonoma Examples of Dystrophic Calcification • **Psammoma bodies[Q]** • **Asbestos bodies[Q]** • **Mönckeberg's sclerosis[Q]**	PRDR (Postgraduate Reads Dr.) • HyperParathyroidism- ▪ Parathyroid tumors ▪ Ectopic PTHRP from malignant tumors • **Resorption of bone tissue-** ▪ **Multiple myeloma[Q]** ▪ Diffuse skeletal metastasis ▪ Accelerated bone turnover-Pagets' disease ▪ Immobilization • Vitamin **D**–related disorders ▪ Vitamin D intoxication, ▪ Sarcoidosis (Macrophages activate vit D precursor) ▪ Idiopathic hypercalcemia of infancy **(Williams syndrome)[Q]** • **Renal failure**-Due to secondary hyperparathyroidism • **Others:** Milk alkali syndrome, Aluminum intoxication • Vitamin A toxicity

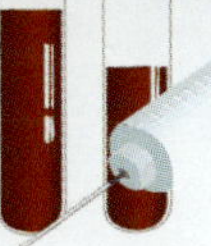

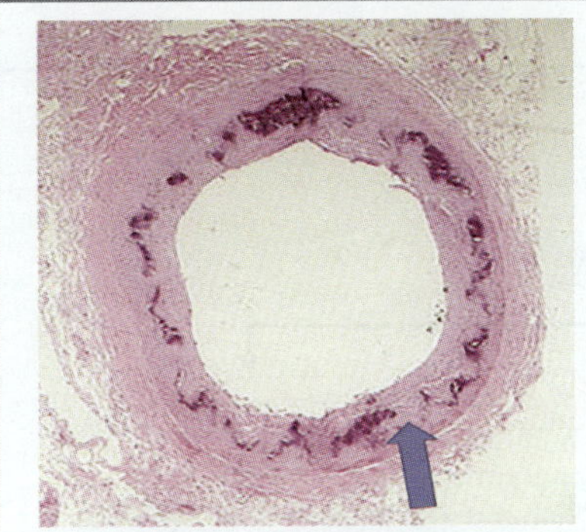
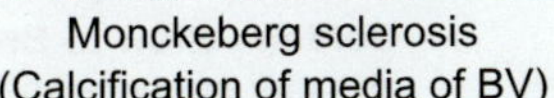

Monckeberg sclerosis
(Calcification of media of BV)

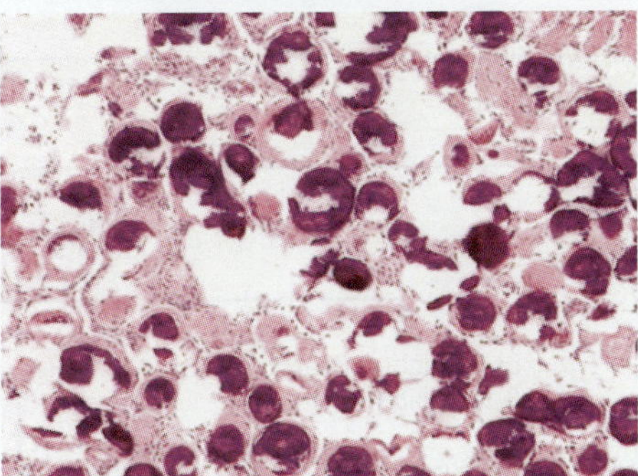

Image showing psammoma bodies

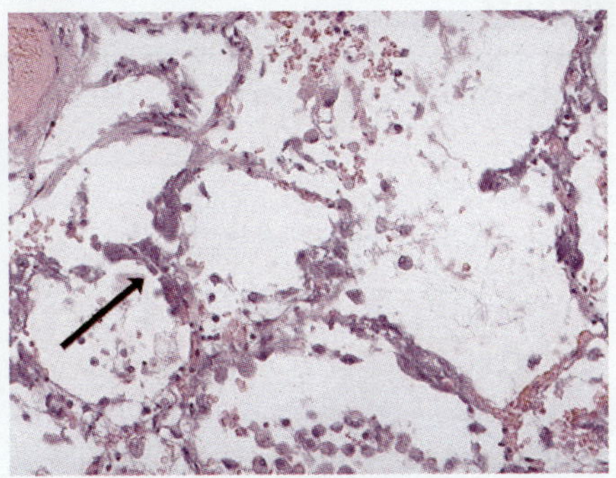

Stains

Most common stain used for
calcium-Von kossa

Von kossa gives black colour to
calcium (arrow)

Most specific stain used for
calcium Alizarin Red

Alizarin Red Stain For Calcium

High Yield Facts

- Calcification **begins** in **mitochondria**[Q]
- **Mönckeberg's sclerosis**[Q] **(medial calcific sclerosis)** i.e it's a type of **dystrophic calcification.**[Q] Calcium deposits are found in **tunica media** of arteries is a misnomer.
- **Internal alkaline environment**[Q] **in tissues** favors **metastatic calcification**
- **Most common site of metastatic calcification is lungs > kidneys**[Q]

Theory

Pigments

```
                          ┌──────────────┐
                          │   Pigments   │
                          └──────────────┘
              ┌────────────────┴────────────────────────┐
       ┌────────────┐                            ┌──────────────┐
       │ Exogenous  │                            │  Endogenous  │
       └────────────┘                            └──────────────┘
        ┌──────┴──────┐              ┌────────────────┼────────────────┐
   ┌─────────┐  ┌──────────┐  ┌──────────────┐ ┌──────────┐ ┌──────────────┐
   │ Carbon  │  │ Tattooing│  │ Lipofuscin   │ │ Melanin  │ │ Hemosiderin  │
   └─────────┘  └──────────┘  │ (Wear &      │ └──────────┘ └──────────────┘
                              │ tear pigment)│
                              └──────────────┘
```

Carbon

- **Most common**[Q] exogenous pigment
- Phagocytosed by **lung macrophages**[Q]

Tattooing

- Localized, exogenous pigmentation of the skin.
- Phagocytosed by **dermal macrophages**[Q]

Lipofuscin (Wear & tear pigment)

- Insoluble pigment
- Also called lipchrome or wear & tear pigment
- Derived by **lipid peroxidation of polyunsaturated lipids of subcellular membranes**[Q]
- **Tell-tale sign** of free radical injury to the cell & lipid peroxidation
- **Yellow brown, Perinuclear**[Q] pigment
- Responsible for **brown atrophy of liver and heart**[Q]
- Seen in **aging**[Q], **protein energy malnutrition**[Q] & **cancer cachexia.**[Q]
- **Stain-long ZN stain**[Q]

Melanin

- Non-heme derived pigment[Q]
- Normally present in hair,[Q] skin, iris, stria vascularis of inner ear,[Q] zona reticularis of adrenal gland[Q] & substantia nigra of brain[Q]
- Only naturally occurring[Q] endogenous black pigment derived from **tyrosine**[Q]
- **Special stain: Masson Fontana**
- IHC stain-S100, **HMB45** (Specific)[Q]
- Albinism-Little or no melanin synthesis
- Tumor of melanocytes-melanoma[Q]

Hemosiderin

- Heme derived pigment[Q]
- **Golden yellow to Brown,** granular or crystalline pigment[Q]
- Seen at sites of – Local hemorrhage or bruise[Q]
- Systemic overload of iron hemosiderin is called hemosiderosis[Q]
- Hemosiderin-aggregates of ferritin micelles[Q]
- **Special stain: Perls Prussian blue stain** – Converts soluble ferrocyanide to ferric ferrocyanide[Q]
- Perls stain detects **Ferric**[Q] **iron** deposits in tissue

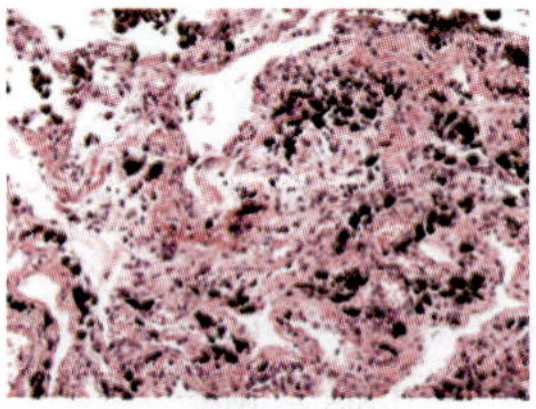

Black carbon pigment inside the cytoplasm of the macrophages in the alveolar wall

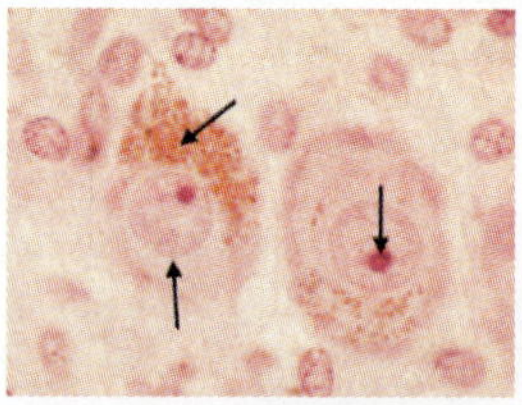

Mic: Perinuclear pigment

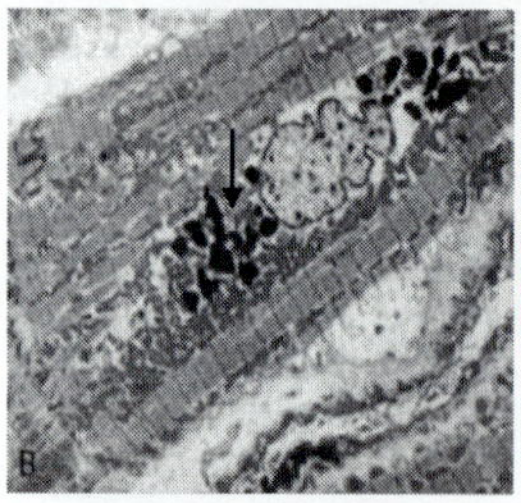

(Electron microscopy showing perinuclear pigment)

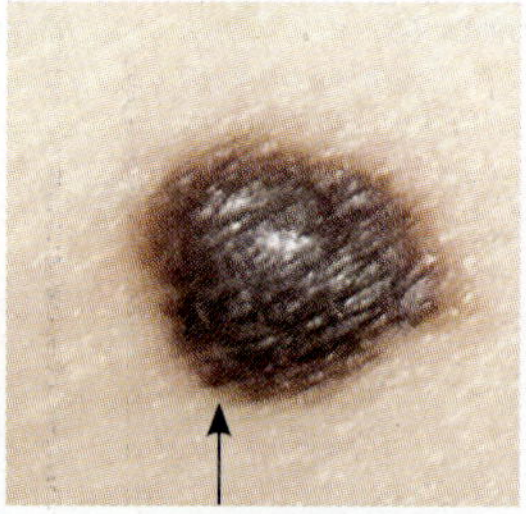

Melanin

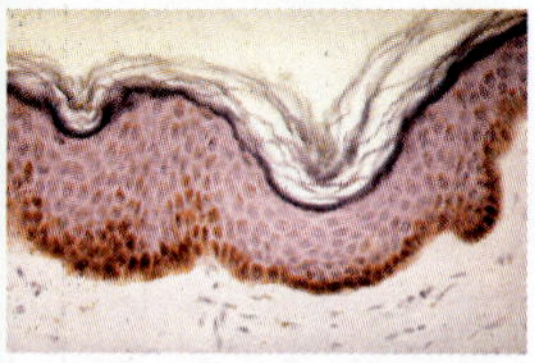

Melanin in **basal** layer or **epidermis**

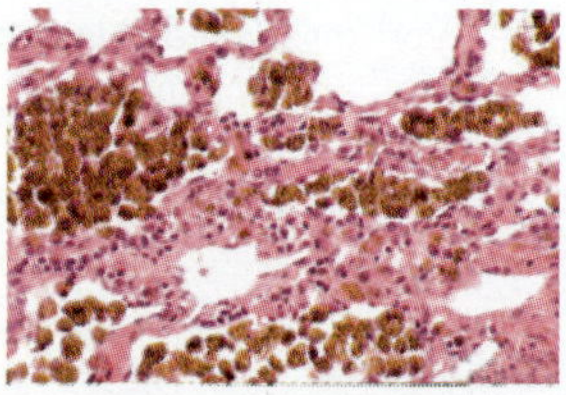

Hemosiderin Laden Macrophages in Lung Alveoli

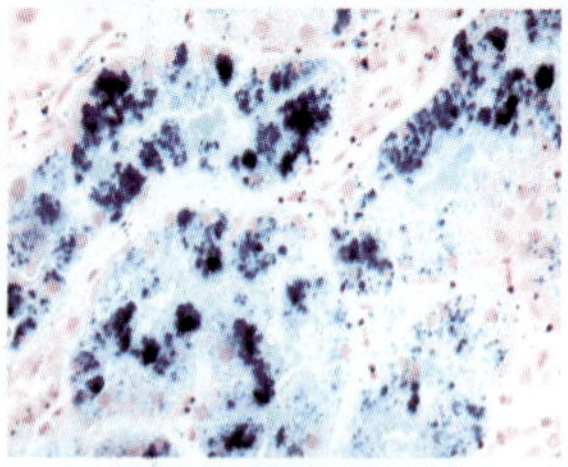

Perls stain showing hemosiderin pigment

High Yield Facts

- The pigments **do not usually evoke any inflammatory response.**[Q]
- Iron is normally **carried with transferrin in circulation.**[Q]
- **In cells**, it is stored in association with a protein, **apoferritin**, to form **ferritin micelles**[Q]
- Whenever there is a local or systemic excess of iron, **ferritin forms hemosiderin granules**[Q]
- Hemosiderin is considered as a **degraded and oxidized form** of ferritin.[Q]
- **Ferritin is soluble** while **hemosiderin is insoluble.**[Q]

Stains

- **Masson Fontana**-melanin
- Remember **Masson trichrome** is not for pigment, it distinguishes collagen from muscle
- **Long ZN stain** for Lipofuscin
- **Perls Prussian blue** for hemosiderin (Fe^{3+})
- The tissue-bound ferric ions subsequently are visualized by treatment with **potassium ferrocyanide** to form bright blue deposits of ferric ferrocyanide or Prussian blue.
- **Lillie's method** is used for picking up ferrous iron

CELLULAR AGING

The major causes of cellular aging are:

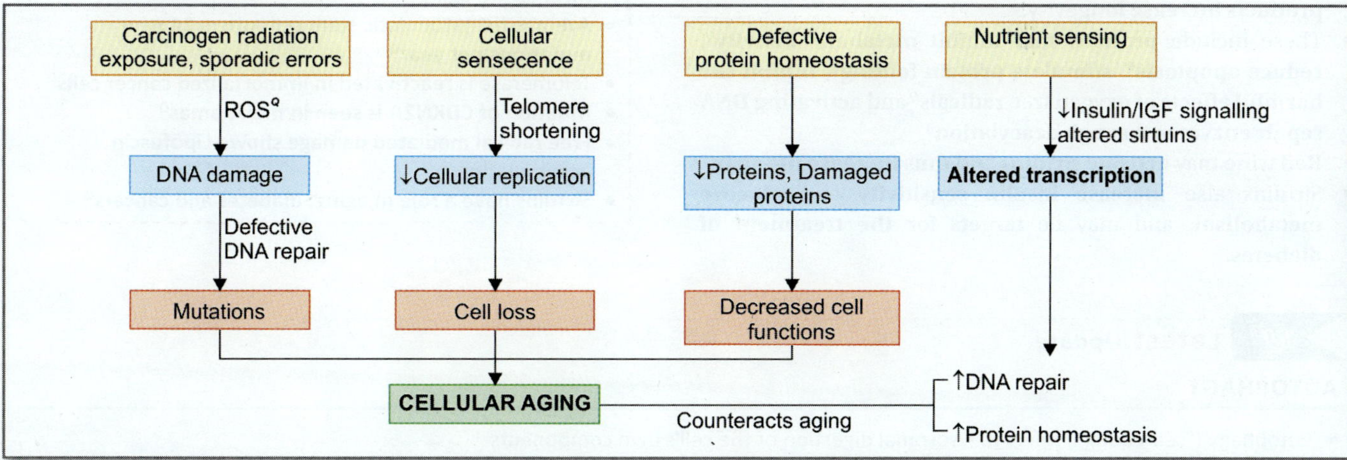

Cellular Senescence

- Normal cells have a limited capacity for replication
- **After a fixed number of divisions,** cells become arrested in a **terminally nondividing state,** known as **"replicative senescence"**[Q]

Two mechanisms are responsible for cellular senescence

Hayflick limit
- Normal cells can undergo 60–70 cell deivisions in their lifetime. This limit is called Hayflick limit.
- Cause of Hayflick limit is progressive telomere shortening with cell division.

Telomere Attrition	Activation of Tumor Suppressor Genes
• Telomeres are short repeated sequences at the ends of DNA which **ensure complete replication of chromosome.**[Q] • Telomere **length is maintained** by enzyme called **telomerase.**[Q] • Telomerase is **RNA dependent DNA polymerase**	**CDKN2A locus encodes a tumor suppressor gene called p16 or INK4a, which controls G1 to S phase progression during the cell cycle**[Q] ↓ Protects the cells from uncontrolled mitogenic signals and pushes cells along the **senescence pathway.**[Q]
• Telomerase is **absent in somatic cells, present only in germ cells and present at low levels in stem cells**[Q] • **Replicative senescence**[Q] -When somatic cells replicate, telomeres become progressively shortened → signals cell cycle arrest	

Defective Protein Homeostasis

- Both normal folding and degradation of misfolded proteins (**by autophagy and ubiquitin-proteasome system**) are impaired with aging
- **Rapamycin** has multiple effects including **promotion of autophagy** and thus increases the life span of middle aged mice

Dysregulated Nutrient Sensing

Caloric restriction increases lon **reducing the signaling intensity of the IGF-1 pathway**[Q] and by increasing sirtuins[Q]

Insulin and insulin-like growth factor 1 (IGF-1) signalling pathway
- **Growth hormone** secretion by the pituitary stimulates **IGF-1 (AKA somatomedin C)**
- IGF1 promotes **anabolic state** as well as **cell growth, replication and aging**
- It has two downstream targets- **AKT and mTOR** (mammalian target of rapamycin)
- **Rapamycin** might **increase the life span** of middle aged mice by **attenuation of IGF-1**

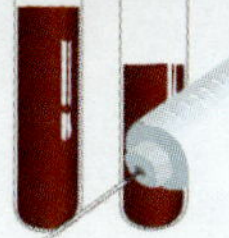

Sirtuins

- Family of **NAD-dependent protein deacetylases.**
- Sirtuin-6^Q promotes the expression of genes whose products increase longevity.
- These include **proteins that inhibit metabolic activity**^{Q}, **reduce apoptosis**^{Q}, **stimulate protein folding**^{Q}, **inhibit the harmful effects of oxygen free radicals**^{Q} and **activating DNA repair enzymes through deacylation**^{Q}
- **Red wine** may **activate sirtuins** and **thus increase life span**
- Sirtuins also **increase insulin sensitivity** and **glucose metabolism**, and may be **targets for the treatment of diabetes.**

High Yield Facts

- **Defective DNA helicase causes Werner's syndrome (premature aging)**
- Average hematopoietic stem cell suffers **14 new mutations per year**^{Q}
- Telomerase is **reactivated in immortalized cancer cells**^{Q}
- **Muation of CDKN2A is seen in melanomas**^{Q}
- **Free radical mediated damage shows-Lipofuscin accumulation**
- **Sirtuins have a role in aging, diabetes and cancers**^{Q}

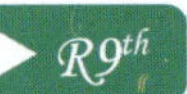

$R9^{th}$ Latest Update

AUTOPHAGY

- Autophagy ("self-eating") refers to lysosomal digestion of the cell's own components
- It is an **adaptation** to nutrient deprivation
- If the stress is too severe for the process to cope with it, it results in cell death by apoptosis
- **Physiological** autophagy is seen in aging and exercise
- **It is of three types:**
  - **Chaperone-mediated**
    - **Direct translocation** through lysosomal membrane by chaperone proteins.
  - **Microautophagy**
    - Inward invagination of lysosomal membrane for delivery.
  - **Macroautophagy**
    - Its **major form** of autophagy
    - It involves sequestration and transportation of cytosol content in a double-membrane bound autophagic vacuole (**autophagosome**).

Autophagy Plays a Role in Human Diseases

- **Cancer:** Autophagy can both promote cancer growth and act as a defense against cancers.
- **Neurodegenerative disorders:**
  - Alzheimer's disease—autophagosomes is **accelerated**
  - Huntington's disease—mutant huntingtin **impairs** autophagy.
- **Infectious diseases:** Macrophage-specific deletion of **Atg5** increases susceptibility to tuberculosis.
- Polymorphisms in a gene involved in autophagy are associated with **inflammatory bowel disease**

High Yield Facts

- Nutrient starvation induces autophagy in eukaryotic cells through **inhibition of TOR** (target of rapamycin)
- Nucleation is started by **Beclin 1**
- **LC3**-useful marker for autophagy

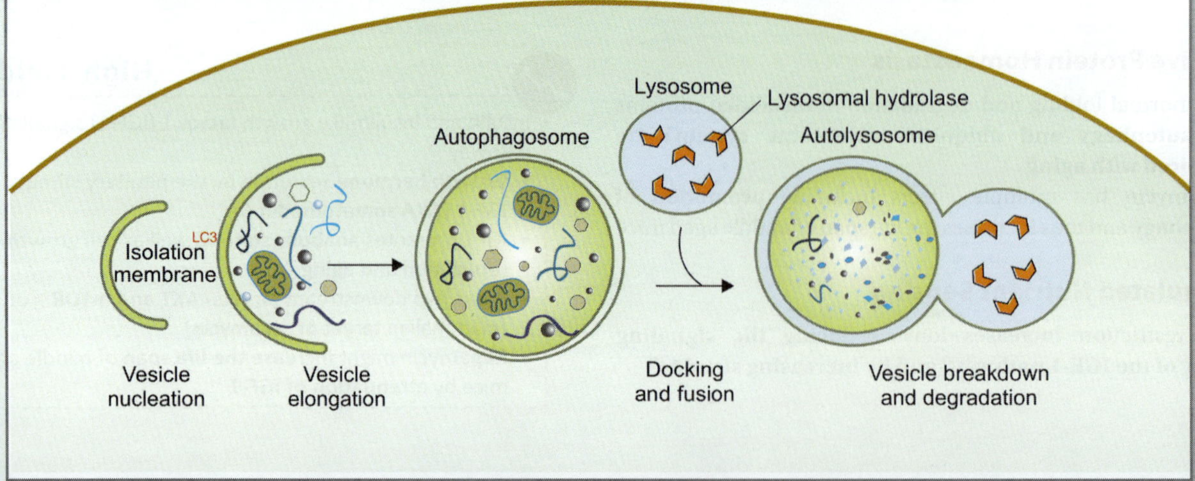

ENDOPLASMIC RETICULUM STRESS

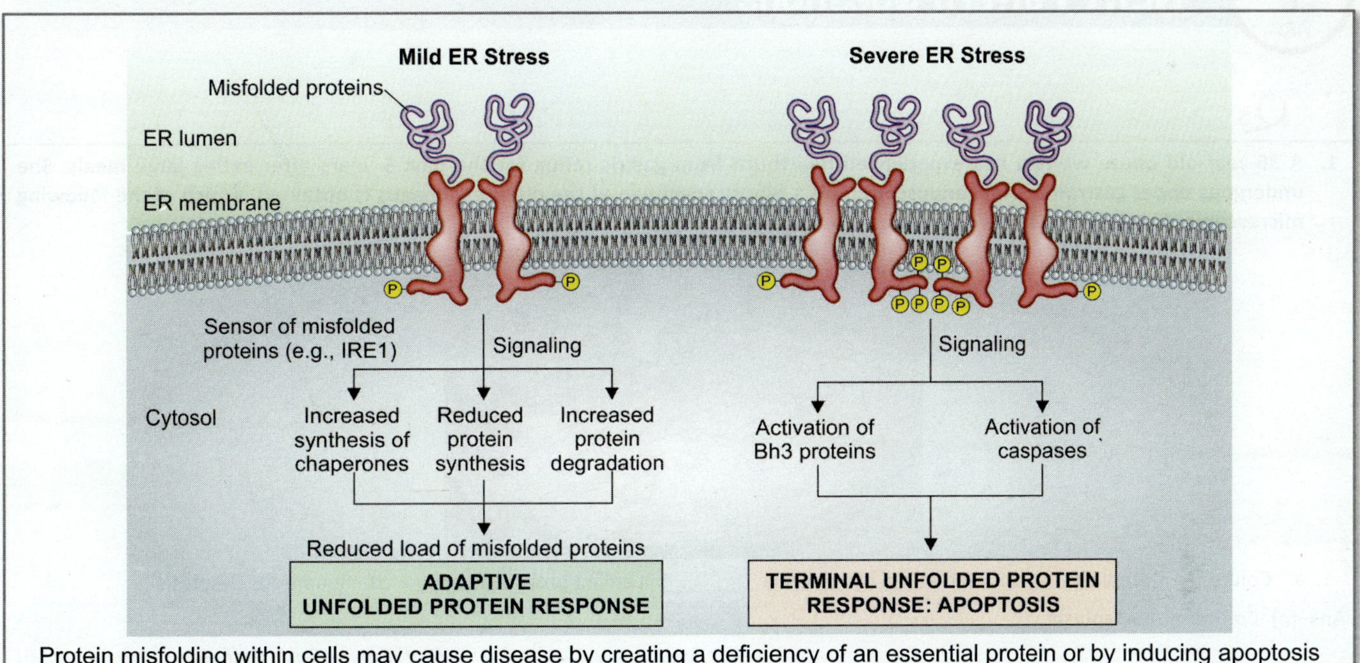

Diseases caused by Misfolded proteins

Disease	Affected Protein	Pathogenesis
Diseases caused by mutant protein that are degraded, leading to their deficiency		
Cystic fibrosis	CFTR	Loss of CFTR leads to defects in chloride transport and death of affected cells
Familial hypercholesterolemia	LDL receptor	Loss of LDL receptor leads to hypercholesterolemia
Tay-Sachs disease	Hexosaminidase β subunit	Lack of the lysosomal enzyme leads to accumulation of GM2 gangliosides in neurons
Diseases caused by Misfolded proteins that result in ER stress-induced cell loss		
Retinitis pigmentosa	Rhodopsin	Abnormal folding of rhodopsin causes photoreceptor loss and cell death, resulting in blindness
Creutzfeldt-Jakob disease	Prions	Abnormal folding of PrPsc causes neuronal cell death
Alzheimer's disease	Aβ	Abnormal folding of Aβ peptide causes aggregation within neurons & apoptosis
Diseases caused by Misfolded protein that result from both ER stress-induced cell loss and functional deficiency of the protein		
Alpha-1-anti-trypsin deficiency	α-1 anti-trypsin	Storage of nonfunctional protein in hepatocytes cause apoptosis; absence of enzymatic activity in lungs causes elastic tissue destruction giving rise to emphysema

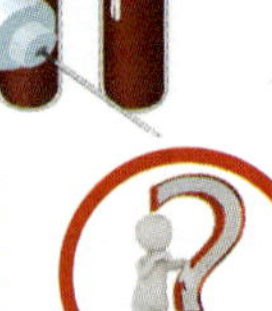

NEXT Pattern Questions

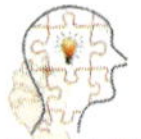

Q's

1. A 36-year-old obese woman has experienced heartburn from gastric reflux for the past 5 years after eating large meals. She undergoes upper gastrointestinal endoscopy, and a biopsy specimen of the distal esophagus is obtained. Which of the following microscopic changes, seen in the figure, has most likely occurred?

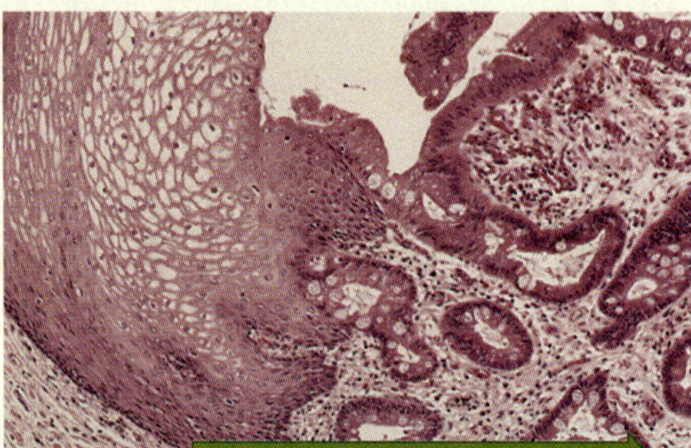

a. Columnar metaplasia   b. Goblet cell hyperplasia   c. Lamina propria atrophy   d. Squamous dysplasia

Ans. (a) Columnar metaplasia

(Ref: Robins Basic Pathology 10th ed/pg 50)

- Inflammation from reflux of gastric acid has resulted in replacement of normal esophageal squamous epithelium by intestinal-type columnar epithelium with goblet cells. Such conversion of one adult cell type to another cell type is called metaplasia, and it occurs when stimuli reprogram stem cells. Goblet cells are not normal constituents of the esophageal mucosa, and they are a minor part of this metaplastic process. The lamina propria has some inflammatory cells, but it does not atrophy. The squamous epithelium does not become dysplastic from acid reflux, but the columnar metaplasia may progress to dysplasia, not seen here, if the abnormal stimuli continue. These cells are not significantly increased in size (hypertrophic).

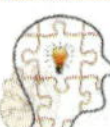

Q's

2. While doing a screening chest radiograph in an asymptomatic 37-year-old man a 3 cm nodule in the middle lobe of his right lung was found. The nodule on sectioning shows a sharply circumscribed mass with a soft, white center. The microscopic appearance is shown in the figure. The serum interferon gamma release assay is positive. Which of the following pathologic processes has most likely occurred in this nodule?

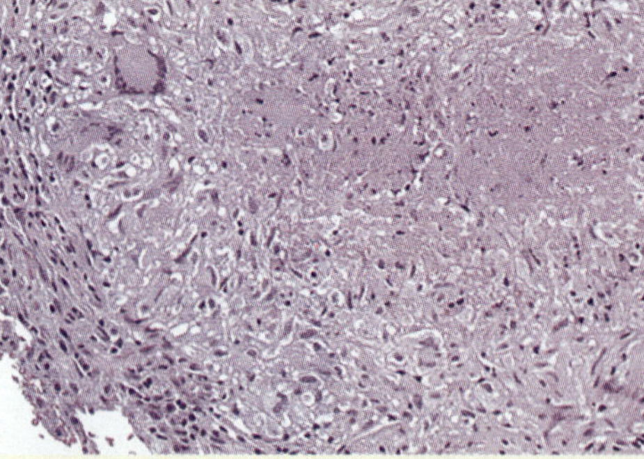

a. Apoptosis   b. Caseous necrosis   c. Coagulative necrosis   d. Fat necrosis

Ans. (b) Caseous necrosis

(Ref: Robins Basic Pathology 10th ed/pg 35)

- The grossly cheese like appearance gives this form of necrosis its name—caseous necrosis. The figure shows amorphous pink acellular material at the upper right surrounded by epithelioid macrophages, and a Langhans giant cell is visible at the upper left. In the lung, tuberculosis and fungal infections are most likely to produce this pattern of tissue injury. Apoptosis involves individual cells, without grossly apparent extensive or localized areas of tissue necrosis. Coagulative necrosis is more typical of ischemic tissue injury. Fat necrosis most often occurs in the breast and pancreas. Fatty change is most often a feature of hepatocyte injury, and the cell integrity is maintained. Gangrene characterizes extensive necrosis of multiple cell types in a body region or organ. Liquefactive necrosis is seen in neutrophilic abscesses or ischemic cerebral injury.

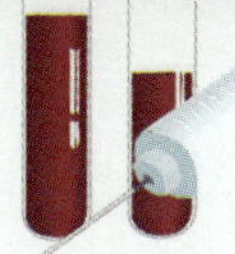

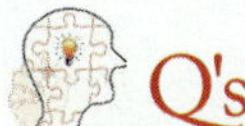 **Q's**

3. **An experiment introduces a knockout gene mutation into a cell line. The frequency of shrunken cells with chromatin clumping, karyorrhexis, and cytoplasmic blebbing is increased compared with a cell line without the mutation. Overall survival of the mutant cell line is reduced. Which of the following genes is most likely to be affected by this mutation?**

   a. BAX   b. BCL2   c. C-MYC   d. FAS

Ans. (b) BCL2

(Ref: Robins Basic Pathology 10th ed/pg 37)

- These histologic findings are typical of apoptosis. The BCL2 gene product inhibits cellular apoptosis by binding to Apaf-1. Hence, the knockout removes this inhibition The BAX gene product promotes apoptosis, and a knockout would protect against apoptosis. The C-MYC gene is involved with oncogenesis. The FAS gene encodes for a cellular receptor for Fas ligand that signals apoptosis. Activity of the p53 (TP53) gene normally stimulates apoptosis, but mutation favors cell survival.

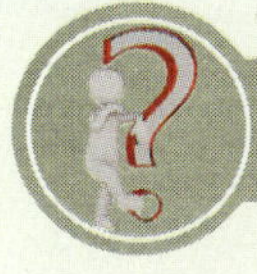

Image-Based Questions

1. **A 45-year-old male had history of hepatitis B infection. On liver biopsy, multiple councilman bodies were seen. Electrophoresis was done to pick up whether he was undergoing apoptosis or necrosis. Identify the pattern in lane 2 and diagnosis.**

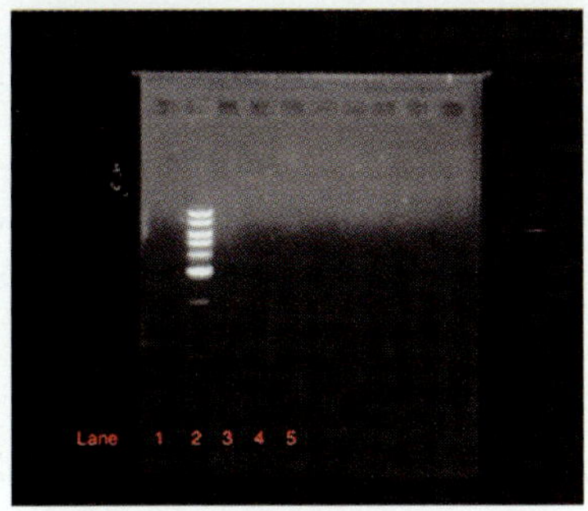

  a. Step ladder pattern, apoptosis
  b. Smeared pattern, necrosis
  c. Step ladder pattern, necrosis
  d. Smeared pattern, apoptosis

3. **A 50-year-old female comes with history of discharge per vaginum. On examination, her squamocolumnar junction of cervix appears erythematous. She underwent cervical biopsy which showed following findings. Describe the change marked by arrow.**

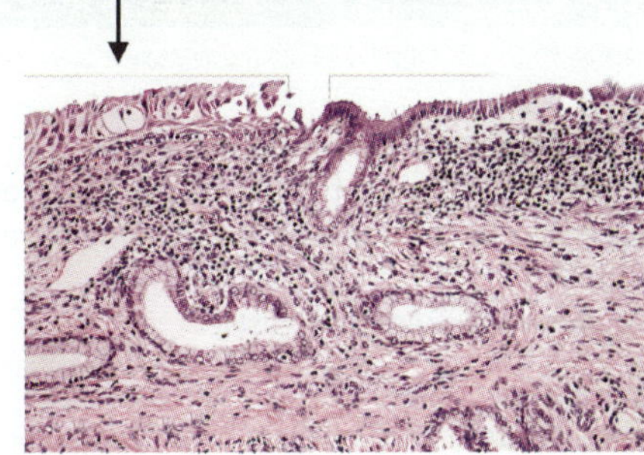

  a. Squamous metaplasia
  b. Columnar metaplasia
  c. Transitional metaplasia
  d. None

2. **Earliest morphological change seen in reversible cellular injury? Inset shows normal hepatocytes as control.**

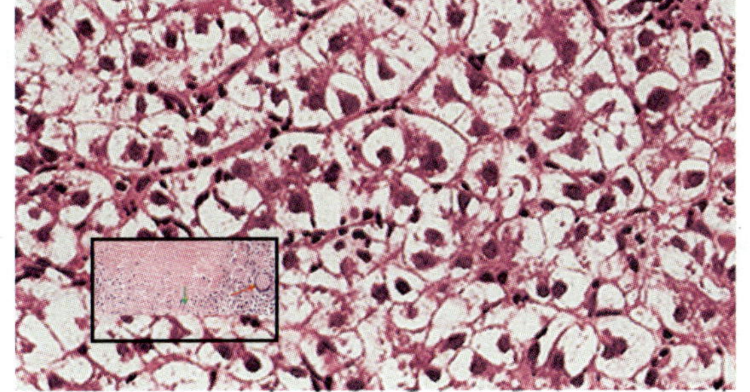

  a. Hydropic change   b. Fatty change
  c. Necrosis   d. None

4. **A 60-year-old asymptomatic female shows following change in tunica media of blood vessels. Diagnosis is:**

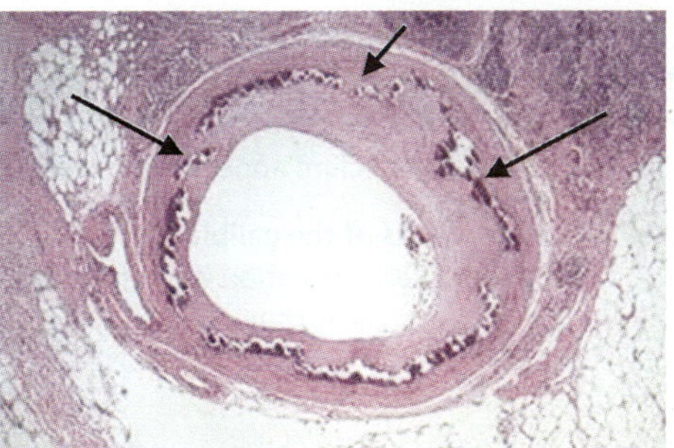

  a. Medial calcification   b. Medial fibrosis
  c. Amyloidosis   d. None

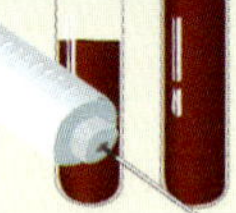

5. **A 50-year-old female underwent cholecystectomy on examination, the lamina propria of gall bladder was seen infiltrated by foam cells. Diagnosis is:**

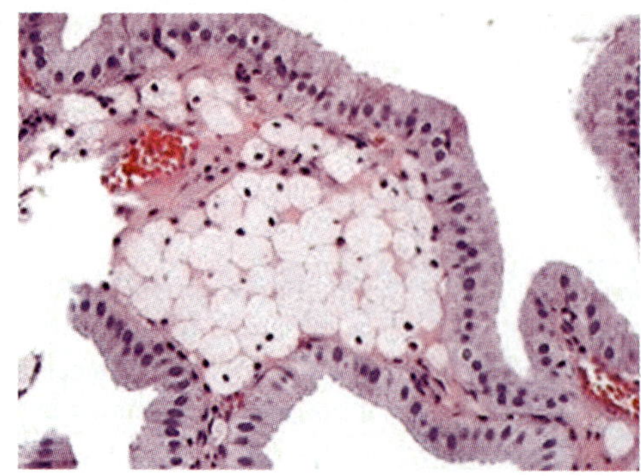

a. Cholestrolosis

b. Atherosclerosis

c. Steatosis

d. None

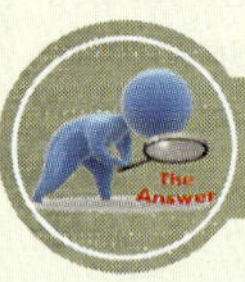

Answers of Image-Based Questions

1. **Ans. (a) Step ladder pattern, apoptosis**
   - This is step ladder pattern which is typically seen in apoptosis, its also called DNA laddering characterized by the activation of endogenous endonucleases with subsequent cleavage of chromatin DNA into internucleosomal fragments of roughly 180-200 base pairs (bp).
   - Smear pattern is seen in necrosis.

2. **Ans. (a) Hydropic change**
   - Cellular swelling is the first manifestation of almost all forms of injury to cells. Cellular swelling appears whenever cells are incapable of maintaining ionic and fluid homeostasis and is the result of failure of energy-dependent ion pumps in the plasma membrane. It is reversible.
   - On microscopic examination, small clear vacuoles may be seen within the cytoplasm; these represent distended and pinched-off segments of the ER. This pattern of nonlethal injury is sometimes called hydropic change or vacuolar degeneration.
   - This is a case of hydropic change in hepatocytes (control normal hepatocytes are seen in inset).

3. **Ans. (a) Squamous metaplasia**
   - Here we are seeing endocervix lined by columnar epithelium. And underlying stroma shows endocervical glands. Here columnar epithelium is being changed to squamous epithelium suggestive of squamous metaplasia. Inciting cause for this metaplasia is chronic cervicitis.

4. **Ans. (a) Medial calcification**
   - Medial artery calcification (MAC) is also known as Mönckeberg's arteriosclerosis, is a nonobstructive condition leading to reduced arterial compliance that is commonly considered as a nonsignificant finding.
   - With the H&E stain, calcium appear deep blue-purple.

5. **Ans. (a) Cholesterolosis of the gallbladder**
   - Here we are seeing accumulation of foam cells in lamina propria of gallbladder suggestive of cholestrolosis

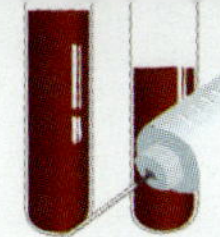

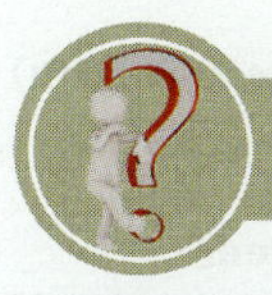

Multiple Choice Questions

ADAPTATIONS

1. True about Metaplasia is: *(JIPMER 2016)*
a. Involves only epithelial cells
b. Is irreversible
c. Occurs at stem cells level
d. Columnar is the most common type

2. An example of metaplasia is? *(Recent Question 2015)*
a. CIN
b. Barrets
c. Adenoma
d. Bronchial carcinoid

3. All the following are true regarding hypertrophy except: *(Recent Question 2015)*
a. Increase in cell size without increase in number
b. DNA content same as in normal cells
c. Increase in cell size is due to synthesize of more cellular proteins
d. Associated with a switch of contractile proteins from adult to fetal or neonatal forms

4. Find the false statement about metaplasia:
a. Reversible *(Recent Question 2015)*
b. No loss of polarity
c. Reprogramming of stem cells
d. Pleomorphism present

5. Increase in the number of goblet cells in the non-respiratory terminal bronchiole is an example of: *(Recent Question 2015)*
a. Anaplasia
b. Dysplasia
c. Metaplasia
d. Hyperplasia

6. In respiratory tract metaplasia occurs from: *(Recent Question 2015)*
a. Squamous to columnar
b. Columanar to cuboidal
c. Columnar to squamous
d. Cuboidal to squamous

7. In Vitamin-A deficiency, cancerous lesions occur due to:
a. Metaplasia
b. Dysplasia *(MH PG 2014)*
c. Aplasia
d. Hyperplasia

8. Definition of hyperplasia is: *(Recent Question 2015)*
a. Increase in number of cells
b. Increase in size of cells
c. Change in type of cell
d. Increase in nuclear:cytoplasmic ratio

9. All are cellular adaptations except: *(Recent Question 2014)*
a. Hypertrophy
b. Hyperplasia
c. Necrosis
d. Metaplasia

10. Decrease in cell size refers to: *(DNB 2012)*
a. Atrophy
b. Metaplasia
c. Hyperplasia
d. Hypertrophy

11. Metaplasia arises from reprograming of *(JIPMER 2012)*
a. Stem cells
b. Stellate cells
c. Squamous cells
d. Columnar cells

CELL INJURY

12. All of the followings are signs of reversible cell injury; except: *(AIIMS May 19)*
a. Loss of microvilli
b. Cell Swelling
c. Bleb formation
d. Dense Mitochondrial deposit

13. Features of irreversible cell injury is/are? *(PGI Nov 2017)*
a. Lysosomal rupture
b. Pyknosis
c. Bleb formation on membrane
d. Severe mitochondrial dysfunction

14. A Patient have acquired syndrome associated with defective breakdown and disposal of intracellular fatty acids. Which intracellular organelle is concerned with this mechanism? *(Recent Questions 2016-17, JIPMER 2014)*
a. Mitochondria
b. Peroxisomes
c. Lysosomes
d. Smooth endoplasmic reticulum

15. In myocardium reperfusion injury is due to? *(Recent Question 2016)*
a. Ca
b. Mg
c. K
d. Mn

16. Which of the following is not a sign of reversible cell injury? *(Recent Question 2015)*
a. ATP depletion
b. Cell shrinkage
c. Fatty acid deposition
d. Reduction of phosphorylation

17. Earliest feature of reversible cell injury is:
a. Cellular swelling *(Recent Question 2015)*
b. Decreased ATP
c. Clumping of chromatin
d. Decreased protein synthesis

18. First manifestation in cell injury *(Recent Question 2015)*
a. Pyknosis
b. Cell swelling
c. Nuclear fragmentation
d. Nuclear lysis

19. The following is not a reversible cell injury *(Recent Question 2015)*
a. Loss of microvilli in plasma membrane
b. Lipid vacuoles in cytoplasm
c. Mitochondrial swelling and small amorphous densities
d. Moth eaten appearance of cytoplasm

20. All are features of reversible injury of cell, except *(Recent Question 2014-15)*
a. Blebs
b. Amorphous densities in mitochondrial matrix
c. Loss of microvlli
d. Cellular swelling

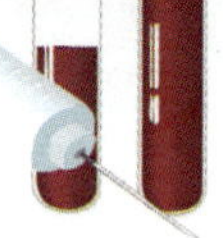

21. **Cells seen in chronic infection of pseudomonas**
    (Recent Question 2014)
    a. Neutrophils
    b. Eosinophils
    c. Lymphocytes
    d. Macrophage

22. **Cells most sensitive to hypoxia are:** *(AIIMS May 2014)*
    a. Myocardial cells
    b. Neurons
    c. Hepatocytes
    d. Renal tubular epithelial cells

23. **Irreversible cell injury:** *(Recent Question 2013)*
    a. Mitochondrial densities
    b. Cellular swelling
    c. Blebs
    d. None

24. **In cell death, myelin figures are derived from:**
    (Recent Question 2013)
    a. Nucleus
    b. Cell membrane
    c. Cytoplasm
    d. Mitochondria

25. **Which finding on electron microscopy indicates irreversible cell injury:** *(AIIMS May 12, Nov 02)*
    a. Dilatation of endoplasmic reticulum.
    b. Dissociation of ribosomes from rough endoplasmic reticulum
    c. Flocculent amorphous densities in the mitochondria
    d. Myelin figures

CELL DEATH

26. **Which of the following is activated by intrinsic or extrinsic pathways?** *(AIIMS Nov 2019)*
    a. Necroptosis
    b. Apoptosis
    c. Necrosis
    d. Ferroptosis

27. **Acute inflammatory response is seen in:**
    (AIIMS May 19)
    a. Pyroptosis
    b. Necroptosis
    c. Necrosis
    d. Autophagy

28. **Which of the following is involved in apoptosis pathway?**
    (JIPMER Dec 19)
    a. Myc
    b. p53 and caspases
    c. APC
    d. VHL

29. **Which of the following statements is false about apoptosis?** *(AIIMS Nov 18)*
    a. No inflammation
    b. Plasma membrane intact
    c. Organelle swelling
    d. Affected by dedicated genes

30. **Which of the following can recognize dead material?**
    (AIIMS Nov 18)
    a. NET
    b. Inflammosome
    c. Necrosis
    d. Toll like receptor

31. **Necrotic cells are recognized by NOD like receptors which then activates inflammosomes. Which of these are anti apoptotic gene?** *(PGI Nov 2018)*
    a. BCL
    b. BCL-2
    c. BAD
    d. BAX
    e. MCL

32. **IL-1 is activated by?** *(Recent Question 2019)*
    a. Caspase 1
    b. Caspase 3
    c. Caspase 5
    d. Caspase 8

33. **Which of the following is an antiapoptotic gene?**
    (Recent Question 2019)
    a. Bcl2
    b. Bcl – XL
    c. BAX
    d. Both a & b

34. **Which of the following type of necrosis is seen in immune complex deposition in blood vessel?**
    (Recent Question 2019)
    a. Coagulative necrosis
    b. Liquefactive necrosis
    c. Fibrinoid necrosis
    d. Caseous necrosis

35. **For programmed cell death type 2 and autophagy, which is apoptotic genes?** *(JIPMER 2017)*
    a. BCL
    b. BAX
    c. BCL-XL
    d. BIM

36. **True about p53 gene?** *(PGI Nov 2016)*
    a. Tumor suppression
    b. Proapoptotic
    c. Antiapoptotic
    d. Cell repair

37. **True about caspases are?** *(PGI Nov 2016)*
    a. They are enzymes starting apoptosis
    b. They inhibit apoptosis
    c. They are receptors of apoptosis
    d. They are proteases which cause cellular death in apoptosis found in irreversible cell damage

38. **About the given image true is?** *(AIIMS May 16)*

    a. C is showing necrosis
    b. C is showing apoptosis
    c. C is showing normal cells
    d. A is showing apoptosis

39. **True about necroptosis is all except?**
    (Recent Question 2016-17)
    a. Caspase 1 & 11 is involved
    b. Caspase independent
    c. Failure of activation of caspase 8
    d. Lipid peroxidation is seen

40. **Which of the following is an antiapoptotic gene**
    (Recent Question 2016-17)
    a. BAX
    b. BAD
    c. BCL-XL
    d. BIM

41. **SMAC/DIAMBLO is a** *(Recent Question 2016-17)*
    a. Anti apoptotic protein
    b. Induces necrosis
    c. Acts both as anti and pro apoptotic protein
    d. Pro-apoptotic protein

42. **Antiapoptotic gene?** *(Recent Question 2016-17)*
    a. FLIP
    b. P53
    c. BAX
    d. BIM

43. **Necrosis seen in chronic pancreatitis is?**
    (Recent Question 2016)
    a. Fatty
    b. Coagulative
    c. Liquifactive
    d. Casseous

44. **False about apoptosis?** *(Recent Question 2015)*
    a. Inflammation present
    b. Program cell death
    c. Normal physiology
    d. Genetically determined by a cell

45. **Earliest change in cell death is?** *(Recent Question 2015)*
    a. Karyolysis
    b. Loss of plasma membrane
    c. Cell swelling
    d. Karyorrhexis

46. **Which of the following induces apoptosis**
    (Recent Question 2015)
    a. Oleic acid
    b. Myristic acid
    c. Glucocorticoid
    d. Isoprenoid

47. **Which of the following is an execution caspase**
    (Recent Question 2015)
    a. Caspase 3
    b. Caspase 5
    c. Caspase 8
    d. Caspase 9

48. **Diabetic foot is an example of** *(Recent Question 2015)*
    a. Dry gangrene
    b. Wet gangrene
    c. Gas gangrene
    d. Necrotizing inflammation

49. **Annexin V is a marker of** *(Recent Question 2015)*
    a. Necrosis
    b. Gangrene
    c. Aging
    d. Apoptosis

50. **Cell organelle which plays a pivotal role in apoptosis**
    (Recent Question 2015)
    a. Nucleus
    b. Mitochondria
    c. Golgi apparatus
    d. Plasma membrane

51. **Fibrinoid necrosis is seen in all except**
    a. Malignant hypertension *(Recent Question 2015)*
    b. Polyarteritis nodosa
    c. Diabetic glomerulosclerosis
    d. Rheumatic heart disease

52. **Ladder pattern of DNA electrophoresis is seen in**
    (Recent Question 2015)
    a. Necrosis
    b. Apoptosis
    c. Cytolysis
    d. Karyorrhexis

53. **The following is not a sensor of apoptosis**
    (Recent Question 2015)
    a. Puma
    b. Noxa
    c. Bax
    d. BAD

54. **Intrinsic pathway of apoptosis is initiated by all the following except** *(Recent Question 2015)*
    a. Growth factor withdrawal
    b. DNA damage
    c. Protein misfolding
    d. Type 1 TNF receptor

55. **Defective apoptosis and increased cell survival is seen in** *(Recent Question 2015)*
    a. Autoimmune disease
    b. Neurodegenerative disease
    c. Viral infections
    d. Ischemic injury

56. **Receptor associated kinases 1 (RIP1) and 3 (RIP3) are involved in** *(Recent Question 2015)*
    a. Necrosis
    b. Apoptosis
    c. Necroptosis
    d. Pyroptosis

57. **Inflammasome is formed in** *(Recent Question 2015)*
    a. Necrosis
    b. Apoptosis
    c. Necroptosis
    d. Pyroptosis

58. **Find the true statement regarding fibrinoid necrosis**
    (Recent Question 2015)
    a. Denaturation of structural proteins
    b. Granuloma formation
    c. Abscess formation
    d. Fibrin deposition

59. **All are true regarding apoptosis except**
    a. Active process *(Recent Question 2015)*
    b. Cell size decreases
    c. Inflammation absent
    d. Smear pattern in electrophoresis

60. **The following is a pro-apoptic factor**
    (WB PGMEE 2016, Recent Question 2015)
    a. Bax
    b. Bcl-2
    c. Bcl-xL
    d. Mci-1

61. **Find the wrong match** *(Recent Question 2015)*
    a. Coagulative necrosis–Tuberculosis
    b. Fat necrosis –Acute pancreatitis
    c. Liquefactive necrosis –Brain
    d. Fibrinoid necrosis –Mlignant hypertension

62. **Fibrinoid necrosis is seen in all the following except**
    a. Malignant hypertension *(Recent Question 2015)*
    b. Aschoff's nodule
    c. Polyarteritis nodosa
    d. Diabetic glomerulosclerosis

63. **Apoptosis is induced by** *(JIPMER 2015)*
    a. Caspases
    b. DNA synthesis
    c. Activation of caspases
    d. Kinase pathway

64. **Hypoxic death of brain tissue results in:**
    (APPGMEE 2015)
    a. Gangrenous necrosis
    b. Liquefactive necrosis
    c. Coagulative necrosis
    d. Fibnrinoid necrosis

65. **True about bcl-2:** *(PGI May 2015)*
    a. ↑ Apoptosis
    b. ↓ Apoptosis
    c. ↑ Resistance of tumour to treatment
    d. Only associated with follicular lymphoma
    e. Cause meningioma

66. **True about Apoptosis are all except**
    a. Inflammation is present *(Recent Question 2014-15)*
    b. Chromosomal breakage
    c. Clumping of chromatin
    d. Cell shrinkage

67. **Not true about apoptosis** *(Recent Question 2014-15)*
    a. Increase in lysosomal enzyme
    b. Increase in caspases
    c. Phosphatidyl serine has important role
    d. Internucleosomal cleavage of nucleus

68. **Apoptotic bodies are** *(Recent Question 2014-15)*
    a. Clumped chromatin bodies
    b. Pyknotic nucleus without organelles
    c. Cell membrane bound with organelles
    d. No nucleus with organelles

69. **"Caspase-independent" programmed cell death**
    (Recent Question 2015)
    a. Necrosis
    b. Necroptosis
    c. Apoptosis
    d. None

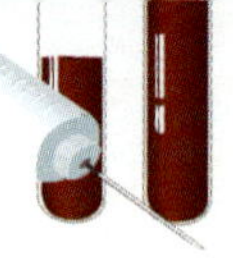

70. **Fibrinoid necrosis is seen in** *(Recent Question 2015)*
    a. Malignant HTN
    b. Benign hypertension
    c. Diabetes
    d. Acute on chronic gangrene

71. **Immune complexes mediated necrosis is of which type?** *(Recent Question 2013)*
    a. Coagulative necrosis
    b. Liquefactive necrosis
    c. Caseous necrosis
    d. Fibrinoid necrosis

72. **Which one of the following is an antiapoptotic protein/ gene?** *(WB PGMEE 2016, Recent Question 2013)*
    a. BAK
    b. BCL-2
    c. BAX
    d. BIM

73. **Coagulative necrosis is due to:** *(Recent Question 2013)*
    a. Denaturation of protein
    b. Enzymatic digestion
    c. Infection
    d. None

74. **Fat necrosis is common in:** *(Recent Question 2013)*
    a. Omentum
    b. Breast
    c. Retroperitoneal fat
    d. All of the above

75. **In apoptosis, cytochrome C acts through:** *(Recent Question 2013)*
    a. Apaf 1
    b. Bcl-2
    c. FADD
    d. TNF

76. **Which of the following is not seen in apoptosis?**
    a. Chromatin condensation *(AIIMS May 2013)*
    b. DNA fragmentation
    c. Inflammation
    d. Cell membrane shrinkage

77. **CD 95 is a marker of:** *(AIIMS May 2013)*
    a. Intrinsic pathway of apoptosis
    b. Extrinsic pathway of apoptosis
    c. Monocyte
    d. Leucocyte

78. **Apoptosis- all are true except?** *(JIPMER 2013)*
    a. Normal physiological process of programmed cell death
    b. Products removed by phagocytosis
    c. Plasma membrane zeiosis
    d. Causes inflammation that damage surrounding cells

79. **Apoptosis does not occur by normal capsase pathway in?** *(DNB Aug. 12 Pattern)*
    a. Liver
    b. Muscle
    c. Neurons
    d. Skin

80. **Type of necrosis in Myocarial Infacrction?** *(JIPMER 2012, UP10)*
    a. Caseous
    b. Coagulative
    c. Liquifactive
    d. Fibrinoid

81. **Which of the following organelles plays a pivotal role in apoptosis?** *(AIIMS May 10, AI 11, 09)*
    a. Mitochondria
    b. Endoplasmic reticulum
    c. Nucleus
    d. Golgi apparatus

82. **Which of the following has a direct role in apoptosis?** *(DNB Dec 11)*
    a. Nitric oxide
    b. Adenylcyclase
    c. cAMP
    d. Cytochrome C

83. **Apoptosis is inhibited by:** *(MH 11)*
    a. p53
    b. nMYC
    c. RAS
    d. Bcl-2

84. **Characteristic feature of apoptosis:** *(AI 10)*
    a. Cell membrane intact
    b. Cytoplasmic eosinophilia
    c. Nuclear moulding
    d. Cell swelling

85. **The characteristic feature of apoptosis on light microscopy is:** *(AI 10)*
    a. Cellular swelling
    b. Nuclear compaction
    c. Intact cell membrane
    d. Cytoplasmic eosinophlia

86. **All of the following are features of apoptosis, except:** *(AI 10)*
    a. Cellular swelling
    b. Nuclear compaction
    c. Intact cell membrane
    d. Cytoplasmic eosinophilia

87. **Coagulative necrosis is seen in:** *(AIIMS May 10)*
    a. T.B.
    b. Sarcoidosis
    c. Cryptococcal infection
    d. Wet Gangrene

88. **Caspases are associated with:** *(AIIMS May 10)*
    a. Organogenesis
    b. Hydropic degeneration
    c. Collagen hyalinization
    d. Morphology

89. **True about apoptosis:** *(PGI May 2010)*
    a. Increase in lysosomal enzyme
    b. Increase in caspases
    c. Phosphatidyl serine has important role
    d. Internucleosomal cleavage of nucleus

90. **In apoptosis, permeabilization of membrane occur in:** *(PGI Nov 2010)*
    a. Nuclear membrane
    b. Cytoplasmic membrane
    c. Lysosome
    d. Ribosome
    e. Mitochondrial membrane

CELLULAR ACCUMULATIONS

91. **Dystrophic calcification is seen in:** *(AIIMS May 19)*
    a. Paget's disease of bone
    b. Lung involvement in sarcoidosis
    c. Immobilized healing fracture
    d. Myositis ossificans

92. **Dystrophic calcification is/are found in?**
    a. Monckeberg's medial sclerosis *(PGI Nov 2017)*
    b. Papillary carcinoma thyroid
    c. Hyperparathyroidism
    d. Meningioma
    e. Vitamin D intoxication

93. **Given below is the histopathology of liver biopsy of hemochromatosis. Which of the following stain is used?** *(AIIMS Nov 16)*

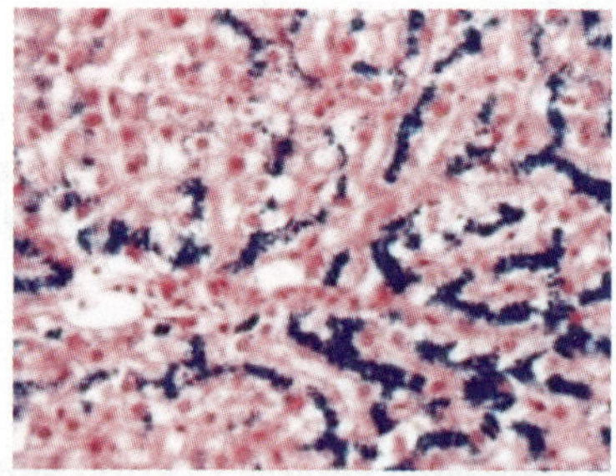

    a. Von kossa
    b. Alcian blue
    c. Prussian blue
    d. Crystal violet

94. **Which of the following stain and the material stained by it is correct?** *(PGI Nov 2016)*
    a. Perl stain-Iron
    b. Collagen- Von kossa
    c. Elastin-VG
    d. Copper-rhodamine

95. Tiggered myocardium is deposition of ?
(Recent Question 2016-17)
a. Fat
b. Hyaline
c. Glycogen
d. Protein

96. Psammoma bodies are absent in?
(MAHA 2016, Recent Question 2015)
a. Meninigioma
b. Papillary ca of ovary
c. Prolactinoma
d. Seminoma

97. Principle of Prussian blue stain:
(Recent Question 2015)
a. Ferrous to ferricyanide
b. Ferrocyanide to ferroferric cyanide
c. Ferroferriccyanide to ferrocyanide
d. Ferrocyanide to ferricferrocyanide

98. Metastatic calcification seen in all except:
(Recent Question 2015)
a. Multiple myeloma
b. Breast cancer
c. Atherosclerosis
d. Renal failure

99. Intracellular calcification begins in
(Recent Question 2015)
a. Nucleus
b. Cytoplasm
c. Golgi complex
d. Mitochondria

100. Most commonly involved organ in metastatic calcification
(Recent Question 2015)
a. Kidney
b. Heart
c. Lungs
d. Aorta

101. The following is not a disease caused by misfolding of proteins
(Recent Question 2015)
a. Cystic fibrosis
b. Parkinsons disease
c. Alzheimer's disease
d. Creutzfeldt-Jacob disease

102. Intracellular calcification begins in
(Recent Question 2015)
a. Nucleus
b. Cytoplasm
c. Golgi complex
d. Mitochondria

103. A patient died of alzheimer's disease. At autopsy, heart contains yellow brown finely granular pigment which are/due to:
(Recent Question 2015)
a. Hemosiderin-iron overload
b. Lipochrome-wear and tear
c. Glcoge-gylgcogen storage disorder
d. Fat-athlerosclerosis

104. Stain for fat all except
(Recent Question 2014-15)
a. Oil red O
b. Sudan black
c. Sudan III
d. Congo red

105. Psammoma bodies features are all except:
a. Seen in meningioma
(Recent Question 2015)
b. Concentric whorled appearance
c. Seen in papillary thyroid carcinoma
d. Seen in teratoma

106. Dystrophic calcification is seen in:
(Recent Question 2014)
a. Dying tissue
b. Hypercalcemia
c. Hyperprathyroidism
d. Calcific metabolic disease

107. Steatosis means:
(Recent Question 2014)
a. Fatty change
b. Accumulation of triglyceride
c. Accumulation of glycogen
d. Accumulation of pigment

108. Dystrophic calcification is seen in all except:
(Recent Question 2014)
a. Lymph node
b. Lungs
c. Kidneys
d. Rheumatic valves

109. Oncocytes are found in all except: *(DNB June 11)*
a. Thyroid
b. Pancreas
c. Pituitary
d. Pineal

110. Which of the following is a pathological calcification?
a. Suprasellar calcification
(DNB June 10)
b. Basal ganglia calcification
c. Pineal body calcification
d. Choroid calcification

CELL AGING

111. Highest telomerase activity is seen in
(Recent Question 2015)
a. Stem cells
b. Somatic cells
c. Germ cells
d. Benign tumors

112. True regarding sirtuin functions
a. Decrease metabolic activity *(Recent Question 2015)*
b. Reduce apoptosis
c. Stimulate protein folding
d. Inhibit harmful effects of oxygen free radicals

113. Werner disease is associated with?
(Recent Question Aug 13)
a. Intestinal polyps
b. Multiple cancer
c. Lax joints
d. Premature ageing

114. Sirtuin is associated with? *(DNB Nov. 12 Pattern)*
a. Cancer
b. Diabetes
c. Ageing
d. All of the above

115. Which of the following is associated with aging
a. Reduced cross linkages in collagen *(AIIMS May 10)*
b. Increased free radical injury
c. Decreased Somatic mutations in DNA
d. Increased superoxide dismutase levels

FREE RADICALS

116. Organelle where H_2O_2 is produced and destroyed is
(Recent Question 2016-17)
a. Peroxisome
b. Lysosome
c. Golgi body
d. Ribosome

117. The enzyme that protects brain from free radical injury:
(Recent Question 2015)
a. Superoxide dismutase
b. Catalase
c. Glutathione peroxidase
d. Monoamine oxidase

118. Which of the following is true about glutathione & glutathione peroxidase: *(PGI May 2015)*
a. Act as scavenger of free radicle
b. Glutathione has anti-oxidant property
c. Reduced glutathione can chemically detoxify H_2O_2
d. Oxidized glutathione can chemically detoxify H_2O_2

119. Which of these is not responsible for removal of free radicals? *(Recent Question 2015)*

a. Catalase
b. Superoxide Dismutase
c. NADPH oxidase
d. Glutathione peroxidase

120. Pathologic Effects of Free Radicals are all except: *(Recent Question 2015)*

a. Lipid peroxidation in membranes.
b. Oxidative modification of proteins
c. Single- and double-strand breaks in DNA
d. Synthesis of new protiens

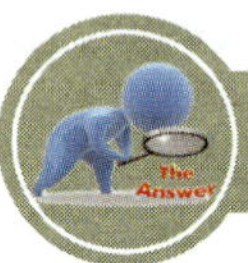

Answers with Explanations

1. Ans. (c) Occurs at stem cells level

Option a & b are-false.
- Cell adaptations are reversible & b both epithelial & mesenchymal

Option c is-true.
- Metaplasia is change in phenotype of cells due to stem cell reprogramming

Option d is-false.
- Most common type of metaplasia is squamous metaplasia

2. Ans. (b) Barrets *(Ref: Robbins 9th/pg 37-38; 8th/pg 10)*

3. Ans. (b) DNA content same as in normal cells

(Ref: Robbins 9th/pg 34; 8th/pg 6, Rev Esp Cardiol. 2006; 59:473-86. - Vol. 59)

Hypertrophy: Characterized by an increment in cardiomyocyte size, with increased protein synthesis and changes in the organization of the sarcomeric structure. DNA content also increases so b is false

4. Ans. (d) Pleomorphism present

(Ref: Robbins 9th/pg 37-38)

Option a-true. All the adaptations are reversible.
Option b-true. loss of polarity is a f/o dysplaia
*Option c-true-***Mechanism of metaplasia: Reprogramming of stem cells**[Q] in normal tissues or of **undifferentiated mesenchymal cells present in connective tissue**.

5. Ans. (c) Metaplasia

(Ref: Robbins 9th/pg 37-38; 8th/pg 10)

Increase in the number of goblet cells in the non-respiratory terminal bronchiole is an example of intestinal metaplasia.

6. Ans. (c) Columnar to squamous *(Ref: R 9th/pg 37-38)*

In smokers, pseudostratified ciliated columnar epithelium of respiratory tract changes to squamous epithelium

7. Ans. (a) Metaplasia

(Ref: Harshmohan Pathology For Dental 4th ed, pg 81)
In Vitamin-A deficiency, squamous metaplasia of conjunctiva leading to xerophthalmia.

8. Ans. (a) Increase in number of cells

(Ref: R 9th/pg 35-36)

9. Ans. (c) Necrosis *(Ref: Robbins 9th/pg 34; 8th/pg 6)*

Necrosis is cell death all others are cell adaptations

10. Ans. (a) Atrophy *(Ref: Robbins 9th/pg 36-37)*

Atrophy: decrease in cell size and number.[Q]

11. Ans. (a) Stem cells *(Ref: 9th/pg 36; 8th/pg 8)*

Mechanism of metaplasia: Reprogramming of stem cells[Q] in normal tissues or of **undifferentiated mesenchymal cells present in connective tissue.**[Q]

12. Ans. (d) Dense Mitochondrial deposit

(Ref: Robbins 9th/pg 42)

13. Ans. (a, b, d); a. Lysosomal rupture; b. Pyknosis; d. Severe mitochondrial dysfunction

Bleb formation on membrane which are cytoplasmic blebs are a feature of reversible injury.

14. Ans. (c) Lysosomes

15. Ans. (a) Ca

(Ref: Gross GJ, Kersten JR, Warltier DC. Mechanisms of postischemic contractile dysfunction. Ann Thorac Surg. 1999; 68: 1898–1904.)

Mediators of reperfusion injury are: *Oxygen Free Radicals, Endothelial Dysfunction and Microvascular Injury, Alterations in Calcium Handling*

16. Ans. (b) Cell shrinkage *(Ref: Robbins 9th/38;8th/pg 17)*

Features of **reversible cell injury** seen in **light microscopy** are **cellular swelling and fatty change.**
Cell shrinkage is a feature of apoptosis (cell death)

17. Ans. (b) Decreased ATP *(Ref: Robbins 9th/38;8th/pg 17)*

Earlier molecular changes in cellular injury are **decreased O_2 to issue leading to decreased oxidative phosphorylation leading to decreased ATP**

18. **Ans. (b) Cell swelling**

(Ref: Robbins 9th/pg 46; 8th/pg 12)

Cloudy swelling^Q **- earliest morphological change** in **reversible cell injury**^{Q} due to **accumulation of water intracellularly**

19. **Ans. (d) Moth eaten appearance of cytoplasm**

(Ref: Robbins 9th/pg 40; 8th/pg 12)

Necrotic cells have a more glassy, homogeneous appearance, mostly because of the loss of glycogen particles.
When enzymes have digested cytoplasmic organelles, the cytoplasm becomes vacuolated and appears "moth-eaten."

20. **Ans. (b) Amorphous densities in mitochondrial matrix**

(Ref: Robbins 9th/pg 40; 8th/pg 12)

Amorphous densities in mitochondria are features of irreversible cell injury-option b is false

21. **Ans. (a) Neutrophils**

(Ref: http://www.hopkinsmedicine.org/mcp/ Education/300.713% 20Lectures/Infectious.pdf)

- Acute response to infection is characterized by neutrophils
- Chronic response to infection is characterized by infiltrate by macrophages and monocytes
- Pseudomonas is an exception in that its chronic response is also characterized by neutrophila

22. **Ans. (b) Neurons** *(Ref: Robbins 9th/pg 130; 8th/pg 129)*

- **Tissue vulnerability to hypoxia-**
- **Neurons** undergo irreversible damage **3 to 4 minutes**^{Q} of ischemia
- **Myocardial cells** die after only **20 to 30 minutes**^{Q} of ischemia
- **Fibroblasts** within myocardium remain viable even after many hours of ischemia

23. **Ans. (a) Mitochondrial densities**

(Ref: R 9th/pg 42; 8th/pg 19)

Features of irreversible injury include:

Severe swelling of mitochondria^Q: **Large, flocculant, amorphous densities**^{Q} develop in mitochondrial matrix **(Increased Ca²⁺ influx)**^{Q}

24. **Ans. (b) Cell membrane** *(Ref: R 9th/pg 42; 8th/pg 9,19)*

Myelin Figures^Q

- Rolled-up or scroll-like arrangement of a **lipid bilayer within a cell**^{Q}
- Derived from **damaged cell membranes**^{Q}

25. **Ans. (c) Flocculent amorphous densities in the mitochondria**

(Ref: Robbins 9th/pg 42; 8th/pg 19; Refer to Ans 29)

Please note: myelin figures first appear in reversible cellular injury and become more pronounced in irreversible cell

injury. Hence if this q was asked in PGI, answer should be both c and d. but if we have to mark one..mark c.

26. **Ans. (b) Apoptosis**

(Ref: Robbins 9th ed/pg 53)

27. **Ans. (c) Necrosis**

(Ref: Robbins 9th ed/pg 50)

28. **Ans. (b) p53 and caspases**

(Ref: to question number 36 and 37)

29. **Ans. (c) Organelle swelling**

Morphology of Apoptosis

- **Cell shrinkage**^{Q}
- **Chromatin condensation: most characteristic feature**^{Q} of apoptosis
- **Formation of cytoplasmic blebs and apoptotic bodies**^{Q}
- **Plasma membrane** remains **intact**^{Q} during apoptosis
- Apoptosis in contrast to necrosis **doesn't elicit inflammation**^{Q}.

30. **Ans. (b) Inflammosome**

31. **Ans. (a, e) a. BCL; e. MCL**

32. **Ans.(a) Caspase 1**

33. **Ans. (d) Both a & b**

34. **Ans. (c) Fibrinoid necrosis**

35. **Ans. (b) BAK**

BAK and BAK are proapoptotic genes.

36. **Ans. (a, b) a. Tumor suppression; b. Proapoptotic**

(Ref: Robbins 9th/pg 53)

P53 is tumor suppressor gene (see neoplasia chaper) and also induces Bax which causes apoptosis

37. **Ans. (a, d) a. They are enzyme starting apoptosis; d. They are proteases which cause cellular death in apoptosis found in irreversible cell damage**

(Ref: Robbins 9th/pg 53)

Caspases are cystiene proteases that cleave after aspartic acid. These protiens have crucial role in apoptosis

38. **Ans. (a) C is showing necrosis** *(Ref: Robbins 9th/pg 53)*

C is showing smudged pattern S/O necrosis

39. **Ans. (b, c) b. Caspase independent; c. Failure of activation of caspase 8** *(Ref: Robbins 9th/pg 59)*

Necroptosis occurs when caspase 8 cannot be activated, in such cases apoptosis is mediated by RIP1 and RIP3 protiens (caspase independent)

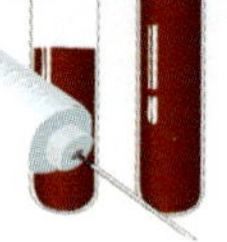

40. **Ans. (c) BCL-XL**

41. **Ans. (d) Pro-apoptotic protein**

42. **Ans. (a) FLIP**

43. **Ans. (a) Fatty** *(Ref: Robbins 9th/pg 43; 8th/pg 15,16)*

Fat necrosis: Seen in **acute pancreatitis, breast, omentum**

44. **Ans. (a) Inflammation present**

(Ref: 9th/pg 53; 8th/pg 25,26)

Apoptosis in contrast to necrosis **doesn't elicit inflammation**[Q]

45. **Ans. (c) Cell swelling** *(Ref: Robbins 9th/pg 46; 8th/pg 12)*

Earliest change in any form of cell injury is cellular swelling due to accumulation of water intracellularly.

46. **Ans. (d) Isoprenoid** *(Ref: Korean J Physiol Pharmacol. 2013 Feb;17(1):43-50.)*

- **Palmitic acid** (PAM), one of the most common saturated fatty acid (SFA) in animals and plants, has been shown to induce **apoptosis**
- Farnesol (FOH) and other **isoprenoid** alcohols induce **apoptosis** in various carcinoma cells and inhibit tumorigenesis in several in vivo models.

47. **Ans. (a) Caspase 3** *(Ref: Robbins 9th/pg 56; 8th/pg 26)*

There are two executionary caspases 3 and 6.
Most important executionary caspase is caspase 3

48. **Ans. (a) Dry gangrene**

(Ref: A Practical Manual of Diabetic Foot Care By Michael E. Edmonds: pg 144)

The combined changes of angiopathy and neuropathy give rise to Diabetic Foot which usually leads to **dry gangrene** in patients of diabetes. In patients with uncontrolled diabetes, however wet gangrene can also ensue.

49. **Ans. (d) Apoptosis**

(Ref: Robbins 9th/pg 53; Robbins 9th/pg 29-30)

Apoptotic cells express **phosphatidylserine/thrombospondin**[Q] on the outer layer of plasma membrane because of which these cells are recognized by the dye **Annexin V**

50. **Ans. (b) Mitochondria**

(Ref: Robbins 9th/pg 38; 8th/pg 17)

51. **Ans. (c) Diabetic glomerulosclerosis** *(Ref: R 9th/pg 44)*

Fibrinoid necrosis: Seen in **PAN, malignant hypertension, acute rheumatic fever**

52. **Ans. (b) Apoptosis**

(Ref: Robbins 9th/pg 53; R 9th/pg 29-30)

DNA breakdown **(Internucleosome cleavage by endonuclease into 200 bp oligonucleosomes is a characteristic)**[Q] at specific sites can be detected by **'step ladder pattern'** on gel electrophoresis or **TUNEL (TdT mediated d-UTP Nick End Labelling) technique**

53. **Ans. (c) Bax** *(Ref: Robbins 9th/pg 55; 8th/pg 28)*

BAD, BIM, BID, Puma, and Noxa are sensors of apoptosis

54. **Ans. (d) Type 1 TNF receptor** *(Ref: Robbins 9th/pg 53)*

Lack of survival signals (option a)and DNA damage (option b and c)trigger intrinsic pathway of apoptosis
Extrinsic pathway is activated by Death receptors are members of the **TNF receptor family**

55. **Ans. (a) Autoimmune disease**

(Ref: AGING, Vol 4, No 5, pp 330-349, Del Puerto HL, Martins AS, Milsted A; et al. (2011)."Canine distemper virus induces apoptosis in cervical tumor derived cell lines". Virol. J. 8 (1): 334)

Inhibition of apoptosis can result in a number of cancers, autoimmune diseases, inflammatory diseases, and viral infections.
Defective Neuronal apoptosis plays an important role in neurodegenerative disorders like **Parkinson's disease (PD), Alzheimer's disease (AD)**

56. **Ans. (c) Necroptosis** *(Ref: Robbins 9th/pg 58-59)*

Necroptosis: Genetically programmed signal transduction event **without caspase activation** → **"caspase-independent" programmed cell death, it is dependent on signaling by the RIP1 and RIP3 complex**

57. **Ans. (d) Pyroptosis** *(Ref: Robbins 9th/pg 58-59)*

Pyroptosis: Promotes the activation of **inflammasome** which activates **Caspase-1**[Q] which releases biologically active form of IL-1 from the precursor.

58. **Ans. (d) Fibrin deposition**

(Ref: R 9th/pg 44; 8th/pg 15,16)

Fibrinoid necrosis: Deposits of **"antigen –antibody complexes"**[Q] & **fibrin** that has leaked out of vessels, result in a bright **pink and amorphous appearance in H & E stains**

59. **Ans. (d) Smear pattern in electrophoresis**

(Ref: R 9th/pg 53)

Smear pattern is seen in necrosis

60. **Ans. (a) Bax** *(Ref: Robbins 9th/pg 55; 8th/pg 28)*

- **Proapoptotic:** Apaf1, cytochrome c, Bak, Bax, Bim, AIF, P53, Caspases, CD95 (FAS), TNF R1 and Smac/Diablo
- **Antiapoptotic:** Bcl2, Bcl_{xL}, Bcl_x, FLIP, McL-1, IAP

61.   **Ans. (a)** **Coagulative necrosis–Tuberculosis**

    (Ref: Robbins 9th/pg 43; 8th/pg 15,16)

62.   **Ans. (d)** **Diabetic glomerulosclerosis** *(Ref: R 9th/pg 44)*

63.   **Ans. (c)** **Activation of caspases** *(Ref: R 9th/pg 52, 53, 56)*

Activation of caspases > caspases alone

64.   **Ans. (b)** **Liquefactive necrosis (Ref: Robbins 9th/pg 43)**

Necrosis in **central nervous system: Liquefactive necrosis**

65.   **Ans. (b, c)** **b. ↓ Apoptosis; c. ↑ Resistance of tumor to treatment** *(Ref: Robbins 9th/pg 55; 8th/pg 28)*

bcl-2: antiapoptotic molecule-option b is true
Option c is true : resistance of tumour cells to therapy can be caused by a failure in the ability to initiate apoptosis
Option d is false: bcl2 mutation though is hallmark of follicular carcinoma but is seen in many other cancers also
Option e is false: tumor suppressor NF2 is disrupted in approximately half of all meningiomas

66.   **Ans. (a)** **Inflammation is present**

    (Ref: R 9th/pg 29, 30, 53)

67.   **Ans. (a)** **Increase in lysosomal enzyme**

    (Ref: Robbins 9th/pg 53; Robbins 9th/pg 29-30)

68.   **Ans. (c)** **Cell membrane bound with organelles**

    (Ref: Robbins 9th/pg 52; 8th/pg 25)

Apoptotic cells break up into fragments, called apoptotic bodies, which contain portions of the cytoplasm and nucleus. The plasma membrane of the apoptotic cell and bodies remains intact, but its structure is altered in such a way that these become "tasty" targets for phagocytes.

69.   **Ans. (b)** **Necroptosis** *(Ref: Robbins 9th/pg 58-59)*

Necroptosis is triggered **by ligation of TNFR1 and Viral proteins of RNA and DNA viruses.**[Q]

70.   **Ans. (a)** **Malignant HTN** *(Ref: 9th/pg 44; 8th/pg 15,16)*

71.   **Ans. (d)** **Fibrinoid necrosis** *(Ref: Robbins 9th/pg 44)*

72.   **Ans. (b)** **BCL-2** *(Ref: Robbins 9th/pg 55; 8th/pg 28)*

Anti-apoptotic.	Pro-apoptotic	Sensors
BCL2, BCL-XL, and MCL1	BAX and BAK	BAD, BIM, BID, Puma, and Noxa

73.   **Ans. (a)** **Denaturation of protein**

(Ref: Robbins 9th/pg 50)

- **Coagulative necrosis: most common type of necrosis**
- **Occurs due to degenerated cytoplasmic proteins**

74.   **Ans. (d)** **All** *(Ref: Robbins 9th/pg 43; 8th/pg 15,16)*

• Fat necrosis	• **Not a specific pattern of necrosis.**[Q] • Signifies focal areas of fat destruction • **Released lipases** split the triglyceride esters contained within fat cells. • The **fatty acids**, so derived, combine with calcium to produce grossly visible **chalky-white areas (fat saponification)**[Q] • Seen in **acute pancreatitis, breast, omentum**[Q]

75.   **Ans. (a)** **Apaf 1**

    (Ref: Robbins 9th/pg 54-55; 8th/pg 29)

Leakage of cytochrome c, other proteins form the inner mitochondrial membrane to cytosol
↓
Cytochrome C binds to **APAF-1**[Q]
↓
Activation of caspase-9-critical initiator caspase of the mitochondrial pathway

76.   **Ans. (c)** **Inflammation**

    (Ref: Robbins 9th/pg 53; 8th/pg 25,26)

- Apoptosis in contrast to necrosis **doesn't elicit inflammation**[Q].

77.   **Ans. (b)** **Extrinsic pathway of apoptosis**

    (Ref: R 9th/pg 53)

The extrinsic pathway of apoptosis is activated by cross-linking members of the tumor necrosis factor (TNF) receptor superfamily, such as **CD95 (Fas) and death receptors DR4 and DR5,** by their receptors, Fas ligand or TRAIL (TNF-related apoptosis-inducing ligand), respectively.

78.   **Ans. (d)** **Causes inflammation that damage surrounding cells** *(Ref: Robbins 9th/pg 53; 8th/pg 25, 26)*

Blebbing or *zeiosis* is the formation of blebs, it is seen in apoptotosis to form apoptotic bodies

79.   **Ans. (c)** **Neurons** *(Ref: The Central Nervous System in Pediatrics Critical Illness page 13)*

80.   **Ans. (b)** **Coagulative**

    (Ref: Robbins 9th/pg 43; 8th/pg 15, 16)

MC type of necrosis in Myocarial Infacrction- coagulative

81.   **Ans. (a)** **Mitochondria**

    (Ref: Essential of apoptosis 2003:245)

Mitochondria is the most important organelle involved in apoptosis initiation and regulation.

82.   **Ans. (d)** **Cytochrome C**
    (Ref: R 9th/pg 53-54; 8th/pg 28, 29)

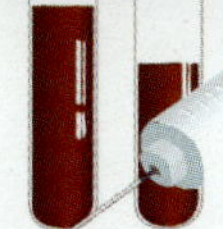

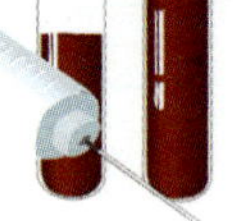

83. **Ans. (d)** **Bcl-2** *(Ref: Robbins 9th/pg 55; 8th/pg 28)*

84. **Ans. (a)** **Cell membrane intact** *(Ref: Robbins 9th/pg 53)*
- Most characteristic feature is condensation of nuclear chromatin
- Intact cell membrane and lack of inflammation differentiates apoptosis from necrosis
- Nuclear molding is seen in small cell carcinoma, lung
- Cytoplasmic eosinophilia- nonspecific finding. Occurs both in necrosis and apoptosis
- If we have to mark one: mark a since that occurs exclusively in apoptosis

85. **Ans. (b)** **Nuclear compaction** *(Ref: Robbins 9th/pg 53)*

Here student gets confused in 2 options b and c..
- On light microscopy, most characteristic feature is condensation of nuclear chromatin and not intactness of cell membrane
- Intact cell membrane and lack of inflammation differentiates apoptosis from necrosis.

86. **Ans. (a)** **Cellular swelling**

(Ref: R 9th/pg 53; 8th/pg 25,26)

Cellular shrinkage and not cellular swelling is a feature of apoptosis

87. **Ans. (a)** **TB** *(Ref: Robbins 9th/pg 43'; 8th/pg 15,16)*

Type of necrosis in **TB: Caseous necrosis.**
Caseous necrosis is a variant of coagulative necrosis

88. **Ans. (a)** **Organogenesis**

(Ref:http://onlinelibrary.wiley.com/doi/10.1002/bdra.10090/abstract)

Caspases are key mediators in the regulation and execution of apoptosis, a crucial part of the morphogenetic process during limb development.

89. **Ans. (b, c, d); b. Increase in caspases; c. Phosphatidyl serine has important role; d. Internucleosomal cleavage of nucleus**

(Ref: Robbins 9th/pg 56; 8th/pg 30)
- In healthy cells, phosphatidylserine is present on the inner leaflet of the plasma membrane, but in apoptotic cells this phospholipid "flips" out and is expressed on the outer layer of the membrane, where it is recognized by several macrophage receptors.
- Apoptosis occurs due to activation of enzymes called **caspases (cysteine proteases that cleave proteins after aspartic residues)**[Q].
- Apoptotic cell exhibit a characteristic breakdown of DNA into large 50 to 300 kilobase piece. Subsequently there is **internucleosomal cleavage**[Q] of DNA into oligonucleosomes, in multiples of 180 to **200 base pairs**[Q], by Ca^{2+} & Mg^{2+} dependent **endonucleases**[Q]. The fragments may be visualized by **agarose gel electrophoresis**[Q] as **DNA ladders**[Q].

90. **Ans. (e)** **Mitochondrial membrane**

(Ref: Robbins 9th/pg 56)

Mitochondrial membrane permeabilization is hallmark of apoptosis

91. **Ans. (d)** **Myositis ossificans**

(Ref: Robbins 9th ed/pg 65)

92. **Ans. (a, b, c); a. Monckeberg's medial sclerosis; b. Papillary carcinoma thyroid; d. Meningioma**

Hyperparathyroidism and Vitamin D intoxication cause hypercalcemia and so are associated with dystrophic calcification.

93. **Ans. (c)** **Prussian blue**

(Ref: Complete review of pathology and Hematology 2nd ed; Praveen Kumar, Vandana Puri Annexure 4)

This is a straight forward question on the **stain used for Iron in tissue** (Hemochromatosis) which is Prussian blue stain.

94. **Ans. (a, c, d) a. Perl stain-Iron; c. Elastin-VG; d. Copper-rhodamine**

(Ref: Complete Review of Pathology and Hematology 2nd ed; Praveen Kumar, Vandana Puri Annexure 4)

95. **Ans. (a)** **Fat** *(Ref: Robbins 9th/pg 62)*

FAT accumulation in myocardium causes fatty change (tigered effect)

96. **Ans. (d)** **Seminoma** *(Ref: Robbins 9th/pg 65; 8th/pg 38)*

Psammoma bodies *are type of dystrophic calcification seen in* -Meningioma, **P**apillary carcinoma of thyroid, ovary (serous carcinoma), prolactinoma, Somatostinoma, mesothelioma

97. **Ans. (b)** **Ferrocyanide to ferroferric cyanide**

(Ref: Dacie and Lewis Practical Haematology 11th ed, pg 338)

Hemosiderin reacts with potassium ferrocyanide to form a blue compound, ferri ferrocyanide; this reaction is the basis of a positive Prussian-blue (Perls') reaction.

98. **Ans. (c)** **Atherosclerosis**

(Ref: Robbins 9th/pg 65; 8th/pg 38)

Atheromatous plaque shows **Dystrophic calcification**
All others are causes of metastatic calcification

99. **Ans. (d)** **Mitochondria**

(Ref: Robbins 9th/pg 62; 8th/pg 33)

Foam cells - cholesterol-laden macrophages

100. **Ans. (c)** **Lungs** *(Ref: Robbins 9th/pg 65; 8th/pg 38)*

Metastaic calcification is seen most commonly in lungs followed by kidneys

101. Ans. (b) Parkinsons disease

(*Ref:* https://en.wikipedia.org/wiki/Proteopathy)

Answer should be **none**; but if we have to mark one go for b. as a, c, d are well known proteinopathies whereas b is still in phase of research.

The proteopathies (also known as **proteinopathies**, **protein conformational disorders**, or **protein misfolding diseases**) include - Alzheimer's disease, Prion diseases, Parkinson's disease, Huntington's disease, Cystic Fibrosis, AL (light chain) amyloidosis

102. Ans. (d) Mitochondria

(*Ref: Robbins 9th/pg 65; 8th/pg 38*)

103. Ans. (b) Lipochrome-wear and tear

(*Ref: Robbins 9th/pg 64; 8th/pg 37*)

- Lipofuschin: **Perinuclear**[Q] brown-coloured pigment, Seen in **aging**[Q], **protein energy malnutrition**[Q] **and cancer cahcexia.**

104. Ans. (d) Congo red (*Ref: Bancroft theory and practice of histological stains 7th ed, pg 165*)

105. Ans. (d) Seen in teratoma (*Ref: R 9th/pg 65; 8th/pg 38*)

- Psammoma bodies (PBs) are concentric lamellated calcified structures, observed most commonly in papillary thyroid carcinoma (PTC), meningioma, and papillary serous cystadenocarcinoma of ovary
- They represent a process of dystrophic calcification

106. Ans. (a) Dying tissue (*Ref: Robbins 9th/pg 65; 8th/pg 38*)

107. Ans. (a, b) a. Fatty change; b. Accumulation of triglyceride (*Ref: Robbins 9th/pg 62; 8th/pg 33*)

Steatosis (Fatty Change): accumulations of triglycerides within parenchymal cells

Organs involved-liver, heart, muscle, and kidney

108. Ans. (b, c) b. Lungs; c. Kidneys (*Ref: Robbins 9th/pg 65*)

Dystrophic calcification occurs in dead and damaged tissues and not in normal organs

109. Ans. (d) Pineal

(*Ref: Rosai and Ackerman's Surgical Pathology 10ed volume 2.. Pathol Annu. 1992; 27(Pt 1):263-304*)

- **Oncocyte** is an epithelial cell characterized by an **excessive amount of mitochondria**
- **Characterized by** abundant acidophilic, granular cytoplasm
- **Other names:** *Oxyphilic cell, Askanazy cell, Hürthle cell* (thyroid gland only), *Apocrine metaplasia* (breast gland only
- They are present in benign tumors of **salivary glands, thyroid, parathyroid, kidney, lung and pitui**

110. Ans. (a) Suprasellar calcification

(*Ref: J Pediatr Neurosci. 2011 Oct; 6 (Suppl1): S46–S55*)

Suprasellar calcifications are always pathological
Other 3 can be physiological as well

111. Ans. (c) Germ cells (*Ref: Robbins 9th/pg 67; 8th/pg 40*)

112. Ans. (a) Decrease metabolic activity

(*Ref: R 9th/pg 67, 68*)

- **Sirutuins:** These include proteins that inhibit metabolic activity[Q], reduce apoptosis[Q], stimulate protein folding[Q], inhibit the harmful effects of oxygen free radicals[Q] and activating DNA repair enzymes through deacylation[Q]

113. Ans. (d) Premature ageing

(*Ref: R 9th/pg 66; 8th/pg 40*)

Syndromes associated with defective DNA repair	
Defective DNA helicase | **Werner syndrome**[Q] **(Premature aging)**	*Defective DNA repair syndromes*[Q] | **BAX-F** Bloom Syndrome[Q] Ataxia Telangiectasia[Q] Xeroderma Pigmentosa[Q] Fanconi Anemia[Q]

114. Ans. (d) All of the above (*Ref: Robbins 9th/pg 67,68*)

Sirutuins

- Family of **NAD-dependent protein deacetylases.**
- Sirtuin-6[Q] promotes the expression of genes whose products increase longevity.
- Since these protiens increase longevity, activate DNA repair enzymes so prevent against cancer
  Sirtuins also increase insulin sensitivity and glucose metabolism, and may be targets for the treatment of diabetes.

115. Ans. (b) Increased free radical injury

(*Ref: Robbins 9th/pg 66-68; 8th/pg 39, 40*)

116. Ans. (a) Peroxisome

117. Ans. (a) Superoxide dismutase

(*Ref: Robbins 9th/pg 48*)

Superoxide dismutase is an antioxidant and known to protect brain from free radical injury

118. Ans. (a, b, c); a. Act as scavenger of free radicle; b. Glutathione has anti-oxidant property; c. Reduced glutathione can chemically detoxify H_2O_2

(*Ref: Robbins 9th/pg 48; 8th/pg 13,14*)

- Glutathione peroxidase: $H_2O_2 + 2GSH \rightarrow GSSG + 2H_2O$
- Reduced glutathione can chemically detoxify H_2O_2

- Intracellular ratio of oxidized glutathione (GSSG) to reduced glutathione (GSH) is a reflection of the oxidative state of the cell
- Important indicator of the cell's ability to detoxify ROS.

119. Ans. (c) NADPH oxidase

(Ref: R 9th/pg 48; 8th/pg 13,14)

Antioxidants

Enzymes	Non enzymes
• **Catalase**- Present in **peroxisomes**[Q] decomposes H_2O_2	**Antioxidants**- vitamins E, A and C glutathione in the cytosol.
• **Superoxidase dismutases:** O_2^- to H_2O_2 • **Manganese**-SOD, which is localized in **mitochondria**, • **Copper-zinc**-SOD, which is found in the **cytosol**.	**Transferrin, ferritin, lactoferrin, and ceruloplasmin**[Q] - Minimise the reactivity of metals by binding with them
Glutathione peroxidase: $H_2O_2 + 2GSH \rightarrow GSSG + 2H_2O$ • **Important indicator of the cell's ability to detoxify ROS**[Q]	

NADPH oxidase

Oxidizes **NADPH**[Q] (reduced nicotinamide-adenine dinucleotide phosphate) and, in the process, **reduces oxygen to superoxide.**[Q]

120. Ans. (d) Synthesis of new proteins *(Ref: R 9th/pg 49)*

Pathologic Effects of Free Radicals are

- Lipid peroxidation in membranes- result in extensive membrane damage.
- Oxidative modification of proteins
- Single- and double-strand breaks in DNA cross-linking of DNA strands, and formation of adducts

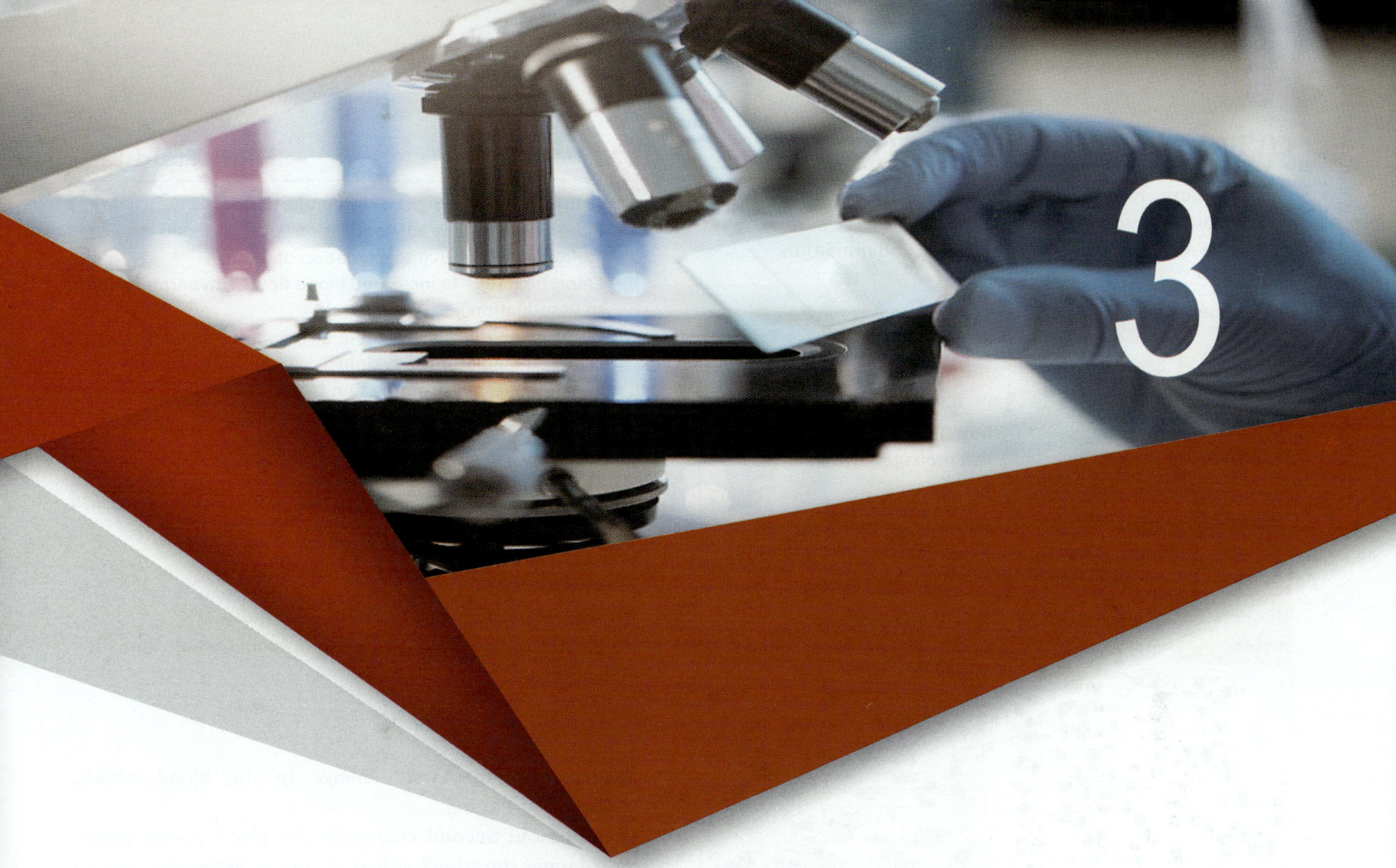

3

Inflammation and Repair

Key Points

» **Hallmark**[Q] of acute inflammation: **Increased vascular permeability**
» Endothelial cell expression **of E-selectin is a hallmark of acute cytokine mediated inflammation**
» **Tissue destruction: Hallmark of chronic inflammation**
» **Granulation tissue**[Q] is the hallmark of the fibrogenic repair.
» **Chemotaxis: Unidirectional movement**[Q] of the leukocytes **towards site of injury** along a **chemical gradient**
» **Opsonisation**: Phagocytosis requires **polymerization of actin filaments**
» Pinocytosis is due to **internalization into clathrin-coated pits**
» **Catarrhal inflammation: Commonest type of inflammation**
» Maximum strength gained 70% of strength of normal skin

Key Recent Updates

» Albumin is **negative** acute phase reactant
» Emperipolesis is seen is Rosai Dorfman disease
» **NETosis** is neutrophil cell death pathway which is protective to body but can sometimes lead to autoimmune diseases.

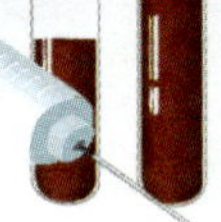

OVERVIEW OF INFLAMMATION

- **Definition:** Response of the vascularized tissues to an injurious stimulus is called inflammation.
- **Types:** Acute inflammation & Chronic inflammation

Features	Acute	Chronic
Onset	Early: minutes to hours	Slow: days to months
Cellular infiltrate	Neutrophils^Q	**Mononuclear cells**-Monocytes/ macrophages, lymphocytes, plasma cells
Exceptions	*Acute typhoid fever (neutropenia)*	Chronic **pseudomonas** infection (neutrophilia)
Tissue injury	Mild and self-limited	Severe and progressive

Neutrophils (arrow)

Lymphocyte (green arrow) and macrophages (yellow arrow)

High Yield Facts

Celsus four cardinal signs of inflammation
- **Rubor:** redness (due to **vasodilation**^{Q} of small blood vessels)
- **Tumor:** swelling (due to exudation of fluid)
- **Calor:** heat (due to increased blood flow i.e **hyperemia due to vasodilation**^{Q})
- **Dolor:** pain (due to stretching of tissue due to edema and chemical mediator **bradykinin**^{Q})
- **Function laesa**-loss of function (Added by Virchow)

ACUTE INFLAMMATION

Three Major Components

1. **Vasodilation**
2. **Increased vascular permeability- the hallmark**^{Q}
3. **Emigration of leucocytes** from microcirculation and their activation

Vascular Changes

- **Vasoconstriction: First**^{Q} change in the blood vessels, **transient**^{Q} in nature.
- **Vasodilation: Second** change in the blood vessels lasting for a **longer duration**^{Q}. It first occurs in **arterioles**. Results in **increased blood flow** → **redness (rubor)** & sensation of **warmth (calor)**
- **Increased permeability: Hallmark**^{Q} of acute inflammation; **M**aximally seen in the venules.^{Q}

Mechanism of Increased Vascular Permeability

Name	Mechanism	Caused by	Affected Vessels
Immediate transient response^Q **(ITR)** Rapid short lived (15–30 min) reversible	*Formation of endothelial gaps*	• Histamine^Q, bradykinin • Contraction of endothelial cell cytoskeleton^Q	Venules
Immediate sustained response^Q **(ISR)** Rapid & long lived	*Direct endothelial injury*	• Burns • Endothelial cell necrosis and detachment^Q	Venules, capillaries and arterioles
Delayed prolonged leakage^Q **(DPL)** (appears after 2–12 hr)	*Mild endothelial damage e.g., Late-appearing sunburn*^{Q}	• Thermal and radiation injury^Q	Venules and capillaries
LMI *(Leukocyte-mediated endothelial injury) late & sustained*	*WBC damage*	• Activated leukocytes • Endothelial injury or detachment^Q	**Venules (mostly);** pulmonary and glomerular capillaries
Increased transcytosis	*Formation of vesiculo-vacuolar organelles*^{Q} *(Intercellular channels)*	• Histamine and VEGF	Venules

Note: Endothelial cell retraction is same as endothelial cell contraction (Robbins 10th ed)

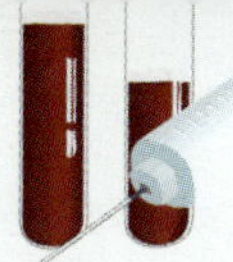

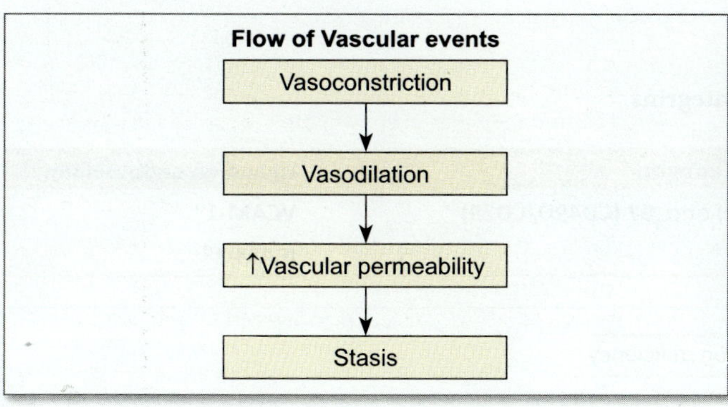

- **In the lumen:** Margination, rolling, and adhesion to endothelium
- **Across lumen: Migration** across the **endothelium and vessel wall**[Q]
- **Outside the lumen: Migration** in the **tissues toward a chemotactic stimulus**[Q]

High Yield Facts

- Formation of endothelial gaps (**Immediate transient response**) is the **most common mechanism**[Q] for **increased permeability.**
- Most important immediate mediator responsible for **Immediate transient response**[Q] is **histamine**[Q]
- The loss of fluid and increased vessel diameter leads to slower blood flow, concentration of red cells in small vessels, and increased viscosity of the blood.

Cellular Changes

Leukocyte recruitment to sites of inflammation from vessel lumen can be divided into the following steps:

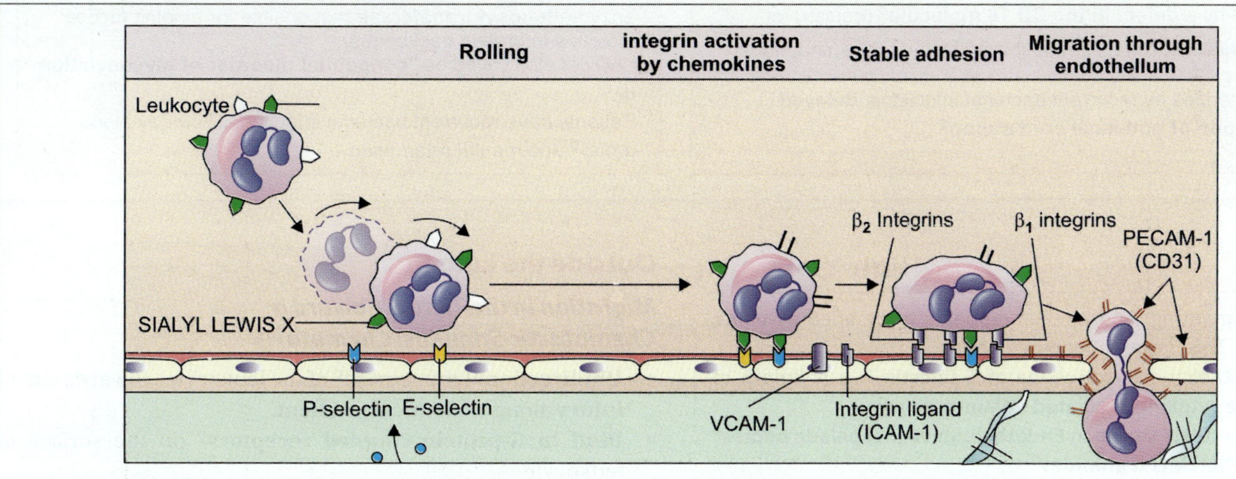

In the Lumen

Margination

- Movement of the leukocytes **principally neutrophils** towards the periphery of the blood vessel
- Occurs due to **increased vascular permeability**[Q]
- **Vasodilatation and selectins** have important role

Rolling

- **Transient adhesion** of **leukocytes** with the **endothelial cells**
  - Mediated by **selectins.**[Q]

Molecule	Distribution	Activated by	Ligand (interact with)
P-selectin (CD62P)	**Platelets**[Q] **and Endothelium**[Q]	(TNF, IL-1), histamine, or thrombin	**Sialyl-Lewis X** expressed on leucocytes
E-selectin (CD62E)	**Endothelium**[Q]	(TNF, IL-1)	**Sialyl-Lewis X** expressed on leucocytes
L-selectin (CD62L)	**Leucocytes**[Q]: Neutrophils, monocytes and T cells (naive and central memory), B cells (naive)	–	**Sialyl-Lewis X/PNAd on** Glycoprotein adhesion molecules (**GlyCAM-1**), CD34, **MAdCAM-1**[Q] expressed on endothelium

Adhesion

- **Firm attachment** of the **leukocytes to the endothelial cells**
- Mediated by **heterodimeric leukocyte surface proteins called integrins**.

Integrin	Molecule of Integrin	Ligand on endothelium
$\beta1$-integrins	VLA molecules (VLA-4 (CD49a/CD29) or α_4B7 **(CD49D/CD29)**	**VCAM-1**[Q].
$\beta2$-integrins	LFA-1 or Mac-1(CD11a/CD18)	**ICAM-1**[Q]

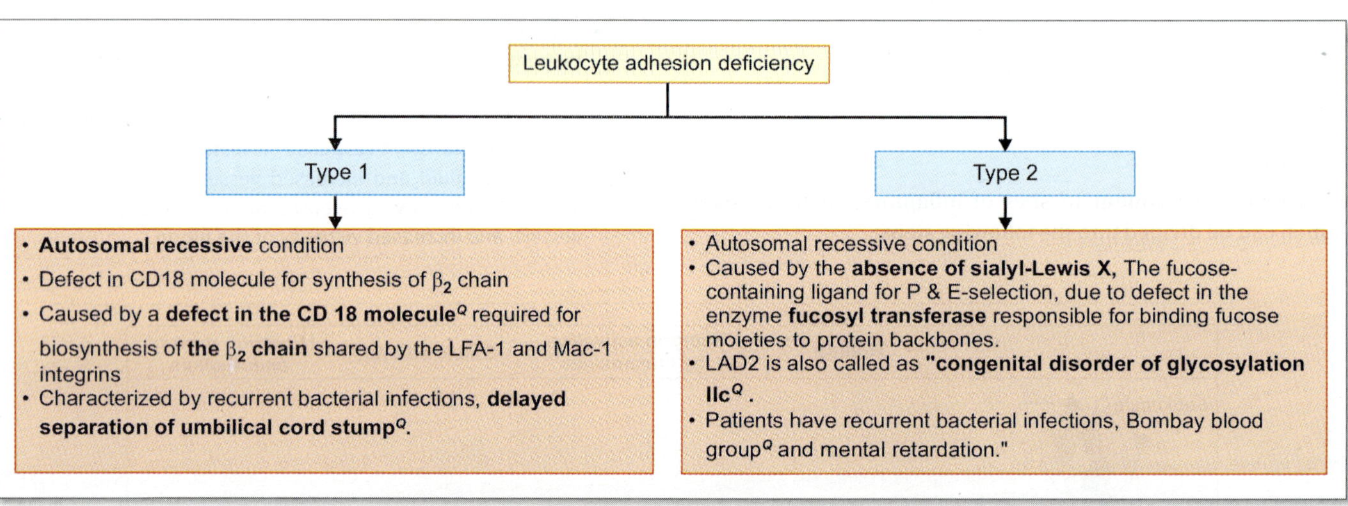

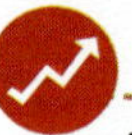

High Yield Facts

- **Pavementing:** Endothelium appears to be lined by white cells. This is due to margination.
- Endothelial cell expression **of E-selectin is a hallmark of acute cytokine-mediated inflammation.**[Q]
- P Selectin is stored in Endothelium weibel palade bodies[Q] and Platelets α granules[Q]
- L-selectin **helps in Lymphocytes homing to high endothelial venules**[Q]

Integrins are transmembrane receptors that are the bridges for cell-cell and cell-extracellular matrix (ECM) interactions. Few ligands for integrins:

- **VCAM & ICAM** – on the endothelium
- **GPIIbIIIa,** an integrin on the surface of blood platelets
- **Fibronectin, vitronectin, collagen, and laminin.**

Across the Lumen

Leukocyte Migration through Endothelium: Transmigration or Diapedesis[Q]

- Occurs mainly in **postcapillary venules.**[Q]
- Most important molecule: **PECAM-1 (platelet endothelial cell adhesion molecule) or CD31.**[Q]
- After traversing the endothelium, leukocytes pierce basement membrane, probably by secreting **collagenases,**[Q] and **enter extravascular tissue.**

Outside the Lumen

Migration in the Tissues Toward a Chemotactic Stimulus: Chemotaxis

- **Unidirectional movement**[Q] of the leukocytes **towards site of injury** along a **chemical gradient**.
- **Bind to G-protein coupled receptors**[Q] on the surface of leukocyte
- Causes **actin polymerization** and all movements.

Chemotactic Agents

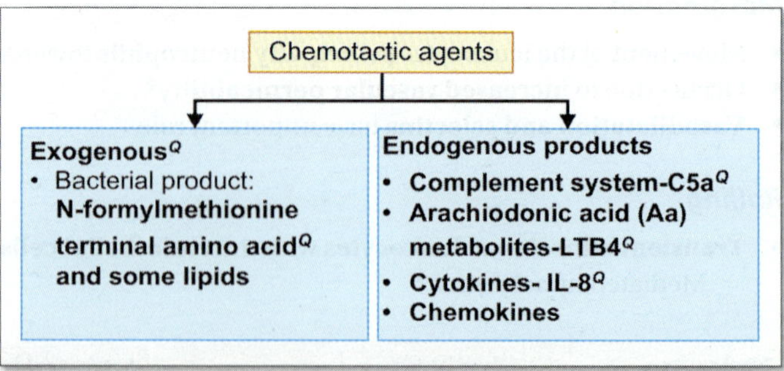

PHAGOCYTOSIS AND CLEARANCE OF THE OFFENDING AGENT

Phagocytosis involves following three sequential steps

Recognition and Attachment

- Particles to be ingested by leukocytes (microbes and dead cells) are **recognized by receptors present on the leucocyte surface like:**[Q]

Mannose receptors	• Recognizes **microbes and not host cells.**[Q] • Part of molecules found on **microbial cell walls**. • Mammalian glycoproteins and glycolipids contain **terminal sialic acid or N-acetylgalactosamine**[Q]
Scavenger receptors	• **Bind microbes and oxidized LDL particles**[Q] that can **no longer bind to LDL receptor**
Macrophage integrins	• Mac-I integrins (**CD11b/CD18**)- bind microbes for phagocytosis

Opsonization

- **Coating of the bacteria** so that they are **easily phagocytosed** by the **leucocytes**.
- Chemicals causing opsonization are called **opsonins**
- Opsonization **increases efficiency** of phagocytosis.
- Phagocytosis can occur without opsonization also.[Q]
- **Opsonins include:**
  - **C3b**[Q], Fc fragment of IgG antibodies[Q], Plasma lectins-mannose-binding lectin[Q] and Fibrinogen[Q], C reactive protein[Q]

Engulfment

- Occurs after the particle is bound to phagocyte receptors
- Leucocyte **cytoplasm** forms pseudopods and leads to formation of phagosome
- Plasma membrane pinches off to form a vesicle
- Fuses with a lysosomal granule, resulting in discharge of the granule's contents into the phagolysosome

High Yield Facts

- Phagocytosis requires **polymerization of actin filaments**[Q]
- Pinocytosis is due to **internalization into clathrin-coated pits**
- Pinocytosis is **not dependent on the actin cytoskeleton.**[Q]

INTRACELLULAR DESTRUCTION OF MICROBES AND DEBRIS

Final step in the elimination of infectious agents and necrotic cells.

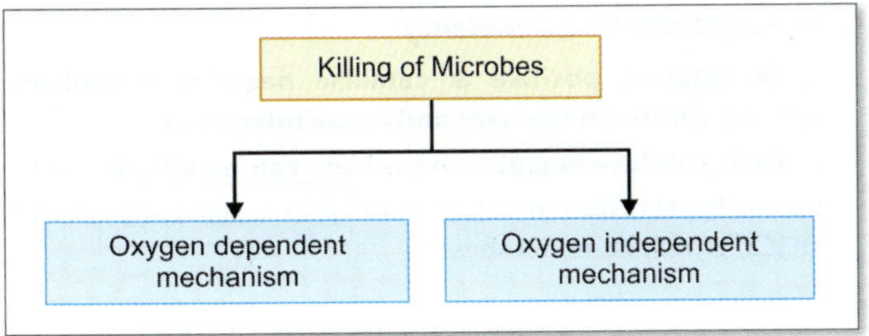

Oxygen-dependent Killing

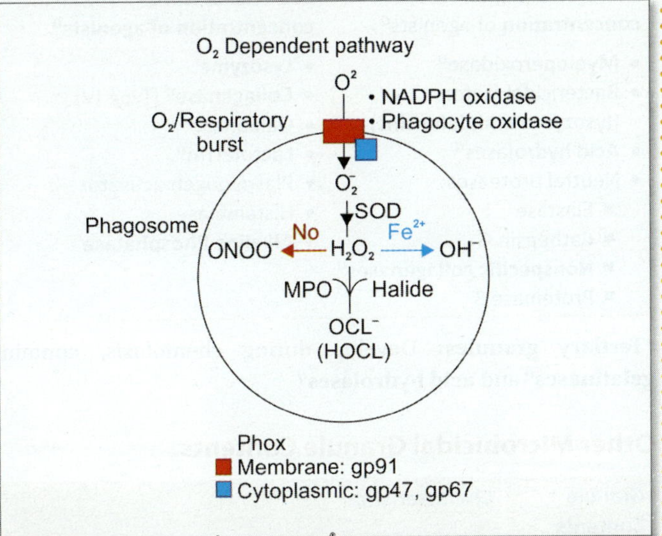

High Yield Facts

- **Respiratory burst** is also called oxidative burst
- **Respiratory burst** results in rapid release of **reactive oxygen species**[Q] from different types of cells
- **NADPH oxidase** is also called **phagocyte oxidase or phagocyte NADPH oxidase" (PHOX)**

Enzymes Involved in Respiratory Burst

Enzyme	Function
NADPH oxidase	**Chiefly**[Q] responsible for the formation of **hydrogen peroxide**[Q]
Catalase (peroxisomes)[Q]	Degrades **hydrogen peroxide into water and oxygen.**[Q]
Superoxide Dismutase (SOD)	Causes conversion of **superoxide ion into hydrogen peroxide.**[Q]
Glutathione peroxidase	Causes conversion of **reduced glutathione to its homodimer.**[Q]

Oxygen Independent Killing

Lysosomal Enzymes and Other Lysosomal Proteins

- **Neutrophils and monocytes** contain **lysosomal granule**[Q] that contribute to **microbial killing**
- Neutrophils have **two main types of granules**

Primary (azurophilic) granules	Secondary (specific) granules
Secreted at **higher** concentration of agonists[Q]	Secreted at **lower** concentration of agonists[Q]

• Myeloperoxidase[Q]
• Bactericidal factors **(lysozyme and defensins)**
• **Acid hydrolases**[Q]
• Neutral proteases:
  ■ Elastase
  ■ Cathepsin G
  ■ **Nonspecific collagenases**[Q]
  ■ Proteinase 3
	• Lysozyme
	• **Collagenase**[Q] (Type IV)
	• Gelatinase
	• **Lactoferrin**[Q]
	• Plasminogen activator
	• Histaminase
	• **Alkaline Phosphatase**

***Tertiary granules:** Develop during chemotaxis, contain **gelatinases**[Q] and **acid hydrolases**[Q]

Other Microbicidal Granule Contents

Granule Contents	Characteristics
Defensins	Cationic **arginine-rich granule peptides**[Q] that are toxic to microbes
Cathelicidins	• Antimicrobial proteins found in neutrophils • **Vitamin D upregulates genetic expression of Human cathelicidin antimicrobial protein (Hcap18)**[Q]
Lysozyme	• Hydrolyzes **muramic acid-N-acetylglucosamine bond,**[Q] • Found in the glycopeptide coat of all bacteria
Lactoferrin	**Iron-binding**[Q] protein present in specific granules
Major basic protein	**Cationic protein of eosinophils,** which has limited bactericidal activity but is cytotoxic to many parasites

DEFECTS IN LEUCOCYTE FUNCTION

Inherited Defect in Phagolysosome Function

A. Chédiak-Higashi Syndrome

- Autosomal recessive
- Defects in the **lysosomal transport protein LYST,**[Q] encoded by the gene *CHS1* at **1q42**[Q]
- **Defective fusion of phagosomes and lysosomes in phagocytes**[Q] (causing susceptibility to infections)
- **Abnormalities in melanocytes**[Q] (leading to **albinism**)
- **Abnormalities in cells of the nervous system**[Q] (associated with **nerve defects)**
- **Abnormalities in platelets**[Q] (causing **bleeding disorders**).

Leukocyte Abnormalities

- **Neutropenia (most common)**[Q]
- Leukocytes contain *giant granules,*[Q] (**characteristic**) result from **aberrant phagolysosome fusion**[Q]

- Defective degranulation, impaired chemotaxis, delayed microbial killing and NK cell function is also impaired

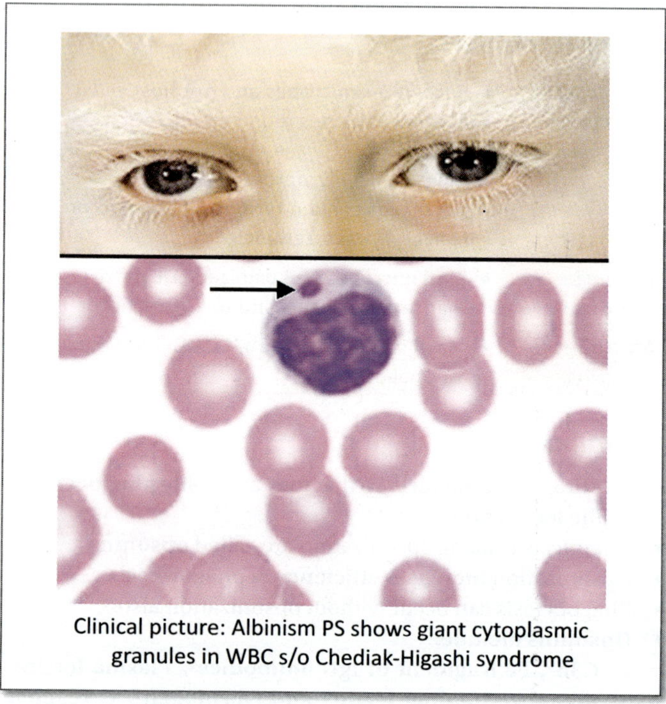

Clinical picture: Albinism PS shows giant cytoplasmic granules in WBC s/o Chediak-Higashi syndrome

B. Chronic Granulomatous Disease

- **Inherited Defect in Microbicidal Activity**
- Inherited defect in genes encoding components of **phagocyte oxidase**[Q]
- **X Linked**: Defect in membrane-bound components **(gp91phox)**[Q]
- **Autosomal recessive** defects: Defect in **(p47phox and p67phox).**[Q]
- Formation of **widespread granulomas**[Q]

Diagnosis

- **Nitroblue-tetrazolium (NBT) test**:
  - Depends upon direct **reduction of NBT** by **superoxide free radical** to form an insoluble **formazan**[Q]
  - **Negative** in chronic granulomatous disease and **positive in normal individuals**.
  - This test tells whether or not PHOX enzymes are present, **not how much they are affected**[Q]
- **Dihydrorhodamine (DHR) test**
- **Cytochrome C reduction assay**:
  - **Quantitative**: Amount of **superoxide a patient's phagocytes can produce**[Q]

C. Myeloperoxidase Deficiency

- **Both catalase positive & catalase negative organisms survive within phagocytes and cause infections**[Q]
- In **CGD catalase negative organisms can be killed**[Q] - H_2O_2 in not broken due to catalase so $\boxed{H_2O_2 + MPO + Cl}$ forms HOCl. Which kills microbes)

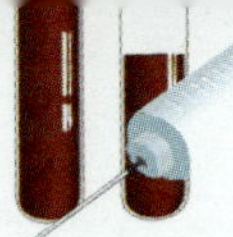

R10ᵗʰ Latest Update

Neutrophil Extracellular Traps (NET)

- **Extracellular fibrillar networks**[Q] that provide a high concentration of antimicrobial substances **at sites of infection**
- **Prevents spread of microbes by trapping them in the fibrils.**[Q]
- **Beneficial suicide:** Neutrophils nucleus undergoing apoptosis to make NETs **(Netosis)**

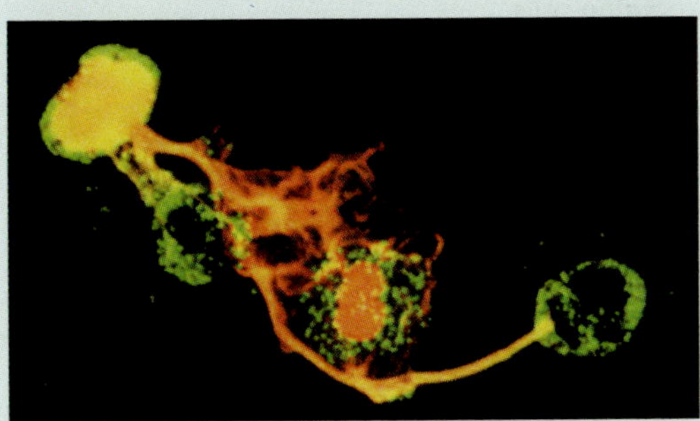

Beneficial suicide Neutrophils

- Consist of a **viscous meshwork of nuclear chromatin which includes histones and associated DNA**[Q]
- **Arginine** is the most important amino acid for NET

- **Nuclear chromatin in the NETs:** Source of nuclear antigens in systemic autoimmune diseases[Q]

Frustrated Phagocytosis

- Seen when phagocytes encounter materials **that cannot be easily ingested**
- Eg immunecomplexes deposited on **immovable flat surfaces (e.g., glomerular basement membrane),**[Q]
- Inability of WBCs to ingest these substances → strong activation & **release of large amounts of lysosomal enzymes into the extracellular environment** → Leukocyte-mediated tissue injury[Q]

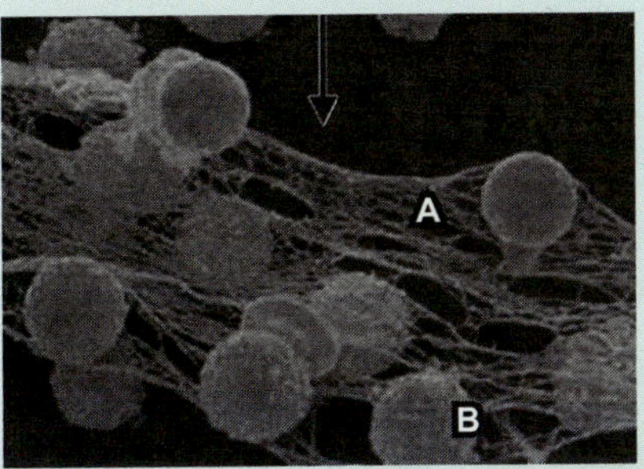

A-NET; B-Cells

D. Acquired Leucocyte Deficiencies

- **Bone marrow suppression:** Tumors, radiation & chemotherapy: Decreased Production[Q] of leukocytes
- **Diabetes,**[Q] malignancy, sepsis, **chronic dialysis: Affects Adhesion and chemotaxis**[Q]
- **Leukemia,**[Q] anemia, sepsis, diabetes, malnutrition: Affects Phagocytosis and microbicidal activity

- **TGF-β**[Q]
- **IL-10**[Q]
- Resolvin and proteins (Derived from **polyunsaturated fatty acids)**[Q]
- **Cholinergic discharge** that **inhibit the production** of TNF in macrophages[Q]

TERMINATION OF THE ACUTE INFLAMMATORY RESPONSE

Anti-inflammatory Mediators

- **Lipoxins**[Q]

MEDIATORS OF INFLAMMATION

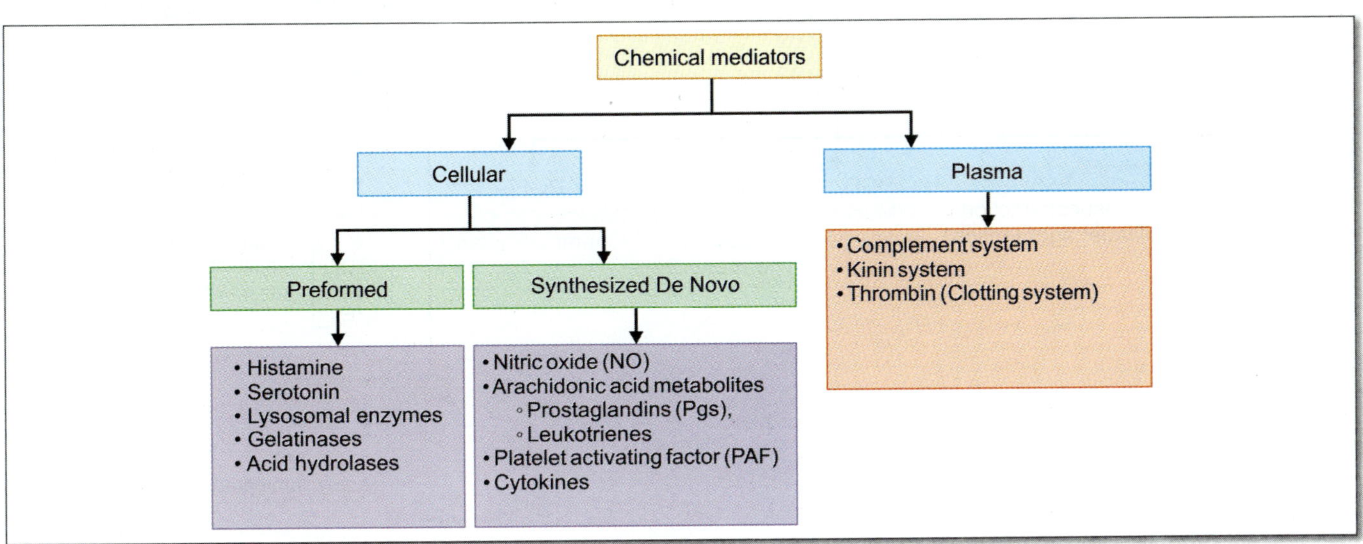

Cellular Mediators

Mediator	Characteristics
Histamine	• Formed from the amino acid '**histidine**' • **Sources: Mast cells (richest source), platelets and basophils** • Causes **vasodilation** (but vasoconstriction of large arteries), **increased permeability** (immediate transient response) & **bronchoconstriction**
Serotonin (5-HT)	• Richest source is **platelets**; also present in enterochromaffin cells. • Its primary function is as a **neurotransmitter** in the **gastrointestinal tract**[Q] • It has actions similar to histamine
Lysosomal Enzymes	• Present in lysosomes of neutrophils and monocytes. • Function: Role in intracellular killing microbes and dead cells
Gelatinase & Acid hydrolases	• Source: Also have tertiary granules or C particles of neutrophils[Q]

Newly Synthesized Cellular Mediators

Nitric Oxide (NO)

Formed from	L-arginine with the help of enzyme nitric oxide synthase (NOS).
Functions	• Intracellular killing of microbes forming peroxynitrite anion • Potent vasodilator, also known as **Endothelium-derived relaxing factor (EDRF)**[Q] • **Reduction of platelet aggregation**[Q]

Arachidonic Acid Metabolites

- Derived from dietary sources or by conversion from the **essential fatty acid: linoleic acid.**
- Released/mobilized from membrane phospholipids (PL) through the action of cellular phospholipases, mainly **phospholipase A2**
- **Hallmark of acute inflammation is increased vascular permeability, thereby most of these mediators increase vascular permeability.**[Q]

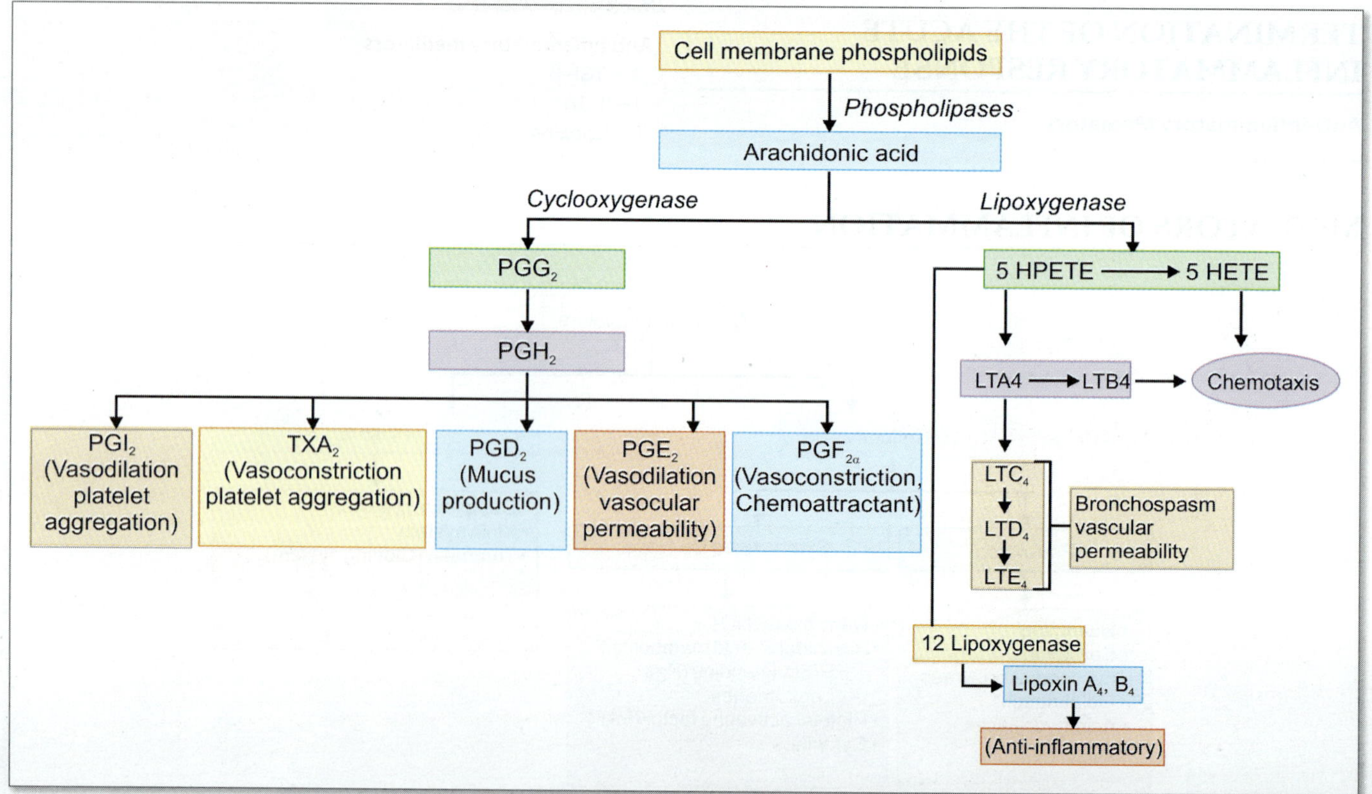

Platelet-Activating Factor (PAF)

- **Produced by:** Platelets, basophils, mast cells, neutrophils, macrophages and endothelial cells
- **Functions**: **Platelet aggregation, vasoconstriction and bronchoconstriction.**[Q]
- At low concentrations, it induces vasodilation and increased venular permeability

Cytokines

- *Produced by:*
  - Activated lymphocytes, macrophages, and **dendritic cells,** but also **endothelial,** epithelial, and connective tissue cells
- *Mediate and regulate:*
  - Immune and inflammatory reactions
- *Action:*
  - Autocrine (same cell), paracrine (close proximity) and endocrine (long distance)
- *Features:*
  - **Pleiotropic:** One cytokine can have different effects on different cells
  - **Redundant:** Different cytokines can have the same effect
  - **Cascade effect**: Cytokines can stimulate the production of other cytokine

High Yield Facts

- Most important cytokine responsible for systemic effects of inflammation are interleukin-**1 (IL-1) and tumor necrosis factor – alpha (TNF- α)**[Q]
- **Intrinsically pyrogenic cytokines**- IL-1α,[Q] IL-1β, TNF-α,[Q] TNF-β, IFN-α, and IL-6.[Q]
- *PLEASE NOTE: IL-18[Q] of IL-1* family is not pyrogenic
- Chemokines mediate their actions through chemokine receptors **(CXCR or CCR).**[Q]
- CXCR4; CCR5- act as co-receptors for binding and entry of **HIV into CD4 cells.**[Q]
- **IL-6**, made by macrophages and other cells, which is involved in **local and systemic reactions**
- **IL-17**, produced mainly by T lymphocytes, which promotes **neutrophil recruitment**.

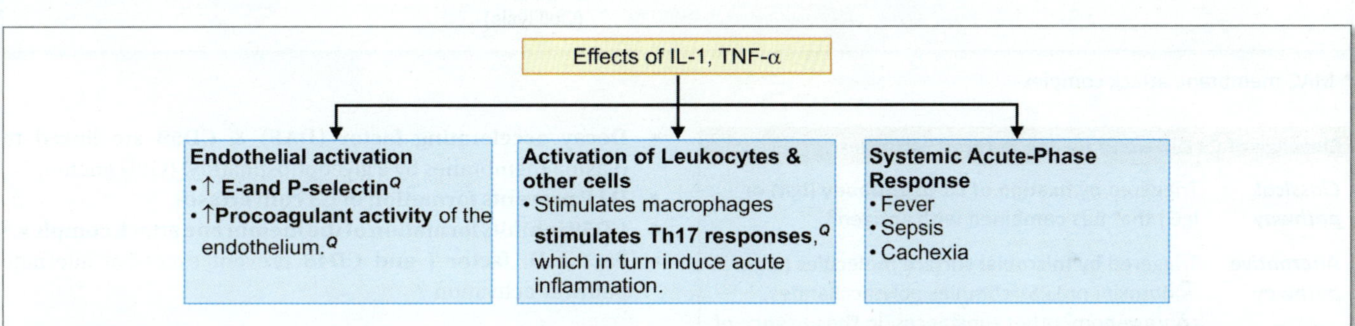

Chemokines

- Family of cytokines that act primarily as **chemoattractant**s for specific types of leukocytes.
- Classified **according to the arrangement of conserved cysteinc residue**[Q] in mature proteins.

Family	α-chemokines (CXC)	β-chemokines (C-C)	γ-chemokines (C chemokines)	CX3C
Description	2 conserved cysteines separated by 1 amino acid	2 conserved cysteines separated by no amino acid	ONE conserved cysteine	2 conserved cysteines separated by 3 amino acid
Action on	Neutrophils	All WBCs **except neutrophils**[Q]	**Lymphocytes**	Monocytes & T cells
Examples	e.g. **IL-8,** IL-l and TNF	• MCP-1 (Monocyte chemoattractant protein • **RANTES**[Q](regulated and normal T-cell expressed and secreted) • **Eotaxin (selectively recruits Eosinophils)**[Q] MlPlα.	Lymphotactin	**Fractalkaline**

Plasma Mediators

Complement System

- This system functions in **both innate and adaptive immunity**[Q]
- The **critical step** in complement activation is the proteolysis of **component C3**

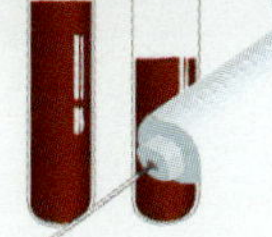

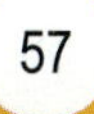

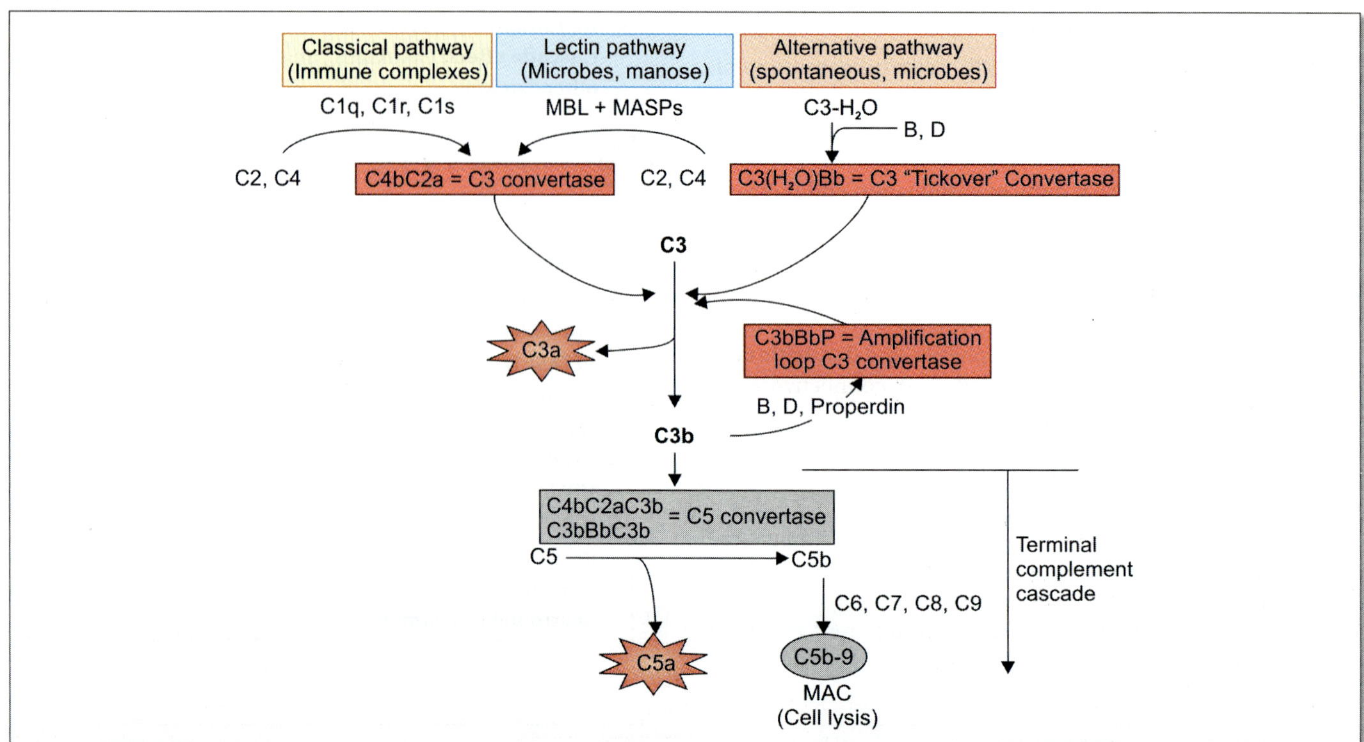

* MAC-membrane attack complex

Cleavage of C3 can occur by one of three pathways	
Classical pathway	Triggered by **fixation of C1 to antibody (IgM or IgG) that has combined with antigen**[Q]
Alternative pathway	Triggered **by microbial surface molecules** (e.g., endotoxin, or LPS), complex polysaccharides, cobra venom, other substances, **in the absence of antibody**
Lectin pathway	Plasma mannose-binding lectin binds to carbohydrates on microbes & directly activates C1.[Q]

All three pathways of complement activation lead to the formation of an active enzyme called the **C3 convertase, which** splits C3 into two functionally distinct fragments, C3a and C3b and finally leads to formation of membrane attack complex **(MAC)**[Q]

The complement system has **three main functions**

Inflammation	• **Anaphylatoxins**[Q]-C3a, C5a, C4a. **Stimulate histamine release from mast cells**[Q] • **Chemotactic**[Q]-C5a
Opsonization & phagocytosis	C_3b, C_4b and C_5b
Cell lysis	• Deposition of MAC on cells makes them permeable to water & ions → death (lysis) of cells

Regulation of Complement System

- **C1 inhibitor(C1 INH)**[Q] blocks binding of C1 to immune complex

- **Decay accelerating factor (DAF) & CD59** are linked to plasma membranes by a glycophosphatidyl (GPI) anchor.
- **DAF prevents formation of C3 convertases**
- **CD59 inhibits formation of the membrane attack complex.**[Q]
- **Factor H, factor I and CD46** prevent excessive alternate pathway activation.[Q]

Disease Associated with Complement System

Refer immunity chapter

Products of Coagulation

- Thrombin activates protease-activated receptors **(PARs)**, which are expressed on platelets and leukocytes play a role in inflammation
- Major role of the PARs is in **platelet activation during clotting**[Q]

Kinins

- Kinins are vasoactive peptides derived from plasma proteins, called **kininogens**, by the action of **kallikreins**.

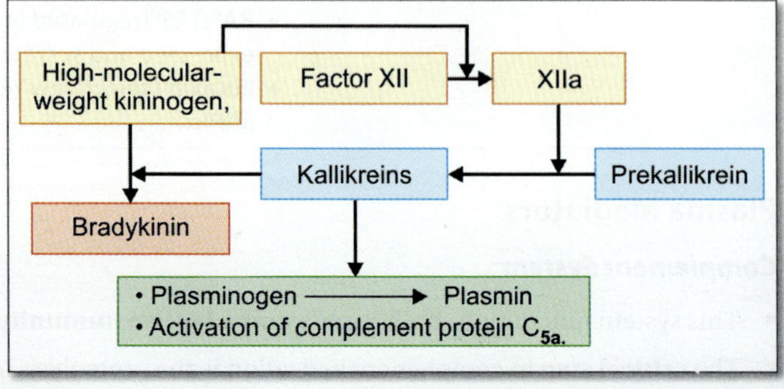

Functions of Bradykinin

- Increases vascular permeability, vasodilation
- Smooth muscle contraction **and pain** when injected into the skin.

ACUTE INFLAMMATION

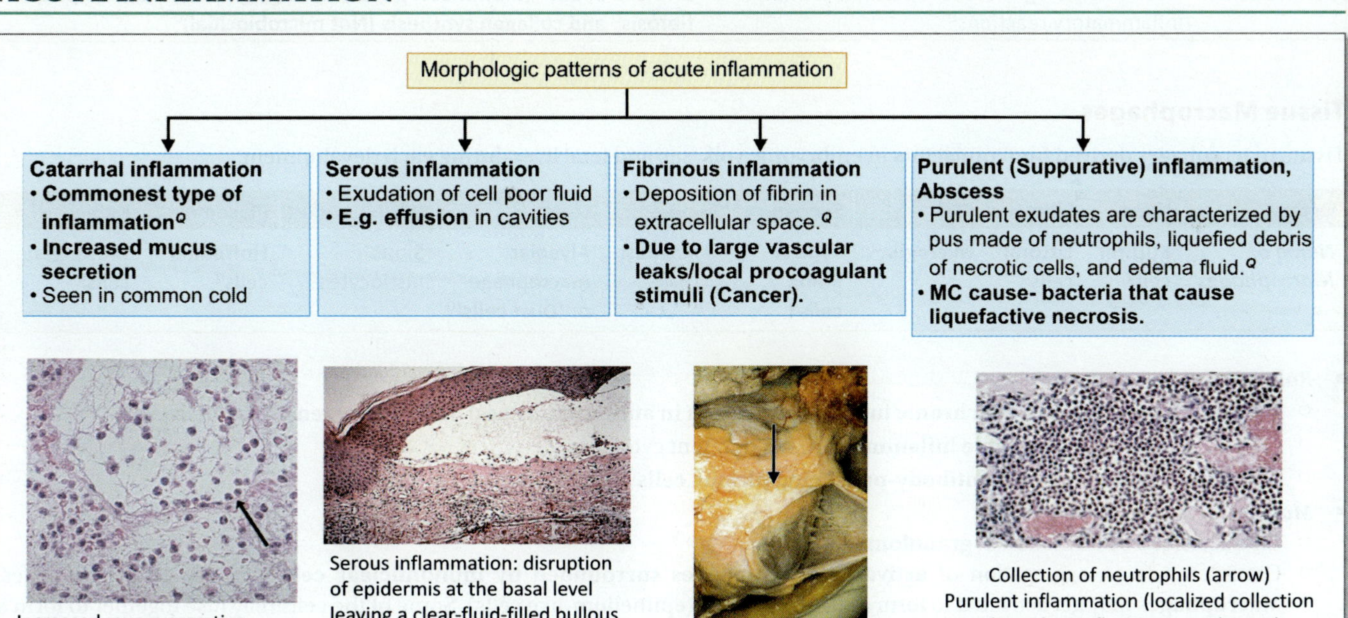

Increased mucus secretion (arrow) Catarrhal inflammation

Serous inflammation: disruption of epidermis at the basal level leaving a clear-fluid-filled bullous lesion

Fibrinous deposition (arrow)

Collection of neutrophils (arrow) Purulent inflammation (localized collection of purulent inflammation: Abscess)

Outcomes of Acute Inflammation

- **Complete resolution**
- **Healing by connective tissue replacement** (scarring, or fibrosis): A **process also called organization.**[Q]
- **Progression** of the response to **chronic inflammation**[Q]

CHRONIC INFLAMMATION

- **Seen in:** Persistent infections, hypersensitivity diseases and prolonged exposure to exogenous or endogenous toxic agents- e.g silicosis, atherosclerosis

- *Characterized by*
  - Infiltration with mononuclear cells-macrophages, lymphocytes, and plasma cells
  - **Tissue destruction- hallmark of chronic inflammation**[Q]
  - **Attempts at healing-via angiogenesis and fibrosis**
- Main Cells in Chronic Inflammation : Macrophages
  - Macrophages are tissue cells **derived from hematopoietic stem cells in the bone marrow and from progenitors in the embryonic yolk sac and fetal liver during early development**[Q]
  - **Half-life of blood monocytes is about 1 day**, whereas the **life span of tissue macrophages is several months or years.**[Q]

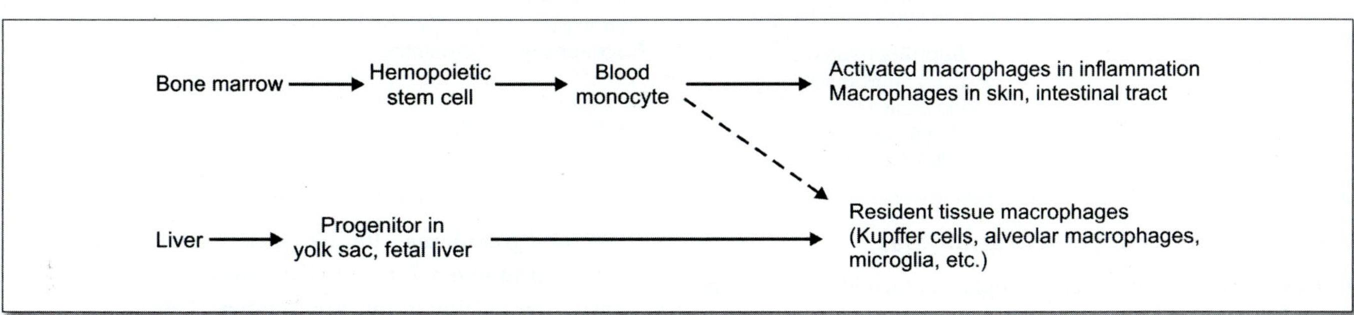

Two types of macrophages:
i. Activated macrophages
ii. Tissue macrophages

Activated Macrophages: 2 Major Types

Type	Classically Activated Macrophages (M1)	Alternatively Activated Macrophages (M2)
Induced by	**IFN-γ**, Microbial products-endotoxin.	**IL-4 and IL-13**: produced by T lymphocytes **(Cytokines other than IFNγ)[Q]**
Releases	**Lysosomal enzymes**, nitric oxide, **IL-1 and IL-12**, reactive oxygen species and NO	**IL-10[Q], TGF-B[Q]**
Involved in	**Host defence against microbes** and in many inflammatory reactions[Q]	Involved in **anti-inflammatory actions, Angiogenesis, Tissue repair, fibrosis[Q] and collagen synthesis (Not microbiocidal)[Q]**

Tissue Macrophages

Tissue macrophages derived from projectors in embryonic yolk sac and fetal liver during each development.

Organs	Liver	Spleen	CNS	Synovium	Bone	Lung	Lymph nodes	Placenta	Kidney
Name of Macrophages	Kupffer cell[Q]	Littoral cells[Q]	Microglia[Q]	Type A lining cells[Q]	Osteoclast	Alveolar macrophage or 'Dust cells'[Q]	Sinus histiocytes	Hoffbauer cells[Q]	Mesangial cells[Q]

- **Role of Lymphocytes**
  - ○ **Dominant population in the chronic inflammation seen in autoimmune and other hypersensitivity diseases[Q]**
  - ○ **CD4+ T lymphocytes promote inflammation[Q]** via different cytokines
  - ○ **Activated B lymphocytes & antibody-producing plasma cells** are also present
- *Morphological pattern*
  - ○ Characterized by formation of **granuloma.**
  - ○ Granuloma is an aggregation of **activated macrophages surrounded by mononuclear cells[Q]** principally lymphocytes. **Macrophages** may get activated to form **epithelioid cells** (epithelium-like cells). Some of the cells may fuse together to form a bigger cell called a **giant cell.**

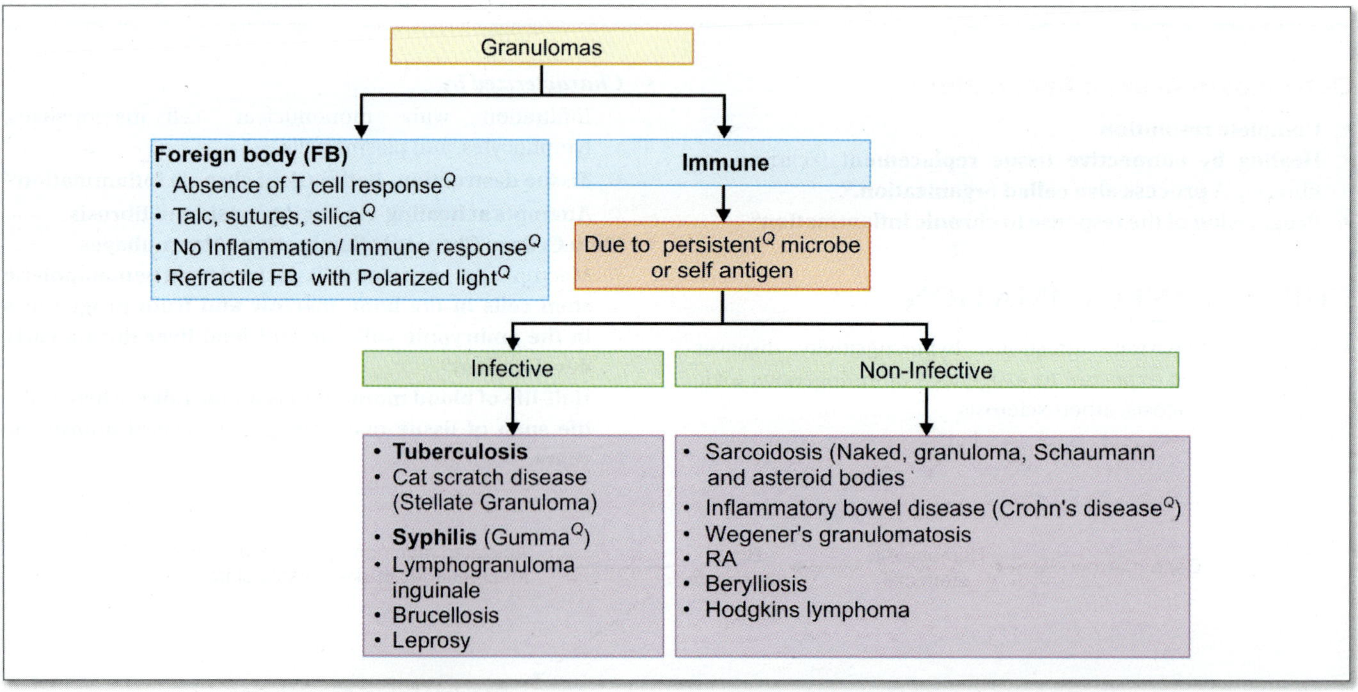

Unique Points of Certain Granulomas

- **Caseating granuloma:** TB, Histoplasma. Coccidioidomycosis, syphilis
- **Noncaseating granuloma:** Sarcoidosis Hodgkin's, TB
- **Naked granuloma:** Granuloma without peripheral rim of lymphocytes e.g. **sarcoidosis**
- **Palisaded granuloma**—RA, Wegener's granulomatosis
- **Stellate granuloma:** Cat scratch diseases
- **Fibrin ring or "doughnut" granulomas:** Q fever
- **Malarial granulomas (Durck's granuloma):** P. falciparum

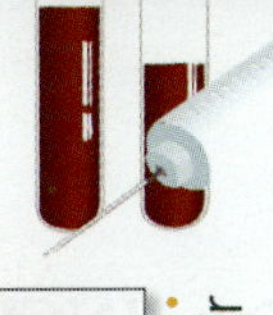

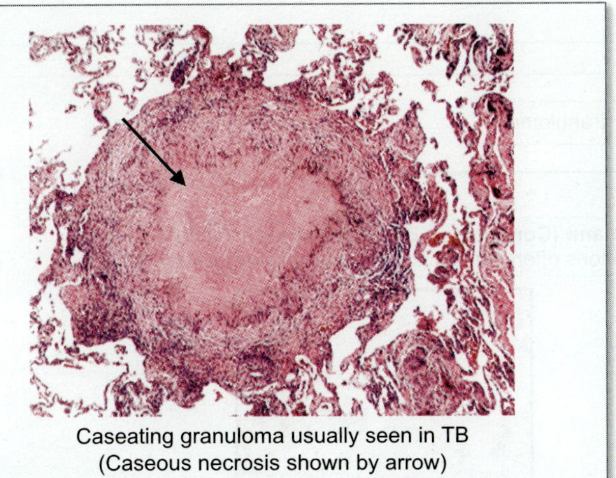

Caseating granuloma usually seen in TB
(Caseous necrosis shown by arrow)

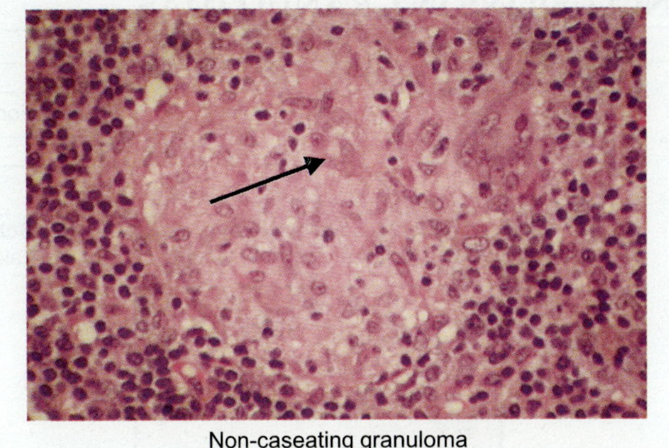

Non-caseating granuloma
(Epithelioid cells shown by arrow)

TYPES OF GIANT CELLS

Giant cells

Pathological

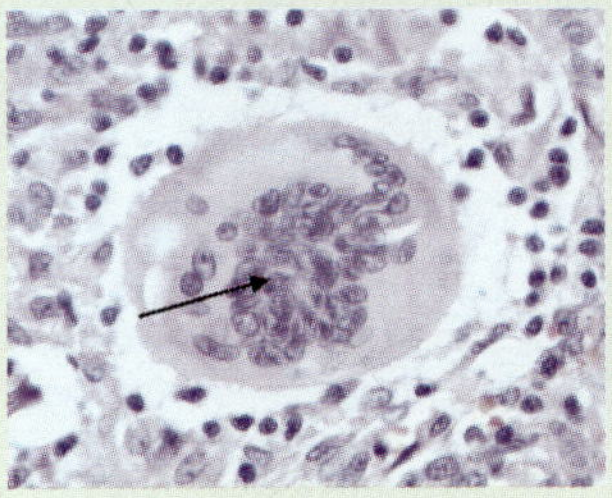

Physiological

Osteoclasts, synctiotrophoblasts, megakaryocytes (*Note:* megakaryocytes have multilobulated nuclei)

Foreign body giant cell
(Haphazardly arranged nuclei shown by arrow)

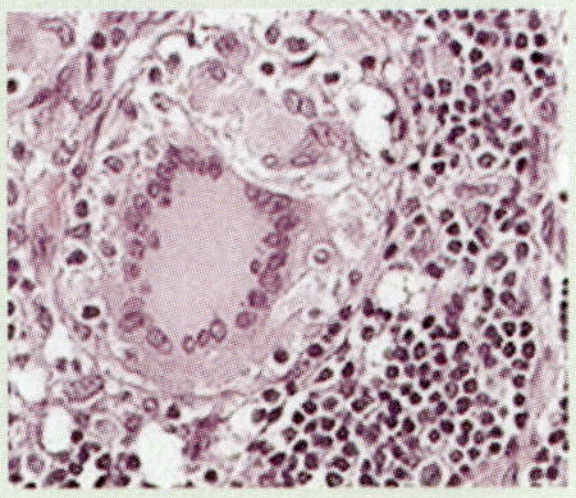

Langhans giant cells
(Nuclei arranged horseshoe-shaped shown by arrow)

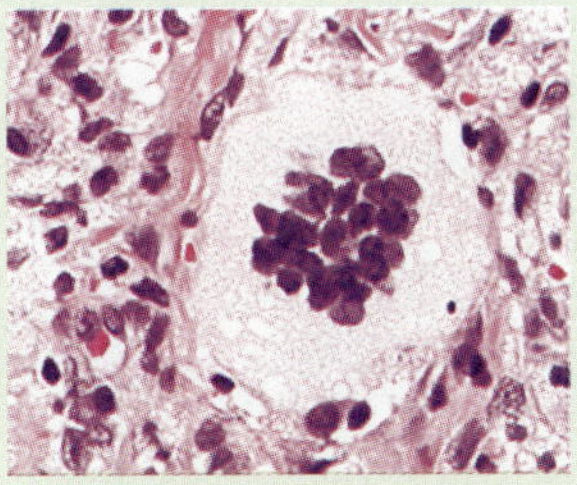

Touton giant cell
(Ring of nuclei surrounded by foamy cytoplasm)

Seen in TB

Seen in xanthomas

Special Type of Giant Cells
- Warthin-Finkeldey syncytial giant cell may have 50 nuclei, many with intranuclear inclusions 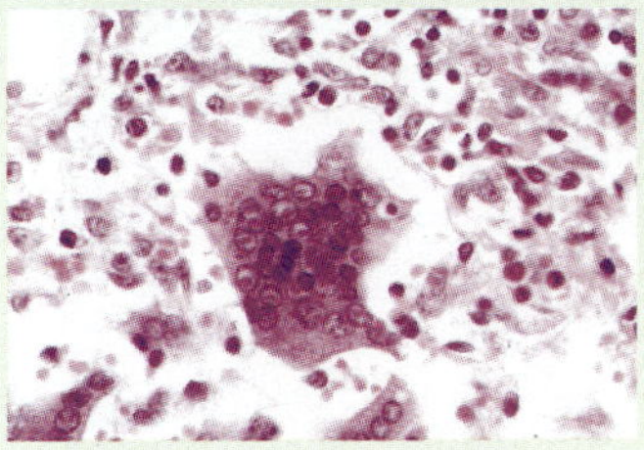
- Reed sternberg cells with eosinophilic nucleoli 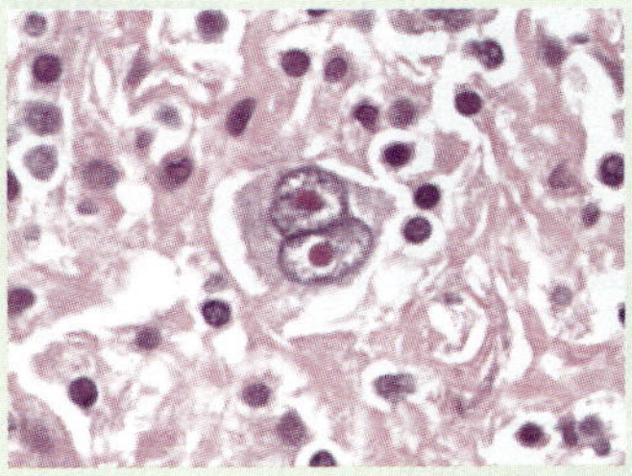
- Aschoff giant cells-Rheumatic heart disease

INCLUSIONS IN GRANULOMAS

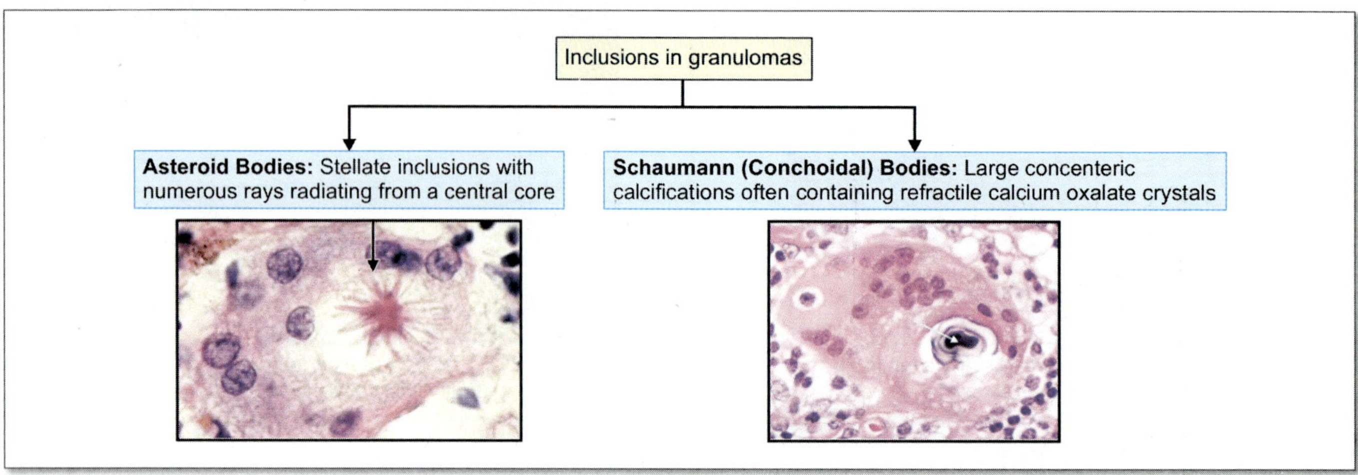

The details about lymphocytes, formation of a granuloma is discussed later in the chapter of 'immunity'.

SPECIAL TYPES OF GRANULOMA

Granuloma Morphology

- **Caseating** epithelioid cell granuloma (Caseous necrosis (green arrow) and Langhans cell (yellow arrow)

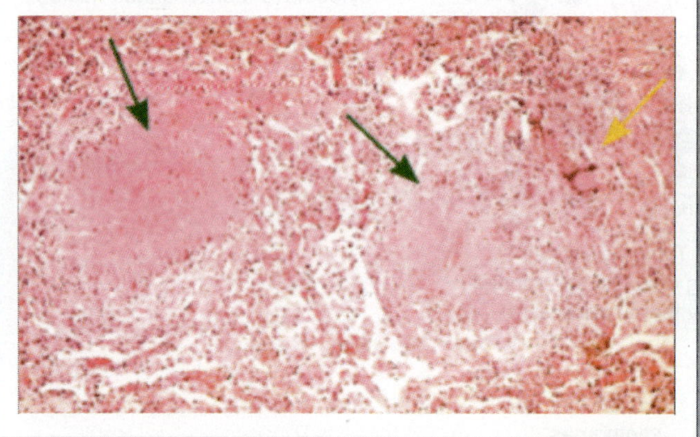

- **Foreign body granuloma:** (Refractile FB seenwith polarized light shown by arrows)

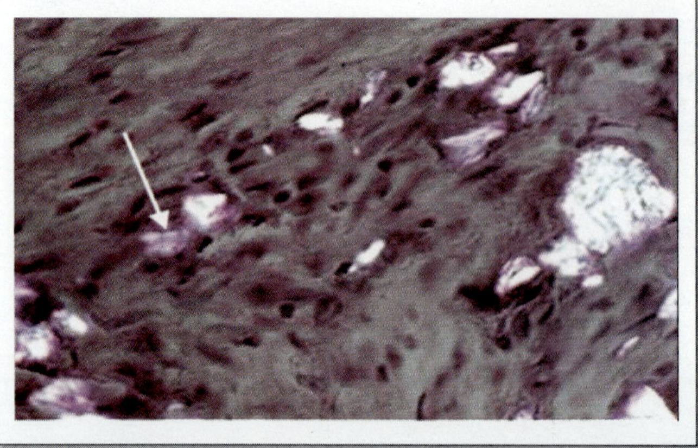

Palisaded granuloma

- Rheumatoid nodule
- Wegeneres granulomatosis

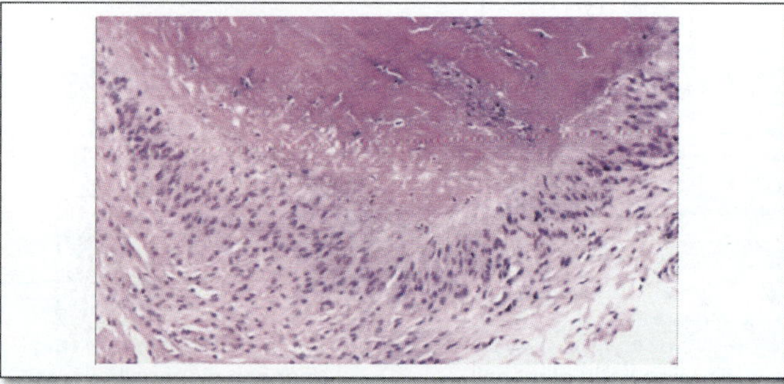

Stellate granuloma

- Stellate granuloma-follicular hyperplasia with central stellate necrosis with neutrophils, surrounded by palisading histiocytes.
- Most commonly found in children
- Benign infectious disease caused by the bacterium Bartonella henselae.
- Seen in cat scratch disease

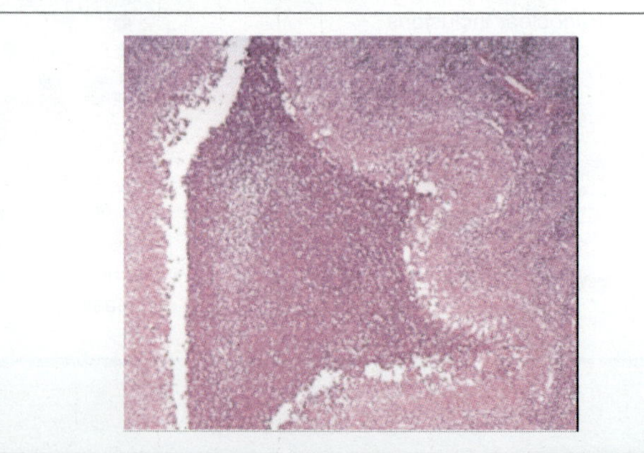

- A **fibrin ring** granuloma, also known as **doughnut** granuloma, is a histopathological finding that is characteristic of **Q fever**

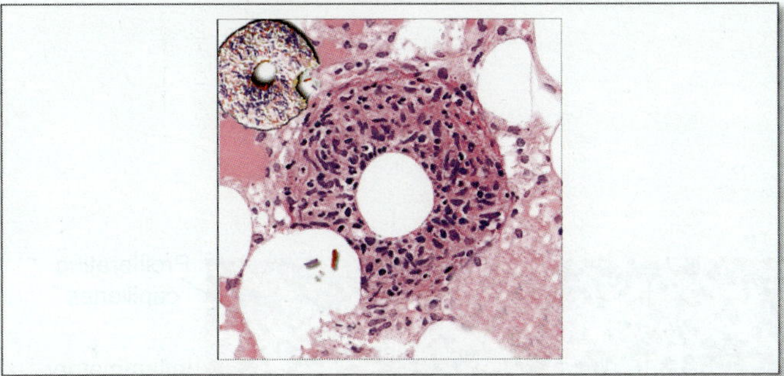

Malarial granulomas (Durck's granuloma)

- Focus of reactive astrocytosis admixed with microglial cells and lymphocytes surrounding a focus of ischemic necrosis or hemorrhage.
- Seen in P. Falciparum

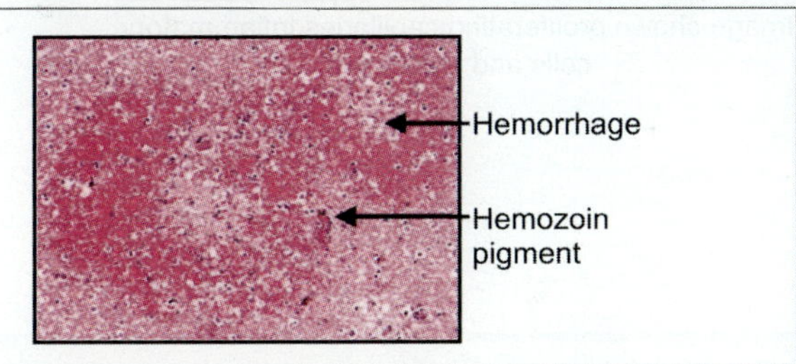

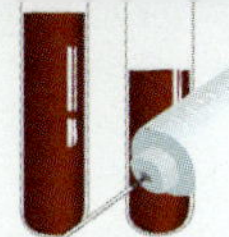

High Yield Facts

- **Granulomas are not seen in ulcerative colitis**[Q]
- **Non Immune granulomas**: Foreign body type granuloma e.g **Silica granulomas**[Q]
- **Necrotic granulomas**: TB, Syphilis, histoplasma, cat scratch disease, Wegners, granulomatosis, necrotizing sarcoidosis, bronchocentric granulomas
- **Tuberculosis can show both caseating and non caseating granulomas**[Q]
- Catscratch disease show stellate granuloma
- Sarcoidosis shows: (Non caseating granuloma, Schaumann and asteroid bodies[Q])
- Caseating granulomas shows langhans cells: TB

TISSUE REPAIR

- **Repair/healing** refers **to the incomplete restoration** of tissue architecture and function **after an injury**[Q]
- **Repair** is often used for **parenchymal and connective tissues,**[Q] healing is used for **surface epithelia**[Q]

Repair of damaged tissues occurs by two types of reactions:

Regeneration

- **Proliferation of cells** and tissues to **replace lost structures**.
- It results in complete restitution of lost or damaged tissue.

On the basis of intrinsic proliferative capacity, tissues are divided into:

Tissue Subtype	Labile (Continuously Dividing) Tissues	Stable Tissues	Permanent Tissues
Features	Continuously being lost and **replaced by maturation from tissue stem cells** and by **proliferation of mature cells**[Q]	Cells are in G_0 stage of the cell cycle. Minimal proliferative activity. However, **capable of dividing in response to injury or loss of tissue mass.**[Q]	Cells are **terminally differentiated and nonproliferative**[Q] in postnatal life.
Examples	• **Hematopoietic cells**[Q] • **Stratified squamous epithelia**[Q] of • **Cuboidal epithelia of** ducts draining exocrine organs • **Columnar epithelium** of the **GIT, FGS** • **Transitional epithelium**	• **Parenchyma of** liver, kidney, and pancreas. • **Endothelial cells, fibroblasts, and smooth muscle cells**[Q]	• **Neurons and cardiac**[Q] **muscle cells**[Q] • **Skeletal muscle**[Q]
Regeneration	**Completely regenerate**[Q]	**Limited capacity to regenerate** after injury **except liver**[Q]	Dominated by **scar formation.**[Q]

Connective Tissue Deposition (Scar Formation)

Occurs by the laying down **of connective (fibrous) tissue:**

- **Fibrosis: extensive deposition of collagen**[Q]
- **Organization: fibrosis develops in a tissue space occupied by an inflammatory exudate**

High Yield Facts

- Proliferation of **endothelial cells, fibroblasts, and smooth muscle cells** is important in **wound healing.**
- **Skeletal muscle** is usually classified as a **permanent tissue**
- **Satellite cells** attached to the **endomysial sheath** provide some **regenerative capacity for muscle.**
- **Granulation tissue**[Q] is the hallmark of the fibrogenic repair.
- Major cytokine involved in fibrosis is **Transforming growth factor- β (TGF- β)**[Q]
- TGF- β is the **most important cytokine**[Q] for the synthesis and deposition of connective tissue proteins
- Central **role in repair** of **TGF- β** is activation of **alternatively activated (M2) macrophages**[Q]

Steps in Scar Formation

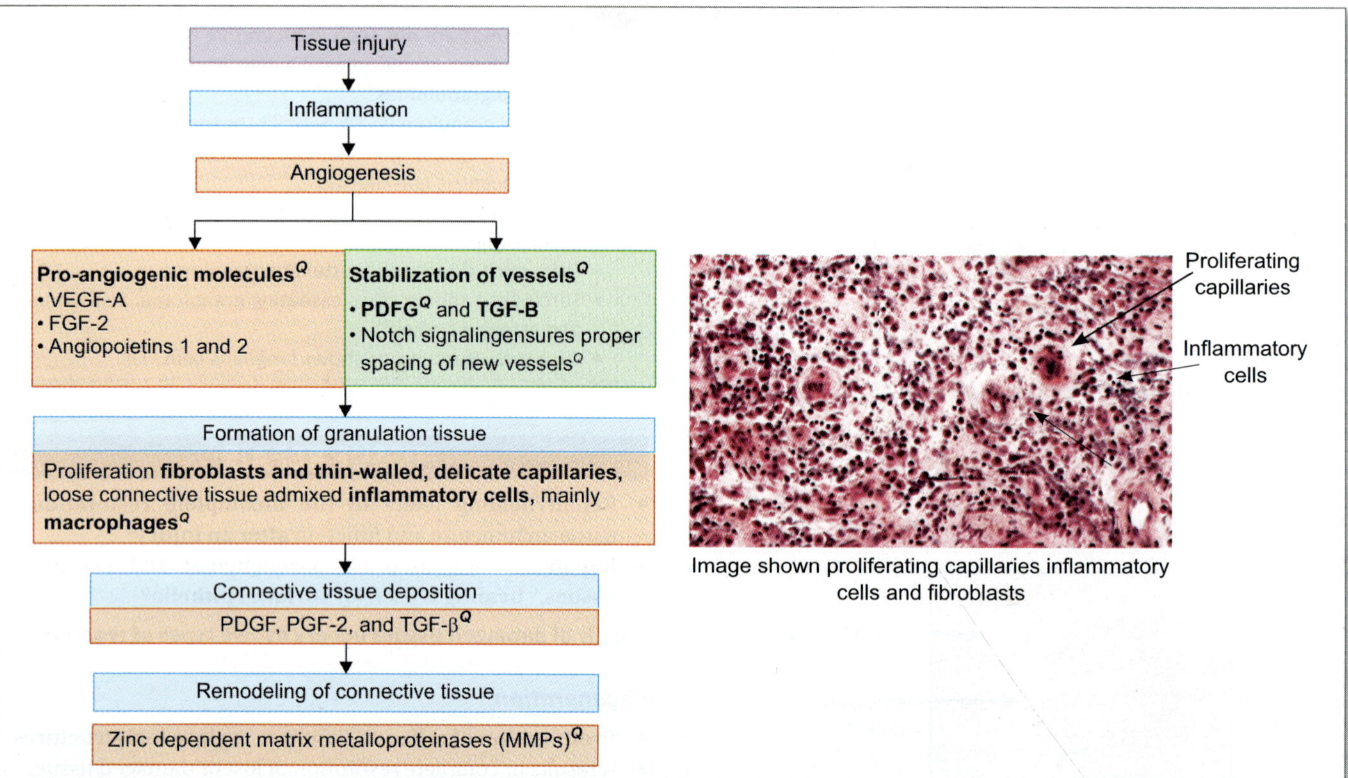

Image shown proliferating capillaries inflammatory cells and fibroblasts

R9th Latest Update

MMPs	Functions
• Interstitial collagenases	Cleave **fibrillar collagen** (MMP-1, -2 and -3);
• **Gelatinases**[Q] (MMP-2 and 9)	**Degrade amorphous collagen and fibronectin**
• **Stromelysins**[Q] (MMP-3, -10, and -11)	**Degrade a variety of ECM constituents**, including proteoglycans, laminin, fibronectin, and amorphous collagen

WOUND HEALING

Cutaneous Wound Healing

Three phases:
• Inflammation (early & late)
• Granulation tissue formation & re-epithelialization
• Wound contraction, ECM deposition & remodeling

Healing occurs in either of two ways:

By First Intention	By Second intention
• **Clean** and **less damage to cell & tissues, uninfected surgical incision**[Q]	• **Extensive loss of cells** and **tissues & infected**[Q]
• **Less intense inflammatory** reaction	• More **intense inflammatory reaction**[Q]
• **Limited granulation tissue** is formed	• Much **larger amounts of granulation tissue** are formed[Q]
	• **Wound contraction is present**[Q]

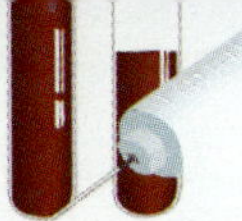

Healing of a Clean Uninfected Wound

Day (hrs)	Finding	
0	**Blood clot** SCAB	
1(24 hrs)	Neutrophils	
2(24–48 hrs)	Continuous thin epithelial layer[Q]	
3	• Macrophages • Appearance of **Granulation tissue**	• Deposition of type III collagen but they **do not bridge the incision**
5	• **Abundant granulation tissue** • **Collagen fibrils bridge the incision**	• **Neovascularization** is maximum • **Full epithelial thickness** with surface keratinization
14 (end of 2 weeks)	• **Accumulation of collagen**; fibroblast proliferation • Disappearance of inflammation • Blanching begins	
1 months	• **Replacement of collagen type III with collagen type I** (has greater tensile strength) • **Dermal appendages are permanantely lost**	

Wound Strength

- **Sutured wounds** have approximately **70% of the strength**[Q] of normal skin due to sutures
- When sutures are removed, **at 1 week,** wound strength is **10%**[Q] of that of unwounded skin[Q]
- Wound strength reaches **approximately 70% to 80% of normal by 3 months**[Q]
- Strength **never reaches 100%**[Q]

Abnormalities in Tissue Repair

Abnormalities in Tissue Repair	Conditions Associated	
Inadequate formation of granulation tissue	**Wound dehiscence and ulceration**[Q]	
Increased abdominal pressure[Q]	Dehiscence or rupture of a wound	
Excessive formation of granulation tissue	**Proud flesh**[Q], **Blocks re-epithelialization of wound**[Q]	
Excessive formation of collagen	**Keloid, hypertrophic scar**[Q]	
Exuberant proliferation of fibroblasts	Desmoids, or aggressive fibromatoses	
Contractures: Exaggerated contraction	• Seen in palms, soles, and the anterior aspect of the thorax • Commonly seen after serious burns • Can compromise the movement of joints	
Delayed wound healing	Due to **foreign body**, ischemia, **diabetes**[Q], malnutrition, hormones **(glucocorticoids)**[Q], **infection,**[Q] **zinc deficiency**[Q] **or scurvy**[Q]	Proud flesh

Disorders of Excessive Collagen	
Hypertrophic Scar	**Keloid**
• Scar **localized** to the wound • Usually regresses	• Scar **beyond the boundaries** of the original wound • **Does not regress**[Q] • **Genetically predisposed** condition, usually in African Americans[Q] • **Favoured sites**- sternum (**most common**), ear lobes[Q]

Hypertrophic scar (scar to localized to wound)

Keloid (scar beyond boundaries)

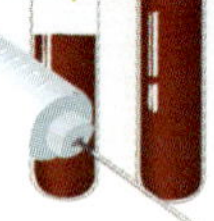

Fibrosis in Parenchymal Organs

- Fibrosis-**excessive deposition of collagen and other ECM components in a tissue**[Q]
- Major cytokine involved in fibrosis is **TGF-β.**[Q]
- Fibrotic disorders into liver cirrhosis

Liver Cirrhosis, systemic Sclerosis (Scleroderma), (idiopathic pulmonary fibrosis, pneumoconioses,), end-Stage Kidney disease and Constrictive Pericarditis.

High Yield Facts

- **Epidermal appendages do not regenerate**[Q]
- In **superficial wounds**, the epithelium is reconstituted and there may be **little scar formation**[Q].
- Predominant collagen in **adult skin is type I**[Q] whereas in **early granulation tissue, it is type III and I**[Q]
- Healing with secondary intension involves formation of a **network of actin-containing fibroblast**[Q] at the edges of the wound.[Q]
- **Permanent wound contraction** requires the **action of myofibroblasts**[Q] seen in healing by **secondary intention**[Q]
- **Myofibroblasts** are **altered fibroblasts** that have ultra-structural characteristics of smooth muscle cells.
- **Contraction of myofibroblasts**[Q] at the wound site **decreases the gap** between the dermal edges of the wound[Q]
- **Fetal cutaneous wounds heal without scar formation**[Q]
- These wounds show **little inflammation** and **practically no fibrosis**[Q].
- **Vitamin C** is required for the **conversion of tropocollagen to collagen**[Q]
- **Vitamin C** helps in **hydroxylation of lysine and proline**[Q] residues providing **stability to collagen molecules**

R10th And Other Latest Update

ACUTE PHASE REACTANTS

Inflammation is associated with cytokine-induced systemic reactions that are collectively called the acute-phase response.

Positive APPs	Negative APPs
- **C-reactive protein** (CRP) - **Serum Amyloid A** (SAA) - **Haptoglobin (Hp)** - **Ceruloplasmin** - α2-Macroglobulin - α1-Acid glycoprotein (AGP) - **Fibrinogen** - **Complement (C3, C4)**	- Albumin - Transferrin - Transthyretin - Retinol-binding protein

EMPERIPOLESIS

- The engulfed cell is viable without physiological or morphological changes
- Unlike in phagocytosis where the engulfed cell is killed by lysosomal enzymes of the macrophage, the cell exists as viable cell within another in emperipolesis and can exit at any time without any structural or functional abnormalities for either of them.

- Seen in:

Rosai—Dorfman disease
- Hematolymphoid disorders[Q] (Hodgkin's disease, leukemia, acute and chronic myeloid leukemia, Non-Hodgkin's lymphoma, myeloproliferative disorders)
- Non-hematological malignancies (neuroblastoma, Rhabdomyosarcoma)

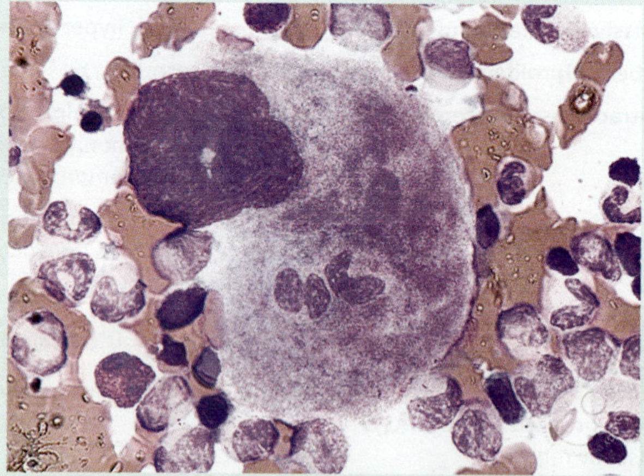
MIC Showing Emperipolesis in megakaryocyte

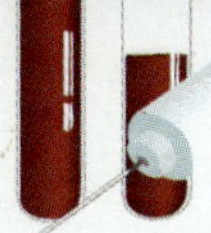

NEXT Pattern Questions

Q's

1. **A 4-year-old child has a history of recurrent infections with pyogenic bacteria. The infections are accompanied by a neutrophilic leukocytosis. Microscopic examination of a biopsy specimen obtained from an area of soft tissue necrosis shows microbial organisms, but very few neutrophils. An analysis of neutrophil function shows a defect in adhesion. This child's increased susceptibility to infection is most likely caused by a defect involving which of the following molecules?**

   a. Complement C3b   b. Integrins   c. Leukotriene B4   d. Selectins

Ans. (b) Integrins

(Ref: Robins Basic Pathology 10th/pg 60)

- Leukocyte rolling is the first step in transmigration of neutrophils from the vasculature to the tissues. Rolling depends on interaction between selectins (P-selectin and E-selectin on endothelial cells, and L-selectin on neutrophils) and their sialylated ligands (e.g., sialylated Lewis X). Integrins (B1 and B2) are involved in the next step of adhesion during which there is firm adhesion between neutrophils and endothelial cells. Complement C3b acts as an opsonin to facilitate phagocytosis. Leukotriene B4 is a chemotactic agent.

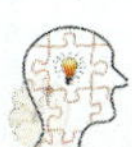

Q's

2. **A 50-year-old woman has had a high fever and cough productive of yellowish sputum for the past 2 days. Her vital signs include temperature of 37.8°C, pulse 103/min, respirations 25/min, and blood pressure 100/60 mm Hg. On auscultation of the chest, crackles are audible in both lung bases. The microscopic appearance of her lung is shown in the figure. Which of the following inflammatory cell types is most likely to be seen in greatly increased numbers in her sputum specimen?**

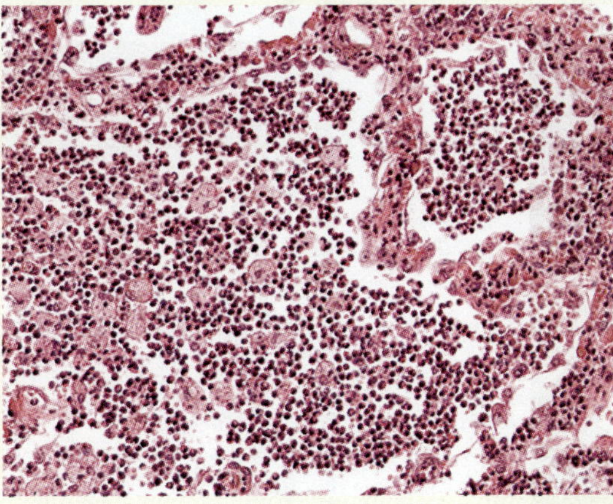

   a. Langhans giant cells   b. Macrophages   c. Mast cells   d. Neutrophils

Ans. (d) Neutrophils

(Ref: Robins Basic Pathology 10th/pg 63)

- These signs and symptoms suggest acute bacterial pneumonia. Such infections induce an acute inflammation dominated by neutrophils that fill alveoli, as shown in the figure, and are coughed up, which gives the sputum its yellowish, purulent appearance. Langhans giant cells are seen with granulomatous inflammatory responses. Macrophages become more numerous after initiation of acute events, cleaning up tissue and bacterial debris through phagocytosis. Mast cells are better known as participants in allergic and anaphylactic responses. Lymphocytes are a feature of chronic inflammation

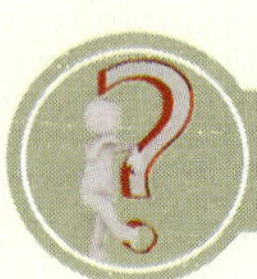

Image-Based Questions

1. A 5-year-old child presented with high grade fever and dyspnea. He also developed pleural effusion. Pleural tapping was done within 24 hours of presentation. Which is the predominant cell population seen?

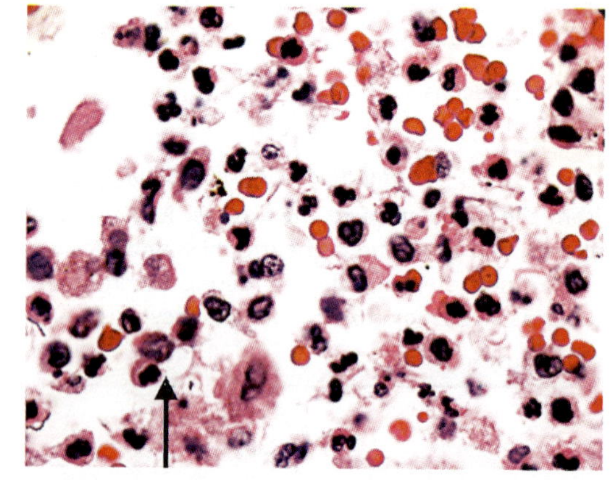

a. Neutrophils
b. Lymphocytes
c. Monocytes
d. Eosinophils

2. Autopsy finding of 25-year-old male who died of chest pain. Diagnosis is:

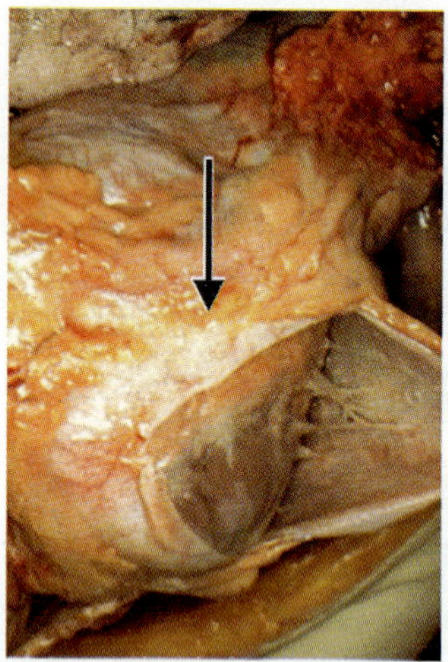

a. Fibrinous pericarditis
b. Serous pericarditis
c. Purulent pericarditis
d. Caseous pericarditis

3. Autopsy finding in a 45-year-old male adrenals. Diagnosis is:

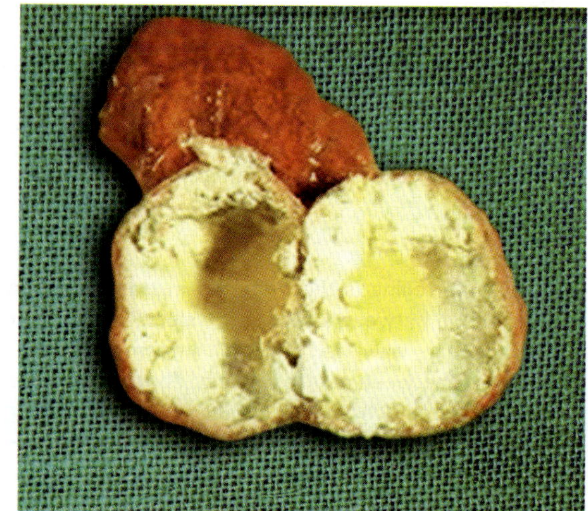

a. Caseous necrosis
b. Fibrinoid necrosis
c. Fat necrosis
d. Liquefactive necrosis

4. A 5-year-old male had fever and cervical lymphadenopathy. Histopathologic examination of cervical lymph nodes shows:

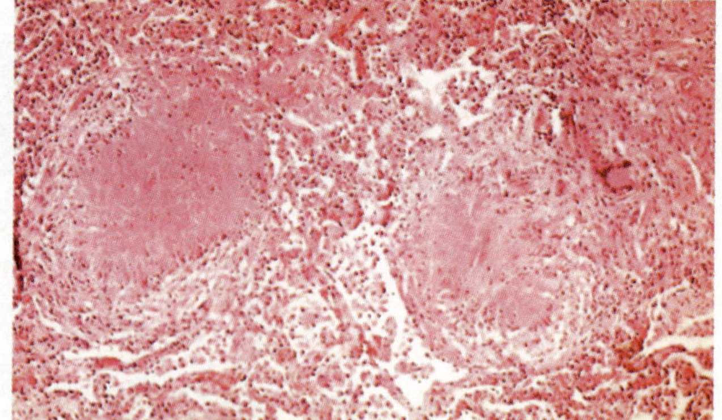

a. Caseating granuloma
b. Non caseating granuloma
c. Stellate granuloma
d. Fat necrosis

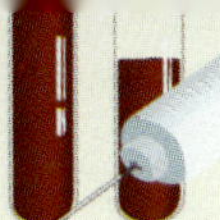

5. A 25-year-old male underwent a blunt trauma. On repair, following changes were noted:

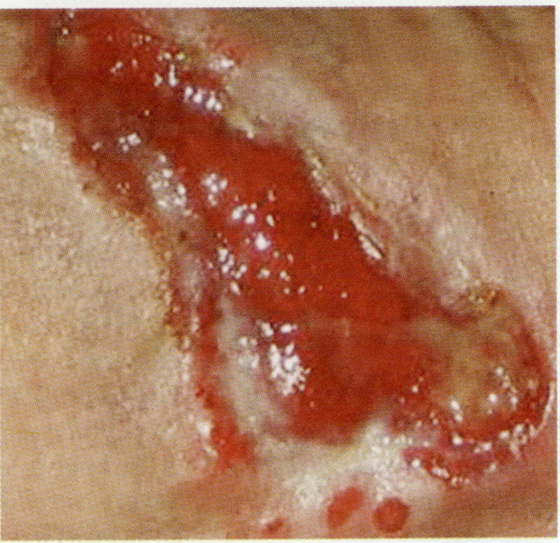

a. Keloid
b. Hypertrophic scar
c. Proud flesh
d. Desmoid

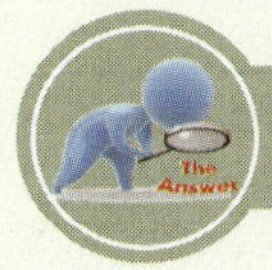

Answers of Image-Based Questions

1. **Ans. (a) Neutrophils**
   - Neutrophils are predominant infiltrate within 24 hours of injury

2. **Ans. (a) Fibrinous pericarditis**
   - Adherent pericardium has been opened to reveal the surface of the heart. There are thin strands of fibrinous exudate that extend from the epicardial surface to the pericardial sac. This is typical for a fibrinous pericarditis.

3. **Ans. (a) Caseous necrosis**
   - We can see cheesy white necrosis, the patient probably died of disseminated tuberculosis

4. **Ans. (a) Caseating granuloma**
   - Caseating granuloma typical granuloma resulting from infection with Mycobacterium tuberculosis showing central area of caseous necrosis, activated epithelioid macrophages, giant cells, and a peripheral accumulation of lymphocytes.. We can also see langhans giant cell at 3, 0 clock position in image

5. **Ans. (c) Proud flesh**
   - Excessive formation of granulation tissue can be seen.

Multiple Choice Questions

ACUTE INFLAMMATION AND MECHANISMS

1. In which of the following condition(s) erythrocyte sedimentation rate is increased: *(PGI May 2019)*
a. Increased serum immunoglobulin level
b. Spherocytosis
c. Increased plasma viscosity
d. Sickle cell anemia
e. Increased level of C-reactive protein

2. Match the following about the endothelial contraction: *(AIIMS May 2019)*

Column-A	Column-B
1. Sunburn less than 24 hrs	a. Immediate sustained
2. Thorn prick and mast release	b. Delayed prolonged
3. Bacterial infection with necrosis	c. Immediate transient

a. 1-a, 2-b, 3-c
b. 1-b, 2-a, 3-c
c. 1-b, 2-c, 3-a
d. 1-a, 2-c, 3-b

3. Which of the following causes vasodilation? *(AIIMS Nov 2019)*
a. TXA2
b. Leukotriene C4
c. Histamine
d. Serotonin

4. Identify the arrow marked cell in the given condition below: *(AIIMS May 16)*

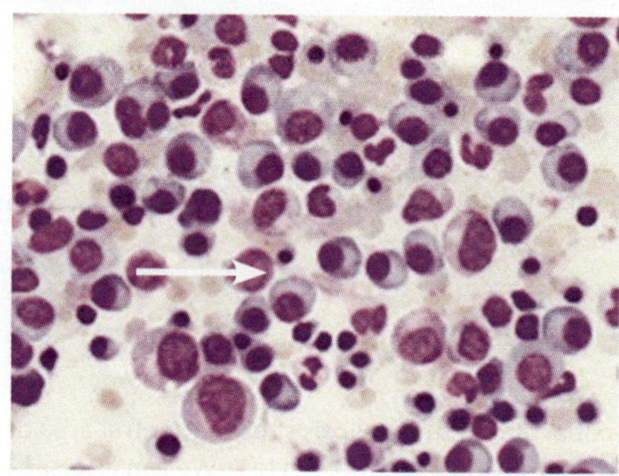

a. Macrophage
b. Lymphocyte
c. Plasma cell
d. Eosinophil

5. Which of the following cells will increase in case of parasite infection? *(AIIMS May 16)*

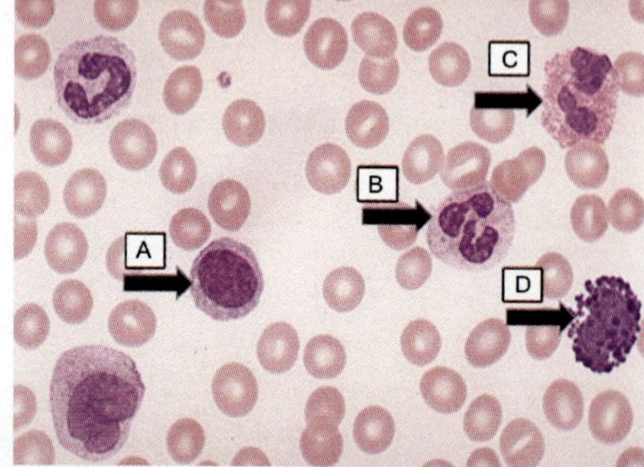

a. A
b. B
c. C
d. D

6. Vasoconstricttion in acute inflammation shown by *(WB PGMEE 2016, Recent Question 2016)*
a. Venules
b. Arterioles
c. Capillaries
d. Vein

7. SIRS diagnostic criteria. Wrong statement is *(Recent Question 2016)*
a. Band >10%
b. Leucocyte >12000 cells/mm³
c. Respi. rate >20
d. Band <5%

8. Eosinophillia is found in: *(Recent Question 2016)*
a. Cryptococcus
b. HPV
c. Stronglyloides
d. Typhoid

9. Severe infection will increase if absolute neutrophil count will become? *(Recent Question 2015)*
a. <500
b. Less than 800
c. Less than 1000
d. Less than 2000

10. Vasodilation in acute inflammation is first shown by: *(Recent Question 2015)*
a. Venules
b. Arterioles
c. Capillaries
d. Vein

11. Cellular infiltrate seen in late pseudomonas infection is formed mainly by *(Recent Question 2014-15)*
a. Neutrophils
b. Lymphocytes
c. Monocytes
d. Plasma cells

12. Which of the following is the mechanism of "late appearing sunburn"? *(Recent Question 2015)*
a. Leucocyte mediated injury
b. Delayed prolonged leakage
c. Early prolonged leakage
d. Delayed transient leakage

13. Increased permeability in acute inflammation is due to- *(Recent Question 2014)*
a. Histamine
b. IL-2
c. TGFβ
d. FGF

14. Sequence of events in acute inflammation-
a. Vasodilatation → Stasis → Transient vasoconstriction → Increased permeability *(Recent Question 2014)*
b. Transient vasoconstriction → Increased permeability → Stasis → Vasodilatation →
c. Transient vasoconstriction → Vasodilatation → Stasis → Increased permeability
d. Transient vasoconstriction → Vasodilatation → Increased permeability → Stasis

15. The following is not an adhesion molecule?
a. Spectrin *(JIPMER 2014)*
b. Integrins
c. Selectins
d. Cadherin

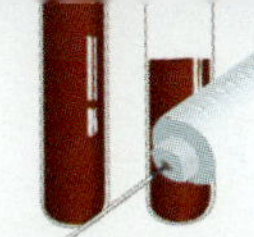

PATHOPHYSIOLOGY OF ACUTE INFLAMMATION

16. The RBCs with schizonts of P. Falciparum are not visible on peripheral blood smear due to which of the following reason? *(AIIMS Nov 16)*

a. Capillary adherence or sequestration of parasitized RBCs

b. ADCC mediated RBC destruction

c. Selective hemolysis of affected RBCs in spleen

d. Cellular lysis due to hemozoin produced by the parasites Erythrocyte Changes in Malaria

17. Amino acid which is useful in Neutrophil extracellular traps (NETs) as to causes lysis of chromatin is? *(JIPMER 2016)*

a. Arginine   b. Alanine

c. Phenyl alanine   d. Valine

18. The following statements are true regarding neutrophil extracellular trap *(Recent Question 2015)*

a. Produced by neutrophils in response to infectious pathogens and inflammatory mediators

b. Provide a high concentration of antimicrobial substances at sites of infection

c. Prevent the spread of the microbes by trapping them in the fibrils

d. All the above

19. All of the following vascular changes are observed in acute inflammation, except: *(Recent Question 2015)*

a. Vasodilation

b. Stasis of blood

c. Increased vascular permeability

d. Decreased hydrostatic pressure

20. Correct sequence in extravasation of leukocytes is: *(Recent Question 2015)*

a. Margination - rolling- adhesion – transmigration

b. Transmigration- margination – rolling-adhesion

c. Rolling- adhesion- transmigration- margination

d. Adhesion- transmigration- margination-rolling

21. Transcytosis is: *(Recent Question 2015)*

a. Transport of fluids and proteins through endothelial cells

b. Migration of neutrophils through endothelial cell

c. Migration of platelets through endothelial cell

d. Locomotion oriented along chemical gradient

22. Transmigration of WBC across the endothelium is called: *(Recent Question 2015)*

a. Margination   b. Rolling

c. Pavementing   d. Diapedesis

23. All the statements are correct in autophagy, except: *(AP 2014)*

a. It is a process in which a cell eats its own contents

b. It is a survival mechanism in times of nutrient deprivation

c. The starved cell lives by cannibalizing itself and recycling the digested contents

d. It is not regulated by any defined set of "genes"

24. Most characteristic feature of acute inflammation: *(AI 11, AIIMS May 10)*

a. Vasoconstriction

b. Vascular stasis

c. Vasodilatation and increased vascular permeability

d. Margination of leucocytes

25. In acute inflammation due to the retraction of endothelial cell cytoskeleton, which of the following results - *(AIIMS Nov 11)*

a. Delayed transient increase in permeability

b. Early transient increase in permeability

c. Delayed prolonged increase in permeability

d. Early permanent increase in permeability

MOLECULAR & CELLULAR PATHOLOGY OF ACUTE INFLAMMATION

26. Which of the following is the correct sequence of cellular events of acute inflammation? *(AIIMS May 18)*

a. Rolling----Stable adhesion---Activation of integrins----migration via endothelium.

b. Rolling ----Activation of Integrins---- Stable Adhesion----migration via endothelium.

c. Stable adhesion---Rolling----Activation of integrins----migration via endothelium.

d. Activation of integrins---- migration via endothelium---stable adhesion--- Rolling.

27. Which of the following involved in leukocyte attachment and emigration during inflammation? *(PGI May 18)*

a. Complement C5a   b. Integrin

c. L-selectin   d. Leukotriene B4

e. Interleukin-8

28. Esterase inhibitor deficiency causes:

a. SLE   *(Recent Question 2015)*

b. MPGN

c. Hereditary angioneurotic edema

d. Omen syndrome

29. Which of the following is an alpha chemokine? *(Recent Question 2015)*

a. IL-8   b. MCP-1

c. Eotaxin   d. Lymphotactin

30. Role of hydroxyl-eicosatetraenoic acid (HETE) in inflammation *(Recent Question 2015)*

a. Vasodilation

b. Vasoconstriction

c. Increased vascular permeability

d. Chemotaxis

31. Leukocyte migration through endothelium is induced by *(Recent Question 2015)*

a. Selectin   b. N CAM

c. CAM   d. PECAM

32. Locomotion across chemical gradient is called

a. Diapedesis   b. Chemotaxis

c. Pavementing   d. Margination

33. Which selectin is stored in weibel palade bodies? *(Recent Question 2015)*

a. Cadherins   b. P-Selectin

c. E-Selectins   d. L-Selectin

34. Which of the following enzymes are responsible for generating 'oxygen burst' within neutrophils for killing intracellular bacteria? *(Recent Question 2014)*

a. Superoxide dismutase   b. Glutathione peroxidase

c. Oxidase   d. Catalase

35. Role of P-selectin in inflammation- *(Recent Question 2013)*

a. Rolling   b. Adhesion

c. Homing   d. Transmigration

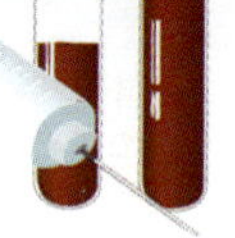

36. Chemotaxis in response to activation of cells results in-
(PGI 2002, AIIMS May 10)
a. Random multidirectional movement
b. Unidirectional motion
c. Adhesion to endothelium
d. Augmeted oxygen dependent bactericidal effect
e. Phagocytosis

37. Which among the following is not an adhesion molecule?
a. Integrin   b. Selectin   *(DNB Dec 10)*
c. Interferon   d. Transferrin

MEDIATORS OF INFLAMMATION

38. Which of the following is/are is endogenous pyrogen?
(Recent Question 2019)
a. IL1   b. TNF
c. Lipopolysaccharride   d. Both a&b

39. Which of the following enzyme is in 1 granule of neutrophil? *(Recent Question 2019)*
a. Alkaline phosphatase
b. Lactoferrin
c. Elastase
d. Lysozyme

40. Which of the following is an Opsonin?
a. C3a   b. C3b   *(Recent exam 2018)*
c. C5a   c. LTC4

41. Which of the cell derived chemical mediators of inflammation is/are preformed in secretory granules?
(PGI Nov 2017)
a. Histamine   b. Lysosomal enzymes
b. Leukotrienes   d. Prostaglandins
e. Serotonin

42. Which of the following is a negative acute phase reactant? *(AIIMS May 2017)*
a. Albumin   b. Haptaglobin
c. Ferritin   d. C reactive protein

43. What decreases during acute inflammation?
(PGI May 2017)
a. Ceruloplasmin   b. Transferrin
c. CRP   d. ESR
e. Albumin

44. Interleukin secreted by Th17 cells   *(JIPMER 2016)*
a. IFN Gamma   b. IL22
c. IL6   d. 1L16

45. 10-year-old male child complains of pain and swelling in the left foot. He gives history of injury while playing. Migration of leukocytes to the site of injury is mediated by:
a. Cytokines   *(JIPMER 2016)*
b. Histamine
c. Chemokines
d. Prostaglandins

46. Which of the following is not an activator of alternate complement system? *(JIPMER 2016)*
a. Factor H   b. IgA
c. Bacteria   d. Immune complex

47. Integrins are involved in: *(JIPMER 2016)*
a. Adhesion   b. Rolling
c. Transmigration   d. Opsonization

48. Complement complex that attacks cell membrane is:
a. C12345   b. C23456   *(AIIMS May 16)*
c. C34567   d. C56789

49. Serotonin, a mediator of inflammation in our body, is secreted/released by: *(PGI May 16)*
a. Leukocytes   b. Endothelial cell
c. Mast cell   d. Platelet
e. Macrophage

50. Th1 cells produce? *(Recent Question 2016-17)*
a. IL-1   b. IL-2
c. IL-4   d. IL-5

51. Primary granule of neutrophil has?
(Recent Question 2016-17)
a. Proteinase 3   b. Alkaline phosphatse
c. Acid protease   d. Lactoferrin

52. Interleukin responsible in surgical trauma.
(Recent Question 2016)
a. IL-1   b. IL-2
c. IL-3   d. IL-4

53. Late complement factor deficiency leads to:
a. Herediatry angioneurotic edema *(Recent Question 2016)*
b. SLE
c. Recurrent infections like Neisseria & Pnemococci
d. HUS

54. Major basic protein is found in? *(Recent Question 2016)*
a. Macrophage   b. Eosinophils
c. Basophil   d. Neutrophil

55. Most important pyogenic Interleukin is?
(Recent Question 2016)
a. IL-2   b. 1L-1
c. IL-6   d. IL-8

56. Membrane attack complex   *(Recent Question 2016)*
a. C5-9   b. C3
c. C2   d. C1

57. Bronchospasm is initiated by?   *(Recent Question 2014)*
a. C5a   b. C3a
c. Leukotrienes   d. Acetylcholines

58. Which of the following is the chief mediator associated with resetting the hypothalamic temperature set point at a higher level, resulting in fever? *(Recent Question 2015)*
a. PGF2 alpha   b. PGE1
c. PGE2   d. PGI2

59. Which of the following is a major pyrogenic cytokine
(Recent Question 2015)
a. IL-12   b. TNF
c. IFN-Y   d. Bradykin

60. The following is not a preformed chemical mediator of inflammation *(Recent Question 2015)*
a. Prostaglandins
b. Histamine
c. Serotonin
d. Lysosomal enzymes

61. Pain during inflammation is mediated by:
a. Nitric oxide   *(Recent Question 2015)*
b. Leukotriene B4
c. Bradykinin
d. Chemokines

62. **The following is not a chemoattactant in acute inflammation** *(Recent Question 2015)*
    a. IL-8
    b. CSa
    c. LTB4
    d. Kinins

63. **The following is not a pyrogenic cytokine** *(Recent Question 2015)*
    a. IL-1
    b. TNF
    c. Substance P
    d. Prostaglandins

64. **Anti-inflammatory cytokine** *(Recent Question 2015)*
    a. IL-1
    b. IL-4
    c. TNF
    d. IFN-Y

65. **All are major cytokines in chronic inflammation except** *(Recent Question 2015)*
    a. IL-6
    b. IL-12
    c. IFN-y
    d. IL-17

66. **The following enzyme is otherwise called TACE (TNF converting enzyme)** *(Recent Question 2015)*
    a. Matrix metalloproteinase
    b. Serine proteinase
    c. ADAM-17
    d. Interstitial collagenase

67. **Most important cytokine for the synthesis and deposition of connective tissue proteins** *(Recent Question 2015)*
    a. TGF-α
    b. TGF-β
    c. FGF-1
    d. FGF-2

68. **Angiogenesis is stimulated by all except** *(Recent Question 2015)*
    a. PDGE
    b. VEGF
    c. FGF
    d. HGF

69. **TNF and IL1 are produced by** *(Recent Question 2014-15)*
    a. Neutrophils
    b. Monocytes
    c. Lymphocytes
    d. Activated Macrophages

70. **Which is not the action of TGF-β**
    a. Anti-inflammatory *(Recent Question 2014-15)*
    b. Proliferation of fibrous tissue
    c. Inhibition of metalloproteinases
    d. Anaphylaxis

71. **Which of the following doesn't belong to Interleukin-2 (IL-2) Subfamily** *(Recent Question 2015)*
    a. IL-2
    b. IL-3
    c. IL-4
    d. IL-1

72. **Which of the following is not endogenous pyrogens?** *(Recent Question 2015)*
    a. IL 6
    b. IL 1 beta
    c. IL 12
    d. TNF alpha

73. **Which of the following is NOT an anaphylatoxin?** *(Recent Question 2014)*
    a. C3a
    b. C4a
    c. C3b
    d. C5a

74. **What is not caused by platelet activating factor?** *(Recent Question 2014)*
    a. Vasoconstriction
    b. Bronchodilation
    c. Causes platelet aggregation
    d. Transmits signals between cells

75. **Which of the following chemical mediator is not a cell derived mediator?** *(JIPMER 2014)*
    a. Leukotrines
    b. Kinins
    c. Cytokines
    d. Prostaglandins

76. **Cytokines responsible for synthesis of acute phase reactant are all except ?** *(Recent Question 2013)*
    a. IL 1
    b. IL 11
    c. IL 6
    d. TNF

77. **Which of the following is anti inflammatory?** *(Recent Question 2013)*
    a. IL-2
    b. IL4
    c. IL-6
    d. IL-10

78. **Which interleukin is required for differentiation of eosinophils?** *(DNB Aug. 12)*
    a. IL-1
    b. IL-3
    c. ITA
    d. IL-5

79. **Important inflammatory mediators is/are:** *(PGI Nov 2011)*
    a. IL-2
    b. IL-6
    c. TNF-alpha
    d. Platelet activating factor
    e. Interferons

80. **Acute phase reactant(s) in acute inflammation is/are:** *(PGI Nov 2011, 08)*
    a. Haptoglobin
    b. C-reactive protein
    c. Alpha-1 acid glycoprotein
    d. Prostaglandins
    e. Fibrinogen

81. **Actions of bradykinin include all of the following, except-**
    a. Vasodilatation *(AI 10)*
    b. Bronchodilatation
    c. Increased vascular permeability
    d. Pain

82. **All of the following are mediators of inflammation except** *(AIIMS May 2005, Nov 10)*
    a. Tumour necrosis factor-a (TNF-a)
    b. Interleukin-l
    c. Myeloperoxidase
    d. Prostaglandins

83. **Resolution of inflammation caused by -**
    a. TNF Alfa, IL-1 and CRP *(DNB Dec 10)*
    b. TN F beta, IL-6 and CRP
    c. TNF Alfa, IL 10 and IL1 receptor antagonist
    d. TNF gamma

84. **Histamine causes all except:** *(DNB June 10)*
    a. Arteriolar dilatation
    b. Increased permeability of venules
    c. Constriction of large arteries
    d. Platelet aggregation

85. **C in CRP stands for -** *(DNB June 10)*
    a. Concanavalin A
    b. Chondroitin sulfate in series with ARP, BRP
    c. Capsular polysaccharide of pneumococcus
    d. Cellular

86. **Endogenous chemoattractants are all except -** *(MH 10)*
    a. C5a
    b. Integrins
    c. LTB4
    d. IL8

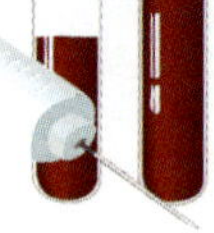

87. Pro inflammatory Cytokines include all of the following except -
   a. Interleukin 1
   b. Interleukin 2
   c. Interleukin 6
   d. TNF- Alpha

MORPHOLOGIC PATTERNS OF ACUTE INFLAMMATION

88. All are true about serous inflammation except
(Recent Question 2015)
   a. A pattern of acute inflammation
   b. Exudation of cell-poor fluid
   c. Fluid in infected by destructive organism
   d. Fluid does not contain large numbers of leukocytes

89. Exudation of cell-poor fluid that is not infected by destructive organisms is characteristic of:
   a. Fibrinous inflammation *(Recent Question 2015)*
   b. Purulent inflammation
   c. Serous inflammation
   d. Chronic inflammation

90. Commonest variety of acute inflammation is
(Recent Question 2014)
   a. Purulent inflammation   b. Serous inflammation
   c. Catarrhal inflammation d. Necrotic inflammation
   e. Fibrinous inflammation

CHRONIC INFLAMMATION

91. Histological picture of a lesion excised from the right cervical region is shown below. What is your diagnosis?
(Recent Pattern Question 2020)

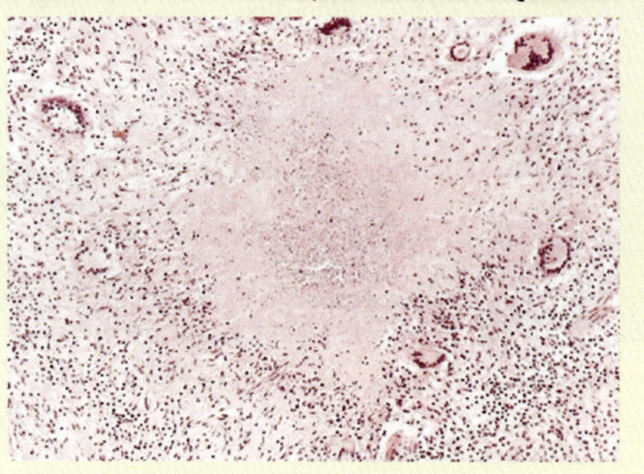

   a. Necrotizing granulomatous inflammation
   b. Neurofibroma
   c. Schwannoma
   d. Hodgkin lymphoma

92. Stellate Granuloma are seen in   *(JIPMER 2016)*
   a. Cat scratch disease   b. Sarcoidosis
   c. LGV   d. Histoplasmosis

93. 9-year-old boy is admitted with acute abdominal pain localized in the right illac fossa. He is pyrexial with localized peritonism in RIF. The causative cell involved here   *(JIPMER 2015)*
   a. Lymphocytes   b. Neutrophil
   c. Macrophages   d. Monocytes

94. True statement about alternative macrophage activation   *(WB PGEE 2016, Recent Question 2015)*
   a. Induced by the cytokine IFN-y
   b. Kill ingested organisms
   c. Secrete cytokines that stimulate inflammation
   d. Main function is in tissue repair

95. Tissue macrophages are called
(Recent Question 2014-15)
   a. Monocytes   b. Histiocytes
   c. Plasma cells d. Epitheloid cells

96. Biopsy of gastronemius muscle in an asymptomatic patient reveals non-caseating granuloma. Diagnosis
(Recent Question 2015)
   a. Tuberculosis b. Syphilis
   c. Sarcoidosis   d. Leprosy

97. The principle cell in granuloma *(Recent Question 2015)*
   a. Fibroblast   b. Epithelioid cell
   c. Giant cell   d. Plasma cell

98. The following factor stimulate angiogenesis
(Recent Question 2015)
   a. Integrins   b. Endostatin
   c. Thrombospondin   d. Tumstatin

99. Durck granuloma is seen in   *(Recent Question 2015)*
   a. Congenital syphilis b. Cat scratch disease
   c. Histoplasmosis   d. Cerebral malaria

100. Hallmark of chronic inflammation
(Recent Question 2015)
   a. Increased vascular permeability
   b. Vasodilation
   c. Granulomas
   d. Tissue destruction

101. Granulomatous inflammation seen in A/E
(Recent Question 2015)
   a. Syphilis   b. Tuberculosis
   c. Sarcoidosis   d. AIDS

102. Stellate granuloma is seen in   *(Recent Question 2015)*
   a. Leprosy   b. Brucellosis
   c. Sarcoidosis   d. Cat-scratch disease

103. Atherosclerosis is a type of?   *(Recent Question 2015)*
   a. Chronic inflammation
   b. Acute inflammation
   c. Tissue repair
   d. Hypertrophy in response to stimuli

104. Macrophages are converted into epithelioid cells by
   a. IFNγ b. IL2 *(Recent Question 2014)*
   c. TNF α d. TGF-β

TISSUE REPAIR

105. True about neutrophils role in wound healing is/are:
(PGI May 2019)
   a. They prevent phagocytosis of bacteria
   b. They are involved in early part of wound healing
   c. Prominent role in chronic inflammation
   d. They produce proteolytic enzymes
   e. Appear within 24 hours on wound margin

106. **A 12-year-old boy had a cut in his forearm 4 days ago. Now the bleeding has been stopped due to granulation tissue formation. While taking a skin biopsy a part of the granulation tissue was also included in the specimen. The histology of granulation tissue is shown below. Which type of collagen is found in this granulation tissue?** *(AIIMS May 18)*
    a. Type 1   b. Type 2
    c. Type 3   d. Type 4

107. **Cytokine involved in epithelial tissue migration and granulation tissue in healing?** *(Recent Question 2016-17)*
    a. TGF-B   b. IL-10
    c. IL-4   d. Inf-gamma

108. **Cell involved in the immediate phase of wound healing** *(Recent Question 2016, JIPMER_May 2015)*
    a. Platelets   b. Fibroblasts
    c. Basophils   d. Macrophages

109. **Scar contraction is caused by?** *(Recent Question 2016-17)*
    a. Fibroblasts   b. Myofibroblasts
    c. Epithelial cells   d. None

110. **Which of the following promotes growth of fibroblasts and recruitment of macrophages in case of angiogenesis process of wound healing?** *(Recent Question 2016)*
    a. EGF   b. PDGF
    c. VEGF   d. FGF

111. **After an incised wound, new collagen fibrils are seen along with growing epithelium. The age of the wound is ?** *(AIIMS May 2015)*
    a. 4-5 days   b. About 1 week
    c. 12-24 hours   d. 24 -72 hours

112. **Wound contraction occurs by the action of?** *(Recent Question 2015)*
    a. Macrophages   b. Myofibroblasts
    c. Endothelial cells   d. Nyictes

113. **Cell involved in the immediate phase of wound healing** *(JIPMER 2015)*
    a. Platelets   b. Fibroblasts
    c. Basophils   d. Macrophages

114. **The following factors impair wound healing except:**
    a. Diabetes mellitus   *(Recent Question 2015)*
    b. Glucocorticoids
    c. Vitamin C deficiency
    d. Clot formation

115. **Not seen in the inflammatory stage of wound healing**
    a. Angiogenesis   *(Recent Question 2015)*
    b. Chemotaxis
    c. Increased vessel permeability
    d. Released of cytokines and chemokines

116. **Find the false statement regarding wound healing** *(Recent Question 2015)*
    a. Macrophages are the key cellular constituents
    b. TGF-β is the most important fibrogenic agent
    c. In remodeling type III collagen replaces type I collagen
    d. Vitamin C is required for the hydroxylation of procollagen

117. **Not true regarding primary union** *(Recent Question 2015)*
    a. Abundant granulation tissue to fill the wound gap
    b. Clear margins
    c. Uninfected
    d. Neat linear scar

118. **Find the false statement about wound healing** *(Recent Question 2015)*
    a. 3 phases in sequence are: Inflammation, proliferation and maturation
    b. In healing by second intention, initially first matrix containing fibrin, plasma fibrin, plasma fibronectin, and type III collagen is formed
    c. 70-80% tensile strength of unwounded skin is obtained in 3 months
    d. After 2 months of wound healing, the increase in tensile strength is due to excess collagen synthesis

119. **Which of the following growth factor in not involved in tissue repair** *(Recent Question 2015)*
    a. VEGF   b. EGF
    c. TNF   d. TGF

120. **In a sutured incised wound, re-epithelialization is complete by** *(Recent Question 2015)*
    a. 24 hours   b. 48 hours
    c. 5 days   d. 2 weeks

121. **Granulation tissue appear at the site of injury by** *(Recent Question 2015)*
    a. <24 hours   b. 24–72 hours
    c. 48–96 hours   d. 5–7 days

122. **Collagen fibres bridge the wound area by** *(Recent Question 2015)*
    a. <24 hours   b. 24–72 hours
    c. 48–96 hours   d. 5–7 days

123. **When suture are removed from an incisional surgical wound at the end of one week, the wound strength of the wounded skin when compared to unwounded skin is approximately** *(Recent Question 2015)*
    a. 1%   b. 10%
    c. 50%   d. 80%

124. **Myofibroblasts are seen in**   *(Recent Question 2015)*
    a. Healing wounds   b. Cancerous site
    c. Adipose tissue   d. Muscle septae

125. **Wound contraction is due to**   *(Recent Question 2015)*
    a. Myocyte
    b. Fibroblast
    c. Myofibroblast
    d. Skeletal muscle fibre

126. **Correct sequence of phases of wound injury** *(Recent Question 2015)*
    a. Inflammation–Maturation–Proliferation–Remodeling
    b. Inflammation–Proliferation–Maturation–Remodeling
    c. Inflammation–Proliferation–Remodeling–Maturation
    d. Inflammation–Maturation–Remodeling–Proliferation

127. **Primary intentional healing which is true** *(Recent Question 2014-15)*
    a. Neovascularization is maximum by day 5
    b. Neovascularization is maximum by day 3
    c. Neutrophils appear at wound margins on day 3
    d. The epidermis recovers its maximum thickness by day 7

128. **Formation of granulation tissue is due to**
    a. Thrombosed vessels   *(MH PG 2014)*
    b. Infiltration of cells
    c. Budding of new capillaries
    d. Mucosal proliferation

129. In wound injury sequence of appearance of cells is-
(Recent Question 2014)
a. Macrophage → Platelet → Neutrophils → Fibrobla
b. Neutrophils → Macrophages → Platelet → Fibroblt
c. Platelet → Neutrophils → Macrophages → Fibroblast
d. Platelet → Macrophages → Neutrophils → Fibroblast

130. Which is not seen in inflammatory stage of wound healing? *(Recent Question 2013)*
a. Angiogenesis
b. Chemotaxis
c. Increased capillary permeability
d. Cytokine and chemotactic factor release

131. During angiogenesis recruitment of pericytes and periendothelial cells is due to- *(Recent Question 2013)*
a. VEGF & PDGF
b. Angiopoietins, TGF & PDGF
c. TGF, VEFG & PDGF
d. VEGF, IL-2, IL-6

132. Wound healing is the summation of following processes except - *(DNB 2012)*
a. Coagulation
b. Matrix synthesis
c. Angiogenesis
d. Fibrolysis

133. Complete restoration of tensile strength of the wound comparable to normal tissue takes as long as:
(DNB Nov 2012)
a. Two weeks
b. Six weeks
c. Six months
d. Two years

134. Cells not involved in healing of clean wound:
a. Macrophages *(PGI Nov 2011)*
b. Platelet
c. Fibroblasts
d. Polymorphonuclear leukocytes
e. MyoFibroblast

TYPES OF CELLS

135. Permanent tissue is? *(Recent Question 2016-17)*
a. Heart
b. Liver
c. Kidney
d. Skeletal muscle

136. The following are labile cells except
(Recent Question 2015)
a. Hepatocytes
b. Bone marrow
c. Intestinal mucosa
d. Epithelium of skin

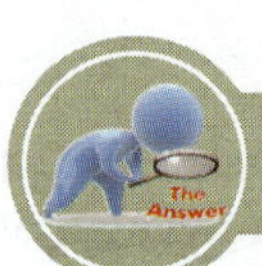

Answers with Explanations

1. **Ans. (a, e); a. Increased serum immunoglobulin level; e. Increased level of C-reactive protein**

(Ref: Robbins 9th/pg 99)

2. **Ans. (c) 1-b, 2-c, 3-a**

3. **Ans. (c) Histamine** *(Ref: to answer number 13)*

4. **Ans. (c) Plasma cell**

(Ref: Wintrobes 13ed/pg 303; Wintrobes Atlas)

Plasma cells are spherical or ellipsoid and range from 5 to 30 μm in size. The cytoplasm is abundant, always is basophilic, and usually is deep blue; it may have a granular char- acter. Plasma cells have a well-defined perinuclear clear zone that contains the Golgi apparatus.

5. **Ans. (c) C** *(Ref: Wintrobes 13th ed. Pg. 303; Wintrobes Atlas)*

Key to the figure:
A: Lymphocyte, B: Neutrophil, C: Eosinophil, D: Basophil

6. **Ans. (b) Arterioles**

(Ref: Essentials of Rubins Pathology 5th ed pg 19)

Transient vasoconstriction of arterioles at the site of injury is the earliest event in acute inflammation. It is usually mediated by neurogenic and chemical mediators and usually resolves within seconds.

7. **Ans. (d) Band <5%**

(Ref: http://www.clevelandclinicmeded.com/ medicalpubs/diseasemanagement/infectious-disease/ sepsis)

The term systemic inflammatory response syndrome (SIRS) describes the host response to a critical illness of infectious or non-infectious cause

Evidence of a systemic inflammatory response is indicated by at least two of the following:

- Fever or hypothermia: core body temperature 38°C or higher or 36°C or lower
- Tachypnea: 20 breaths/min or more, or need for mechanical ventilation for an acute process
- Tachycardia: heart rate 90 beats/min or more, unless the patient has a preexisting tachycardia
- White blood cell count:12,000 cells/mm³ or higher, 4,000 cells/mm3 or less, or more than 10% bands on differential

8. **Ans. (c) Stronglyloides**

(Ref: dacie and lewis practical ematology, 11th ed, pg 102)

Moderate eosinophilia occurs in allergic conditions; more severe eosinophilia (20–50 × 10⁹/L) may be seen in parasitic infections

9. **Ans. (a)** **<500** (*Ref: Robbins 9th/pg 582*)

Neutropenia is denoted as ANC (absolute neutrophil count)

$$ANC = \frac{(\%\text{neutrophils} + \%\text{bands}) \times (WBC)}{100}$$

- Mild neutropenia (1000 ≥ ANC < 1500): minimal risk of infection
- Moderate neutropenia (500 ≥ ANC < 1000): moderate risk of infection
- Severe neutropenia (ANC < 500): severe risk of infection.
- Agranulocytosis refers to a virtual absence of neutrophils in peripheral blood. It is usually applied to cases in which the ANC is lower than 100/μL

10. **Ans. (b)** **Arterioles** (*Ref: Robbins 9th/pg 74; 8th/pg 47*)

Vasodilation first involves the arterioles and then leads to opening of new capillary beds in the area.

The result is *increased blood flow*, which is the cause of heat and redness (*erythema*) at the site of inflammation.

11. **Ans. (a)** **Neutrophils** (*Ref: 9th/pg 71; 8th/pg 44*)

12. **Ans. (b)** **Delayed prolonged leakage** (*Ref: R 9th/pg 74*)

Mechanism of increased vascular permeability:

Mechanism	Caused by	Blood vessels affected	Type of response
Mild endothelial damage	• Thermal and radiation injury[Q] • Late-appearing Sunburn[Q]	Venules and capillaries	Reversible, **Delayed & prolonged**

13. **Ans. (a)** **Histamine** (*Ref: Robbins 9th/pg 74; 8th/pg 47*)

Increased vascular permeability
- Formation of endothelial gaps (**Immediate transient response**) is the **most common mechanism**[Q] for **increased permeability.**
- Most important immediate mediator responsible for **Immediate transient response**[Q] is **histamine**[Q]
- ***Other immediate*** mediators: bradykinin, leukotriene, substance P
- ***Somewhat*** delayed mediators: TNF, IL-1,1FN-γ

Option b: IL2: IL-2 is known to activate T-cells, especially CD4+ T-helper cells. Other minor function of IL2 are: IL2 can activate lipoxygenase pathway with release of lipoxygenase metabolites which play a role in pulmonary vascular permeability. (*Cytokines and Inflammation By Edward S. Kimball, pg 215*)

Option c and d: are mediators of chronic inflammation

Here the answer is definitely histamine >> IL2

14. **Ans. (d)** **Transient vasoconstriction → Vasodilatation → Increased permeability → Stasis** (*Ref: R 9th/pg 73-74*)

15. **Ans. (a)** **Spectrin** (*Ref: Robbins 9th/pg 75-76; 8th/pg 48-49*)

Families of CAMs
- Ig (immunoglobulin) superfamily
- Integrins
- Cadherins
- Selectins.

16. **Ans. (a)** **Capillary adherence or sequestration of parasitized RBCs**

- In *P. falciparum* infections, **membrane protuberances** appear on RBC surface 12–15 h after the cell's invasion. These **"knobs" extrude a** membrane adhesive protein **(PfEMP1)** that mediates **attachment to receptors on venular and capillary endothelium—an event termed** *cytoadherence.*
- They result in the **sequestration of RBCs containing mature forms of the parasite in vital organs (particularly the brain), where they interfere with microcirculatory flow and metabolism.**

17. **Ans. (a)** **Arginine** (*Ref: R 9th/pg 81*)

NETs contain a framework of nuclear chromatin with embedded granule proteins, such as antimicrobial peptides and enzymes. The nuclear chromatin in the NETs, includes histones and associated DNA.Histone modification by peptidylarginine deiminase 4 (PAD4) is necessary for NET release.

18. **Ans. (d)** **All the above** (*Ref: Robbins 9th/pg 81*)

Neutrophil extracellular traps (NETs) are extracellular fibrillar networks that provide a high concentration of antimicrobial substances at sites of infection and prevent the spread of the microbes by trapping them in the fibrils. They consist of a viscous meshwork of of nuclear chromatin that binds and concentrates granule proteins such as antimicrobial peptides and enzymes

19. **Ans. (d)** **Decreased hydrostatic pressure**

(*Ref: R 9th/pg 73-75*)

20. **Ans. (a)** **Margination - rolling- adhesion – transmigration** (*Ref: Robbins 9th/pg 73-75*)

Cellular events of inflammation is characterized by: **Margination - rolling- adhesion – transmigration**

21. **Ans. (a)** **Transport of fluids and proteins through endothelial cells** (*Ref: Robbins 9th/pg 74*)

Increased transport of fluids and proteins, called transcytosis, through the endothelial cell.

This process may involve intracellular channels that may be stimulated by vascular endothelial growth factor (VEGF)

22. **Ans. (d)** **Diapedesis** (*Ref: Robbins 9th/pg 76-77*)

Migration of the leukocytes through the endothelium, is called transmigration or diapedesis.

It is mediated by PECAM-1

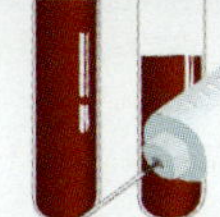

23. **Ans. (d) It is not regulated by any defined set of "genes"**

(Ref: Dev Cell. 2008 Sep; 15(3): 344–357)

24. **Ans. (c) Vasodilatation and increased vascular permeability** *(Ref: Robbins 9th/pg 74; R8"47)*

25. **Ans. (b) Early transient increase in permeability**

(Ref: Robbins 9th/pg 74; 8th/pg 47)
Contraction of endothelial cell cytoskeleton leads to Formation of endothelial gaps. This response is called Immediate transient response.

26. **Ans. (b) Rolling---Activation of Integrins---Stable Adhesion--- migration via endothelium**

27. **Ans. (b, c) b. Integrin; c. L-selectin**

28. **Ans. (c) Hereditary angioneurotic edema**

(Ref: Harrison 18:2666-67, 17th ed 2030, 2031)

Deficiency of complement component	Disease/Syndrome
1. C1 esterase Inhibitor	Hereditary angioneurotic edema

29. **Ans. (a) IL-8** *(Ref: Robbins 8th/pg 62)*
α Chemokines-IL8, IL, TNF

30. **Ans. (d) Chemotaxis** *(Ref: Robbins 9th/pg 84)*
Chemotaxis, leukocyte adhesion is mediated by Leukotrienes B4, HETE

31. **Ans. (d) PECAM** *(Ref: Robbins 9th/pg 76; 8th/pg 49-50)*
Leukocyte Migration through Endothelium: Transmigration or diapedesis[Q]
- Occurs mainly in **postcapillary venules.**[Q]
- Most important molecule: **PECAM-1 (platelet endothelial cell adhesion molecule) or CD31.**[Q]

32. **Ans. (b) Chemotaxis** *(Ref: Robbins 8th/pg 62)*
Migration in the tissues toward a chemotactic stimulus: Chemotaxis:
- **Unidirectional movement**[Q] of the leukocytes **towards site of injury** along a **chemical gradient.**

33. **Ans. (b) P-Selectin** *(Ref: Robbins 9th/pg 74-75; 8th/pg 48-49)*
P-selectin (CD62P): Is stored in Platelets α granules[Q] and endothelium weibel palade bodies[Q]

34. **Ans. (c) Oxidase** *(Ref: Robbins 9th/pg 79; 8th/pg 53)*
- **REACTIVE OXYGEN SPECIES (ROS)** - Produced by the rapid assembly and activation of a multicomponent oxidase, **NADPH oxidase**, which oxidizes **NADPH**[Q] and, in the process, **reduces oxygen to superoxide.**

- **NADPH oxidase** is also called **phagocyte oxidase or phagocyte NADPH oxidase" (PHOX**) and is responsible for oxidative burst
- **All others options are antioxidants**

35. **Ans. (a) Rolling** *(Ref: Robbins 9th/pg 74-75; 8th/pg 48-49)*

36. **Ans. (b) Unidirectional motion**

(Ref: 9th/pg 77; 8th/pg 50)
Unidirectional movement[Q] of the leukocytes **towards site of injury** along a **chemical gradient.**

Exogenous[Q]	Bacterial products : N-formylmethionine terminal amino acid[Q] and some lipids
Endogenous products	• Complement system-C5a[Q] • Arachidonic acid (AA) metabolites-LTB4[Q] • Cytokines- IL-8[Q]

37. **Ans. (d) Transferrin**

(Ref: Robbins 9th/pg 74-75; 8th/pg 48-49)
Transferrin is iron carrying protein

38. **Ans. (d) Both a and b**

39. **Ans. (c) Elastase**

40. **Ans. (b) C3b** *(Ref: Robbins 9th ed p 78)*
The major opsonins are IgG antibodies, the C3b breakdown product of complement, and certain plasma lectins, notably mannosebinding lectin, all of which are recognized by specific receptors on leukocytes.

41. **Ans. (a, b, e); a. Histamine; b. Lysosomal enzymes; e. Serotonin**

42. **Ans. (a) Albumin** *(Ref. R9th/ 99)*

43. **Ans. (b, e); b. Transferrin; e. Albumin**

44. **Ans. (b) IL22** *(Ref: Immunity 2008 Apr. 28(4): 454–467)*
IL-22 is one of the IL-10 family cytokines, which also include IL-10, IL-19, IL-20, IL-24, and IL-26, as well as more distally related IL-28 and IL-29.
It has a role in autoimmune diseases, tissue-repair and wound-healing apart from being proinflammatory

45. **Ans. (c) Chemokines** *(Ref: Robbins 9th/pg 87)*

46. **Ans. (d) Immune complex**

Alternative pathway	• Triggered **by microbial surface molecules** (e.g., endotoxin, or LPS), complex polysaccharides, cobra venom, and other substances, **in the absence of antibody** • IgA can directly activate this pathway

47. **Ans. (a) Adhesion** *(Ref: Robbins 9th/pg 85)*

48. **Ans. (d) C56789**

(Ref: Robbins and Cotran: Pathological basis of disease 8/e p64)

- Deposition of MAC **(C5-C9)** on cells makes them permeable to water & ions → death (lysis) of cells

49. **Ans. (d) Platelet** *(Ref: Robbins 9th/pg 88)*

50. **Ans. (b) IL-2**

(Ref: Inflamm Bowel Dis. 1999 Nov;5(4):285-94)

Type 1 T helper (Th1) cells produce interferon-gamma, interleukin (IL)-2, and tumour necrosis factor (TNF)-beta, which activate macrophages and are responsible for cell-mediated immunity and phagocyte-dependent protective responses. By contrast, type 2 Th (Th2) cells produce IL-4, IL-5, IL-10, and IL-13, which are responsible for strong antibody production, eosinophil activation, and inhibition of several macrophage functions, thus providing phagocyte-independent protective responses.

51. **Ans. (c) Acid protease** *(Ref: R 9/88 Harrison)*

52. **Ans. (a) Il-1** *(Ref: Immunol Today, 1994;15:74-80)*

The response starts at the trauma site where macrophages and monocytes stimulate cytokine release, especially IL-1 and TNF, which are considered primary interleukins.

By themselves, they cause further cytokine release, especially IL-6, which has been considered a major acute phase liver protein stimulator and organic defense response mediator.

53. **Ans. (c) Recurrent infections like Neisseria and Pnemococci**

(Ref: Harrison 18:2666-67, 17th ed 2030, 2031)

Refer immunity chapter
- Deficiency of the terminal components of complement predisposes to **Neisseria infections**[Q]

54. **Ans. (b) Eosinophils**

(Ref: Robbins 9th/pg 204, Ref: Anderson 10thed: 397)

Eosinophils produce:

1. Major basic protein	4. PAF	6. Eosinophilic cationic protein
2. Peroxidase	5. Leukotrienes	7. Reactive oxygen species
3. Neurotoxin		

55. **Ans. (b) 1L-1**

(Ref: J Infect Dis. (1999) 179 (Supplement 2): S294-S304. doi: 10.1086/513856, Harrison 18th ed:2666)

Following cytokines are intrinsically pyrogenic in that they produce a rapid-onset fever by acting directly on the hypothalamus without the requirement for the formation of another cytokine:

> **IL-1α, TNF-α, TNF-β, IFN-α, and IL-6.**

PLEASE NOTE : *IL-18 of IL-1 family* is not pyrogenic

56. **Ans. (a) C5-9** *(Ref: Harrison 18:2666-67, 17th ed 2030, 2031)*

57. **Ans. (c) Leukotrienes** *(Ref: Robbins 9th/pg 89)*

- LTE4 cause intense vasoconstriction, bronchospasm (importantin asthma), and increased permeability of venules.
- C3a, C5a, and, to a lesser extent, C4a stimulate histamine release from mast cells and thereby increase vascular permeability and cause vasodilation. They are called anaphylatoxins

58. **Ans. (c) PGE2** *(Ref: Robbins 9th/pg 99)*

The increase in body temperature is caused by prostaglandins that are produced in the vascular and perivascular cells of the hypothalamus.

In the hypothalamus, the prostaglandins, especially PGE2, stimulate the production of neurotransmitters that reset the temperature set point at a higher level.

59. **Ans. (b) TNF**

(Ref: J Infect Dis. (1999) 179 (Supplement 2): S294-S304. doi: 10.1086/513856, Harrison 18th ed:2666)

60. **Ans. (a) Prostaglandins** *(Ref: Robbins 9th/pg 84)*

61. **Ans. (c) Bradykinin** *(Ref: Robbins 9th/pg 65, 89)*

Functions of bradykinin:
- Increases vascular permeability, vasodilation
- Smooth muscle contraction **and pain** when injected into the skin.

62. **Ans. (d) Kinins** *(Ref: Robbins 9th/pg 89, 65)*

As weknow: **LTB4,** -C5a and IL8 are strong chemotactic agents

Kinins are vasoactive peptides derived from plasma proteins, called **kininogens**, by the action of **kallikreins – not chemotactic**

63. **Ans. (c) Substance P**

(Ref: J Infect Dis. (1999) 179 (Supplement 2): S294-S304. doi: 10.1086/513856, Harrison 18th ed:2666)

IL1 AND TNF are well known pyrogenic cytokines

In the hypothalamus, the prostaglandins, especially PGE2, stimulate the production of neurotransmitters that reset the temperature set point at a higher level, hence pyrogenic

64. **Ans. (b) IL-4** *(Ref: Robbins 9th/pg 94,95)*

Anti-inflammatory cytokines are-**IL-10, TGF-B, Lipoxins, IL-4**

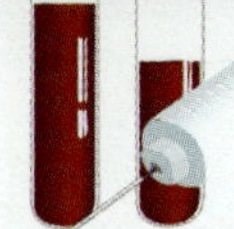

65. **Ans. (a)** **IL-6**

(Ref: Fundamental immunology by William E Paul:1030, Koj –chapter 3)
Il6 IS INVOLVED IN ACUTE FRBRILE RESPONSES
Others are involved in chronic inflammation

66. **Ans. (c)** **ADAM-17**

(Ref: Immunology: Mucosal and Body Surface Defences, 4.8)
ADAM metallopeptidase domain 17 (ADAM17), also called TACE (tumor necrosis factor-α-converting enzyme), is a 70-kDa enzyme that belongs to the ADAM protein family of disintegrins and metalloproteases.

67. **Ans. (b)** **TGF-β** *(Ref: Robbins 9th/pg 105)*

Transforming growth factor-β (TGF-β) is the most important cytokine for the synthesis and deposition of connective tissue proteins.

68. **Ans. (d)** **HGF**

(Ref: Angiogenesis: An Integrative Approach from Science to Medicine, pg 82)
Pro- angiogenesis molecules

Stimulator	Mechanism
FGF	Promotes proliferation & differentiation of endothelial cells, smooth muscle cells, and fibroblasts
VEGF	Affects permeability
Ang1 and Ang2	Stabilize vessels
PDGF (BB-homodimer) and PDGFR	Recruit smooth muscle cells
TGF-β, endoglin and TGF-β receptors	↑extracellular matrix production
Integrins αVβ3, αVβ5 and α5β1	Bind matrix macromolecules and proteinases
VE-cadherin and CD31	Endothelial junctional molecules
Ephrin	Determine formation of arteries or veins
Plasminogen activators	Remodels extracellular matrix, releases and activates growth factors
Plasminogen activator inhibitor-1	Stabilizes nearby vessels

69. **Ans. (d)** **Activated Macrophages** *(Ref: R 9th/pg 86-87)*

70. **Ans. (d)** **Anaphylaxis**

(Ref: Robbins 9th/pg 86-87, 105, Immunology: Mucosal and Body Surface Defences, 4.8)
Transforming growth factor-β (TGF-β) is the most important cytokine for the synthesis and deposition of connective tissue proteins. Other functions: Angiogenesis. Anti-inflammatory cytokine
Up-regulation of tissue inhibitor of metalloproteinases-3 gene expression is done by TGF-beta in articular chondrocytes

71. **Ans. (d)** **IL-1**

(Ref: Curr. Opin. Immunol. 23 (5): 598–604, Harrison 18th ed:2666)

Interleukin-2 (IL-2) Subfamily[Q]:
- **Interleukins:** IL-2, IL-3, IL-4, IL-5, IL-6, IL-7, IL-9, IL-11, IL-12, IL-13, IL-15, IL-21, IL-23
- **Not called interleukins:** Colony-stimulating factor-1 (CSF1), granulocyte–macrophage colony-stimulating factor (CSF2) erythropoietin (EPO), thrombopoietin (THPO), leukocyte inhibitory factor (LIF)
- **Not interleukins:** Growth hormone (GH1), prolactin (PRL), leptin (LEP), **cytokine receptor-like factor 1[Q]** (CLC or CLF)
- **Interferon (IFN) subfamily:** IFN-β, IFN-α
- **IL-10 subfamily[Q]:** IL-10, IL-19, IL-20, IL-22, IL-24 and IL-26 IL-1 does not belong to IL2 family

72. **Ans. (c)** **IL 12**

(Ref: J Infect Dis. (1999) 179 (Supplement 2): S294-S304. doi: 10.1086/513856, Harrison 18th ed:2666)

73. **Ans. (c)** **C3b** *(Ref: Robbins 9th/pg 83; 8th/pg 57)*
Anaphylatoxins-C3a, C5a, C4a.

74. **Ans. (b)** **Bronchodilation** *(Ref: R 9th/pg 89; 8th/pg 59)*
PAF
- **Produced by:** platelets, basophils, mast cells, neutrophils, macrophages, and endothelial cells
- **Functions: platelet aggregation, vasoconstriction and bronchoconstriction.[Q]**
- At low concentrations it induces vasodilation and increased venular permeability
- Transmits signals between cells

75. **Ans. (b)** **Kinins** *(Ref: Robbins 9th/pg 82; 8th/pg 57)*

Plasma Derived	Cell Derived
Fibrin split products	Histamine
Kinins (bradykinin)	Serotonin
C3a, C5a	Prostaglandins, Leukotrienes
	Nitric oxide
	Platelet-activating factor

76. **Ans. (b)** **IL 11** *(Ref: Robbins 9th/pg 86-87)*

IL-6, tumour necrosis factor-alpha (TNF-alpha) and IL-1 are thought to be the key mediators of the acute phase response *(Ref: Clin Exp Immunol. 1995 Oct; 102(1): 217–223.)*
Coming to option b:

IL-11	gp 130	Bone marrow stromal cells	Megakaryocytes,	Induces megakaryocyte colony formation^Q

77. Ans. (d) 1L-10

(Ref: Jolanta Jura and Aleksander Koj –chapter 3)

Anti inflammatory cytokines
IL-10, IL-13, 1L-4 and TGF-β
Please note, both IL-4 and IL-6 are pro as well as anti inflammatory cytokines

78. Ans. (d) IL-5

79. Ans. (a, b, c, e); a. IL-2; b. IL-6; c. TNF-alpha; e. Interferons

(Ref: Fundamental immunology by William E Paul :1030, chapter 3)

80. Ans. (a, b, e,); a. Haptoglobin; b. C-reactive protein; e. Fibrinogen

(Ref: http://www.uptodate.com/contents/acute-phase-reactants)

Acute phase reactants are

CRP	Ferritin
Fibrinogen	Hepcidin
Serum Amyloid A	Alpha-1 antitrypsin
Haptoglobulin	Ceruloplasmin
Procalcitonin	

81. Ans. (b) Bronchodilatation *(Ref: Robbins 9th/pg 65, 89)*

Functions of bradykinin:
- Increases vascular permeability, vasodilation
- Smooth muscle contraction **and pain** when injected into the skin.

82. Ans. (c) Myeloperoxidase

(Ref: Robbins 9th/pg 83; 8th/pg 57)

MPO- lysosomal protein stored in azurophilic granules of the neutrophil.

83. Ans. (c) TNF Alfa, IL 10 and IL1 receptor antagonist

(Ref: Fundamental immunology by William E Paul:1030, chapter 3)

Ans none but if to mark one, go for c. 2 options in c are correct and 1 wrong
Resolution of infection is by:
- IL10- anti inflammatory cytokine–CORRECT
- IL1- pro inflammatory cytokine and IL1 receptor antagonist will cause resolution of inflammation–CORRECT
- TNF- pro inflammatory cytokine–WRONG

84. Ans. (d) Platelet aggregation *(Ref: R 9th/pg 82; 8th/pg 57)*

Mediator	Characteristics
Histamine	• Formed from the amino acid **'histidine'** • Sources: Mast cells (richest source), platelets and basophils • Causes **vasodilation** (but vasoconstriction of large arteries), **increased permeability** (immediate transient response) & **bronchoconstriction**

85. Ans. (c) Capsular polysaccharide of pneumococcus

(Ref: Essential of pathology, 8th ed: 781)

86. Ans. (b) Integrins *(Ref: Robbins 9th/pg 77; 8th/pg 50)*

87. Ans. (b) Interleukin 2

(Ref: Robbins 9th/pg 85-86; 8th/pg 58)

All are Pro inflammatory Cytokines but if to mark one go for b. Since all other 3 are major Pro inflammatory Cytokines.

88. Ans. (c) Fluid in infected by destructive organism

(Ref: Robbins 9th/pg 90)

Serous Inflammation

A pattern of acute inflammation
Marked by the exudation of cell poor fluid into spaces created by cell injury or into body cavities lined by the peritoneum, pleura, or pericardium
Typically, the fluid in serous inflammation is not infected by destructive organisms
Does not contain large numbers of leukocytes

89. Ans. (c) Serous inflammation *(Ref: Robbins 9th/pg 90)*

90. Ans. (c) Catarrhal inflammation

(Ref: Chandrasoma taylor: 3ed: 45)

Catarrhal inflammation
- **Commonest type of inflammation^Q**
- **Increased mucus secretion**
- Seen in **common cold**

91. Ans. (a) Necrotizing granulomatous inflammation

(Ref: Robbins 9th ed/pg 98)

92. Ans. (a) Cat scratch disease

(Ref: Anderson 10th/pg 582)

93. Ans. (b) Neutrophil

(Ref: Robbins 9th/pg 71; 8th/pg 44)

This is a case of acute appendicitis
The principal inflammatory cell in this case of acute appendicitis is the neutrophil.

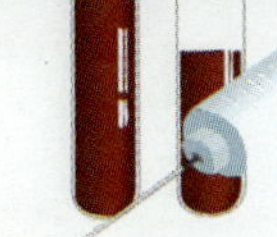

94. Ans. (d) Main function is in tissue repair

(Ref: Robbins 9th/pg 94)

95. Ans. (b) Histiocytes *(Ref: Anderson 10th ed pg 583)*

- Macrophages are tissue cells **derived from hematopoietic stem cells in the bone marrow and from progenitors in the embryonic yolk sac and fetal liver during early development**[Q]
- Circulating cells of this lineage are known as monocytes. Tissue macrophages are called **histiocytes**
Activated macrophages are called epithelioid cells

96. Ans. (c) Sarcoidosis *(Ref: Robbins 9th/pg 94; 8th/pg 71)*

Leprosy and TB- Caseating granuloma
Syphilis- plasma cell rich granuloma (gumma)
Sarcoidosis- non caseating granuloma

97. Ans. (b) Epithelioid cell *(Ref: Anderson 10th ed pg 583)*

- Macrophages (also known as **histiocytes**) are the cells that define a granuloma
- The macrophages in granulomas are often referred to as "epithelioid"
- Epithelioid macrophages differ from ordinary macrophages in that they have **elongated nuclei** that often resemble the sole of a slipper or shoe.
- These changes are thought to be a consequence of **"activation" of the macrophage by the offending antigen.**

98. Ans. (a) Integrins

*(Ref: Angiogenesis: An Integrative Approach from Science to Medicine, pg 123; **Angiogenesis molecules have been described at Ans no 82.** Also students must know anti angiogenesis molecules)*

Antiangiogenic molecules are

1. Endostation
2. Thrombospondin
3. Tumstation
4. Restin
5. Endorepellin
6. Fibulin 5
7. Canstatin

99. Ans. (d) Cerebral malaria *(Ref: Malaria - Page 76)*

In malignant cerebral malaria caused by Plasmodium falciparum, brain vessels are plugged with parasitized red cells, causing ring hemorrhage which is accompanied by necrosis of surrounding parenchyma.
The damage leads to formation of Durck's granuloma – collection of microglial cells surrounding area of demyelination

100. Ans. (d) Tissue destruction *(Ref: Robbins 9th/pg 494)*

101. Ans. (d) AIDS *(Ref: Robbins 9th/pg 494; 8th/pg 500)*

102. Ans. (d) Cat-scratch disease *(Ref: Robbins 9th/pg 494)*

103. Ans. (a) Chronic inflammation

(Ref: Robbins 9th/pg 494)

Atherosclerosis as a **chronic inflammatory and healing response** of the arterial wall to **endothelial injury**.

104. Ans. (a) IFNγ *(Ref: Anderson 10th ed pg 583)*

- Epithelioid macrophages differ from ordinary macrophages in that they have **elongated nuclei** that often resemble the sole of a slipper or shoe.
- *IFN*-γ is important in activating macrophages and transforming them into epithelioid cells and multinucleate giant cells

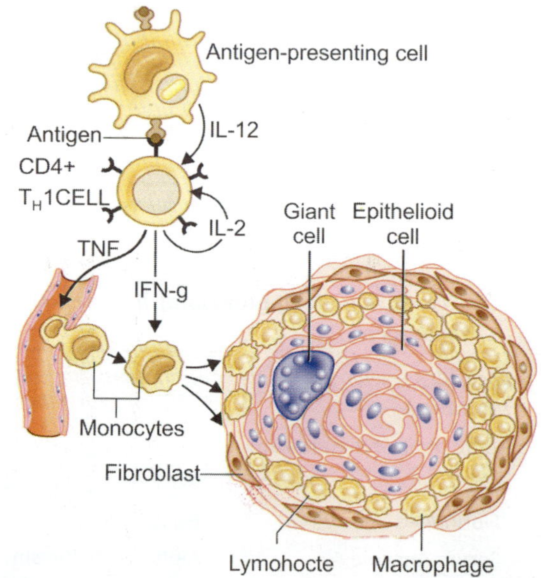

105. Ans. (b, d, e); b. They are involved in early part of wound healing; d. They produce proteolytic enzymes; e. Appear within 24 hours on wound margin

(Ref: Robbin's 9th ed/pg. 107)

106. Ans. (c) Type 3

The early granulation tissue mainly has collagen type 3 >1

107. Ans. (a) TGF-B *(Ref: Robbin's 9th ed/pg. 107)*

108. Ans. (a) Platelets *(Ref: Robbin's 9th ed/pg. 104)*

Ist phase is clot form action which involves platelets

109. Ans. (b) Myofibroblasts

- **Permanent wound contraction** requires the **action of myofibroblasts**[Q] *seen in healing by **secondary intention**[Q]*
- **Myofibroblasts** are **altered fibroblasts** that have ultra-structural characteristics of smooth muscle cells.

110. Ans. (d) FGF *(Ref: Robbin's 9th ed/pg. 104)*

- Fibroblast growth factors (FGFs), mainly FGF-2, stimulates the proliferation of endothelial cells. It also promotes the migration of macrophages and fibroblasts to the damaged area, and stimulates epithelial cell migration to cover epidermal wounds.

- PDGF-recruits smooth muscle cells
- TGF-β suppresses endothelial proliferation and migration, and enhances the production of ECM proteins.
- Vascular endothelial growth factors (VEGFs), mainly VEGF-A, stimulates both migration and proliferation of endothelial cells

111. Ans. (d) 24 -72 hours *(Ref: Robbin's 9th ed/Pg 107)*

112. Ans. (b) Myofibroblasts *(Ref: R 9th/pg 108; 8th/pg 106)*

113. Ans. (a) Platelets *(Ref: Robbin's 9th ed/pg 107)*

The earliest feature in wound repair is Presence of **blood clot** in the incision. This clot is formed by the initial effort of platelets and then the coagulation factors.

114. Ans. (d) Clot formation *(Ref: Robbin's 9th ed/pg 106)*

Factors Impairing Healing

Infection
Diabetes
protein deficiency, vitamin C deficiency
Glucocorticoids (steroids)
Mechanical factors such as increased local pressure or torsion may cause wounds to dehisce
Poor perfusion, due either to arteriosclerosis and diabetes or to obstructed venous drainage (e.g., in varicose veins)
Foreign bodies
Blood clot formation is the earliest event in wound repair

115. Ans. (a) Angiogenesis

(Ref: Robbins 9th/pg 103; 8th/pg 101)

Three phases of wound healing:
- Inflammation (early & late)- option b, c, d
- Granulation tissue formation & re-epithelialization- option a
- Wound contraction, ECM deposition & remodeling

116. Ans. (c) In remodeling type III collagen replaces type I collagen *(Ref: Robbins 9th/pg 107; 8th/pg 102-5)*

In remodeling type I collagen replaces type III collagen

117. Ans. (a) Abundant granulation tissue to fill the wound gap (Ref: Robbins 9th/pg 108; 8th/pg 106)

118. Ans. (d) After 2 months of wound healing, the increase in tensile strength is due to excess collagen synthesis

(Ref: Robbins 9th/pg 108; 8th/pg 106)

Option a-true-Three phases of wound healing- Inflammation (early & late), Granulation tissue formation & re-epithelialization and Wound contraction, ECM deposition & remodeling
- Strength **never reaches 100%**[Q] Option d- The recovery of tensile strength results from the excess of collagen
- Synthesis over collagen degradation during the first 2 months of healing, and, at later times, from **structural modifications** of collagen fibers (cross-linking, increased fiber size) option D.

119. Ans. NONE > TNF *(Ref: Robbins 9th/pg 107)*

In Granulation tissue formation phase: Migration of fibroblasts to the site of injury is driven by chemokines, TNF, PDGF, TGF-β, and FGF. Their subsequent proliferation is triggered by multiple growth factors, including PDGF, EGF, TGF-β, and FGF, and the cytokines IL-1 and TNF.

120. Ans. (c) 5 days *(Ref: Robbins 9th/pg 107; 8th/pg 102-5)*

121. Ans. (b) 24–72 hours *(Ref: R 9th/pg 107; 8th/pg 102-5)*

122. Ans. (d) 5–7 days *(Ref: Robbins 9th/pg 107)*

123. Ans. (b) 10% *(Ref: Robbins 9th/pg 108; 8th/pg 106)*

124. Ans. (a) Healing wounds *(Ref: 9th/pg 108)*

125. Ans. (c) Myofibroblast *(Ref: R 9th/pg 108; 8th/pg 106)*

126. Ans. (b) Inflammation–Proliferation–Maturation– Remodeling *(Ref: Robbins 9th/pg 108; 8th/pg 106)*

127. Ans. (a) Neovascularization is maximum by day 5

(Ref: Robbins 9th/pg 107; 8th/pg 102-5)

128. Ans. (c) Budding of new capillaries *(Ref: R 9th/pg 106)*

129. Ans. (c) Platelet → Neutrophils → Macrophages → Fibroblast *(Ref: Robbins 9th/pg 107; 8th/pg 102-5)*

Blood clot → neutrophils → macrophages → collagen → fibroblast

130. Ans. (a) Angiogenesis

(Ref: Robbins 9th/pg 103; 8th/pg 101)

Three phases of wound healing:
- Inflammation (early & late)- option b, c, d
- Granulation tissue formation & re-epithelialization- option a
- Wound contraction, ECM deposition & remodeling

131. Ans. (b) Angiopoietins, TGF & PDGF

(Ref: R 9th/pg 104)

Factors involved in angiogenesis:

Growth factors.	Structural maturation of new vessels	Stabilisation of vessels	• **Notch signaling**
• Mainly **VEGF-A**	**Angiopoietins 1 and 2 (Ang 1 and Ang 2)**	**PDGF and TGF-β**	• Regulates the sprouting and branching of new vessels
• Fibroblast growth factors mainly FGF-2			• Ensures proper spacing of vessels.

Newly formed vessels need to be stabilized by the recruitment of pericytes and smooth muscle cells and by

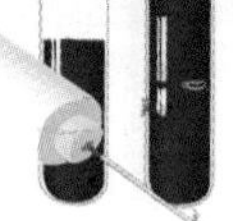

the deposition of connective tissue-**Angiopoietins, PDGF and TGF-β.**

132. Ans. (d) Fibrolysis *(Ref: R 9th/pg 107; 8th/pg 102-105)*

133. Ans. (c) Six months *(Ref: Robbins 9th/pg 108; 8th/pg 106)*

Ans should be none. But if to mark one, it should be close to 3 months.

134. Ans. (e) MyoFibroblast *(Ref: R 9th/pg 108; 8th/pg 106)*

Permanent wound contraction requires the **action of myofibroblasts**[Q] *seen in healing by **secondary** intention*[Q]
- **Myofibroblasts** are **altered fibroblasts** that have ultra-structural characteristics of smooth muscle cells.

135. Ans. (d) Skeletal muscle *(Ref: Robbins 9th/pg 101)*

Permanent Tissues
- **Neurons and cardiac**[Q]
- **Muscle cells**[Q]
- **Skeletal muscle**[Q]

136. Ans. (a) Hepatocytes

(Ref: Robbins 9th/pg 101; 8th/pg 81)

Labile Tissues
- **Parenchyma of** liver, kidney, and pancreas.
- **Endothelial cells, fibroblasts, and smooth muscle cells;**[Q]

Labile (Continuously Dividing) Tissues
- **Hematopoietic cells**[Q]
- **Stratified squamous epithelia**[Q]
- **Cuboidal epithelia of** ducts draining exocrine organs (salivary glands, pancreas, biliary tract);
- **Columnar epithelium** of the **GIT, uterus**, and fallopian tubes;
- **Transitional epithelium** of the urinary tract.[Q]

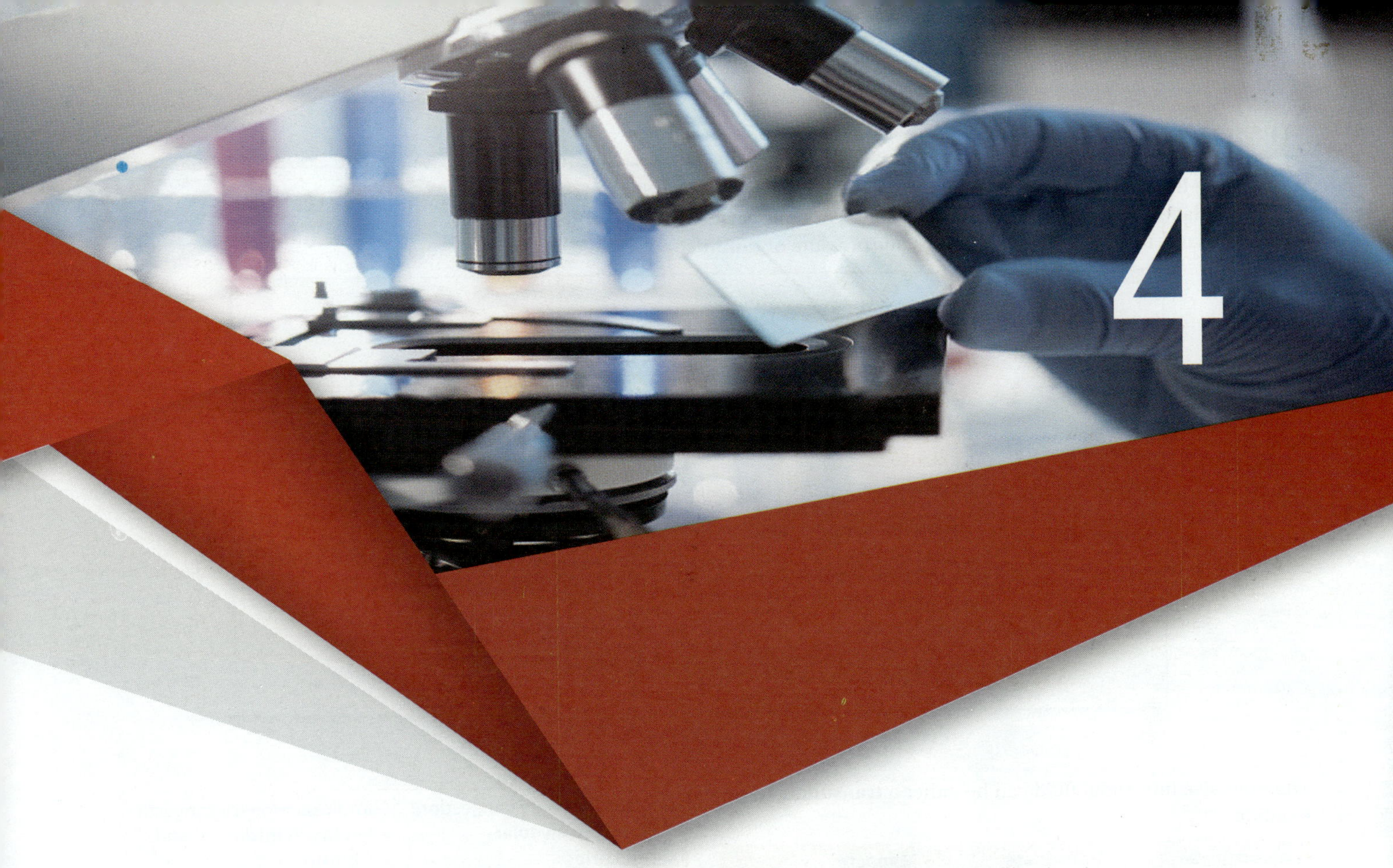

Hemodynamics

Key Points

- **Hyperemia** is an **active** process
- **Nutmeg liver** is seen in chronic passive hepatic congestion
- Hemosiderin-laden macrophages **(heart failure cells)** are seen in chronic pulmonary congestion
- **Line of Zahn**-distinguish antemortem clots from the bland non-laminated postmortem[Q] clots
- Fat embolism syndrome is characterized by pulmonary insufficiency, neurologic symptoms, **anemia** & thrombocytopenia (petechial rash)
- Arterial occlusions cause **white infarcts** whereas venous occlusion cause **red Infarcts[Q]**
- Primary initiating factor in septic shock: **cytokine release**
- Most common cytokine involved in Septic shock is **TNF-α**

Key Recent Updates

- **Procalcitonin** is marker of sepsis
- Most common cause of septic shock is **gram positive bacteria** (PAMP)
- **Endotoxin** [lipopolysaccharide] and lipoteichoic acids are PAMPs (pathogen associated molecular patterns).

HEMODYNAMICS

- **Vascular hydrostatic pressure** is **balanced** by **plasma colloid osmotic pressure**[Q]
- Accumulation of fluid in tissues is called **edema** or body cavities is called **effusions**.[Q]
- It occurs due to either **elevated**[Q] hydrostatic pressure or **diminished**[Q] colloid osmotic pressure

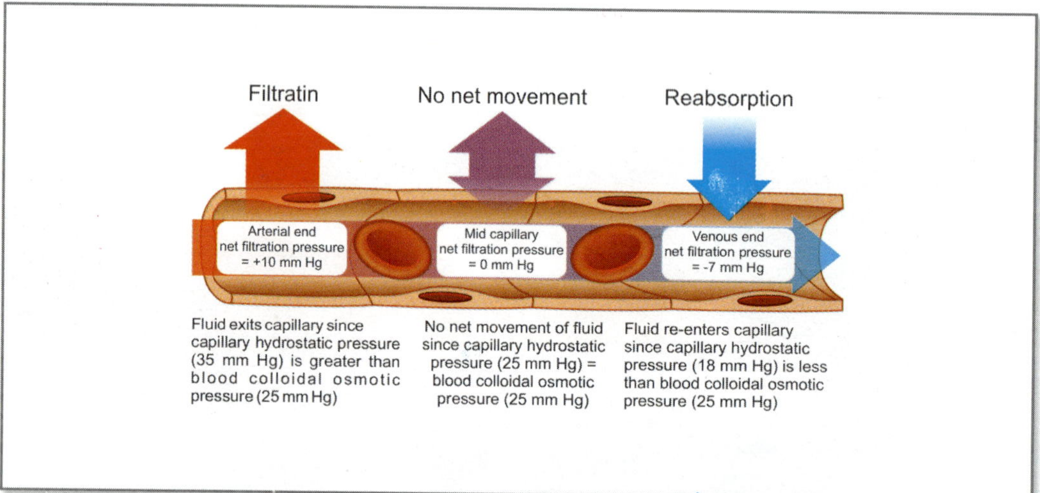

The excessive interstitial fluid can be either a **transudate** or an **exudate**

Characteristic	Transudate	Exudate
Appearance	Clear, Colorless	Yellow, turbid, purulent, bloody
Specific gravity	< 1.015[Q]	> 1.015[Q]
Protein	< 3 g/dL	> 3 g/dL
LDH	< 200 IU	> 200 IU
Cell count	< 1000/uL[Q]	> 1000/uL[Q]
Permeability	Normal[Q]	Altered[Q]
Conditions	Congestive Heart Failure	Infections, Malignancies

HYPEREMIA AND CONGESTION

- **Increased volume of blood**[Q] within dilated vessels of tissue or organ.

Features	Hyperemia	Congestion
Process	Active process[Q]	Passive process[Q]
Cause	Arteriolar dilation	Impaired venous outflow
Edema	Absent	Present[Q]
Colour of the tissues	Red color[Q]	Blue red color[Q] (deoxyhemoglobin)
Seen in	Inflammation[Q]	Right heart failure

Acute pulmonary congestion:
- **Engorged alveolar capillaries**[Q]
- Alveolar **septal edema**[Q]
- **Focal intraalveolar hemorrhage**[Q]

Acute hepatic congestion:
- **Centrilobular** hepatocytes: **ischemic necrosis**[Q]
- **Periportal** hepatocytes - **fatty change**[Q]

Chronic pulmonary congestion:
- Septa are **thickened and fibrotic**[Q]
- **Hemosiderin-laden macro-phages (heart failure cells)**[Q] **(Fig. 1)**

Chronic passive hepatic congestion:
- **Nutmeg liver**[Q]: centrilobular regions are red-brown against surrounding zones of uncongested tan liver **(Fig. 2)**
- Initially **centrilobular necrosis & hemosiderin laden macrophages.**[Q]
- Later: hepatic fibrosis called **cardiac cirrhosis.**[Q]

High Yield Facts

- CVC liver—**Nutmeg liver**
- CVC spleen shown **Gamna Gandy Bodies**. (organized hemorrhage with dystrophic calcification and hemosiderin pigment in spleen)

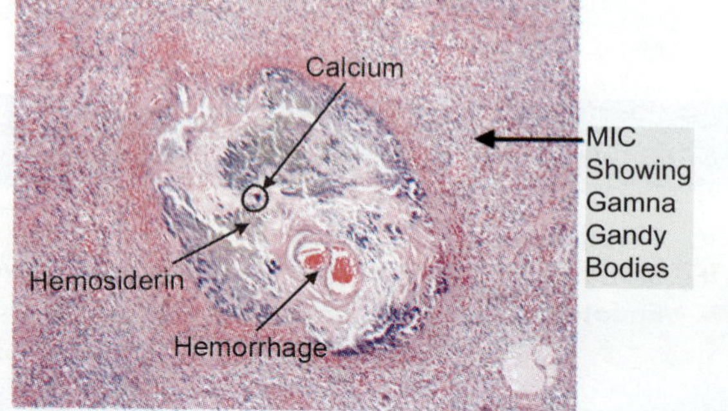

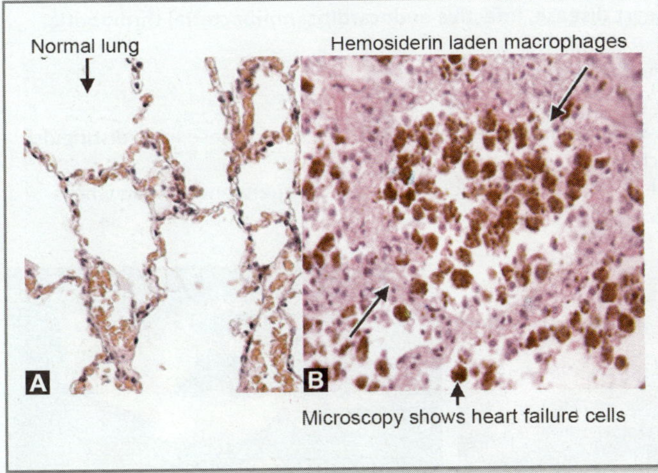

Figs 1A and B: A. Normal lung; B. Microscopy showing heart failure cells s/o chronic pulmonary congestion

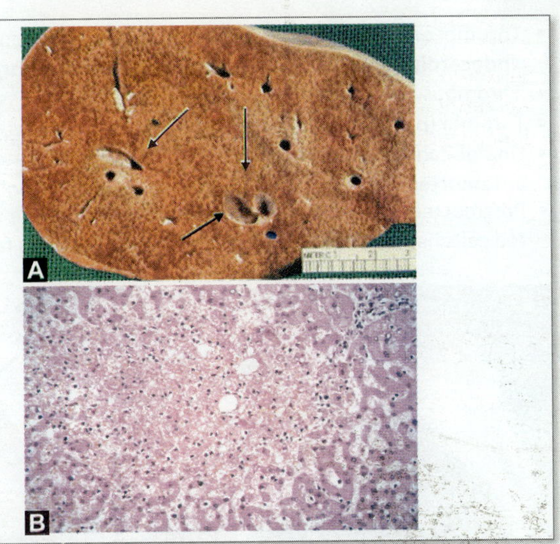

Figs 2A and B: Chronic passive hepatic congestion. A. Gross appearance: Liver shows dilated congested centrilobular regions s/o nutmeg liver B. Microscopic preparation shows centrilobular hepatic necrosis.

HEMOSTASIS

Explained in detail in Chapter Bleeding and its disorders (Chapter 11)

THROMBOSIS

- **Pathologic formation of intravascular thrombus**
- **Virchow's triad** is required for **thrombus formation.**[Q]

Explained in detail in Chapter 11

Types

There are three types of thrombosis

Thrombosis

Mural thrombosis

- **Mural thrombi:** arterial thrombus originate in heart or aorta & adhere to wall of underlying structure.

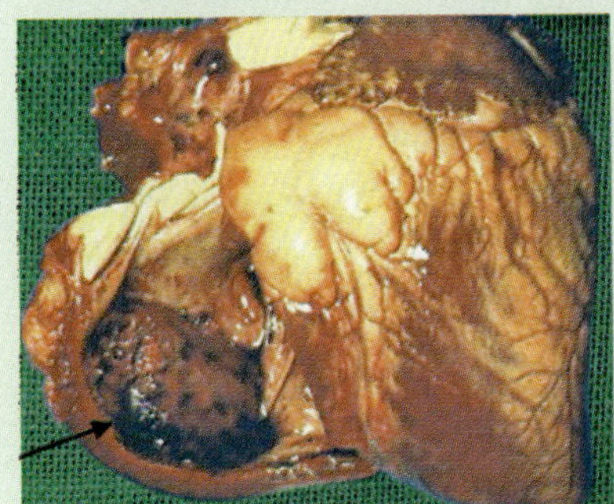

Gross appearance of heart showing mural thrombi

Arterial thrombosis

- **Occurs in rapidly flowing blood**[Q] **of arteries & heart**[Q]
- **Sites: Coronary > cerebral > femoral arteries**[Q]
- **Cause: Atherosclerosis**[Q] **is a major cause**
- **Ulcerated atherosclerotic plaque and aneurysmal dilation**[Q] are the precursors of aortic thrombi[Q]
- **Propagation: Retrograde**[Q] direction from the point of attachment
- **Occlusion:** Usually **mural,** does **not occlude**[Q] the lumen completely
- **Gross: White thrombi.**[Q]
- **Microscopy:** Contain **more platelets**[Q]
- **Embolization: Less common**[Q]

Venous thrombosis

- **Occurs in slow moving blood**[Q] **in veins**[Q]
- **Sites:** Phlebothrombosis (**lower extremities M.C**)
  - Upper limbs, periprostatic plexus, ovarian and periuterine veins
- **Cause: Stasis**[Q]
- **Propagation: Extend in the direction**[Q] of blood flow (i.e., toward the heart).
- **Occlusion:** Almost **always occlusive**[Q]
- **Gross: Red, or stasis, thrombi.**[Q]
- **Microscopy:** Contain **more erythrocytes**[Q]
- **Embolization: More common**[Q]

- Thrombi on heart valves are called **vegetations**: seen in **Rheumatic heart disease, infective endocarditis; nonbacterial thrombotic endocarditis and verrucous (Libman-Sacks) endocarditis**[Q] **(Fig. 3)**.
- Thrombus has a **firm attachment**[Q] to underlying vessel or heart wall, which is **not seen in clot**[Q]
- Thrombi **(both arterial & venous)**[Q] have laminations, called **line of Zahn**[Q]
- Line of Zahn are due to **alternate pale layers of platelets with fibrin & darker layers with more RBCs (Fig. 4)**. These lines **distinguish antemortem clots** from the bland non-laminated clots postmortem[Q] **clots**
- Postmortem clot: Gelatinous & **not attached**[Q] to the underlying wall (in contrast to thrombus[Q]), **Dark red dependent portion** where red cells have settled by gravity and yellow **"chicken fat"**[Q] upper portion **(Fig. 5)**.

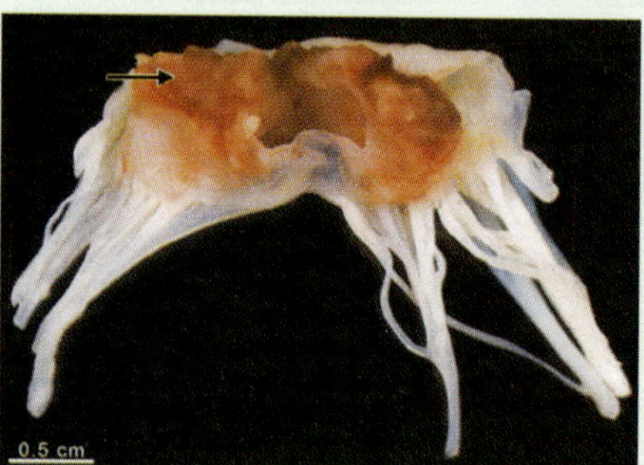
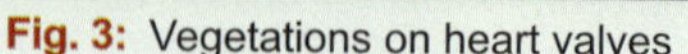

Fig. 3: Vegetations on heart valves

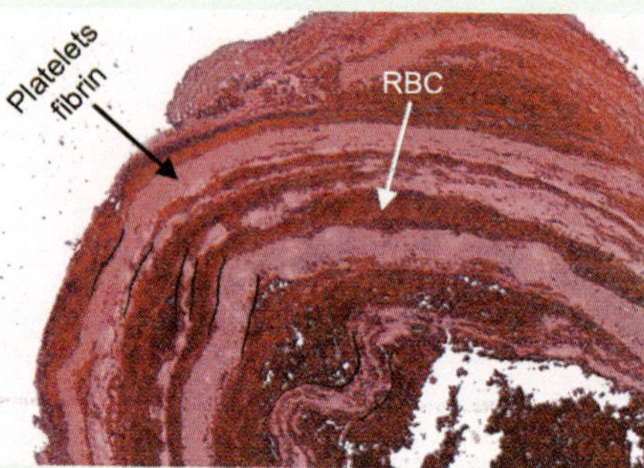

Fig. 4: Line of Zahn

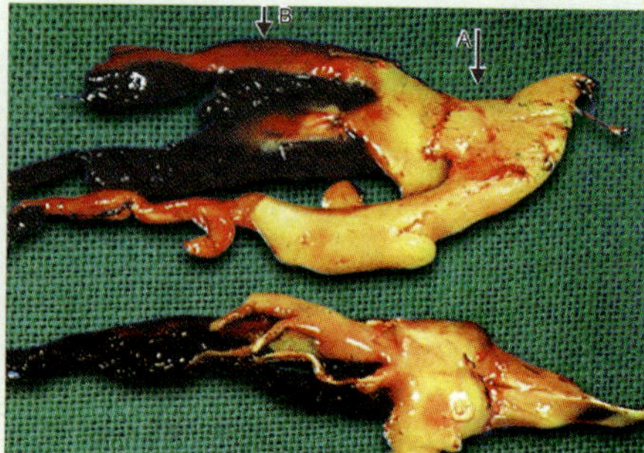

Fig. 5: Postmortem clot

Fate of the Thrombus

Thrombus undergoes four events in the ensuing days to weeks: **possible fates** DOPE:[Q]

- **D**issolution-is the result of **fibrinolysis**
- **O**rganization & repair-in older thrombi; by ingrowth of fibroblasts, endothelial & smooth muscle cells
- **P**ropagation-by accumulation of additional platelets and fibrin
- **E**mbolization-Thrombi dislodge and travel to other sites in the vasculature

DISSEMINATED INTRAVASCULAR COAGULATION (DIC)/CONSUMPTION COAGULOPATHY

Discussed in Chapter 11.

EMBOLISM

- **'Embolus'** is a **detached intravascular solid, liquid, or gaseous mass** that is carried by the blood **from its point of origin to a distant site**[Q],
- **The vast majority of emboli are dislodged thrombi, hence the term thromboembolism.**[Q]

Pulmonary Emboli (Fig. 6)

- **Most common form of thromboembolic disease.**[Q]
- Most arise in the **deep leg veins above the level of knees.**[Q]
- 80% are **clinically silent**[Q] because of **dual circulation and small size**
- **Multiple emboli over time cause pulmonary hypertension and right ventricular failure**[Q]
- >60% obstruction in pulmonary circulation → sudden death or corpulmonale
- **Paradoxical embolus**[Q] **can pass through interatrial/interventricular defect, thus entering the systemic circulation.**[Q]

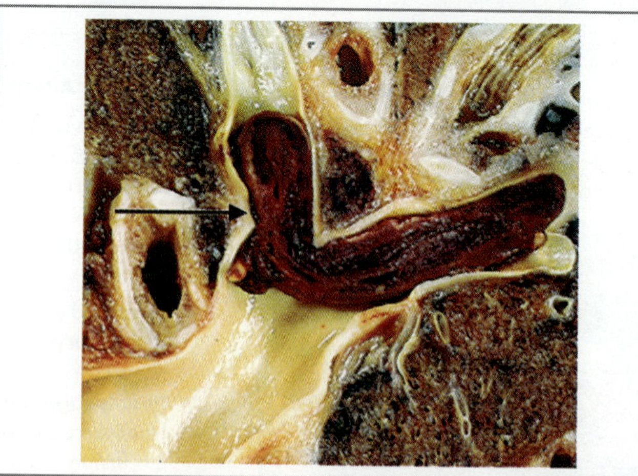

Fig. 6: Pulmonary emboli : Gross appearance

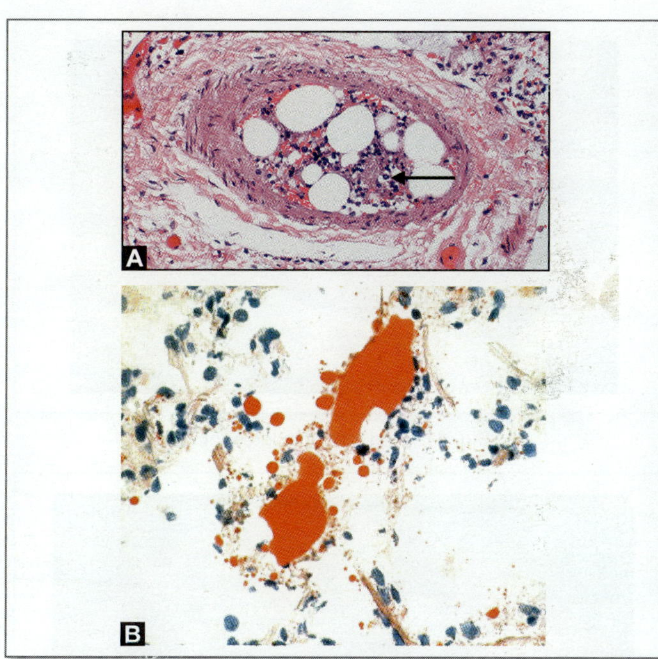

Figs 7A and B: A. Mic showing fat and hematopoietic elements;
B. Fat emboli highlighted by oil red 0

Systemic Thromboembolism or Arterial Emboli

- Most systemic emboli (80%) arise from **intracardiac mural thrombi**[Q]
- 2/3rd associated with **left ventricular wall infarcts** and 1/4th with **left atrial dilation and fibrillation**
- **Major sites: lower extremities** (75%) > brain (10%) > intestines > kidneys > spleen

Fat and Marrow Embolism (Figs 7A and B)

- Occurs in **90% of individuals** with severe skeletal injuries
- MC cause is Fractures of **long bones (which contain fatty marrow)**
- Fat embolism syndrome is characterized by pulmonary insufficiency, neurologic symptoms, anemia & thrombocytopenia (petechial rash) typically seen **1 to 3 days after injury**
- Mechanical obstruction & free fatty acids causing **local toxic injury to endothelium.**[Q]
- **Lab findings-** thrombocytopenia[Q], anemia, fat **microglobulinemia**[Q] (not **macroglobulinemia**[Q]) & fat globules in urine[Q]

Mnemonic

Fat embolism: findings
"Fat, Bat, Fract"
- Fat in urine, sputum
- Bat-wing lung x-ray
- Fracture history
  Also, fracture of FEMur causes Fat EMboli.

Air Embolism

- **>100 cc**, is necessary to produce a clinical effect in the **pulmonary circulation**
- **Decompression sickness** occurs when **there is sudden decreases in atmospheric pressure.**
- Characterized by **pends and chokes:**
  - **Bends: painful condition**[Q] due to rapid gas bubble formation within skeletal muscles & supporting tissues around joints
  - **Chokes:** Respiratory distress due to gas bubbles in vessels causing edema, hemorrhage & focal atelectasis or emphysema
- **Caisson disease (chronic form of decompression sickness)-** persistence of gas emboli in the skeletal system causes multiple foci of ischemic necrosis[Q]; the **more common sites are the femoral heads, tibia, and humeri.**[Q]

Amniotic Fluid Embolism (Fig. 8)

- **Fifth most common cause of maternal mortality** worldwide[Q]
- Ominous complication of **labor and immediate postpartum period.**
- Due to infusion of amniotic fluid or fetal tissue into the maternal circulation via **a tear in the placental membranes or rupture of uterine veins**
- Lead to severe dyspnea and pulmonary edema

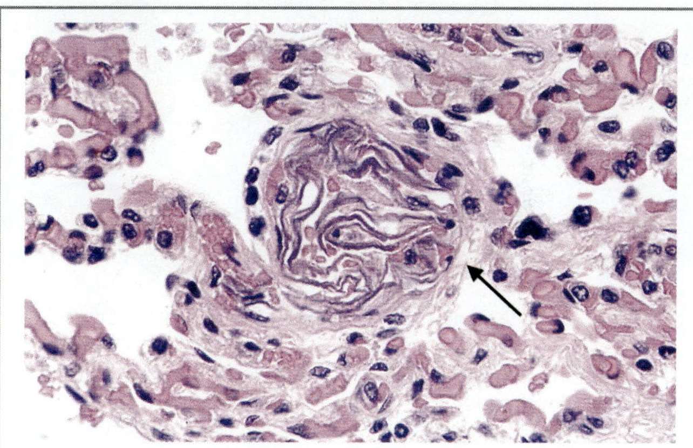

Fig. 8: Mic shows amniotic membranes s/o amniotic fluid embolism in lung alveoli

INFARCT

- An infarct is an area of **ischemic necrosis** due to occlusion of either arterial supply or venous drainage
- Nearly 99% of all infarcts result from **thrombotic or embolic events,**[Q]
- More in organs with a **single venous outflow** like testis and ovary
- The infarcts may be either red (hemorrhagic) or white (anemic) and may be either septic or bland.

Feature	Red Infarcts[Q]	White infarcts[Q]
Cause	• **Dual circulations** (e.g., lung & small intestine) • **Venous occlusion**[q] (ovarian torsion) • Loose, spongy tissues (e.g., lung) • **Tissues previously congested by sluggish venous flow**[q] • When flow is **reestablished**[q] to a site of previous arterial occlusion and necrosis (e.g., **following angioplasty**)	• **End Arterial Circulation** • **Arterial occlusions** • **Solid organs** e.g., heart, spleen, and kidney • **Solid tissue**[Q] -tissue density limits the **seepage**[Q] of blood from adjoining capillary beds into the necrotic area.
Organs	**Loose organs**[Q] like **Lung and small intestine (Figs 9 to 11)**	**Solid organs**[Q] **(heart, spleen, kidney) (Figs 12 to 14)**
Color	Hemorrhagic	Pale[Q] & progressively paler with time
Margins	**Ill-defined hemorrhagic margins,**[Q] brown in color	**Well defined margins**
Edema	Usually **present**[Q]	Usually **absent**[Q]

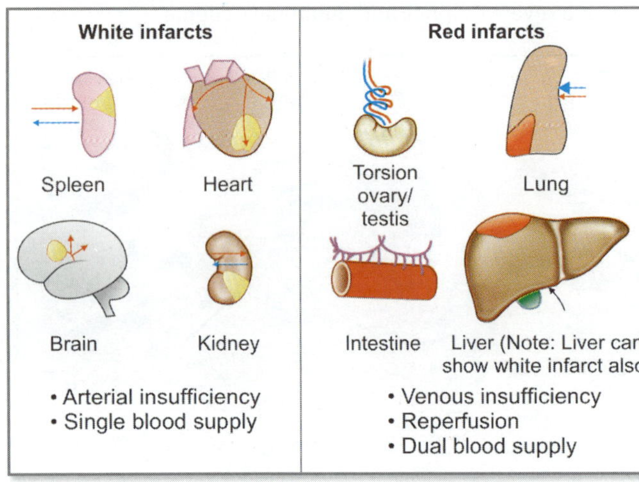

Fig. 9: White and red infarcts sites in different body organs

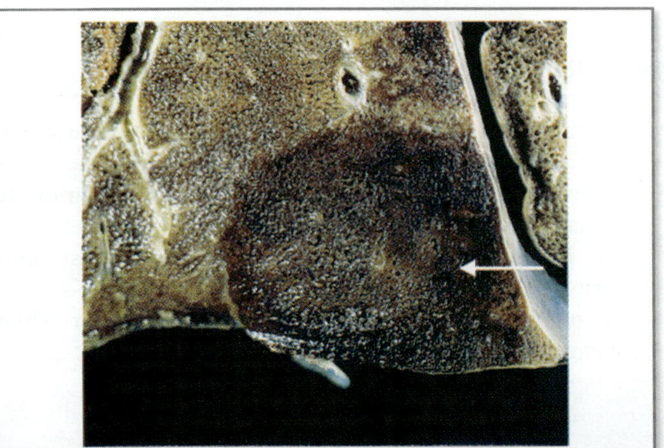

Fig. 10: Red infarct in lung : Gross appearance

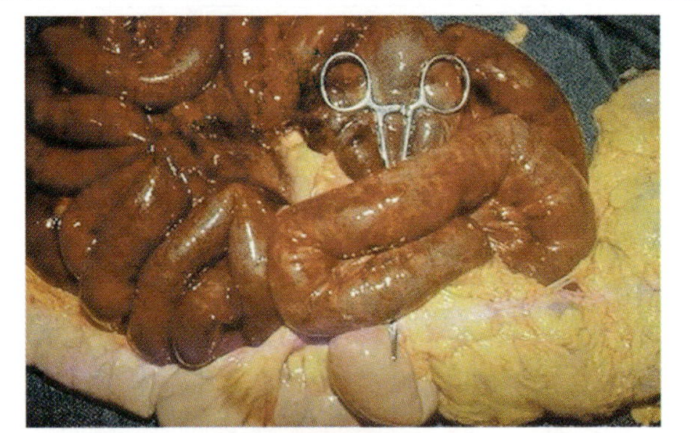

Fig. 11: Red infarct in intestine

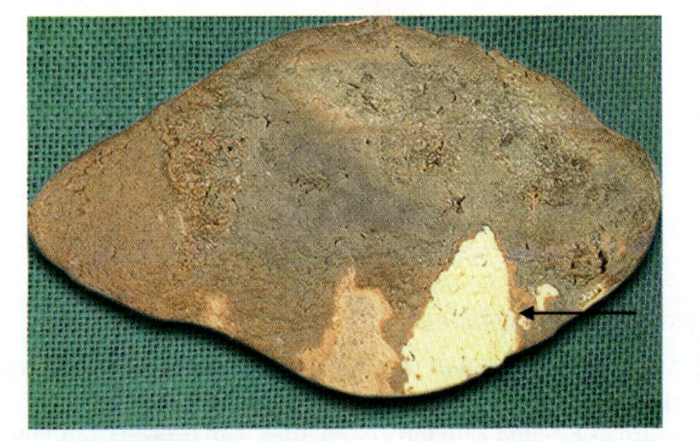

Fig. 12: Gross showing white infarct in spleen

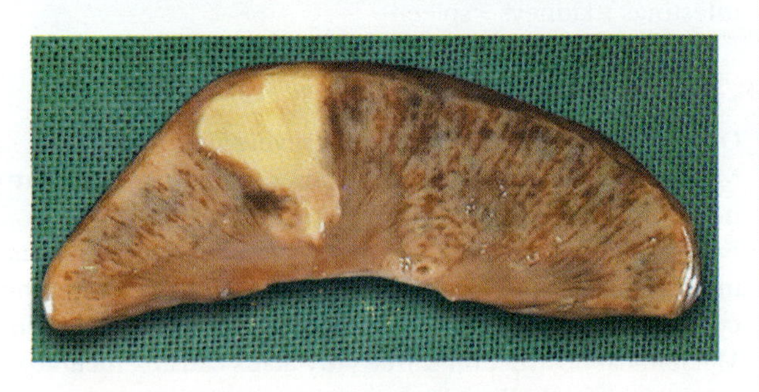

Fig. 13: White infarct in kidney

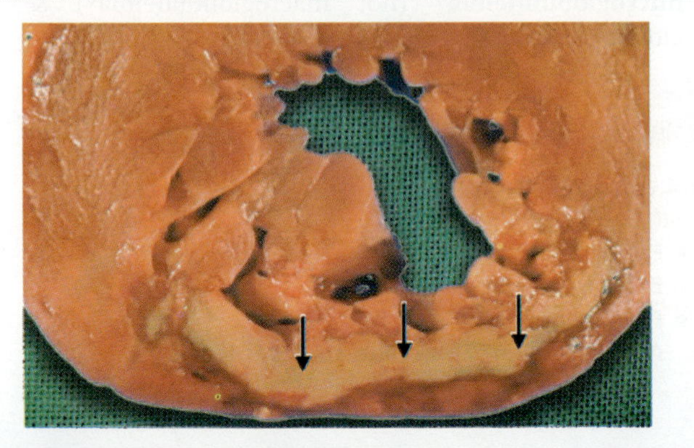

Fig. 14: White infarct in myocardium

- Liver can show both white as well as red infarcts
- Infarcts are **wedge-shaped**[Q], with **occluded vessel at the apex and the periphery of the organ forming the base**[Q]
- All infarcts microscopically has features of **ischemic coagulative necrosis.**[Q] except brain (**liquefactive necrosis**[Q])

Coralline thrombus

In veins thrombi form coral-like system with framework of platelets, fibrin and trapped white blood cells

Septic infarctions

- Occur when infected **cardiac valve vegetations embolize or when microbes seed necrotic tissue**
- In these cases, the **infarct is converted into an abscess**, with a correspondingly greater inflammatory response

SHOCK

A state in which **diminished cardiac output** or **reduced effective circulating blood volume impairs tissue perfusion** and leads to **cellular hypoxia**.

Types

These are three main types of shock

Types of shock	Cardiogenic shock	Hypovolemic shock	Shock associated with systemic inflammation
Cause	Cardiac pump failure	Inadequate blood or plasma volume	Activation of **cytokine cascade**[Q]; peripheral vasodilation and pooling of blood[Q]; endothelial activation/injury;[Q] leukocyte-induced damage[Q], disseminated intravascular coagulation[Q]
Associated conditions	MI, cardiac arrhythmia, cardiac tamponade and pulmonary embolism	Hemorrhage, severe burns and severe dehydration	Microbial infections, burns, trauma, and or pancreatitis

Other Types

- Neurogenic shock: seen with **anesthetic accident or a spinal cord injury**[Q]
- Anaphylactic shock: Due to generalized vasodilation (**type I hypersensitivity)**[Q]

Stages of Shock

Stages	Phase	Features
I	**Non-progressive**	**Reflex compensatory mechanisms activated**[Q] & perfusion of vital organs **maintained**
II	**Progressive**[Q]	**Tissue hypoperfusion, worsening circulatory & metabolic imbalances, lactic acidosis**[Q]
III	**Irreversible**[Q]	Having **irreversible tissue injury**[Q] and multiple organ failure[Q]

- **Primary initiating factor** in **septic shock: cytokine release** → **endothelial damage** → systemic inflammatory response → vasodilation, increased permeability & DIC
- Most common cause of septic shock is Gram-positive bacterial infections, followed by Gram-negative bacteria & fungi.
- Most common cytokine involved in Septic shock is **TNF-α**

Pathogenesis of Septic Shock

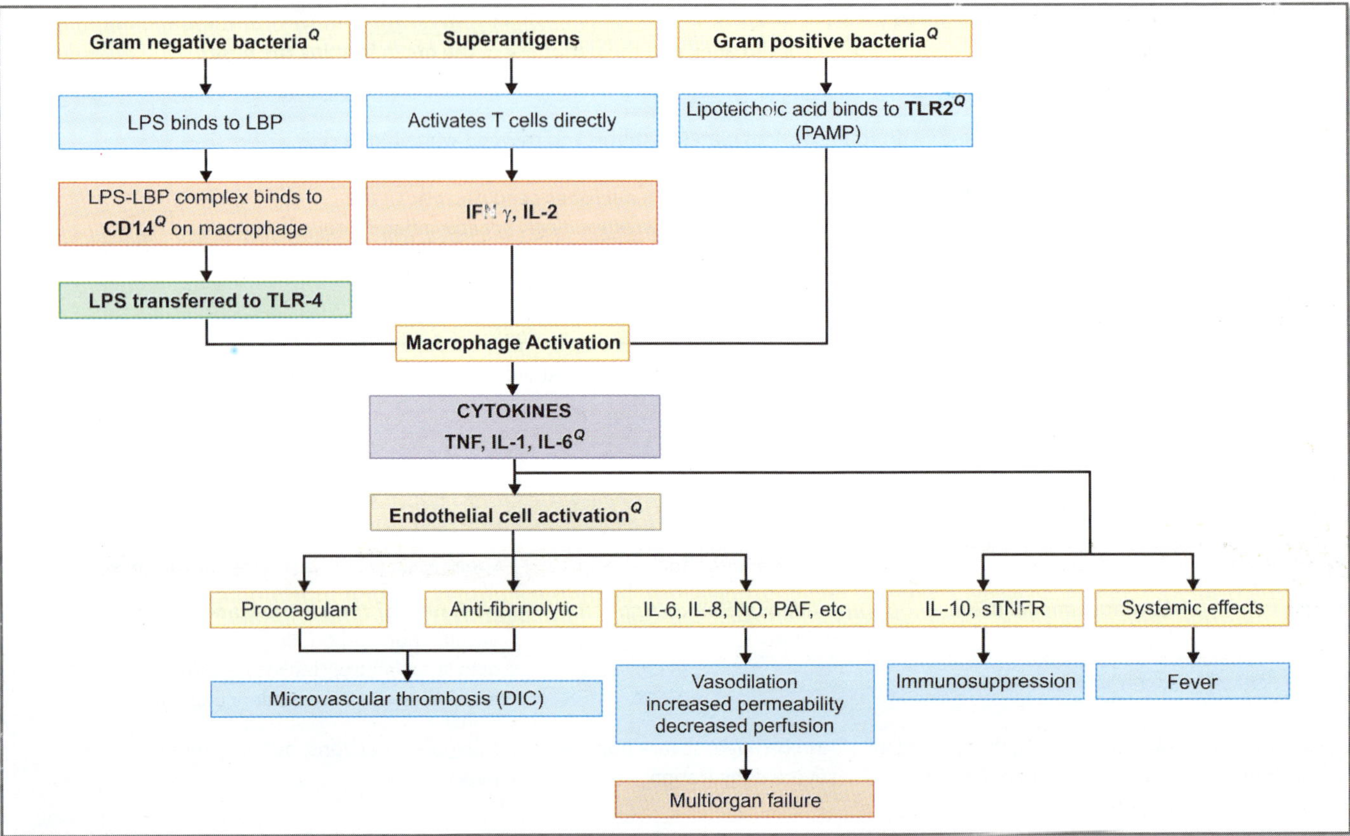

Features of Shock

Changes can manifest in any tissue–**Particularly evident in brain^Q, heart^Q, lungs^Q, kidneys^Q, adrenals, and gastrointestinal tract.**

Adrenal	Kidneys	Heart	Brain	Liver	GIT
↓	↓	↓	↓	↓	↓
Cortical cell lipid depletion^Q	**Acute tubular necrosis^Q**	Coagulative necrosis or **contraction band necrosis^Q**	Ischemic encephalopathy^Q	Fatty change with hemorrhagic central necrosis; **'shock liver'^Q**	**Hemorrhagic Enteropathy^Q**

Histological Features of Shock

Organ	Changes
Adrenal	**Cortical cell lipid depletion.^Q**
Kidneys	**Acute tubular necrosis^Q**
Lungs	**Diffuse alveolar damage (DAD)^Q**
Heart	**Contraction band necrosis^Q**
Brain	Ischemic encephalophathy^Q
Liver	Fatty change with hemorrhagic central necrosis
GIT	**Hemorrhagic Enteropathy^Q**

R10^{th} **Latest** Update

- LPS and lipoteichoic acids are PAMPs
- Procalcitonin is acute phase reactant → MARKER OF SEPSIS

Definitions of sepsis

Criteria for SIRS[a]

Two or more of the following are required:

- Body temperature >38°C or <36°C
- Heart rate >90 beats/min
- Respiratory rate >20 breaths/min (or arterial pCO_2 <32 mmHg, indicating hyperventilation)
- White blood cell count >12.0×10^9/L or <4.0×10^9/L (or >10% immature forms)

Sepsis = Infection + SIRS

Severe sepsis = Sepsis + evidence of organ dysfunction

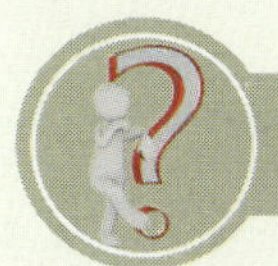

Image-Based Questions

1. A 50-year-old male presents with chronic right heart failure. The succumbs to his illness. On autopsy, liver shows following changes:

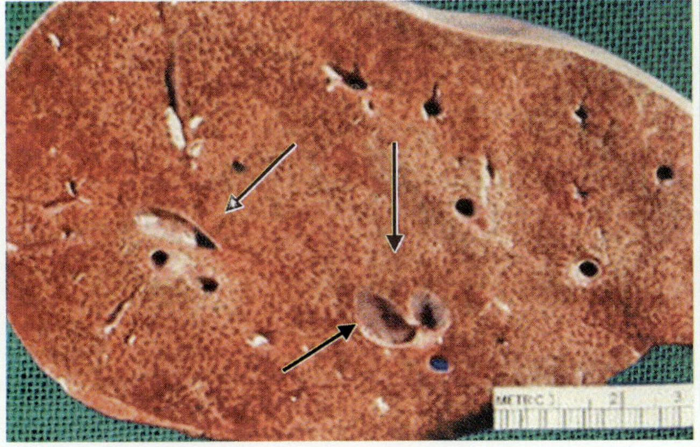

a. Nutmeg liver
b. Normal liver
c. Hemosiderosis liver
d. Liver failure

3. A 64-year-old male died due to RTA. On examination, his vessels showed following clots. Diagnosis is:

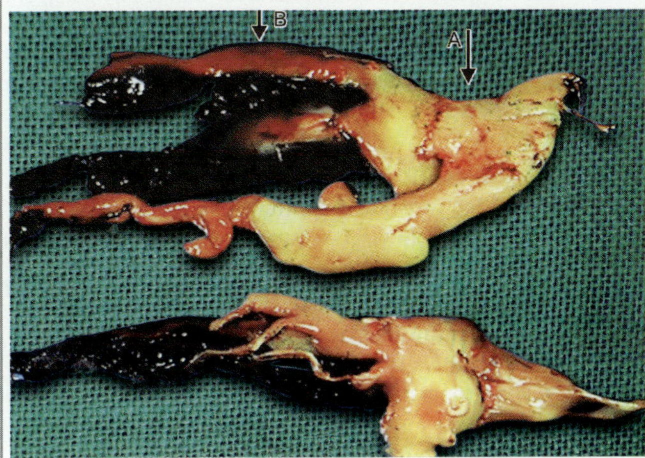

a. Lines of Zahn
b. Chicken fat thrombus
c. Red cells
d. White cells

2. A 20-year-old male was found dead in his home. Family claimed it as dead due to sudden MI. What is the best test to distinguish antemortem from post-mortem clot?

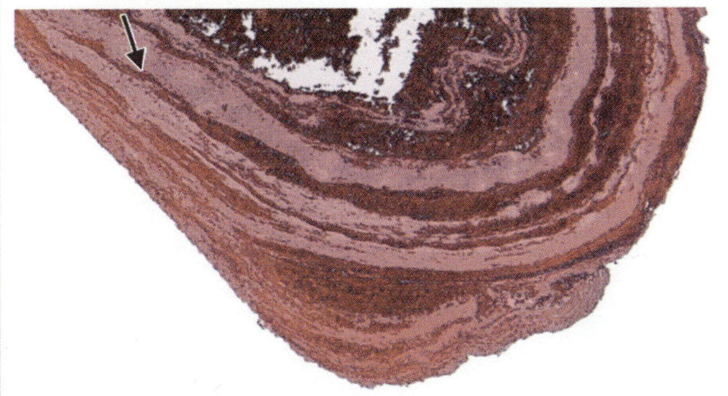

a. Lines of Zahn
b. Chicken fat
c. Red cells
d. White cells

4. A 34-year-old male patient presented with left-upper-quadrant abdominal pain. On CT with contrast, diagnosis of splenic infarct was made. Identify the type of infarct.

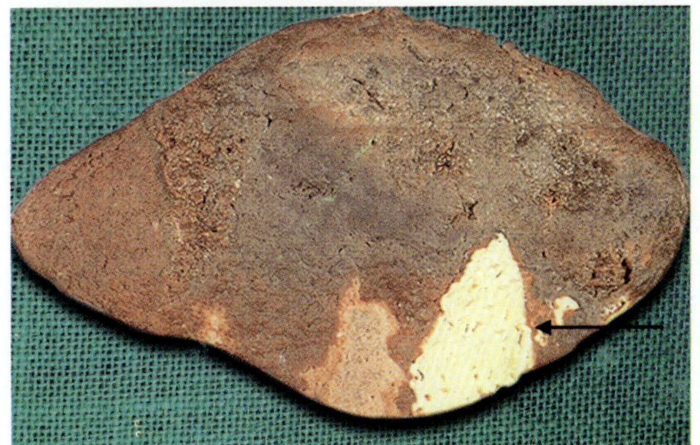

a. White infarct
b. Red infarct
c. Both
d. None

Image-Based Questions

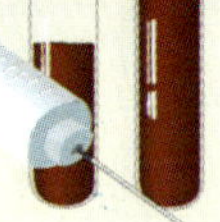
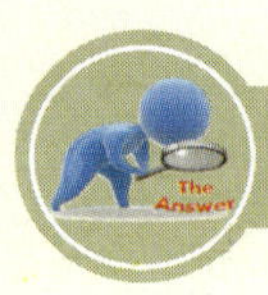

Answers of Image-Based Questions

1. **Ans. (a) Nutmeg liver**
   - Pathologically, the term nutmeg liver refers to the speckled appearance of the cut liver in chronic venous congestion, due to dilated and congested red central veins surrounded by paler, unaffected liver tissue (resembling a grated nutmeg kernel)
   - Note the dark red congested regions that represent accumulation of RBC's in centrilobular regions
   - Microscopically, the nutmeg pattern results from congestion around the central veins
   - Nutmeg liver is **most frequently** seen in **right heart failure**[Q]
   - If the passive congestion is pronounced, then there can be centrilobular necrosis
   - If chronic hepatic passive congestion continues for a long time, a condition called **"cardiac cirrhosis"**[Q]

2. **Ans. (a) Lines of Zahn**
   - Line of Zahn are due to **alternate pale layers of platelets with fibrin & darker layers (marked with arrow)with more RBCs.**
   - These lines **distinguish antemortem clots** from the bland non-laminated clots postmortem[Q] **clots**

3. **Ans. (b) Chicken Fat Thrombus/ Postmortem Clot**
   A. Chicken fat
   B. Current jelly (red cells)
     - Postmortem clots are not attached to vessel walls
     - Show separation of red cells and plasma so that the clotted plasma resembles "chicken fat" layered on top of a rubber gelatinous dark red mass of erythrocytes resembling "current jelly"

4. **Ans. (a) White Infarct**
   - **Wedge-shaped**[Q], **with occluded vessel at the apex and the periphery of the organ forming the base**[Q]
   - **It is usually seen in solid organs** e.g., heart, spleen, and kidney
   - **Solid tissue**[Q] density **limits the seepage**[Q] of blood from adjoining capillary beds into the necrotic area.

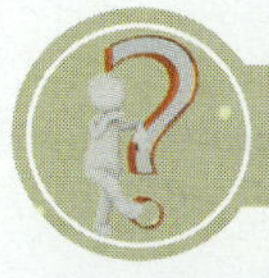

Multiple Choice Questions

HYPEREMIA AND CONGESTION

1. **Edema is due to:** *(JIPMER 2016, Recent Question 2015)*
    a. Lymphatic obstruction
    b. Decreased hydrostatic pressure
    c. Increased oncotic pressure
    d. Increased plasma proteins

2. **Liver biopsy in chronic RHF shows:**
    a. Shrinking *(Recent Question 2015)*
    b. Greasy fatty liver
    c. Hypertrophy
    d. Congestion

3. **Heart failure cells are** *(Recent Question 2015)*
    a. Foam cells
    b. Lipid laden macrophages
    c. Hemosiderin laden macrophages
    d. Type 1 pneumocytes

4. **The given figure shows which of the following?**
    (AIIMS Nov 2015)

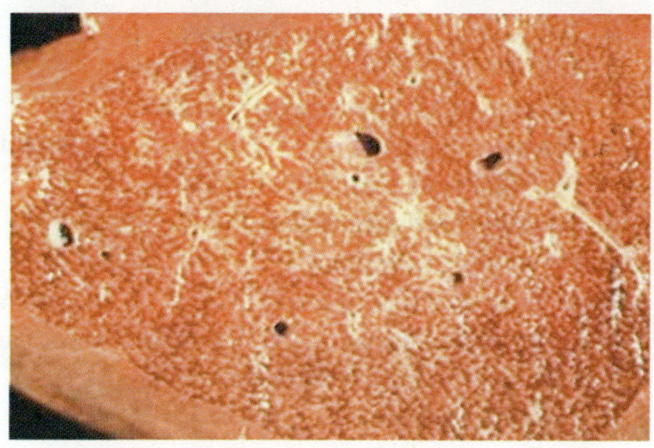

    a. Amyloidosis-grew; viable white necrotic
    b. Nutmeg liver-red areas are viable pericentral areas; white areas are periportal necrotic areas
    c. Red areas are necrotic areas near central vein, white areas are viable, fibrotic periportal area
    d. Amyloidosis-necrotic white periportal viable gray pericentral areas

5. **Nutmeg liver seen in** *(Recent Question 2014-15)*
    a. Alcoholic liver disease
    b. Chronic venous congestion
    c. Hepatoma
    d. Secondary carcinoma deposits in liver

6. **Heart failure cells are seen in**
    (Recent Question 2014-15)
    a. Heart   b. Lungs
    c. Kidney   d. Liver

7. **Edema occurs when plasma protein level is below:**
    (Recent Question 2015)
    a. 8 g/dL   b. 2 g/dL
    c. 5 g/dL   d. 10 g/dL

THROMBOSIS

8. **Which of the following has a major role in thrombus formation?** *(Recent Pattern Question 2020)*
    a. Endothelial injury   b. Vasoconstriction
    c. Platelet activation   d. Coagulation cascade

9. **All the following are features of arterial thrombus except:** *(Recent Question 2015)*
    a. Associated with endothelial injury
    b. Lines of zahn present
    c. Also called white thrombi
    d. Grows in an anterograde manner from the point of attachment

10. **Lines of Zahn are seen in:** *(PGI Nov 2015)*
    a. Antemortem clots
    b. Postmortem clots
    c. Coralline thrombus
    d. Line of Zahn are due to alternate pale layers of platelets with fibrin & darker layers with more RBCs
    e. Lines of Zahn are thrombi (both arterial & venous) with laminations

11. **True about thrombus formation:** *(PGI May 2015)*
    a. Arterial thrombus grow in direction toward heart
    b. Venous thrombus grow in direction toward heart
    c. Venous thrombus form chicken fat
    d. Line of Zahn is seen microscopically in red thrombi

12. **Virchow's triad for thrombosis include all EXCEPT:**
    a. Endothelial injury
    b. Stasis *(MH PG 2014)*
    c. Platelet aggregation
    d. Hypercoagulability

13. **All are predisposing factors of Deep Vein thrombosis, except:** *(Recent Question 2015)*
    a. HIT
    b. Polycythemia
    c. Malignancy
    d. Hyperlipidemia

14. **All are hypercoagulable states, except:**
    a. Protein C resistance *(AIIMS June 12)*
    b. Protein S deficiency
    c. Antiphospholipid antibody
    d. Polycythemia

15. **Which of the following DOES NOT present with recurrent episodes of upper limb thrombosis:**
    a. Prostatic Ca. *(AIIMS June 11)*
    b. Pancreatic Ca,
    c. Osteosarcoma
    d. Acute pro myelocytic leukemia

16. **Both arterial and venous thrombosis occur in:**
    a. Antiphospholipid antibodies *(PGI Nov 2011)*
    b. Antithrombin III deficiency
    c. Hyperhomocysteinemia
    d. Protein C deficiency
    e. Mutation in factor V gene

17. Hypercoagulability due to defective factor V gene is called

a. Lisbon mutation *(AIIMS May 10)*
b. Leiden mutation
c. Antiphospholipid syndrome
d. Inducible thrombocytopenia syndrome

EMBOLISM

18. Patient after trauma has respiratory discomfort. Ventilation tried but not helpful histopath of lung given.
(AIIMS Nov 2016)

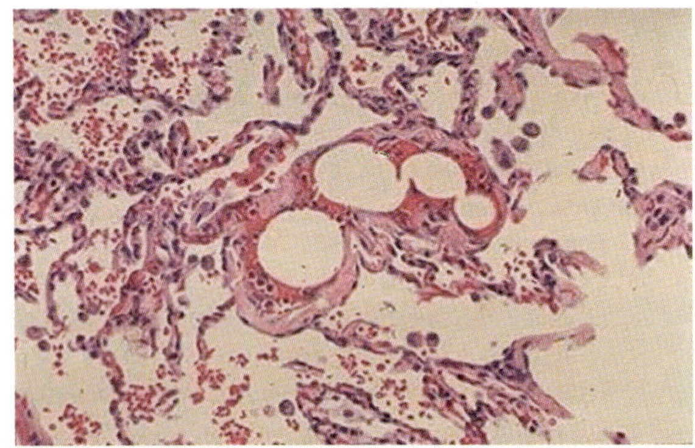

a. Diffuse alveolar hmg with pul edema
b. Diffuse damage due to ventilation pressure
c. FAT embolism
d. None

19. Least affected organ in arterial thromboembolism is?
(MH PG 2016, Recent Question 2015)

a. Liver
b. Kidney
c. Heart
d. Brain

20. Minimum quantity of air in pulmonary circulation to cause clinical effects *(Recent Question 2015)*

a. 10 mL
b. 50 mL
c. 100 mL
d. 500 mL

21. The most common source of embolism:
(Recent Question 2014)

a. DVT
b. Trauma
c. Infection
d. Surgery

INFARCT

22. White infarcts are seen in all the following organs except: *(Recent Question 2015)*

a. Lung
b. Heart
c. Spleen
d. Kidney

23. Red infarct is seen in: *(Recent Question 2015)*

a. Lung
b. Heart
c. Kidney
d. Spleen

24. Red infarct occur in: *(PGI May 2015)*

a. In tissues with dual circulations
b. Occur only when both arterial and venous obstruction occurs simultaneously
c. Organs which are previously congested
d. Organs with loose tissue

25. White infarct is seen in: *(Recent Question 2015)*

a. Lung
b. Intestine
c. kidney
d. Ovary

26. Pale infarcts are seen at all of the following sites except: *(AIIMS Nov 10/ AI 97)*

a. Heart
b. Spleen
c. Kidney
d. Lung

SHOCK

27. Endothelium activation refers to:
(Kerela PG 2016, Recent Question 2014-15)

a. Aberration of anatomy of vessel wall
b. Irreversible changes in functional state of vessel wall
c. Smooth muscle proliferation
d. Increased expression of adhesion molecules for leukocyte recruitment

28. Septic Shock is due to: *(Recent Question 2015)*

a. Vasodilatation
b. Decreased Cardiac output
c. Endothelial damage
d. All of the above

29. MC endogenous pyrogen and shock manifestation are: *(Recent Question 2015)*

a. IL-6
b. IL-8
c. IL 1beta
d. TNF alpha

30. Procalcitonin is used as a marker for?

a. Sepsis *(DNB Aug 12)*
b. Medullary carcinoma of thyroid
c. Vitamin D resistant rickets
d. Parathyroid adenoma

31. Endotoxin shock is initiated by: *(AIIMS Nov 10)*

a. Endothelial injury
b. Peripheral vasodilation
c. Increased vascular permeability
d. Cytokines action

MISCELLANEOUS

32. In cornea stem cell present at?
(Recent Question 2016-17)

a. Limbus
b. Descments membrane
c. Basement membrane
d. Rods and cones

33. Weibel-palade bodies are present in: *(AP 2012)*

a. Vascular endothelial cells
b. Warthin finkeldey cells
c. Leydig cells
d. Dendritic cells

34. Which one of the following factors is labelled as cytokine in the pathogenesis of systemic inflammatory response syndrome: *(Recent Question 2014)*

a. Nitric oxide
b. Complements
c. Leukotrienes
d. Tumor Necrosis factor

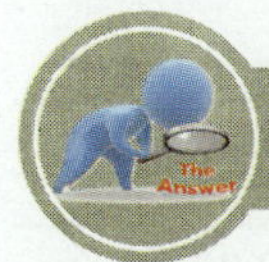

Answers with Explanations

1. **Ans. (a) Lymphatic obstruction** *(Ref: Robbins 9th/pg 114)*

2. **Ans. (d) Congestion** *(Ref: Robbins 9th/pg 115; 8th/pg 113)*

3. **Ans. (c) Hemosiderin laden macrophages**

   (Ref: Robbin's 9th/pg 115)

   Chronic pulmonary congestion: shows **Hemosiderin-laden macrophages (heart failure cells)[Q]**

4. **Ans. (c) Red areas are necrotic areas near central vein, white areas are viable, fibrotic periportal area**

   (Ref: Robbin's 9th/129)

   The given picture shows **Chronic passive hepatic congestion,** the centrilobular regions are red-brown & slightly depressed (because of cell death) & are prominently visible against surrounding zones of uncongested tan liver (**nutmeg liver**).

5. **Ans. (b) Chronic venous congestion** *(Ref: R 9th/ 129)*

6. **Ans. (b) Lungs** *(Ref: Robbin's 9th/pg 115; 8th/pg 113)*

7. **Ans. (c) 5 g/dL** *(Ref: Harshmohan 5th pg 97)*

   When total plasma proteins <5 gm/dl (normal 6-8 gm/dl) or albumin <2.5 gm/dl (normal 3.5-5 gm/dl) edema takes place

8. **Ans. (a) Endothelial injury**

   (Refer to answer 12)

9. **Ans. (d) Grows in an anterograde manner from the point of attachment**

   (Ref: Robbins 9th/pg 122; 8th/pg 121)

10. **Ans. (a, c, d, e) a. Antemortem clots; c. coralline thrombus; d. Line of Zahn are due to alternate pale layers of platelets with fibrin and darker layers with more RBCs; e. Lines of Zahn are thrombi (both arterial and venous) with laminations**

    (Ref: Robbins 9th/pg 122; 8th/pg 121)

    - Thrombi (**both arterial & venous**)[Q] have laminations, called **line of Zahn**[Q]
    - Line of Zahn are due to **alternate pale layers of platelets with fibrin & darker layers with more RBCs**.
    - These lines **distinguish antemortem clots** from the bland non-laminated clots that occur post-mortem

- In veins thrombi form coral-like system with framework of platelets, fibrin and trapped white blood cells this is a coralline thrombus. Lines of zahn are seen in this.

11. **Ans. (b) Venous thrombus grow in direction toward heart** *(Ref: Robbins 9th/pg 122; 8th/pg 121)*

12. **Ans. (c) Platelet aggregation** *(Ref: Robbin's 9th/pg 122)*

13. **Ans. (d) Hyperlipidemia** *(Ref: R 9th/pg 122; 8th/pg 121)*

14. **Ans. (d) Polycythemia**

    (Ref: Robbin's 9th/pg 122; 8th/pg 121)

    Polycythemia is cause of hyperviscosity and not hypercoagulability

15. **Ans. (c) Osteosarcoma** *(Ref: Robbin's 8th/pg 673)*

    Cancers causing thrombosis

Pancreas	Acute promyelocytic leukemia	Breast	Brain
Lung	Stomach	Prostate	

    Peripheral venous thrombosis with visceral carcinoma esp pancreatic carcinoma is called trousseau syndrome or migratory thrombophlebitis.

16. **Ans. (a, c); a. Antiphospholipid antibodies; c. Hyperhomocysteinemia** *(Ref: Harrison 17th pg 367)*

    Risk factor for thrombosis

	ARTERIAL + VENOUS
Inherited	Homocystinuria, Dysfibrinogenemia
Acquired	• Cancer • Disseminated intravascular coagulation • Heparin-induced thrombocytopenia • Antiphospholipid antibody syndrome • PNH, TTP • ET (essential thrombocythemia) • PV (polycythemia vera)
Inherited + acquired	Hyperhomocystienemia

17. **Ans. (b) Leiden mutation**

    Ref: Robbins 9th/pg 122; 8th/pg 121

    - **Factor V mutation (called as leiden mutation,** after the city in the Netherlands where it was discovered) is **most important cause** of primary hypercoagulability.

- The mutation results in a **glutamine to arginine** substitution at **position 506** that renders factor V **resistant to cleavage by protein C.**

18.   Ans. (c) FAT embolism *(Ref: Robbin's 9th/pg/130)*

19.   Ans. (a) Liver

(Ref: Robbins 9th/pg 127; 8th/pg 126, MD Guidelines-Arterial Embolism and Thrombosis by Presley Reed, MD)

Arterial emboli often occur in the legs and feet. Some may occur in the brain, or heart.

Less common sites include the Liver, intestines, and eyes

20.   Ans. (c) 100 mL *(Ref: Robbins 9th/pg 127; 8th/pg 126)*

- **>100 cc**, is necessary to produce a clinical effect in the **pulmonary circulation**

21.   Ans. (a) DVT *(Ref: Robbins 9th/pg 127; 8th/pg 126)*

- MC cause of venous embolism is DVT
- Most arise in the **deep leg veins above the level of the knee.**[Q]

22.   Ans. (a) Lung *(Ref: Robbins 9th/pg 129; 8th/pg 128)*

A.   Red infarct- Lung, Ovary, Intestine

B.   White infact – **kidney, heart, spleen and brain**

Liver infarctions are rare because of liver's dual blood supply. Its infarction is described as dichotomic, i.e. it can show overlap between red to white infarct.

23.   Ans. (a) Lung *(Ref: Robbin's 9th/pg 129; 8th/pg 128)*

24.   Ans. (a, c, d) a. In tissues with dual circulations; c. Organs which are previously congested; d. Organs with loose tissue *(Ref: Robbins 9th/pg 129; 8th/pg 128)*

25.   Ans. (c) Kidney *(Ref: Robbins 9th/pg 129; 8th/pg 128)*

26.   Ans. (d) Lung *(Ref: Robbin's 9th/pg 129; 8th/pg 128)*

27.   Ans. (d) Increased expression of adhesion molecules for leukocyte recruitment

(Ref: Thromb Res 123 (Suppl 4): S30–4)

Endothelial activation is a proinflammatory and procoagulant state of the endothelial cells lining the lumen of blood vessels. It is most characterized by **Increased expression of adhesion molecules for leukocyte recruitment**

28.   Ans. (d) All of the above *(Ref: R 9th/pg 131-132; 8th/pg 131)*

29.   Ans. (d) TNF alpha *(Ref: R 9th/pg 131-132; 8th/pg 131)*

30.   Ans. (a) Sepsis *(Ref: Critical care forum.com)*

- Measurement of procalcitonin can be used as a **marker of severe sepsis** caused by bacteria and generally grades well with the degree of sepsis.

31.   Ans. (d) Cytokines action *(Ref: Robbin's 9th/pg 131-132)*

32.   Ans. (a) Limbus *(Ref: Robbins 9th/pg 28)*

33.   Ans. (a) Vascular endothelial cells

*(Ref: Weibel ER, (October 1964). J. Cell Biol. **23** (1): 101–12)*

Weibel–Palade bodies are the storage granules of endothelial cells. They store and release von Willebrand factor and P-selectin.

34.   Ans. (d) Tumor Necrosis factor *(Ref: R 9th/pg 131-132)*

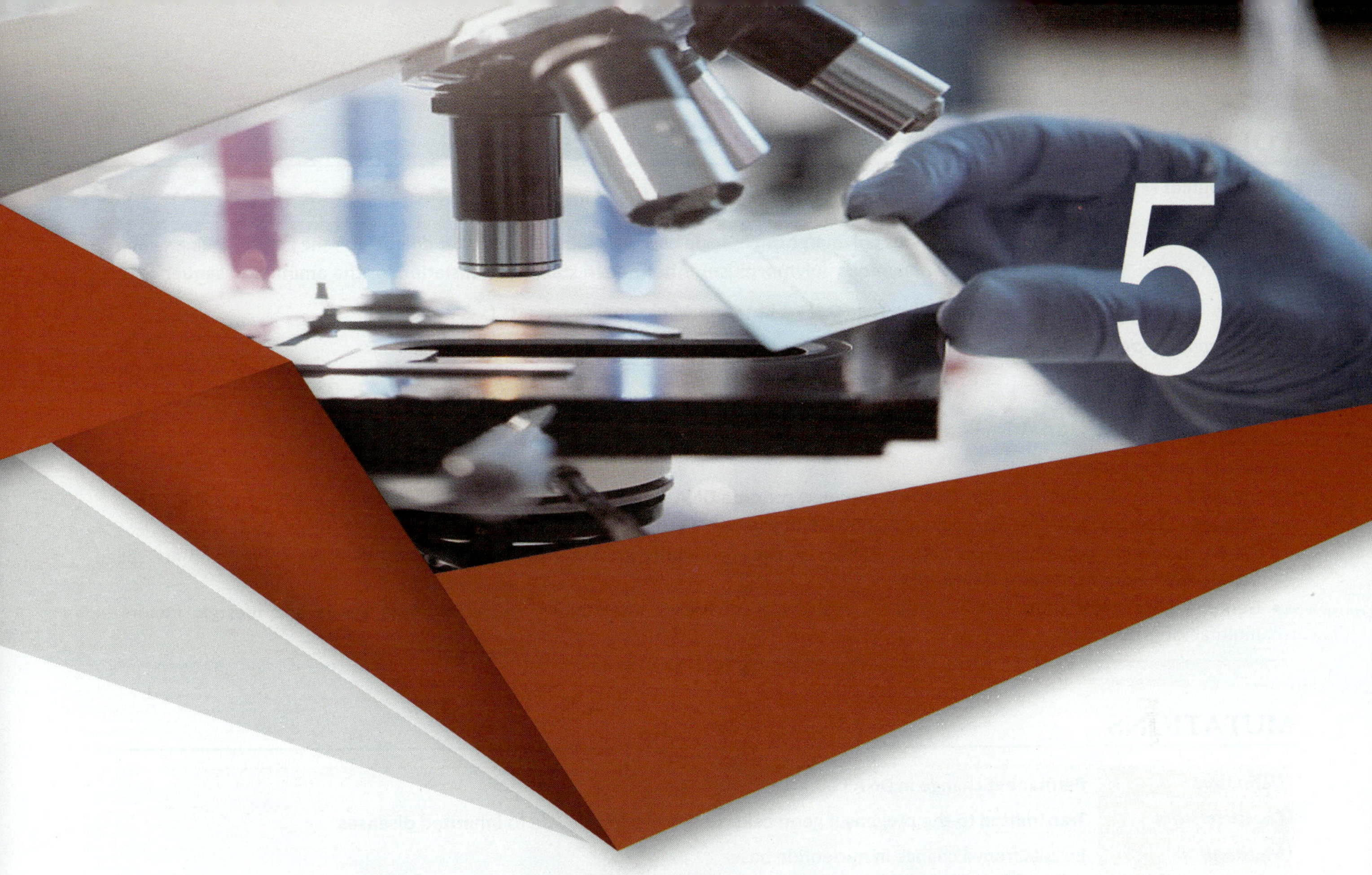

Genetic Disorders

5

Key Points

» An **observed trait** is referred to as a **phenotype**[Q]
» **Genetic information** defining the phenotype is called the **genotype**[Q]
» **Locus** is the **position of gene** on a chromosome
» **Alternative forms** of a gene or a genetic marker are referred to as **alleles**[Q]
» The **normal** or common allele is usually referred to as **wild type**[Q]
» When alleles at a given locus are **identical**, the individual is **homozygous**[Q]
» If alleles are different on maternal and paternal copy of the gene; individual is **heterozygous**[Q]
» If **two different mutant alleles** are inherited **at a given locus**, the individual is said to be a **compound heterozygote**[Q]
» **Hemizygous**[Q] is used to describe males with a mutation in an X gene or a female with a loss of one X locus.

Key Recent Updates

» **CRISPR**—Knock out technology
» Gaucher's disease is strongly linked with **Parkinson's disease**
» **Zebra Bodies** are seen in Niemann Pick disease, metachromatic leukodystrophy and mucopolysaccharidoses.

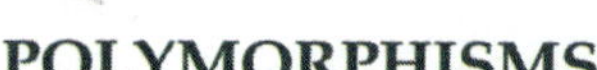

POLYMORPHISMS

Physiological sequence variations[Q], have a frequency of at least 1%.

Types depending on protein coding sequence alteration	• **Synonymous polymorphism[Q]**: Single **base-pair substitutions[Q]** that **do not** alter the protein coding sequence • **Non-synonymous polymorphism**: Alter mRNA stability, translation, or the amino acid sequence[Q]
Types of Repeat length	**Microsatellite repeats (< 1 kb)[Q]** and **Mini-satellite repeats (1-3 kb)[Q]**
Polymorphisms detected by	**Linkage analysis[Q] or GWAS[Q]**

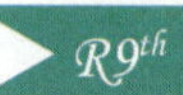

R9th Latest Update

Human Genome Project
- Initiated in the mid-1980s to characterize the **human genome DNA sequence.**[Q]
- **23 pairs** of human chromosomes encode 23,000–**30,000 genes**[Q] (3 billion bp)
- **Single nucleotide polymorphisms (SNPs)** that are in **close proximity** are **inherited together (i.e., they are linked)** and are called **haplotypes[Q]**, hence the name **HapMap[Q]**
- **Genome-wide association studies (GWAS)[Q]** explains the complex **interactions** among **multiple genes** and **lifestyle factors** in multifactorial disorders.

MUTATIONS

Definition	**Permanent change in DNA[Q]**
Characteristics	**Transmitted to the progeny** if germ cells are affected;[Q] give rise to **inherited diseases**
Mechanisms	Results from a change in nucleotide base- • **Transitions** - One **purine** is replaced by **another purine[Q]** base (A → G) or a **pyrimidine** is replaced by **another pyrimidine** (C → T) • **Transversions**- Changes from a **purine to pyrimidine[Q]**, or vice versa

Flowchart 1: Types of mutation

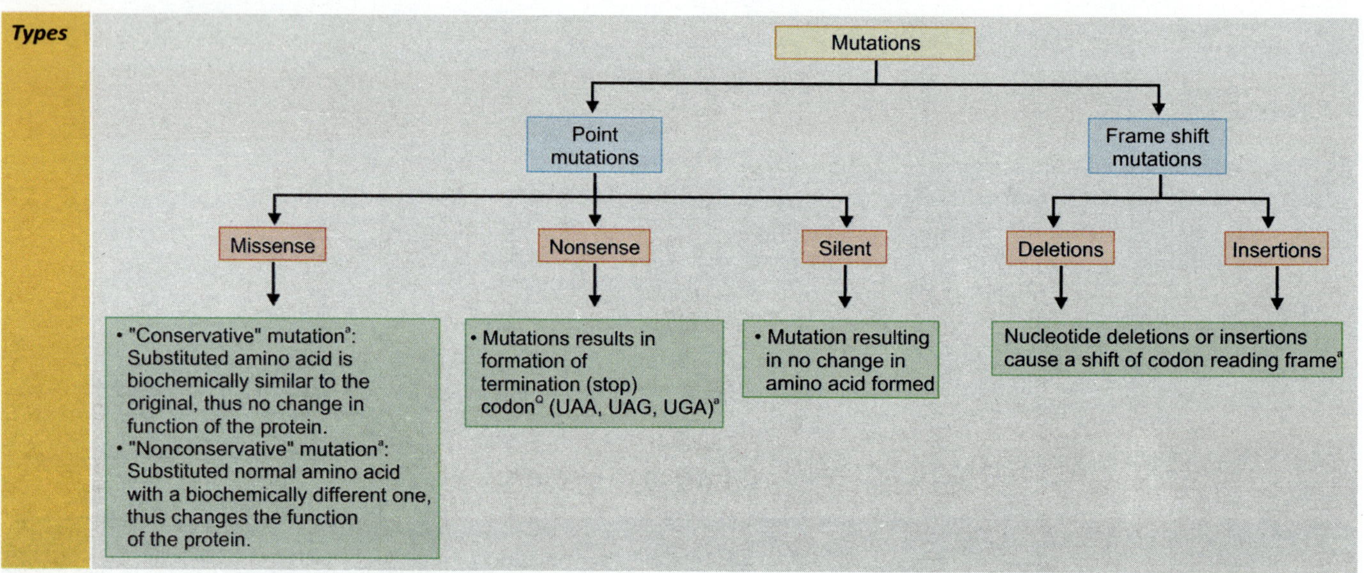

Flowchart 2: Classification of genetic disorders

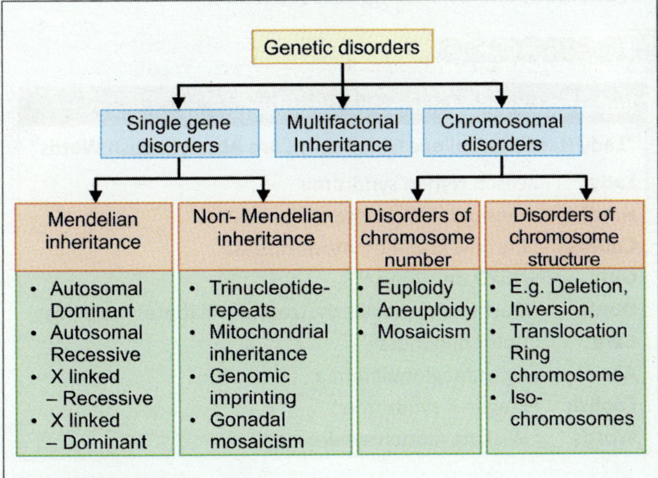

MENDELIAN DISORDERS

Autosomal Dominant Disorders

- Manifestation of an allele in even **heterozygous**[Q] state
- Its called **vertical inheritance** because of transmission from parent to offspring.

Characteristics

- When an **affected person** marries an **unaffected one**, every child has **50% chance of having the disease**[Q]
- Incomplete **penetrance and variable expressivity**[Q]
- Age of onset may be **delayed until adulthood**[Q]
- May be **loss-of-function (more common)** or **gain-of-function mutations**

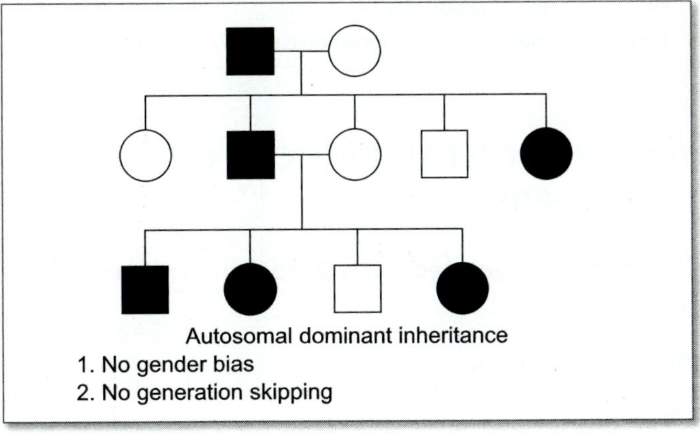
Autosomal dominant inheritance
1. No gender bias
2. No generation skipping

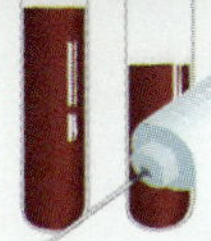

Important Autosomal Dominant Diseases
"HEAVY DOMINANT"

H : Hypercholestrolemia[Q], Hereditary spherocytosis[Q], HNPCC[Q]

E : **E**hler Danlos syndrome (except type VI)

A : **A**denomatous polyposis coli

V : **V**on willebrand disease[Q]

Y : Pseudoh**y**poparathyroidism

D : **D**ystrophia myotonica[Q]

O : **O**steogenesis imperfecta[Q]

M : **M**arfan's syndrome[Q]

I : **I**ntermittent porphyria

N : **N**eurofibromatosis 1 and 2[Q]

A : **A**chondroplasia[Q], Adult polycystic kidney disease

N : **N**oonan's syndrome

T : **T**uberous sclerosis

High Yield Facts

- **Codominance**[Q]: When **both alleles** of a gene pair contribute to the phenotype. E.g., Blood group 'AB' and histocompatibility complex
- **Pleiotropism**[Q]: **Many end effects** due to a **single mutant gene**
- **Genetic heterogeneity**[Q]: Same trait produced by mutations at several loci
- **Penetrance**: **% of individuals** carrying the gene **who express the trait**[Q]
- **Variable expressivity**[Q]: Variable expression (severe or mild) of a disease, among individuals who carry the **same mutant**
- **Dominant negative**[Q]: When a **mutant allele impairs the function of a normal allele**, causing profound deficiency of the final product. E.g.: Osteogenesis imperfecta
- **Gain of function** mutation: Huntingtons disease

Autosomal Recessive Disorders

They occur only when **both alleles** at a given gene locus are **mutated (homozygous)**[Q]

- It is called **horizontal inheritance** : single generation affected.

Features:

- Siblings have **one in four chance** of having the trait (**25% for each birth**)[Q]
- If **mutant gene** is **uncommon**, affected individual can be the product of a **consanguineous marriage**[Q]
- **Complete penetrance** is **common** with **onset early in life**[Q]
- Uniform expression.
- All inborn errors of metabolism are the example.

Mnemonic

Important Autosomal Recessive Diseases
"ABCDEFGHI"
A : **A**lbinism[Q], **A**lkaptonuria[Q], **A**taxia Telengiectasia[Q]
B : **B**eta (thalassemia[Q], Sickle cell anemia[Q])
C : **C**ystic fibrosis[Q], **C**ongenital adrenal hyperplasia
D : **D**eafness (Sensorineural)
E : **E**mphysema (α1-antitrypsin deficiency)
F : **F**riedrich's Ataxia[Q]
G : **G**aucher disease[Q], **G**alactosemia
H : **H**omocystinuria, **H**emochromatosis[Q]
I : **I**nborn errors of metabolism[Q]

R9th Latest Updates

Mutations within noncoding sequences
- Mutations in **promoter and enhancer** sequences which interfere with binding of transcription factors and thus lead to a marked reduction in, or total lack of transcription. E.g. Thalassemias
- **Point mutations within introns** lead to **defective splicing of intervening sequences** → **failure** to form **mature mRNA**.

X-linked Disorders

- All **sex-linked disorders are X-linked**, and almost all are **recessive.**[Q]
- **Males** with **mutations affecting the Y-linked genes** are usually **infertile**, and hence there is **no Y-linked inheritance**[Q]

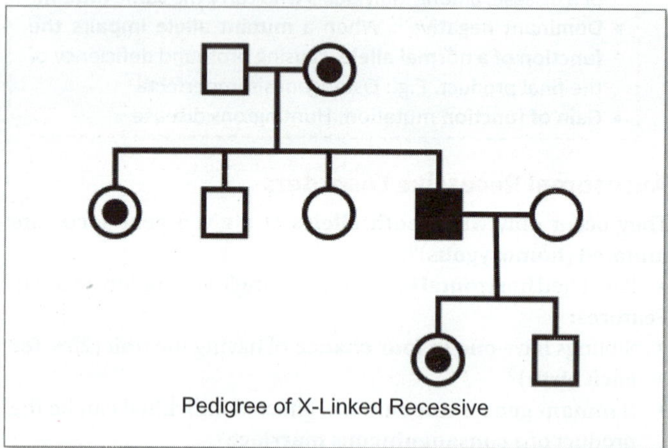

Pedigree of X-Linked Recessive

X-Linked Recessive Disorders

Features

- **Affected male transmits** the disorder to **all his daughters (carriers)**[Q]
- Heterozygous female usually **does not express** the phenotype because of one normal X chromosome[Q]

- **Heterozygous female** transmits the disorder to **50% sons (affected)** and **50% daughters (carrier)**[Q]

Mnemonic

Important X-linked Recessive Disorders
"Lady Hardinge College Girls Don't Care About Foolish Words"
Lady : Lesch Nyhan syndrome
Hardinge : Hemophilia[Q], Hunter syndrome[Q]
College : Chronic granulomatous disease
Girls : G6PD deficiency[Q]
Don't : Duchene muscular dystrophy[Q], Diabetes insipidus
Care : Color blindness[Q]
About : Agammaglobulinemia
Foolish : Fragile X syndrome[Q]
Words : Wiskott Aldrich syndrome[Q]

X-Linked Dominant

Features

- **Affected heterozygous female** transmits to **50% sons** and **50% daughters**
- **Affected male** transmits the disease to **all his daughters (100%)** but **none of his sons**

Mnemonic

Important X-linked Dominant Disorders
"Red Rose For All Children"
Red : X-linked hypophosphatemic **R**ickets[Q]
Rose : **R**ett's syndrome[Q]
For : **F**ragile X syndrome[Q] ($X_R > X_D$)
All : **A**lport syndrome[Q]
Children : **C**harcot–Marie–Tooth disease

SOME IMPORTANT SINGLE GENE DISORDERS

Disorders Associated with Defect in Structural Proteins

Marfan's Syndrome

R9th Latest Updates

Protein	Fibrillin-1	Fibrillin-2
Gene (chr)	FBN1(Chr 15q21.1)	FBN2 (Chr 5q23.31)
Disease	Marfan's syndrome	Congenital contractural arachnodactyly

Mnemonic

Features of Marfan's syndrome

"M-A-R-F-A-N-S"

- **M**itral valve prolapse[Q]
- **A**ortic aneurysm[Q]
- **R**etinal detachment
- **F**ibrillin deficiency[Q]
- **A**rachnodactyly (long, tapering fingers)[Q]
- **N**egative Nitroprusside test
- **S**uperotemporal subluxation of lens (ectopia lentis)[Q]
- **S**keletal changes (Tall with long extremities, pectus excavatum/carinatum, kyphoscoliosis, dolichocephaly)[Q]

Ehlers-Danlos Syndrome (EDS)

Results from some **defect in the synthesis or structure of fibrillar collagen; joint hyperextensibility and laxity**[Q]

Classification of Ehlers-Danlos Syndromes

EDS Type	Clinical Findings	Inheritance	Gene Defects
Classic (I/II)	Skin and joint hypermobility, atrophic scars, easy bruising	Autosomal dominant	COL5A1, COL5A2
Hypermobility (III)	Joint hypermobility, pain, dislocations	Autosomal dominant	Unknown
Vascular (IV)	Thin skin, arterial or uterine rupture, bruising, small joint hyperextensibility	Autosomal dominant	COL3A1
Kyphoscoliosis (VI)	Hypotoria, joint laxity, congenital scoliosis, ocular fragility	Autosomal recessive	Lysyl hydroxylase
Arthrochalasia (VIIa,b)	Severe joint hypermobility, skin changers (mild), scoliosis, bruising	Autosomal dominant	COL1A1, COL1A2
Dermatosparaxis (VIIc)	Severe skin fragility, cutis laxa, bruising	Autosomal recessive	Procollagen *N*-peptidase

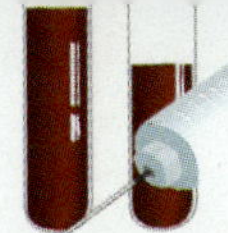

High Yield Facts

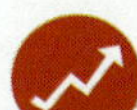

- All types are of **Ehlers-Danlos Syndromes** are **autosomal dominant except types VI and VIIc**
- **Ehlers-Danlos Syndromes Type IV: most dangerous**[Q] and **type III: Most common**[Q]
- **Fibrillin** is found in **aorta, ligaments and ciliary zonules** that support the lens
- **Cardiovascular lesions:** Aortic dissections are most common cause of mortality in Marfan's syndrome
- **Cystic medial necrosis** leads to **ascending aorta aneurysm**[Q] and **aortic dissection in Marfan's syndrome**
- Waardenburg syndrome is due to mutation of **PAX-3 gene**

Disorder with Defect in Receptor Proteins

Familial Hypercholesterolemia

Familial hypercholesterolemia is a "**receptor disease**" that is the consequence of a mutation in the gene encoding the receptor for LDL, which is involved in the transport and metabolism of cholesterol.

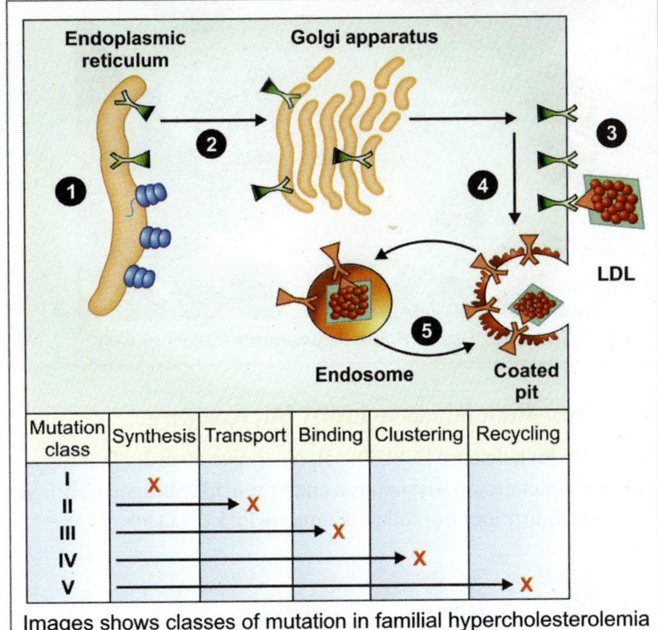

Mutation class	Synthesis	Transport	Binding	Clustering	Recycling
I	X				
II		X			
III			X		
IV				X	
V					X

Images shows classes of mutation in familial hypercholesterolemia

LYSOSOMAL STORAGE DISEASES

Disease	Enzyme def.	Cherry-red spot	Hepatosplenomegaly	Skeletal lesions
GM1 Gangliosidosis[Q]	**Beta galactosidase**[Q]	+	+	+
Gaucher's disease[Q]	**Glucocerebrosidase**[Q]	–	+	+
Niemann Pick disease	**Sphingomyelinase**[Q]	+	+	–
Tay Sachs disease	**Hexosaminidase A**[Q]	+	–	–

Gaucher's Disease

Most common lysosomal storage disease[Q]

Basic defect	Accumulation of **cerebroside**[Q] inside **mononuclear phagocytic cells**[Q]
Inheritance	**Autosomal recessive**[Q]
Clinical features	• 3 types, of which **type I is most common**[Q] • **Splenohepatomegaly,**[Q] Bone pains/pathologic fractures,[Q] Bruising (thrombocytopenia) and Anemia[Q] • Neurological features ±/- (present in types II and III)[Q]
Diagnosis	• **Def. glucocerebrosidase**[Q] in leukocytes/fibroblasts • **Gaucher cells**[Q] (**wrinkled paper appearance** of cytoplasm) in bone marrow • X Ray long bones: **'Erlenmeyer flask deformity'**[Q]
Treatment	Enzyme Replacement therapy ± Stem Cell transplantation

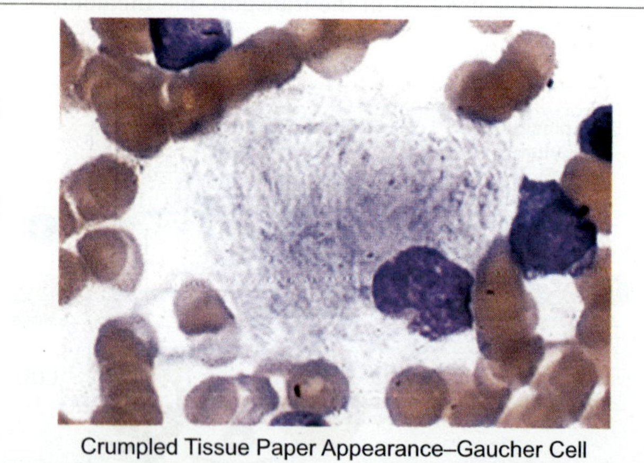

Crumpled Tissue Paper Appearance–Gaucher Cell

Niemann-Pick Disease Light Microscopy

Niemann-Pick disease (NPD) is a lipid storage disorder that results from the deficiency of a lysosomal enzyme, acid sphingomyelinase. Compare foamy looking cell in Niemann-Pick disease.

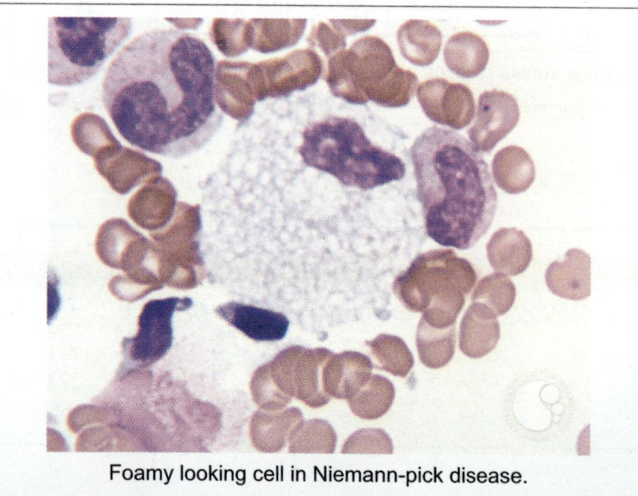

Foamy looking cell in Niemann-pick disease.

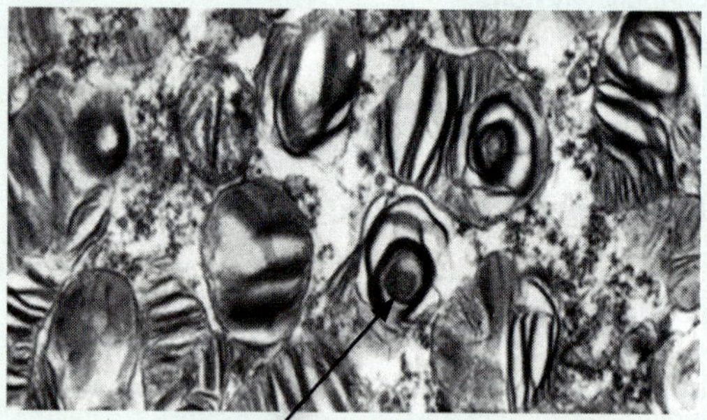

R10th Latest Updates

Zebra bodies

Membrane-bound granules containing lamellae found in Schwann cells and macrophages. They are associated with **metachromatic leucodystrophy** and storage diseases such as **Niemann-Pick and mucopolysaccharidoses**. The storage diseases result in an accumulation of sphingomyelin and other phospholipids in the reticuloendothelial system.

Image shows Zebra bodies

Mucopolysaccharidoses

All Mucopolysaccharidoses are Autosomal recessive[Q] **except Hunter's disease which is inherited as X linked recessive**[Q]

Type	Name	Clinical features
I	Hurler-Scheie	**Coarse face, Corneal Clouding,**[Q] **Mental retardation, Hepatosplenomegaly, Dysostosis multiplex**
II	Hunter	Same as above but **No corneal clouding**[Q]
III	San Fillipo	Only Mental Retardation present
IV	Morquio	**Bony abnormalities most severe**[Q] and corneal clouding may be present
VI	Maroteaux-Lamy	Same as Morquio + Coarse facies + Visceromegaly
VII	Sly	Hepatosplenomegaly + Bony abnormalities

COMPLEX MULTIGENIC DISORDERS

- Disorders caused by interactions between variant forms of **genes and environmental factors**.
- Occur when many polymorphisms, each with a modest effect and low penetrance, are co-inherited

Representative Diseases Associated with Multifactorial Inheritance	
Adults	**Children**
Hypertension	Pyloric stenosis
Atherosclerosis	Cleft lip and palate
Diabetes type 2	Congenital heart disease
Allergic diathesis	Meningomyelocele
Psoriasis	Anencephaly
Schizophrenia	Hypospadias
Ankylosing spondylitis	Congenital hip dislocation
Gout	Hirschsprung's diseases

CHROMOSOMAL DISORDERS

Numerical Abnormalities of Chromosomes

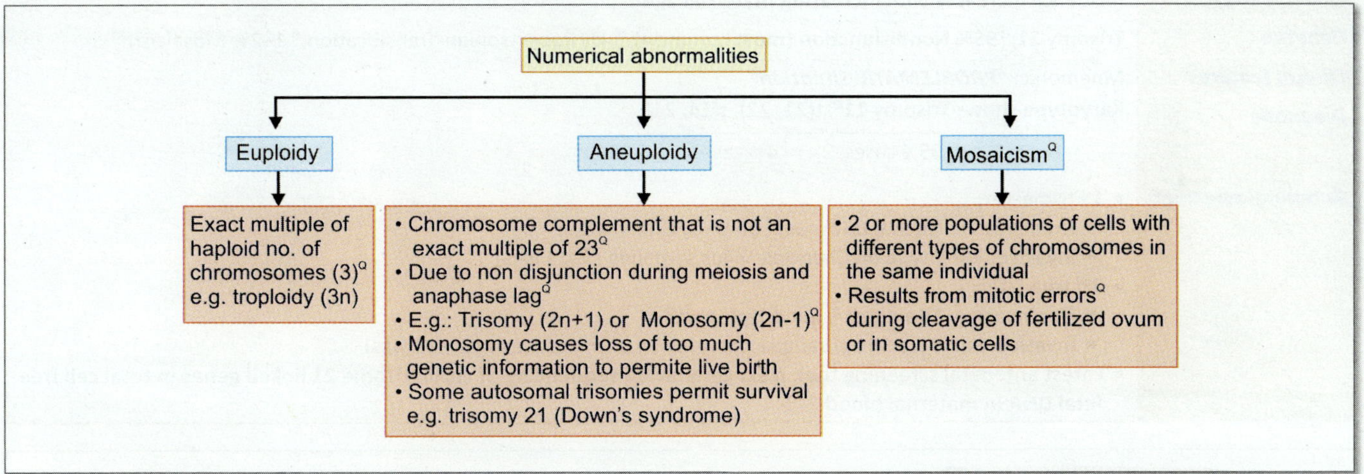

Structural Abnormalities of Chromosomes

Deletion	Loss of a portion[Q] of a chromosome. E.g.: 46, XY, del(15)(p11.2p13.1) describes breakpoints in short arm of chromosome 15 at 15p11.2 and 15p13.1	
Ring chromosome	Due to **break at both ends**[Q] of a chromosome with **fusion** of the damaged ends. **E.g.: 46, XY, r(10)**	
Inversion	Rearrangement that involves **two breaks within a single** chromosome with re-insertion of the inverted, intervening segment • **Paracentric**: inversion involving **only one arm** of the chromosome • **Pericentric**: if the breaks are **on opposite sides** of the centromere	
Iso-chromosome[Q]	1 arm of a chromosome is lost and the remaining arm is duplicated or when the axis of division occurs **perpendicular to the normal axis**[Q] of division	
Translocation	Segment of one chromosome is transferred to another. • **Balanced reciprocal**: Single breaks in two chromosomes, with exchange of material (**without any loss** of genetic material)[Q] E.g. **46, XX, t(9;22)(q34;q11)** • **Robertsonian translocation (or centric fusion)**: a translocation between **two acrocentric chromosomes,** leading to **one very large chromosome** and one **extremely small one**, along with **small product being lost.**[Q]	

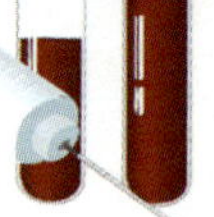

IMPORTANT CYTOGENETIC DISORDERS INVOLVING AUTOSOMES

Down's Syndrome

Epidemiology	Incidence increases with **increasing maternal age**[Q]
Genetics	**Trisomy 21;**[Q] **95% Nondisjunction (most common),**[Q] 4% Robertsonian-Translocation,[Q] 1–2% Mosaicism[Q]
Clinical features	Mnemonic: **"PROBLEMATIC Situation"**
Diagnosis	**Karyotype** shows **Trisomy 21**[Q], t(21, 22), t(14, 21) 95% cases · 4% cases
Antenatal screening	• **1st trimester:** ■ **Noninvasive: Nuchal thickness**[Q] on USG, Dual marker ■ **Invasive:** Karyotype on Chorionic villus sampling (9–11 wks) • **2nd trimester:** ■ **Noninvasive- Triple test**[Q]**, quadruple test**[Q] ■ **Invasive:** Karyotype from sample obtained by amniocentesis (14–16 wks) • **Latest antenatal screening tool: Next generation sequencing of chromosome 21 linked genes in total cell free fetal DNA in maternal blood**

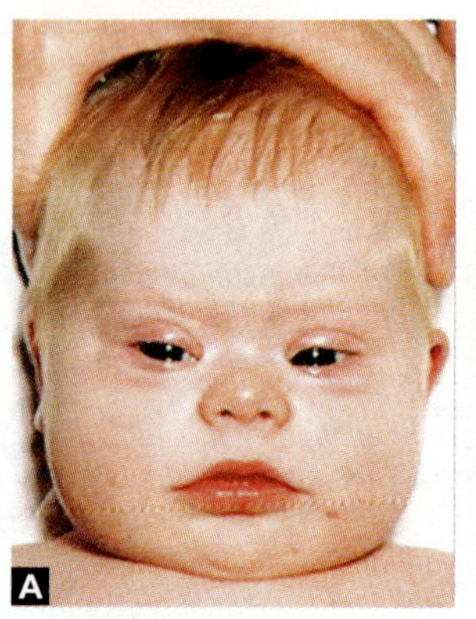
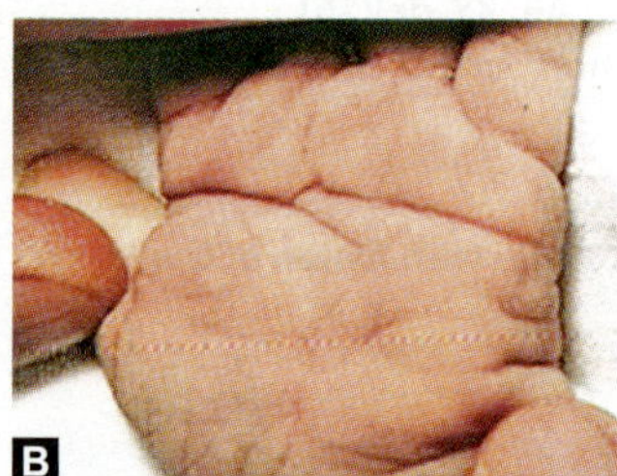
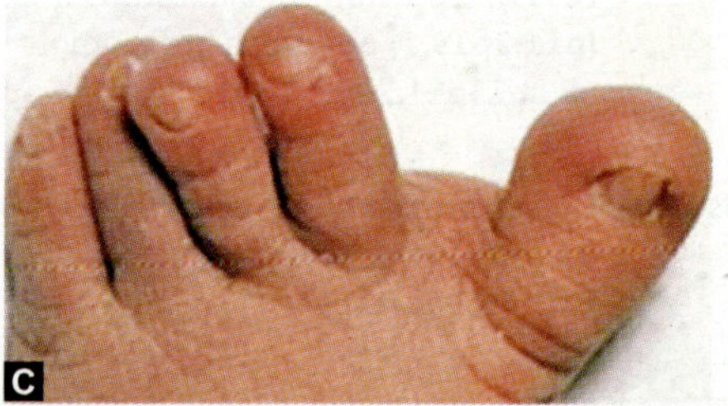

Clinical features S/o Down's syndrome

Mnemonic

Important clinical features of Down's syndrome: "PROBLEMATIC Situation"

- **P**rotruding tongue
- **R**ound face
- **O**cciput flat/**O**pen, wide fontanele[Q]
- **B**rushfield spots in iris[Q]/**B**rachycephaly/**B**rachydactyly/**B**ehavioural difficulties
- **L**ow (depressed) nasal bridge/**L**anguage problem/less tone (hypotonia)
- **E**picanthic fold[Q]/**E**ars low-set and dysplastic[Q] ± hearing problem
- **M**ongoloid slant[Q] (**o**blique palpebral fissure)/**M**ental retardation[Q]/**M**yoclonus
- **A**cute Leukemia (AML>ALL)/**A**lzheimer's disease[Q]/**A**tlantoaxial instability[Q]/**A**tresia of duodenum
- **T**risomy 21/thyroid problem (hypothyroidism)
- **I**ncurved 5th finger (**clinodactyly**)[Q]/**I**ntellectual disability
- **C**ongenital heart disease[Q]/**C**ataracts
- **S**andle gap[Q] (Increased gap between 1st and 2nd toes)/**S**imian palmar crease[Q]

High Yield Facts

- **Down's syndrome is the most common chromosomal abnormality**[Q]
- **Most common genetic cause of mental retardation**[Q] is Down syndrome
- **Down** Syndrome is **most commonly caused by maternal nondisjunction**[Q]
- **Klinefelter** syndrome is **most commonly caused by paternal nondisjunction**[Q]
- The most common **congenital heart disease** in Down syndrome is **Endocardial cushion Defect**[Q] > VSD, ASD, PDA and PAH
- The most common cause of intestinal obstruction in Down's syndrome is **Duodenal atresia**[Q]
- MC hematological abnormality in Down's syndrome is **TAM (Transient Abnormal Myelopoiesis)**
- MC leukemia in Down's syndromes < 4 yrs is **AML M7**
- MC leukemia in Down's syndromes > 4 yrs is **ALL**
- In cases of **translocation or mosaic** Down's syndrome, **maternal age is of no importance**.
- If a child with Down's syndrome has translocation (21; 21) recurrence risk is next child is 100%

> **Other Trisomies**
> - Trisomy 13: Patau syndrome[Q] (**T**hirteen – Pa**T**au)
> - Trisomy 18: Edward syndrome[Q] (**E**ighteen – **E**dward)

Important Deletions

A. **22q11.2 deletion gives rise to: CATCH 22**[Q] (**C**ardiac anomaly, **A**nomalous face, **T**hymus hypoplasia/aplasia, **C**left palate, and **H**ypocalcemia)

   Previously classified as: (now considered part of same spectrum)

   - **Di-George syndrome** (thymic hypoplasia with diminished T-cell immunity, parathyroid hypoplasia with hypocalcemia) and

   - **Velocardiofacial**[Q] **syndrome** (congenital heart disease, dysmorphism, developmental delay).

B. **Cri du Chat syndrome**[Q]: **5p deletion**[Q]; Characteristic cry, developmental delay and behavioral problems.

CYTOGENETIC DISORDERS INVOLVING SEX CHROMOSOMES

Genetic diseases involving the sex chromosomes are more common than autosomal aberrations.

Lyon Hypothesis (Lyonisation)[Q]

- **Only one** of the **X chromosomes** is genetically **active**
- The **other X** of **either maternal or paternal** origin undergoes **heteropyknosis** and is rendered **inactive**[Q]
- Inactivation of either the maternal or paternal X **occurs at random**[Q] among all the cells of the blastocyst on or about **day 5.5**[Q] of embryonic life, and
- Inactivation of the same X chromosome **persists in all the cells**[Q] derived from each precursor cell
- The molecular basis of X inactivation involves a unique gene called **XIST**[Q]
- **21% of genes on Xp, and a smaller number (3%) on Xq escape X inactivation SRY (sex-determining region on Y chromosome): dictates testicular development**[Q]

Turner's Syndrome (45, XO)[Q]

Always seen in FEMALES[Q]

Karyotype

- Missing X chromosome in 57% **(45, XO) (most common)**
- **Mosaics** in 29% (e.g. 45, XO/ 46, XX)
- Partial monosomy of X chromosome in 14%

> **Features of Turners Syndrome**
>
> **"C-L-O-W-N-S"**
> - **C**ardiac abnormalities (**coarctation of aorta**)[Q], **Cubitus valgus**[Q]
> - **L**ymphedema
> - **O**varies underdeveloped: **"streak ovaries"**[Q] (causing infertility, amenorrhea)
> - **W**ebbed neck
> - **N**ormal intelligence[Q]/**N**ipples widely spaced
> - **S**hort stature[Q]/Short 4th metacarpal[Q]

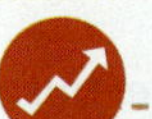

High Yield Facts

- Most important cause of **primary amenorrhea**[Q]: Turner's Syndrome
- **Infertility**[Q] due to rudimentary uterus and **streak ovaries**[Q] (ovaries are reduced to **atrophic fibrous strands without ova and follicles**)
- Reduced ovarian feedback results in significantly **elevated FSH and LH levels**[Q]
- **Most common** CVS abnormality in Turner's syndrome: **Bicuspid aortic valve (50%)**[Q] > Coarctation of Aorta
- In Turner's syndrome, there is increased incidence of **cystic hygroma and gonadoblastoma**[Q]
- **Noonan's** syndrome: **AD**, seen in **males as well as females; Mental retardation present**[Q]
- **Most common** CVS abnormality in **Noonan's syndrome** is **hypertrophic pulmonary stenosis**[Q]

Klinefelter's Syndrome: 47, XXY (Seen in Males)

Male hypogonadism that occurs when there are ≥ 2 X chr and ≥ 1Y Chr[Q]

Genetic Abnormality

- **47, XXY karyotype (90%)**[Q]: results from **nondisjunction during the meiotic division**
- Maternal age is increased in the cases associated with errors in oogenesis.
- **Mosaic patterns (46, XY/47, XXY) (15%)**[Q] and 47, XXY/48, XXXY[Q]

> **"K-L-I-N-E-F-E-L-T-S" syndrome**
>
> - **K**aryotype, most common is 47, XXY[Q]
> - **L**ong stature with long legs[Q]
> - **In**fertility[Q], **In**cidence: 1 in 1000 men
> - **N**on-disjunction of **paternal**[Q] sex chromosomes
> - **E**unuchoid[Q] body proportions
> - **F**SH elevated[Q], scanty **F**acial and axillary hair
> - **E**stradiol/testosterone ratio elevation → Gynecomastia[Q]
> - **L**H elevated, **L**eukemias (increased risk for AML)[Q] and breast tumors, **L**earning disability
> - **T**estosterone reduced, small **T**estes and penis[Q]
> - **S**econdary sexual characters absent

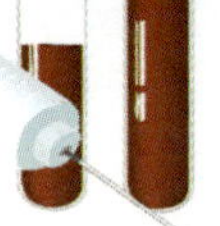

Hermaphroditism and Pseudohermaphroditism

1. Hermaphrodite
2. Pseudohermaphrodite

RECENT EXAM[Q]

1. The term true *hermaphrodite* implies the presence of both ovarian and testicular tissue. In contrast, a pseudohermaphrodite represents a disagreement between the phenotypic and gonadal sex.
2. Female pseudohermaphrodite has ovaries but male external genitalia.
3. Male pseudohermaphrodite has testicular tissue but female-type genitalia.

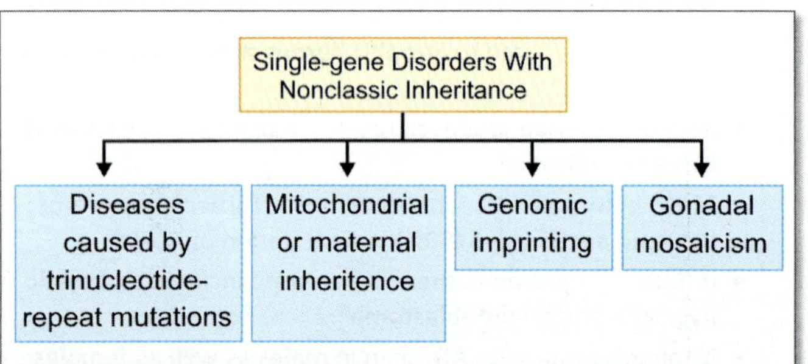

DISEASES CAUSED BY TRINUCLEOTIDE-REPEAT MUTATIONS

- Disorder with expansion of Trinucleotides
- Can occur is coding or noncoding region.

Trinucleotide Repeat Disorders

Region	Disease	Repeat	Inheritance	Gene Product
Coding region	X-chromosomal spinobulbar muscular atrophy	CAG[Q]	XR	Androgen receptor
	Huntington's disease (HD)	CAG[Q]	AD	Huntingtin
	Spinocerebellar ataxia type 1 (SCA1)	CAG	AD	Ataxin 1
Noncoding region	Fragile X-syndrome (FRAXA)	CGG[Q]	XR	FMR-1 protein[Q]
	Dystrophia Myotonica (DM)	CTG[Q]	AD	Myotonin protein kinase
	Friedreich's ataxia (FRDA1)	GAA[Q]	AR	Frataxin[Q]

Fragile X Syndrome

- ***Caused by:*** A trinucleotide mutation in familial mental retardation-1 **(FMR1) gene**[Q]
- ***Epidemiology:* Second most common genetic cause of mental retardation**[Q] after Down's syndrome.
- ***Clinical features:***
  - ○ **Long face** with a **large mandible**, **large ears**, **large testicles**[Q] (macro-orchidism), hyperextensible joints, a high arched palate, and mitral valve prolapse
  - ○ Most distinctive feature is **post-pubertal macro-orchidism**[Q]
- ***Anticipation***[Q]
  - ○ Clinical features **worsen with each successive** generation,[Q] as the number of repeats increases with successive generations:
    - • **Normal population**: 29–55 CGG repeats in the FMR1 gene.
    - • **Carrier** males and females: Carry **pre-mutations**[Q] 55-200 CGG repeats that can expand during **oogenesis.**
    - • **Full mutation** (fragile X syndrome): 4000 repeats
- ***Diagnosis of choice:*** PCR-detection of repeats

High Yield Facts

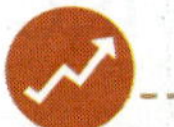

Fragile X Tremor/Ataxia
- Toxic gain of function of CGG containing mRNA
- 20% –premature ovarian failure
- 50%–Progressive neurodegenerative illness

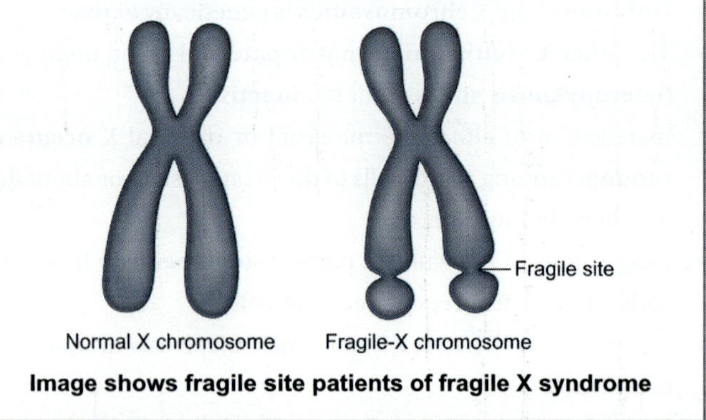

Image shows fragile site patients of fragile X syndrome

Mutation in Mitochondrial DNA (mtDNA): Maternal Inheritance[Q]

Mechanism

- **mtDNA** complement of the zygote is derived **entirely from the ovum**[Q]
- Thus, mutation in **mother's** mtDNA will be **transmitted** to **all her off springs**[Q]
- mtDNA encodes enzymes involved in **oxidative phosphorylation**

- Mutations of mtDNA primarily affect **organs** most dependent on **oxidative phosphorylation** such as **CNS, skeletal and cardiac muscles, liver, and kidneys.**[Q]

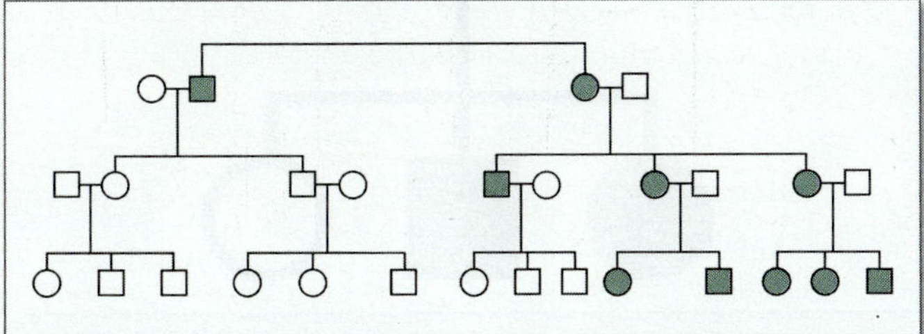

Pedigree shows all progeny of an affected male (shaded squares) are normal, but all children, male and female, of the affected female (shaded circles) manifest diseases

Important Features of Mitochondrial Diseases

- **Heteroplasmy**[Q]: An individual may harbor **both wild-type and mutant**[Q] mt-DNA
- **Threshold effect: Minimum percentage** of mutant mtDNA that must be present in a cell **for the disease to occur**

Important Mitochondrial Diseases: "K-L-M-N-O-P"

Disease	Phenotype
Kearn-Sayre syndrome (KSS)[Q]	External ophthalmoplegia, heart block, retinal pigmentation, ataxia
Leber Hereditary Optic Neuropathy (LHON)[Q]	Bilateral subacute or acute painless optic atrophy
MELAS[Q]	**M**itochondrial **e**ncephalomyopathy, **l**actic **a**cidosis, and **s**troke like episodes; may manifest only as diabetes
MERRF	**M**yoclonic **e**pilepsy, **r**agged **r**ed **f**ibers in muscle, ataxia, increased CSF protein, sensorineural deafness, dementia
NARP[Q]**, Leigh disease**	Neurogenic weakness, ataxia, and retinitis pigmentosa (NARP)
Chronic progressive external ophthalmoplegia (CPEO)[Q]	Late-onset bilateral ptosis and ophthalmoplegia, proximal muscle weakness, and exercise intolerance
Pearson syndrome	Pancreatic insufficiency, pancytopenia, lactic acidosis

Genomic Imprinting

- **Definition**
  - Inheritable **preferential expression**[Q] of **one**[Q] of the **parental alleles**.
- **Types**
  - **Maternal imprinting** refers to transcriptional **silencing of the maternal** allele[Q]
  - **Paternal imprinting** implies that the **paternal allele is inactivated**[Q]
- **Site and Time**
  - Imprinting occurs **in the ovum or sperm, before fertilization**, and then is stably **transmitted** to all somatic cells through **mitosis**
- **Mechanism**
  - DNA **methylation** at CG nucleotides
  - Histone H4 **de-acetylation**
  - **Methylation**
- **Examples**
  - Prader-Willi syndrome, Angelman syndrome

Mechanism of Imprinting: Epigenetic Alterations

Definition	Study of **heritable** chemical **modification of DNA or chromatin** that **do not alter the DNA sequence**[Q] itself.
Examples	**Methylation**[Q] of DNA, and methylation and acetylation of **histones**[Q]

High Yield Facts

- Affected gene in Angelman syndrome = **UBE3A** (imprinted on paternal chromosome. Expressed on maternal chromosome especially is brain).
- Affected genes in Prader Willi syndrome = **SNORP** family of gene (encode small nuclear RNA → modifies ribosomal RNA)
  - Imprinted on material chromosome expressed on paternal chromosome
- Epigenetics play role in X chromosome inactivation and
- imprinting

Prader-Willi Syndrome

- Characterized by **mental retardation**, short stature, **hypotonia**, profound hyperphagia, **obesity**, small hands and feet, and **hypogonadism**[Q]
- del(15)(q11.2q13); deletion affects the paternally derived chromosome 15

Angelman syndrome: Mnemonic: "M-A-S-T"

Mentally retarded, **A**taxic gait, **S**eizures, and inappropriate laughter "happy puppe**T**s."

Mnemonic

Mechanisms in Prader Willi and Angelman syndrome:[Q]		
PRADER WILLI	**MECHANISM**	**ANGELMAN**
PATERNAL	DELETION (70%)	MATERNAL
MATERNAL	DISOMY (20-25%)	PATERNAL

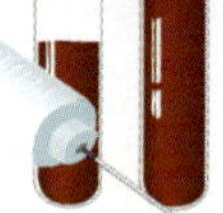

Gonadal Mosaicism

Mechanism	• Mutation that **occurs post-zygotically**[Q] during early (embryonic) development. • Mutation **affects only cells destined to form the gonads**, the **gametes carry the mutation**[Q], therefore the somatic cells of the individual are completely normal.
Effect	In some **autosomal dominant** disorders, like by **osteogenesis imperfecta**[Q], **phenotypically normal parents** have **more than one affected child**.

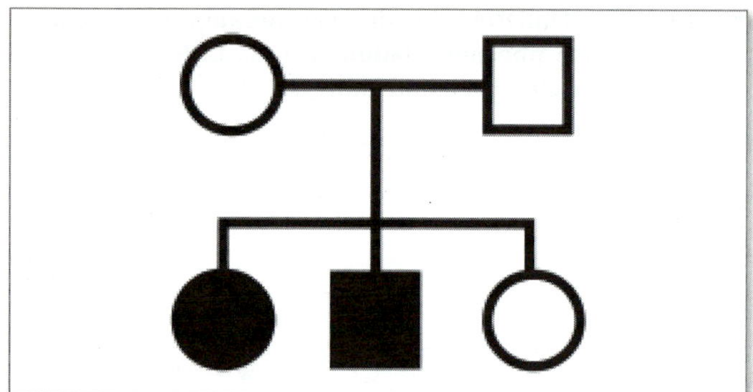

DIAGNOSTIC TOOLS IN GENETICS

Karyotype

Obtained by	Arranging each pair of autosomes **according to length**[Q], followed by sex chromosomes.			
Normal	**46, XX (females)**[Q] **and 46, XY (males)**[Q]			
Method	Chromosomes are examined after **arresting dividing cells** in **metaphase**[Q] with mitotic spindle inhibitors (e.g., N-diacetyl-N-methyl**colchicine**), followed by staining			
Samples used[Q]	**Antenatal**		**Postnatal**	
	• **Chorionic villi sampling (11-13 weeks)**[Q] • **Amniocentesis (14-16 weeks)**[Q] • Fetal umbilical blood • **Circulating fetal DNA in maternal blood**		• **Peripheral blood lymphocytes**[Q] **(Best) (not monocytes)**[Q] • Bone marrow • **Skin fibroblasts**[Q] • Lymph node tissue, Solid tumor sample	
Resolution	2 to 5 million base (mb) pairs[Q] (in light microscope), Max resolution in prophase[Q]			
Staining methods		**G-Banding**[Q]	**R-Banding**	**Q- Banding**	**C-Banding**
	Pre-treatment	Digestion with Trypsin	Heat Denaturation	None	Chemically extract DNA
	Stain used	**Giemsa**[Q]	Giemsa	**Quinacrine mustard**[Q]	Giemsa
	Microscopy	Light	Light	Fluorescent	Light

Description of a Karyotype

- **Total number** of chromosomes with **sex** chromosome
- Arrange chromosomes in **ascending**[Q] numerical order
- **Short arm** of a chromosome is designated **p (for petit)**[Q] **and long arm** is referred to as **q**[Q]
- The **regions** are numbered (e.g., 1, 2, 3) from the centromere outward
- Each region is further subdivided into **bands and sub-bands**, and these are ordered numerically
- E.g. 6p12.3= short arm of chromosome 6, region 1, band 2, and sub-band 3

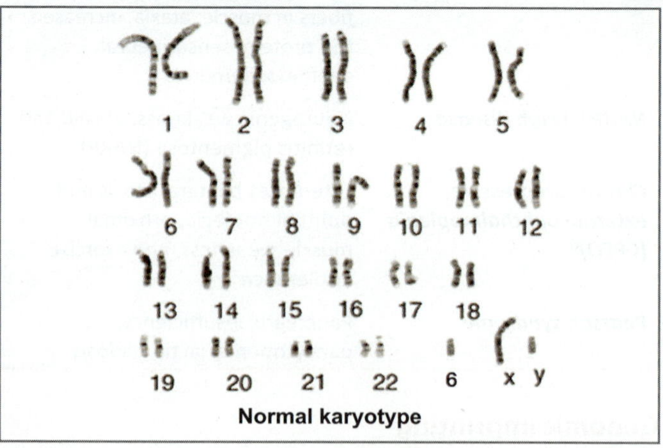

Normal karyotype

Classification of Chromosomes

Group	Size and centromere position	Ideogram number
A or I	Large : Metacentric/submetacentric	1–3
B or II	Large : Submetacentric	4, 5
C or III	Medium : Submetacentric	6 – 12 and X

Contd...

D or IV	Medium : Acrocentric	13-15
E or V	Small : Metacentric/ Submetacentric	16-18
F or VI	Small : Metacentric	19-20
G or VII	Smallest : Acrocentric	21, 22 and Y

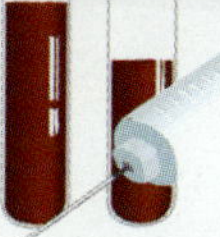

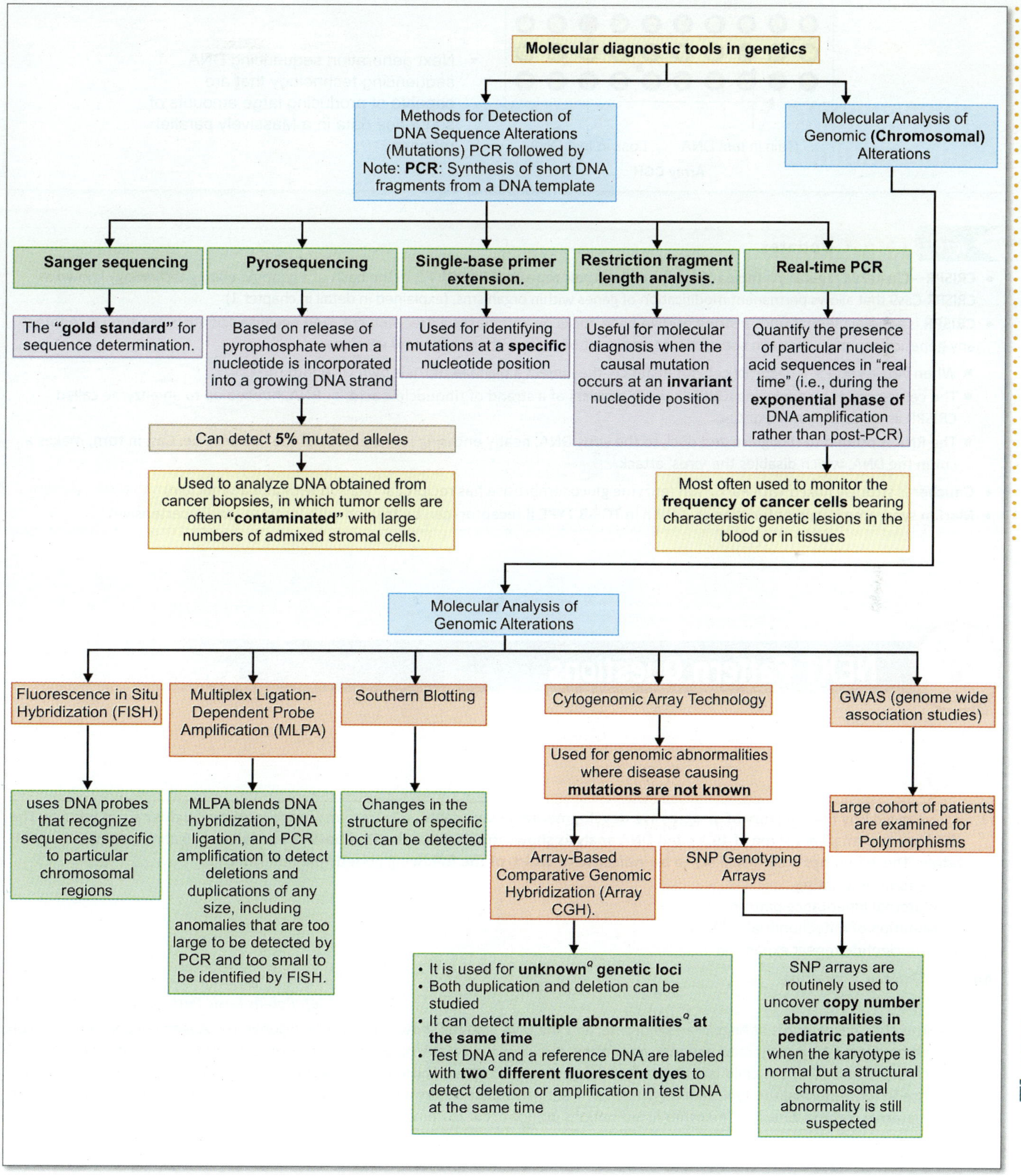

Molecular diagnostic tools in genetics

Methods for Detection of DNA Sequence Alterations (Mutations) PCR followed by
Note: **PCR**: Synthesis of short DNA fragments from a DNA template

Molecular Analysis of Genomic (Chromosomal) Alterations

Sanger sequencing

The **"gold standard"** for sequence determination.

Pyrosequencing

Based on release of pyrophosphate when a nucleotide is incorporated into a growing DNA strand

Can detect **5%** mutated alleles

Used to analyze DNA obtained from cancer biopsies, in which tumor cells are often **"contaminated"** with large numbers of admixed stromal cells.

Single-base primer extension.

Used for identifying mutations at a **specific** nucleotide position

Restriction fragment length analysis.

Useful for molecular diagnosis when the causal mutation occurs at an **invariant** nucleotide position

Real-time PCR

Quantify the presence of particular nucleic acid sequences in "real time" (i.e., during the **exponential phase of** DNA amplification rather than post-PCR)

Most often used to monitor the **frequency of cancer cells** bearing characteristic genetic lesions in the blood or in tissues

Molecular Analysis of Genomic Alterations

Fluorescence in Situ Hybridization (FISH)

uses DNA probes that recognize sequences specific to particular chromosomal regions

Multiplex Ligation-Dependent Probe Amplification (MLPA)

MLPA blends DNA hybridization, DNA ligation, and PCR amplification to detect deletions and duplications of any size, including anomalies that are too large to be detected by PCR and too small to be identified by FISH.

Southern Blotting

Changes in the structure of specific loci can be detected

Cytogenomic Array Technology

Used for genomic abnormalities where disease causing **mutations are not known**

Array-Based Comparative Genomic Hybridization (Array CGH).

- It is used for **unknown[a] genetic loci**
- Both duplication and deletion can be studied
- It can detect **multiple abnormalities[a] at the same time**
- Test DNA and a reference DNA are labeled with **two[a] different fluorescent dyes** to detect deletion or amplification in test DNA at the same time

SNP Genotyping Arrays

SNP arrays are routinely used to uncover **copy number abnormalities in pediatric patients** when the karyotype is normal but a structural chromosomal abnormality is still suspected

GWAS (genome wide association studies)

Large cohort of patients are examined for Polymorphisms

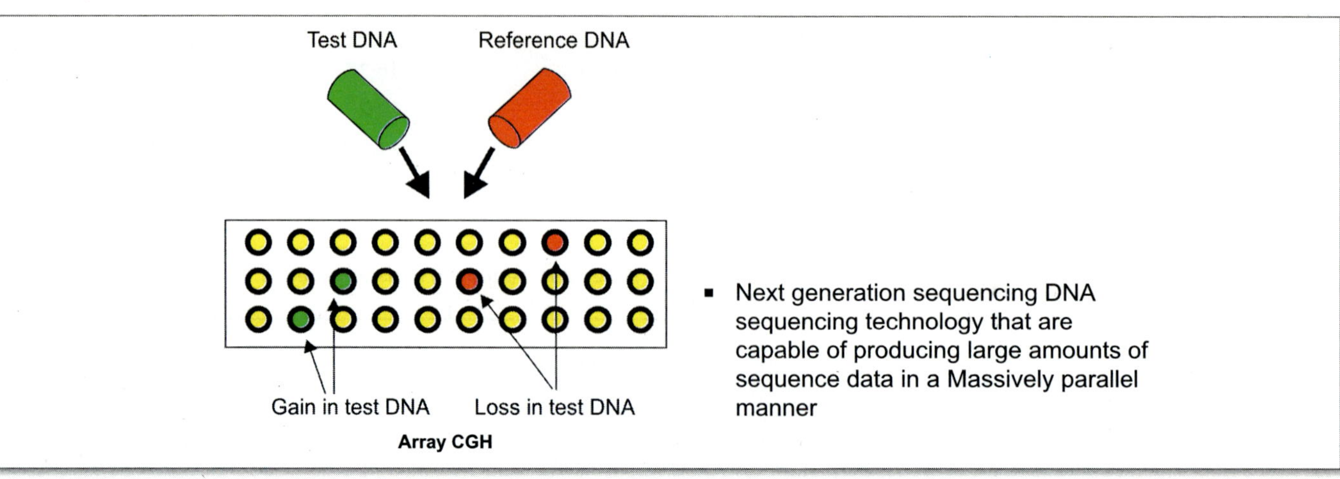

- Next generation sequencing DNA sequencing technology that are capable of producing large amounts of sequence data in a Massively parallel manner

R10ᵗʰ Latest Updates

- **CRISPR—Clustered regularly interspaced short palindromic repeats (CRISPR):** Form the basis of a genome editing technology known as CRISPR-Cas9 that allows permanent modification of genes within organisms. (explained in detail in chapter 1)
- **CRISPR** is a molecule that finds a string of DNA code, locks on and makes a precision cut. And because scientists can tune it to target any genetic sequence, they can use it to turn genes off or replace them with new versions.
  - When viruses attack a bacterial cell, for instance, they inject a payload of their own DNA into the cell.
  - The cell responds by deploying CRISPR, which consists of a strand of ribonucleic acid, or RNA, hooked up to an enzyme called CRISPR associated protein, or Cas.
  - The RNA is primed to recognise and dock to the virus DNA, neatly encasing it in a pocket of the Cas enzyme. Cas, in turn, makes a cut in the DNA, which disables the virus' attack.
- **Gaucher** is strongly linked with Parkinson (enzyme glucocerebrosise has reciprocal relation with alpha synuclein)
- **Marfan** syndrome is gain of function mutation in TGF-B TYPE II receptor- can be treated with losartan (antihypertensive)

NEXT Pattern Questions

Q's

1. **A 3-year-old boy has a history of progressive developmental delay, ataxia, seizures, and inappropriate laughter since infancy. The child has a normal karyotype of 46,XY, but DNA analysis shows that he has inherited both of his number 15 chromosomes from his father. These findings are most likely to be indicative of which of the following genetic mechanisms?**
   a. Genomic imprinting
   b. Maternal inheritance pattern
   c. Mutation of mitochondrial DNA
   d. Trinucleotide repeat expansion

Ans. (a) Genomic imprinting

(Ref: Robins Basic Pathology 10th ed/pg 271)

- This child has features of Angelman syndrome, and the DNA analysis shows uniparental disomy. The Angelman gene encoded on chromosome 15 is subject to genomic imprinting. It is silenced on the paternal chromosome 15, but is active on the maternal chromosome 15. If the child lacks maternal chromosome 15, there is no active Angelman gene in the somatic cells. This gives rise to the abnormalities typical of this disorder. The same effect occurs when there is a deletion of the Angelman gene from the maternal chromosome 15. The other listed options do not occur in uniparental disomy.

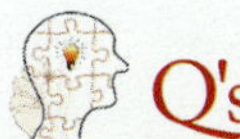 **Q's**

2. A 15-year-old girl has developed multiple nodules on her skin over the past 10 years. On physical examination, there are 20 scattered, 0.3–1 cm, firm nodules on the patient's trunk and extremities. There are 12 light brown macules averaging 2–5 cm in diameter on the skin of the trunk. Slit-lamp examination shows pigmented nodules in the iris. A sibling and a parent are similarly affected. Genetic analysis shows a loss-of-function mutation. Which of the following inheritance patterns is most likely to be present in this family?
   a. Autosomal dominant
   b. Autosomal recessive
   c. Mitochondrial
   d. X-linked recessive

Ans. (a) Autosomal dominant

(Ref: Robins Basic Pathology 10th ed/pg 245)

- Neurofibromatosis type 1 (NF-1) is characterized by the development of multiple neurofibromas and pigmented skin lesions. Neurofibromas are most numerous in the dermis but also may occur in visceral organs. Patients with NF-1 also may develop a type of sarcomatous neoplasm known as a *malignant peripheral nerve sheath tumor (MPNST)*. NF-1 is a tumor suppressor that appears with an autosomal dominant pattern of inheritance, though some cases result from spontaneous new mutations (no prior family members with the mutation). NF-1 exhibits variable expressivity, because the manifestations (location and types of neoplasms) are not the same in all patients. The other forms of inheritance listed are not associated with tumor suppressor genes.

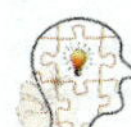 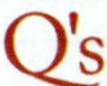 **Q's**

3. An 8-year-old girl experiences sudden severe dyspnea. On examination, she has upper airway obstruction from soft tissue swelling in her neck. A radiograph shows a hematoma compressing the trachea. She was then diagnosed to have hemophilia A. Both parents and two female siblings are unaffected by this problem, but a male sibling has experienced a similar episode. Which of the following genetic abnormalities is most likely to account for the findings in this girl?
   a. Autosomal dominant mutation
   b. Genomic imprinting
   c. Germline mosaicism
   d. Random X inactivation

Ans. (d) Random X inactivation

(Ref: Robins Basic Pathology 10th ed/pg 267)

- This girl has features of hemophilia A. This X-linked recessive condition is expected to occur in males who inherit the one maternal X chromosome with the genetic mutation, and they do not have another X chromosome with a normal functional allele, as is the case in her brother. Hemophilia in a female can be explained by the Lyon hypothesis, which states that only one X chromosome in a female is active (the "turned off" X chromosome is the Barr body) for most genes, but this inactivation is a random event. Some unlucky females are out on the tail end of the Poisson distribution of random events and have few active X chromosomes with the normal allele, leading to markedly diminished factor VIII activity. The other choices do not explain this phenomenon.

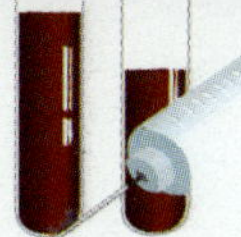

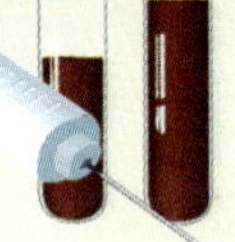
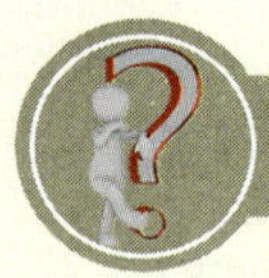

Image-Based Questions

1. The given pedigree shows which type of inheritance?

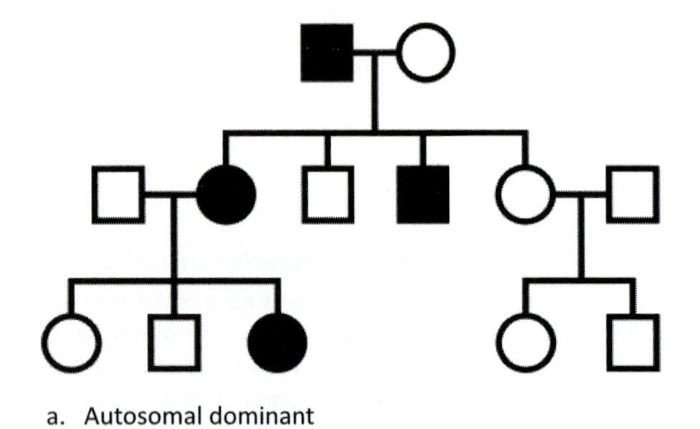

- a. Autosomal dominant
- b. Autosomal Recessive
- c. X-linked Dominant
- d. X-linked Recessive

2. The given pedigree shows which type of inheritance?

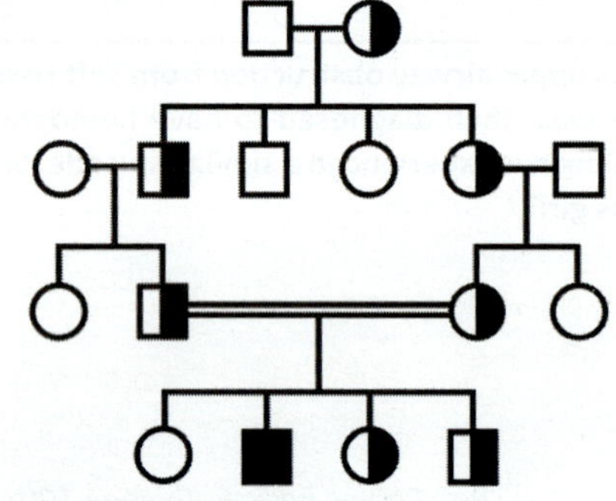

- a. Autosomal dominant
- b. Autosomal Recessive
- c. X-linked Dominant
- d. X-linked Recessive

3. Resolution of light microscope when viewing this is?

- a. 5 Kb
- b. 5 Mb
- c. 500 Kb
- d. 500 Mb

4. What is the locus of the gene marked as arrow in the given chromosome?

- a. 1p3.2
- b. 1q3.2
- c. 1q2.3
- d. 1q23.0

5. Identify the abnormality in the given karyotype?

- a. Normal
- b. Aneuploidy
- c. Triploidy
- d. Trisomy

6. Identify the chromosome in the given sequence?

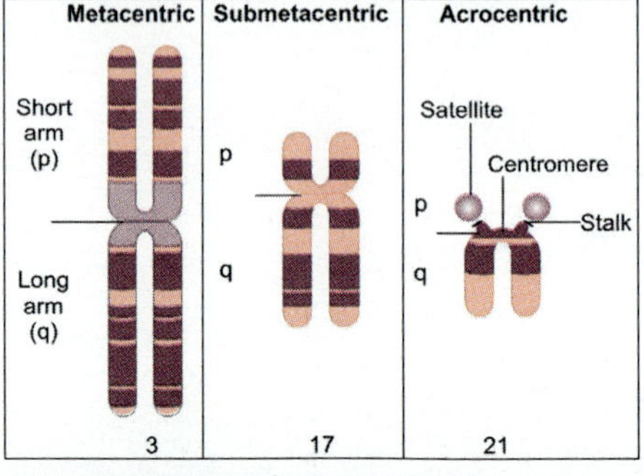

- a. Telocentric, Metacentric, Acrocentric
- b. Telocentric, Acrocentric, Metacentric
- c. Metacentric, Sub-metacentric, Telocentric
- d. Telocentric, Metacentric, Acrocentric

7. The given figure shows a technique important for diagnosing chromosomal aberrations. What is the technique and abnormality seen?

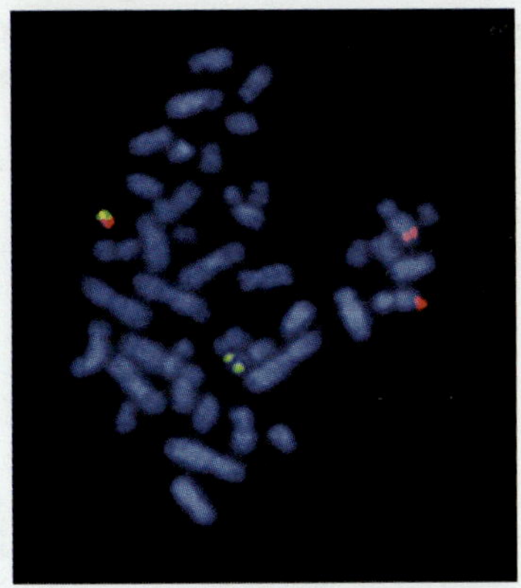

a. Fluorescence in-situ hybridization, Deletion
b. Fluorescence in-situ hybridization, Translocation
c. Comparative genomic hybridization, Deletion
d. Chromosomal painting, Translocation

8. Identify the technique used?

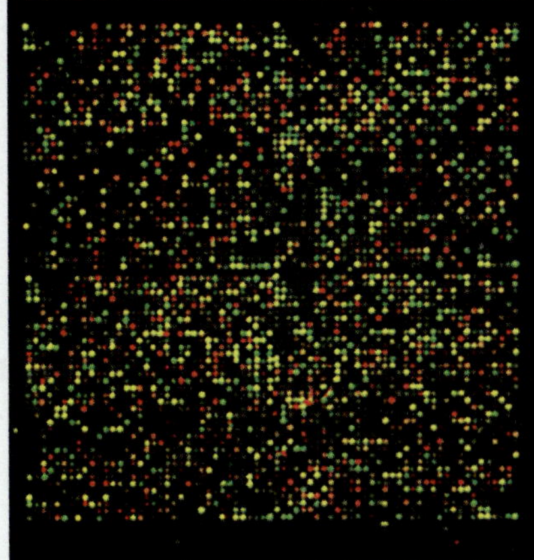

a. CGH
b. FISH
c. Microarray
d. Next gen sequencing

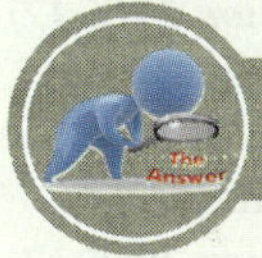

Answers of Image-Based Questions

1. **Ans. (a) Autosomal dominant**
   - One affected parent causing 50% affected progeny suggests autosomal dominant pattern

2. **Ans. (b) Autosomal Recessive**
   - Both carrier parents have 25% affected child, 50% carrier suggests autosomal recessive pattern

3. **Ans. (b) 5Mb**
   - Karyotype is study of chromosomes in which each pair of autosomes are arranged according to length, followed by sex chromosomes.

4. **Ans. (c) 1q2.3**
   - Locus of a gene is number, arm, region and band

5. **Ans. (c) Triploidy**
   - Triploidy is condition in which each set of chromosome has 3 chromosomes, so total is 23 × 3 = 69

6. **Ans. (c) Metacentric, Sub-metacentric, Telocentric**
   - The category of chromosome is according to centromere position, middle is metacentric, needle to middle is submetacentric while near to one end is telocentric

7. **Ans. (b) Fluorescence in-situ hybridization, Translocation**
   - The given image shows study of chromosomes by tagging them with fluorescent probes called FISH. In this condition you can notice two colors coming together (left upper) which suggests a translocation among two different chromosomes with different colored probes.

8. **Ans. (c) Microarray**
   - This technique involves study/detection of genes, proteins, DNA or tissue by micro probes attached to a chip and causing reverse hybridization to it called microarray.

Multiple Choice Questions

1. **Which of the following tumor(s) is/are related to DICER1 Gene mutation:** *(PGI May 2019)*
   a. Retinoblastoma
   b. Pleuropulmonary blastoma
   c. Cystic nephroma
   d. Thyroid carcinoma
   e. Sertoli-Leydig cell tumor

2. **Which of the following is/are chromosomal disorder(s):** *(PGI May 2019)*
   a. Noonan syndrome
   b. Turner syndrome
   c. Klinefelter's syndrome
   d. Fragile-X syndrome
   e. Prader-Willi syndrome

3. **In Down syndrome which is/correct?** *(PGI May 2018)*
   a. Most common cause of death is congenital heart disease
   b. 95% have an extra 21st chromosome
   c. Increased nuchal fold thickness on USG
   d. Karyotyping is required in all cases for prenatal diagnosis
   e. Advanced paternal age (>35 years) is a risk factor

4. **Which chromosome is responsible for the production of MIF?** *(Recent Question 2018)*
   a. Chromosome 16
   b. Chromosome 22
   c. X Chromosome
   d. Y Chromosome

5. **Which of the following is/are true about Turners Syndrome?** *(AIIMS May 2017)*
   a. Most common viable aneuploidy
   b. Long stature
   c. High hair line
   d. Narrow chest
   e. Mental retardation present

6. **Which of the following is/are not feature of Turner syndrome?** *(PGI Nov 2017)*
   a. Tall stature
   b. Associated with celiac disease
   c. 45XO karyotype
   d. 45XO/46XY karyotype
   e. Hypertension

7. **Chromosome 21 is which type of chromosome?** *(JIPMER 2016)*
   a. Metacentric
   b. Submetacentric
   c. Short acrocentric
   d. Medium acrocentric

8. **Karyotype of a male patient shows the following, what is the clinical abnormality that is expected?** *(Recent Question 2016)*

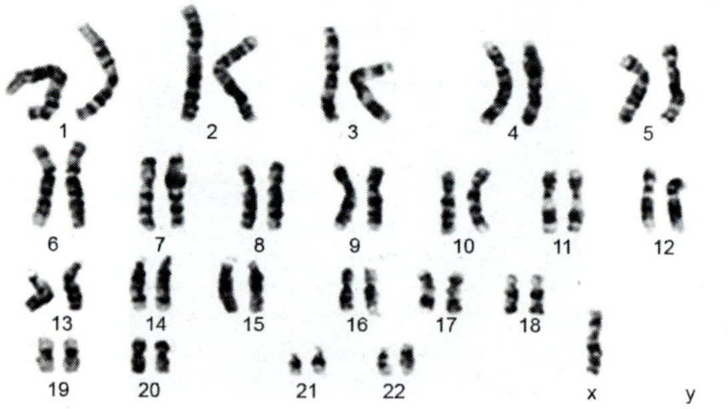

   a. Turner syndrome
   b. Kallman syndrome
   c. Androgen insensitivity syndrome
   d. Down syndrome

9. **Velocardiofacial defect is due to mutation in:** *(Recent Question 2016-17)*
   a. Chr 11   b. Chr 13
   c. Chr 22   d. Chr 3

10. **Presentation of Pierre-Robin syndrome includes:** *(Recent Question 2016-17)*
    a. Retrognathia   b. Low set ear
    c. Prominent forehead   d. Isolated cleft palate
    e. Glossoptosis

11. **Karyotype of a patient shows the following, what is the clinical abnormality that is expected?** *(AIIMS May 2015)*

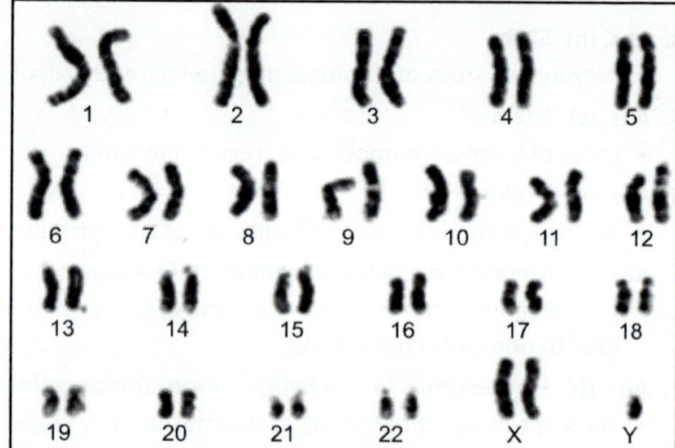

    a. Gynecomastia with long thin limbs
    b. Short stature with polydactyly
    c. Webbed neck with widely spaced nipples
    d. Rocker bottom feet

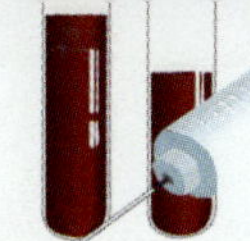

12. In Downs syndrome there is? *(Recent Question 2016)*
a. Translocation
b. Mutations
c. Paternal nondisjunction
d. Maternal nondisjunction

13. A female presents with karyotype 45, XO and absent gonads. What is your diagnosis? *(Recent Question 2015)*
a. Klinefelter's syndrome
b. Androgen insensitivity syndrome
c. Turner syndrome
d. Kallman's syndrome

14. Streak gonads are seen in - *(Recent Question 2014)*
a. Turner syndrome
b. Klinefelter's syndrome
c. Patau's syndrome
d. Down's syndrome

15. True statement regarding chromosomes *(JIPMER 2015)*
a. In females both X chromosomes are activated
b. Klinefelter syndrome results due to an extra Y chromosome in males
c. Germinal cells contain 23 chromosomes
d. Turner syndrome results due to an extra X chromosome in females

16. Cri du chat syndrome is: *(Recent Question 2015)*
a. 22q-
b. 5q-
c. 22p-
d. 5p-

17. Most common cause of primary amenorrhoea with secondary sexual character development is?
a. Turner syndrome *(WBPG 16)*
b. Kallmann syndrome
c. Androgen insensitivity syndrome
d. Down syndrome

18. The following karyotype in female is seen in which of the following syndromes? *(AIIMS Nov 14)*

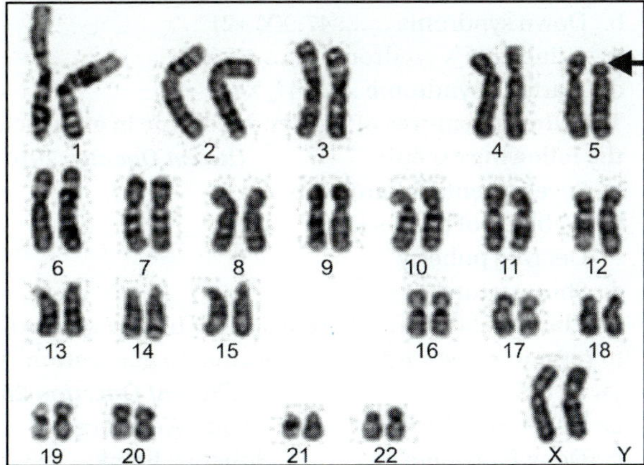

a. Bloom syndrome
b. Fragile X syndrome
c. Angelman syndrome
d. Cri du chat syndrome

19. The structural abnormality of chromosome in which one arm is lost and remaining arm is duplicated is called: *(MA 2016)*
a. Ring chromosome
b. Isochromosome
c. Translocation
d. Mutation

20. A 16-year-old female presents with primary amenorrhea and raised FSH. On examination, her height was 58 inches. What would be the histopathological finding in the ovary? *(AIIMS Nov 2013)*
a. Absence of oocytes in the ovaries (streak ovaries)
b. Mucinous cystadenoma
c. Psamomma bodies
d. Hemorrhagic Corpus Leuteum

21. If a chromosome divides in an axis perpendicular to usual axis of division it is going to form:
a. Ring chromosome *(AIIMS May 2013)*
b. Isochromosome
c. Acrocentric chromosome
d. Subtelocentric chromosome

22. Condition not associated with increased risk of Cancer are all except? *(JIPMER 2013)*
a. NF-1
b. Turners syndrome
c. Down syndrome
d. Chr 13 deletion

23. Most common microdeletion syndrome is? *(DNB Aug 2012)*
a. WAGR syndrome
b. Velo-cardio-facial syndrome
c. PraderWilli syndrome
d. Angelman syndrome

24. Down's syndrome increases risk of: *(PGI May 2011)*
a. Hirschprung's disease
b. Leukemia
c. Sensorineural hearing loss
d. Hyperthyroidism
e. Atlanto-occipital dislocation

25. Which of the following is not associated with Down's syndrome? *(AIIMS Nov 11)*
a. Trisomy 21
b. Mosaic 21
c. Translocation t (15;21), t (21;21)
d. Deletion of 21

26. The chromosomal karyotype in Patau syndrome is - *(DNB Dec 2008/ Karn 2011)*
a. 47XX, +21
b. 46XX/47XX,+18
c. 45XX, der(14;21)
d. 47XX,+13

27. All the following are characteristic of Turner Syndrome EXCEPT- *(DNB Dec 10)*
a. Webbing of Neck
b. Cubitus valgus
c. Umbilical Hernia
d. Coarctation of Aorta

MENDELIAN / SINGLE GENE DISORDERS

28. All of the following statement(s) is/are true about Marfan syndrome except: *(PGI May 2019)*
a. It is autosomal dominant inheritance
b. Defect in type-1 collagen
c. Defect in type-2 collagen
d. Occur due to mutation in fibrillin 1 gene
e. There is defect in lysyl hydroxylase enzyme

29. CGG repeat sequence is found in: *(JIPMER 2019)*
a. Fragile X syndrome
b. Huntington's chorea
c. Dentatorubropallidoluysian atrophy
d. Machado–Joseph disease

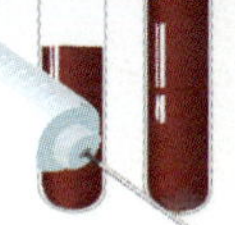

30. **Identify the inheritance pattern?** *(AIIMS Nov 2018)*

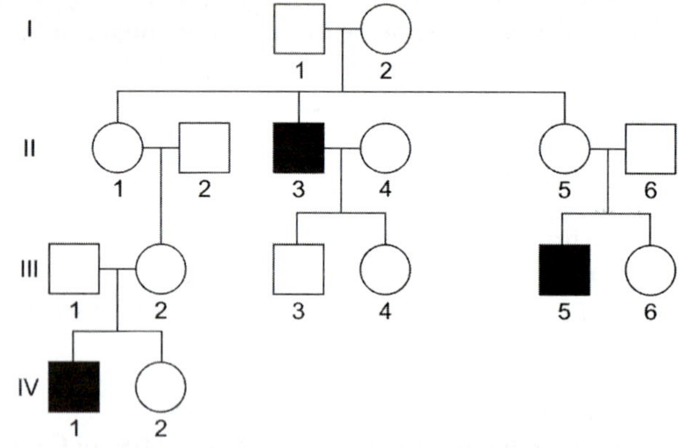

   a. Y linked recessive   b. Y linked dominant
   c. X linked recessive   d. X linked dominant

31. **Which of following dyads are correct ?** *(PGI May 2018)*
   a. Marfan syndrome: Autosomal recessive
   b. Phenylketonuria: Autosomal dominant
   c. Vit. D resistant rickets: Autosomal dominant
   d. Alkaptonuria: Autosomal recessive
   e. Duchene muscle dystrophy: X-linked recessive

32. **Which of the following is Autosomal dominant disorder?** *(JIPMER 18)*
   a. Bests disease
   b. Laurence-Moon Biedl syndrome
   c. Bassen-Kornzweig syndrome
   d. Usher syndrome

33. **Which of the following disease is X- linked?**
(Recent Question 2018)
   a. Thalassemia   b. Color blindness
   c. Sickle cell anemia   d. Galactosemia

34. **All of the following are autosomal dominant, except?**
   a. Familial hypercholesterolemia *(Recent Question 2018)*
   b. Congenital adrenal hyperplasia
   c. Achondroplasia
   d. Acute intermittent porphyria

35. **Which of the following is true regarding ataxia telangiectasia?** *(Recent Question 2018)*
   a. It is X linked recessive disease
   b. It is autosomal recessive disorder
   c. It is associated with increased levels of IgM
   d. None of the above

36. **Which of the following is the gene for Duchenne muscular dystrophy?** *(Recent Exam 2018)*
   a. DMPK gene   b. STK11 gene
   c. PTCH gene   d. Dystrophin gene

37. **Xeroderma pigmentosa all true except:**
   a. Autosomal dominant
   b. Onset of squamous cell ca by 2nd-3rd decade
   c. Develops non melanotic cancer by the age of 9yrs
   d. Nucleotide excision repair defect

38. **An obese women with T2 diabetes and hypertension had endometrial ca.Which of the following gene is involved?** *(JIPMER 2017)*
   a. PTEN   b. P53
   c. B catenin   d. SMAD

39. **Locations of gene which codes for alpha 1 anti-trypsin deficiency?** *(JIPMER 2017)*
   a. 14q   b. 13p
   c. 17p   d. 14p

40. **Find Correct match among the following?**
(PGI May 2017)
   a. Hypophosphatemic rickets- X linked dominant
   b. Duchenne muscular dytrophy- X linked recessive
   c. Sickle cell: AR
   d. Osteogenesis imperfecta-1 :AR
   e. Achondroplasia : AR

41. **Autosomal recessive disease(s) is/are:** *(PGI May 2016)*
   a. Sickle cell anaemia   b. Phenylketonuria
   c. Tuberous scelerosis   d. Familial polyposis coli
   e. Marfan syndrome

42. **Chromosomal abnormalities in Down syndrome is/are due to:** *(PGI May 2016)*
   a. Nondisjunctional of maternal chromosome
   b. Nondisjunctional of paternal chromosome
   c. Translocations between chromosome 21 & 14
   d. Disjunction of paternal chromosome
   e. Mosaicism

43. **True about Lyonization of X chromosome:**
(Recent Question 2016-17)
   a. Inactivation of X chromosome only in somatic cell
   b. Inactivation of X chromosome only in germ cell
   c. Inactivation of X chromosome in somatic & germ cell both
   d. Maximum number of Barr body is equal to X chromosome

44. **Which of the following pairs is not correctly matched?**
(Recent Question 2016-17)
   a. Turner's syndrome .... 45, XO
   b. Down syndrome .... 47, XY, +21
   c. Klinefelter's syndrome .... 47, XXY
   d. Marfan's syndrome .... 47, XYY

45. **The clinical features of Turner Syndrome in girls include the following except:** *(Recent Question 2016-17)*
   a. Severe mental retardation
   b. Webbing of the neck
   c. Delayed puberty
   d. Short stature

46. **The law "Relative frequencies of each gene allele tends to remain constant from generation to generation", was given by?** *(Recent Question 2015)*
   a. Henry Sigerist   b. Hardy Weinberg
   c. Doug Engelberg   d. Johanna Frank

47. **ABO blood group is an example of ?** *(AIIMS May 2015)*
   a. Co-dominance
   b. AD
   c. AR
   d. Mitochondrial inheritance

48. **A 48-year-old lady presented with hepatosplenomegaly with pancytopenia. On bone marrow examination, a tissue paper crumpled appearance is seen. Which is the most likely product to have accumulated ?**
(AIIMS May 2015)
   a. Glucocerebroside   b. Sphingomylin
   c. Sulfatide   d. Ganglioside

49. Frameshift mutation occurs due to?
(Recent Question 2016)
a. Transition
b. Transversion
c. Insertion
d. Point mutation

50. Hypophosphatemic Vit D Resistant Rickets is?
(Recent Question 2016)
a. AD
b. AR
c. XD
d. XR

51. Which of the following is X-linked recessive?
(Recent Question 2016)
a. Duchenne muscular dystrophy
b. Hypophostemic rickets
c. Marfans syndrome
d. Downs syndrome

52. All the following are Autosomal Dominant EXCEPT
a. Cronkhite Canada syndrome *(Recent Question 2015)*
b. Bannayan Ruvalcaba Riley syndrome
c. Peutz Jegher's syndrome
d. Gardner's syndrome

53. Waardenburg syndrome is due to mutation of
(Recent Question 2015)
a. PAX2 gene
b. PAX3 gene
c. PAX6 gene
d. PAX9 gene

54. Which among the following subtypes of Osteogenesis imperfecta is not associated with blue sclera?
(Recent Question 2015)
a. Type I
b. Type II
c. Type III
d. Type IV

55. Globoid cells is a diagnostic feature of
(Recent Question 2015)
a. Krabbe's disease
b. Progressive multifocal leukoencephalopathy
c. Tay Sach's disease
d. Metachromatic leukodystrophy

56. Von Recklinghausen's disease of the bone is caused by
(Recent Question 2015)
a. Paget's disease
b. Severe hyperparathyroidism
c. Renal osteodystrophy
d. Severe osteomalacia

57. Which of the following is not due to defect in type II collagen?
(Recent Question 2015)
a. Achondrogenesis II
b. Hypochondrogenesis
c. Stickler's syndrome
d. Multiple epiphyseal dysplasia

58. Which of the following is inherited autosomal recessive?
(Recent Question 2015)
a. Achondroplasia
b. Tuberous sclerosis
c. Hemochromatosis
d. Osteogenesis imperfecta

59. RET proto-oncogene is located on which chromosome:
(Recent Question 2015)
a. 9
b. 10
c. 11
d. 12

60. Which of the following is autosomal recessive inherited cancer syndrome?
(Recent Question 2015)
a. Ataxia telangiectasia
b. Cowden syndrome
c. Retinoblastoma
d. HNPCC

61. Inheritance of Beckers muscular dystrophy is?
(Recent Question 2016)
a. X-linked recessive
b. X-linked dominant
c. Autosomal recessive
d. Autosomal dominant

62. Which of the following is an autosomal dominant metabolic disorder? *(Recent Question 2016)*
a. Hereditary hypercholesterolemia
b. Tay sachs disease
c. Gaucher's disease
d. Tyrosinemia

63. Gene responsible for embryogenesis of eye
(Recent Question 2016)
a. PAX 6
b. PAX 2
c. PAX 5
d. RAX

64. PRSS1 gene is on ? *(Recent Question 2016)*
a. Chr20q
b. Chr 17p
c. Chr 7q
d. Chr1p

65. BRCA1 is the most common gene mutated in familial breast cancer. This gene is located on which chromosome? *(Recent Question 2015)*
a. 13
b. 17
c. 20
d. 21

66. A 20-year-old male presents with mental retardation, large mandible, large everted ears and large testes. What is the most likely diagnosis?
(Recent Question 2015)
a. Down syndrome
b. Patau syndrome
c. Fragile X syndrome
d. Klinefelter syndrome

67. Y chromosome is ? *(Recent Question 2015)*
a. Metacentric
b. Submetacentric
c. Acrocentric
d. Telocentric

68. Chromosome involved in friedreisch ataxia
(Recent Question 2015)
a. 9q
b. 19q
c. 17p
d. X chromosome

69. For karyotyping, the dividing cells are arrested by the addition of colchicines in the following mitotic phase
(Recent Question 2015)
a. Prophase
b. Metaphase
c. Anaphase
d. Telophase

70. The best suited nucleated cell for chromosomal study
(Recent Question 2015)
a. Polymorphs
b. Lymphocytes
c. Epithelial cells
d. Langerhan's cell

71. F body is *(Recent Question 2015)*
a. Y chromatin
b. X chromatin
c. Chromosome 1
d. Chromosome 21

72. An example for gain of function mutation is?
(Recent Question 2015)
a. Osteogenesis imperfecta
b. Ehler danlos syndrome
c. Marfan syndrome
d. Huntington's disease

73. All are true about Angelman syndrome except
(Recent Question 2015)
a. Microdeletion on maternal chromosome 15
b. Obesity
c. Mental retardation
d. Happy puppets

74. Banding technique most commonly employed for cytogenetic analysis *(Recent Question 2015)*
a. G banding
b. Q banding
c. R banding
d. C banding

75. Germline mosaicism is seen in *(Recent Question 2015)*
a. Fragile X syndrome
b. Angelman syndrome
c. Mitochondrial myopathy
d. Osteogenesis imperfecta

76. Approximate number of genes in human genome *(Recent Question 2015)*
a. 10000–15000
b. 20000–25000
c. 40000–50000
d. 100000

77. Most lethal karyotype is? *(Recent Question 2016)*
a. 45, XO
b. 45, YO
c. 47, XXY
d. 48, XYYY

78. All the following are true regarding autosomal dominant inheritance except *(Recent Question 2015)*
a. Usually defects of structural proteins or receptors
b. Many new mutations seem to occur in germ cells of relatively older fathers
c. Complete penetrance
d. Variable expressivity

79. Arterial or uterine rupture occurs in which type of Ehlers Danlos syndrome *(Recent Question 2015)*
a. Type I
b. Type II
c. Type III
d. Type IV

80. The following feature is not common in 22q11.2 deletion syndrome *(Recent Question 2015)*
a. Mental retardation
b. Schizophrenia
c. ADHD
d. Congenital heart defects

81. Protein affected in spinocerebellar ataxia type 6 *(Recent Question 2015)*
a. Ataxin
b. α1A-Voltage-dependent calcium channel subunit
c. Atrophin
d. Androgen receptor

82. Not a true statement about fragile X ataxia tremor syndrome *(Recent Question 2015)*
a. Females carrying the premutations may have premature ovarian failure
b. Premutation carrying males cannot transmit the disease
c. Males exhibit a neurodegenerative syndrome characterized by intention tremors and cerebellar ataxia
d. May progress to parkinsonism

83. The following technique is used to analyze DNA obtained from cancer biopsies, in which tumor cells are often contaminated with large numbers of admixed stromal cells
a. Sanger sequencing *(Recent Question 2015)*
b. Single base primer extension
c. Pyrosequencing
d. Amplicon length analysis

84. Submicroscopic deletions of any size can be detected by? *(Recent Question 2015)*
a. Multiplex ligation-Dependent probe amplification (MLPA)
b. Southern blotting
c. Cytogenomic array technology
d. Chromosome painting

85. True about autosomal dominant type of inheritance: *(PGI May 2015)*
a. 25% affected & 50% carrier if one parent affected
b. 50% affected & 75% carrier if both parent affected
c. 75% affected if both parent affected
d. 50% affected if one parent affected
e. All carrier irrespective of either one parent affected or both parent affected

86. Accumulation of cerebral gangliosides occurs due to deficiency of: *(Recent Question 2015)*
a. β glucocerebrosidase
b. β galactosidase
c. Hexosaminidase A
d. Sphingomyelinase

87. If parents are carrier for an autosomal recessive disorder. What are the chances of offspring to get affected- *(Recent Question 2014)*
a. 1 : 1
b. 1 : 2
c. 1 : 3
d. 1 : 4

88. Type of inheritance in Tuberous sclerosis - *(Recent Question 2014) (WB PG 2012)*
a. Autosomal dominant
b. Autosomal recessive
c. X-linked dominant
d. X-linked recessive

89. Enzyme deficiency in Hunter disease is: *(WB PG 2014)*
a. L-iduronidase
b. Iduronate sulfatase
c. Heparan sulfamidase
d. Hyaluronidase

90. Which of the following disease is caused by point mutation? *(PGI May 2013, May 2012)*
a. Colon cancer
b. Diabetes mellitus type II
c. Cystic fibrosis
d. Sickle cell disease
e. Gauchers disease

91. In Xeroderma Pigmentosum, defect is in?
a. Base pair defect *(Recent Question 2013)*
b. Nucleotide excision Repair
c. Mismatch repair defect
d. Protein folding

92. Hemophilia is associated with- *(Recent Question 2014)*
a. X chromosome
b. Y chromosome
c. Chromosome 3
d. Chromosome 16

93. If both parents have sickle cell anemia, then the likelihood of children having the disease is- *(Recent Question 2015)*
a. 10%
b. 25%
c. 50%
d. 100%

94. In an Autosomal Dominant disorder, mother is affected but is heterozygous. Father is normal. What are the chance of disease in children? *(Recent Question 2014)*
a. 50% affected
b. 25% affected
c. 75% affected
d. All affected

95. True statement about inheritance of an X linked recessive trait is - *(Recent Question 2015)*
a. 50% of boys of carrier mother are affected
b. 50% of girls of diseased fathers are carriers
c. Father transmits disease to the son
d. Mother transmits the disease to the daughter

96. In Marfan syndrome, the defect is in - *(Recent Question 2014, 2012), (DNB June 11)*
a. Fibrillin I
b. Fibrillin II
c. Collagen
d. Elastin

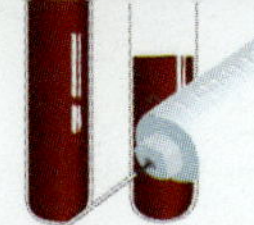

97. Which of the following is not X linked condition?
a. Duchenne muscular dystrophy *(Recent Question 13)*
b. Emery-Dreifuss muscular dystrophy
c. Fascio-scapulo-humeral muscular dystrophy
d. Becker muscular dystrophy

98. In a X-linked recessive condition, what is the chance of an offspring being affected with an affected mother and normal father? *(Recent Question 2012)*
a. 50% of daughters are carriers
b. 50% of sons are asymptomatic carriers
c. 50% of the off-springs are carriers
d. Males will never be affected

99. A normal couple has one daughter affected with Cystic fibrosis. They are now planning to have another child. What is the chance of siblings being affected by the disease - *(AI PGMEE 2010)*
a. 0   b. 50%
c. 25%   d. 75%

100. Disease having autosomal recessive inheritance –
a. Cystic fibrosis *(PGI May 10)*
b. Hydrocephalus
c. Duchene muscular dystrophy
d. Albinism
e. Vitamin D resistant rickets

101. Which is the most common tumor associated with type I neurofibromatosis?
a. Optic nerve glioma
b. Meningioma
c. Acoustic schwannoma
d. Low grade astrocytoma

102. Identify the inheritance pattern? *(JIPMER 2017)*

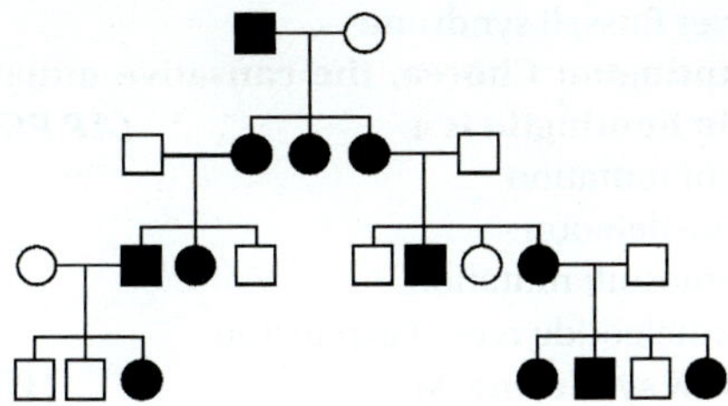

a. AD   b. AR
c. XD   d. XR

103. A 1-year-old boy presented with hepatosplenomegaly and delayed milestones. The liver biopsy and bone marrow biopsy revealed presence of histiocytes with PAS-positive Diastase resistant material in the cytoplasm. Electron microscopic examination of these histiocytes is most likely to reveal the presence of -
a. Birbeck granules in the cytoplasm
b. Myelin figures in the cytoplasm
c. Parallel rays of tubular structures in lysosomes
d. Electron dense deposit in the mitochondria

104. Which of the following is inherited as autosomal recessive form? *(DNB June 2010)*
a. Sickle cell anemia
b. Hemophilia
c. Hereditary spherocytosis
d. Glucose 6-PO4 dehydrogenase deficiency

DISORDERS WITH NONCLASSIC INHERITANCE

105. Mutation in DNA Helicase causes: *(Recent Pattern Question 2020)*
a. Wermer syndrome
b. Werner syndrome
c. Sipple syndrome
d. Autoimmune lymphoproliferative syndrome

106. Which of the following mode of inheritance is shown below? *(Recent Pattern Question 2020)*

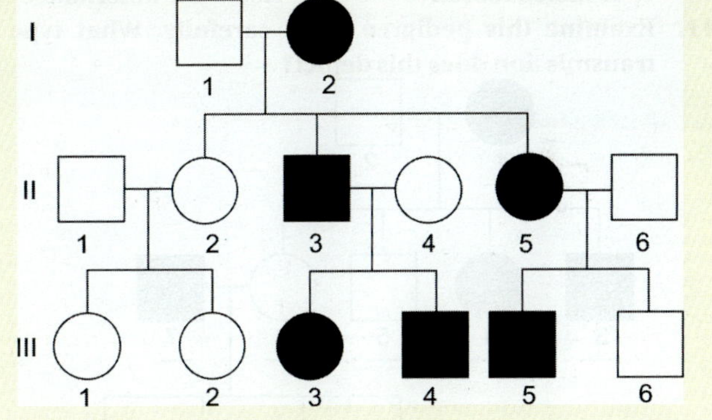

a. AD   b. AR
c. X linked dominant   d. X linked recessive

107. An 8-year-old child presented with history of recurrent infections. The child had rashes. Investigations revealed low platelets. What could be the probable cause? *(Recent Pattern Question 2020)*
a. Job syndrome
b. Wiskott-Aldrich syndrome
c. Henoch–Schönlein purpura
d. Hyper IgM syndrome

108. True statement(s) about Mitochondrial Inheritance: *(PGI May 2019)*
a. Only girls are affected
b. Mutation cause MELAS
c. Disease transfers from mother only
d. Commonly affects brain, heart, muscle, liver
e. Doesn't follow typical Mendelian inheritance pattern

109. An affected male does not have affected children but an affected female always has affected children. Type of inheritance? *(AIIMS May 2019)*
a. X linked recessive   b. Autosomal recessive
c. X linked dominant   d. Mitochondrial

110. **Examine this pedigree chart carefully. What type of transmission does it depict?**

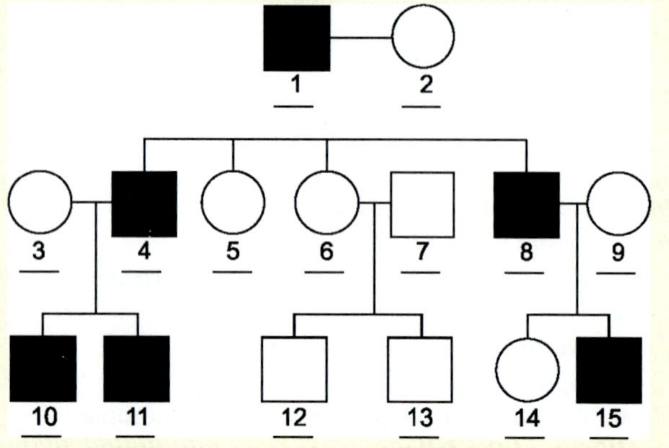

a. AD inheritance   b. AR inheritance
c. X-linked recessive   d. Holandric inheritance

111. **Examine this pedigree chart carefully. What type of transmission does this depict?**

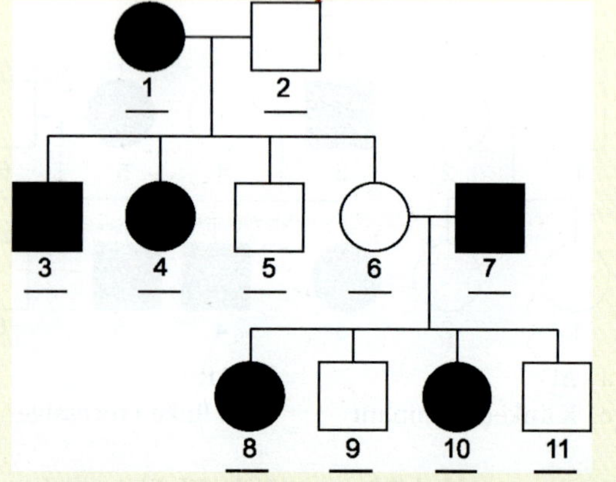

a. Autosomal dominant   b. Autosomal recessive
c. X-linked recessive   d. X-linked dominant

112. **%of Gene's in mitochondria ?** *(PGI Nov 2018)*
a. 1.5   b. 3.5
c. 6   d. 10

113. **Child with growth retardation came with Tripod skull and clinodactyly?** *(JIPMER 2017)*
a. Silver russel syndrome
b. Beckwith wideman syndrome
c. Angelman syndrome
d. Prader willi syndrome

114. **Which of the following can change the gene expression by methylation and acetylation without changing content of the gene?** *(AIIMS May 2017)*
a. Translocation   b. Inversion
c. Mutation   d. Epigenetics

115. **True about mammalian mitochondrial DNA:** *(PGI May 2016)*
a. Contains around 16500 nucleotide sequence
b. Makes up around 3% total cellular DNA
c. Makes up around 10% total cellular DNA
d. Makes up around 0.3% total cellular DNA
e. Makes up around 1% total cellular DNA

116. **% of individual who inherited the gene and will express the trait is known as?** *(Recent Question 2016)*
a. Penetrance   b. Inheritance
c. Co-dominance   d. Pleiotropism

117. **Trinucleotide repeat disorder is?**
a. Mitochondrial myopathy   *(Recent Question 2016)*
b. Myotonia dystrophica
c. Inflammatory myopathy
d. Duchene's dystrophy

118. **Anticipation is a feature of** *(Recent Question 2016)*
a. Tri nucleotide repeats
b. Genomic imprinting
c. Trisomy
d. Mosaicism

119. **True about mitochondrial DNA:** *(PGI May 2015)*
a. Linear   b. Circular
c. Transmitted by mother only
d. Transmitted by both parents
e. Contains less gene than nuclear DNA

120. **The phenomenon where subsequent generations are at risk of earlier and more severe disease is known as?** *(AIIMS May 2015)*
a. Anticipation   b. Dominance
c. Pleiotropy   d. Dominance

121. **Type of inheritance in MELAS-** *(Recent Question 2014)*
a. AD   b. AR
c. Mitochondrial   d. X-linked

122. **Paternal 15 chromosome deletion is seen in-**
a. Angelman syndrome   *(Recent Question 2014)*
b. PraderWilli syndrome
c. Down syndrome
d. Turner syndrome

123. **Uniparental disomy is seen in all except?** *(AIIMS May 2014, Nov 2013)*
a. Angelman syndrome
b. Praderwilli syndrome
c. Bloom's syndrome
d. Silver Russell syndrome

124. **In Huntington Chorea, the causative mutation in the protein huntingtin is a** *(AP PGMEE 2014)*
a. Point mutation
b. Gene deletion
c. Frameshift mutation
d. Trinucleotide repeat expansion

125. **Fragile X syndrome is:** *(WB PG 2014)*
a. AD   b. AR
c. X-linked   d. Multifactorial

126. **All are mitochondrial disorders EXCEPT:** *(MH 2016)*
a. Pearson Syndrome
b. MERRF (Myoclonic Epilepsy Ragged Red Fibre)
c. MELAS (Mitochondrial Encephalopathy Lactic Acidosis and Stroke-like episode)
d. Fragile X Syndrome

127. **True about Mitochondrial inheritance is/are:** *(PGI May 2013)*
a. Mothers transmit their mtDNA to both their sons and daughters
b. Both parents can transmit their mtDNA to both their children
c. Mitochondrial DNA codes for 37 genes
d. Mitochondrial disease commonly affect neuromuscular system
e. Mutation cause Leber hereditary optic neuropathy

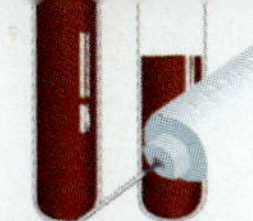

128. True about mitochondrial DNA: *(PGI May 2011)*
   a. Maternal inheritance
   b. Same evolutionary origin
   c. Not highly conserved and has high mutation rate
   d. Mitochondrial disease is associated mostly with mutation and some have deletion in mt-DNA
   e. Mostly encodes membrane protein

129. Mitochondrial DNA (mt- DNA) is known for all except-
   a. Maternal inheritance *(DPG 11)*
   b. Heteroplasmy
   c. Leber hereditary optic neuropathy is the prototype
   d. Nemaline myopathy results due to mutations in mt-DNA

130. True about genomic imprinting - *(PGI Nov 10)*
   a. Different expression of gene depending on parent of origin
   b. Prader- Willi syndrome is due to maternal deletion of chromosome 15
   c. Angelman syndrome is due to paternal deletion of chromosome 15
   d. Uniparental disomy is other name of genomic imprinting

131. Two siblings with osteogenesis imperfecta, but their parents are normal. Mechanism of inheritance is -
   a. Anticipation *(AIIMS May 10)*
   b. Genomic imprinting
   c. Germ line mosaicism
   d. New mutation

132. Analyze the following pedigree and give the mode of inheritance: *(PGI May 10)*

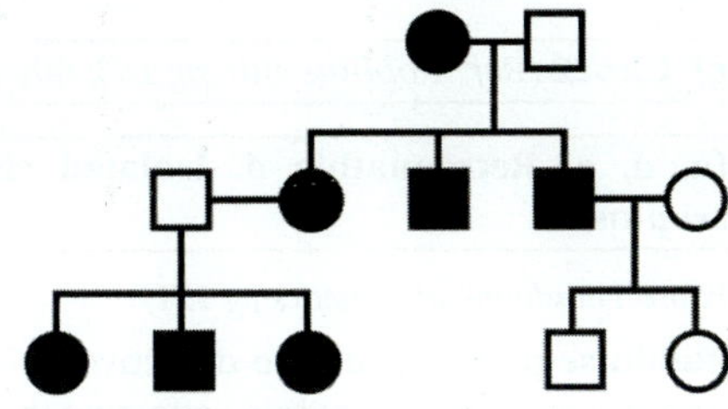

   a. Autosomal recessive
   b. Autosomal dominant
   c. Mitochondrial inheritance
   d. X linked dominant

133. Which of the following disorders is due to maternal disomy of chromosome 15? *(AIIMS Nov 10)*
   a. PraderWilli syndrome   b. Angelman syndrome
   c. Hydatidiform mole   d. Klinefelter's syndrome

134. True about mitochondrial diseases - *(PGI Nov 10)*
   a. Paternal inheritance
   b. LHON & CPEO are typical examples
   c. Most common abnormality shown is neurological
   d. Li-Fraumeni syndrome is a mitochondrial disease
   e. Common mode of inheritance

135. Mitochondrial abnormalities are seen in - *(PGI May 10)*
   a. Oncocytoma   b. Kearn-Sayre syndrome
   c. Faber disease   d. Mitochondrial myopathy
   e. Leigh's disease

DIAGNOSTIC TOOLS IN GENETICS

136. Karyotyping is/are not necessary in which of the following conditions? *(PGI May 18)*
   a. Recurrent abortions
   b. Child with multiple malformation
   c. Pregnancy in advance maternal age with previous pregnancy with an abnormal chromosomal complement
   d. Child with seizure
   e. Down syndrome

137. Gene silencing means a gene which would be expressed under normal circumstances is switched off by cell machinery. Which one of the following cellular components is not involved in gene silencing? *(UPSC 2016)*
   a. Micro-RNA   b. Double stranded RNA
   c. Ribosomal RNA   d. Si RNA

138. With reference to "DNA Microarray" technology, which of the following statements is/are correct? *(UPSC 2016)*

   1. It helps in identifying the genes involved in a disease by comparing the gene expressions between the tissues from a healthy and an infected person.
   2. It allows visualizing the activity of hundreds of genes simultaneously.

   Select the correct answer using the code given below:
   a. 1 only   b. 2 only
   c. Both 1 and 2   d. Neither 1 nor 2

139. True about array CGH is/are all except:
   a. Used for known Genetic loci *(PGI Nov 2014)*
   b. Both duplication and deletion can be studied
   c. Uses 2 colour label
   d. Can detect multiple abnormalities at the same time
   e. Uses array hybridization technology

140. Known gene loci is can be diagnosed by:
   a. FISH *(AIIMS Nov 2013)*
   b. Comparative gene hybridization
   c. PCR
   d. Chromosomal painting

141. Resolution of light microscope of viewing chromosome
   a. 5 Kb   b. 500 kb *(AIIMS Nov 2013)*
   c. 5 mb   d. 50 mb

142. Real time polymerase chain reaction is done for:
   a. DNA detection only *(AIIMS May 2013)*
   b. RNA detection only
   c. Both RNA and DNA detection
   d. Monitoring amplification of target nucleic acid

143. Karyotyping is done in which phase of cell cycle: *(Recent Question 2014)*
   a. Anaphase   b. Metaphase
   c. Telophase   d. S phase

144. Microarray is - *(Recent Question 2014)*
   a. Study of multiple genes
   b. Study of diseases
   c. Study of organisms
   d. Study of blood group

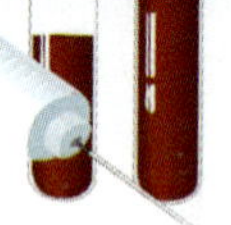

145. Which of the following procedures is routine technique for karyotyping using light microscopy -
(DNB Dec 2010, AI PGMEE 2003)
a. C-banding
b. G-banding
c. Q-banding
d. Brd V-staining

146. Karyotyping is done with all, except:
(AIIMS May 2011, June 98)
a. Blood lymphocyte
b. Blood monocyte
c. Amnion
d. Fibroblast

MISCELLANEOUS

147. BRCA 1 and BRCA 2 is responsible for all these Cancers except:
(Recent Question 2015)
a. Breast
b. Ovary
c. Intestinal lining cancer
d. Prostate

148. Multifactorial inheritance is most likely to play a role in-
(Recent Question 2014)
a. Cleft lip
b. Marfan's syndrome
c. Down's syndrome
d. Erythroblastosis fetalis

149. HOX gene mutation can cause all except-
(Recent Question 2014)
a. Syndactyly
b. Polydactyly
c. Fused carpal bones
d. VSD

150. Technique(s) used detecting for Gene Mutation is/are:
a. Real-time PCR
(PGI May 2012)
b. Denaturing gradient gel electrophoresis
c. DNA sequencing
d. Restriction fragment polymorphism (RFLP)
e. Single-strand conformational polymorphism

151. Which of the following is a DNA repair defect?
(DNB Dec 2010)
a. Bloom syndrome
b. Incontinentia pigmenti
c. Aplastic anemia
d. Tuberous sclerosis

152. Karyopyknotic index is a method for?
a. Ovarian carcinoma
(DNB Aug 2012)
b. Hormonal evaluation
c. Dysplasia measurement
d. Measurement of cells in active replication

153. Regarding 'Davidson body', all are correct EXCEPT:
a. Present in males
(MH 2016)
b. Present in neutrophils
c. Present in 4 – 6 % of cells
d. Drumstick appearance

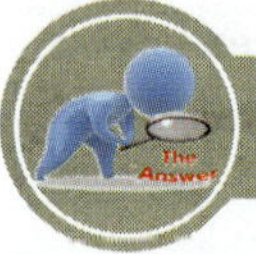

Answers with Explanations

1. **Ans. (b, c, d, e)** b. **Pleuropulmonary blastoma; c. Cystic nephroma; d. Thyroid carcinoma; e. Sertoli-Leydig cell tumor**

2. **Ans. (b, c)** b. **Turner syndrome; c. Klinefelter's syndrome** *(Ref: Robbins 9th/pg 165)*

3. **Ans. (a, b, c)** a. **Most common cause of death is congenital heart disease; b. 95% have an extra 21st chromosome; c. Increased nuchal fold thickness on USG**

4. **Ans. (d) Y Chromosome**

5. **Ans. (e) Mental retardation present**

6. **Ans. (a) Tall stature** *(Ref: Robbins 9/e pg 166)*

Left-sided cardiovascular abnormalities, particularly pre-ductal coarctation of the aorta and bicuspid aortic valve, are seen. Hypertension may be a feature of coarctation of aorta.

7. **Ans. (c) Short acrocentric** *(Ref: Emery Genetics)*

8. **Ans. (a) Turner syndrome** *(Ref: R 9th/pg 166; 8th/pg 165)*

In the given karyotype, we can observe that there is only 1 X chromosomes and no Y chromosome. This suggests the karyotype of patient as 45 XO (Turners Syndrome)

9. **Ans. (c) Chr 22** *(Ref: Robbins 9th/pg 163; 8th/pg 162)*

10. **Ans. (a, d, e) Retrognathia d. Isolated cleft palate e. Glossoptosis**

(Ref: Oxford Handbook of Genetics pg 171)

Pierre Robin sequence is due to defective DNA near the SOX9 gene is a set of abnormalities affecting the head and face, The three main features are **cleft palate, retrognathia** and **glossoptosis**.

11. **Ans. (a) Gynecomastia with long thin limbs**

(Ref: Robbins 9th/pg 166; 8th/pg 165)

In the given karyotype, we can observe that there are two X chromosomes and single Y chromosome. This suggests the karyotype of patient as 47 XXY (Klinefelter Syndrome) Male hypogonadism that occurs when there are ≥ 2 X chrand ≥ 1Y Chr.

12. **Ans. (d) Maternal nondisjunction** *(Ref: R 9th/pg 161)*

Down's syndrome is most commonly caused by **Maternal nondisjunction[Q] > Translocation> Mosaicism**

13. **Ans. (c) Turner syndrome** *(Ref: Robbins 9tth/pg 166-167)*

14. **Ans. (a) Turner syndrome** *(Ref: Robbins 9th/pg 166-167)*

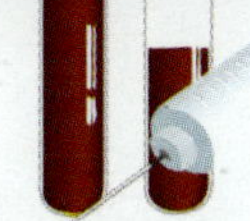

15. **Ans. (b) Klinefelter syndrome results due to an extra Y chromosome in males**

(Ref: Robbins 9th/pg 166; 8th/pg 165)

a. False: O*nly one of the X chromosomes is genetically active, the otherX of either maternal or paternal origin undergoes heteropyknosisand is rendered inactive called* Barr body, so females have one activated chromosome

b. **True:** Klinefelter syndrome is best defined as male hypogonadism that occurs when there are **two or more X chromosomes and one or more Y chromosomes**

c. False: Germs cells have haploid set of 23 chromosomes

d. False: Turners is due to missing X chr.

16. **Ans. (d) 5p-** *(Ref: Robbins 9th/pg 163; 8th/pg 162)*

17. **Ans. (c) Androgen insensitivity syndrome**

18. **Ans. (d) Cri du chat syndrome** *(Ref: Robbins 9th/pg 163)*

This is karyotype showing an arrow on **deleted part of short arm of chromosome 5**, which is suggestive of **Cri du Chat syndrome: Chromosome 5p deletion**[Q]

Features: Characteristic **cry, developmental delay, behavioral problems**.

19. **Ans. (b) Isochromosome** *(Ref: R 9th/pg 160; 8th/pg 160)*

20. **Ans. (a) Absence of oocytes in the ovaries (streak ovaries)**

(Ref: Robbins 9th/pg 166-167; 8th/pg 165-166)

In this question, the patient is presenting with **primary amenorrhea** and **raised FSH**, along with **short stature** (Given Height = 58 inches, which is less than 5th percentile of expected at 16 years age). All these features are suggestive of Turner Syndrome.

Infertility[Q] due to **rudimentary uterus** and **streak ovaries** is an important feature[Q], as ovaries are reduced to **atrophic fibrous strands without ova and follicles** in Turner syndrome

21. **Ans. (b) Isochromosome** *(Ref: R 9th/pg 160; 8th/pg 160)*

22. **Ans. (b) Turners syndrome**
(Ref: Robbins 9th/pg 166-167)

- Down Syndrome has increased risk of Leukemia
- **Turner syndrome has very low risk of Wilms tumor and colorectal Ca**

So, it seems that the answer should be none, but to choose 1 of the answers, I would choose the least common one which is Turner syndrome.

23. **Ans. (b) Velo-cardio-facial syndrome**
(Ref: R 9th/pg 163)

24. **Ans. (a, b, c, e); a. Hirschprung's disease; b. Leukemia; c. Sensorineural hearing loss; e. Atlanto-occipital dislocation**

(Ref: Robbins 9th/pg 161; 8th/pg 161)

25. **Ans. (d) Deletion of 21**

(Ref: Robbins 9th/pg 161; 8th/pg 161)

26. **Ans. (d) 47XX,+13** *(Ref: Robbins 9th/pg 161; 8th/pg 161)*

27. **Ans. (c) Umbilical Hernia** *(Ref: Robbins 9th/pg 166-167)*

Umbilical Hernia is usually not seen in Turner syndrome, but is commonly seen in Down syndrome

28. **Ans. (b, c, e); b. Defect in type-1 collagen; c. Defect in type-2 collagen; e. There is defect in lysyl hydroxylase enzyme** *(Ref: Robbins 9th/pg 144)*

29. **Ans. (a) Fragile X syndrome** *(Refer to answer 64)*

30. **Ans. (c) X linked recessive**

In the given pedigree, male are prominently affected so it goes in favour of X linked disease. Now since there is generation skip, so it will be recessive. So its, X-linked recessive.

31. **Ans. (d, e) d. Alkaptonuria: Autosomal recessive; e. Duchene muscle dystrophy: X-linked recessive**

32. **Ans. (a) Bests disease**

33. **Ans. (b) Color blindness**

(Ref: Robbins 9th ed and NCERT)

The most common cause of color blindness is an inherited fault in the development of one or more of the three sets of color sensing cones in the eye. Males are more likely to be color blind than females, as the gene responsible for the most common forms of color blindness are on the X chromosome.

34. **Ans. (b) Congenital adrenal hyperplasia**

(Ref: Robbins 9th ed 1128)

Congenital adrenal hyperplasia stems from several autosomal recessive, inherited metabolic errors, each characterized by a deficiency or total lack of a particular enzyme involved in the biosynthesis of cortical steroids, particularly cortisol.

35. **Ans. (b) It is autosomal recessive disorder**

(Ref: Robbins 9th ed p 315)

Several rare autosomal recessive cancer syndromes have been described that are characterized by hypersensitivity to certain kinds of DNA-damaging agents, such as ionizing radiation (Bloom syndrome and ataxia-telangiectasia), or DNA cross-linking agents, such as many chemotherapeutic drugs (Fanconi anemia). The phenotype of these diseases is complex and includes, in addition to predisposition to cancer, features such as neural symptoms (ataxia-telangiectasia), bone marrow aplasia (Fanconi anemia), and developmental defects (Bloom syndrome).

Answers with Explanations

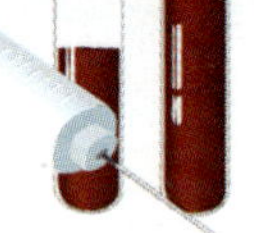

36. **Ans. (d)** **Dystrophin gene** *(Ref: Robbins 9th ed p 1242)*

Duchenne and Becker muscular dystrophy are caused by loss-of-function mutations in the dystrophin gene on the X chromosome. Dystrophin is one of the largest human genes, spanning 2.3 million base pairs and composed of 79 exons. The encoded protein, dystrophin, is a key component of the dystrophin glycoprotein complex (DGC)

37. **(a)** **Autosomal dominant**

Xeroderma pigmentosa is autosomal recessive disease.

38. **Ans. (a)** **PTEN**

39. **Ans. (a)** **14q**

SERPINA1 gene provides instructions for making a protein called alpha-1 antitrypsin, which is a type of serine protease inhibitor (serpin). Cytogenetic Location: 14q32.13, which is the long (q) arm of chromosome 14 at position 32.13

40. **Ans. (a, b, c)** **a. Hypophosphatemic rickets- X linked dominant b. Duchenne muscular dytrophy- X linked recessive d. Sickle cell: AR**

41. **Ans. (a, b)** **a. Sickle cell anaemia b. Phenylketonuria**

(Ref: Robbins 9th/141)

42. **Ans. (a, b, c, e)** **a. Nondisjunctional of maternal chromosome b. Nondisjunctional of paternal chromosome c. Translocations between chromosome 21 & 14 e. Mosaicism**

(Ref: Robbins (SEA) 9th/ 161-63)

43. **Ans. (a)** **Inactivation of X chromosome only in somatic cell**

(Ref: Robbins 9th/ 164-65; Genetics in Medicine by Thompson 8th/91)

44. **Ans. (d)** **Marfan's syndrome.. 47, XYY**

45. **Ans. (a)** **Severe mental retardation**

(Ref: R 9th/pg 166-167)

Turners syndrome has normal intelligence and not mental retardation.

46. **Ans. (b)** **Hardy weinberg**

(Ref: Modern Biology, pg 1-108)

47. **Ans. (a)** **Co-dominance** *(Ref: R 9th/pg 141; 8th/pg 141)*

When **both alleles** of a gene pair contribute to the phenotype.E.g.: Blood group 'AB'

48. **Ans. (a)** **Glucocerebroside**

(Ref: R 9th/pg 151; 8th/pg 151)

The clinical feature and bone marrow feature is typical of Gauchers disease. This results due to accumulation of cerebroside[Q] inside **mononuclear phagocytic cells** due to deficiency of β-**glucocerebrosidase.**

49. **Ans. (c)** **Insertion** *(Ref: Robbins 9th/pg 160; 8th/pg 160)*

NF1 is associated with hamartomas of the iris termed Lisch nodules.

50. **Ans. (c)** **XD** *(Ref: Robbins 9th/pg 142; 8th/pg 142)*

Frame shift mutations occur due to nucleotide **deletions or insertions** cause a **shift of codon reading frame.**

51. **Ans. (a)** **Duchenne muscular dystrophy**

(Ref: R 9th/pg 142)

a. Duchenne muscular dystrophy	X-linked recessive
b. Hypophostemic rickets	X-linked dominant
c. Marfans syndrome	Autosomal dominant
d. Downs syndrome	Chromosomal trisomy

52. **Ans. (a)** **Cronkhite Canada syndrome** *(Ref: R 9th/pg 140)*

Cronkhite Canada syndrome is non-inherited condition occurring in old age with features of loss of taste, intestinal polyps, hair loss and nail growth problem.

53. **Ans. (b)** **PAX3 gene** *(Ref: Robbins 9th/pg 140; 8th/pg 140)*

Waardenburg syndrome (WS):

- Autosomal dominant inherited condition
- Hypopigmentation of hair, skin, and/or iris of both eyes (partial albinism); and/or congenital deafness.
- 4 types: **Types I and II are the most common** forms of Waardenburg syndrome, while types III and IV are rare.
- Mutations in the **EDN3, EDNRB, MITF, PAX3, SNAI2, and SOX10** genes can cause Waardenburg syndrome.

54. **Ans. (d)** **Type IV** *(Ref: Robbins 9th/pg 140; 8th/pg 140)*

Classification of Osteogenesis Imperfecta (OI)

Type	Bone Fragility	Blue Sclera	Abnormal Dentition	Hearing Loss	Inherit-ance
I	Mild	Present	Present in some	Present in most	AD
II	Extreme	Present	Present in some	Unknown	S, rarely AR
III	Severe	Bluish at birth	Present in some	High incidence	AD, rarely AR
IV	Variable	Absent	Absent in IVA, present in IVB	High incidence	AD
V	Moderate to severe	Absent	Absent		AD
VI	Moderate to severe	Absent	Absent		Unknown
VII	Moderate	Absent	Absent	Absent	AR

55. **Ans. (a)** **Krabbe's disease**

(Ref: Harrison Chap 363)

Globoid cells are a unique and diagnostic feature of Krabbe disease which is actually an aggregation of engorged macrophages in the brain parenchyma and around blood vessels.

56. **Ans. (b)** **Severe hyperparathyroidism**

(Ref: R 9th/pg 141)

57. **Ans. (d)** **Multiple epiphyseal dysplasia**

(Ref: R 9th/pg 140)

Diseases Caused by Mutations in Collagen Genes

Gene or Enzyme	Disease
COL1A1/1A2	Osteogenesis imperfecta, type 1 Osteoporosis Ehlers-Danlos syndrome type VII
COL2A1	Severe chondrodysplasias • Achondrogenesis II • Hypochondrogenesis • Stickler's syndrome Osteoarthritis
COL3A1	Ehlers-Danlos syndrome type IV
COL4A3–COL4A6	Alport syndrome
COL7A1	Epidermolysis bullosa, dystrophic
COL10A1	Schmid metaphysial chondrodysplasia
Lysyl hydroxylase	Ehlers-Danlos syndrome type VI
Procollagen N-proteinase	Ehlers-Danlos syndrome type VII
Lysyl hydroxylase	Menkes disease

58. **Ans. (c)** **Hemochromatosis**

(Ref: R 9th/pg 141; 8th/pg 141)

59. **Ans. (b)** **10** *(Ref: Robbins 9th/pg 166; 8th/pg 166)*

60. **Ans. (a)** **Ataxia telangiectasia**

(Ref: R 9th/pg 141; 8th/pg 141)

61. **Ans. (a)** **x linked recessive** *(Ref: R 9th/pg 142; 8th/pg 142)*

62. **Ans. (a)** **Hereditary hypercholesterolemia**

(Ref: Robbins 9th/pg 140; 8th/pg 140)

Inheritance pattern of Progressive Muscular Dystrophies

Type	Inheritance
Duchenne's	XR
Becker's	XR
Limb-girdle	AD/AR
Emery-Dreifuss	XR/AD
Congenital	AR
Myotonia dystrophica	AD
Facioscapulohumeral	AD
Oculopharyngeal	AD

63. **Ans. (a)** **PAX 6** *(Ref: Emery genetics)*

The PAX-6 gene locus is a transcription factor for the various genes and growth factors involved in eye formation. Eye formation in the human embryo begins at approximately 3 weeks into embryonic development and continues through the tenth week.

64. **Ans. (c)** **Chr 7q** *(Ref: Robbins 9th/pg 166; 8th/pg 166)*

- Hereditary pancreatitis is characterized by recurrent attacks of severe acute pancreatitis often beginning in childhood and ultimately leading to chronic pancreatitis.
- The disorder is genetically diverse, but **the shared feature of most forms is a defect that increases or sustains the activity of trypsin.** Three genes implicated in hereditary pancreatitis are *PRSS1, SPINK1,* and *CFTR.*
- Most hereditary cases are due to gain-of-function mutations in the *trypsinogen* gene (also known as *PRSS1*) on chr 7q34

65. **Ans. (b)** **17** *(Ref: Robbins 9th/pg 141; 8th/pg 141)*

66. **Ans. (c)** **Fragile X syndrome**

(Ref: R 9th/pg 170; 8th/pg 170)

67. **Ans. (c)** **Acrocentric** *(Ref: Emery Genetics) Refer to ans 1)*

68. **Ans. (a)** **9q** *(Ref: Robbins 9th/pg 168; 8th/pg 168)*

69. **Ans. (b)** **Metaphase** *(Ref: Robbins 9th/pg 158; 8th/pg 159)*

70. **Ans. (b)** **Lymphocytes**

(Ref: Robbins 9th/pg 161; 8th/pg 161)

71. **Ans. (a)** **Y chromatin** *(Ref: Emery Genetics)*

Quinacrine, a fluorescence dye, binds strongly to the Y chromosome forming a bright fluorescent spot (F body). This is clearly visible in stained interphase cells from various tissues from the human male and in mature spermatozoa

72. **Ans. (d)** **Huntington's disease**

- In Huntington disease, the trinucleotide repeat mutation affecting the Huntington gene gives rise to an abnormal protein, called *huntingtin,* that is toxic to neurons causing neurologic deficit

73. **Ans. (b)** **Obesity**

(Ref: Clinical Embryology: A Color Atlas and Text; p 34)

Contd...

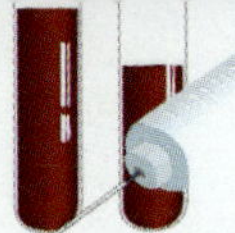

74. **Ans. (a) G banding** *(Ref: Robbins 9th/pg 160; 8th/pg 160)*

75. **Ans. (d) Osteogenesis imperfecta**
(Ref: Robbins 9th/pg 160)

In some **autosomal dominant** disorders, like **osteogenesis imperfecta**[Q], phenotypically normal parents have more than one affected child. This is due to germline mosaicism.

76. **Ans. (b) 20000–25000**

(Ref: Robbins 9th/pg 160; 8th/pg 160)

77. **Ans. (b) 45,YO** *(Ref: Robbins 9th/pg 160; 8th/pg 160)*

Karyotype 45, YO is never found in live born infants, presumably because the X chromosome carries genetic information essential for life.

78. **Ans. (c) Complete penetrance** *(Ref: Robbins 9th/pg 140)*

Complete penetrance is shown by autosomal recessive.

79. **Ans. (d) Type IV** *(Ref: Robbins 9th/pg 140; 8th/pg 140)*

80. **Ans. (a) Mental retardation** *(Ref: Robbins 9th/pg 163)*

Individuals with the 22q11.2 deletion syndrome have high risk for psychotic illnesses, such as **schizophrenia** (25% cases) and **bipolar disorders**.
In addition, **attention deficit hyperactivity disorder** is seen in 30–35% of affected children.

81. **Ans. (b) a1A-Voltage-dependent calcium channel subunit** *(Ref: 19th[a]/pg 451)*

Spinocerebellar ataxia type 6 is due to CACNA2A gene on chromosome 19p13.3, which codes for α1A-Voltage-dependent calcium channel subunit protein.

82. **Ans. (b) Premutation carrying males cannot transmit the disease** *(Ref: Robbins 9th/pg 140; 8th/pg 140)*

83. **Ans. (c) Pyrosequencing** *(Ref: R 9th/pg 140; 8th/pg 140)*

Pyrosequencing:
- **Highly sensitive** than Sanger sequencing and can detect even 5% mutated DNA
- For this reason, it is be used to analyze DNA obtained from cancer biopsies, in which tumor cells are often "contaminated" with large numbers of admixed stromal cells.

84. **Ans. (a) Multiplex ligation-Dependent probe amplification (MLPA)**

(Ref: Robbins 9th/pg 177; 8th/pg 179)

Multiplex Ligation-Dependent Probe Amplification (MLPA):
MLPA is a technique which mixes DNA hybridization, DNA ligation, and PCR amplification to detect deletions and duplications of any size, including anomalies that are too large to be detected by PCR and too small to be identified by FISH.

85. **Ans. (d) 50% affected if one parent affected**

(Ref: Robbins 9th/pg 140; 8th/pg 140)

86. **Ans. (b) β galactosidase** *(Ref: Robbins 9th/pg 151-154)*

GM1-gangliosidosis:
- Caused by a genetic deficiency of lysosomal acid β-galactosidase (β-gal); autosomal recessive inheritance;
- There is accumulation of **cerebral gangliosides**
- Manifests either as an **infantile, juvenile or adult form.**

87. **Ans. (d) l:4** *(Ref: Robbins 9th/pg 141; 8th/pg 141)*

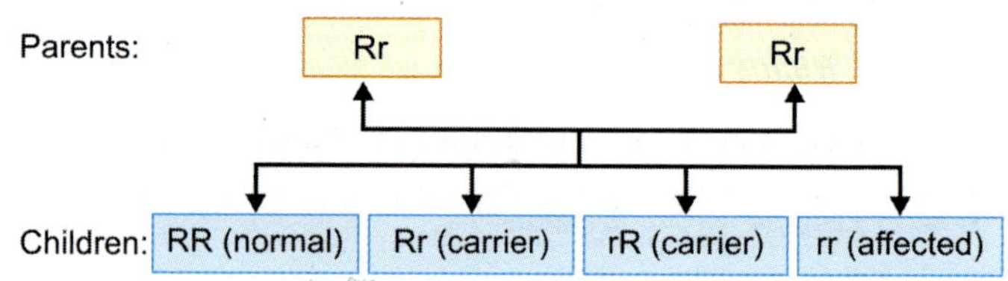

Therefore, if parents are carriers for an autosomal recessive disorder, the chances of offspring to get affected is 1:4 or 25%

88. **Ans. (a) Autosomal dominant** *(Ref: Robbins 9th/pg 140)*

89. **Ans. (b) Iduronate sulfatase**

(Ref: Robbins 9th/pg 154-155)

All Mucopolysaccharidoses are autosomal recessive except Hunter's disease which is X linked recessive[Q]

90. **Ans. (c, d, e); c. Cystic fibrosis; d. Sickle cell disease; e. Gauchers disease** *(Ref: Robbins 9th/pg 140; 8th/pg 140)*

Discussing the options one by one:

A. Colon cancer –Mostly sporadic, can be Autosomal dominant
B. **Diabetes** mellitus type II –**Multifactorial** inheritance
C. **Cystic fibrosis –Point mutation on CFTR gene**
D. **Sickle cell disease- Point mutation at 6th position of β-chain of haemoglobin**
E. **Gaucher** disease- **Autosomal recessive** inheritance due to mutations in the GBA gene. Mutations can be point mutations or deletion in GBA gene

91. **Ans. (b) Nucleotide Excision Repair**

(Ref: Harrison 18th/Chapter 61)

Patients with **xeroderma pigmentosum** have **defects in DNA damage recognition or in the nucleotide excision and repair pathway.** Exposed **skin is dry and pigmented** and is extraordinarily sensitive to the mutagenic effects of ultraviolet irradiation.

92. **Ans. (a) X chromosome** *(Ref: Robbins 9th/pg 141)*

93. **Ans. (d) 100%** *(Ref: Robbins 9th/pg 141; 8th/pg 141)*

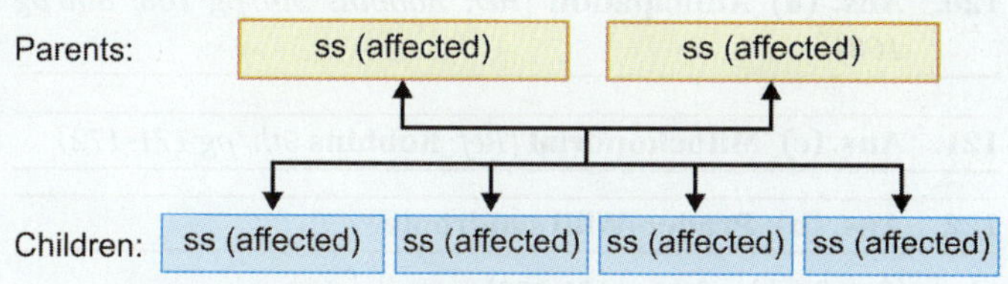

Therefore, if both parents have sickle cell anemia, then the likelihood of children having the disease is 100%

94. Ans. (a) 50% affected

(Ref: Robbins 9th/pg 140; 8th/pg 140)

In an Autosomal Dominant disorder, mother is affected but is heterozygous and father is normal.

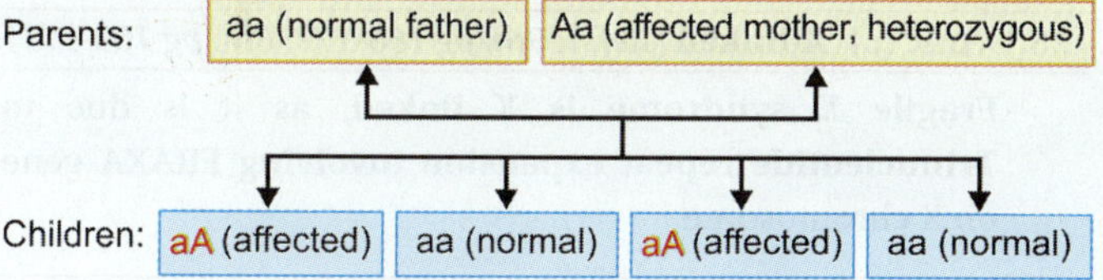

Therefore, the chances of disease in children is 50%

95. Ans. (a) 50% of boys of carrier mother are affected

(Ref: Robbins 9th/pg 141; 8th/pg 141)

In a X linked recessive disorder, if father is normal & mother is a carrier:

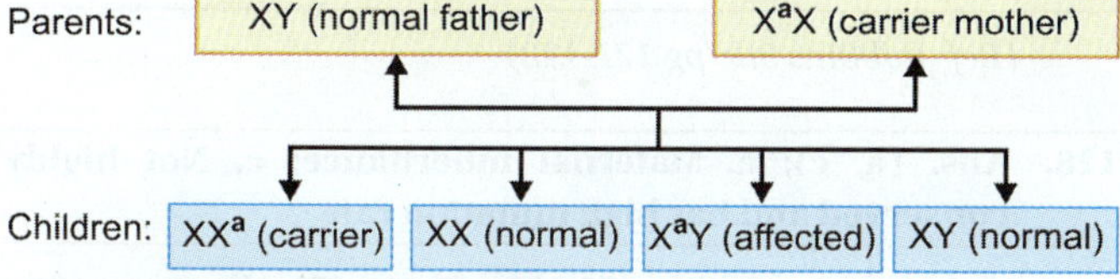

In such a situation,
- 50% of the sons are affected
- 50% of daughters are carriers, but none of the daughters are affected
- Mother transmits the disease to the sons

In a X linked recessive disorder, if father is affected & mother is normal:

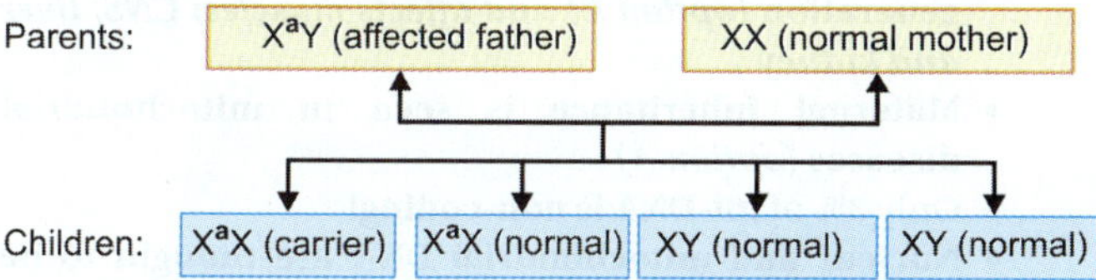

In such scenario,
- 100% of daughters are carriers
- Father transmits the disease to the daughters and not to sons, as all sons of an affected father are normal

96. Ans. (a) Fibrillin I

(Ref: R 9th/pg 144-145; 8th/pg 144-145)

Marfan syndrome
- Due to an inherited defect in an extracellular glycoprotein called **fibrillin-1**[Q]
- Affects **connective tissues**, manifested principally by changes **skeleton, eyes & cardiovascular system**.

- **Inheritance: Autosomal dominant (75%)**[Q], new mutations (25%)

97. Ans. (c) Fascio-scapulo-humeral muscular dystrophy

(Ref: Robbins 9th/pg 141; 8th/pg 141)

98. Ans. (c) 50% of the off-springs are carriers

(Ref: Robbins 9th/pg 141; 8th/pg 141)

In a X-linked recessive condition, if the father is normal & mother is affected:

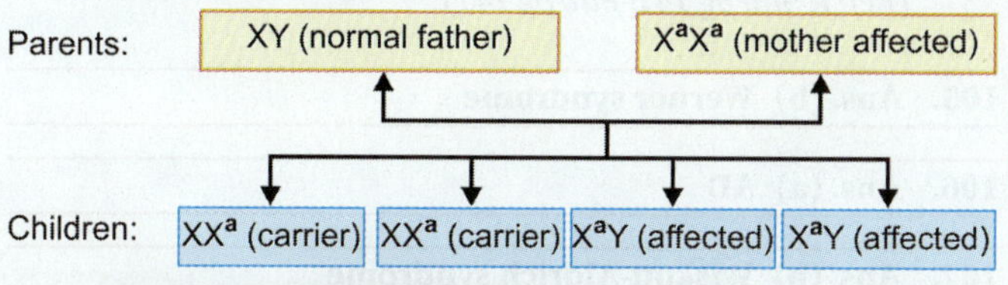

50% of the off-springs are carriers (all daughters) & 50% of them are affected (all sons)

99. Ans. (c) 25% *(Ref: Robbins 9th/pg 141; 8th/pg 141)*

- **Cystic fibrosis** is an **autosomal recessive** condition.
- If one daughter is affected, genotype will be cc
- Therefore, both parents must have been carriers of cystic fibrosis.

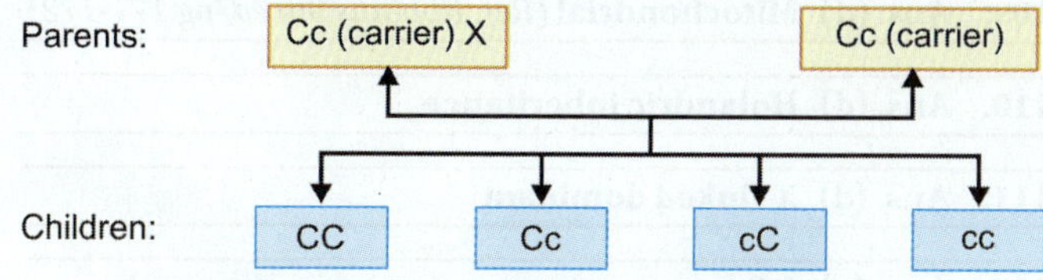

Thus each child (other sibling) has a 1 in 4 (25%) chance of being affected.

100. Ans. (a, d); a. Cystic fibrosis; d. Albinism

(Ref: Robbins 9th/pg 141; 8th/pg 141)

Disease	Inheritance
A. Cystic fibrosis[Q]	Autosomal Recessive
B. Hydrocephalus	Sporadic
C. Duchene muscular dystrophy[Q]	**X-linked recessive**[Q]
D. Albinism[Q]	**Autosomal Recessive**[Q]
E. Vitamin D resistant rickets[Q]	Autosomal Dominant

101. Ans. (a) Optic nerve glioma *(Ref: Robbins 9th/pg 298)*

- NF1 patients have **increased risk** of **Meningioma**[Q], **Pheochromocytoma**[Q] & **Wilm's Tumor**[Q]
- Most common **tumor** in NF1 is **optic nerve glioma**[Q]
- **Most common Leukemia** in NF1 is **JMML**[Q] (Juvenile Myelomonocytic Leukemia)

102. Ans. (c) XD

The pattern of inheritance is X linked as males are not transmitting to sons and its dominant because there is no generation skipping.

103. Ans. (c) Parallel rays of tubular structures in lysosomes

(Ref: Robbins 9th/pg 153-154; 8th/pg 153-154)

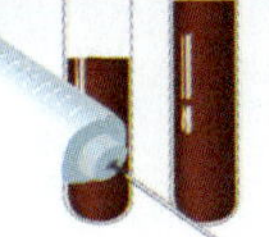

This clinical scenario of a **1-year-old** boy with **hepato-splenomegaly** and **delayed milestones (neurological** involvement) and liver biopsy and bone marrow biopsy showing histiocytes with **PAS-positive Diastase -resistant** material in the cytoplasm is s/o **Gaucher disease**. In Gaucher disease, electron microscopic examination of histiocytes show parallel rays of tubular structures in lysosomes.

104. Ans. (a) Sickle cell anemia

(Ref: R 9th/pg 141; 8th/pg 141)

105. Ans. (b) Werner syndrome

106. Ans. (a) AD

107. Ans. (b) Wiskott-Aldrich syndrome

(Ref: Robbins 9th ed/pg 242)

108. Ans. (b, c, d, e); b. Mutation cause MELAS; c. Disease transfers from mother only; d. Commonly affects brain, heart, muscle, liver; e. Doesn't follow typical Mendelian inheritance pattern *(Ref: Robbins 9th ed/pg 171-172)*

109. Ans. (d) Mitochondrial *(Ref: Robbins 9th ed/pg 171-172)*

110. Ans. (d) Holandric inheritance

111. Ans. (d) X-linked dominant

112. Ans. (a) 1.5a

113. Ans. (a) Silver russel syndrome

Russell Silver Syndrome which included short stature, relative macrocephaly, triangular facies and bilateral clinodactyly.

114. Ans. (d) Epigenetics *(Ref: Robbins 9/e pg 5)*

115. Ans. (a, e) a. Contains around 16500 nucleotide sequence e. Makes up around 1% total cellular DNA

(Ref: Robbins 9th/ 171-72; Genetic Medicine by Thomson 8th/246; Molecular Biology of Cell by Alberts 6th/802)

116. Ans. (a) Penetrance

(Ref: Robbins 9th/pg 140; 8th/pg 140)

117. Ans. (b) Myotonia dystrophica *(Ref: Robbins 9th/pg 140)*

118. Ans. (a) Tri nucleotide repeats

(Ref: Robbins 9th/pg 168)

119. Ans. (b, c, e); b. Circular; c. Transmitted by mother only; e. Contains less gene than nuclear DNA

(Ref: Robbins 9th/pg 170; 8th/pg 170)

120. Ans. (a) Anticipation *(Ref: Robbins 9th/pg 168; 8th/pg 168)*

121. Ans. (c) Mitochondrial *(Ref: Robbins 9th/pg 171-172)*

122. Ans. (b) Prader–Willi syndrome

(Ref: Robbins 9th/pg 171-172)

123. Ans. (c) Bloom's syndrome *(Ref: Robbins 9th/pg 172-173)*

Bloom syndrome is an **AR disorder** due to **defective DNA repair**

124. Ans. (d) Trinucleotide repeat expansion

(Ref: Robbins 9th/pg 168-171; 8th/pg 168-171)

125. Ans. (c) X-linked *(Ref: R 9th/pg 168-171; 8th/pg 168-171)*

Fragile X syndrome is X linked, as it is due to **Trinucleotide repeat expansion involving** FRAXA gene on X chromosome

126. Ans. (d) Fragile X Syndrome *(Ref: R 9th/pg 171-172)*

127. Ans. (a, c, d, e) a. Mothers transmit their mtDNA to both their sons and daughters; c. Mitochondrial DNA codes for 37 genes; d. Mitochondrial disease commonly affect neuromuscular system; e. Mutation cause Leber hereditary optic neuropathy

(Ref: Robbins 9th/pg 171-172)

128. Ans. (a, c); a. Maternal inheritance; c. Not highly conserved and has high mutation rate

(Ref: Robbins 9th/pg 171-172; 8th/pg 171; Harrison 18th/ chapter 61)

Mitochondrial DNA
- 16.6 kbp **circular dsDNA**
- Codes for **37 genes**: 2 rRNA, 22 tRNA & 13 protein **enzymes** that are components of the **respiratory chain** involved in **oxidative phosphorylation and ATP generation *(option E)* and affects muscles; CNS, liver and kidney**
- **Maternal inheritance is seen in mitochondrial diseases *(option A)***
- Only **3% of mt-DNA is non-coding!**
- **Nuclear and mitochondrial DNA are thought to be of separate evolutionary origin,** with the mtDNA being derived from the circular genomes of the bacteria that were engulfed by the early ancestors of today's eukaryotic cells. This theory is called the **endosymbiotic theory *(option B)***
- **mtDNA is not highly conserved and has a rapid mutation rate, (*option C*)**
- **Mitochondrial diseases are sometimes (about 15% of the time) caused by mutations in the mitochondrial DNA.** Other causes of mitochondrial disease are mutations in genes of the nuclear DNA, whose gene products are imported into the Mitochondria as well as acquired mitochondrial conditions. *(option D)*

129. Ans. (d) Nemaline myopathy results due to mutations in mt-DNA

(Ref: Robbins 9th/pg 171-172; 8th/pg 171)

130. Ans. (a) Different expression of gene depending on parent of origin

(Ref: R 9th/pg 172-173; 8th/pg 172-173)

Genomic imprinting refers to **different expression of gene depending on parent of origin**

131. Ans. (c) Germ line mosaicism *(Ref: Robbins 9th/pg 174)*

Germ Line/ Gonadal Mosaicism

- Mutation that **occurs post-zygotically** during early (embryonic) development.
- If the mutation affects only cells destined to form the gonads, the **gametes carry the mutation, but the somatic cells of the individual are completely normal.**
- **Effect:** In some **autosomal dominant** disorders, e.g. **osteogenesis imperfecta, phenotypically normal parents** have **more than one affected child.**

132. Ans. (c) Mitochondrial inheritance

(Ref: Robbins 9th/pg 171-172)

The given pedigree shows:
All children of the affected mother have the disease: a characteristic of **Mitochondrial inheritance**

133. Ans. (a) Prader–Willi syndrome

(Ref: Robbins 9th/pg 172-173; 8th/pg 172-173)

Discussing the options one by one:
A. **Prader Willi syndrome**: Uniparental disomy of maternal chromosome 15
B. **Angelman syndrome:** Uniparental disomy of paternal chromosome 15
C. **Hydatidiform mole**: Contains a normal number of diploid chromosomes, but they are all of **paternal** origin.
The opposite situation occurs in **ovarian teratoma**, with 46 chromosomes of **maternal** origin.
Note that **Hydatidiform mole & ovarian Teratoma are also due to uniparental disomy**
D. **Klinefelter's syndrome: 47, XXY**

134. Ans. (b, c); b. LHON & CPEO are typical examples; c. Most common abnormality shown is neurological

(Ref: Robbins 9th/pg 171-172; 8th/pg 171)

- **Mitochondrial diseases** have **maternal inheritance: LHON & CPEO** are typical examples
- Most commonly involves **neuromuscular system**
- **Li-Fraumeni syndrome: p53 mutation; Most common mutation** associated with human cancers.

135. Ans. (a, b, d, e); a. Oncocytoma; b. Kearn-Sayre syndrome; d. Mitochondrial myopathy; e. Leigh's disease

(Ref: Robbins 9th/pg 171-172 & 953; 8th/pg 171 & 964)

Oncocytoma
- **Benign tumors** with cells showing intense eosinophilia due to **characteristic accumulation of mitochondria;**
- May involve **salivary glands, thyroid, parathyroid, kidney, pituitary and lung**
- **Mitochondrial abnormality is seen, though it does not have mitochondrial inheritance.**

136. Ans. (d) Child with seizure

137. Ans. (c) Ribosomal RNA *(Ref: Robbins 9th/pg 172-173)*

- Two of the leading methods of gene silencing are RNA interference (RNAi), Si RNA and antisense oligonucleotides (ASOs), ds RNA
- It does not affect ribosomal RNA

138. Ans. (c) Both 1 and 2 *(Ref: Robbins 9th/pg 177-178)*

- In Microarray, there is study of multiple genes, based on reverse hybridization technology. So it is highly possible to compare the DNA of patient and Normal DNA.
- Detects genomic abnormalities without prior knowledge of the genes involved, using microarray

139. Ans. (a) Used for known Genetic loci

(Ref: Robbins 9th/pg 177-178; 8th/pg 179-180)

In Array CGH (**Array-Based Comparative Genomic Hybridization**):
- Test DNA and a reference DNA are labeled with **two different fluorescent dyes**
- It is **used for unknown Genetic loci**
- **Primers for genes to be studied are hybridized on the chip;**
- **Both duplication and deletion** can be studied at the same time.
- It can **detect multiple abnormalities at the same time, by detecting difference in signal with duplication, deletion and normal genes;**

140. Ans. (a) FISH

(Ref: Robbins 9th/pg 177; 8th/pg 179)

141. Ans. (c) 5 mb

(Ref: Robbins 9th/pg 158; 8th/pg 159)

Resolution of light microscope of viewing chromosome (Karyotype): 5 mb
Resolution of FISH: 200 Kilobases (more sensitive than karyotype)

142. Ans. (d) Monitoring amplification of target nucleic acid

(Ref: Robbins 9th/pg 175-176; 8th/pg 174)

Real time polymerase chain reaction is done for:
- **Monitoring amplification of target nucleic acid**
- **Quantitate amount of DNA in sample**

143. Ans. (b) Metaphase

(Ref: Robbins 9th/pg 158; 8th/pg 159)

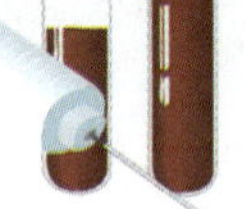

In Karyotype

- Chromosomes are examined after **arresting dividing cells** in **metaphase** with mitotic spindle inhibitors (e.g. N-diacetyl-N-methyl**colchicine**), followed by staining
- **Resolution of Karyotyping: 2 to 5 million base pairs^Q**

144.　Ans. (a)　Study of multiple genes

(Ref: R 9th/pg 177-178)

In Microarray, there is study of multiple genes, based on reverse hybridization technology.

Detects genomic abnormalities **without prior knowledge of the genes involved, using microarray.**

145.　Ans. (b)　G-banding

(Ref: Robbins 9th/pg 158; 8th/pg 159)

146.　Ans. (b)　Blood monocyte

(Ref: R 9th/pg 158; 8th/pg 159)

- To produce a karyotype, **cells capable of growth and division is used**, as karyotyping is done by arresting mitosis in dividing cells in metaphase.
- None of the leukocytes in blood normally divide, but **lymphocytes can readily be induced to proliferate, providing a very accessible source of metaphase cells; but monocytes cannot be used.**

147.　Ans. (c)　Intestinal lining cancer

(Ref: Robbins 9th/pg 291)

Genes	Protein	Function	Associated Cancers
BRCA1 (17q21)	Breast cancer-1	Tumor suppressor, Transcriptional regulation, Repair of double-stranded DNA breaks	**Ovarian, male breast cancer (but lower than BRCA2), prostate, pancreas, fallopian tube**
BRCA2 (13q12-13)	Breast cancer-2		Ovarian, male breast cancer, prostate, pancreas, **stomach, melanoma, gallbladder, bile duct, pharynx**

148.　Ans. (a)　Cleft lip *(Ref: Robbins 9th/pg 158; 8th/pg 157)*

149.　Ans. (d)　VSD

HOX gene mutation can cause A. Syndactyly, B. Polydactyly, C. Fused carpal bones

HOX genes (also known as 'homeotic' genes)	
Properties	Their protein product is a **transcription factor** They **contain a DNA** sequence known as the **homeobox**
Physiologic Role	In the **development of the central nervous system, axial skeleton, limbs, gut, urogenital tract and external genitalia,**
Examples	**HOXD13 is mutated in synpolydactyly and HOXA13 in Hand-Foot-Genital syndrome.**

150.　Ans. (a, b, c, d, e) a.　Realtime PCR; b. Denaturing gradient gel electrophoresis; c. DNA sequencing; d. Restriction fragment polymorphism (RFLP); e. Single-strand conformational polymorphism

(Ref: R 9th/pg 177)

Techniques used detecting for Gene Mutation is/are given in pretexts

151.　Ans. (a)　Bloom syndrome

(Ref: R 9th/pg 314; 8th/pg 312)

152.　Ans. (b)　Hormonal evaluation

'Karyopyknotic index' is a method for **Hormonal evaluation; Has nothing to do with karyotyping** Karyopyknotic index is % of **intermediate and superficial cells of squamous epithelium of vagina** which have pyknotic nuclei.

153.　Ans. (a)　Present in males

(Ref: Concepts of Genetics 7th ed/pg 208)

Davidson bodies are small nuclear buds of chromatin found in neutrophil leucocytes in females. Often shaped like a drumstick, they are found in up to six percent of cells. These bodies are absent in males (compare with Barr bodies)

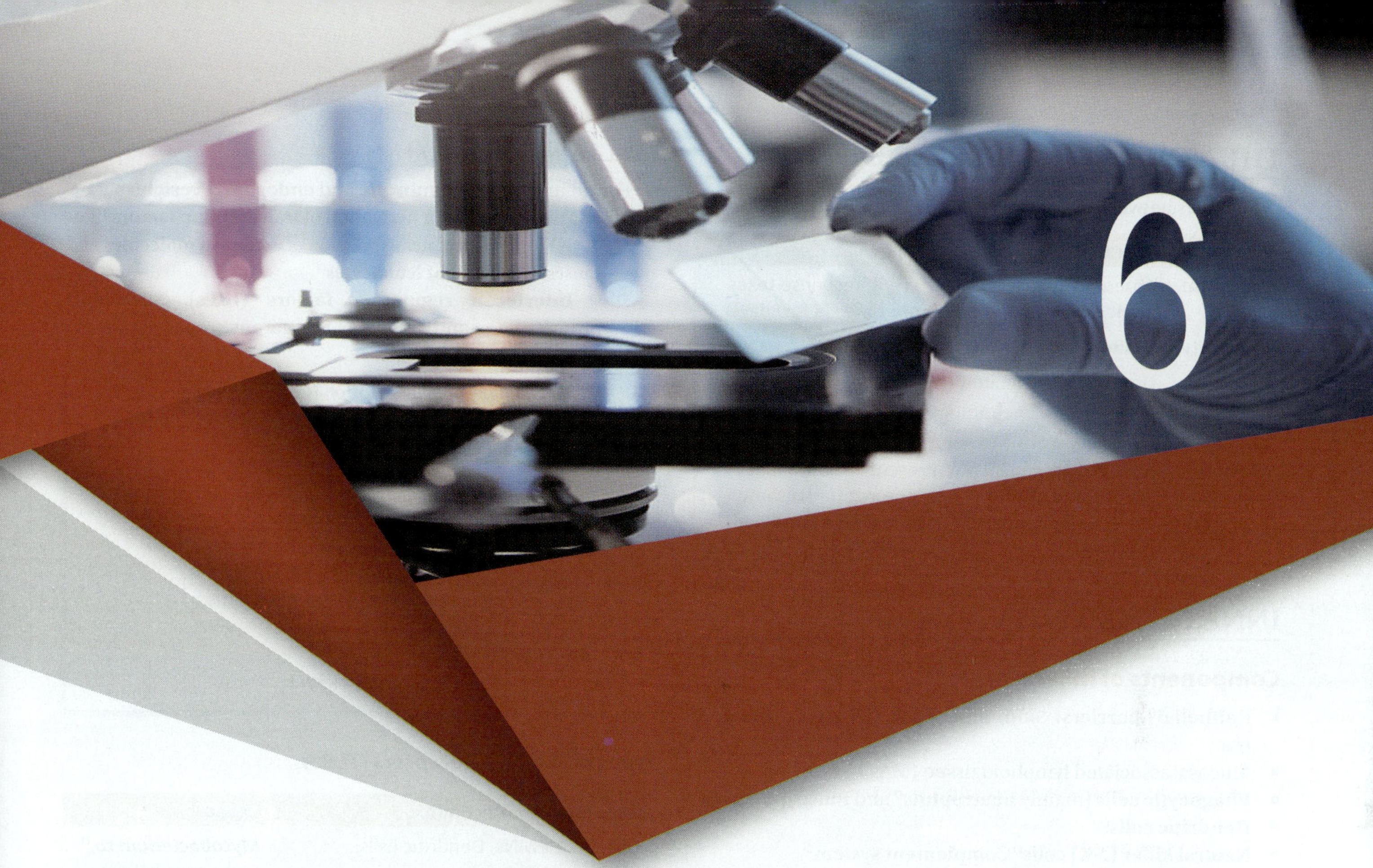

6

Diseases of the Immune System

Key Points

- **Innate immune** response is **immediate**, limited, **nonspecific, short lived** while **adaptive response** takes time, **specific** & **long lived**
- Toll-like-receptors are pattern recognition receptors act by transcription of **NF-κβ from nucleus**
- NOD-like-receptors (NLRs) and the Inflammasome act via **caspase-1**
- B-lymphocytes arise and develop in bone marrow while T-lymphocytes arise from **bone marrow** and develop in **Thymus**
- **CD4** molecules bind to **class II^Q** MHC ($4 \times 2 = 8$) and **CD8** molecules bind to class I^Q MHC ($8 \times 1 = 8$) **"Rule of 8"**
- **Innate lymphoid cells are lymphocytes that lack TCRs** but produce **cytokines similar T cells**
- Hypersensitivity is poorly controlled, **excessive, or misdirected effector mechanisms** of defense against infectious pathogens
- Substances secreted by **Mast cells** are Histamine, Heparin and Neutrophil chemotactic factor
- LE or hematoxylin bodies^Q strongly indicative of SLE
- **Class I Lupus Nephritis is the least common^Q and class IV is the most common pattern^Q**
- **In transplant immunology, 50%** HLA alleles matching is required for kidney while 0% for cornea, liver and heart.
- **The most Common Primary immunodeficiency** is **Isolated IgA immunodeficiency**
- **HIV in CNS** infects macrophages and microglia, while **Neurons are not infected**
- **Rectal biopsy** is **most specific** and **best site** for Amyloidosis diagnosis

Key Recent Updates

- β_2 microglobulin of MHC I is coded by chromosome 15
- **Natural IgM** antibodies are responsible for hyperacute rejection.

THE NORMAL IMMUNE RESPONSE

Differences between Innate and Adaptive Immunity

Features	Innate	Adaptive
Lag phase	Absent, response is **immediate**[Q]	Present, response **takes more time**[Q] (a few days)
Specificity	Limited	**More specific**[Q]
Diversity	**Limited**, hence limited specificity	**Extensive,**[Q] a wide range of antigen receptors present
Memory	**Absent**, subsequent exposure to agent generate the same response	**Present,**[Q] subsequent exposures to the same agent induce **amplified response**[Q]

INNATE IMMUNITY

Components of Innate Immunity

- **Epithelial**[Q] **barriers: Skin, mucosa** of GIT and respiratory tract
- Mucosa-associated lymphoid tissue (**MALT**)
- **Phagocytic cells** (mainly **neutrophils**[Q] and **macrophages**[Q])
- **Dendritic cells**[Q]
- **Natural killer (NK) cells**[Q] **Complement system**[Q]
- **C-reactive protein**
- **Innate lymphoid cells** [R9th]
- **Mannose-binding lectin** [R9th]
- **Lung surfactant** [R9th]

Cellular Receptors (Pattern Recognition Receptors)[Q]

Innate immunity cells are capable of recognizing certain microbial components that are often essential for infectivity.

Types of pattern	• **Pathogen-associated molecular patterns**[Q]- recognize **microbial** components • **Damage-associated molecular patterns** - recognize **injured and necrotic cells**
Location of receptor	• **Plasma membrane** receptors detect **extracellular** microbes • **Endosomal** receptors detect **ingested**[Q] microbes • **Cytosolic** receptors detect **microbes in the cytoplasm**
Classes (examples)	• **Toll-like receptors (TLR)**[Q] • **NOD-Like Receptors (NLR)** • **C-type lectin** receptors (CLRs) detect **fungal glycans**[Q] • **RIG-like receptors** (RLRs) detect **nucleic acids of viruses** [R9th] • **G protein–coupled** receptors- recognize bacterial peptides with **N-formyl-methionyl residues**[Q] • **Mannose** receptors- recognize **microbial sugars**[Q]

Toll-Like Receptors (TLR)

- Found in **plasma membrane** and **endosomal vesicles**[Q]
- **Mechanism of action:** Activation of transcription factors like-
  - ○ **NF-κB:**[Q] stimulates expression of **adhesion molecules** and causes **activation of leukocytes**[Q]
  - ○ **Interferon regulatory factors (IRFs)**: Stimulates production of antiviral type I interferons

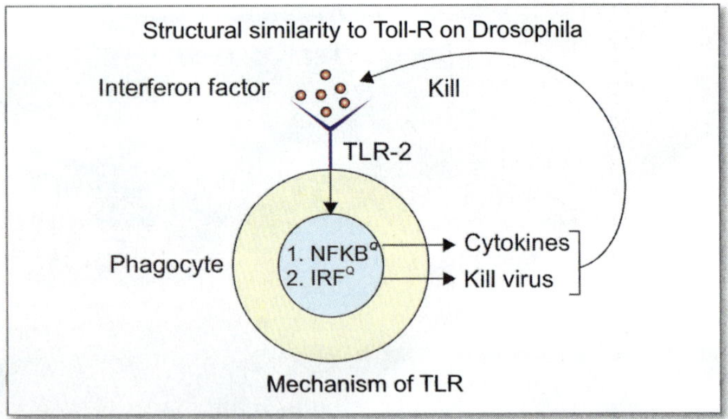

Mechanism of TLR

Types of Toll-Like Receptors (TLRS)

Receptor	Cellular Source	Ligand
TLR2	**PMNs**, Dendritic cells, Monocytes	**Mycobacterium tb,**[Q] Gram +ve bacteria
TLR3	Dendritic cells & **NK cells**	dsRNA of **viruses**[Q]
TLR4	**Macrophages**, Dendritic cells, Epithelial cells	**E. coli LPS**[Q] (Gram-negative), **Chlamydia**
TLR5	Monocytes, immature Dendritic cells, Epithelial cells, NK, T cells	**Flagellin**[Q], **Toxoplasma**
TLR7/8	B cells, plasmacytoid precursors dendritic cells	ssRNA, Imidazoquinolines
TLR9	Plasmacytoid precursor dendritic cells, B cells, macrophages, PMNs, NK cells, & microglia cells	CpG DNA

R9th Latest Update

NOD-Like Receptors (NLRs) and the Inflammasome	
Location	**Cytosolic receptors**
Recognize	Necrotic cells, ion disturbances (e.g., loss of K⁺), urate crystal & some microbial products.
Mechanism of action	Activates Caspase-1 → activates IL-1 → recruits leukocytes & induces fever.
Role in diseases	• **Periodic fever syndromes**[Q] (**'autoinflammatory' syndromes**): Due to Gain-of-function mutations • **Obesity-associated type 2 diabetes & Atherosclerosis:** due to activation bylipids and cholesterol crystals • **Inflammation in Gout:** Due to recognition of urate crystals by a class of NLRs

Macrophages: A Part of Mononuclear-Phagocyte System

Functions

- **Antigen-presenting cells**[Q] in T-cell activation.
- **Cell-mediated immunity**[Q]
- **Efficiently phagocytose**[Q] and destroy microbes that are opsonized (coated) by IgG or C3b.

Natural Killer Cells: 5–10% of Oeripheral Lymphocytes[Q]

- *Derived from:* **Large granular lymphocytes**[Q]
- *Markers*
  - ○ ○ **CD16**[Q] - An **Fc receptor for IgG**, makes NK cells lyse IgG-coated target cells: known as **'antibody-dependent cell-mediated cytotoxicity' (ADCC)**[Q]
  - ○ ○ **CD56**[Q] - NCAM (Natural Killer Cell Adhesion Molecule)
- *Function:* Destroy irreversibly stressed, **virus-infected**[Q] cells & **tumor cells**[Q] without prior exposure
- *Activating Receptors:* **NKG2D receptors: recognize surface molecules induced by** various kinds of **stress**, such as infection & DNA damage
- *Inhibiting Receptors:* **Recognize self class I MHC**[Q] molecules, **prevent NK cells from killing normal cells**[Q] (MHC Nonrestricted)
- *Cytokines secreted*
  - ○ ○ **IL-2**[Q] and **IL-15** stimulate proliferation of **NK cells**

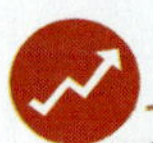

High Yield Facts

- NK cell is a **large granular lymphocyte**[Q]
- The primary function of **Toll-like Receptors** is **activation of immune system**[Q]
- As NK cells neither have B nor T-cell markers, hence called **'Null Cells'**[Q]
- **Super antigens** bind directly to **both MHC II and T cell receptor** causing T cell activation and bind T cells directly to lateral aspect of T cell receptor **irrespective of antigen specificity** of TCR[Q]
- **Toll-like receptors** types **II and IV** are involved in action against **bacterial endotoxins**
- **Interleukin** characteristically produced in a **Th1 response** is **IL-2**[Q]
- Interleukin secreted by **macrophages**, stimulating lymphocytes is **IL-1**[Q]
- Dendritic cell expresses **MHC 2**[Q]

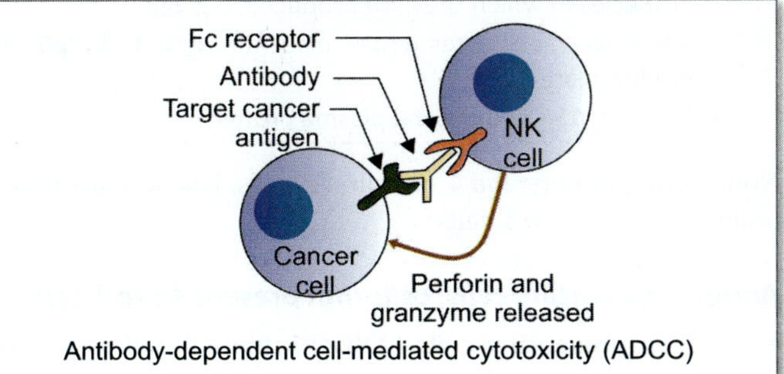

Antibody-dependent cell-mediated cytotoxicity (ADCC)

ADAPTIVE IMMUNITY

Types of Adaptive Immunity

Cell-mediated Immunity	Humoral Immunity
• Protects against **intracellular**[Q] microbes • Mediated by **T lymphocytes**[Q]	• Protects against **extracellular**[Q] microbes & their toxins • Mediated by **B – lymphocytes** and **Immunoglobulins**[Q]

Cells of Adaptive Immune System

T Lymphocytes (T Cells): 60 – 70% of Lymphocytes

- Arise from **bone marrow** (Hematopoietic stem cells) and develop in **Thymus**[Q]
- 60% of mature T cells are CD4+ and 30% are CD8+ ; so, **CD4:CD8 ratio is 2:1**[Q]

Type of T cell	Characteristics/functions
Helper T cells	Stimulate **B cells**[Q] to make **antibodies** & activate phagocytes to destroy microbes.
Naive CD4+ T cells	Recognize peptides displayed by dendritic cells → secrete IL-2 (autocrine growth factor) → stimulates proliferation of T cells → differentiation of T cells to Th1 or Th17 cells
Cytotoxic T cells	Kill **virus infected and tumor** cells[Q]

R9th Latest Update

Other types of T-cells

- *Regulatory T cells:* **Limit immune responses & prevent reactions against self-antigens.** *R9th* They are CD4+, CD25+, Fox P_3+.
- *NK-T cells:* T cells that **express markers are also found on NK cells** *R9th*
- *γ δ T cells:* **Aggregate at epithelial surfaces** of skin & mucosa of GIT & genitourinary tract *R9th*

T-cell Receptor (TCR)

- **Antigen-specific**
- **95% of TCR have a** α and β **polypeptide chain**[Q]
- **MHC restriction:** αβ TCR **recognizes** peptide antigens that are **presented by major histocompatibility complex**[Q] (MHC) molecules on the surfaces of antigen-presenting cells
- **CD3 complex and** ζ chain dimer – also involved in **signal transduction**

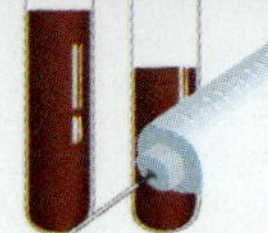

Helper T cells

Types of Helper T Cells

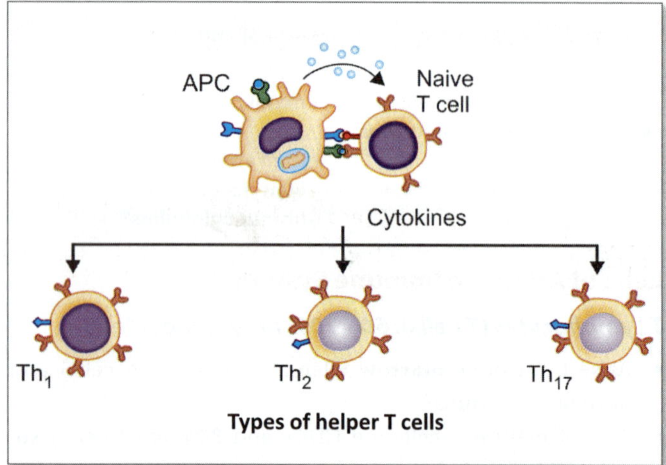

Types of helper T cells

Characteristics	TH₁ cells	TH₂ cells	TH₁₇ cells
Activated by	IFNγ, IL-12^Q	IL-4	TGFβ,^{Q}IL-6, IL-1, IL-23
Cytokines produced	IFNγ^Q	**IL-4, IL-5, IL-13**^{Q}	IL-17, IL-22
Functions	**Activates Macrophages,**^{Q} stimulates IgG production	Stimulates **IgE**^{Q} production, activates **mast cells & eosinophils**^{Q}	Recruitment of **neutrophils, monocytes**^{Q}
Defense against	Intracellular microbes	Helminthic parasites	Extracellular bacteria, fungi
Role in disease	**Autoimmune** diseases e.g. IBD, psoriasis & Chronic inflammation (granuloma)	**Allergies**	**Autoimmune & chronic inflammatory** diseases (e.g. IBD, psoriasis, MS)

High Yield Facts

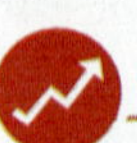

- **CD4** molecules bind to **class II**^{Q} MHC (4X2=8) & **CD8** molecules bind to **class I**^{Q} MHC (8X1=8) **"Rule of 8"**
- γδ TCR does not require MHC^Q for antigen recognition
- **Epstein-Barr virus (EBV)** enters B cells via CR2^Q
- **RBCs lacks HLA antigen**^{Q}

High Yield Facts

- **By CD40L- and helper T-cell actions, antibodies of different classes (IgG, IgA, IgE) produced**
- **Isotype switching is induced by IFN-γ and IL-4.**^{Q}
- **Helper T cells** also stimulate **affinity maturation**, that improves **quality of humoral immune** response^Q
- As these helper T-cells migrate to and **reside in the germinal centers**: called **follicular helper T cells (TFH)**

Humoral Immunity: Activation of B Lymphocytes

Acts against	**Extracellular** Microbes^Q
Mechanism	**On Activation** → B cells proliferate & differentiate into **plasma cells** → secrete **Antibodies**

B Lymphocytes: 10% – 20% of Lymphocytes

Arise from	Bone marrow (Hematopoietic stem cells)^Q
Mature in	Bone marrow
Found in	**Peripheral lymphoid tissues** such as **lymph nodes, spleen** & **mucosa-associated lymphoid tissues**
Functions	Mediates Humoral Immunity, Stimulation by Antigen → B cells develops into **plasma cells**^{Q} → produce **antibodies**
Components of B-cell antigen receptor	• **Ig receptors: IgM** and **IgD** Isotypes^Q • **Igα** (CD79a) and **Igβ** (CD79b) • **Type 2 complement receptor** (CR2 or CD21): recognize complement products • **CD40**-receives signals from **helper T cells.**

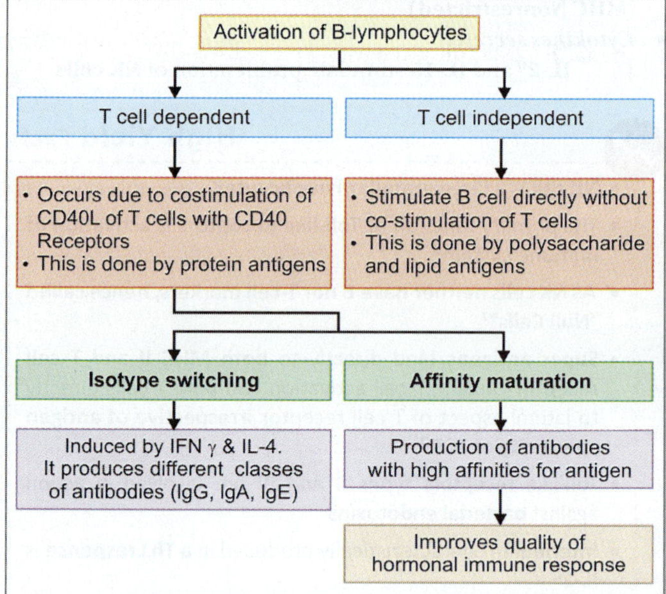

High Yield Facts

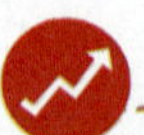

- **Homocytotropic Ab:** Higher affinity for receptors of cells in species in which they are produced, e.g. **IgE**
- All 4 IgG subclasses cross placenta, **IgG 1** & **IgG 3** predominate
- IgG form **15–18%** of total plasma protein

Now, having understood T cells and B cells, lets now see how is antigen presented to T cells?

Antigen Presenting cells; cells that present Ag to T-cells

- **Antigen-presenting cells (APCs)** initiate T-cell responses against protein antigens^Q
- **Mature dendritic cells** are the **most potent**^{Q} stimulator of **Naive T-cells**

Types of Antigen Presenting Cells

Professional APC	Non-professional APC
Express **MHC class II**	Express **MHC class I**
Macrophages, dendritic cells and B-cells	**Fibroblasts**, thymic epithelial cells, thyroid epithelial cells, **glial cells, pancreatic beta cells & vascular endothelial cells**.

Dendritic Cells: Professional Antigen-Presenting Cells

Why do dendritic cells have a key role in antigen presentation?

- Immature dendritic cells (Langerhans cells) within the epidermis are **at perfect site** to capture antigens
- **Express many receptors like TLRs and lectins**[Q]- for capturing and responding to microbes.
- In response to microbes, they are **recruited to the T-cell zones** of lymphoid organs to present antigens to T cells.

- Dendritic cells **express high levels of MHC**[Q] for presenting antigens to and activating T cells.

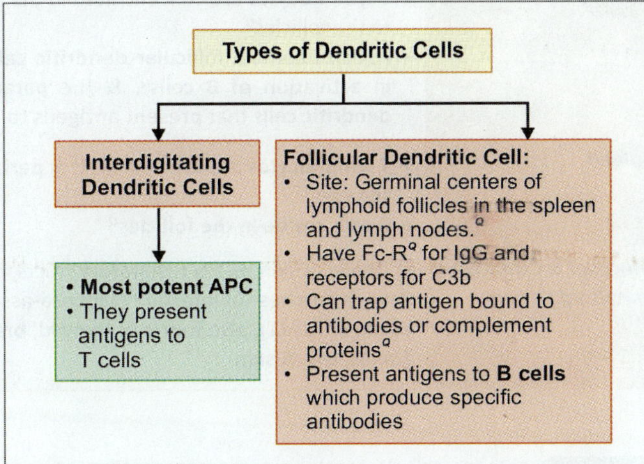

CELL-MEDIATED IMMUNITY: ACTIVATION OF T LYMPHOCYTES

Activation of T-cell Requires Three Signals

- **Signal 1:** TCR on T-cell with **MHC on APC**[Q]
- **Signal 2:** CD28[Q] on T-cell with **B7-1 (CD80) /B7-2(CD86) on APC**
- **Signal 3:** Cytokine IL-1 from APC stimulates T-cell which in turn secretes **IL-2**[Q] (which has **autocrine** effect)

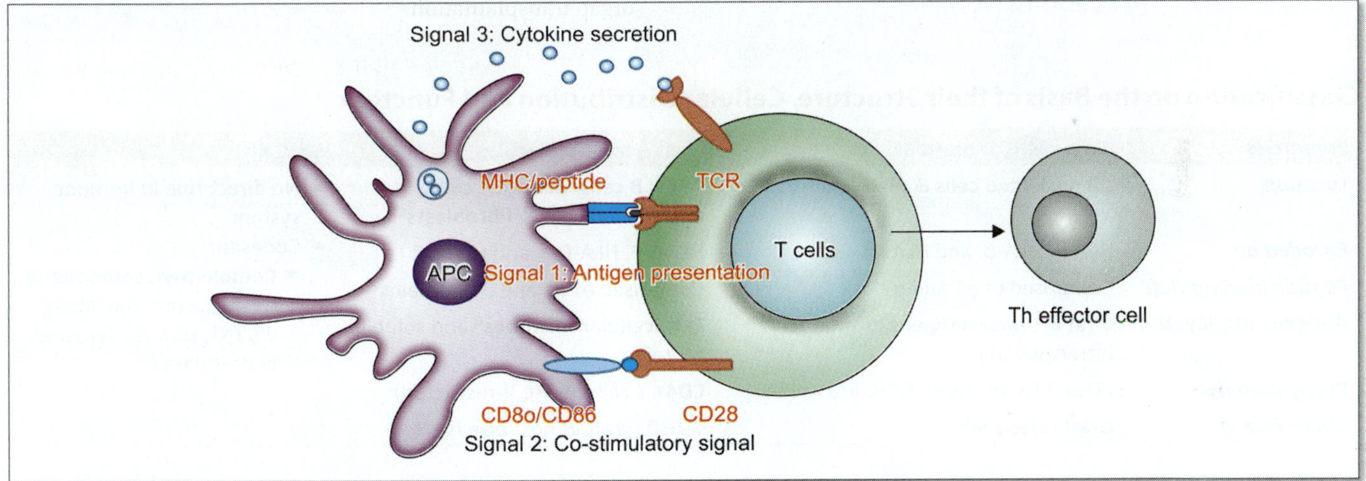

R9th Latest Update

- M cells (microfold cells) are APC

Innate Lymphoid Cells (ILCs)
- Lymphocytes that lack TCRs but produce **cytokines similar to those that are made by T cells**
- Example: NK cells

- **Cytokines** produced: IFN-γ, IL-5, IL-17, and IL-22.
- **Functions:**
  - Early defense against infections
  - Recognition and elimination of stressed cells (so-called stress surveillance)[Q]
  - Providing cytokines that influence the differentiation of T lymphocytes.

TISSUES OF THE IMMUNE SYSTEM

Generative (Central) Lymphoid Organs

- **Thymus:** Site of development of **T cells**[Q]
- **Bone marrow:** Site of maturation of **B lymphocytes**[Q]

Peripheral Lymphoid Organs

In which adaptive immune responses to microbes are initiated.

Lymph nodes	• **B cells** are concentrated in **follicles**, located in **cortex** of lymph node[Q] • **T lymphocytes** are concentrated in the **paracortex**, adjacent to the follicles[Q] • Follicles contain **follicular dendritic cells** that are involved in **activation of B cells[Q]**, & the **paracortex** contains the **dendritic cells** that **present antigens** to T lymphocytes.
Spleen	• **T lymphocytes** are concentrated in **periarteriolar lymphoid sheaths[Q]** • **B cells reside in the follicles[Q]**
Mucosal & Cutaneous lymphoid tissues	Epithelia of skin, GIT & respiratory tracts, pharyngeal tonsils & **Peyer's patches[Q]** of intestine (**Mucosa-associated lymphoid tissue or MALT**), also found in thyroid, breast, lung, salivary glands, eye & skin

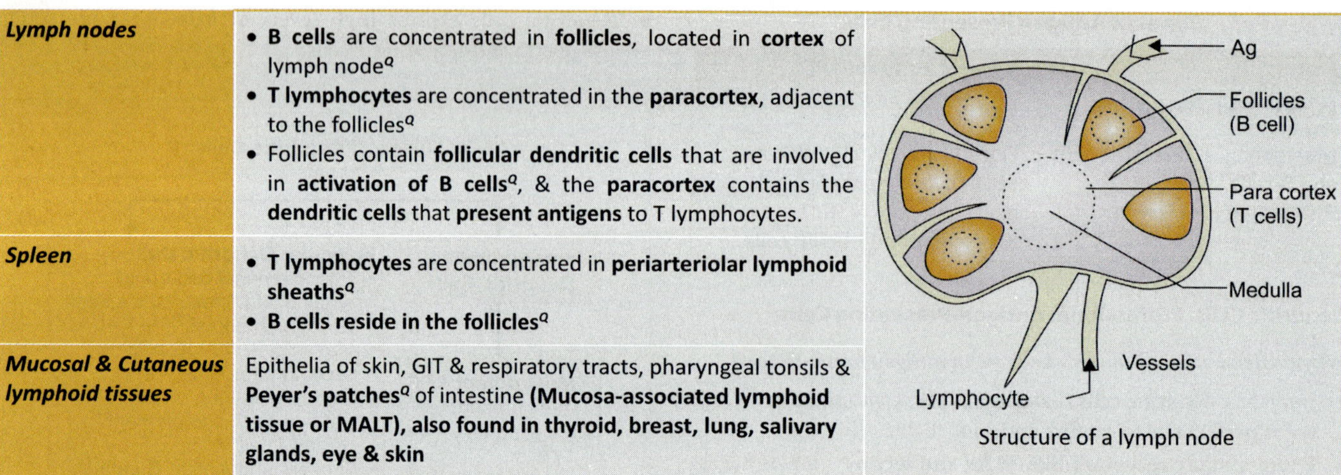

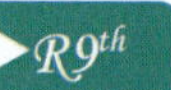

R9th **Latest** Update

Lymphocyte Recirculation
• **Naive T** lymphocytes traverse the **peripheral lymphoid organs like lymph nodes through specialized postcapillary venules called high endothelial venules (HEVs)** where **immune responses are initiated**, and **effector lymphocytes** migrate to **sites of infection and inflammation.**

MAJOR HISTOCOMPATIBILITY COMPLEX (MHC)

- Display peptide fragments of protein antigens for recognition by antigen-specific T cells
- **On short arm of Chromosome 6 (6p)[Q]**
- Also called **human leukocyte antigens (HLA)[Q]** - detected on leukocytes by the binding of antibodies.
- **Highly polymorphic[Q]** so constitutes a formidable barrier in organ transplantation.

Classification on the Basis of their Structure, Cellular Distribution and Function

Properties	Class I MHC molecules	Class II MHC molecules	MHC III
Location	**All nucleated cells & platelets[Q]**	**APCs: B cells, dendritic cells, endothelial cells & fibroblasts[Q]**	• **No direct role in immune system[Q]** • Codes for: ▪ **Complement components** C2, C4, properdin, factor B[Q], TNF, HSP-70, Tyrosine hydroxylase
Encoded by	HLA-**A**, HLA-**B**, and HLA-**C[Q]**	HLA-**DP**, HLA-**DQ**, and HLA-**DR**	
Peptide binding cleft	Comprised of α1 and α2	Comprised of α1 and β1 domains	
Antigens displayed	**Viral & tumor antigens** located **intracellularly[Q]**	**Extracellular microbes[Q]** and soluble proteins.	
Recognized by	**CD8+** T lymphocyte (MHC I-restricted)	**CD4+** T cells (MHC II-restricted)	
Major role in	**Graft rejection[Q]**	**GVHD** (graft vs host disease)[Q]	

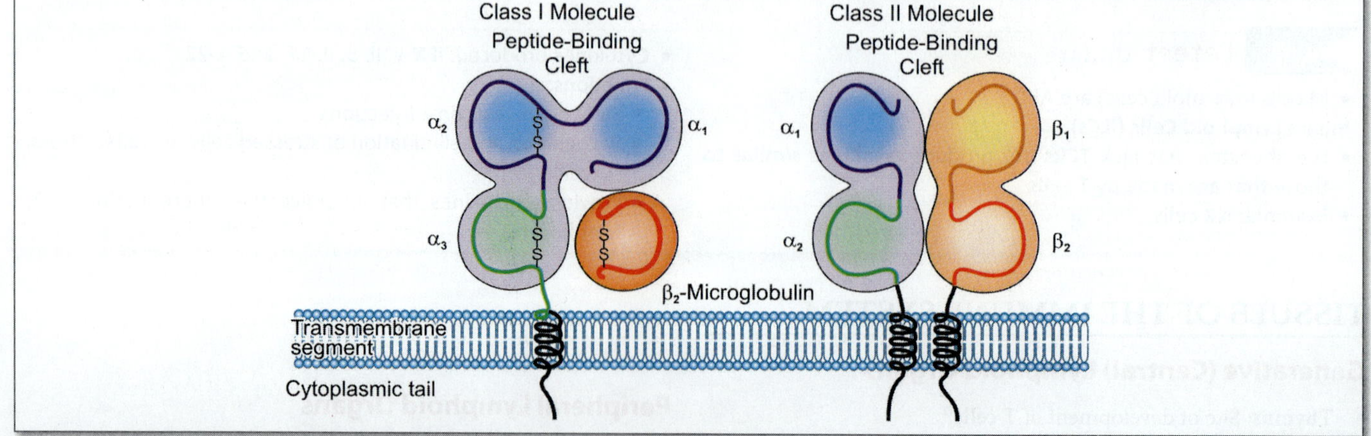

HLA Typing & HLA Matching

Methods of HLA typing	Uses of HLA matching
• **Mixed lymphocyte reaction**[Q] • Serological **detection of HLA**[Q] • Molecular detection methods: 　■ Sequence specific primer PCR (SSP-PCR) 　■ Sequence specific oligonucleotide probes (SSOP) 　■ Direct DNA sequencing	• **Organ & stem cell transplantation**[Q] • Disease association studies • **Disputed paternity**[Q]

HYPERSENSITIVITY (HSN)

General Features

- Elicited by **exogenous antigens** (microbial or nonmicrobial) or **endogenous self-antigens**
- Results from an **imbalance** between the effector and the control mechanisms
- Often associated with the **inheritance** of particular susceptibility genes
- Poorly controlled, **excessive, or misdirected effector mechanisms** of defense against infectious pathogens

Immediate (Type I) Hypersensitivity

What is it	Rapid immunologic reaction occurring in a **previously sensitized**[Q] individual	
Triggered by	Binding of an **antigen to IgE antibody** on the surface of **mast cells.**[Q]	
Also called	**Allergy,** and the **antigens** that elicit them are **allergens.**[Q]	
2 Phases	*Immediate reaction*	*Late-phase reaction*
Time taken	Within **minutes to hours**[Q]	Sets in 2 to 24 **hours to days**[Q]
Characterized by	**Vasodilation, vascular leakage,** and depending on the location, smooth muscle spasm or glandular secretions	Infiltration of tissues with **eosinophils**[Q], neutrophils, basophils, monocytes & **CD4+T cells**[Q], causing **tissue destruction** & **mucosal epithelial cell damage**
Mediators	A. Preformed Mediators: 　• Vasoactive amines, e.g. **Histamine** 　• Enzymes: e.g. **Chymase, tryptase** B. Lipid Mediators: 　• Arachidonic acid–derived products: **Leukotrienes B4, C4 & D4, Prostaglandin D2** 　• **Platelet-activating factor (PAF)**[Q] C. Cytokines: **TNF, IL-1, IL-4**[Q]	• **Eotaxin** • **IL-5** • **MPB (Major Basic Protein)**[Q] • **ECP (Eosinophil Cationic Protein)**
Examples of type I HSN	• **Local:** Urticaria, angioedema, allergic rhinitis (hay fever), **bronchial asthma, eczema**[Q] • **Systemic: anaphylactic shock**[Q] (Initiated by histamine) • **Others: Theobald Smith** phenomenon, **Prausnitz Kusnter** reaction,[Q] **Casoni's test,**[Q] Schultz-Dale phenomenon	

Mechanism of Immediate Reaction

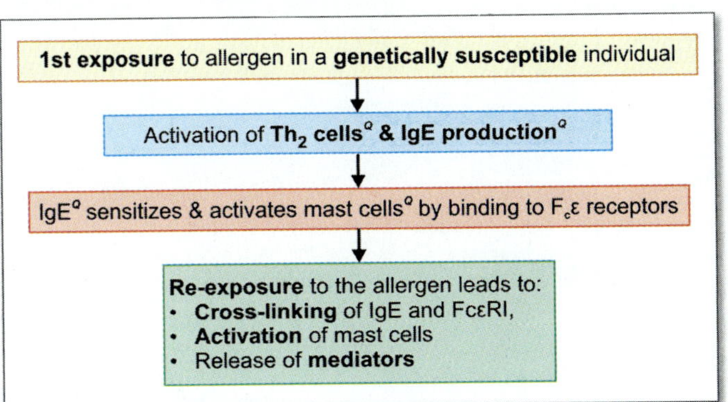

Mechanism of Late-phase Reaction

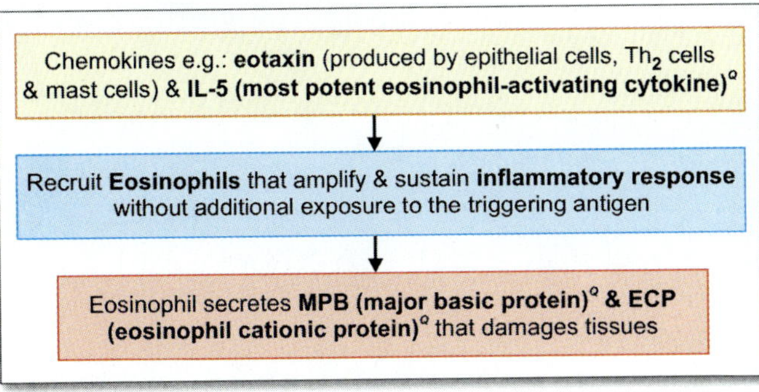

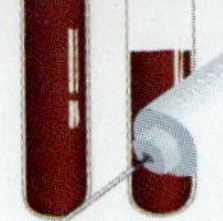

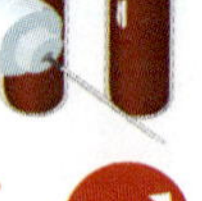

- **Histamine** causes **smooth muscle contraction, increased vascular permeability & increased mucus secretion**[Q] by nasal, bronchial & gastric glands.
- **Leukotrienes C4 & D4** are the **most potent**[Q] vasoactive & spasmogenic agents
- **Leukotriene B4** is highly **chemotactic**[Q] for neutrophils, eosinophils, and monocytes.
- **Prostaglandin D2** is the **most abundant**[Q] mediator produced in mast cells

- **Platelet-activating factor (PAF)**[Q] causes platelet aggregation, release of histamine, bronchospasm, increased vascular permeability & vasodilation.
- **TNF, IL-1, chemokines**: promote **leukocyte recruitment**[Q]
- **IL-4**: increases **TH2 response**[Q]
- **IL-2** is a **growth & survival factor** for **activated & regulatory T cells**[Q]

Antibody-Mediated (Type II) Hypersensitivity

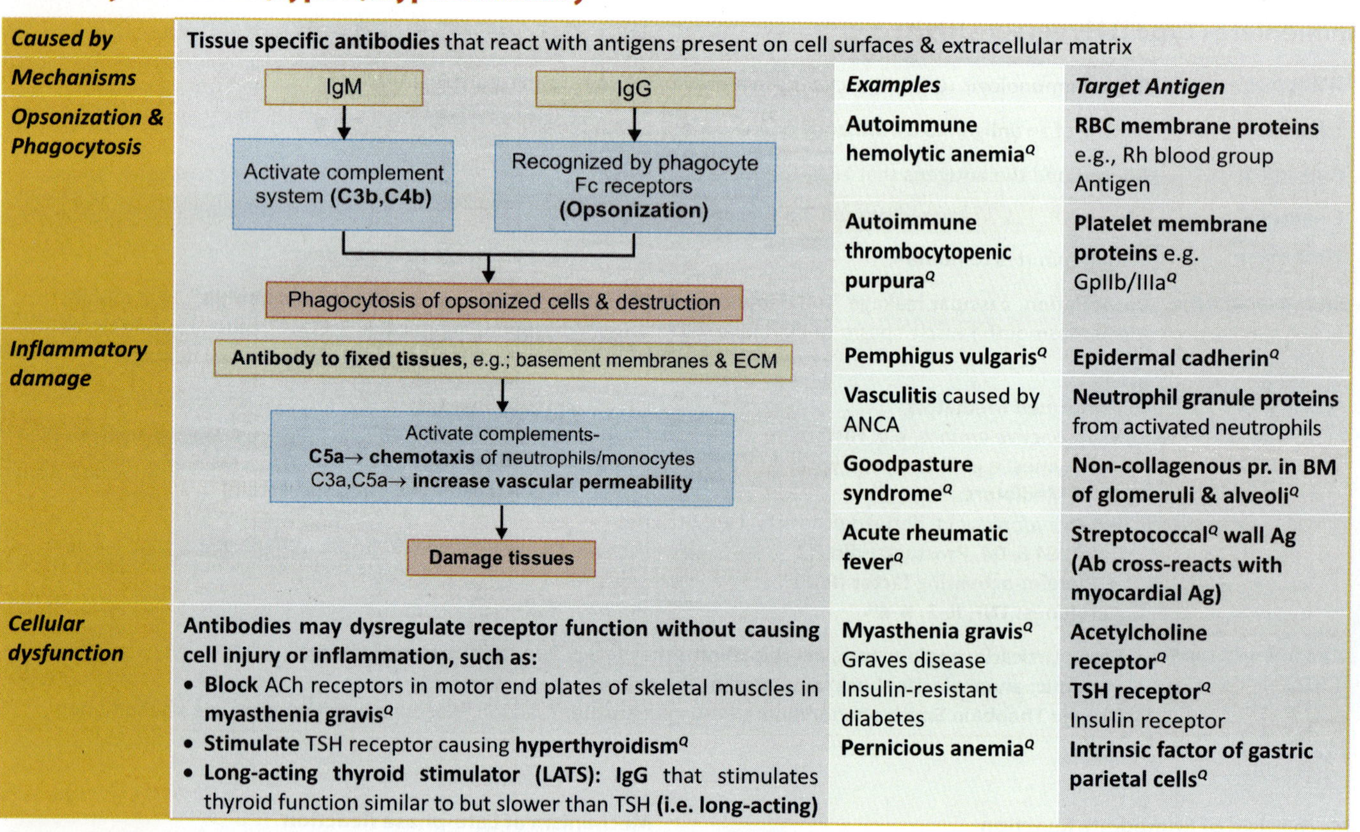

		Examples	Target Antigen
Caused by	Tissue specific antibodies that react with antigens present on cell surfaces & extracellular matrix		
Mechanisms	IgM / IgG		
Opsonization & Phagocytosis	Activate complement system (C3b, C4b) — Recognized by phagocyte Fc receptors (Opsonization) → Phagocytosis of opsonized cells & destruction	Autoimmune hemolytic anemia[Q]	RBC membrane proteins e.g., Rh blood group Antigen
		Autoimmune thrombocytopenic purpura[Q]	Platelet membrane proteins e.g. GpIIb/IIIa[Q]
Inflammatory damage	Antibody to fixed tissues, e.g.; basement membranes & ECM → Activate complements- C5a→ chemotaxis of neutrophils/monocytes C3a,C5a→ increase vascular permeability → Damage tissues	Pemphigus vulgaris[Q]	Epidermal cadherin[Q]
		Vasculitis caused by ANCA	Neutrophil granule proteins from activated neutrophils
		Goodpasture syndrome[Q]	Non-collagenous pr. in BM of glomeruli & alveoli[Q]
		Acute rheumatic fever[Q]	Streptococcal[Q] wall Ag (Ab cross-reacts with myocardial Ag)
Cellular dysfunction	Antibodies may dysregulate receptor function without causing cell injury or inflammation, such as: • **Block** ACh receptors in motor end plates of skeletal muscles in **myasthenia gravis**[Q] • **Stimulate** TSH receptor causing **hyperthyroidism**[Q] • **Long-acting thyroid stimulator (LATS): IgG** that stimulates thyroid function similar to but slower than TSH **(i.e. long-acting)**	Myasthenia gravis[Q] Graves disease Insulin-resistant diabetes Pernicious anemia[Q]	Acetylcholine receptor[Q] TSH receptor[Q] Insulin receptor Intrinsic factor of gastric parietal cells[Q]

Immune Complex–Mediated (Type III) Hypersensitivity

Initiated by	**Nonspecific antibody** towards an antigen		
Morphology	• Principal morphologic manifestation of immune complex injury is **acute vasculitis**[Q] • **Fibrinoid necrosis**[Q] of vessel wall & intense neutrophilic infiltration		
Mechanism	Interaction of antigen and antibody ↓ Formation of **immune complexes**[Q] **(phase I)** (locally at the site of injury or systemically in the circulation) ↓ **Deposition of immune complexes (phase II)** ↓ Activates **complement**[Q] ↓ **Acute inflammation**[Q] **and injury (phase III) starts 10 days after antigen entry**		
Examples	**Infections** • **Subacute infective endocarditis**[Q] • **Post-streptococcal glomerulonephritis**[Q] • Syphilis	**Autoimmune diseases** • **Systemic lupus erythematosus**[Q] • **Rheumatoid arthritis**[Q]	• Polyarteritis nodosa • Hashimoto's disease (thyroiditis)
	Malignant diseases • Leukemias • Hodgkin's disease[Q]	**Drug reactions**[Q] • Serum sickness (systemic)	• Penicillamine toxicity • **Arthus reaction (localized)**

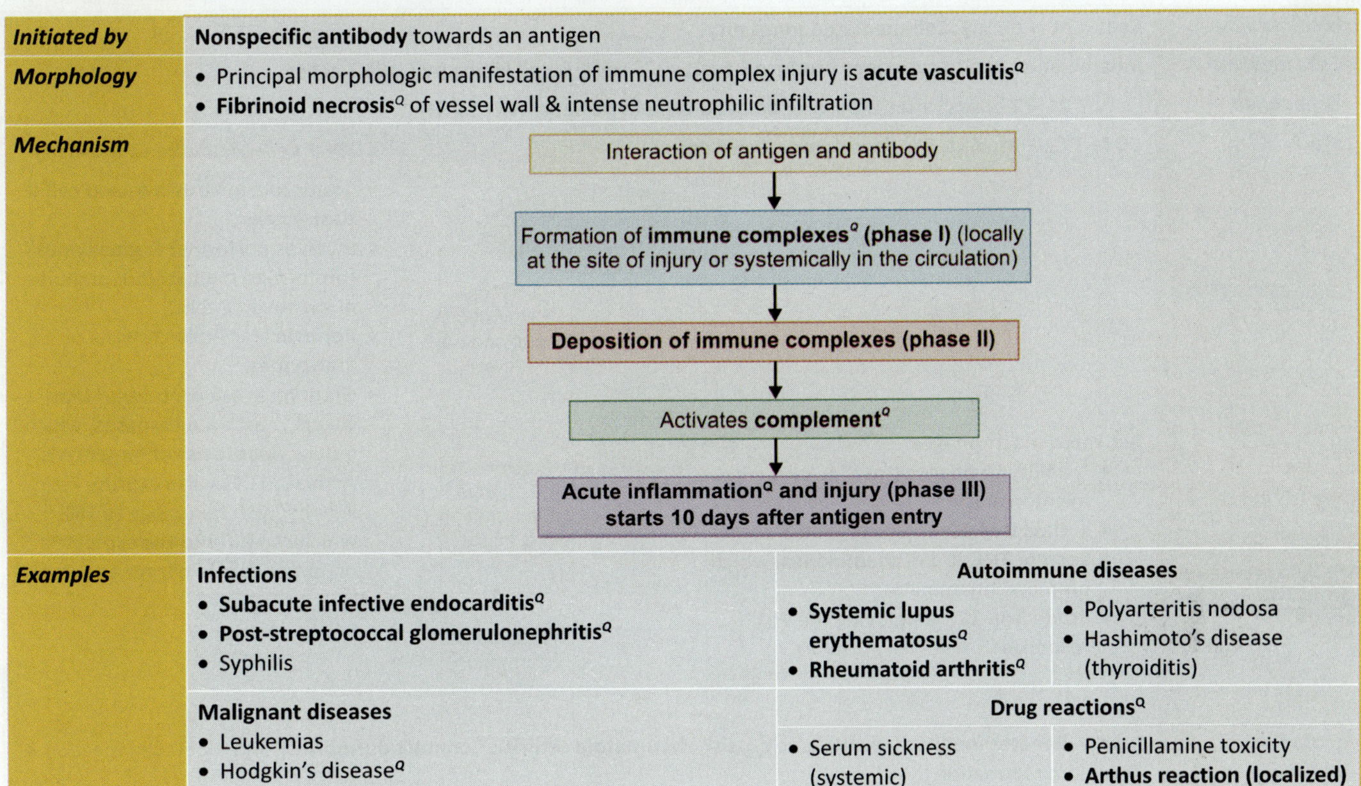

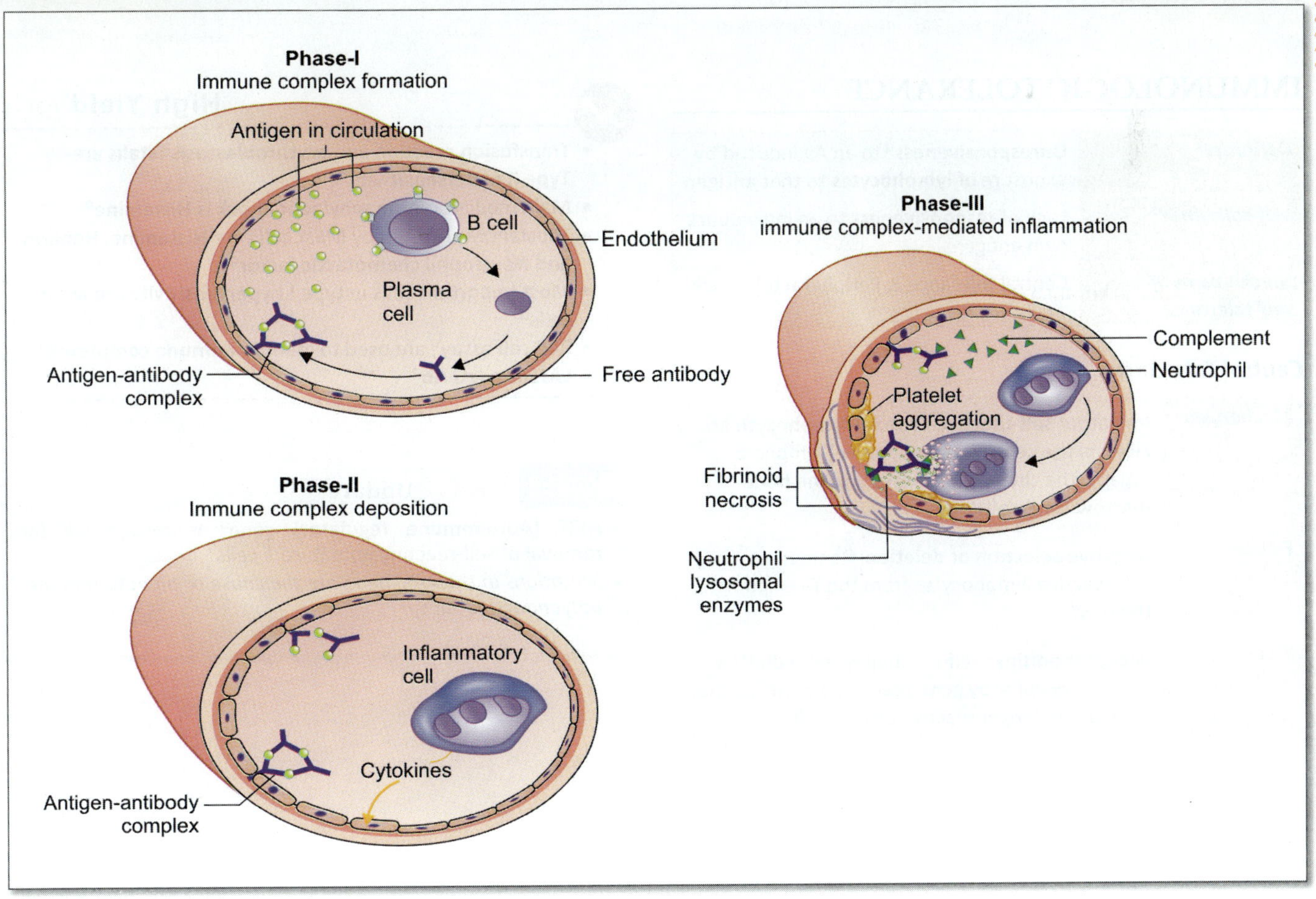

Theory

T Cell–Mediated (Type IV) Hypersensitivity

Mediated by	Cells, not antibody: **Cell-mediated immunity**
Cells involved	Inflammation due to **cytokines produced by CD4+ T cells**[Q] & cell killing by **CD8+ T cells**[Q]
Time taken	Occurs **24–72 hours**[Q] after exposure: **delayed-type hypersensitivity (DTH)**[Q]

Mechanism

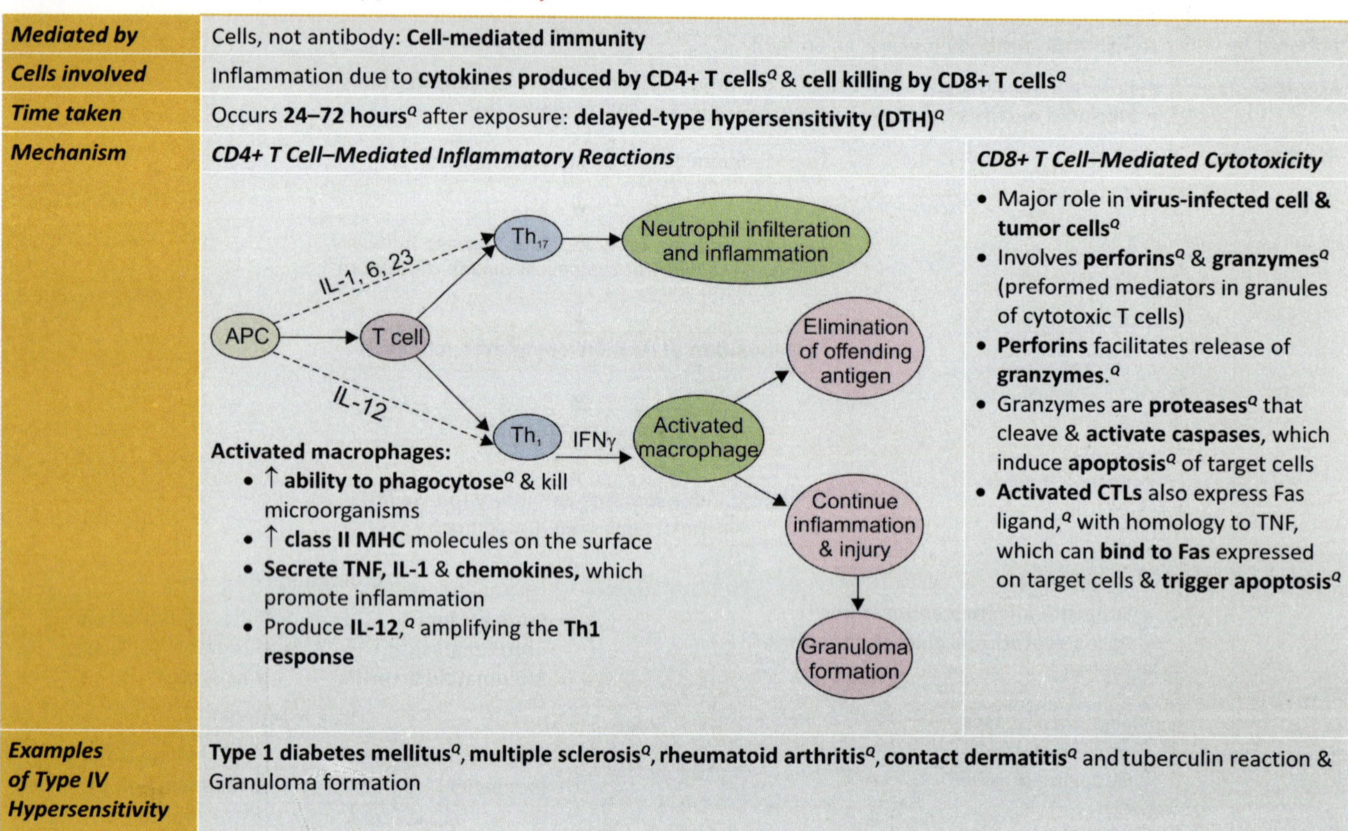

CD8+ T Cell–Mediated Cytotoxicity

- Major role in **virus-infected cell & tumor cells**[Q]
- Involves **perforins**[Q] & **granzymes**[Q] (preformed mediators in granules of cytotoxic T cells)
- **Perforins** facilitates release of **granzymes.**[Q]
- Granzymes are **proteases**[Q] that cleave & **activate caspases**, which induce **apoptosis**[Q] of target cells
- **Activated CTLs** also express Fas ligand,[Q] with homology to TNF, which can **bind to Fas** expressed on target cells & **trigger apoptosis**[Q]

Examples of Type IV Hypersensitivity	**Type 1 diabetes mellitus**[Q], **multiple sclerosis**[Q], **rheumatoid arthritis**[Q], **contact dermatitis**[Q] and tuberculin reaction & Granuloma formation

IMMUNOLOGIC TOLERANCE

Definition	**Unresponsiveness**[Q] to an Ag induced by exposure of **lymphocytes to that antigen**
Self-tolerance[Q]	**Lack of responsiveness** to an individual's own antigens
Mechanisms of self-tolerance	Central tolerance & Peripheral tolerance

Central Tolerance

Mechanism	Immature **self-reactive T- and B-lymphocyte** are killed in the **central** (or generative) lymphoid organs (the **thymus for T cells** and the **bone marrow for B cells**)[Q]
T-cells	**Negative selection or deletion**: Removal of self-reactive lymphocytes from the T-cell pool in **thymus**[Q]
B-cells	**Receptor editing**: Self-reacting B-cells edit their antigen receptor by **gene rearrangement**[Q] so that they are no longer reactive against self.

High Yield Facts

- **Transfusion reaction** and **erythroblastosis fetalis** are- Type II hypersensitivity[Q]
- Main mediator in **Anaphylactic shock** is Histamine[Q]
- Substances secreted by **Mast cells** are Histamine, Heparin and Neutrophil chemotactic factor[Q]
- **Most important** cells in **type I hypersensitivity** are Mast cells[Q]
- **Raji cell assay**[Q] are used to identify **immune complexes**[Q]
- **LATS is a IgG Ab**[Q]

Latest Update (R9th)

- **AIRE (Autoimmune regulator)** gene[Q] is responsible for removal of self-reacting immature T cells
- *Mutations in the AIRE gene are the cause of an **autoimmune-polyendocrinopathy**[Q]*

Peripheral Tolerance

Definition	**Silencing of potentially auto-reactive T and B cells in peripheral tissues (Mainly for T cells)[Q]**

Mechanisms (S-A-D mnemonic)	**Suppression by regulatory T cells. Regulatory T-cells[Q]**
	functions to prevent immune reactions against self-antigens. Regulatory T cells may play a role in the acceptance of the fetus.
	Regulatory T cells are CD4+ cells that express:
	• **CD25:** α chain of the IL-2 receptor[Q]
	• **FOXP3:** transcription factor of the forkhead family[Q]
	• **CD25 & FOXP3** → **Development & maintenance of functional CD4+ regulatory T cells**
	• FOXP3 mutations causes systemic autoimmune disease - **IPEX** (an acronym for Immune dysregulation, Polyendocrinopathy, Enteropathy, X-linked)[Q]
	
	Anergy[Q]
	• Inhibition of self-reacting T-lymphocytes by certain receptors
	  Mechanism: CTLA-4 & PD-1 are inhibitory receptors & are structurally homologous to CD28 which are the coreceptors for antigen recognition
	• Helper T cell have **CTLA-4**[Q] (cytotoxic T-lymphocyte-associated protein 4) receptors which transmits an **inhibitory signal to T** cells. (CTLA-4 has higher affinity for B7 molecules than does CD28).
	• **PD-1 (programmed Death-1)**[Q] receptor are upregulated on activated CD4 T-cells which binds to PD-L1 expressed on monocytes to induce IL-10 production for **immunosuppression.**
	
	Deletion by apoptosis
	• Self reacting T-cells are destroyed by apoptosis by either:
	  ■ **Overexpression of pro**apoptotic factor **BIM**[Q]
	  ■ **FAS**-FAS Ligand pathway[Q]
	
	Mutations in the FAS gene results in **autoimmune lymphoproliferative syndrome (ALPS)**[Q]

AUTOIMMUNITY

Definition	**Activation** of **self-reactive lymphocytes**[Q] by combination of inheritance of **susceptibility genes** and **environmental triggers** such as infections & tissue damage
Mechanisms	• **Defective tolerance or regulation:** failure of mechanisms that maintain self-tolerance[Q] • Abnormal display of self-antigens[Q] • **Inflammation** or an initial innate immune response which may induce autoimmunity

High Yield Facts

Immune-privileged sites:[Q]
- **Testis, eye, and brain**[Q]
- Tissues in which these antigens are located **do not communicate** with the blood and lymph
- **Difficult to induce immune responses** to antigens introduced into these sites
- Prolonged tissue inflammation on injury & release of antigen from these sites: **post-traumatic orchitis & uveitis**[Q]

Role of Susceptibility Genes: Association of HLA Alleles with Disease

Association of non-MHC genes with Diseases

Gene	Diseases	Function of encoded protein & role in Disease
Genes involved in immune regulation		
PTPN 22[Q]	• **Rheumatoid Arthritis**[Q] • **Type I Diabetes**[Q] • **Inflammatory Bowel Ds**[Q]	**Protein tyrosine phosphatase,**[Q] affects signaling of lymphocytes & alter negative selection or activation of self- reactive T cells
IL23R	• Inflammatory Bowel Ds • Psoriasis & Ankylosing spondylitis	**Receptor for T$_H$ 17-induces IL-23;**[Q] alters differentiation of CD4+T cell into pathogenic T$_H$ 17 effector cells
CTLA4	• Type I Diabetes • Rheumatoid Arthritis	**Inhibits T cells responses**[Q] by terminating activation & promoting activity of regulatory T cells; Interferes with self-tolerance
IL2RA	• Multiple sclerosis • Type I Diabetes	α chain of receptors for IL-2 may affect development of **effector cells** and/or regulation of immune responses

Contd...

Gene	Diseases	Function of encoded protein & role in Disease
Genes involved in immune response to microbes		
NOD2[Q]	Inflammatory Bowel Disease	**Cytoplasmic sensor of bacteria**[Q] expressed in paneth & other intestinal epithelial cells; controls resistance to gut commensals
ATG 16	Inflammatory Bowel Disease	Involved in **autophagy;**[Q] Role in defense against microbes & maintenance of epithelial barrier function
IRF5, IRH1	Systemic Lupus Erythematosus	Role in **type 1 IFN**[Q] production, which is involved in the pathogenesis of SLE

Role of Infections

- Infections may **up-regulate** the expression of **costimulators on APCs**
- **Molecular mimicry**[Q]: Some infections may express antigens that have the same amino acid sequences as self antigens. Immune responses against the microbial antigens may result in the activation of self-reactive lymphocytes.

AUTOIMMUNE DISEASES

Systemic Lupus Erythematosus (SLE)

- Caused by **deposition of immune complexes** and **binding of antibodies** to various cells and tissues.
- **Characteristic lesions due to** immune complex **deposition in:** blood vessels, kidneys, connective tissue, skin
- **Blood Vessels:** Acute necrotizing vasculitis with **fibrinoid deposits**[Q]

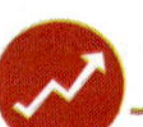

High Yield Facts

Renal Involvement in SLE

Classification of Lupus Nephritis (International Society of Nephrology)

- **Class I** : **Minimal Mesangial**[Q]
- **Class II** : **Mesangial Proliferative**
- **Class III** : **Focal** Lupus Nephritis[Q]
- **Class IV** : **Diffuse** Lupus Nephritis[Q]
- **Class V** : **Membranous** Lupus Nephritis[Q]
- **Class VI** : **Advanced** Sclerotic Lupus Nephritis

High Yield Facts

Drug Induced Lupus

- Less female predilection than SLE
- Anti histone Ab: Common
- Rarely involves kidney & brain
- Anti-ds DNA ±

R10th Latest Update

Systemic lupus international collaborating clinic criteria for classification of systemic lupus erythematosus

Clinical manifestations	Immunologic manifestations
<ul><li>Skin, acute, subacute cutaneous LE and chronic cutaneous LE</li><li>Oral ulcers</li><li>Alopecia</li><li>Synovitis (nonerosive)</li><li>Renal: Prot/Cr ≥ 0.5, RBC casts and biopsy*</li><li>Neurologic: Seizures, psychosis, mononeuritis, myelitis</li><li>Hemolytic anemia: Leukopenia (< 4000) or, lymphopenia (<1000) and thrombocytopenia (< 100, 000)</li></ul>	<ul><li>ANA > reference negative value</li><li>Anti-ds DNA</li><li>Anti-Sm</li><li>Antiphospholipid</li><li>Low serum complement</li><li>Positive direct Coombs test</li></ul>
*Renal biopsy read as systemic lupus qualities for classification as SLE even if none of the other above features are present	

Interpretation: Presence of any 4 criteria (must have at least 1 in each category) qualifies patient to be classified as having SLE with 93% specificity and 92% sensitivity.

Autoantibodies in Systemic Lupus Erythematosus (SLE)[Q]

Antibody	Antigen Recognized	Clinical Utility
Antinuclear antibodies[Q]	Multiple nuclear	**Best screening test/ Most sensitive[Q]**
Anti-dsDNA[Q]	DNA (double-stranded)	**Specific,[Q]** correlate with disease activity, nephritis, vasculitis
Anti-Sm[Q]	U1 RNA	**Most Specific for SLE[Q]**
Anti-RNP	U1 RNA	Not specific for SLE
Anti-Ro/La (SS-A)[Q]	hY RNA,	Sicca syndrome, neonatal lupus with congenital heart block[Q]
Anti-histone[Q]	Histones	**Drug-induced lupus[Q]**

High Yield Facts

- **50%** patients with SLE have clinically significant **renal involvement[Q]**
- **Class I Lupus Nephritis is least common[Q]** and **class IV is the most common pattern[Q]**
- **"Wire loop lesions"[Q]** are characteristically seen in **Class IV[Q] Lupus Nephritis** due to **sub-endothelial** immune complex deposits, on **light microscopy**-Also seen in **Class III/V Lupus nephritis[Q]**

Sjogren Syndrome

- *Characterized by:* Dry eyes (**keratoconjunctivitis sicca**)[Q] and **dry mouth (xerostomia)[Q]** due to immunologically mediated destruction of the lacrimal and salivary glands.
- *Two forms*
  - ○ **Primary form (sicca syndrome)[Q]**: as an isolated disorder
  - ○ **Secondary form**: in association with other autoimmune disease (e.g. RA, SLE, scleroderma)
- *Autoantibodies*
  - ○ **Anti SS-A (Ro)** and **SS-B (La)[Q]**: Most important, present in 90% patients
  - ○ High titers of Anti SS-A → more likely to have **early disease onset, longer disease duration, and extraglandular manifestations** (e.g. cutaneous vasculitis and nephritis)
- *Morphology:*
  - ○ **Main targets:** Lacrimal and salivary glands[Q]
  - ○ **Earliest histologic finding:** Periductal and perivascular **lymphocytic infiltration**
  - ○ **Lymphoid follicles** with **germinal centers** in larger salivary glands may be seen
  - ○ **Late changes: atrophy** of acini, fibrosis, and hyalinization;
  - ○ At high risk for development of **B-cell Marginal zone lymphoma[Q]**
- *Diagnosis:* **Biopsy of the lip** (to examine minor salivary glands) is required for diagnosis

Scleroderma (Systemic Sclerosis) (SSc)

Characterized by	• **Chronic inflammation,[Q]** as a result of autoimmunity • **Widespread damage** to small blood vessels • **Progressive interstitial** & perivascular **fibrosis[Q]** in skin & multiple organs.	
2 major categories	**Limited Cutaneous SSc**	**Diffuse Cutaneous SSc**
Skin involvement	**Limited** to fingers, forearms, face[Q]	Diffuse: fingers, extremities, face, trunk;[Q]
Onset & course	Indolent & slow	Rapid
Visceral involvement	Late	Early
Auto-antibodies seen	**Anti-centromere[Q]**	Anti-topoisomerase I (Scl-70),[Q] anti-RNA polymerase III[Q]
Crest syndrome	**More common[Q]**	Less common[Q]

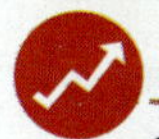

High Yield Facts

- **CREST syndrome**: **C**alcinosis, **R**aynaud's phenomenon, **E**sophageal dysmotility, **S**clerodactyly & **T**elangiectasia[Q]
- *Mikulicz syndrome* refers to lacrimal & salivary gland enlargement from any cause, including sarcoidosis, lymphoma & other tumors[Q]
- **Most common organ involved in Scleroderma is Skin[Q]**
- **Antitopoisomerase I(Scl-70)[Q]** is **most specific[Q]** for Scleroderma
- **ANA positivity is seen in virtually all patients with SSc (Systemic sclerosis)**

Mixed Connective Tissue Disease

- Clinical features are a mixture of the features of **SLE, systemic sclerosis, and polymyositis[Q]**
- Elevated **anti-U1 ribonucleoprotein Ab[Q]**
- Presentation: Synovitis of fingers, Raynaud phenomenon, mild myositis, renal involvement

REJECTION OF TISSUE TRANSPLANTS

Types of grafts[Q]	• **Autografts[Q]**: Transplant of individual own organ • **Isograft**: Graft from identical twin • **Allografts[Q]**: Between individuals of the same species • **Xenografts[Q]**: Grafts from one species to another species
Types of Rejection Pathway	• **Direct pathway**: **CD4 & CD8-T** cells[Q] of the transplant recipient recognize allogenic (donor) MHC molecules on the surface of APCs in the graft. • **Indirect pathway**: Recipient **CD4-T lymphocytes[Q] recognize MHC antigens** of the graft donor after they are presented by the recipient's own APCs.

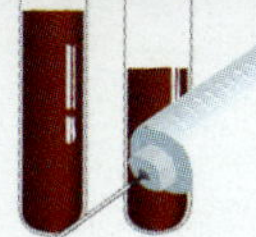

- In kidney transplants, polymorphic HLA alleles are **at least 50% matched** (HLA-A, -B & DR)[Q]
- HLA matching is NOT required for Cornea transplant[Q]
- HLA matching is usually **NOT done for** transplants of **liver, heart, and lungs**, because other considerations, such as

anatomic compatibility, severity of the underlying illness, and the **need to minimize the time** of organ storage, **override the potential benefits** of HLA matching
- "000 mismatcch" means no mismatch in HLA-A, B, D
- Most important HLA is HLA DRB1 for transplant survival

Types of Renal Graft Rejection: *(On the Basis of the Morphology & Underlying Mechanism)*

Features	Hyperacute rejection	Acute Rejection	Chronic Rejection
Time to occur	**Minutes to hours**[Q]	**Days** (months or even years)[Q]	**Months or even years**[Q]
Mechanism (Type of hypersensitivity)	• **Type 2 HSN:**[Q]due to preformed antibodies • Type 3 HSN	• **Type 4 HSN**-Cellular rejection[Q] • Type 2-mediated by anti-donor antibodies	• **Type 4-HSN** Cellular rejection[Q]
Histology	• **Neutrophillic infiltration**[Q] & thrombotic occlusion of capillaries • **Fibrinoid necrosis** occurs in arterial walls. Showing fibrin thrombi in glomerulus along with ischemic necrosis	In **cell-mediated rejection**: • Tubulo-interstitial pattern **(tubulitis)** • Vascular pattern **(endotheliitis)** In **antibody mediated rejection**: Inflammation of glomeruli & peritubular capillaries with **deposition of C4d**[Q] Showing C_4d deposition in peritubular capillaries	**Intimal thickening** with inflammation; Glomerulopathy; **peritubular capillaritis**[Q] **Interstitial fibrosis**[Q] & tubular atrophy

IMMUNODEFICIENCY SYNDROMES

Types

- **Primary (or congenital)** : Genetically determined[Q]

- **Secondary (or acquired)**: Complications of **cancers, infections, malnutrition**, or side effects of immunosuppression, **irradiation, or chemotherapy** for cancer and other diseases[Q]

Primary Immunodeficiency Diseases

Defects in Innate Immunity

Disease	Defect
Defects in Leukocyte function	
Leukocyte adhesion deficiency 1	Defective WBC adhesion because of **mutations in β chain of CD11/CD18 integrins**[Q]
Leukocyte adhesion deficiency 2	Defective WBC adhesion due to **mutations in fucosyltransferase**[Q] required for synthesis of sialylated oligosaccharide (receptor for selectins)
Chediak – Higashi syndrome	Decreased **leukocyte functions** due to mutations of **protein involved in lysosomal membrane traffic**[Q]
Chronic granulomatous disease • X-linked • Autosomal recessive	Decreased **oxidative burst**[Q] Phagocyte oxidase (membrane component) Phagocyte oxidase (cytoplasmic components)
Myeloperoxidase deficiency	Decreased microbial killing because of **defective MPO-H_2O_2 system**[Q]

Complement Deficiencies & Associated Diseases

Component	Associated Diseases
Classic Pathway	
Clq, Clr, Cls, C4, C2	Immune-complex syndromes[Q], pyogenic infections
C1 esterase Inhibitor	Hereditary angioneurotic edema[Q]
C3 and Alternative Pathway C3	
C3	Immune-complex syndromes, pyogenic infections
D	Pyogenic infections[Q]
Properdin	*Neisseria* infections[Q]
I	Pyogenic infections[Q]
H	Hemolytic uremic syndrome[Q]
Membrane Attack Complex	
C5, C6, C7, C8	Recurrent *Neisseria* infections,[Q] immune-complex disease
C9	Rare *Neisseria* infections

Primary immunodeficiency mechanism

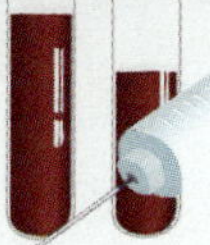

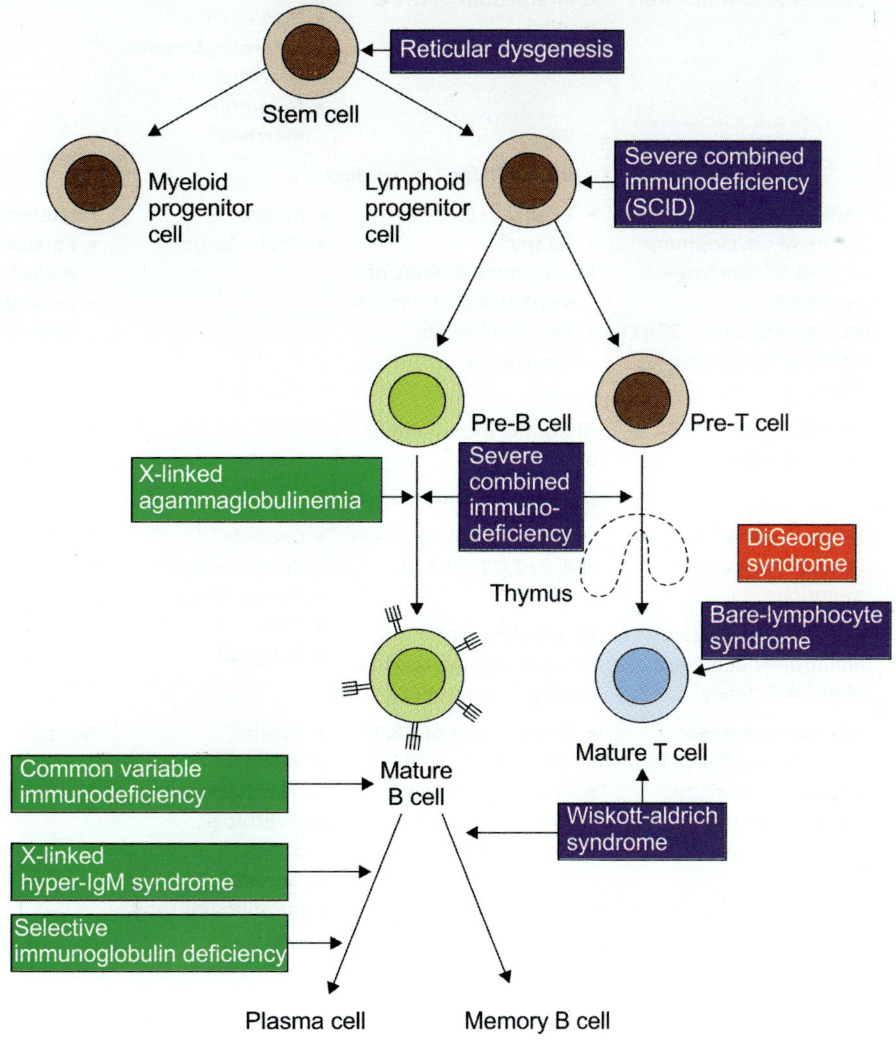

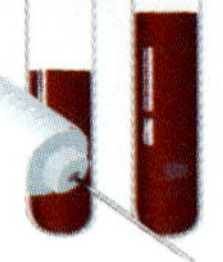

Defects in Adaptive Immune System: (Primary Immunodeficiency Disorders)

Disease	Primary Defect	Secondary Defect	Infections/Features	Morphology
B cell (Humoral) defects				
Bruton's X-Linked Agammaglobulinemia	Bruton tyrosine kinase(Btk); Xq21.22 gene mutations[Q]	• Failure of pro B-cells to mature • **Plasma cells absent**[Q] • T-cells normal	*H. influenzae,* *S. pneumoniae,* *S. aureus*	Underdeveloped: • **Germinal centers** of L. nodes[Q] • **Peyer's patches** of appendix[Q] • **Tonsils**[Q]
Hyper-IgM Syndrome	**X-linked:** Mutations in CD40L (Xq26)[Q] **Autosomal recessive:** Mutations in CD40 & AID (activation-induced cytidine deaminase)	• **Defect in Ig class switching**[Q] and affinity maturation • Inability to produce IgG, IgA, and IgE Antibodies	• Recurrent • **Pyogenic** infections[Q] • *Pneumocystis jiroveci*[Q]	Normal
Isolated IgA Deficiency	**Impaired differentiation** of naive B cells to IgA-producing plasma cells	• **Deficient IgA** • Concomitant defect in **IgG2 and IgG4**[Q]	• Infections • Respiratory tract **allergy**[Q] • Autoimmune: **SLE and RA**[Q]	Normal
Common Variable Immunodeficiency	Defect in receptor for a cytokine called **BAFF**[Q] Defect in **ICOS**[Q] **(inducible costimulator)**	Defect in survival and differentiation of **B cells** Defect in **T-cell** activation & **interactions** b/w **T & B cells**[Q]	• Recurrent **sino-pulmonary** & pyogenic infections • Herpes virus • Enteroviral menin-goencephalitis • **G. lamblia diarrhea**[Q]	B-cell areas of the lymphoid tissues are **hyperplastic**[Q]
Predominant T cell defect				
DiGeorge Syndrome (Thymic Hypoplasia)[Q]	**Familial cases:** failure of development of **3rd & 4th pharyngeal pouches**[Q] **Nonfamilial cases:** 22q11 **deletion**[Q] syndrome (50%)	• T-cell defect • **Tetany**[Q] • Congenital **defects of heart** and great vessels • Mucocutaneous Candidiasis	• Fungal • Viral infections	**Depleted:**[Q] • **Paracortical areas** of L. nodes[Q] • Periarteriolar sheaths of spleen
Bare lymphocyte syndrome	Defect in **class II MHC gene expression.**	Abnormal development of CD4+ T cells.		Normal
Combined T and B cell defect				
Severe Combined Immunodeficiency	**X-linked:**γ-chain (γc) of cytokine receptor mutations **Autosomal recessive:** adenosine deaminase **(ADA) deficiency**[Q]	Defect in signaling of IL-2, 4, 7, 9, 11, 15 &21 Accumulation of deoxyadenosine-toxic to rapidly dividing WBCs	• *Candida*[Q] • *Pneumocystis*[Q] • *Pseudomonas* • *CMV* • *Varicella*	**Thymus is small**[Q] and devoid of lymphoid cells
Ataxia Telangiectasia	**Autosomal-recessive** mutation in **ATM gene**[Q] (ataxia telangiectasia mutated) on **chr 11**	• Combination of T & B cell defects • Defective isotype switching • Low IgA & IgG-2	• **Ataxia** • **Vascular telangiectases**[Q] • **Neurologic deficits**[Q] • **Tumors**[Q] • Immunodeficiency	Normal

Contd...

Disease	Primary Defect	Secondary Defect	Infections/Features	Morphology
Hyper IgE syndrome	**Autosomal dominant:**[Q] mutation in **STAT3** gene: Defective signaling pathways	• **Elevated serum IgE** levels • **Defective TH17** effector responses[Q]	• **Recurrent skin abscesses**[Q] • Lung infections & **pneumatoceles**[Q] • **Pyogenic bacteria & fungi** • Dysmorphism • Defective teeth • Hyperextensibility • Scoliosis, Osteoporosis.	Normal
X-linked Lymphoproliferative disease	Mutations in **SLAM-associated protein (SAP)**[Q]	Activation of NK, T & B cells, including Signalling Lymphocyte Activation Molecule (SLAM)	Epstein-Barr virus **(EBV)**	
Wiskott-Aldrich Syndrome	**X-linked:**Mutations in Wiskott-Aldrich syndrome protein **(WASP), Xp11.23**[Q]	• **CD8+T-cell deficiency** • **IgM-low**[Q] • **IgA & IgE-↑ed**[Q] • **IgG-normal**[Q]	**Thrombocytopenia**[Q] **Eczema**[Q] **Recurrent infection**[Q]	Normal

Immune Regulatory Defects	
Innate immunity	• **Autoinflammatory** syndromes (outside the scope of this chapter) • **Severe colitis**
Adaptive immunity	• **Hemophagocytic lymphohistiocytosis (HLH)** • **Autoimmune lymphoproliferation syndrome (ALPS)**[Q] • **Autoimmunity** and inflammatory diseases (IPEX, APECED)

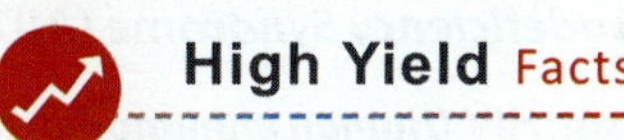

High Yield Facts

SCID
- Most severe immunodeficiency in children
- Presents soon after Birth
- Graft rejection not seen
- Risk of severe GVHD with non-irradiated blood products

Hemophagocytic Lymphohistiocytosis (HLH)

- ■ *Characterized by:*
  - ○ **Activation of CD8+ T lymphocytes and macrophages** leading to organ damage
  - ○ Impaired T and NK lymphocyte cytotoxicity.
- ■ *Triggered by:* **Viruses (Most commonly: EBV)Q**
- ■ *Clinical features*
  - ○ Fever
  - ○ Edema
  - ○ Hepatosplenomegaly
  - ○ Neurologic diseases
  - ○ **Blood cytopenia**
  - ○ **Hypofibrinogenemia**
  - ○ Increased liver enzymes
  - ○ **High triglyceride levels**
- ■ *Lab findings*
  - ○ Elevated markers of T cell activation
  - ○ Hemophagocytic features in the bone marrow or cerebrospinal fluid
  - ○ **Functional assays** of post-activation cytotoxic granule exocytosis (**CD107** fluorescence at cell membrane) can suggest **genetically** determined HLH.
- ■ *Subsets of HLH*
  - ○ **Familial** HLH (A.R)
    - • **Perforin** deficiency[Q]
    - • Munc13-4 deficiency
    - • Syntaxin 11 deficiency
  - ○ HLH with partial **albinism**
    - • **Chediak-Higashi syndrome**[Q]
    - • **Griscelli syndrome**[Q]
    - • Hermansky Pudlak syndrome type II.
  - ○ **X-linked** proliferative syndrome
  - ○ Following EBV infection
  - ○ **Main Defects include:**
    - • SH2DIA gene
    - • Low 2B4-mediated NK cell cytotoxicity
    - • **Impaired differentiation of NK T cells**
    - • Defective antigen-induced T cell death
    - • Defective T cell helper activity for B cells

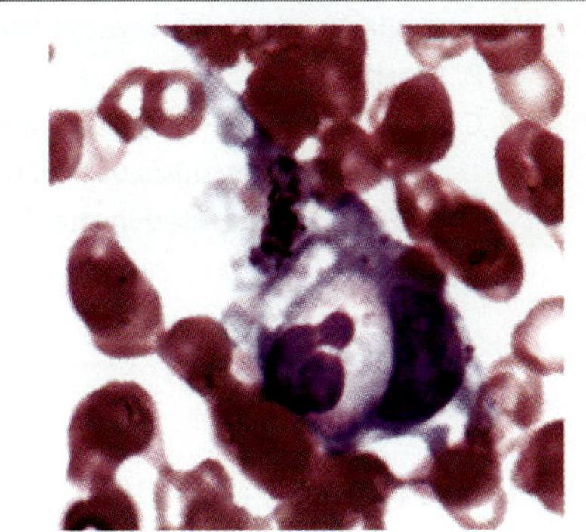

Hemophagocytosis in bone marrow aspirate

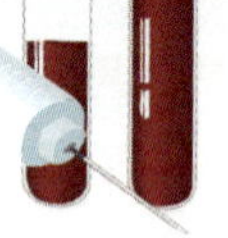

- Nitrobluetetrazolium test^Q is used for Phagocytes
- The **commonest Primary immunodeficiency** is **Isolated IgA immunodeficiency**^{Q}
- In **agammaglobulinemia** there is loss of germinal centre in lymph node^Q
- **Commonest fungal infection in neutropenia** is **Candida**^{Q}
- HIV was isolated in **1983**
- HIV-2: 1st case in **1987**

Secondary (Acquired) Immunodeficiencies

Cause	Mechanism
Human immunodeficiency virus (HIV) infection^Q	**Depletion of CD4+** helper T cells
Irradiation & chemotherapy^Q *treatments for cancer*	**Decreased** bone **marrow precursors**^{Q} for all leukocytes
Involvement of bone marrow by cancers^Q *(Metastases, Leukemias)*	Reduced site of leukocyte development
Protein- calorie malnutrition	Metabolic derangements **inhibit lymphocyte maturation & function**
Removal of spleen	**Decreased phagocytosis** of microbes

Acquired Immunodeficiency Syndrome (AIDS)

Causative Organism: HIV (Human Immunodeficiency Virus)

Family	Non-transforming human **retrovirus** of **lentivirus family**^{Q}	
Classification	Two types: HIV-1 & HIV-2	
Groups of HIV1	3 Groups: • **Major group** (HIV-1 M)-**Most common world wide**^{Q} • **Outlier group** (HIV-1 O) • New/Neither M nor O group (HIV-1 N)	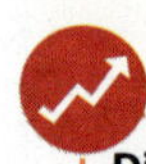
Subtypes/clades of HIV-1 M group	HIV-1 M group is further classified into subtypes or clades: A through H, J and K • **HIV-1 group M subtypes C predominant in India, fastest spreading**^{Q} • HIV-1 group M subtypes B predominant in U.S	
Structure of HIV	**Viral core** is surrounded by a **matrix protein (p17)**^{Q} followed by **host cell derived lipid envelope**^{Q}	Structure of HIV virus

A. **Core protein**
- **Major Capsid protein (p24) (most abundant)**^{Q}
- **Nucleocapsid** protein (p7/p9)
- **Two copies of single stranded RNA**
- Viral **enzymes:**^{Q} Reverse transcriptase (p51), Integrase (p31) & Protease (p9)

B. **Matrix (p17)**^{Q}

C. **Lipid Envelope** with **gp 120 and gp 41**^{Q}
- **gp-120: Protrudes out** on the surface of the virus^Q **& binds to CD4** molecule & co-receptors^Q
- **gp-41: Embedded** in the lipid matrix **& helps in fusion** with target cells^Q

Difference between HIV-1 and 2:
HIV-2 Infection:
- **Not transmitted as efficiently** as HIV-1^Q
- Progression to AIDS **takes longer**
- **Slower rate of CD4 cell decline** and viral replication
- Rarely causes vertical transmission

Genetics of HIV

Structural Genes

High Yield Facts

AIDS defining illness CDC stage 3 Includes:

Infection
- Esophageal candidiasis
- Extrapul cryptococcosis
- CMV Retinitis
- Diss. Histoplasmosis 1B (any site)
- MAC
- Pneumocystis jiroveci
- Toxoplasmosis of brain

Neoplasms
- Invasive cervical Ca
- Kaposi sarcoma
- Burkitt's lymphoma
- Primary CNS lymphoma
- Immunoblastic lymphoma

Regulatory/Accessory Genes

Pathogenesis of HIV Infection and AIDS (Steps)

- **gp120 binds to host CD4 receptors** on[Q] **T-cells, Macrophages, Dendritic cells** & other Antigen presenting cells
- Binding to **co-receptor molecules CCR-5/CXCR4**[Q]
  - ○ ○ **R5 strains** use CCR5: **M-tropic**, preferentially infects monocyte/macrophages **(MC in EARLY infection)**[Q]
  - ○ ○ **X4 strains** use CXCR4: **T-tropic**, preferentially infects T-cells **(MC in LATE infection)**
  - ○ ○ R5X4 strains: Dual tropic
- Exposure of **gp-41** leading to **fusion of the virus with the host cell**
- **Uncoating** of viral genome
- **Reverse transcription** of ssRNA to dsDNA
- ds DNA along with enzymes **(Pre-integration complex)**[Q] transported to nucleus
- **Viral DNA gets integrated** with host cell DNA **(provirus)**[Q]
- Direct **viral protein synthesis** (transcription & translation)
- **Virus assembly and budding**

High Yield Facts

Modes of Transmission of HIV
- **Sexual** contact – heterosexual/homosexual[Q]
- Receipt of **infected blood** and its products[Q]
- **Mother to child (vertical)** transmission[Q]
- **Percutaneous/mucosal exposures** to blood and body fluids of HIV infected
- Accidental – **occupational** (health care workers)
- I/V drug abuse

High Yield Facts

- **Most common fungal** infection in patients with AIDS: **Candida**[Q]
- **Most common sites of Candida** infection in HIV: **oral cavity, vagina, and esophagus**[Q]
- In asymptomatic HIV, **oral candidiasis** is a sign of **immunologic decompensation**[Q]
- **Invasive candidiasis** is INFREQUENT in patients with AIDS[Q]
- Majority (50%) of **CNS mass lesions** is caused by: **Toxoplasma gondii**[Q]

T-cell defects in HIV

Mechanisms of T-Cell Depletion in HIV Infection[Q]
- **Direct cytopathic** effects of the replicating virus[Q]
- Apoptosis of uninfected cells by **activation-induced cell death**[Q]
- **Inflammasome** pathway leading to **pyroptosis**[Q]
- **Loss of immature precursors** by direct infection or cytokines essential for CD4+ T-cell maturation
- **Syncytia (giant cells formation) and cell death**

Mechanisms of Qualitative defects of T cells in HIV/AIDS
- Reduction in antigen-induced T-cell proliferation
- **Decrease in TH1-responses:** increased susceptibility to infections[Q]
- Defects in intracellular signaling,
- **Loss of the memory subset of CD4+ helper T cells**[Q]

High Yield Facts

- **Most common malignancy** in patients with AIDS: **Kaposi Sarcoma**[Q]
- **HHV-8 (Kaposi sarcoma virus)** causes **Kaposi sarcoma, primary effusion lymphoma and multicentric Castleman's disease** in HIV[Q]
- **Most common hematologic abnormality** in HIV-infected patients: **Anemia**[Q]
- **Most common lymphoma** seen in HIV: **Immunoblastic lymphoma (DLBCL)**[Q] **>Burkitt's lymphoma> primary CNS lymphoma**
- **Most common Kidney** biopsy finding in HIV is : **Collapsing variant of FSGS**[Q]
- CD4 T cells <200 cells/nm³ predispose to **P. jirovecii**
- CD4 T cells <100 cells/nm³–**cryptococcus**
- CD4 T cells <50 cells/nm³–**CMV, MAC., IRIS**
- CD4 T cells >300 cells/nm³–**TB**.

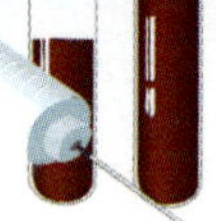

Natural History of HIV Infection

- **Acute retroviral syndrome- 3-6 wks** after infection, usually resolves spontaneously[Q]
- **Middle, chronic phase (clinical latency)**[Q]
- **Clinical AIDS**

Immune Reconstitution Inflammatory Syndrome (IRIS)

- **Paradoxical worsening**[Q] of clinical condition is seen following the initiation of ART (antiretroviral therapy)
- Occurs weeks to months **following the initiation of antiretroviral therapy**[Q]

- Is **most common in** patients starting therapy with a **CD4+ T cell count < 50/uL**[Q]
- Is frequently seen in the setting of **tuberculosis**[Q]
- Can be fatal

Morphology-Lymph node Biopsy in HIV infection

- **Early HIV:** Marked **hyperplasia of follicles** with attenuated mantlezones[Q]
- **Late HIV: Atrophic Lymph nodes**[Q] with depletion of lymphocytes and disruption of follicular dendritic cells

AMYLOIDOSIS

Definition	Amyloidosis is a pathological proteinaceous substance deposited between cells[Q] in various tissues and organs of the body in a variety of clinical settings.
Sites of biopsy	• **Rectal biopsy**-Most specific and best site • **Abdominal fat aspirate:** Most sensitive & easy site • Gingival biopsy • Organ specific biopsy for localized amyloidosis
Diagnosis	• **Grossly:** Affected organ is **enlarged** and grey with a waxy, firm consistency • **Histologically: Extracellular pink** homogenous deposit • On special staining:

Technique	Stain	Feature
Light microscope	**Congo red**	**Salmon-red** color amyloid deposits[Q]
Polarized light	**Congo red**	**Apple-green birefringence**[Q]
Fluorescent staining	**Thioflavin T**	**Yellow color**[Q]
Electron microscope	—	**Non-branching fibrils**[Q], 7.5 to 10 nm[Q] diameter
X-ray crystallography & infrared spectroscopy	—	Characteristic **cross-β-pleated sheet**[Q]

Classification of Amyloidosis

Clinicopathologic category	Associated Diseases	Fibril protein	Precursor protein
Systemic (Generalized) Amyloidosis			
• *Primary amyloidosis*	Multiple myeloma	**AL**	Immunoglobulin light chain (λ)
• *Secondary amyloidosis*	Chronic inflammatory conditions	AA	SAA
• *Hemodialysis- associated amyloidosis*	Chronic renal failure	A β₂ m	β₂-microglobulin
Localized Amyloidosis			
• *Senile cerebral*	Alzheimer's disease	A β	APP
• *Medullary carcinoma of thyroid*		A Cal	Calcitonin
• *Islets of Langerhans*		AIAPP	Islet amyloid peptide
• *Isolated atrial amyloidosis*		AANF	Atrial natriuretic factor
Hereditary Amyloidosis			
• *Familial Mediterranean fever*		AA	SAA
• *Familial amyloidotic neuropathies*		ATTR	Transthyretin
• *Systemic senile amyloidosis*		ATTR	Transthyretin

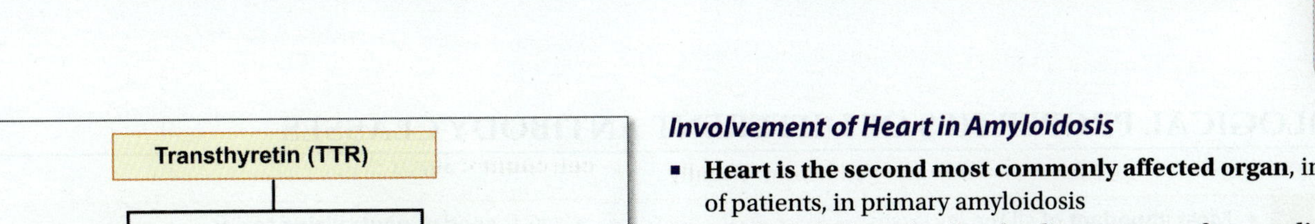

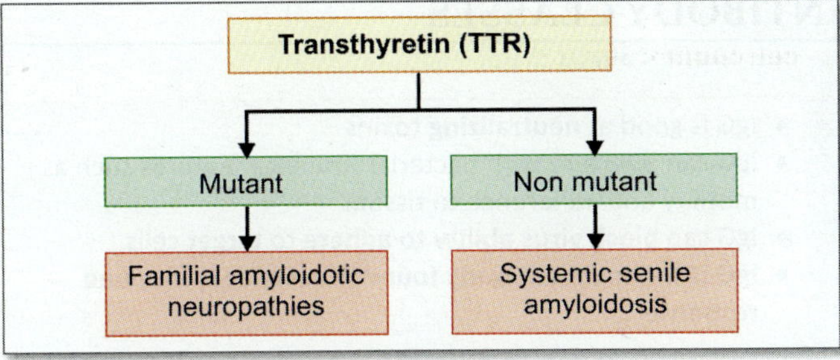

AA (Amyloid Associate Protein)

- It is unique **non-immunoglobulin protein** synthesized by reticuloendothelial cells of liver[Q].
- Associated with **secondary amyloidosis** & **reactive systemic amyloidosis**[Q].

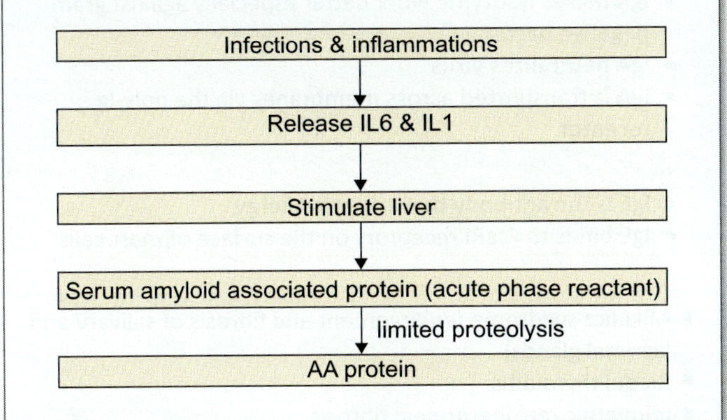

- Seen in:

Connective tissue disorders	Nonimmune derived tumors
• Rheumatoid Arthritis (MC)[Q]	• Renal cell carcinoma[Q]
• Ankylosing spondylitis[Q]	• Hodgkin's lymphoma[Q]
• Primary biliary cirrhosis[Q]	

Individual organ Amyloidosis	
Kidney	1st deposits in mesangium
Spleen	Sago → deposit in follicles Lardaceous-deposit in red pulp
Heart	1st deposit in subendocardial areas of atrium
Liver	1st deposit in space of Disse
Blood	Deposit inactivate factor X

Hemodialysis-Associated Amyloidosis

- Patients on long-term dialysis for renal failure develop amyloidosis due to deposition of β2-microglobulin
- This protein is present in high concentrations in the serum of persons with renal disease and is retained in the circulation because it **cannot be filtered through dialysis membranes**.
- Patients often present with carpal tunnel **syndrome because of β2-microglobulin deposition.**
- In some patients on long-term dialysis, amyloid deposits in the **synovium, joints, or tendon sheaths**.

Involvement of Heart in Amyloidosis

- **Heart is the second most commonly affected organ**, in 50% of patients, in primary amyloidosis
- **Cardiac failure is the leading cause of mortality in Amyloidosis.**
- Early on, the electrocardiogram may show low voltage in the limb leads, with a **pseudo-infarct pattern.**
- Eventually, the echocardiogram will display **concentrically thickened ventricles and diastolic dysfunction**, leading to a **restrictive cardiomyopathy**; systolic function is preserved until late in the disease.

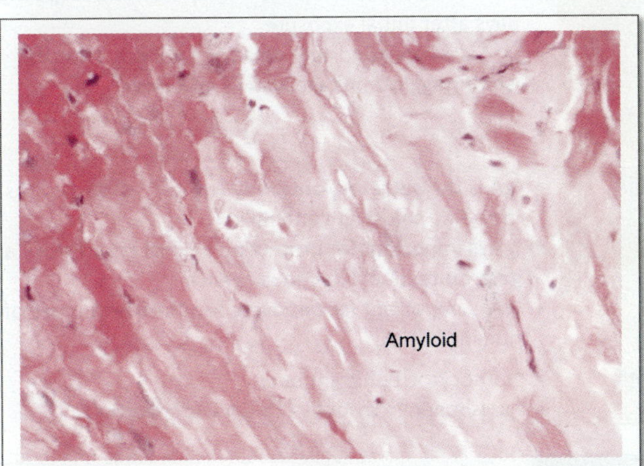

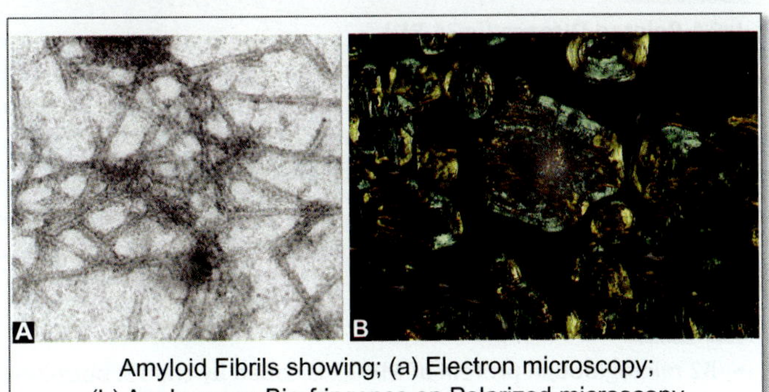

Amyloid Fibrils showing; (a) Electron microscopy; (b) Apple green Birefringence on Polarized microscopy

Amyloidosis of Kidney

- It is the **most common (affected in 70%) and potentially the most serious** form of organ involvement.
- Amyloid is deposited primarily in glomeruli, it starts first in mesangium.
- Interstitial peritubular torne arteries and arterioles are affected.
- Usually manifests as **proteinuria, often in nephrotic range** and associated with significant hypoalbuminemia, secondary hypercholesterolemia, and edema or anasarca.
- Tubular rather than glomerular deposition of amyloid can produce **azotemia** without significant proteinuria

High Yield Facts

Scintigraphy with radiolabeled serum amyloid P is rapid and specific test. It can tell extent of amyloidosis

BIOLOGICAL PROPERTIES OF DIFFERENT ANTIBODY CLASSES

IgG	• **Most abundant** of all the Ig classes • **Longest half-life** of all the Ig classes • Agglutinates particulate antigens & Precipitates soluble antigens • The only antibody class that **crosses the placenta** • IgG bound to cells or aggregated in antigen-antibody complexes can **activate complement**.	• IgG is good at **neutralizing toxins** • IgG can interfere with bacterial virulence features such as motility and adherence to tissues • IgG can **block virus ability to adhere to target** cells • IgG is the main antibody found in secondary immune response
IgM	• IgM monomer is the **B-cell receptor** of the mature B-cell • **First antibody made in a primary immune response**, 7-10 days after initial exposure • IgM is a very good agglutinating antibody (**Natural isohemagglutinins are also of IgM class**)	• IgM is the **first antibody made in life** (about 5 months in utero) • IgM is the antibody made to T-independent antigens polysaccharides • IgM attached to antigen is a very **good activator of complement** • IgM **does not cross** the placenta
IgA	• IgA is the **secretory antibody** found in all secretions including colostrum and milk. • IgA is important for protection against **respiratory and gastrointestinal** infectious agents. • IgA is important for **passively acquired immunity** of nursing baby.	• IgA makes lysozyme work better especially against gram-negative bacteria • IgA **neutralizes virus** • IgA is transported across membranes via the poly-Ig receptor
IgE	• Homocytotrophic antibody • IgE is made in response to **parasitic worms**.	• IgE is the antibody that **triggers allergy** • IgE binds to FcεRI receptors on the surface of mast cells

R10th Latest Update

IgG4-Related Disease (IgG4-RD)

• A **newly recognized** constellation of disorders characterized by **tissue infiltrates by IgG4 antibody-producing plasma cells** and lymphocytes, particularly T cells, **storiform fibrosis**, **obliterative phlebitis**, and usually **increased serum IgG4.**
• Spectrum includes:

■ Mikulicz syndrome (enlargement and fibrosis of salivary and lacrimal glands)
■ Riedel thyroiditis
■ Idiopathic retroperitoneal fibrosis
■ Autoimmune pancreatitis
■ Inflammatory pseudotumors of the orbit, lungs and kidneys

Note: IgG4 levels may or may not be high.

R10th Latest Update

• B2 microglobulin protein of MHC 1 is coded by chr 15. beta-2-microglobulin (coded chromosome 15) which plays an important role in the structural support of the heavy chains
• Natural IgM antibodies are also responsible for hyperacute reaction

HLA Typing

Serology	• Complement Dependent Cytotoxicity (CDC) • Microlymptiocycitotoxic test
Molecular methods (Diagnosis of choice)	• PC-I SSP (Sequence Specific Priming) • PCR SSOP (Sequence Specific Oligonudeoticle Probes) • Sequence Based Typing (BT) Reference Strand Conformational Analysis (RSCA) Luminex technology-SSOP Based Method

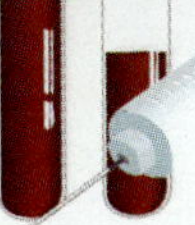

NEXT Pattern Questions

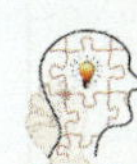

Q's

1. **Scenario Type Question**
   1. CD8+ cells
   2. Dendritic cells
   3. Natural killer cells
   4. Neutrophils
   5. Plasma cells
   6. CD4+ lymphocyte
   7. Mast cell

Scenario A. An epidemiologic study is conducted to determine riskfactors for HIV infection. The study documents that individuals with coexisting sexually transmitted diseases such as chancroid are more likely to become HIV-positive. It is postulated that an inflamed mucosal surface is an ideal location for the transmission of HIV during sexual intercourse. Which of the following cells in these mucosal surfaces is most instrumental in transmitting HIV to CD4+ T lymphocytes?

Scenario B. A 48-year-old woman has fingers that are tapered and claw-like, with decreased motion at the small joints. There are no wrinkle lines on her facial skin. The microscopic appearance of the skin is shown in the figure. The patient also has diffuse interstitial fibrosis of the lungs, with pulmonary hypertension and cor pulmonale. Which of the following dermal inflammatory cells is the most likely initiator of the process that is the cause of her skin disease?

Ans. A-2, B-6

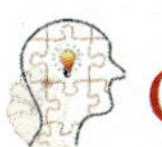

Q's

2. **A 40-year-old man complains of cough with sputum and evening rise of temperature for the past 3 months. The lung lesions were biopsied and the following image was obtained. What is the type of hypersensitivity reaction occurring in this patient?**

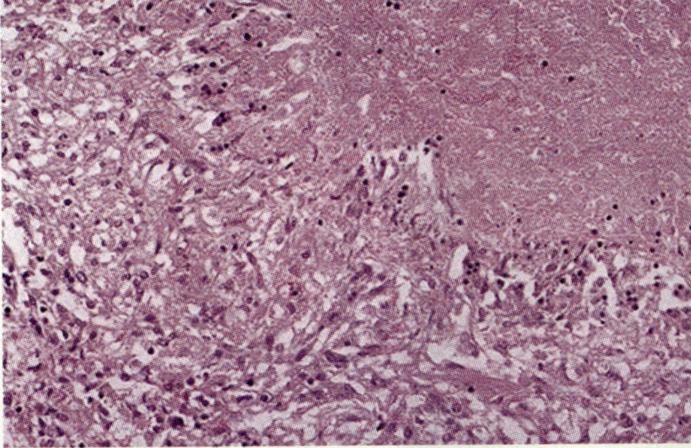

a. Hypersensitivity Type I   b. Hypersensitivity Type II   c. Hypersensitivity Type III   d. Hypersensitivity Type IV

Ans. (d) Hypersensitivity Type IV

(Ref: Robins Basic Pathology 10th ed/pg142)

Picture given: Caseating granulomatous inflammation → Tuberculosis
Examples of:
- **Type I HS:** Anaphylaxis, allergy, bronchial asthma
- **Type II HS:** Autoimmune hemolytic anemia, Good pasture syndrome
- **Type III HS:** SLE, serum sickness, Arthus reaction
- **Type IV HS:** Contact dermatitis, multiple sclerosis, type I diabetes, tuberculosis

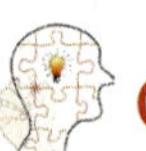

Q's

3. The type of WBC shown in the picture plays a major role in which of the following hypersensitivity reactions?

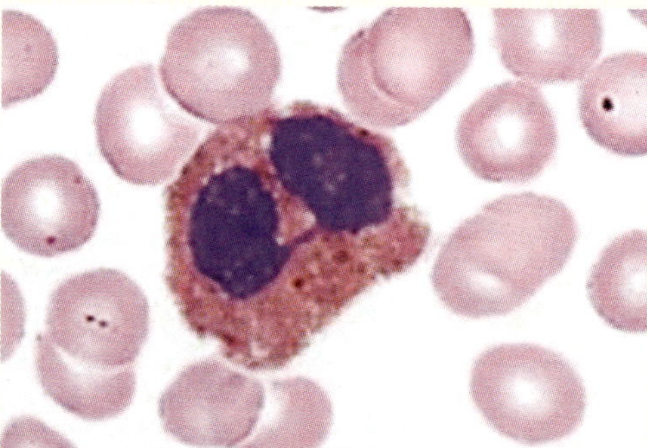

a. Hypersensitivity Type I   b. Hypersensitivity Type II   c. Hypersensitivity Type III   d. Hypersensitivity Type IV

Ans. (a) Hypersensitivity Type I

(Ref: Robins Basic Pathology 10th ed/ pg 136)

Picture – orange red granules and a spectacle shaped nucleus → Eosinophil

- **Type I—Immediate hypersensitivity:** Production of IgE antibody – release of vasoactive amines from mast cells. TH2 response occurs in late phase → IL5 release → Eosinophil activation
- **Type II—Antibody mediated hypersensitivity:** Production of IgG and IgM – binds to target and leads to phagocytosis; recruitment of WBCs
- **Type III—Immune-complex mediated hypersensitivity:** Deposition of antigen- antibody complexes – complement activation
- **Type IV—Cell mediated hypersensitivity:** Activated T lymphocytes – release of cytokines, inflammation and macrophage activation

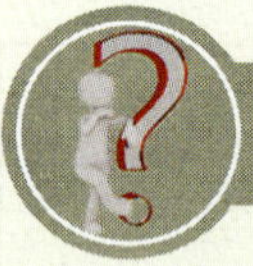

Image-Based Question

1. The following are features of which disease?

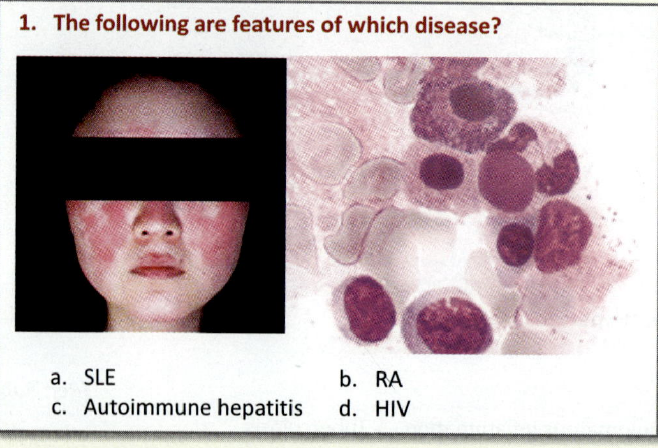

a. SLE   b. RA
c. Autoimmune hepatitis   d. HIV

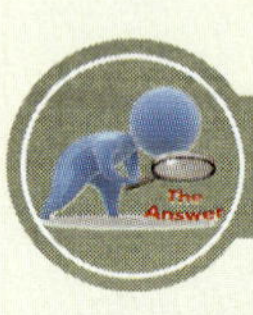

Answer of Image-Based Question

1. **Ans. (a) SLE**
   - The first figure shows butterfly malar rash and the second one shows a neutrophil engulfing a lymphocyte (L.E body) which are highly suggestive features of SLE.

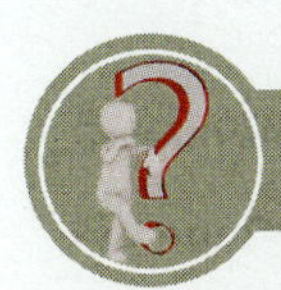

Multiple Choice Questions

1. **Antibody independent cell mediated toxicity is seen in:**
    (AIIMS Nov 18)
    a. NK cell
    b. NK cell only
    c. Macrophage
    d. NK cells, neutrophils & macrophages

2. **Gama Delta-T cells have role in?** **(AIIMS May 18)**
    a. First line of defence against bacterial peptide.
    b. CD 5
    c. CD 4
    d. CD 8

3. **Macrophage engulfs different cells as shown in the image, the process is called:** **(AIIMS Nov 18)**

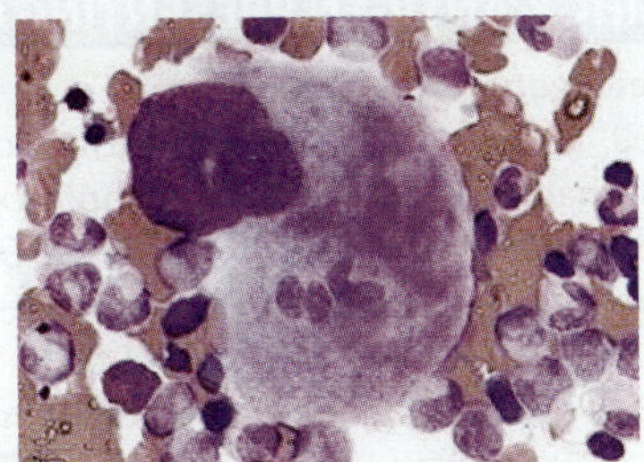

    a. Necrosis
    b. Phagocytosis
    c. Emperipolesis
    d. Autophagy

4. **Immune privilege site is:** **(AIIMS Nov 18)**
    a. Seminiferous tubule
    b. Optic nerve
    c. Area postrema
    d. Spinal canal

5. **CD markers for natural killer cells is/are:**
    a. CD 16
    b. CD 117 **(PGI Nov 2017)**
    c. CD 56
    d. CD 1
    e. CD 4

6. **Which CD molecule is important for presentation of lipid antigen?** **(JIPMER 2016)**
    a. CD4
    b. CD8
    c. CD1
    d. CD16

7. **Interleukin secreted by Th1 cells include?**
    a. IL-2
    b. IL-4 **(JIPMER 2016)**
    c. IL-10
    d. IL-13

8. **Which of the following is a secondary lymphoid organ?**
    a. Liver
    b. Spleen **(JIPMER 2016)**
    c. Bone marrow
    d. Thymus

9. **Which of the following are/is not an activator of alternate complement system?** **(JIPMER 2016)**
    a. Factor H
    b. IgA
    c. Bacteria
    d. Toxin

10. **Which antibody indicates intrauterine infection in baby?** **(Recent Question 2016-17)**
    a. IgA
    b. IgM
    c. IgG
    d. IgD

11. **Which antibody protects from intestinal infection?**
    (Recent Question 2016-17)
    a. IgA
    b. Ig M
    c. Ig G
    d. IgE

12. **Immunoglobulins differ with each other in all except**
    (Recent Question 2016-17)
    a. Heavy chain
    b. Light chain
    c. Electrophoresis
    d. Molecular weight
    (Recent Question 2016-17)

13. **Stellate Granuloma are seen in**
    (Recent Question 2016-17)
    a. Cat scratch disease
    b. Sarcoidosis
    c. LGV
    d. Histoplasmosis

14. **Castleman syndrome is associated with?**
    (Recent Question 2016-17)
    a. EBV
    b. CMV
    c. HHV 8
    d. Herpes virus

15. **Role of macrophages in antibody production is?**
    (Recent Question 2016-17)
    a. Antigen presentation
    b. B cell production
    c. Class switching
    d. B cell activation

16. **Which virus causes abnormal proliferation of B cells?**
    (Recent Question 2016-17)
    a. CMV
    b. HHV-8
    c. HTLV
    d. EBV

17. **Which of the following immunoglobulin is called homocytotropic antibody?** **(Recent Question 2015)**
    a. IgA
    b. IgG
    c. IgM
    d. IgE

18. **Which Antibody crosses placenta?** **(Recent Question 2016)**
    a. IgG1
    b. IgG4
    c. IgA
    d. IgD

19. **IgG is what % of total plasma proteins?**
    (Recent Question 2016)
    a. 5-10
    b. 10-15
    c. 15-20
    d. 25-30

20. **EBV enters the cells through** **(Recent Question 2016)**
    a. CR1
    b. CR2
    c. CR3
    d. CR4

21. **About Natural killer cells, all are true except?**
    a. Large granular cells **(PGI NOV 2015)**
    b. Have perforins
    c. Need thymus for development
    d. CD16 is FcR of IgG
    e. Kills intracellular bacteria

22. **Conditions with high ESR and normal CRP is/are?**
    (PGI Nov 2015)
    a. Pregnancy
    b. Tuberculosis
    c. Multiple myeloma
    d. Polycythemia
    e. SLE

23. **Which is a large granular lymphocyte?**
    (Recent Question 2015)
    a. NK cell
    b. B-lymphocyte
    c. T-lymphocyte
    d. Macrophage

24. **Which of these is CD marker of cytotoxic cells?**
    (Recent Question 2015/2014)
    a. CD8
    b. CD4
    c. CD1a
    d. CD1

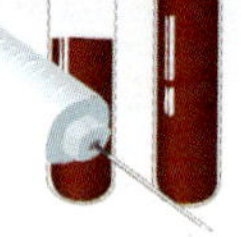

25. **Cells involved in humoral immunity:**
(Recent Question 2014)
   a. B-cells
   b. T-cells
   c. Helper cells
   d. Dendritic cells

26. **Macrophages are converted to epithelioid cells by which cytokine:** *(Recent Question 2014)*
   a. IL-2
   b. IFN-ɣ
   c. TNF-alpha
   d. TGF-beta

27. **Which cytokine activate macrophages:**
(Recent Question 2014)
   a. IL-8
   b. IFN-ɣ
   c. PAF
   d. Leukotriene B4

28. **Phagocytosis is the function of:**
(Recent Question 2014)
   a. Astrocytes
   b. Oligodendrocytes
   c. Microglia
   d. Schwan cells

29. **MALT is most commonly present in** *(AIIMS Nov 14)*
   a. Duodenum
   b. Jejunum
   c. Ileum
   d. Stomach

30. **Which of the following are examples of innate immunity?** *(PGI MAY 2014)*
   a. NK cells
   b. Macrophages
   c. B-cell
   d. T cell
   e. Complements

31. **Null cells constitute what percentage of peripheral lymphocytes?** *(JIPMER 2014)*
   a. 0-1
   b. 2-5
   c. 5-10
   d. 15-20

32. **All of the following are true about type 1 HLA except?**
(Recent Question 2016)
   a. Present on APC
   b. Activate cytotoxic T cell and kill virus infected cell
   c. Present on nucleated cells
   d. First line defense mechanism

33. **EBV action in nasopharynx through?**
(Recent Question 2015)
   a. CD 3
   b. CD 4
   c. CD 8
   d. CD 21

34. **Macrophages- false statement is?** *(JIPMER 2013)*
   a. Derived from monocytes
   b. Harbor Mycobacteria
   c. Involved in Type 3 HSN
   d. Produces TNF and interleukins

35. **Antibody that is produced rapidly and in high amounts during secondary response?** *(JIPMER 2013)*
   a. IgM
   b. IgG
   c. IgA
   d. IgE

36. **Cells that are identified by presence of immunoglobulins on the surface are?** *(JIPMER 2013)*
   a. Neutrophils
   b. B-cells
   c. NK cells
   d. Monocytes

37. **Not true regarding NK cells is?** *(JIPMER 2013)*
   a. Active against malignant cells
   b. Involve MHC antigen for killing micro-organisms
   c. First line defense against viral infections
   d. No prior sensitization required

38. **Which of the following are activators of T lymphocyte:**
(PGI May 12)
   a. CD 79b
   b. CD 3
   c. CD 28
   d. CD 14
   e. LCK

39. **All of the following are functions of CD4 helper cells, except:** *(AIIMS May 11, 10, AI 09)*
   a. Immunogenic memory
   b. Produce immunoglobulins
   c. Activate macrophages
   d. Activate cytotoxic cells

40. **B-cell markers are:** *(PGI Nov 2011)*
   a. CD-15
   b. CD-19
   c. CD-20
   d. CD-56
   e. CD-79a

41. **Virus infected cells die by the help of:** *(WB PG 2011)*
   a. IL1
   b. BIL-2
   c. B cell with antibody
   d. Cytotoxic T cell

HLA, MHC & ANTIGEN PRESENTING CELLS

42. **Naive T cell gets activated by?** *(AIIMS Nov 18)*
   a. NK cell
   b. Dendritic cell
   c. Macrophage
   d. B- lymphocytes

43. **MHC-II is present on?** *(Recent Question 2019)*
   a. All nucleated cells
   b. Antigen presenting cells
   c. RBCs
   d. CD4T cells

44. **Which of the following cells have MHC class II?**
   a. RBC *(AIIMS MAY 2017)*
   b. B cells, Dendritic cells, NK cells
   c. All nucleated cells
   d. Platelets

45. **Antigen presenting cells are?** *(AIIMS May 2017)*
   a. Langerhans cells of skin
   b. Kupffer
   c. Macrophages
   d. Monocytes
   e. Thymocytes

46. **Complement complex that attacks cell membrane is:**
(AIIMS Nov 2016)
   a. C12345
   b. C23456
   c. C34567
   d. C56789

47. **HLA is absent in** *(AIIMS Nov 2016)*
   a. RBC
   b. Monocyte
   c. Neutrophils
   d. Thrombocytes

48. **Which of the following is not an antigen presenting cell?**
(AIIMS May 2016)
   a. M cell
   b. Thymocyte
   c. Macrophage
   d. Langerhans cells

49. **Which hepatitis virus is associated with spontaneous remission with HLA DR4 ?** *(JIPMER 2016)*
   a. HAV
   b. HBV
   c. HCV
   d. HDV

50. **Dendritic cell expresses?** *(Recent Question 2015)*
   a. MHC 1
   b. MHC 2
   c. MHC 3
   d. MHC 4

51. **MHC III codes for** *(Recent Question 2015)*
   a. TNF alpha
   b. IL 1
   c. HLA A
   d. HLA B

52. **The professional antigen presenting cells are:**
(Recent Question 2014)
   a. B cells
   b. Dendritic cells
   c. T cells
   d. NK cells

53. **HLA is located on**
(Recent Question 2014/AIIMS Nov 09, 08)
a. Short arm of chr-6
b. Long arm of chr-6
c. Short arm of chr-3
d. Long arm of chr-3

54. **True about MHC:** *(Recent Question 2014)*
a. Present on chromosome 5
b. Class II comprises A,B,C
c. Class III codes for complement
d. Class I is involved in mixed leucocyte reaction

55. **The role played by Major Histocompatibility Complex-1 and -2:** *(AIIMS Nov 14/MAY 2012)*
a. Transduce the signal to T cells following antigen recognition
b. Mediate immunogenic class switching
c. Present antigens for recognition by T cell antigen receptors
d. Enhance the secretion of cytokines

56. **Class II MHC is expressed in all except?** *(JIPMER 2013)*
a. Activated T cells
b. Dendritic cells
c. Langerhans cells
d. Neutrophils

57. **MHC II is/are presented by:** *(PGI May 12)*
a. Macrophage
b. Dendritic cells
c. Lymphocyte
d. Epithelial cell
e. Platelets

HYPERSENSITIVITY REACTIONS

58. **B cells are induced to produce IgE by which of the following?** *(Recent Pattern Question 2020)*
a. IL–2
b. IL–4
c. IL–1
d. IL–6

59. **Basophils are activated by:** *(AIIMS Nov 2019)*
a. IL–5
b. IgE fixed cell
c. Complement factor
d. TNF

60. **Variation-2: Basophils are activated by:**
(AIIMS Nov 2019)
a. IL–1
b. IL–2
c. IL–4
d. IL–10

61. **Interleukin involved in early phase of hematopoiesis is:** *(JIPMER 2019)*
a. IL–1
b. IL–2
c. IL–3
d. IL–4

62. **Which of the following is secreted by TH-1 helper cells?** *(JIPMER 2019)*
a. IL–1
b. IL–2
c. IL–4
d. IL–3

63. **Which of the following is a major cell infiltrate in rheumatoid arthritis?** *(Recent exam 2018)*
a. CD4+ helper cell
b. Macrophage
c. Lymphocyte
d. Dendritic cells

64. **Rh incompatibility is an example of**
a. Immune complex reaction *(Recent Question 2016)*
b. Ag Ab reaction
c. Delayed hypersensitivity
d. Immediate type

65. **IgE receptor present on ?** *(AIIMS May 2015)*
a. Mast cell
b. NK cell
c. B cell
d. T cell

66. **A 45-year-old patient presents with fever, night sweats, weight loss. On X ray a mass in apical lobe of lung is seen. On histopathology found to have caseous necrosis. What is the underlying process?** *(AIIMS May 2015)*
a. Enzymatic degeneration
b. Hypersensitivity reaction with modified macrophages, lymphocytes and giant cells
c. Acute decrease in blood supply
d. decreased growth factors

67. **Delayed hypersensitivity is initiated by** *(MH PG 2014)*
a. CD3+T cells
b. CD4 + T cells
c. CD8+Tcells
d. CD1O+Tcells

68. **Schwartzman reaction is an example of:**
a. None of the options *(APPGMEE 2015)*
b. Type I hypersensitivity reaction
c. Type III hypersensitivity reaction
d. Type II hypersensitivity reaction

69. **Which factor is secreted by macrophage and acts on neutrophil and endothelium in hypersensitivity reaction?** *(Recent Question 2015)*
a. IL-1
b. Tumor necrosis factor
c. Insulin like Growth factor
d. Thromboxane A2

70. **Type V hypersensitivity reaction is a subtype of:**
(Recent Question 2015)
a. Type I
b. Type II
c. Type III
d. Type IV

71. **Major basic protein is found in?** *(Recent Question 2015)*
a. Macrophage
b. Eosinophils
c. Basophil
d. Neutrophil

72. **Most important mediator of late phase of immediate type of hypersensitivity reaction is:**
a. Histamine *(Recent Question 2015)*
b. Major basic protein
c. Platelet activating factor
d. PGE2

73. **Antibodies in ITP are:** *(Recent Question 2014)*
a. IgG
b. IgM
c. IgE
d. IgD

74. **Transfusion reaction and erythroblastosis fetalis are:**
(Recent Question 2014, DNB June 11)
a. Type I hypersensitivity
b. Type II hypersensitivity
c. Type III hypersensitivity
d. Type IV hypersensitivity

75. **48 hours after taking penicillin, a patient complains of body ache. He gives no history of any oldallergy to penicillin. Blood tests show anti penicillin antibody and hemolysis. Which type of hypersensivity reaction is this?** *(AIIMS Nov 14)*
a. Type 1HSN
b. Type II HSN
c. Type III HSN
d. Type 1V HSN

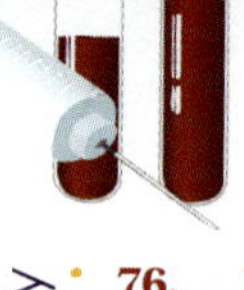

76. Which is the example of type 2 hypersensitivity reaction?
a. Serum sickness   b. PAN   *(WB PG 2014)*
c. SLE   d. Rh incompatibility

77. An adult develops swelling of tongue and neck after ingestion of peanut. What is your diagnosis?
(JIPMER 2014)
a. Foreign body larynx
b. Angioneurotic edema
c. Parapharyngeal abscess
d. Inflammatory response

78. Type I lepra reaction is an example of which type of hypersensitivity according coombs and gel classification?
(JIPMER 2014), (MAHA 2016)
a. I   b. II
c. III   d. IV

79. Which of the following immune hypersensitivity reaction is responsible for Myasthenia Gravis: *(AI 12)*
a. Type I Hypersensitivity
b. Type II Hypersensitivity
c. Type III Hypersensitivity
d. Type IV Hypersensitivity

80. LATS is a?   *(DNB Aug 12 Pattern)*
a. IgMAb   b. IgGAb
c. Glycoprotein   d. IgA Ab

81. Substance that can cause Anaphylactic shock is?
(Recent Question 12)
a. Histamine   b. Adrenaline
c. Nor-adrenaline   d. Glucocorticoids

82. Raji cell assay are used to identify?   *(DPG 11)*
a. Complement levels   b. Immune complexes
c. T- cells   d. IFN levels

AUTOIMMUNE SYSTEM

83. Which of the following is/are involved in etiopathogenesis of SLE: *(PGI May 2019)*
a. Interferon-1 (IFN-1)
b. Interferon-1 (IFN-β)
c. Exposure to UV rays
d. Deficiency of early complement factors
e. Failure of self-tolerance in B cells

84. A 29-year-old female with history of polyarthalgia and back ache was investigated. She had nucleolar pattern in IF. Which of the following is the best fit in her case?
a. Glomerlonephritis and heart failure *(AIIMS MAY 2017)*
b. Raynaud phenomenon and sclerodactyly
c. Genital and oral painful ulcers
d. Joint pains with nodules on skin.

85. During development, all the antigens of self are introduced to thymic cells in-order to be removed to prevent autoimmunity. Which of the following genes is involved in the process?   *(AIIMS MAY 2017)*
a. NOTCH1   b. AIRE
c. RB gene   d. CPK gene

86. Which of the following gene is responsible for Autoimmune polyendocrinopathy which gene?
a. FOX P3   b. AIRE   *(JIPMER 2016)*
c. CD 25   d. PD-1

87. Schaumann bodies are not seen in :
a. Sarcoidosis   *(Recent Question 2016-17)*
b. Histoplasmosis
c. Cryptococcosis
d. Hypersensitivity pneumonitis
e. Tuberculosis

88. Which of the following is a Immune privileged region?
(AIIMS May 2015)
a. Area postrema   b. Seminiferous tubules
c. Kidney   d. Optic nerve

89. Which of the following is not an auto immune disorder?
(AIIMS May 2015)
a. Ulcerative colitis   b. Grave's disease
c. Rheumatoid arthritis   d. SLE

90. Most sensitive antibody for SLE *(Recent Question 2015)*
a. Anti-nuclear   b. Anti-ds DNA
c. Anti-Smith   d. Anti-histone

91. Antibody in drug induced lupus
(Recent Question 2015)
a. Anti-nuclear   b. Anti-ds DNA
c. Anti-Smith   d. Anti-histone

92. All of the following are features of SLE except
a. Shrinking lung syndrome   *(Recent Question 2015)*
b. Erosive arthritis
c. Libman sack's endocarditis
d. Cognitive dysfunction

93. Site of biopsy in Sjogren syndrome
(Recent Question 2015)
a. Kidney   b. Abdominal fat
c. Lip   d. Rectum

94. Antibody in diffuse scleroderma
a. Anti-DNA topoisomerase   *(Recent Question 2015)*
b. Anti-Centromere
c. Anti-RNA polymerase
d. Anti-Smith

95. Most common antibody in sjogren syndrome
(Recent Question 2015)
a. Anti-DNA topoisomerase
b. Anti-Centromere
c. Anti-RNA polymerase
d. Anti-Ribonucleoprotein

96. Class IV lupus nephritis   *(Recent Question 2015)*
a. Mesangial lupus nephritis
b. Proliferative lupus nephritis
c. Membranous lupus nephritis
d. Diffuse sclerosing lupus nephritis

97. Shrinking lung syndrome is a feature of
(Recent Question 2015)
a. Systemic lupus erythematosus
b. Systemic sclerosis
c. AIDS
d. ARDS

98. Anti-smith antibody is specific for
a. Systemic sclerosis   *(Recent Question 2015)*
b. Sjogren syndrome
c. Systemic lupus erythematosus
d. Drug induced lupus

99. Commonest renal lesion in SLE is:
(Recent Question 2015)
   a. Focal proliferative   b. Diffuse Proliferative
   c. Membranous   d. Minimal change disease

100. Joint erosions are typically absent in
   a. Rheumatoid arthritis   *(Recent Question 2015)*
   b. Systemic lupus erythematosus
   c. Psoriatic arthritis
   d. Osteoarthritis
   e. Mesangial Proliferative

101. Antibody seen in neonatal lupus with congenital heart block   *(Recent Question 2015)*
   a. Anti-ribosomal   b. Anti-Ro (SS-A)
   c. Anti-neuronal   d. Anti-histone

102. Most severe form of lupus nephritis
(Recent Question 2015)
   a. Mesangial lupus lomerulonephritis
   b. Focal proliferative glomerulonephritis
   c. Diffuse proliferative glomerulonephritis
   d. Membranous glomerulonephritis

103. Anti-histone antibodies are specific for
(Recent Question 2015)
   a. CNS lupus
   b. Drug induced lupus
   c. Neonatal lupus
   d. Cutaneous lupus

104. False statement regarding musculoskeletal manifestations of SLE   *(Recent Question 2015)*
   a. Intermittent polyarthritis
   b. Commonly involves hands, wrist, knees
   c. Erosions seen on X-rays
   d. Ischemic necrosis of bone can occur, when the patient is on glucocorticoids

105. All are true about limited cutaneous systemic sclerosis except   *(Recent Question 2015)*
   a. Anti-Topoisomerase I antibody
   b. Digital ischemia
   c. Calcinosis
   d. Isolated pulmonary arterial hypertension

106. Most common cause of death in SLE after first few years of diagnosis   *(Recent Question 2015)*
   a. CNS disease
   b. Opportunistic infections
   c. Accelerated atherosclerosis
   d. Nephritis

107. All the following about drug induced SLE are true except
   a. More common in females   *(Recent Question 2015)*
   b. Renal and CNS involvement is uncommon
   c. Complement level are normal
   d. The disease remits after withdrawal of the offending drug

108. Most common autoimmune disease associated with sjogren syndrome   *(Recent Question 2015)*
   a. Scleroderma
   b. Rheumatoid arthritis
   c. Inflammatory bowel disease
   d. SLE

109. Which part of GIT is most severely affected in systemic sclerosis   *(Recent Question 2015)*
   a. Esophagus   b. Jejunum
   c. Sigmoid colon   d. Rectum

110. Digital ischemia is common in   *(Recent Question 2015)*
   a. Diffuse scleroderma
   b. Diffuse cutaneous scleroderma
   c. Limited scleroderma
   d. Systemic lupus erythematosus

111. Match the above HLA associationsand choose the best match: *(APPGMEE 2015)*

p	HLA DR2	w	Dermatitis herpetiformis
q	HLA DR3	x	Celiac disease
r	HLA DR4	y	Dermatitis herpetiformis
s	HLA DQ2	z	Pemphigus vulgaris

   a. pqrs = wxzy   b. pqrs = ywzx
   c. pqrs= xwys   d. pqrs = zxwy

112. Which is not included in Mixed connective tissue disorder?   *(Recent Question 2015)*
   a. Systemic sclerosis   b. SLE
   c. Rheumatoid arthritis   d. Polymyositis

113. Which antibody is associated with Mixed connective tissue disease (MCTD)?   *(Recent Question 2015)*
   a. Anti U1-RNP Ab   b. Anti DNA Ab
   c. Anti histoneAb   d. Anti ds-DNA Ab

114. Band test is done in: *(Recent Question 2014)*
   a. RA   b. SLE
   c. Scleroderma   d. PAN

115. Antinuclear antibody specific for SLE is:
   a. Anti ds DNA   *(Recent Question 2014)*
   b. Anti nuclear antibodies
   c. Anti centromere antibody
   d. Anti histoneAb

116. HLA associated with psoriasis:
(Recent Question 2014, 2013)
   a. HLA-B27   b. HLA-DR4
   c. HLA-CW6   d. HLA-B8

117. Drug induced lupus antibodies are:
(Recent Question 2014)
   a. Anti-Rho   b. ds-DNA
   c. Anti-Sm   d. Anti-histone antibody

118. HLA marker of Bechet's syndrome:
(Recent Question 2014)
   a. HLA-B27   b. HLA-DR5
   c. HLA-B51   d. HLA-CW6

119. HLA associated with rheumatoid arthritis:
(Recent Question 2014, 2013)
   a. HLA-B27   b. HLA-DR4
   c. HLA-CW6   d. HLA-B8

120. Thromboangitis obliterans is associated with:
(Recent Question 2014)
   a. HLA-B27   b. HLA-DR4
   c. HLA-B5   d. HLA-DR2

121. ANA (antinuclear antibody) is seen in all except:
(Recent Question 2014)
   a. SLE   b. RA
   c. Sjogren's syndrome   d. Systemic sclerosis

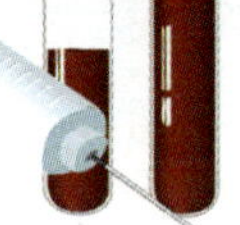

122. HLA B-27 has > 90% association with? *(AIIMS Nov 14)*
a. Enteropathic
b. Reactive arthritis
c. Rheumatoid arthritis
d. Ankylosing spondylitis

123. Miller-Fisher syndrome associated with: *(WB PG 2014)*
a. HLA DQBI
b. Antibodies to GQ1B
c. Antibodies to peroxidase
d. HLAB5

124. Thrombosis is seen in which stage of lupus nephritis? *(Recent Question 2013)*
a. Class I
b. Class II
c. Class III
d. Class IV

125. A 30-year-old lady presents to the outpatient department with an erythematous butterfly rash on her cheeks. Which of the following antibodies should be assayed initially for her suspected condition: *(AI 12)*
a. Anti-ds-DNA
b. Anti-Ro-Antibody
c. Anti-Centromere-Antibody
d. Anti-mitochondrial-Antibody

126. In SLE, active nephritis is/are characterized by:
a. Proliferation of endothelium *(PGI Nov 2011)*
b. Glomerular leukocyte infiltration
c. Mesangial cell proliferation
d. Epithelial cell proliferation
e. Tubulitis

127. In SLE, pulmonary involvement is characterized by:
a. Interstial Fibrosis *(PGI Nov 2011)*
b. Shrinking lung syndrome
c. Alveolar hemorrhage
d. Pulmonary arterial hypertension
e. Cavitation

128. Nucleolar pattern on immunofluorescence is seen in: *(PGI May 2011)*
a. Antibody to DNA
b. Antibody to RNA
c. Antibody to histone
d. Systemic sclerosis
e. SLE

129. Biopsy of the parotid gland in a patient with Sjogren's syndrome shows: *(Jipmer 11)*
a. Neutrophils
b. Lymphocytes
c. Eosinophils
d. Basophils

130. HLA associated with rheumatoid arthritis:
a. DRB1
b. DR1 *(PGI May 10)*
c. DR2
d. DR3
e. DR4

131. Best marker of SLE? *(DNB June 10)*
a. Anti Sm antibodies
b. Anti-ds DNA antibodies
c. Anti-Histone antibodies
d. Anti Ro (SS-A) antibodies

REJECTION OF TISSUE TRANSPLANTS

132. Graft between identical twins is: *(Recent Pattern Question 2020)*
a. Allograft
b. Xenograft
c. Isograft
d. Autograft

133. Organ transplantation between mother to child is a type of?
a. Autograft
b. Isograft
c. Allograft
d. Xenograft

134. Cells involved in GVHD are? *(JIPMER 2017)*
a. Recipient B cells
b. Recipient T cells
c. Donor B cells
d. Donor T cells

135. Hyperacute rejection occurs within:? *(Recent exam 2018)*
a. 12 hours
b. 2 weeks
c. 1 month
d. 3 months

136. A patient of cirrhosis with liver failure comes to you for stem cell transplantation your method will be? *(PGI Nov 2016)*
a. Transfer of stem cells from other persons liver
b. Taking patient skin stem cell and transferring into liver
c. Tranfer hepatocytes from the same person for regeneration
d. Transfer hepatic progenitor cells (HPCs) of same person for regeneration

137. Graft vs Host reaction can be reduced by?
a. Irradiation *(JIPMER 2016)*
b. Leuckoreduction/leuckofiltration
c. Immunosuppression
d. Buffy coat removal

138. After a solid organ transplantation, which of the following is responsible for acute graft rejection.? *(AIIMS May 2016)*
a. C3a
b. C3b
c. C5a
d. C4d

139. For transplantation which HLA requires minimum matching is required *(Recent Question 2016-17)*
a. HLA A
b. HLA B
c. HLA DR
d. HLA DP

140. In a case of kidney allograft rejection, what is the best diagnostic feature ? *(Recent Question 2016-17)*
a. Increased neutrophil
b. Increased basophils
c. Biopsy
d. Complements levels

141. A patient requires liver transplant. He plans to receive it from his brother. They are not twins. On HLA typing, HLA is matched at the A, B, and DRB1 loci. Siblings are:
a. Matched, unrelated donors *(Recent Question 2016)*
b. Matched, related donors
c. Mismatched, related donors
d. Mismatched, unrelated donors

142. For a successful transplantation how many HLA should be matched? *(Recent Question 2016)*
a. 1-4
b. 5-10
c. 11-15
d. 15-20

143. Which of the following is not a characteristic feature of GVHD? *(Recent Question 2015)*
a. Skin involvement
b. Renal involvement
c. Liver involvement
d. Intestinal involvement

144. "000" mismatch in graft transplanatation means?
(Recent Question 2016)
   a. Partial mismatched
   b. Completely mismatched
   c. Matched
   d. Partially matched

145. True about hyperacute rejection in renal transplant:
   a. Occur within few days of transplant   *(PGI May 2015)*
   b. T cell involvement
   c. Blood vessel thrombosis
   d. Eosinophilic infiltration
   e. B cell infiltration

146. Graft rejection is: *(Recent Question 2014)*
   a. Cell mediated   b. Humoral
   c. Both   d. None

147. HLA-I is present on: *(Recent Question 2014)*
   a. All nucleated cells
   b. Only on cells of immune system
   c. Only on B-cells
   d. Only on T-cells

148. In acute transplant after 6 months, the rejection is because of?   *(Recent Question 2015)*
   a. Neutrophil
   b. T-lymphocyte
   c. B-lymphocyte
   d. Macrophage

149. Following conditions must be fulfilled in a person before taking him as a kidney donor EXCEPT   *(APPGMEE 14)*
   a. ABO compatibility with recipient
   b. Presence of two normally functioning kidneys
   c. No HIV infection
   d. Zero HLA mismatch with recipient

150. Allograft rejection is an example of?   *(JIPMER 2014)*
   a. GVHD
   b. Delayed types hypersensitivity
   c. Immediate hypersensitivity
   d. Acute rejection

151. Hyperacute rejection is due to: *(AIIMS May 2013)*
   a. Preformed antibodies   *(AIIMS Nov 2012)*
   b. Cytotoxic T-lymphocyte medicated injury
   c. Circulating macrophage mediated injury
   d. Endothelitis caused by donor antibodies

152. Most commonly involved organs in graft versus host disease are all except: *(Recent Question 12)*
   a. Gut
   b. Liver
   c. Skin
   d. Kidney

153. Graft from identical twin is defined as: *(WB PG 2012)*
   a. Allograft   b. Isograft
   c. Xenograft   d. Autograft

154. In GVH disease all are involved except:
(WB PG 2011, AIIMS May 07)
   a. Liver   b. Lungs
   c. Intestine   d. Skin

155. In the given below flow cytometry graphs; If A and B are normal scatter plots for B cells. Interpret images C and D and come to diagnosis.   *(AIIMS Nov 2019)*

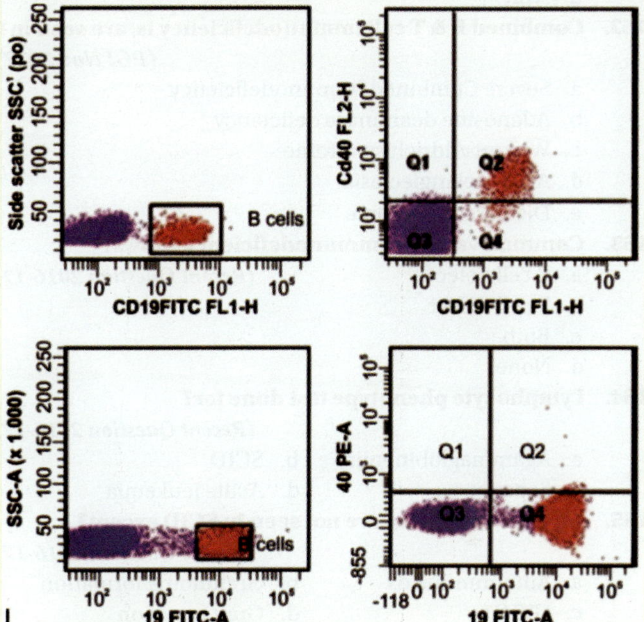

   a. Bare lymphocyte syndrome
   b. SCID
   c. Hyper IgM syndrome
   d. Chronic granulomatous disease

156. Which is not a cause/involved in SCID? *(AIIMS Nov 2019]*
   a. ZAP70   b. IL2R
   c. JAK3   d. BTK

157. Which is not a feature of Lofgren syndrome?
(JIPMER 2019)
   a. Uveitis
   b. Erythema nodosum
   c. Polyarthralgia
   d. Bilateral hilar adenopathy

158. Which of the following is/are results from defect in innate immunity: *(PGI May 2019)*
   a. DiGeorge syndrome
   b. Severe combined immunodeficiency
   c. Common variable immunodeficiency
   d. Chediak-Higashi syndrome
   e. Bruton agammaglobulinemia

159. True regarding 'Bare lymphocytes syndrome'?
   a. Autosomal recessive   *(PGI May 2018)*
   b. Part of SCID
   c. MHC overexpression
   d. Leads to abnormal CD4T cell development

160. Feature(s) of DiGeorge syndrome is/are all except?
(PGI Nov 2017)
   a. Results from failure of development of the third and fourth pharyngeal pouches
   b. Absent thyroid
   c. Absent parathyroid glands
   d. B cell defect
   e. Enhanced susceptibility of bacterial infection

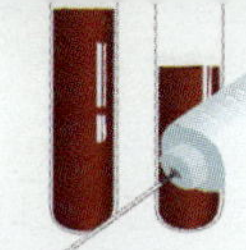

161. In SCID which DNA mechanism is defective?
a. Non homologous disjunction repair *(AIIMS Nov 2017)*
b. Homologous disjunction repair
c. Base excision repair
d. NER

162. Combined B & T cell immunodeficiency is/are seen in?
(PGI Nov 2017)
a. Severe Combined Immunodeficiency
b. Adenosine deaminase deficiency
c. Wiskott-Aldrich syndrome
d. Ataxia telangiectasia
e. DiGeorge syndrome

163. Common variable immunodeficiency shows?
a. B cell defect *(Recent Question 2016-17)*
b. T cell defect
c. Both
d. None

164. Lymphocyte phenotype test done for?
(Recent Question 2016-17)
a. Agammaglobinemia   b. SCID
c. Sepsis   d. Acute leukemia

165. All of the following are not seen in SCID except?
(Recent Question 2016-17)
a. Autoimmune ds   b. Granuloma formation
c. GVHD   d. Graft rejection

166. Both B and T cell defect is present in: *(PGI May 12)*
a. SCID
b. Common Variable immunodeficiency
c. Wiskott-Aldrich syndrome
d. X-linked Agammaglobulinemia
e. Chronic mucocutaneous candidiasis

167. Chediak Higashi syndrome is characterised by the following except: *(MH 11)*
a. Neutrophilia
b. Defective degranulation
c. Delayed microbial killing
d. Giant granules

HIV/AIDS

168. Identify the parasite in the intestinal biopsy of a HIV positive patient. *(Recent Pattern Question 2020)*

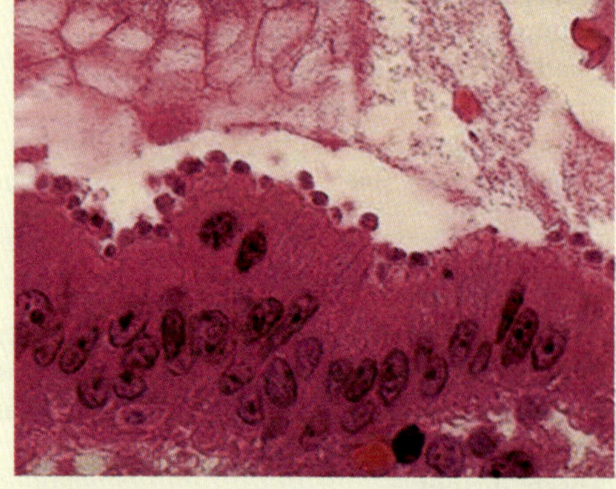

a. Giardia   b. CMV
c. Amoebic colitis   d. Cryptosporidium

169. HIV-1 differs with HIV-2 in? *(PGI Nov 2016)*
a. HIV-2 is more dangerous than HIV-1
b. Enfuvirtide is not active against HIV-2
c. HIV-2 is more common than HIV-1 in India
d. More commonly transmitted from mother to child
e. HIV-1 worsens faster than HIV-2

170. Which of the following malignancy is commonly found in AIDS patients ? *(MH PG 2014)*
a. Kaposi's sarcoma   b. Fibrosarcoma
c. Cavernous hemangioma   d. Melanoma

171. HIV was discovered in which year? *(AIIMS Nov 2014)*
a. 1983   b. 1979
c. 1969   d. 1990

172. A person died of HIV infection. Lung Autopsy performed in this person showed intranuclear basophilic inclusions. His CD4 count was less than 100/ uL. Which is the most probable diagnosis? *(AIIMS May 2014)*
a. CMV
b. Herpes infection
c. ARDS
d. Pneumocystis carinii

173. Which of the following are AIDS defining cancers?
a. Burkitt's lymphoma *(PGI May 2014)*
b. Non Hodgkin's Lymphoma
c. Ca esophagus
d. Primary lymphoma of brain
e. Invasive cancer of uterine cervix

174. HIV affects? *(JIPMER 2014)*
a. B-cells
b. Helper T cells
c. Suppressor T-cells
d. Cytotoxic T-cells

175. Immunity in HIV true is? *(Recent Question 2016)*
a. Cellular immunity is lost
b. Antibody mediated is lost
c. Not lost
d. Both lost

176. Family of HIV virus *(Recent Question 2016)*
a. Lentivirus
b. Alpha retrovirus
c. Beta retro virus
d. none

177. What is false about HIV? *(Recent Question 2016)*
a. HIV 2 is more pathogenic than HIV 1'
b. HIV 2 was discovered in 1987
c. HIV 1 is the most common type
d. HIV-1 group M subtype C is predominant in India

178. WHO AIDS stage III criteria are all except?
a. Candidiasis of esophagus *(PGI Nov 2015)*
b. Kaposi's sarcoma
c. Pneumocystis jirovecii
d. Cryptococcosis, extrapulmonary
e. Ankylostoma duodenale infection

179. Most common HIV subtype in India is?
(Recent Question 2013)
a. HIV-1 M   b. HIV-1 N
c. HIV-2   d. HIV-1 O

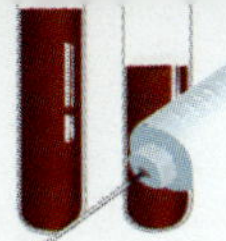

AMYLOIDOSIS

180. Amyloidosis is/are associated with which of the following feature(s)? *(PGI May 2019)*
a. Hepatosplenomegaly
b. Congestive heart failure
c. Proteinuria
d. Lytic bone lesions
e. Large fiber neuropathy in initial presentation

181. True or false regarding amyloidosis: *(AIIMS May 2019)*
a. SAA is most common Mediterranean fever
b. On Congo red staining, amyloid shows apple green birefringence
c. AL has kappa light chain.
d. Senile amyloidosis is due to β2-microglobulin

182. Secondary amyloidosis is seen in? *(PGI Nov 2018)*
a. Bronchiectasis
b. Pulmonary TB
c. Lung abscess
d. Malignancy
e. Myeloma

183. Congo Red stains due to ? *(Recent Question 2016-17)*
a. B pleated sheets
b. α helix
c. Isoelectric Ph
d. Amyloid fibrils

184. Characteristic feature of amyloid on staining *(Recent Question 2015)*
a. Apple green birefringence on infrared microscopy
b. Apple green birefringence on X-ray crystallography
c. Apple green birefringence on polarizing microscopy
d. Apple green birefringence on light microscopy

185. Most widely used stain for amyloidosis: *(Recent Question 2015)*
a. Oil red O
b. Congo red
c. PAS
d. Thioflvavin T

186. Chemical nature of amyloid in hemodialysis associated amyloidosis *(Recent Question 2015)*
a. AA
b. AL
c. Aβ2
d. TTR

187. True regarding familial amylodotid polyneuropathy *(Recent Question 2015)*
a. Autosomal recessive
b. Mutation in pyrin gene
c. Mutant form transthyretin is deposited
d. Deposited in the heart

188. Site of biopsy in amyloidosis *(Recent Question 2015)*
a. Kidney
b. Abdominal fat
c. Lip
d. Rectum

189. Amyloid deposited in the heart of aged *(Recent Question 2015)*
a. Normal transthyretin
b. Mutant transthyretin
c. Beta 2 microglobulin
d. Amyloid light chain

190. A 70-year-old patient presents with features of cardiac failure. Abdominal fat aspirate is stained with congo red and on examination with polarizing microscope exhibit apple green birefringence, Diagnosis
a. Marfan syndrome *(Recent Question 2015)*
b. Familial hypercholesterolemia
c. Amyloidosis
d. SLE

191. Which is the most striking and specific test to diagnose amyloid in tissue? *(APPGMEE 2015)*
a. Congo red + polarized microscopy
b. Congo red stain+ light microscopy
c. Toluidine stain
d. Methyl violet stain

192. All of the following statements are true about properties of amyloid, except: *(AP 2012)*
a. By electron microscope, it is made up largely continuous non-branching fibrils with a diameter of approximately 7.5 to 10 nm.
b. This electron microscope structure is not identical in all types of amyloid.
c. X-ray crystallography and infrared spectroscopy demonstrates a characteristic cross-beta-pleated sheet conformation
d. Congo red staining shows apple green birefringence under polarizing microscope

193. Which thyroid carcinoma is associated with calcitonin amyloid deposition? *(Recent Question 2014)*
a. Papillary
b. Follicular
c. Anaplastic
d. Medullary

194. Which one of the following stains is specific for Amyloid?
a. Periodic Acid schif (PAS) *(Recent Question 2014)*
b. Alzerian red
c. Congo red
d. Von – Kossa

195. Gingival biopsy is used for diagnosis of: *(Recent Question 2014)*
a. Scurvy
b. Sarcoidosis
c. Amyloidosis
d. SLE

196. Major fibril protein in Primary Amyloidosis is? *(Recent Question 2014)*
a. AL
b. AA
c. Transthyretin
d. Procalcitonin

197. False statement about Amyloidosis is? *(JIPMER 2013)*
a. Extracellular eosinophillic hyaline material
b. Made of calcified proteins
c. Apple green birefringence
d. Complication of chronic infection

198. Which of the following amyloid forms is seen in secondary amyloidosis associated with chronic diseases:
a. Amyloid Associated Protein *(AI 12)*
b. Amyloid light chain
c. Beta 2 Amyloid
d. ATTR

199. Amyloid deposition in patients with long term hemodialysis usually takes place in? *(JIPMER 2012)*
a. Renal vessels
b. Peripheral nerve
c. Knee joint
d. Carpal tunnel

200. Pinch purpura is seen in? *(JIPMER 2012)*
a. Primary systemic amyloidosis
b. Vitamin C deficiency
c. Purpura fulminans'
d. Kawasaki disease

201. A 60-year-old female is suffering from renal failure and is on hemodialysis since last 8 years. She developed carpal tunnel syndrome. Which of the following will be associated? *(AIIMS Nov 11)*
a. AL
b. AA
c. ATTR
d. Beta 2 microglobulin

202. Protein deposited in familial amyloid neuropathy: *(PGI May 2011)*
a. Mutated transthyretin
b. Normal transthyretin
c. Mutated beta-1
d. Mutated beta-2
e. Mutated beta-3

203. Most common cause of death in primary amyloidosis is? *(DNB June 11)*
a. Respiratory failure
b. Cardiac failure
c. Renal failure
d. Septicemia

204. Deposition of protein A beta 2 microglobulin is seen in which clinico-pathologic category of amyloidosis:
a. Familial Mediterranean fever *(Karnataka 11)*
b. Hemodialysis associated
c. Senile cerebral'
d. Systemic senile

205. Best investigation for diagnosing amyloidosis: *(AIIMS May 10, AI 07, DNB 10)*
a. Rectal biopsy
b. Colonoscopy
c. CT scan
d. Upper GI endoscopy

206. Which of the following is/are Heredofamilial amyloidosis
a. Alzheimer's disease *(PGI May 10)*
b. Multiple myeloma
c. Familial Mediterranean fever
d. RA
e. Systemic senile amyloidosis

207. Stains used in amyloidosis: *(PGI May 10)*
a. Congo red
b. Thioflavin
c. Reticulin
d. Grams Iodine
e. PAS

Answers with Explanations

1. **Ans. (d) NK cells, neutrophils and macrophages**

Antibody-dependent cell-mediated cytotoxicity (ADCC) is the killing of an antibody-coated target cell by a cytotoxic effector cell through a non-phagocytic process, characterised by the release of the content of cytotoxic granules or by the expression of cell death-inducing molecules. ADCC is triggered through interaction of target-bound antibodies (belonging to IgG or IgA or IgE classes) with certain Fc receptors (FcRs), glycoproteins present on the effector cell surface that bind the Fc region of immunoglobulins (Ig). Effector cells that mediate ADCC include natural killer (NK) cells, monocytes, macrophages, neutrophils, eosinophils and dendritic cells

2. **Ans. (a) First line of defence against bacterial peptide**

3. **Ans. (c) Emperipolesis**

Emperipolesis is the active penetration of one cell by another which remains intact." It differs from phagocytosis in that an engulfed cell exists temporarily within another cell and with an intact normal structure while in phagocytosis, the engulfed cell is destroyed by the protective action of lysosomal enzymes.

4. **Ans. (a) Seminiferous tubules**

In testis, there occurs segregation of antigens in the seminiferous tubules from immune cells in the interstitial space by a layer of Sertoli cells connected by impermeable tight junctions which form a blood-testis barrier.

High Yield Facts

- **Immune-privileged sites:**[Q]
- **Testis, eye and brain**[Q]
- Tissues in which these antigens are located **do not ommunicate** with the blood and lymph
- **Difficult to induce immune responses** to antigens introduced into these sites
- Prolonged tissue inflammation on injury & release of antigen from these sites: **post-traumatic orchitis & uveitis**[Q]

5. **Ans. (a, c); a. CD 16; c. CD 56**

6. **Ans. (c) CD1** *(Ref: Wintrobes 13th/2499)*

Expression of CD1 in foam cells of atherosclerotic plaques may present lipid antigens to CD1-restricted T cells and contribute to inflammation of these lesions

7. **Ans. (a) IL-2** *(Ref: Robbins 9th/198)*

Cells of the TH1 subset secrete IL-2 for self activation & cytokine IFN-γ, which is a potent macrophage activator.

8. **Ans. (b) Spleen** *(Ref: Robbins 9th/193)*

9. **Ans. (a) Factor H** *(Ref: Robbins 9th/pg 162-164)*

- The alternative pathway, can be triggered by microbial surface molecules (e.g., endotoxin, or LPS), complex polysaccharides, cobra venom, and other substances, in the absence of antibody
- **Factor I and H inhits complement activation**

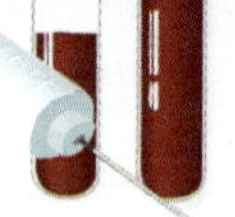

10. **Ans. (b) IgM** *(Ref: Robbins 9th/pg 199)*

Since IgM is a pentameric Ig, Maternal IgM will not pass through the placenta into the fetus. However in case of fetus being infected, it will produce its own IgM molecule against the infection.

11. **Ans. (a) IgA** *(Ref: Kuby immunology pg 419)*

IgA antibodies are found in circulation, they are the major isotype found in secretions, including mucus in the gut, milk from mammary glands, tears, and saliva. In these secretions, IgA can neutralize both toxins and pathogens, continually interacting with the resident (commensal)bacteria that colonize our mucosal surfaces and preventing them from entering the bloodstream

12. **Ans. (b) Light chain** *(Ref: Kubys Immunology pg 84)*

- All antibodies share a common structure of four polypeptide chains consisting of two identical **light (L) chains** and two identical **heavy (H) chains**.
- The two major light chain constant region sequences are referred to as **(kappa) or (lambda) chains** common in all the Antobodies.

13. **Ans. (a) Cat scratch disease** *(Ref: Robbins 9th/98)*

Cat-scratch disease causes rounded or stellate granuloma containing central granular debris and recognizable neutrophils; giant cells

14. **Ans. (c) HHV 8** *(Ref: Harrison 19th/697)*

Human herpesvirus 8 is associated with primary effusion lymphoma in HIV-infected persons and multicentric Castleman's disease, a diffuse lymphadenopathy associated with systemic symptoms of fever, malaise, and weight loss.

15. **Ans. (a.) Antigen presentation** *(Ref: Robbins 9th/198)*

Macrophages that have phagocytosed microbes and protein antigens process the antigens and present peptide fragments to T cells. **Upon activation, B lymphocytes proliferate and then differentiate into plasma cells that secrete different classes of antibodies with distinct functions**

16. **Ans. (d) EBV** *(Ref: Robbins 9th/pg 192-194)*

17. **Ans. (d) IgE** *(Ref: Kuby Immumology pg 298)*

Homocytotropic antibodies are antibodies which have a higher affinity to Fc-receptors of the cells of the animal species in which they are produced than to Fc-receptors of the cells of other animal species.

In humans, IgE antibodies belong to this group.

18. **Ans. (a) IgG1**

(Ref: Maternal, Fetal, & Neonatal Physiology: A Clinical Perspective; pg 484)

- All four **IgG subclasses cross**, although the IgG1 and IgG3 subclasses are predominate.
- IgG1 crosses earliest in pregnancy & is the primary immunoglobulin transferred before 28 weeks.
- IgG3 crosses later & does not reach maternal levels until after 32-33 weeks

19. **Ans. (c) 15-20**

(Ref: Chemical and Cellular Architecture edited by N.S. Abel Lajtha pg 423)

- Albumin constitutes 52-67% of serum protein
- IgG accounts for 15-18% of total plasma proteins but only 5-12% of total CSF protein

20. **Ans. (b) CR2** *(Ref: Robbins 9th/pg 191; 8th/pg 186)*

Epstein-Barr virus (EBV) enters B cells via CR2 (CD21)

21. **Ans. (b, c, e); b. Have perforins; c. Need thymus for development; e. Kills intracellular bacteria**

(Ref: Robbins 9th/pg 191; 8th/pg 186)

a. True, because of its morphology
b. False, CD8 T cells have perforins
c. False, T lymphocytes need thymus for development
d. True, CD16 is FcR of IgG
e. False, NK cells kill viruses & tumor infected cells

22. **Ans. (a, c, d, e); a. Pregnancy c. Multiple myeloma d. Polycythemia e. SLE** *(Ref: Harrison 19th)*

Patients with a high ESR (erythrocyte sedimentation rate) and normal C-reactive protein are those conditions without systemic inflammation such as malignancy.

- Some low-grade bone and joint infections by coagulase negative staphylococci)
- Systemic lupus erythematosus. (high levels of type 1 interferons which inhibit the production of C-reactive protein in hepatocytes)

Other conditions: Leukaemia, anaemia, polycythaemia, viral infection, ulcerative colitis, pregnancy, oestrogens or steroids.

23. **Ans. (a) NK cell**

(Ref: Wintrobe's clinical hematology - 12th ed, pg 300; Robbins 9th/pg 192; 8th/pg 188)

- Most lymphocytes in blood are small (≤10 μm), while some are large, known as **large granular lymphocytes (LGL),** as they contain **azurophilic granules** in their cytoplasm.
- These cells are LGL type of **natural killer (NK) cells.**

24. **Ans. (a) CD8** *(Ref: Robbins 9th/pg 191; 8th/pg 186)*

CD8

- Is a marker for **cytotoxic T cells**
- Acts as a **co-receptor** for TCR
- Binds to HLA-I to cause **cytotoxic effect** on **virus infected and tumor cells**

25. **Ans. (a) B-cells** *(Ref: Robbins 9th/pg 191; 8th/pg 187)*

26. **Ans. (b) IFN-ϒ** *(Ref: Robbins 9th/pg 210; 8th/pg 207)*

- **TH1 secrete IFN-γ → activates macrophages** ("classically activated"). Macrophages transform to **epithelioid cells which are** large epithelium-like cells with abundant cytoplasm.

27. **Ans. (b) IFN- ϒ** *(Ref: Robbins 9th/pg 210; 8th/pg 207)*

28. **Ans. (c)** **Microglia** *(Ref: Robbins 9th/pg 192; 8th/pg 188)*

Microglial cells are **modified macrophages of CNS**, hence they take part in **phagocytosis.**

29. **Ans. (c)** **Ileum**

(Ref: Wheater's Functional Histology: A Text and Colour Atlas 6th ed Pg 216)

- **MALT is most commonly** present in Peyer's patches in lamina propria of **ileum** & throughout small intestine

Components of MALT are sometimes subdivided into:

GALT	Gut-associated lymphoid tissue; Eg Peyer's patches found in the lining of the small intestines
BALT	Bronchus-associated lymphoid tissue
NALT	Nasal-associated lymphoid tissue
CALT	Conjunctival-associated lymphoid tissue
O-MALT	Organized mucosa-associated lymphatic tissue; Eg tonsils of Waldeyer's tonsillar ring
D-MALT	Diffuse mucosa-associated lymphatic tissue
LALT	Larynx-associated lymphoid tissue
SALT	Skin-associated lymphoid tissue

30. **Ans. (a, b, e);** **a. NK cells; b. Macrophages; e. Complements**

(Ref: Robbins 9th/pg 186-188; 8th/pg 184)

31. **Ans. (c)** **5-10** *(Ref: Robbins 9th/pg 192; 8th/pg 188)*

- **Natural Killer Cells or Null cells** constitute **5% to 10%** of peripheral lymphocytes[Q]
- As NK cells neither have B nor T-cell markers, hence also called **Null Cells**
- NK cells destroy irreversibly stressed, virus-infected cells & tumor cells **without prior exposure**

32. **Ans. (d)** **First line defense mechanism** *(Ref: R 9th/pg 191)*

a. True; It is present on all nucleated cells including antigen presenting cells as well as platelets
b. True; It activates cytotoxic T cell and kill virus infected cell
c. True; It is present on platelets also, which are non-nucleated cells
d. False; It is a part of adaptive immunity (second line defense mechanism)

33. **Ans. (d)** **CD21** *(Ref: Robbins 9th/pg 191; 8th/pg 186)*

34. **Ans. (c)** **Involved in Type 3 HSN**

(Ref: Robbins 9th/pg 210)

A. True	Monocytes in tissues are known as Macrophages
B. True	Macrophages engulf Mycobacteria but are not able to kill it; So they harbor Mycobacteria
C. False	Macrophages are involved in Type 4 Hypersensitivity & not type 3, which is immune-complex mediated
D. True	• Macrophages **secrete TNF, IL-1,** and **chemokines,** which promote inflammation • Macrophages also produce **IL-12,** thereby amplifying the **TH1 response**

35. **Ans. (b)** **IgG** *(Ref: Kuby Immunology)*

36. **Ans. (b)** **B-cells** *(Ref: Robbins 9th/pg 191; 8th/pg 187)*

B-cells have IgM and IgG on the surface of cells, which are used to identify them

37. **Ans. (b)** **Involve MHC antigen for killing micro-organisms** *(Ref: Robbins 9th/pg 192; 8th/pg 188)*

- **Natural Killer Cells Destroy** virus-infected cells and tumor cells **without prior exposure;**
- **NK cells do not require MHC for killing micro-organisms**
- **Surface molecules of NK cells are CD16 & CD56**

38. **Ans. (b, c, e);** **b. CD 3; c. CD 28; e. LCK**

(Ref: Robbins 9th/pg 191; 8th/pg 186)

A. CD 79b	**B-cell** development and B-cell function
B. CD 3	Activates **T cells** & helps in signal transduction
C. CD 28	Co-stimulatory receptor for T cells
D. CD 14	LPS-induced **activation of monocytes;** innate immunity
E. LCK	Tyrosine phosphorylation causing **T Cell Receptor stimulation & activation**

The table suggests that the activators of lymphocyte are: **CD3, CD28 and LCK**

39. **Ans. (b)** **Produce immunoglobulins** *(Ref: R 9th/pg 210)*

40. **Ans. (b, c, e)** **b. CD-19; c. CD-20; e. CD-79a**

(Ref: Robbins 9th/pg 191; 8th/pg 187)

B cell markers are **CD19 (most specific),** CD20, CD21, CD22, CD23, CD24, CD10, CD79a

41. **Ans. (d)** **Cytotoxic T cell** *(Ref: Robbins 9th/pg 191)*

Cytotoxic T lymphocytes (CTLs) kill **virus infected and tumor** cells

42. **Ans. (b)** **Dendritic cell**

Antigen Presenting cells; cells that present Ag to T-cells

- **Antigen-presenting cells (APCs) for initiating T-cell responses against protein antigens**[Q]
- **Mature dendritic cells are the most potent**[Q] **stimulator of Naive T-cells**

43. **Ans. (b)** **Antigen presenting cells**

44. **Ans. (b)** **B cells, Dendritic cells, NK cells**

(Ref: R 9/p 191)

45. **Ans. (a, c);** **a. Langerhan cells of skin; c. Macrophages**

46. **Ans. (d)** **C56789**

(Ref: Robbins and Cotran: Pathological basis of disease 8/e p64,89)

The deposition of the MAC (C5-C9) on cells makes these cells permeable to water and ions and results in death (lysis)

47.   **Ans. (a)**   **RBC**

As RBC lacks nucleus so lacks HLA

48.   **Ans. (b)**   **Thymocyte** *(Ref: Robbins 9th / pg 195-196)*

Actually thymic epithelial cells are Antigen presenting cells not thy mocytes
About M cells (in gut mucosa) or microfold (M) cells
- Unique morphological features include:
  - Presence of a **reduced glycocalyx**
  - Irregular brush border and reduced microvilli.
  - Highly specialized for the **phagocytosis and transcytosis** of gut lumen macromolecules, particulate antigens and patho genic or commensal microorganisms across epithelium

49.   **Ans. (b)**   **HBV**

(Ref: Harrison 19th/2010; J Med Virol. 2016 Mar; 88(3):371-9)

This Question is based on the concept that HBV-HLA-specific cytolytic T cell responses of the adaptive immune system are felt to be responsible for recovery from HBV infection
The observed findings from various studies are:
- *HLA-DR*03* and *HLA-DR*07* were associated with an increased risk of persistent HBV infection
- *HLA-DR*04* and *HLA-DR*13* were associated with clearance of HBV infection.

50.   **Ans. (b)**   **MHC 2** *(Ref: Robbins 9th/pg 192; 8th/pg 187)*

- **Dendritic cells** are the **most important antigen-presenting cells (APCs) for initiating T-cell responses against protein antigens**[Q], they express MHC-II

51.   **Ans. (a)**   **TNF alpha** *(Ref: Robbins 9th/pg 195; 8th/pg 191)*

MHC III: No direct role in immune system[Q]
- Codes for:
- **complement components** C2, C4, properdin, factor B[Q]
- TNF, HSP-70, Tyrosine hydroxylase

52.   **Ans. (b)**   **Dendritic cells (Ref: Robbins 9th/pg 192)**

53.   **Ans. (a)**   **Short arm of chr-6** *(Ref: Robbins 9th/pg 195)*

54.   **Ans. (c)**   **Class III codes for complement**

(Ref: Robbins 9th/pg 195)

55.   **Ans. (c)**   **Present antigens for recognition by T cell antigen receptors** *(Ref: Robbins 9th/pg 195; 8th/pg 191)*

HLA I and II display peptide fragments of protein antigens for recognition by antigen-specific T cells.

56.   **Ans. (d)**   **Neutrophils**

(Ref: Robbins 9th/pg 195; 8th/pg 191)

57.   **Ans. (a)**   **Macrophage; b. Dendritic cells; d. Epithelial cell** *(Ref: Robbins 9th/pg 195-196; 8th/pg 191-192)*

58.   **Ans. (b)**   **IL–4**

(Ref: Robbins 9th ed/pg 201)

59.   **Ans. (b)**   **IgE fixed cell**

(Ref: Robbins 9th ed/pg 201)

60.   **Ans. (c)**   **IL–4**

(Ref: Robbins 9th ed/pg 201)

61.   **Ans. (c)**   **IL–3**

(Ref: Robbins 9th ed/pg 198)

62.   **Ans. (b)**   **IL–2**

(Ref: Robbins 9th ed/pg 198)

63.   **Ans. (a)**   **CD4+ helper cell** *(Ref: Robbins 9th ed p 1209)*

CD4+ T helper (TH) cells may initiate the autoimmune response in Rheumatoid arthritis by reacting with an arthritogenic agent, perhaps microbial or a self-antigen. The T cells produce cytokines that stimulate other inflammatory cells to effect tissue injury.

64.   **Ans. (b)**   **Ag Ab reaction** *(Ref: Robbins 9th/205-206)*

65.   **Ans. (a)**   **Mast cell** *(Ref: Robbins 9th/pg 200; 8th/pg 198)*

Mast cells have Fc receptor for IgE; Antigen binding to it results in the activation of mast cells leading to type I hypersensitivity.

66.   **Ans. (b)**   **Hypersensitivity reaction with modified macrophages, lymphocytes and giant cells**

(Ref: Robbins 9th/pg 208-211; 8th/pg 204-208)

The given clinical features and radiological findings are suggestive of Tuberculosis in which histopathology of the affected organ shows granuloma, that consists of modified macrophages, lymphocytes and giant cells.

67.   **Ans. (b)**   **CD4 + T cells**

(Ref: Robbins 9th/pg 208; 8th/pg 204)

68.   **Ans. (a)**   **None of the options** *(Ref: Robbins 9th/pg 208)*

Shwartzman reaction is a **non-immunologic** phenomenon in which **endotoxin (lipopolysaccharide)** induces local & systemic reactions; It can either be local or systemic type.

69.   **Ans. (b)**   **Tumor necrosis factor**

(Ref: Robbins 9th/pg 198)

- **TNF and IL-1** are two of the major cytokines that mediate inflammation & are produced mainly by **activated macrophages.**

70.   **Ans. (b)**   **Type II**

(Ref: Textbook of Microbiology & Immunology by Subhash Chandra Parija, 2nd edition, 2012, pg 155)

- **Type V hypersensitivity** reaction is a **subtype of type II** hypersensitivity
- In type V hypersensitivity, antibodies combine with antigens on cell surface which induce cells to proliferate & enhances activity of effector cells; **E.g., Graves disease.**

71.   **Ans. (b)   Eosinophils**

(Ref: Robbins 9th/pg 200; 8th/pg 198)

72.   **Ans. (b)   Major Basic Protein**

(Ref: Robbins 9th/pg 200-204)

Out of the given options, most **important mediator of late phase of immediate type of hypersensitivity reaction is Major basic protein.**

73.   **Ans. (a)   IgG**   *(Ref: Robbins 9th/pg 205-206)*

- Antibodies in Immune thrombocytopenic purpura are of IgG type directed against gp Ib/IX and IIb/IIIa.
- These antibodies cause Type II hypersensitivity reaction.

74.   **Ans. (b)   Type II hypersensitivity**

(Ref: R 9th/pg 205-206)

Transfusion reaction and erythroblastosis fetalis are examples of Type II (antibody) mediated reactions.

75.   **Ans. (b)   Type II HSN**   *(Ref: Robbins 9th/pg 205-206)*

In the question, there are some clues to the diagnosis:

- Reaction **started 48 hrs after** taking penicillin: Rules out Immediate type I HSN
- **No prior history of allergy**: Again rules out Immediate HSN
- **Anti-penicillin antibody**: Shows Antibody (Humoral) type of reaction
- There are two type of HSN based on Antibodies: Type II and Type III
- **Hemolysis occurs in Type II HSN**
- So, clearly the answer is Type II HSN

76.   **Ans. (d)   Rh incompatibility**

(Ref: Robbins 9th/pg 205-206)

Examples of Antibody-Mediated Diseases (Type II Hyper-sensitivity) *Refer to pretext of this chapter*

77.   **Ans. (b)   Angioneurotic edema**   *(Ref: R 9th/pg 200-204)*

Hereditary angioedema or Angioneurotic edema

- **Autosomal dominant** disorder due to an underlying **deficiency of C1 inhibitor**
- C1 inhibitor is a protease inhibitor whose target enzymes are C1r & C1s of complement cascade, factor XII of the coagulation pathway, and the kallikrein system.
- Patients have episodes of edema affecting skin and mucosal surfaces such as larynx & GIT, swelling of lips
- May result in life-threatening asphyxia or nausea, vomiting & diarrhea after minor trauma or emotional stress.

78.   **Ans. (d)   IV**   *(Ref: Harrison 18th/chapter 166)*

Type 1 Lepra Reactions (Downgrading and Reversal Reactions)

- When type 1 lepra reactions **precede the initiation of antimicrobial therapy,** they are termed '**downgrading**' reactions, and the case becomes histologically more lepromatous;

- When they occur **after the initiation of therapy**, they are termed '**reversal' reactions**, and the case becomes more tuberculoid.
- **Edema** is the most characteristic microscopic feature of type 1 lepra lesions
- **Reversal reactions** are typified by a TH1 cytokine profile, with an influx of **CD4+ T helper cells** and increased levels of **IFNγ & IL-2; So it is an example of type IV hypersensitivity**

Type 2 Lepra Reactions: Erythema Nodosum Leprosum

- It is **immune complex mediated (type III hyper-sensitivity)**
- Occurs exclusively in patients near the **lepromatous** end of the leprosy spectrum (**BL-LL**)

79.   **Ans. (b)   Type II Hypersensitivity**

(Ref: R 9th/pg 205-206)

80.   **Ans. (b)   IgG Ab**   *(Ref: Robbins 9th/pg 200-204)*

Long-acting thyroid stimulator (LATS): IgG that stimulates thyroid function similar to but slower than TSH (i.e. long-acting)

81.   **Ans. (a)   Histamine**   *(Ref: Robbins 9th/pg 200-204)*

Histamine can cause Anaphylactic shock

82.   **Ans. (b)   Immune complexes**

Raji cell assay:

- A sensitive test for **detection & quantitation of soluble complement fixing immune complexes** in sera of patients.
- **Raji cells lack membrane-bound immunoglobulin** but have **receptors for IgG Fc, AHG** is used as an in vitro model of human immune complexes.
- The uptake by Raji cells is quantitated by I^{125}-**radiolabeled antihuman IgG.**

83.   **Ans. (a, b, c, d, e)   a. Interferon-1 (IFN-1); b. Interferon-1 (IFN-1); c. Exposure to UV rays; d. Deficiency of early complement factors; e. Failure of self-tolerance in B cells** *(Ref: Robbins 9th ed/pg 218)*

84.   **Ans. (b)   Raynaud phenomenon and sclerodactyly**

(Ref: R9/p 226)

Patterns in Anti-Nuclear Antibody (ANA) testing

Diffuse or homogenous	dsDNA, histone	SLE, DLE
Rim/peripheral	Ds DNA	SLE
Speckled	Sm	SLE
	SS-A, SS-B	Sjogren syndrome
Nucleolar	Nucleolar RNA	Scleroderma

85.   **Ans. (b)   AIRE**   *(Ref: R 9/p 213)*

The process in the questions refers to Central tolerance, where the self reacting T cells are presented to the thymus to prevent autoimmunity. A protein called AIRE (autoimmune regulator) stimulates expression of few "peripheral tissue-restricted" self antigens in the thymus. This causes deletion of immature T cells specific for these antigens and so is able to prevent autoimmunity.

86.   Ans. (b)   AIRE *(Ref: Robbins 9th/216)*

Mutations in the AIRE gene are the cause of an autoimmune-polyendocrinopathy

87.   Ans. (b, c) b. Histoplasmosis c. Cryptococcosis

(Ref: Harshmohan 7th/155; Robbins (SEA) 9th/ 693)

Schaumann bodies are calcium and protein inclusions inside of Langhans giant cells as part of a granuloma.
Seen in:
- Sarcoidosis,
- Hypersensitivity pneumonitis, and
- Berylliosis.
- Crohn's disease and tuberculosis

88.   Ans. (b)   Seminiferous tubules

(Ref: Robbins 9th/pg 214)

89.   Ans. (a)   Ulcerative colitis *(Ref: Robbin 9th/pg 214-215)*

90.   Ans. (a)   Anti-nuclear *(Ref: Robbins 9th/pg 218-221)*

91.   Ans. (d)   Anti-histone *(Ref: Robbins 9th/pg 218-221)*

92.   Ans. (b)   Erosive arthritis *(Ref: Robbin 9th/pg 218)*

Non-erosive arthritis is a feature of SLE

93.   Ans. (c)   Lip *(Ref: Robbins 9th/pg 218; 8th/pg 213)*

94.   Ans. (a)   Anti-DNA topoisomerase

(Ref: Robbins 9th/pg 218)

95.   Ans. (d)   Anti-Ribonucleoprotein

(Ref: Robbins 9th/pg 218; 8th/pg 213)

Autoantibodies in Sjogren's syndrome:
- **Anti SS-A (Ro)** and **SS-B (La)^Q:** Most important, present in 90% patients;
- High titers of Anti SS-A → more likely to have **early disease onset, longer disease duration**, and **extra-glandular manifestations** (eg cutaneous vasculitis and nephritis)
- **Rheumatoid factor** (an antibody reactive with self IgG): in 75%^{Q}, **ANA:** in 50% to 80%

96.   Ans. (d)   Diffuse sclerosing lupus nephritis

(Ref: Robbins 9th/pg 218; 8th/pg 213)

97.   Ans. (a)   Systemic lupus erythematosus

(Ref: R 9th/pg 218)

98.   Ans. (c)   Systemic lupus erythematosus

(Ref: Robbins 9th/pg 218)

99.   Ans. (b)   Diffuse Proliferative *(Ref: Robbins 9th/pg 218)*

100.   Ans. (b)   Systemic lupus erythematosus

(Ref: Robbins 9th/pg 218; 8th/pg 213)

101.   Ans. (b)   Anti-Ro (SS-A) *(Ref: Robbins 9th/pg 218)*

102.   Ans. (c)   Diffuse proliferative glomerulonephritis

(Ref: Robbins 9th/pg 218; 8th/pg 213)

103.   Ans. (b)   Drug induced lupus *(Ref: Robbins 9th/pg 218)*

104.   Ans. (c)   Erosions seen on X-rays

(Ref: Robbins 9th/pg 218)

105.   Ans. (a)   Anti-Topoisomerase I antibody

(Ref: Robbins 9th/pg 218; 8th/pg 213)

106.   Ans. (d)   Nephritis

(Ref: Robbins 9th/pg 218; 8th/pg 213)

Nephritis is usually the most serious manifestation of SLE, particularly because nephritis and infection are the leading causes of mortality in the first decade of disease.

107.   Ans. (a)   More common in females

(Ref: Robbins 9th/pg 218; 8th/pg 213)

Drug-Induced Lupus

- It is a syndrome of positive ANA associated with symptoms such as fever, malaise, arthritis or intense arthralgias/myalgias, serositis, and/or rash.
- It appears during therapy with certain medications like antiarrhythmics procainamide, disopyramide, and propafenone; antihypertensive hydralazine; antithyroid propylthiouracil; antipsychotics chlorpromazine and lithium; anticonvulsants carbamazepine and phenytoin; antibiotics isoniazid, minocycline & nitrofurantoin; antirheumatic sulfasalazine; diuretic hydrochlorothiazide;
- It is predominant in whites & has less female predilection than SLE
- It rarely involves kidneys or brain, is rarely associated with anti-dsDNA, is commonly associated with antibodies to histones
- It usually resolves over several weeks after discontinuation of the offending medication.

108.   Ans. (b)   Rheumatoid arthritis *(Ref: Robbins 9th/pg 218)*

109.   Ans. (a)   Esophagus *(Ref: Robbins 9th/pg 218; 8th/pg 213)*

110.   Ans. (c)   Limited scleroderma *(Ref: Robbins 9th/pg 228)*

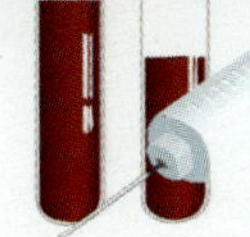

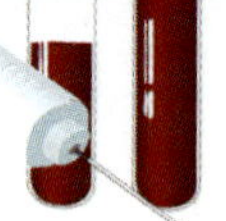

111. Ans. (b) pqrs = ywzx

(Ref: Robbins 9th/pg 228; 8th/pg 223)

112. Ans. (c) Rheumatoid arthritis *(Ref: Robbins 9th/pg 231)*

Mixed connective tissue disease
- Clinical features are a mixture of the features of **SLE, systemic sclerosis, and polymyositis.**
- Elevated **anti-U1 ribonucleoprotein Ab**[Q]
- Presentation: Synovitis of fingers, Raynaud phenomenon, mild myositis, renal involvement

113. Ans. (a) Anti U1-RNP Ab (Ref: Robbins 9th/pg 231)

114. Ans. (b) SLE *(Ref: Dubois' Lupus Erythematosus pg 542)*

Lupus Band test
- A diagnostic procedure used **to detect deposits of immunoglobulins and complement** components along the **dermo-epidermal junction** in patients with SLE & cutaneous lupus
- It is **positive in about 70%–80% of sun-exposed** & 55% of sun-protected **non-lesional skin specimens** obtained from patients with SLE

115. Ans. (a) Anti ds DNA *(Ref: Robbins 9th/pg 218-221)*

116. Ans. (c) HLA-CW6 *(Ref: Robbins 9th/pg 215)*

Role of Susceptibility Genes: Association of HLA Alleles with Disease; Refer to pretext of this chapter

Disease	Marker
• Ankylosing spondylitis[Q]	**B27**[Q]
• Reiter's syndrome[Q]	**B27**[Q]
• Acute anterior uveitis	B27
• Reactive arthritis[Q]	**B27**[Q]
• Psoriatic spondylitis	B27
• Juvenile arthritis, pauciarticular	DR8, DR5
• **Rheumatoid arthritis**[Q]	**DR4** (DRB1*04)[Q]
• **Sjögren's syndrome**[Q]	**DR3**[Q]
• (celiac disease)[Q]	**DQ2/DQ8**[Q]
• Chronic active hepatitis	DR3
• Dermatitis herpetiformis	DR3
• Psoriasis vulgaris	**Cw6**[Q]
• Pemphigus vulgaris	**DR4, DQ1**[Q]
	DQ7
• Type 1 diabetes mellitus	**DQ8, DR4, DR3,**
• Hyperthyroidism (Graves')	**DR2**[Q]
• Adrenal insufficiency	B8, DR3
	DR3
• Myasthenia gravis	**B8, DR3**[Q]
• Multiple sclerosis	DR2
• Behçet's disease	B51
• Congenital adrenal hyperplasia	B47
• **Good-pasture's syndrome**	**DR2**[Q]
• Thromboangitis obliterans	B5

117. Ans. (d) Anti-histone antibody *(Ref: R 9th/pg 218-221)*

118. Ans. (c) HLA-B51 *(Ref: Robbins 9th/pg 215)*

119. Ans. (b) HLA-DR4 *(Ref: Robbins 9th/pg 215)*

HLA-DR4 (DR4) is an HLA-DR serotype that recognizes the DRB1*04 gene products.

120. Ans. (c) HLA-B5 *(Ref: Robbins 9th/pg 215)*

121. Ans. (b) RA *(Ref: Harrison 18th/chapter 321, 323)*

Antibodies seen **in RA** are **rheumatoid factors** (RFs) and **anti–cyclic citrullinated peptides** (CCP) antibodies
ANA is seen in:
- Almost **all (>95%) cases of SLE**
- In virtually **all patients with SSc** (Systemic sclerosis)
- **50% to 80% cases of Sjogren** syndrome

122. Ans. (d) Ankylosing spondylitis

(Ref: Harrison 18th/chapter 325)
Prevalence of HLA B27 is 90% in patients with Ankylosing Spondylitis, independent of disease severity.

123. Ans. (b) Antibodies to GQ1B

(Ref: Harrison 18th/chapter 385)

Miller Fisher syndrome (MFS)
- It is a **variant of GBS**, which presents as **rapidly evolving ataxia and areflexia** of limbs **without weakness**
- **Ophthalmoplegia, often with pupillary paralysis** is present.
- Accounts for **5% of all cases of GBS (Guillain Barre syndrome)**
- Is strongly associated with **antibodies to the ganglioside GQ1b**

124. Ans. (c) Class III *(Ref: Robbins 9th/pg 222-223)*

Focal proliferative glomerulonephritis (class III lupus nephritis)
- It is seen **in 20-35% of patients**, and is defined by **fewer than 50% involvement of all glomeruli.**
- Lesions **may be segmental** (affecting only a portion of glomerulus) or **global** (involving entire glomerulus).
- Affected glomeruli may exhibit **crescent** formation, **fibrinoid necrosis, proliferation of endothelial & mesangial** cells, infiltrating **leukocytes**, and **eosinophilic deposits** or **intracapillary thrombi**, which often correlate with **hematuria and proteinuria.**

125. Ans. (a) Anti-ds-DNA *(Ref: Robbins 9th/pg 218-221)*

The given clinical features are suggestive of SLE;
- **Specific test** for diagnosis of SLE is **anti ds DNA;**
- This antibody also **correlates with disease activity, nephritis, vasculitis.**
- So Anti-dsDNA should be initially assayed in this case.

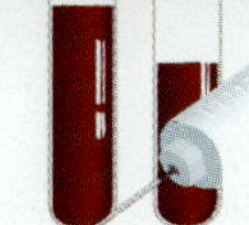

126. Ans. (a, b, d); a. Proliferation of endothelium; b. Glomerular leukocyte infiltration; d. Epithelial cell proliferation (Ref: Harrison 18th/chapter 319)

Active nephritis in SLE includes:
- **Focal proliferative** lupus nephritis
- **Diffuse segmental proliferative** lupus nephritis &
- **Diffuse global proliferative** lupus nephritis
- So, **proliferation of endothelium, glomerular leukocyte infiltration & epithelial cell proliferation** are **features of active nephritis;**
- Mesangial alterations may or may not be present;
- **Tubulitis is not a feature of lupus nephritis;**

127. Ans. (a, b, c, d); a. Interstial Fibrosis; b. Shrinking lung syndrome; c. Alveolar hemorrhage; d. Pulmonary arterial hypertension

(Ref: Robbins 9th/pg 218; 8th/pg 214) Refer to pretexts.

128. Ans. (b, d) b. Antibody to RNA; d. Systemic sclerosis

(Ref: Robbins 9th/pg 219; 8th/pg 215)

Antinuclear antibodies:
- They are **directed against nuclear antigens**.
- The most widely used method for detecting ANAs is **indirect immunofluorescence**, which can identify antibodies that bind to a variety of nuclear antigens, including **DNA, RNA, and proteins**
- The **pattern of nuclear fluorescence suggests the type of antibody present** in the patient's serum.

Four basic patterns are recognized:

Staining Pattern	Antibodies & their Characteristics
Homogeneous or diffuse nuclear staining	Antibodies to **chromatin, histones & occasionally, double-stranded DNA**.
Rim or peripheral staining	Antibodies to **double-stranded DNA**
Speckled pattern	Presence of uniform or variable-sized speckles. Antibodies to **non-DNA nuclear constituents**. Eg Antibody to **Sm antigen, ribonucleoprotein, SS-A & SS-B antigens**.
Nucleolar pattern	Presence of a few discrete **spots of fluorescence within the nucleus** Represents **antibodies to RNA** Seen most often in patients with **systemic sclerosis**.

129. Ans. (b) Lymphocytes *(Ref: Robbins 9th/pg 226-227)*

130. Ans. (a, b, e) a. DRB1; b. DR1; e. DR4

(Ref: Harrison 18th/chapter 321)

In **Rheumatoid Arthritis**, some of the **HLA-DRB1 alleles** bestow a **high risk of disease (*0401)**, whereas others confer a more **moderate risk (*0101, *0404, *1001 & *0901)**.
HLA-DR4 (DR4) is a **HLA-DR serotype that recognizes the DRB1*04** gene products.

131. Ans. (b) Anti-ds DNA antibodies

(Ref: Harrison 18th/chapter 319)

- **Anti dsDNA** is **specific for SLE**, only **in high titers;**
- But still, **anti ds DNA is the best marker for SLE** because its **prevalence in SLE is 70%;**
- Whereas, **Anti Sm antibody**, which is **specific for SLE**, but is **seen in only 25% patients with SLE**

132. Ans. (c) Isograft

133. Ans. (c) Allograft

Transplantation between same species is allograft

134. Ans. (d) Donor T cells

Immunocompetent Donor T cells destroy immunosuppressed recipient cells in GVHD

135. Ans. (a) 12 hours *(Ref: Robbins 9th ed p 233)*

Hyperacute rejection occurs when preformed antidonor antibodies are present in the circulation of the recipient. This form of rejection occurs within minutes or hours after transplantation. A hyperacutely rejecting kidney rapidly becomes cyanotic, mottled, and flaccid, and may excrete a mere few drops of bloody urine. Immunoglobulin and complement are deposited in the vessel wall, causing endothelial injury and fibrin-platelet thrombi.

136. Ans. (d) Transfer hepatic progenitor cells (HPCs) of same person for regeneration

(Ref: Nature Cell Biology 17, 971–983 (2015)

Hepatocytes and cholangiocytes self-renew following liver injury. But after severe injury like **cirrhosis** and **acute liver failure** hepatocytes are increasingly senescent. In this case there are two options: first diseased-donor liver and living-donor transplantation, in which a just portion of a healthy donor's liver is used for transplantation or second hepatic progenitor cells (HPCs), which contribute significantly to restoration of liver parenchyma, regenerating hepatocytes and biliary epithelia, highlighting their *in vivo* lineage potency. The best option is D among the options.

137. Ans. (a) Irradiation *(Ref: Wintrobes 13th/704-705)*

- Irradiation with a dose of 2,500 cGy at the center of the irradiation field, with a minimum dose of 1,500 cGy at any point in the field **inhibits proliferation of donor lymphocytes** but has no significant adverse effect on red cell, platelet, or granulocyte function.
- It should be noted that though the other options are also effectice in reducing the leukocytes but they do not completely deplete the lymphocytes and so can cause GVHD.

138. Ans. (d) C4d *(Ref: Robbins 9th/234)*

Acute antibody-mediated rejection is manifested mainly by damage to glomeruli and small blood vessels. Typically, the lesions consist of inflammation of glomeruli and peritubular capillaries, associated with deposition of the complement breakdown product C4d, which is produced during activation of the complement system by the antibody dependent classical pathway

139. Ans. (d) HLA DP *(Ref: Harrison 18th/chapter 282)*

- **In kidney transplants, polymorphic** HLA alleles are at **least 50 % matched** (HLA-A, -B & DR)

140. Ans. (c) Biopsy *(Ref: Harrison 18th/chapter 282)*

141. Ans. (b) Matched, related donors

(Ref: AIIMS, Transplant immunology Protocol; Kidney transplant principle & practise pg 156)

Important terminologies for Donors in transplant immunology:
- **Matched Donor:** HLA allelic identity at HLA A, B, C and DRB1 loci which is referred as 8/8match. (These 4 HLA antigens have 2 alleles each that makes it 8)
- **Related Donor:** Siblings from same parents who is HLA matched for HLA A, B, DRB1 minimum at the antigen level.

So obviously, the answer here is matched related donor.

142. Ans. (b) 5-10

(Ref: AIIMS, Transplant immunology Protocol)

For different types of transplantation, different criteria are followed for HLA matching:

Organs	Minimum Matching	Matching done at
Bone Marrow	100% (8/8)	A,B,C DRB1
Kidney	50% (3/6)	A,B,DR
Liver/Heart	0% (0/6)	–
Cornea	0% (0/6)	–

Note: In liver, heart transplantation; practical considerations (ischemic times, availability of donors, clinical need of recipients) makes HLA matching less important.
- **HLA-DR mismatches** are the **most important** in the **first 6 months** after transplantation.
- **HLA-B** effect emerges in the **first 2 years.**
- **HLA-A** mismatches have a deleterious effect on **long-term graft survival**.

143. Ans. (b) Renal involvement *(Ref: Robbins 9th/pg 231)*

144. Ans. (c) Matched

(Ref: AIIMS, Transplant immunology Protocol)

Best tissue matches are **HLA A, B, DR** identical referred to as **"000 mismatch"** (100% matching which is 6/6 match). Any mismatch is referred to as **1 like "100, 010, 110"**

145. Ans. (c) Blood vessel thrombosis

(Ref: Robbins 9th/pg 231; 8th/pg 221); Refer to pretexts

146. Ans. (c) Both *(Ref: Robbins 9th/pg 231-234)*

147. Ans. (a) All nucleated cells *(Ref: Robbins 9th/pg 195)*

Properties	Class I MHC Molecules	Class II MHC Molecules
Location	**All nucleated cells and platelets**[Q]	**APCs**: B cells, dendritic cells, endothelial cells & fibroblasts[Q]

148. Ans. (b) T-lymphocyte *(Ref: Robbins 9th/pg 189)*

149. Ans. (d) Zero HLA mismatch with recipient

(Ref: Harrison 18th/chapter 282)

Donor for kidney transplantation:
- Donors can be **deceased or volunteer living donors**.
- Living donors are usually family members who have **at least partial compatibility for HLA** antigens.
- **At least 50% HLA match (3/6) is a must requirement** for kidney transplant
- Living volunteer donors should be **normal on physical examination**
- Should have the **same major ABO blood group**, because crossing major blood group barriers prejudices survival of the allograft.
- Should have **two normally functioning kidneys**
- Donor **should be free of malignant neoplastic disease, hepatitis, and HIV**

150. Ans. (b) Delayed type hypersensitivity

(Ref: Robbins 9th/pg 231-234; 8th/pg 221-229; Refer Ans 200)

Types of Rejection Pathway:
- **Direct pathway**: **CD4 and CD8-T** cells of the transplant recipient recognize allogeneic (donor) MHC molecules on the surface of APCs in the graft.
- **Indirect pathway:** recipient **CD4-T lymphocytes** recognize MHC antigens of the graft donor after they are presented by the recipient's own APCs.

As both the pathways are **cell mediated**, hence they are **delayed hypersensitivity** reactions.

151. Ans. (a) Preformed antibodies *(Ref: R 9th/pg 231-234)*

152. Ans. (d) Kidney *(Ref: Robbins 9th/pg 236; 8th/pg 230)*

In Acute GVH disease:
Immune system and epithelia of the skin, liver & intestines are mainly involved.

153. Ans. (b) Isograft *(Ref: Robbins 9th/pg 231-234)*

***Types of grafts*[Q]**
- **Autografts**[Q]: transplant of individual own organ
- **Isograft:** Graft from identical twin
- **Allografts**[Q]: between individuals of the same species
- **Xenografts**[Q]: grafts from one species to another species

154. Ans. (b) Lungs *(Ref: Robbins 9th/pg 236)*

155. Ans. (c) Hyper IgM syndrome

(Ref: Robbins 9th/pg 241; Wintrobe 13th/pg 342)

156. Ans. (d) BTK

(Ref: Robbins 9th/pg 239)

157. **Ans. (a) Uveitis**

158. **Ans. (d) Chediak-Higashi syndrome**

   (Ref: Robbins 9th/pg 237)

159. **Ans. (a, b, d) a. Autosomal recessive; b. Part of SCID; d. Leads to abnormal CD4T cell development**

   Bare lymphocyte syndrome is a condition caused by mutations in certain genes of the major histocompatibility complex or involved with the processing and presentation of MHC molecules, so there is abnormal T cell development. It is a form of severe combined immunodeficiency

160. **Ans. (d) B cell defect** *(Ref: R 9TH/P 24)*

   DiGeorge syndrome is a T-cell deficiency that results from failure of development of the third and fourth pharyngeal pouches.

161. **Ans. (a) Non homologous disjunction repair**

   (Ref: Wintrobes 14th/pg 333)
   DNA-PK (DNA-dependent protein kinase) complex consists of a catalytic subunit (DNA-Pkcs) and a DNA-binding complex called Ku, which binds altered DNA structures such as double-strand breaks, nicks, or hairpin loops. Recombination of broken DNA strands occurs either between strands that have long stretches of homology (homologous recombination) or between DNA strand breaks without relying on the presence of considerable homology between them. This recombination is known as nonhomologous end joining (NHEJ). Mutations in this system result in the accumulation of V(D)J-specific double-strand breaks, indicating a defective repair mechanism, which causes SCID.

162. **Ans. (a, b, c, d) a. Severe combined immunodeficiency; b. Adenosine deaminase deficiency; c. Wiskott-Aldrich syndrome; d. Ataxia telangiectasia**

163. **Ans. (c) Both**

   (Ref: Robbins 9th/pg 239-240; 8th/pg 234-235)
   Defect in Common Variable Immunodeficiency is mainly Defect in receptor for a cytokine called BAFF causing defect in survival and differentiation of B cells defect in T-cell activation & interactions b/w T & Bcells

164. **Ans. (b) SCID**

   (Ref: HENRY'S Clinical Diagnosis and Management by Laboratory Methods; 22ned ed/ pg 944-945)

   Lymphocyte phenotyping for assessing immune deficiency includes CD3 (pan T cell), CD4 (T helper subset), CD8 (T cytotoxic/suppressor subset), CD19 (pan B cell), CD 16/56 (pan NK cell) and other cell surface markers as required based on clinical data. This analysis is indicated in diagnosis and monitoring of immunodeficiencies and immunotherapy in children and adults

165. **Ans. (c) GVHD** *(Ref: Robbins 9th/pg 236; 8th/pg 230)*

   - Patients with SCID have the most severe immunodeficiency.

- Affected infants also lack the ability to reject foreign tissue and are therefore at risk for severe or fatal graft-versus host disease (GVHD) from T lymphocytes in non-irradiated blood products or in allogeneic stem cell transplants.

166. **Ans. (a) SCID; c. Wiskott-Aldrich syndrome**

   (Ref: Robbins 9th/pg 239-240; 8th/pg 234-235)

   Mucocutaneous candidiasis is seen in DiGeorge Syndrome (Thymic Hypoplasia), which is a predominant T cell defect;

167. **Ans. (a) Neutrophilia**

   (Ref: Nelson 19 pg 744; Robbins 9th/pg 238; 8th/pg 55)

   Neutropenia rather than neuprophilia is seen in Chediak Higashi Syndrome

168. **Ans. (d) Cryptosporidium**

169. **Ans. (b) Enfuvirtide is not active against HIV-2, (d) More commonly transmitted from mother to child, (e) HIV-1 worsens faster than HIV-2**

   (Ref: Robbins 9th/pg 243)

   In the United States, the first case of HIV-2 infection was diagnosed in 1987 in a West African woman who presented with central nervous system toxoplasmosis

   Difference between HIV-1 and 2: HIV-2 infection –
   - **Not transmitted as efficiently** as HIV-1ℚ
   - Progression to AIDS **takes longer**
   - **Slower rate of CD4 cell decline** and viral replication
   - Rarely causes vertical transmission

170. **Ans. (a) Kaposi's sarcoma** *(Ref: Robbins 9th/pg 253)*

171. **Ans. (a) 1983** *(Ref: Robbins 9th/pg 243; 8th/pg 236)*

   History of HIV:

Year	HIV linked developments
1981	AIDS was first recognized in the United States by U.S. Centers for Disease Control and Prevention (CDC).
1983	HIV isolated from a patient with lymphadenopathy (HIV 1st discovered)
1984	HIV demonstrated as causative agent of AIDS
1985	Enzyme-linked immunosorbent assay (ELISA) was developed to diagnose HIV

172. **Ans. (a) CMV** *(Ref: Robbins 9th/pg 246; 8th/pg 239)*

   In HIV infection with:
   CD4+ T cell counts <200/uL → high risk of disease from *P. jiroveci*
   CD4+ T cell counts <50/uL → high risk of disease from CMV, *M. avium* complex (MAC), and/or *T. gondii*
   Intramuclear parophillic incluria is seen with CMV

173. **Ans. (d, e); d. Primary lymphoma of brain; e. Invasive cancer of uterine cervix** *(Ref: Robbins 9th/pg 253)*

The neoplastic diseases considered to be AIDS-defining conditions are **Kaposi's sarcoma, non-Hodgkin's lymphoma, and invasive cervical carcinoma.**

In addition, there is also an increase in the incidence of a variety of **non-AIDS-defining malignancies:**

- Hodgkin's disease;
- Multiple myeloma;
- Leukemia;
- Melanoma; and
- Cervical, brain, testicular, oral, lung, gastric, liver, renal, and anal cancers

174. Ans. (b) Helper T cells *(Ref: Robbins 9th/pg 246-249)*

gp120 receptors on HIV binds to host cell receptors (CD4) on[Q]
- **T-Lymphocytes (helper T cells)**
- **Macrophages**
- **Dendritic cells**
- Other Antigen presenting cells

175. Ans. (d) Both lost *(Ref: Robbins 9th/pg 246)*

176. Ans. (a) Lentivirus *(Ref: Robbins 9th/pg 246; 8th/pg 240)*

177. Ans. (a) HIV 2 is more pathogenic than HIV 1

(Ref: Robbins 9th/pg 246; 8th/pg 240)

178. Ans. (e) Ankylostoma duodenale infection

(Ref: Harrison 19th/pg 1215)

179. Ans. (a) HIV-1M *(Ref: Robbins 9th/pg 246-249)*

Causative organism: HIV (*Human immunodeficiency virus*)
- **HIV-1 group M subtypes C predominant in India, fastest spreading[Q]**
- HIV-1 group M subtypes B predominant in U.S

180. Ans. (a, b, c, d); a. Hepatosplenomegaly; b. Congestive heart failure; c. Proteinuria; d. Lytic bone lesions

(Ref: Robbins 9th/pg 257-60)

181. Ans. (a, b, c, d); a. True, b. True, c. True, d. False, it shows wild type of ATTR.

(Ref: Robbins 9th/pg 257-60)

182. Ans. (a, b, c, d,) a. Bronchiectasis; b. Pulmonary TB; c. Lung abscess; d. Malignancy

183. Ans. (d) Amyloid fibrils

(Ref: Histopathology Guy Orchard, Brian Nation ; pg 70)

Congo Red dye forms non-polar hydrogen bonds with amyloid and red to green birefringence occurs when viewed by polarised light due to parallel alignment of the dye molecules on the linearly arranged amyloid fibrils.

184. Ans. (c) Apple green birefringence on polarizing microscopy *(Ref: Robbins 9th/pg 257-260; 8th/pg 250-253)*

185. Ans. (b) Congo red *(Ref: Robbins 9th/pg 257-260)*

186. Ans. (c) Aβ2

(Ref: Robbins 9th/pg 257-260; 8th/pg 250-253)

187. Ans. (c) Mutant form transthyretin is deposited

(Ref: Robbins 9th/pg 257-260; 8th/pg 250-253)

188. Ans. (d) Rectum *(Ref: Robbins 9th/pg 257-260)*

Sites of biopsy for diagnosis of Amyloidosis:
- **Rectal biopsy**-Most specific and best site
- **Abdominal fat aspirate**
- Gingival biopsy
- Organ specific biopsy for localized amyloidosis

189. Ans. (a) Normal transthyretin *(Ref: R 9th/pg 257-260)*

This is an example of senile amyloidosis in which unmutated (normal) transthyretin is deposited.

190. Ans. (c) Amyloidosis *(Ref: Robbins 9th/pg 257-260)*

191. Ans. (a) Congo red + polarized microscopy

(Ref: Robbins 9th/pg 257-260; 8th/pg 250-253)

192. Ans. (b) This electron microscope structure is not identical in all types of amyloid.

(Ref: Robbins 9th/pg 257-260; 8th/pg 250-253)

193. Ans. (d) Medullary *(Ref: Robbins 9th/pg 260; 8th/pg 253)*

Microscopically, medullary carcinomas:

- Composed of polygonal to spindle-shaped cells, which may form nests, trabeculae, and even follicles.
- Acellular **amyloid deposits**, derived from altered calcitonin polypeptides, are present in the adjacent stroma in many cases.
- Calcitonin is readily demonstrable within the cytoplasm of the tumor cells as well as in the stromal amyloid by immunohistochemical methods.

194. Ans. (c) Congo red *(Ref: Robbins 9th/pg 257-260)*

195. Ans. (c) Amyloidosis *(Ref: Robbins 9th/pg 257-260)*

196. Ans. (a) AL *(Ref: Robbins 9th/pg 257-260)*

- **AL** protein is made of complete **Ig light chains**, amino-terminal fragments of light chains, or both.
- Most of the AL proteins are composed of λ light chains or their fragments, but in some cases κ chains
- The amyloid fibril protein of the AL type is produced from free Ig light chains secreted by a monoclonal population of plasma cells, like multiple myeloma.

197. Ans. (b) Made of calcified proteins

(Ref: Robbins 9th/pg 257-260; 8th/pg 250-253)

- **Amyloid is a pathological proteinaceous substance deposited between cells** in various tissues and organs of the body in a variety of clinical settings.

In polarized light, amyloid shows Apple-green birefringence on Congo Red staining

- **Chronic infections like Tuberculosis & Osteomyelitis may show Amyloidosis**

198.   Ans. (a)   Amyloid Associated Protein

(Ref: Harrison 18th/chapter 112)

- In **secondary amyloidosis associated with chronic diseases**, there is deposition of **SAA** or AA
- **AA does not have structural homology to immuno-globulins**.
- **Derived by proteolysis** from a larger precursor in the serum called **SAA (serum amyloid–associated)** protein that is **synthesized in liver** and circulates in association with high density lipoproteins.
- Production of SAA protein is **increased in inflammatory states** as part of the **"acute phase response,"** and is often called **secondary amyloidosis.**

199.   Ans. (d)   Carpal tunnel *(Ref: Harrison 18th/chapter 112)*

200.   Ans. (a)   Primary systemic amyloidosis

(Ref: Harrison 18th/chapter 112)

- **Cutaneous lesions** associated with **primary systemic amyloidosis** are often **pink** in color and translucent.
- Common locations are **face, especially periorbital** and **perioral** regions, and **flexural areas.**
- On biopsy, **homogeneous deposits of amyloid are seen in the dermis** and in the **walls of blood vessels;**
- These deposits lead to an **increase in vessel wall fragility.**
- As a result, petechiae and purpura develop in clinically normal or abnormal skin following minor trauma, hence the term **pinch purpura.**

201.   Ans. (d)   Beta 2 microglobulin

(Ref: Harrison 18th/chapter 112)

202.   Ans. (a)   Mutated transthyretin

(Ref: Robbins 9th/pg 259; 8th/pg 252)

203.   Ans. (b)   Cardiac failure *(Ref: Harrison 18th/chapter 112)*

204.   Ans. (b)   Hemodialysis associated *(Ref: R 9th/pg 259)*

205.   Ans. (a)   Rectal biopsy *(Ref: Robbins 9th/pg 257-260)*

206.   Ans. (c)   Familial Mediterranean fever; e. Systemic senile amyloidosis *(Ref: Harrison 18th/chapter 112)*

Familial forms of amyloidosis: Familial Mediterranean fever:
- **Autosomal recessive** condition
- **"Autoinflammatory"** syndrome associated with abnormally high production of the cytokine IL-1
- **Attacks of fever** accompanied by inflammation of serosal surfaces (peritoneum, pleura & synovial membrane).
- The gene for familial Mediterranean fever encodes **a protein called *pyrin*** (for its relation to fever)
- The amyloid fibril proteins are made up of **AA proteins**, suggesting that this form of amyloidosis is related to the recurrent bouts of inflammation.

Familial amyloidotic polyneuropathies:
- **Autosomal dominant** familial disorder
- Characterized by deposition of amyloid predominantly in **peripheral and autonomic nerves**.
- In these genetic disorders, the fibrils are made up of **mutant TTRs**

207.   Ans. (a)   Congo red; b. Thioflavin; e. PAS

(Ref: Robbins 9th/pg 257-260; 8th/pg 250-253)

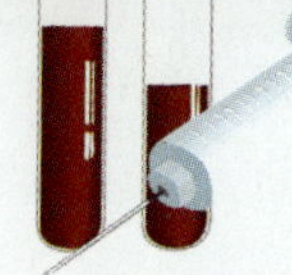

Note

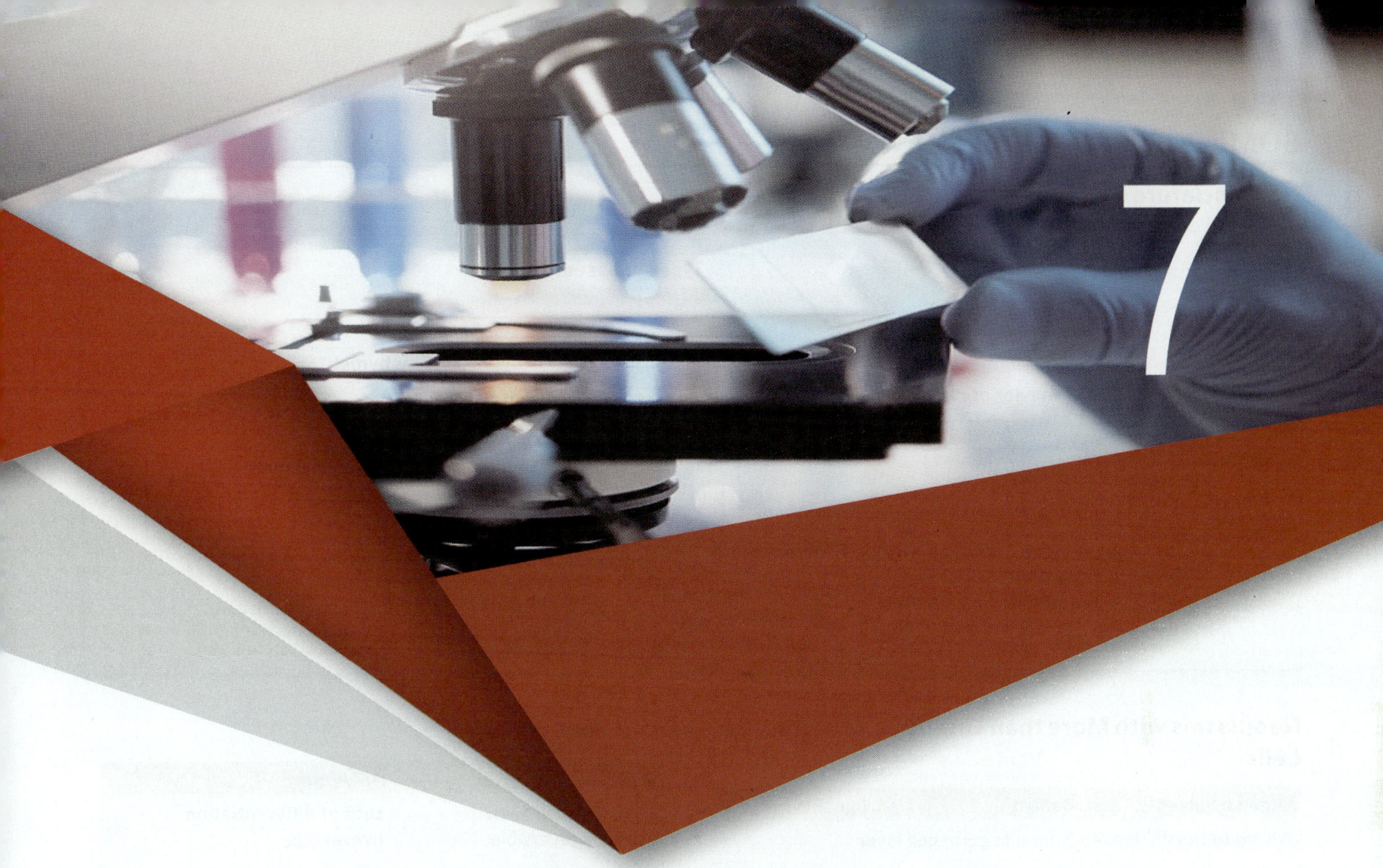

7

Neoplasia

SOME IMPORTANT TERMINOLOGIES

Nomenclature of Neoplasms of Differentiated Cells

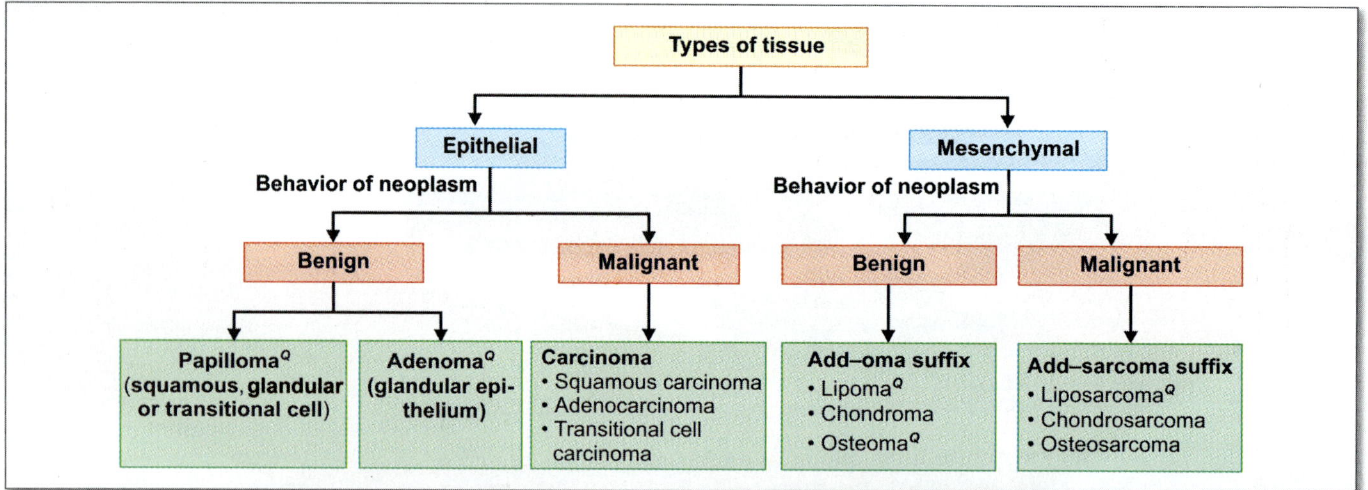

Neoplasms with More than One Type of Neoplastic Cells

Organ involved	Benign	Malignant
Mixed tumors[Q]: Derived from **one germ cell layer**		
• Salivary glands	Pleomorphic adenoma[Q]	Malignant mixed tumor
• **Renal anlage[Q]**	–	Wilms tumor[Q]
Teratomas[Q]: Derived from **more than one germ cell layer**		
Totipotential cells in embryonic rests	Mature teratoma,[Q] Dermoid cyst	Immature teratoma, Terato-carcinoma

Basic Component Soft Tumors

- **Neoplastic Cells:** Constitute the tumor parenchyma
- **Reactive Stroma:** Made up of connective tissue, blood vessels and cells of the immune system.

CHARACTERISTICS OF BENIGN AND MALIGNANT NEOPLASMS

Comparison between Benign and Malignant Tumors

Characteristics	Benign	Malignant
Differentiation	**Well** differentiated[Q]	**Poorly** differentiated (anaplasia)[Q]
Rate of growth	Slow	Erratic and rapid
Mitotic figures	**Rare and normal**[Q]	**Numerous and abnormal**[Q]
Local invasion	**Do not invade**[Q] or infiltrate surrounding tissue	**Locally invasive,** infiltrating surrounding tissue[Q]
Metastasis	**Absent**[Q]	**Frequently present**[Q]

Differentiation

Dysplasia	Anaplasia
Disordered growth Partially reversible	**Lack of differentiation Irreversible**
Common features	
• Pleomorphism • Nuclear irregularity • Hyperchromatism	• High N:C ratio • Loss of polarity • Atypical, increased Mitosis

- When dysplasia is severe and involves full epithelial thickness without penetrating basement membrane, it is called carcinoma in situ
- Once the tumor cells breach the basement membrane, the tumor is said to be invasive
- **ANAPLASIA is the hallmark of malignancy**

First let's understand the cell cycle

Cell Cycle

- *Definition:* Cell cycle is the **sequence of events that results in cell division**[Q]
- *Sequence:*

$$G0 \rightarrow G1 \rightarrow S \rightarrow G2 \rightarrow M$$

Cells can enter G1 either from G0 quiescent cell pool, or after completing a round of mitosis

- *Phases*

G1	Pre-synthetic growth[Q]
S	DNA synthesis[Q] (**most radioresistant phase**)[Q]
G2	Pre-mitotic growth
M	Mitotic phase (**most radiosensitive phase**)[Q]
G0	**Quiescent** cells that are **not actively** cycling are said to be in G0 state

- **G_1/S checkpoint:**
  - Checks for **DNA damage before replication in S phase** → **arrests cell cycle if damage is present** → **activates DNA repair mechanisms**
  - DNA can be **repaired** only as long as the **chromatids have not separated.**[Q]
- **G_2/M checkpoint:**
  - Monitors the **completion of DNA replication**[Q]
  - Checks whether the cell can safely initiate mitosis and separate sister chromatids.
  - Defects in this checkpoint give rise to **chromosomal abnormalities.**[Q]
  - Cells exposed to **ionizing radiation** → Cell cycle **arrested in G_2** and **repair mechanisms activated**[Q]

Components of Cell Cycle Cyclins and Cyclin-dependent Kinases (CDK)[Q]

- ***Cyclins*[Q]: Proteins** (with **cyclic production and degradation**) that **drive cell cycle progression**
- ***Cyclin-dependent kinases (CDKs):*** **Cyclin-associated enzymes** that acquire the ability to **phosphorylate** protein substrates by **forming complexes with the relevant cyclins**[Q]
- ***CDK inhibitors (CDKIs):*** Proteins that **block the cell cycle** by **binding to cyclin-CDK complexes**.

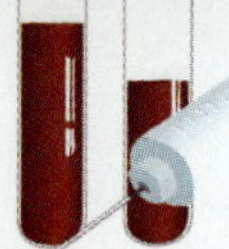

Check Points	Cyclin	CDK
G_1-S	Cyclin D	**CDK4/CDK6**[Q]
	Cyclin E	CDK2
G_2-M	Cyclin A	**CDK2/CDK1**[Q]
	Cyclin B	CDK1[Q]

Cell Cycle Inhibitors[Q]

Family	Checkpoints	Proteins	Functions
CIP/KIP (CDKN1)	G1-S & G2-M	p21 p27 p57	• **p21 is induced by p53**[Q] • **p27** responds to**TGF-β**[Q]
INK4/ARF (CDKN2)	G1-S	p15 p16 p18 p19	• **p16/INK4a** binds to CyclinD-CDK4 & promotes inhibitory effects of RB[Q] • **p14/ARF increases p53 levels** by **inhibiting MDM2**[Q]

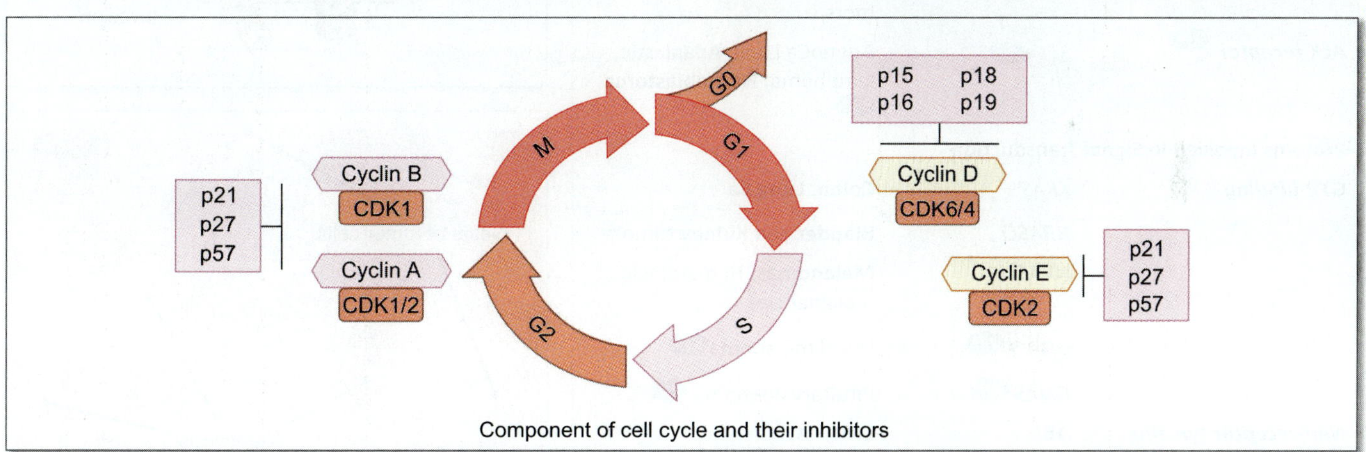

Component of cell cycle and their inhibitors

Hallmarks of Cancer ("S-T-E-A-L A-T-M")

- ***Self-sufficiency*[Q]** in growth signals
- ***Tumor suppressor gene inactivation:*** Insensitivity to growth inhibitory signals[Q]
- ***Evasion of apoptosis***
- ***A***ltered cellular metabolism (**aerobic glycolysis-Warburg effect**)[Q]
- ***Limitless replicative potential*** (immortality)
- Sustained ***Angiogenesis*[Q]**
- Evasion of immuni***T***y
- ***Metastasis***

Self-sufficiency in Growth Signals (By Genetic Mutations and Oncogene Activation)

- **Proto-oncogenes: Unmutated counterparts** of oncogenes found **normally in a cell**
- **Functions of Proto-oncogenes: Cell growth**[Q], **inhibition of apoptosis**[Q] and **nuclear transcription**[Q]
- **Oncogenes**[Q]: **Mutated or over expressed** version of **proto-oncogenes** that **function autonomously**
- **Oncogenes have no**[Q] **dependence** on normal growth promoting signals and **growth factors**

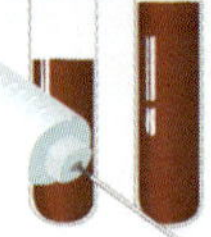

- **Proto-oncogenes can be activated to oncogene by translocation (Most common in hematologic neoplasms), amplification and point mutation**
- **Proto-oncogenes** can be **activated by virus**^{Q} to **oncogenes**
- **Oncoproteins: Proteins encoded by oncogenes** that promote **cell growth** in **absence** of **growth promoting signals**

Oncogenes and Associated Tumors

Category	Proto-oncogene	Associated Human Tumor
Growth Factors		
PDGF-β chain	*SIS*^{Q} (*PDGFB*)	**Astrocytoma**^{Q}
Fibroblast growth factors (FGF)	HST1	**Osteosarcoma**
	INT2 (*FGF3*)	Stomach, Bladder
TGF-α	*TGFA*	**Astrocytomas**
HGF	*HGF*	Hepatocellular Carcinoma, Thyroid cancer
Growth Factor Receptors		
EGF-receptor family	***ERBB1 (EGFR)*** ***ERBB2 (HER)***	**Adenocarcinoma Lung** **Breast Ca**
FMS-like tyrosine kinase3	FLT3	**Leukemia (ALL)**
Receptor for neurotrophic factors	*RET*^{Q}	**MEN 2A & 2B, medullary thyroid**^{Q}
PDGF receptor	***PDGFRB***^{Q}	**Gliomas,**^{Q} **Leukemias**^{Q}
Receptor for KIT	*KIT*^{Q}	Gastrointestinal stromal tumors,
ALK receptor	ALK	AdenoCa Lung, Anaplastic lymphoma, **Neuroblastoma**
Proteins Involved In Signal Transduction		
GTP-binding	*KRAS*^{Q}	**Colon, Lung Ca**
	HRASQ	**Bladder** and **Kidney** tumors
	NRASQ	**Melanomas**, Hematologic malignancies
	GNAQ	Uveal melanoma
	GNAS	Pituitary adenoma
Non-receptor tyrosine kinase	**ABL**	**CML,**^{Q} ALL
RAS signal transduction	**BRAF**^{Q}	**Melanoma, Hairy Cell Leukemia, ColonCa**
Notch signal transduction	NOTCH1	Leukemias,
JAK/STAT signal transduction	JAK2	Myeloproliferative disorders, **ALL**
WNT signal transduction	β-catenin^Q	Hepatoblastomas, hepatocellular carcinoma
Nuclear-Regulatory Proteins		
Transcriptional activators	**C-MYC**^{Q}	**Burkitt lymphoma**^{Q}
	N-MYC^Q	**Neuroblastoma, small-cell Ca lung**^{Q}
	L-MYC	**Small-cell of lung**^{Q}

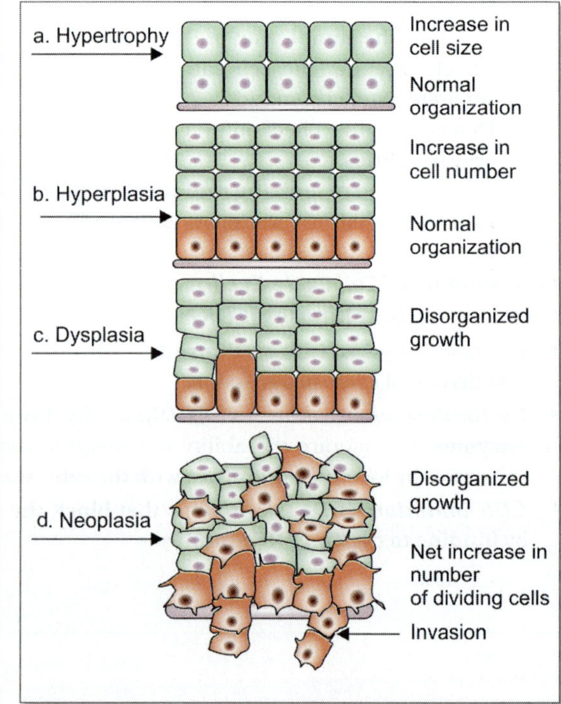

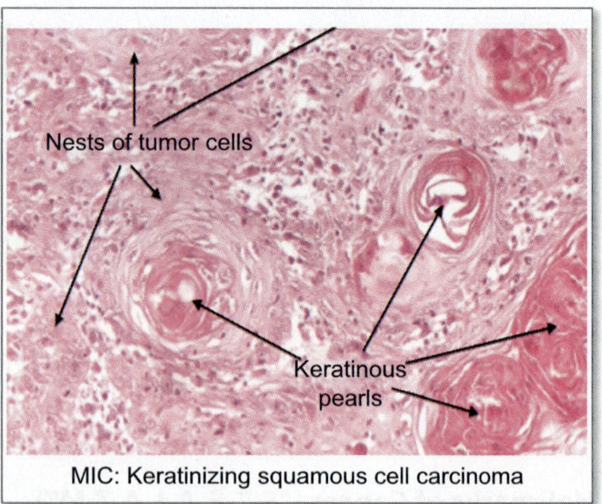

MIC: Keratinizing squamous cell carcinoma

High Yield Facts

Oncogene Addiction
- Tumor cells are highly dependent on the activity of one or more oncogenes Seen in CML. Hence inhibition of its activity is a highly effective therapy.

Contd...

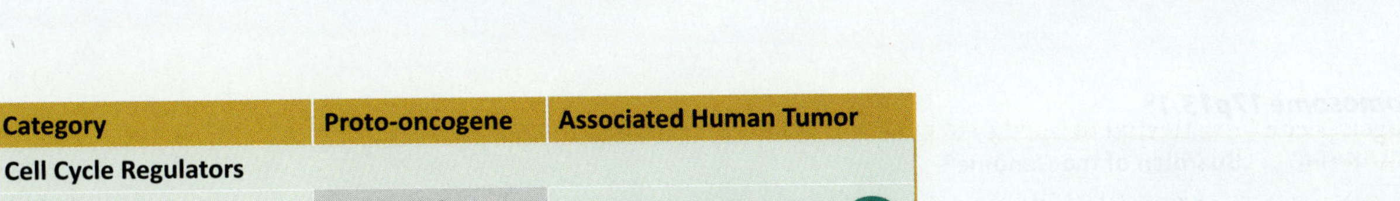

Category	Proto-oncogene	Associated Human Tumor
Cell Cycle Regulators		
Cyclins	**Cyclin D1**[Q] (CCND1)	**Mantle cell lymphoma**[Q],
Cyclin-dependent kinase	*CDK4*	Glioblastoma, Melanoma

Tumor Suppressor Genes

Genes that prevent uncontrolled proliferation of cell We will discuss few important ones

RB (Retinoblastoma) Gene: on Chromosome13q14[Q]

- *Also called:* **Governor of proliferation**[Q]
- *Function:* Key **negative**[Q] **regulator** of **G1/S**[Q] **cell cycle** transition
- *Tumors associated:* **Retinoblastoma,**[Q] **Osteosarcoma,**[Q] Glioblastomas, Small-cell Ca of lung, Breast Ca & Bladder Ca

- *Knudson's "2 hit"*[Q] *hypothesis of Oncogenesis for Retinoblastoma:*
  - In **sporadic** form, **mutations** in **both RB genes** in the retinal cell are **acquired**[Q]
  - In **familial** form, all somatic cells **inherit one mutated copy** of RB gene (heterozygous), and **one additional RB mutation** is required for complete loss of RB function. **(loss of heterozygosity)**[Q]

Regulation of Cell Cycle by RB Gene

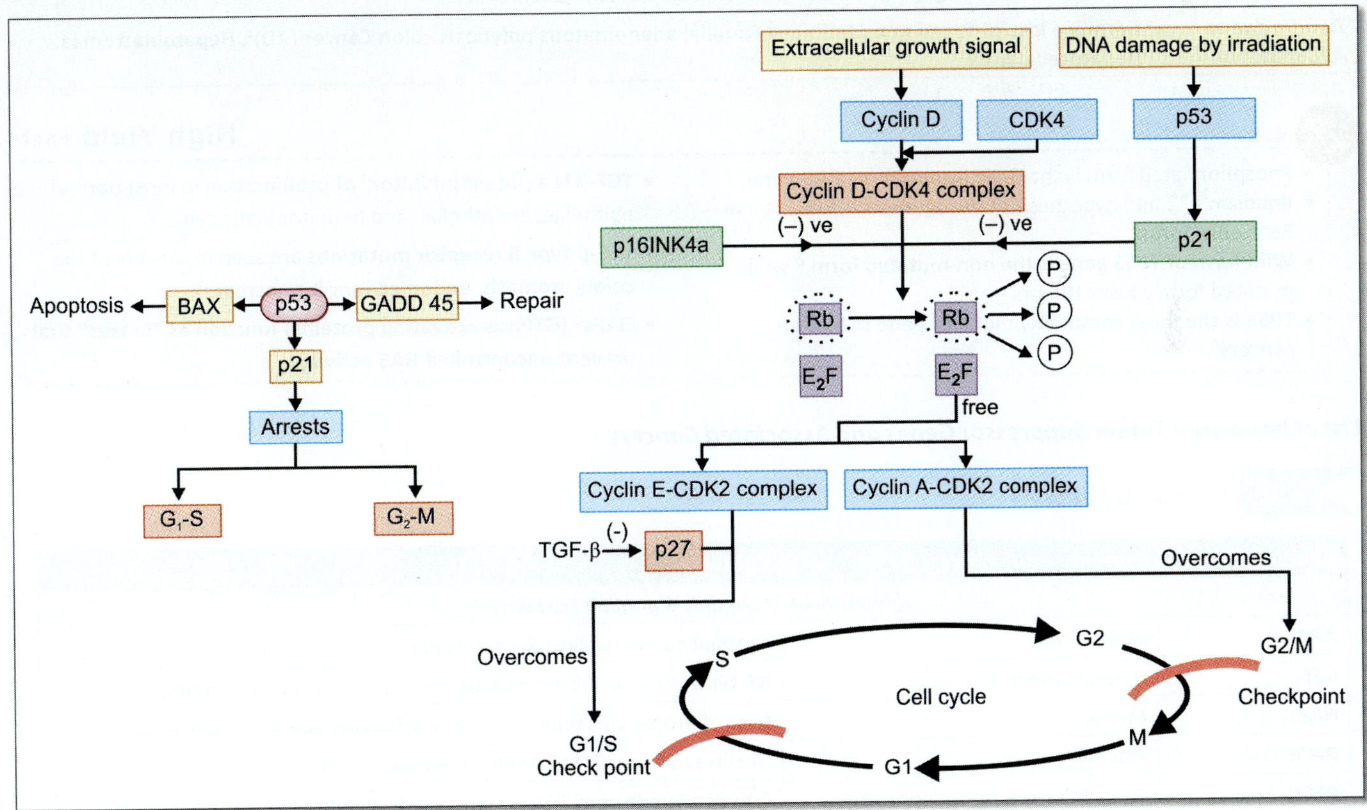

TP53: on chromosome 17p13.1[Q]

Also called	Guardian of the Genome[Q]
Functions	• p53 is **universally expressed** in all cells & **encodes a 53 kDa protein**[Q] • Regulates cell cycle progression, DNA repair, cellular senescence & apoptosis • p53 activates CDK inhibitor (p21) → inhibits cyclin-CDK complexes & hence **inhibits phosphorylation of RB** → arrests cell-cycle at G1-S phase.
TP53 mutation causes	Brain Tumors, Breast Ca,[Q] Leukemia, Adrenal Ca, Sarcomas,
Other members of P53 family	• **p63** is essential for the differentiation of **stratified squamous epithelia** [R9th] • **p73** has strong **pro-apoptotic effects** after DNA damage by **chemotherapeutic agents** [R9th]
Li-Fraumeni syndrome[Q]	• Individuals who have **inherited one mutated TP53 allele**[Q] • **Predisposed to malignancy**[Q] as only 1 additional "hit"[Q] in the lone normal allele is **needed** • Have 25-fold greater chance of developing a malignancy by age 50 • Develop cancer at younger ages[Q] and may develop multiple[Q] primary tumors • **Common** Tumors: Sarcomas, Breast cancer,[Q] Leukemias,[Q] Brain tumors,[Q] Adrenal Ca.[Q]

Adenomatous Polyposis Coli (APC) Gene: Chr 5q21[Q]

Also called	Gate-keeper of Colonic Neoplasia[Q]
Functions	• Component of the **WNT signaling pathway**[Q] • Controls cell fate, adhesion & cell polarity during embryonic development. • It also **controls oncogenic effects of β-catenin** so prevents carcinomas
Tumors due to APC mutation	• Germline **loss-of-function** mutation → **Familial adenomatous polyposis colon Cancer (AD)**[Q], **Hepatoblastomas, Hepatocellular Ca**

High Yield Facts

- Phosphorylated form is the deactivated form of RB gene
- Knudson's "2 hit" hypothesis of oncogenesis is for Retinoblastoma
- **Wild form of TP53 gene is the non-mutated form,**[Q] while mutated form causes tumors
- TP53 is the most commonly mutated gene in human cancers[Q]

- **TGF-β is a potent inhibitor**[Q] **of proliferation** in most normal epithelial, endothelial, and hematopoietic cells.
- **TGF-β type II receptor mutations** are seen in cancers of the **colon, stomach, endometrium & pancreas.**[Q]
- **GAPs**[Q] (GTPase-activating proteins) function as "brakes" that **prevent uncontrolled RAS activity.**

List of Important Tumor Suppressor Genes and Associated Cancers

R9th Latest Update

Gene	Protein	Cancers
Inhibitors of Mitogenic Signaling Pathways		
APC	APC protein	**Familial colonic polyps & Carcinoma**[Q]
NFI	Neurofibromin 1	**NF type 1**[Q] (Neurofibromas & peripheral nerve sheath tumors)
NF2	Merlin	Neurofibromatosis type 2 (acoustic **schwannoma & meningioma**)[Q]
PTCH	Patched	**Gorlin syndrome**[Q] (Basal cell Ca, Medulloblastoma)
PTEN	Phosphatase & tensin homologue	**Cowden Syndrome**[Q] (Breast, endometrial, and prostate carcinoma)
SMAD2, SMAD4	SMAD2, SMAD4	**Juvenile polyposis**[Q], *pancreatic Ca*
Inhibitors of Cell Cycle Progression		
RB	Retinoblastoma (RB) Protein	**Familial retinoblastoma syndromes** (Retinoblastoma[Q] & Osteosarcoma[Q])
CDKN2A	P16/INK4 a and p14/ARF	**Familial melanoma**[Q]
Inhibitors of "pro-growth" Programs of Metabolism and Angiogenesis		
VHL	VHL protein	**Von Hippel-Lindau syndrome**

Contd...

STK11	Liver kinase B1 (LKB1) or STK11	**Peutz-Jeghers syndrome**[Q] (GI polyps, GI cancers, pancreatic carcinoma)[Q]
SDHB, SDHD	Succinate dehydrogenase B & D	Familial paraganglioma, pheochromocytoma
	Inhibitors of Invasion and Metastasis	
CDH1	**E-cadherin**[Q]	**Familial gastric cancer**[Q]
	Enablers of Genomic Stability	
TP53	P53 protein	**Li–Fraumeni syndrome**[Q] (see above)
	DNA Repair Factors	
BRCA1, BRCA2	BRCA1 and BRCA2	**Familial breast and ovarian Ca;**[Q]
	Unknown Mechanisms	
WT1	Wilms tumor-1 (WT1)	**Familial Wilms' tumor**[Q]
MEN1	Menin	**MEN1**[Q] **syndrome**

Warburg Effect: Aerobic Glycolysis/Glucose Hunger[Q]

- Otto Warburg was awarded Nobel Prize in 1931 for this theory
- Cancer cells tend to convert most glucose to lactate[Q] even in presence of ample oxygen (aerobic glycolysis)[Q]
- Even though **ATP production is low** with formation of lactate compared to mitochondrial oxidative phosphorylation, it **provides metabolic intermediates** that are needed for the synthesis of **cellular components**.
  - Warburg Effect is the Basis of Positron Emission Tomography (PET)[Q]
- Patients are injected with **18F-fluorodeoxyglucose (FDG)**, a non-metabolizable derivative of glucose, that is **preferentially taken up into tumor cells** (due to glucose hunger), which can be detected by PET scanning

Evasion of Programed Cell Death (Apoptosis)

- **Intrinsic apoptotic pathway** (mitochondrial pathway) **most frequently disabled in cancer.**[Q]
- **BCL-2**: mutated in **85% of follicular B-cell lymphomas**[Q]
- **Autophagy: Tumor cells** in **severe nutrient deficiency**, arrest their growth and also **cannibalize** their own **organelles, proteins, and membranes** as carbon sources for **energy production.**[Q]

Limitless Replicative Potential

- **Cancer stem cells**: Stem cell–like cells that are **immortal** and have limitless replicative potential, seen in all cancers.
- May arise through **transformation of a normal stem cell** or through **acquired genetic lesions**
- **Immortality of cancer cells is due to**:
  - **Evasion of senescence**: By disruption of **RB-dependent G1/S cell cycle checkpoint**[Q]
  - **Evasion of mitotic crisis**: By **telomere maintenance,**[Q] **up-regulation of telomerase**[Q] or **alternative lengthening** of telomeres

- **Capacity for self-renewal**[Q]: Self-renewal means that **each time a stem cell divides at least one of the two daughter cells remains a stem cell** (also called **Asymmetric cell division)**[Q]

Angiogenesis

- Tumor cannot enlarge beyond **1–2 mm**[Q] in diameter unless it has the capacity to **induce angiogenesis**.
- **Angiogenesis** is an important requirement for tumors to **undergo metastasis**

Pro-angiogenic factors	Anti-angiogenic factors
• **Angiogenin**	• Endostatin[Q]
• **Vascular Endothelial Growth Factor (VEGF)**[Q]	• Angiostatin[Q]
• **Fibroblast Growth Factor (FGF)**[Q]	• **Interferon**-Alfa
• **Transforming Growth Factor-β (TGF- β)**[Q]	• Thrombospondin-1[Q]
• Platelet activating factor (PAF)	

Metastasis

- *Definition:* **Spread** of a tumor **to sites** that are **physically discontinuous** with primary tumor.
- *Pathways of metastasis:*
  - **Direct** seeding of body cavities or surfaces, e.g., ovarian Ca
  - **Lymphatic** spread e.g., Carcinomas[Q]
  - **Hematogenous** spread e.g., sarcomas[Q]
- *Steps involved:*
  - Invasion of the extracellular matrix (ECM):
    - "**Loosening up**" of tumor cell–tumor cell interactions: **E-cadherin mutations**
    - **Degradation of ECM: Metalloproteinases** (MMPs type **2 and 9**)[Q] also known as **Type IV collagenase**[Q], cathepsin D, & urokinase plasminogen activator
    - **Attachment** to novel ECM components by **Fibronectin**[Q]
    - **Migration** and **invasion** of tumor cells

○ Vascular Dissemination and Homing of Tumor Cells:
- Expression of **CD44**[Q] in solid tumors which binds to **hyaluronate** on high endothelial venules which enhances their spread to lymph nodes and other metastatic sites.

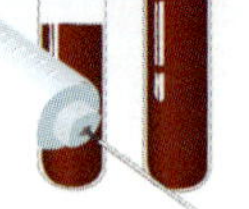

R10ᵗʰ Latest Update

Metastasis oncogenes:
- **SNAIL & TWIST**: encode transcription factors which promote **epithelial-to-mesenchymal transition (EMT)**
- **EMT: Down-regulation of epithelial** markers (e.g., E-cadherin) and **up-regulation of mesenchymal** markers (e.g., vimentin and smooth muscle actin)
- **Pro-migratory phenotype** is essential for metastasis.

Evasion of Host-Immune Defense

Mechanisms by which immune system is evaded in immune-competent hosts:

- Selective outgrowth of **antigen-negative**[Q] variants
- Loss or **reduced** expression of **histocompatibility antigens**[Q]
- **Immunosuppression**[Q] mediated by expression of certain factors (e.g., **TGF-β, PD-1 ligand, galectins**) by the tumor cells

RECENT EXAM[Q]

- The 2018 Nobel Prize in Physiology or Medicine has been awarded jointly to two cancer immunotherapy researchers, James P. Allison, PhD, of The University of Texas MD Anderson Cancer Center, and Dr. Tasuku Honjo of Kyoto University in Japan.
- In his laboratory at the University of California, Berkeley, Allison studied the T cell protein CTLA-4. When this protein attaches to another protein (called B7) found on the surface of some cancer cells, it signals the T cell that this cell is functioning properly. As long as a regular or cancer cell is sending the message that it is functioning well, the immune system will not destroy the cell. By blocking the CTLA-4 protein and thereby the message that the cell is working as it should, the immune system can recognize cancer cells and attack them. This discovery eventually led to the drug Yervoy (ipilimumab), which is used to treat melanoma skin cancer and some other cancers.
- Honjo at Kyoto University in Japan discovered PD-1, which is another protein found on the surface of some T cells. When this protein attaches to a protein called PD-L1 on cancer cells, it can prevent the T cells from recognizing the cancer cells, so the immune system won't destroy them. Blocking the PD-L1 protein on cancer cells, or the corresponding PD-1 protein on immune cells, allows the immune system to recognize the cancer cells as foreign and attack them.
- Drugs that target PD-1 include Keytruda (pembrolizumab) and Opdivo (nivolumab), while drugs that target PD-L1 include atezolizumab (Tecentriq), avelumab (Bavencio), and durvalumab (Imfinzi). These drugs are now used to treat people with many different cancer types, including melanoma skin cancer, non-small cell lung cancer, kidney cancer, bladder cancer, head and neck cancers, and Hodgkin lymphoma.

High Yield Facts

- **All malignant tumors can metastasize except Gliomas and Basal cell Ca**[Q]
- **Decrease of telomerase activity** cause **antitumor effects**[Q]
- **Most common site of metastasis is Lungs > Liver**[Q]
- **'Anoikis' is apoptosis stimulated by detachment of epithelial cells from basement membranes & from cell-cell interactions**[Q]
- **Immunosuppressed patients** have **increased risk** for development of **cancer,** particularly caused by **oncogenic DNA viruses.**
- **Fibromatoses** are apparently **autonomous proliferation** of **myofibroblasts,** occasionally forming **tumor like** masses

GENETIC BASIS OF CANCERS

- Genetic aberrations that **increase mutation rates** fastens **driver mutations** that are required for transformation and subsequent tumor progression
- Selection of fittest cells can explain not only tumor evolution but also changes is tumor behaviour following therapy

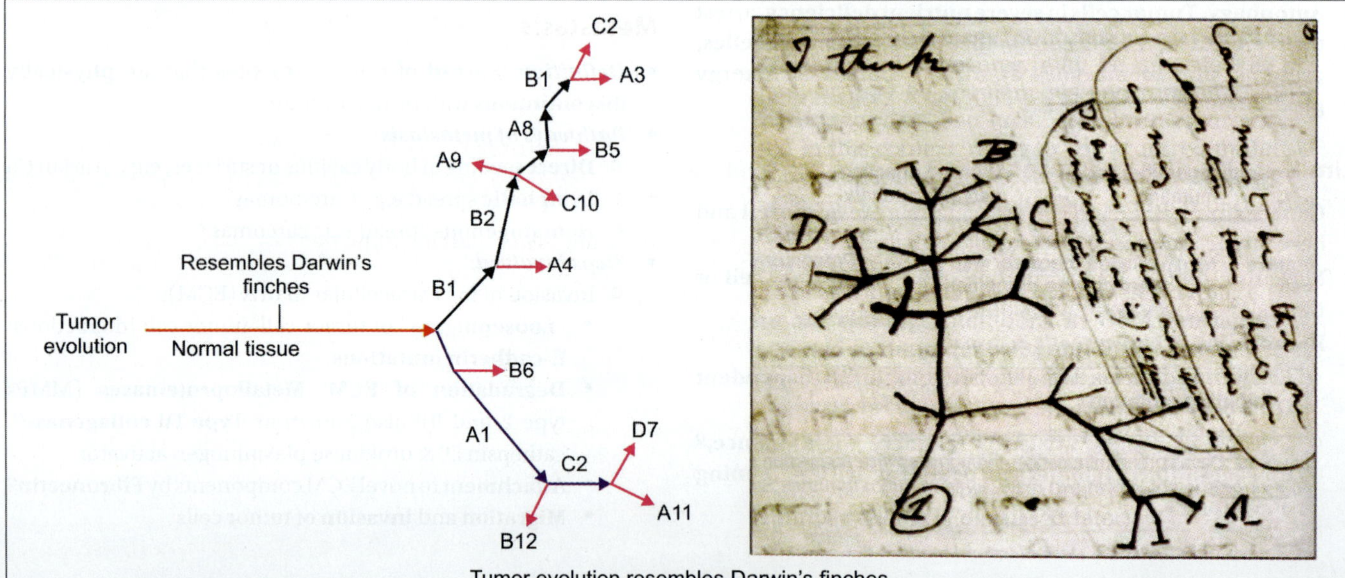

Tumor evolution resembles Darwin's finches

Dysregulation of Cancer-Associated Genes

Chromosomal Abnormalities like deletions, translocation, gene amplifications can cause cancer (Refer to annexures)

Defect in DNA Repair Mechanism

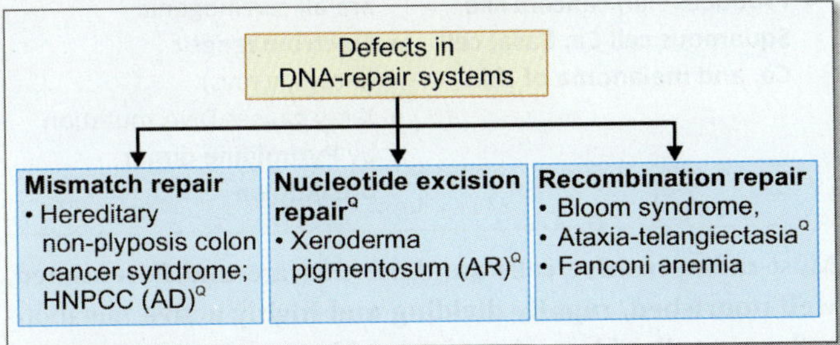

Ataxia Telangiectasia

- *Immunodeficiency:* Thymic hypoplasia[Q] (**most consistent defect**) with **cellular and humoral (IgA and IgG2)**[Q] immunodeficiency
- *Clinical features:* Recurrent pulmonary infections,[Q] premature aging, Type 1 diabetes mellitus
- *Tumors seen:* Lymphomas,[Q] Hodgkin's disease,[Q] T cell ALL & Breast cancer
- *Neuropathologic changes:*
  - **Loss of Purkinje, granule, and basket cells** in the **cerebellar cortex**[Q] (**most striking change**) & deep cerebellar nuclei.

Epigenetic Changes

Epigenetic Changes are factors other than the sequence of DNA that regulate gene expression
Play major role in:

- **Expression of cancer genes**[Q], **Control of differentiation,** Self renewal, Drug sensitivity and drug resistance

Epigenetic Alterations in Cancers

- Exhibiting **abnormal DNA methylation**: hypomethylation[Q] or hypermethylation[Q]
- **Silencing of tumor suppressor genes**[Q] by **local hypermethylation** of DNA
- Changes in histones near genes that **influence cellular behavior**[Q]

Examples of Epigenomic Regulatory Genes that are Mutated in Cancer

Gene(s)	Tumor
ARID1A	Ovarian clear cell Ca (60%), Endometrial Ca
SNF5	**Malignant rhabdoid tumor (100%)**
DNMT3A	AML (20%)
MLL1	**ALL**
MLL2	**Follicular lymphoma (90%)**[Q]
CREBBP/EP300	Diffuse large B Cell lymphoma (40%)

MicroRNAs (miRs) and Cancer

- *What are miRs?*
  - **MicroRNAs (miRs)** are small non-coding, ssRNA, approx 22 nucleotides in length
- *Function:*
  - Mediate sequence-specific **inhibition of messenger RNA (mRNA) translation** through the action of the **RNA-induced silencing complex (RISC)**
- *Mechanism of Oncogenesis:*
  - **Decreased expression of** tumor suppressive mIRs → increases oncogenic mRNA translation
  - **Overexpression of** oncogenic miRNAs) → repress the expression of tumor suppressor genes
- *Examples:*
  - **OncomiRs** (oncogenic miRNAs)
    - miR-200- promote epithelial-mesenchymal transitions, invasiveness & metastasis
    - miR-155- upregulates genes that promote proliferation (MYC) → B cell lymphomas
  - Tumor suppressive miRs:
    - miR-15 and miR-16 upregulates BCL-2 in CLL
  - **Tumor suppressive properties of miR processing factors**
    - DICER: a gene that encodes an endonuclease that is required for the processing and production of functional miRs.
    - Ovarian and testicular tumors

> **R10ᵗʰ Latest Update**
>
> **Some other Non-coding RNAs**
>
> | Type | Full name | Function |
> | --- | --- | --- |
> | piRNA | piwi-interacting RNA | **Most common type of small noncoding RNA,** have a role in post-transcriptional gene silencing |
> | snoRNA | small nucleolar RNA | **Maturation of rRNA** and the assembly of ribosome |
> | l ncRNA | long intervening non-codingRNA | **Regulate histones** and thereby control gene expression |

Chromothryipsis

Literally means, **chromosome shattering**.

- Single event in which several **chromosome breaks** occur within a single chromosome or multiple chromosomes.
- Later **DNA repair mechanisms**[Q] are activated in affected cells that **stitch the pieces** together in a **disorganized** way
- This may create **chromosome rearrangements**[Q] and also result in the **loss of some chromosome** segments.
- This may also **activate oncogenes** and **inactivate tumor suppressors,**
- Finally these changes **accelerate the process of carcinogenesis.**[Q]

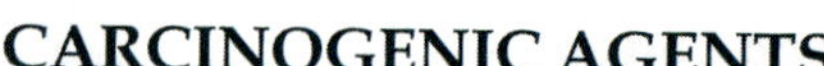

CARCINOGENIC AGENTS

Chemical Carcinogens (Occupational Cancers)

Major Chemical Carcinogens

Chemical	Types of Cancer
Polycyclic hydrocarbons	
Soot (benzopyrene, dibenzanthracene)	**Skin; scrotal cancer**
Tobacco	**Lung**, bladder, **oral cavity, larynx**, esophagus
Aromatic amines	
Benzidine, 2–naphthylamine	**Bladder[Q]**
Aflatoxins	**Liver[Q]**
Nitrosamines	Esophagus, stomach
Cancer chemotherapeutic agents	
Cyclophosphamide,[Q] chlorambucil, busulfan	Leukemias
Asbestos[Q]	**Lung cancer, mesothelioma[Q]**
Heavy metals	
Nickel, chromium, cadmium	Lung
Arsenic	Skin
Vinyl chloride[Q]	**Liver (angiosarcoma)[Q]**

Radiation Carcinogenesis

Ultraviolet B Rays	Ionizing Radiation
• Leads to **formation of pyrimidine dimers in DNA[Q]** • **Produces skin cancers like Squamous cell Ca, Basal cell Ca, and melanoma of skin**	• **Particulate** radiation (α & β particles, protons, neutrons) are all carcinogenic • **Electromagnetic** (x-rays, γ rays) • X-ray causes DNA mutation by **Pyrimidine dimer breakdown**

Most **radiosensitive** cells are those that are **undifferentiated, well nourished, rapidly dividing and highly active** metabolically. e.g., **cells of buccal mucosa > skin**

High Yield Facts

- **Lethal dose** of radiation for humans is **250–400 rads[Q]**
- **Most radiosensitive** tissue are **spermatogonia[Q]**, erythroblasts, epidermal & GI stem cells
- **Least radiosensitive** are Cartilage[Q] > Bone, nerve cells and muscle fibers.
- **Radiation increases** the risk of leukemias[Q] and solid tumors in several organs eg thyroid,[Q] breast, and lungs.[Q]
- In thyroid, papillary Ca of thyroid is common due to radiation[Q]

Microbial Carcinogenesis

Organism	Gene	Mechanism	Tumor
Oncogenic RNA Viruses			
HTLV–1	Tax[Q]	Increased **pro growth signaling & cell survival** & genomic instability.	**Adult T cell leukemia[Q]/ Lymphoma[Q]**
Hep C	HCV core protein	Activates growth-promoting signal transduction pathways	**Hepatocellular carcinoma[Q]**
Oncogenic DNA Viruses			
HPV Low risk (6,11) High risk (16,18)	E6[Q]	Degradation of **p53[Q]** & stimulation of **TERT**	**Low risk:** Genital warts[Q] **High risk:** Squamous cell Ca cervix, Ca Oropharynx, anus, head/neck **(laryngeal papilloma)[Q]**, Esophagus
	E7[Q]	**Inactivates RB[Q] & CDKI** (p21 & p27)	
EBV (Epstein–Barr virus)	LMP1[Q]	Activates **NF-kB** & **JAK/STAT** pathway	**Lymphoma:** Burkitt's,[Q] Hodgkin, T-cell & NK cell **Carcinoma:** Nasopharyngeal[Q] & gastric
	EBNA2	Activates **cyclin D**	
	vIL-10	B cell activation	
Hep B	HBx	Activates transcription factors	**Hepatocellular carcinoma[Q]**
Bacteria			
H.pylori	Cag-A	Growth factor stimulation	**Gastric adenocarcinomas[Q]** & gastric **MALToma[Q]**

CLINICAL ASPECTS OF NEOPLASIA

Cancer Cachexia

- **Progressive loss of body fat and lean body mass**[Q] with profound weakness, anorexia & anemia, seen in cancer.
- **TNF**[Q] is the **major contributor** to cachexia with advanced cancer.
- Equal loss of both **fat and lean muscle**[Q]
- **Elevated basal metabolic rate**
- Evidence of **systemic inflammation** (e.g., an increase in acute phase reactants)

Paraneoplastic Syndromes

- Signs and symptoms that **cannot be** readily be explained by the **anatomic distribution** of the tumor or by the **elaboration of hormones** indigenous to the tissue from which the tumor arose.
- Seen in 10% of persons with cancer

Paraneoplastic Syndromes are Important to Recognize, for Several Reasons:

- Can be the **earliest** manifestation of an occult neoplasm.
- Can cause significant **clinical problems** and may even be **lethal**.
- May **mimic metastatic disease** and therefore confound treatment.

Paraneoplastic Syndrome

Clinical syndrome	Major forms of underlying cancer
Vascular and Hematologic changes	
Trousseau phenomenon[Q]	**Pancreatic**[Q], **Bronchogenic**[Q] **& Colon Ca**[Q]
DIC	**APML, prostatic carcinoma**
Nonbacterial thrombotic endocarditis	**Advanced cancers**[Q]
Red cell aplasia[Q]	**Thymic neoplasms**[Q]
Nerve and Muscle syndrome	
Myasthenia	**Bronchogenic Ca**[Q], thymic neoplasms
Dermatologic, soft tissue & osseous changes	
Acanthosis nigricans (EGF)	**Gastric**[Q], lung & uterine carcinoma
Dermatomyositis	**Bronchogenic & Breast carcinoma**[Q]
Clubbing ± Hypetrophic osteoarthropathy	Bronchogenic Ca, **Thymic neoplasms**[Q]
Endocrinopathies	
Cushing syndrome (ACTH)	Pancreatic, **Small-cell Ca lung**[Q], Neural tumors
Syndrome of inappropriate antidiuretic hormone secretion (SIADH) (ADH)	**Small-cell Ca lung**, Pancreas, **Thymoma**[Q], Mesothelioma, Bronchial adenoma, **Carcinoid**[Q], **Ewing's sarcoma**[Q]
Hypercalcemia (Pthrp)	**Squamous cell Ca lung**, Breast Ca, Renal Ca
Hypoglycemia (Insulin)	Ovarian carcinoma, **fibrosarcoma**[Q]
Polycythemia (Crythropoetin)	**RCC, HCC, cerebellar hemangioma**

Tumor Lysis Syndrome (TLS)

- Caused by the **destruction** of a large number **of rapidly proliferating neoplastic cells.**[Q]
- **Hyperuricemia**[Q], **hyperkalemia**[Q] **(life threatening), hyperphosphatemia**[Q], and **hypocalcemia**[Q] **± Acidosis** seen.
- Hyperphosphatemia[Q] (due to release of intracellular phosphate) produces a decrease in serum calcium.
- Deposition of **calcium phosphate in the kidney** and **hyperphosphatemia** may cause **acute renal failure**.
- Often seen during treatment of **Burkitt's lymphoma**[Q], ALL, **chronic leukemias**[Q] & rarely, solid tumors

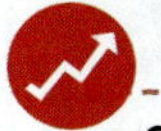

High Yield Facts

- **Cushing's syndrome** is the **most common** paraneoplastic endocrinopathy[Q]
- **Hypercalcemia** is the **most common** paraneoplastic syndrome[Q]
- Cancer-associated hypercalcemia is due to production of parathyroid hormone-related protein **(PTHRP)**[Q]
- **Most common tumors in men arise in the prostate**[Q] **> lung, and colon/rectum.**[Q]
- **In women, cancers of the breast**[Q], **lung, and colon/rectum are the most frequent**
- **Sacrococcygeal teratoma (SCT)**[Q] **is the most frequent tumor in the neonatal period.**

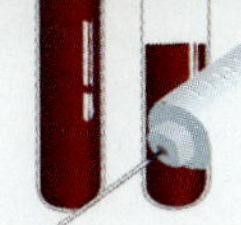

LABORATORY DIAGNOSIS OF CANCERS

Tissue Specimen

- ***Histologic and Cytologic Methods***
  Sampling may be done by:
  - Excision or biopsy, Needle aspiration, and Cytologic smears
- ***Exfoliative Cytology***
  - **Cells are collected** after they have been either **spontaneously shed**[Q] by the body ("spontaneous exfoliation") or **manually scraped/brushed off** of a surface in the body ("mechanical exfoliation")
  - Used in diagnosis of **Carcinoma stomach, bronchus, cervix**[Q] (PAP smear)
- ***Immunohistochemistry***
  Using **specific antibodies**[Q]
  - **Categorization** of undifferentiated malignant tumors
  - Determination of **site of origin of metastatic** tumors.
  - Detection of molecules that have **prognostic or therapeutic significance**.

Marker	Tumors
Cytokeratin (CK)	Carcinoma (Squamous cell Ca, Adenocarcinoma)
Vimentin	**Sarcoma**[Q]
Neurofilament	Neural tumors
GFAP	**Gliomas e.g., Astrocytoma**[Q]
Desmin	**Muscle tumors e.g., Rhabdomyosarcoma**[Q]
S-100	**Melanoma,**[Q] **Neuroendocrine Tumor, Schwannoma, Histiocytoma LCH**[Q]
HMB 45[Q]	**Melanoma**[Q]
Leucocyte common antigen (CD 45)	Lymphoma[Q]

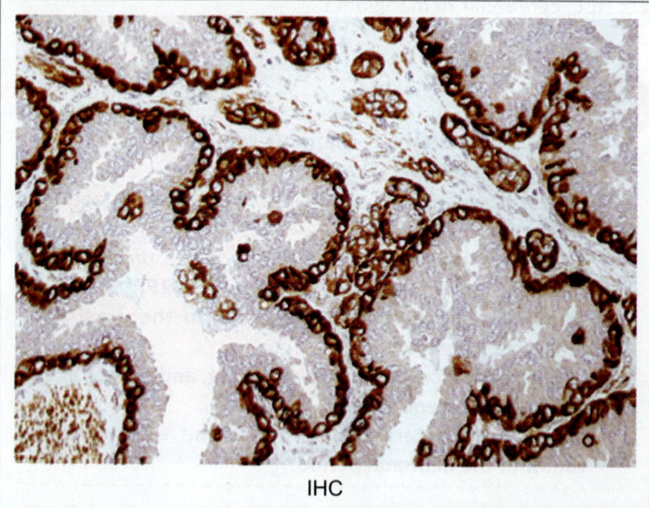
IHC

Tumor Markers

Biomarker found in the blood, urine, or body tissues that can be **elevated in cancer**, among other tissue types. Uses of tumor markers: (**not used for confirmatory diagnosis**)

- **Screening**[Q] for common cancers
- **Monitoring of cancer**[Q] survivors after treatment
- **May help in diagnosis**[Q] of specific tumor types

Important Tumor Markers

Tumor Markers	Tumor Types
Glycoproteins	
• *CA-125*[Q]	**Ovarian**[Q] cancer
• *CA-19-9*[Q]	**Colon** cancer, **pancreatic** cancer
• *CA-15-3*	**Breast**[Q] cancer
• *CA 72-4*	**Gastric**[Q] carcinoma
Enzymes	
• *Prostatic acid phosphatase (PAP)*	**Prostate cancer**[Q]
• *Neuron-specific enolase (NSE)*	**Small-cell** cancer of lung, **Neuroblastoma**[Q]
• *Alkaline phosphatase (ALP)*	**Osteosarcoma**[Q]
• *Lactate Dehydrogenase (LDH)*	**Prostate Ca**[Q], **testicular tumors, Lymphoma, Ewing's sarcoma**[Q]
• *Tyrosinase*	**Melanoma**[Q]
• *Gastrin*	**Pancreatic neuroendocrine tumor (Gastrinoma, ZES)**[Q]
Specific proteins	
• *Immunoglobulins (Ig)*	Multiple myeloma and other gammopathies
• *Beta 2 microglobulin*[Q] ($\beta_2 M$)	**Multiple myeloma**[Q]
• *Prostate-specific antigen (PSA)*	Prostate cancer
Hormones	
• *Human chorionic gonadotropin (HCG)*	Germ cell tumor, **non-seminomatous**[Q] testicular tumors
• *Calcitonin*[Q]	**Medullary carcinoma of thyroid**[Q]
• *Catecholamine metabolites*	**Pheochromocytoma**[Q]
Oncofetal antigens	
• *α – Fetoprotein (AFP)*	**Liver cancers**[Q], **non-seminomatous** germ cell tumors of testis
• *Carcinoembryonic antigen (CEA)*[Q]	**Colon, pancreas, lung, stomach & breast Ca**

Molecular Diagnosis (Discussed in Genetics Chapter)

- **PCR (Polymerase Chain Reaction)**
  - Used to produce **large amounts of target DNA fragment**, provided that the **DNA sequence of that region is known**[Q]
- **Array CGH (Comparative Genomic Hybridization)**[Q]
- **SNP** (Single Nucleotide Polymorphism) Array
- **Next gen Sequencing**: term used to describe several **newer DNA sequencing technologies**[Q] that are capable of sequencing entire human genome in few hours.[Q]

Others

- **Flow Cytometry (Refer to Chapter 23)**
  - **Rapid & quantitative** measure of cellular antigens expressed by "liquid" tumors,
  - Advantage of flow cytometry over IHC is that **simultaneous identification of multiple antigens**[Q] on individual cells possible
- **Circulating Tumor Cells**
  - Detection, quantification, and **characterization of rare solid tumor cells**[Q] (e.g., carcinoma, melanoma) circulating in the blood

---

R10th **Latest** Update

Gompertzian growth

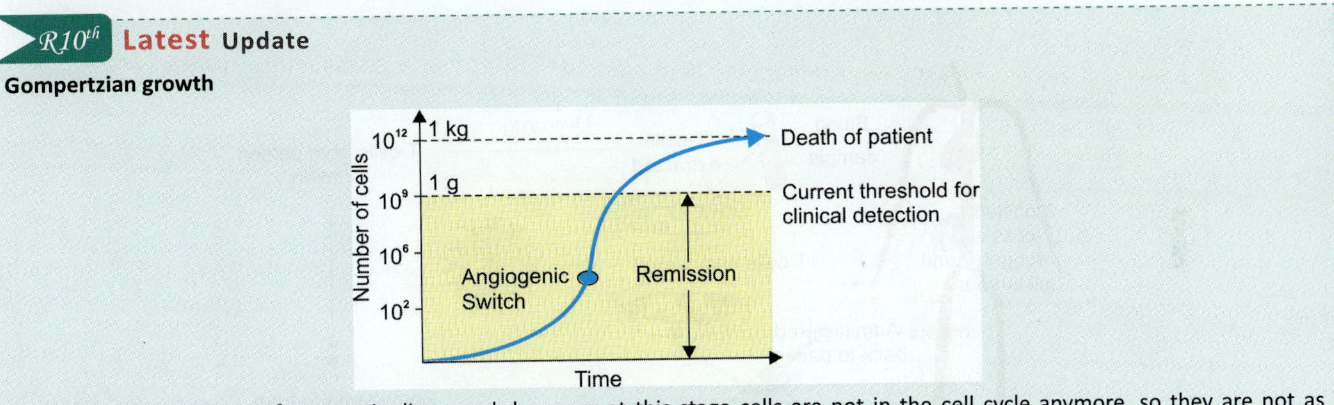

Gompertzian growth. A 10^9, cancer is diagnosed; however at this stage cells are not in the cell cycle anymore, so they are not as responsive to treatment. 10^{12} levels are not compatible with life (death).

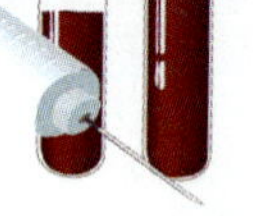

CARs have extracellular domains consisting of antibodies that bind tumor antigens and intracellular domains that delivered signals that activate CTLs following their engagement with antigen on the surface of tumor cells.

Tisagenlecleucel (KymriahTm) is FDA approved for the treatment of patients up to 25 years of age with B-cell precursor acute lymphoblastic leukemia (ALL) that is refractory or in second or later relapse. It is a CD19-directed genetically modified autologous T cell immunotherapy.

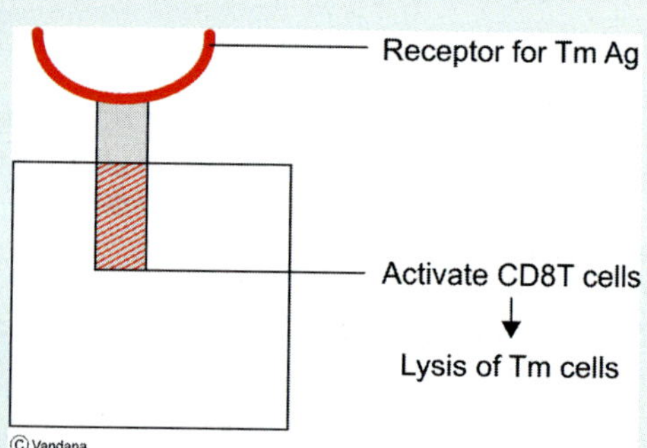

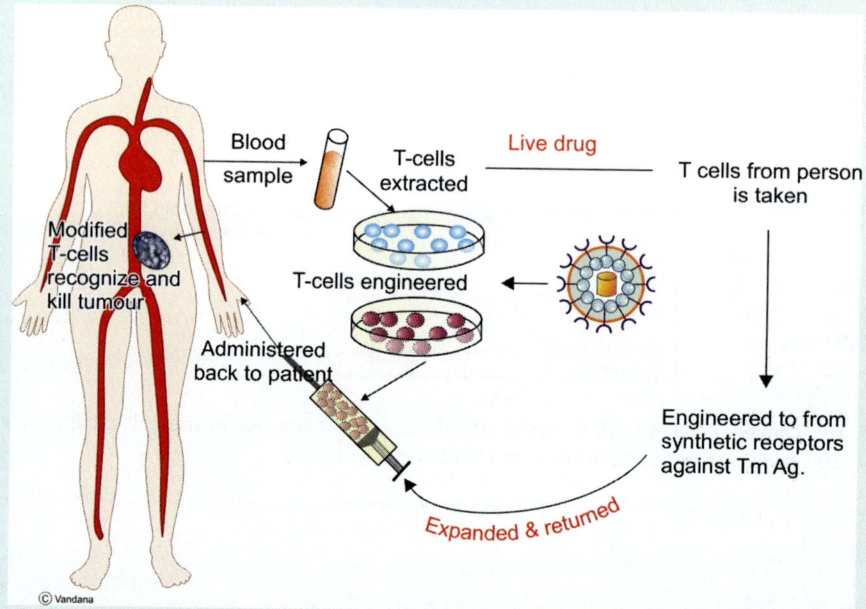

Neoplasia
- Mc gene mutated is P53 (>75%)
- Temporary cell cycle arrest is caused by P53 by inducing p21 that blocks cyclin D 1 and stops the cell cycle
- Mutated Isocitrate dehydrogenase (IDH) produces 2 hydroxy-glutarate which is called **oncometabolite**. Thus enzymes of krebbs cycle play a role in **oncometabolism**. Isocitrate dehydrogenase 1 and 2 (IDHI and IDH2) are key metabolic enzymes, converting isocitrate to α-ketoglutarate (αKG). IDH1 and IDH2 mutations have been identified in multiple tumor types, including gliomas, cholangiocarcinoma and myeloid malignancies such as acute myeloid leukemia (AML) and myelodysplastic syndromes (MDS).

Immunotherapy
- Personalised vaccines—against tumor antigens
- Adoptive immunotherapy—developing cell having **chimeric antigen receptors** have 2 domains—extracellular domain which has antibody that bind to tumor antigen and intracellular domain has a signal that activate cytotoxic T cells.

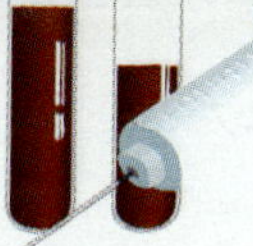

NEXT Pattern Questions

Q's

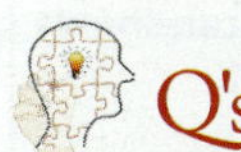

1. The overall survival is increased by screening procedure in which of the following cancer?
   a. Prostate cancer   b. Lung cancer   c. Colon cancer   d. Ovarian cancer

Ans. (c) Colon cancer

(Ref: Robbins Basic Pathology 10th ed/pg 235)

"Colorectal cancer is an ideal candidate for screening strategies".
Because:
- It is common
- Has precursor lesion
- It is slow growing
- Testing is available

So, its detection by screening well increase survival.

Tumors in which screening is done are:

Cancer	Technique
Ovarian cancer	Ca–125, transvaginal sonography
Cervical cancer	Pap smear
Breast cancer	Mammography
Prostate cancer	Digital rectal examination, prostate specific antigen
Lung	Chest X-ray, sputum cytology

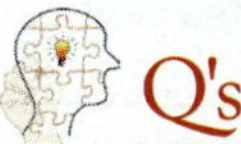

Q's

2. All of the following are features of malignant transformation by cultured cells except:
   a. Increased cell density
   b. Increased requirement for growth factors
   c. Alterations of cytoskeletal structures
   d. Loss of anchorage

Ans. (b) Increased requirement for growth factors

(Ref: Robbins Basic Pathology 10th ed/pg 205)

Changes shown by cultured cells which suggest the malignant transformation are:
- **Alterations of morphology:** Transformed cells often have a much rounder shape than control cells.
- **Increased cell density (loss of contact inhibition of growth):** Transformed cells often form multilayer, while control cells usually form a *monolayer*.
- **Loss of anchorage dependence:** Transformed cells can grow without attachment to the surface of the culture dish and will often grow in agar.
- **Loss of contact inhibition of movement:** Transformed cell grow over one another, while normal cells stop moving when they come into contact with each other.
- *A variety of biochemical changes*, including an increased rate of glycolysis, alterations of the cell surface (e.g., changes in the composition of glycoproteins or glycosphingolipids), and secretion of certain proteases. Alterations of cytoskeletal structures, such as actin filaments.

Diminished requirement for growth factors and, often, increased secretion of certain growth factors into the surrounding medium

NEXT Pattern Questions

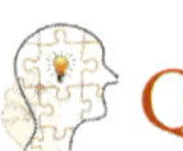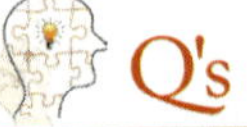

Q's

3. A 50-year-old man experiences an episode of hemoptysis. On physical examination, he has puffiness of the face, pedal edema, and systolic hypertension. A chest radiograph shows an irregular perihilar 5 cm mass of the right lung. Laboratory studies show normal serum electrolytes. A transbronchial biopsy is performed, and the microscopic findings are shown in the figure. A bone scan shows no metastases. Immunohistochemical staining of the tumor cells is most likely to be positive for which of the following?

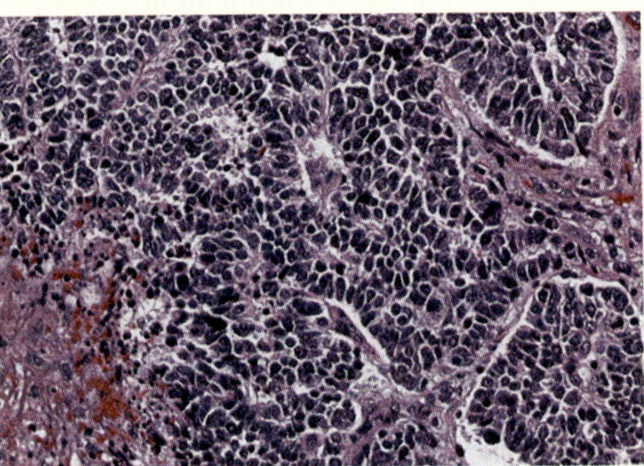

   a. Antidiuretic hormone
   b. Corticotropin
   c. Erythropoietin
   d. Parathyroid hormone-related peptide

Ans. (b) Corticotropin

(Ref: Robbins Basic Pathology 10th ed/pg 228)

The small cells have scant cytoplasm but marked hyperchromatism, consistent with small cell carcinoma. This patient has Cushing syndrome resulting from ectopic corticotropin production by the tumor, a form of paraneoplastic syndrome common to small cell carcinomas of the lung. Such small cell carcinomas are of neuroendocrine derivation. A syndrome of inappropriate antidiuretic hormone (SIADH) secretion from small cell carcinomas is also common, but leads to hyponatremia as well as edema. Erythropoietin production with polycythemia is more likely to be associated with a renal cell carcinoma. Insulin and gastrin production are most often seen in islet cell tumors of the pancreas. Hypercalcemia from a parathyroid hormone-related peptide (PTHrP) is more typically associated with pulmonary squamous cell carcinomas.

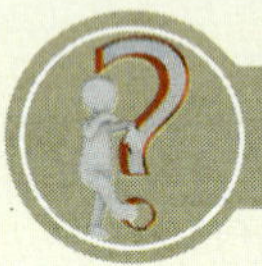

Image-Based Questions

1. The given biopsy from intestine suggests:

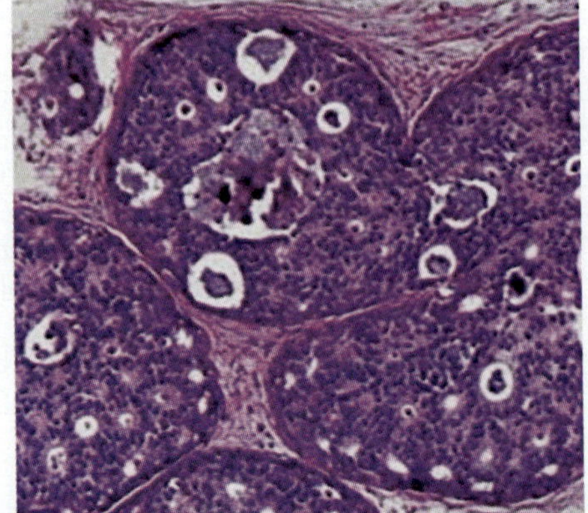

   a. Squamous cell Ca   b. Adenocarcinoma
   c. Adenoma   d. Colorectal Ca

2. Biospy from a lesion of breast mass is suggestive of:

   a. Lobular Ca   b. Medullary Ca
   c. Fibroadenoma   d. Carcinoma in situ

3. **Given below is the biopsy from cervix of 45/F who presented with cervical discharge and occasional bleeding. Compare to the normal biopsy of left side (green circle), what is your interpretation of lesion on the right (red circle)?**

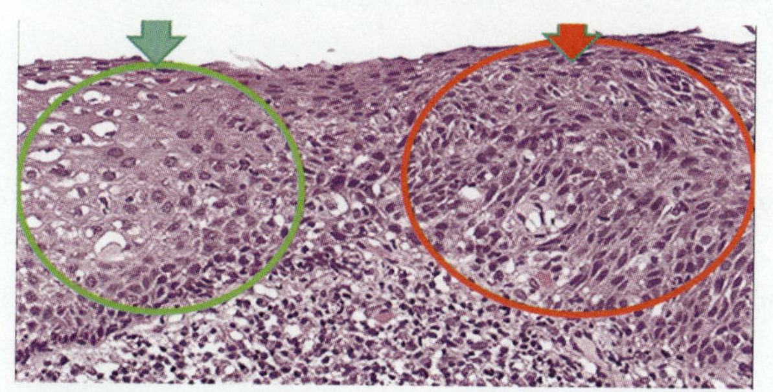

   a. Carcinoma in situ
   b. Cervical anaplasia
   c. Cervical dysplasia
   d. CMV infection

5. **The given figure shows:**

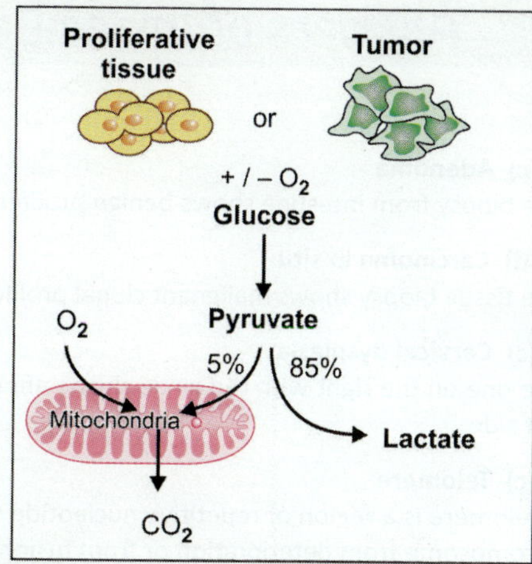

   a. Aerobic glycolysis-Warburg effect
   b. Anaerobic glycolysis-Warburg effect
   c. TCA Cycle in tumor cells
   d. Angiogenesis in tumor cells

4. **The given figure shows a very important component in chromosome of tumor cells for their replication potential. Identify?**

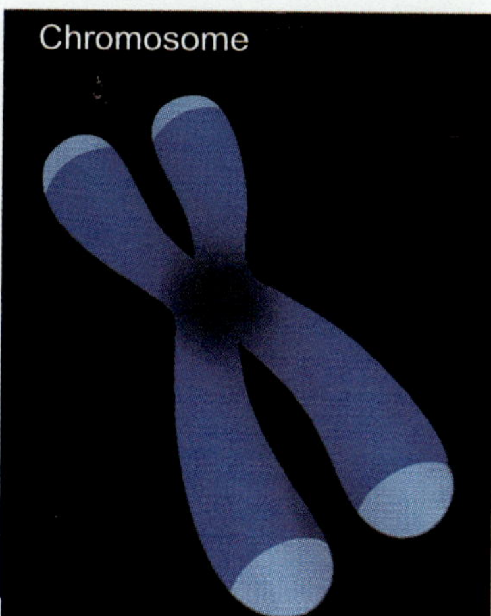

   a. Angiogenic gene
   b. Telomerase
   c. Telomere
   d. Chromosome lethality

6. **A 31-year-old woman has had dull, constant abdominal pain for 6 months. CT scan of the pelvis shows a 7 cm circumscribed mass that involves the right ovary and contains irregular calcifications. The right fallopian tube and ovary are surgically excised. The gross appearance of the ovary, which has been opened, is shown in the figure. What is the most likely diagnosis?**

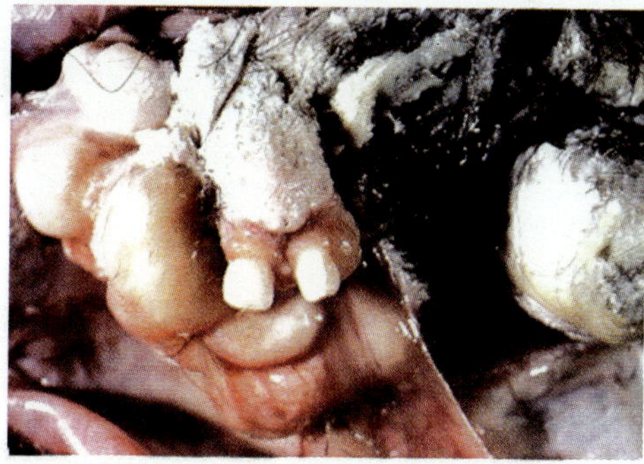

   a. Mucinous cystadenoma
   b. Choriocarcinoma
   c. Dysgerminoma
   d. Mature cystic teratoma

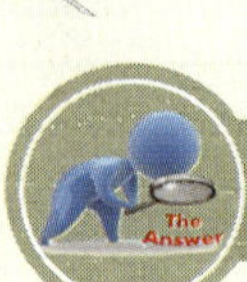

Answers of Image-Based Questions

1. **Ans. (c) Adenoma**
   - The biopsy from intestine shows benign proliferation of glandular tissue without any infiltration into deeper layers.

2. **Ans. (d) Carcinoma in situ**
   - The tissue biopsy shows malignant clonal proliferation of epithelial cells limited to ducts and lobules by the basement membrane

3. **Ans. (c) Cervical dysplasia**
   - The one on the right with red circle shows abnormal proliferation, architecture and arrangement of cells compared to normal on left side.

4. **Ans. (c) Telomere**
   - A telomere is a region of repetitive nucleotide sequences (TTAGGG) at each end of a chromosome, which protects the end of the chromosome from deterioration or from fusion with neighboring chromosomes.

5. **Ans. (a) Aerobic glycolysis-Warburg effect**
   - Cancer cells preferred to aerobic glycolysis than to oxidative phosphorylation to produce lactate .

6. **Ans. (d) Mature cystic teratoma**
   - Characteristically they are unilocular cysts containing hair and sebaceous material along with hair shafts. Within the wall, tooth structures and areas of calcification are seen.

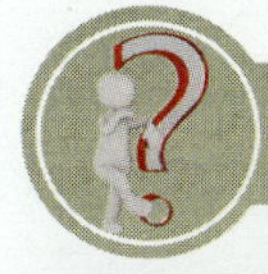

Multiple Choice Questions

TYPES OF NEOPLASMS

1. Which of the following are features of anaplasia?
   a. Metaplasia   *(PGI May 18)*
   b. Pleomorphism
   c. Loss of cell polarity
   d. Abnormal nuclear morphology
   e. Abnormal mitosis

2. Lack of differentiation is called? *(Recent exam 2018)*
   a. Anaplasia   b. Metaplasia
   c. Dysplasia   d. Carcinoma

3. Which of the following is the most common malignant tumor in adult males in India?
                                    (Recent Question 2016-17)
   a. Lung cancer   b. Oropharyngeal carcinoma
   c. Gastric carcinoma   d. Colorectal carcinoma

4. Two most common cancer in Indian woman is:
                                    (Recent Question 2016-17)
   a. Carcinoma breast   b. Carcinoma cervix
   c. Carcinoma colon   d. Carcinoma stomach
   e. Carcinoma lung

5. C-KIT mutations are seen in: *(Recent Question 2015)*
   a. Gastrointestinal stromal tumors
   b. Ovarian cancers
   c. Neuroblastoma
   d. Small-cell carcinoma of lung

6. Most common cancer in the world
                                    (Recent Question 2015)
   a. Lung   b. Breast
   c. Prostate   d. Cervix

7. Most common cancer in females *(Recent Question 2015)*
   a. Lung   b. Breast
   c. Stomach   d. Cervix

8. Most common cancer in males *(Recent Question 2015)*
   a. Lung   b. Prostate
   c. Stomach   d. Colorectum

9. Most common cause of cancer death
                                    (Recent Question 2015)
   a. Breast   b. Liver
   c. Lung   d. Brain

10. Hamartoma is: *(Recent Question 2015)*
   a. Malignant tumor
   b. Metastatic tissue
   c. Development malformation
   d. Hemorrhage in vessel

11. Choristoma is: *(Recent Question 2015)*
   a. Dilated vascular malformation
   b. Malignant stroma of stem cells
   c. Normal tissue at abnormal site in the body
   d. Benign tumor in which normal elements become abnormally owergrown

12. Choristoma is a: *(AP PGMEE 2015)*
   a. Heterotopic (ectopic) rest of cells
   b. Example of hamartoma
   c. Benign tumor of trophoblastic cell
   d. Benign tumor of cartilaginous tissue

13. Next to metastasis, which is the most reliable feature to differentiate benign from malignant tumors:
                                    (Recent Question 2015)
   a. Anaplasia   b. Dysplasia
   c. Local invasion   d. Loss of polarity

14. Number of cancer cells present in the smallest clinically detectable mass *(Recent Question 2015)*
   a. 10^3cell   b. 10^6cell
   c. 10^9cell   d. 10^{12}cell

15. Overgrowth of a bile duct at localized region is?
                                    (Recent Question 2013)
   a. Hamartoma   b. Malignant tumor
   c. Choriostoma   d. Polyp

16. Example of autonomous hyperplasia? *(JIPMER 2012)*
   a. Choristoma   b. Hamartoma
   c. Fibromatosis   d. Endometrial hyperplasia

17. Features(s) of hamartoma is/are: *(PGI Nov 2011)*
   a. Benign   b. Malignant
   c. Malformation   d. Mostly symptomatic
   e. Neoplasms

18. High risk of malignancy is seen in? *(DNB June 11)*
   a. Simple hyperplasia with atypia
   b. Simple hyperplasia without atypia
   c. Complex hyperplasia with atypia
   d. Complex hyperplasia without atypia
   e. Intraductal carcinoma in situ

TUMOR SUPPRESOR GENES

19. A 75-year-old male, known smoker presented to pulmonology department with history of cough. Biopsy was taken which showed the following. What is the change shown? *(Recent Pattern Question 2020)*

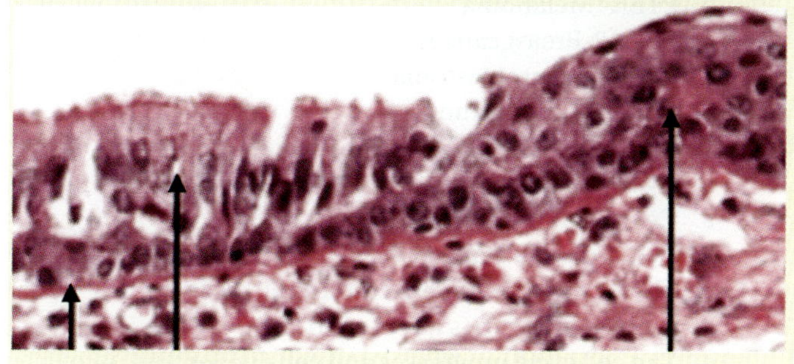

   a. Dysplasia   b. Metaplasia
   c. Hyperplasia   d. Atrophy

20. If DNA is damaged in the cell cycle, which gene causes cell cycle arrest? *(AIIMS May 2019)*
   a. Rb   b. MYC
   c. p53   d. K-RAS

21. Arrange the sequence of the event of the cell cycles:
                                    (AIIMS May 2019)
   a. Cyclin D-CDK4   b. Cyclin A-CDK1
   c. Cyclin B-CDK2   d. Cyclin E-CDK2

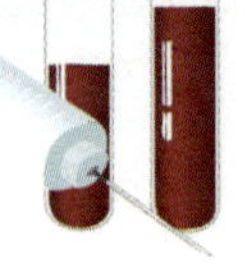

22. **Proto-oncogenes to oncogenes transformation occurs by:** *(AIIMS Nov 2019)*
1. Point mutation
2. Promoter insertion
3. Amplification
4. Enhancer insertion
a. 1 and 2 are correct
b. 1 and 3 are correct
c. 1, 3 and 4 are correct
d. All are correct

23. **True about p53 Gene:** *(PGI May 2019)*
a. Most common gene mutation found in human cancers
b. Causes cell cycle arrest at G1/S check point
c. Promote transcription of cell cycle inhibitors
d. Known as guardian of genome
e. Regulate cellular senescence

24. **Characteristics of proto-oncogenes?** *(PGI Nov 2018)*
a. One mutation is enough for causing tumors
b. Two mutations are needed for causing tumors
c. Mutations of proto oncogenes is in somatic cells
d. Mutations can be transferred through germ line

25. **Which of the following mutation is seen in Cowden syndrome?** *(Recent Question 2018)*
a. PTEN mutation
b. STK11 mutation
c. PTCH mutation
d. SMAD4 mutation

26. **Which is not a tumour suppressor gene?** *(PGI May 2017)*
a. p53
b. CD 95
c. RAS
d. PTEN
e. Stk 7/Stk11

27. **On which cell cycle checkpoints BRCA-2 acts?** *(PGI Nov 2017)*
a. G2-M
b. G1-M
c. M phase
d. G1 phase
e. S phase

28. **Which of the following Dyads are correctly matched?** *(PGI Nov 2017)*
a. RB1-retinoblastoma
b. PTEN- Melanoma
c. BRCA2-Breast cancer
d. n-MYC-Neuroblastoma
e. WT1 = Wilms' tumor

29. **If the RB gene phosphorylation is defective which of the following will happen?** *(AIIMS May 2017)*
a. Cell cycle will stop at G2
b. Cell cycle will stop at G1
c. There will be no effect on cell cycle as RB gene phosphorylation is not needed
d. The cell cycle progresses and cell divides

30. **All are true regarding Retinoblastoma except?** *(JIPMER 2017)*
a. Play major role in cell cycle regulation
b. Require deletion of both Rb genes
c. Autosomal Dominant
d. Located on chr 13p14

31. **Which of the following statement is true about p53 gene?**
a. Has tyrosine kinase activity *(PGI Nov 2016)*
b. Has pro-apoptotic activity present
c. A tumor suppressor protein
d. Has anti-apoptotic activity

32. **Homozygous loss of the VHL tumor suppressor protein;**
a. Clear cell carcinomas *(JIPMER 2016)*
b. Papillary renal cell carcinomas
c. Chromophobe
d. Belini duct Ca

33. **Most common gene involved in endometrial ca is?** *(JIPMER 2016)*
a. PTEN
b. BRAF mutation
c. KRAS
d. Mismatch repair genes

34. **BRAF mutation is seen in?** *(Recent Question 2016-17)*
a. LCH
b. Colon Ca
c. Hairy cell leukemia
d. AML M7

35. **There are different check points in cell growth and regulation. Which one is the primary point for regulation of cell growth?** *(AIIMS Nov 2015)*

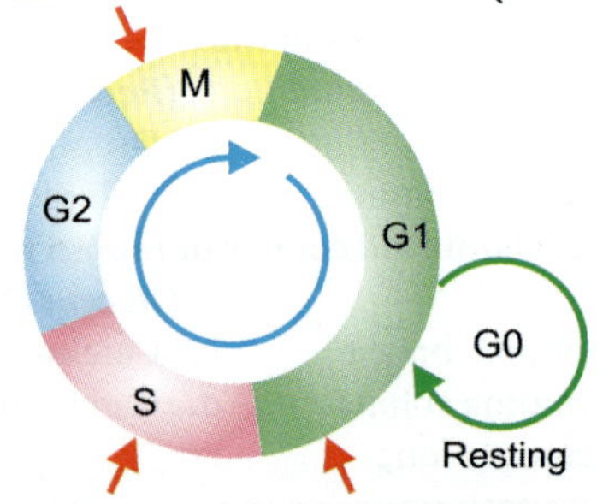

a. End of G1
b. Start of G2
c. End of S
d. End of M

36. **K-RAS protooncogene is associated with** *(Recent Question 2015)*
a. Colon cancer
b. Breast cancer
c. Bladder cancer
d. Melanoma

37. **RET protooncogene is associated with**
a. MEN1 *(Recent Question 2015)*
b. Medullary carcinoma of thyroid
c. Small cell carcinoma of lung
d. Melanoma

38. **The following protein is called "Governor of proliferation"** *(Recent Question 2015)*
a. RB
b. TP53
c. APC
d. Patched

39. **E6 protein of high risk human papilloma viruses bind to the following protein and there by promotes carcinogenesis** *(Recent Question 2015)*
a. RB
b. TP53
c. APC
d. MDM2

40. **The following protein is called "Gatekeeper of colonic neoplasia"** *(Recent Question 2015)*
a. APC
b. STK11
c. SMAD2
d. PTEN

41. **Hall mark mechanism of tumor suppressor gene inactivation** *(Recent Question 2015)*
a. Loss of heterozygosity
b. DNA hypermethylation
c. DNA hypomethylation
d. Histone deacetylation

42. **Protooncogene involved in GIST** *(Recent Question 2015)*
a. KIT
b. RAS
c. RET
d. MYC

43. **Tumor suppressor gene mutated in familial gastric cancer** *(Recent Question 2015)*
    a. APC
    b. CDKN2A
    c. E-cadherin
    d. PTEN

44. **All are associated with BRCA mutation except** *(Recent Question 2015)*
    a. Ovarian carcinoma
    b. Prostate carcinoma
    c. Endometrial carcinoma
    d. Papillary serous cancer of peritoneum

45. **SIS proto-oncogene over-expression is seen in:** *(Recent Question 2015)*
    a. Astrocytoma
    b. Breast carcinoma
    c. Melanoma
    d. Gastric carcinoma

46. **Tumor suppressor gene associated with pancreatic carcinoma** *(Recent Question 2015)*
    a. p53
    b. P16/INK4a
    c. PTEN
    d. PTCH1 and PTCH

47. **BRCA 1 and BRCA 2 genes are located on chromosomes** *(Recent Question 2015)*
    a. 13 and 17
    b. 17 and 22
    c. 17 and 13
    d. 13 and 22

48. **The following is not a cell cycle inhibitor**
    a. p21 *(Recent Question 2015)*
    b. p27
    c. p16/INK4a
    d. Cyclin D-CDK4 complex

49. **The following is not one of the 4 key cell cycle regulators which are dysregulated in vast majority of human cancers** *(Recent Question 2015)*
    a. p16/INK4a
    b. Cyclin D
    c. p21
    d. RB

50. **The cell cycle check point which is important in cells exposed to ionizing radiation** *(Recent Question 2015)*
    a. G0-G1 check point
    b. G1-S check point
    c. G2-M check point
    d. S-G2 check point

51. **Which of the following is a Tumor suppressor gene?**
    a. RB
    b. MYC *(JIPMER 2015)*
    c. RAS
    d. RET

52. **AKT-1 gene mutation is associated with?** *(Recent Question 2015)*
    a. Stomach
    b. Breast
    c. Ovary
    d. Pancreas

53. **CDK4 positive tumors are?** *(PGI Nov 2015)*
    a. Melanomas
    b. Sarcomas
    c. Glioblastomas
    d. Lobular Ca breast
    e. Prostate Ca

54. **Gain of function in RAS gene mutation is equal to loss of function mutation in which of the following?** *(Recent Question 2015)*
    a. Rb
    b. bcr-tyrosine kinase
    c. bcl-2
    d. c-myc
    e. GAP protein

55. **Cyclin D dependent proteins are?** *(PGI May 2014)*
    a. CDK-1
    b. CDK-2
    c. CDK-3
    d. CDK-4
    e. CDK-6

56. **Cells are most radio-resistant in** *(AP PGMEE 14)*
    a. S phase
    b. M phase
    c. G2 phase
    d. G1 phase

57. **MYC gene is:** *(Recent Question 2013)*
    a. Protein kinase inhibitor
    b. Growth factor inhibitor
    c. GTPase
    d. Transcription activator

58. **The most radiosensitive phase of cell cycle is:**
    a. G1
    b. G2 *(MH 16)*
    c. S
    d. M

59. **Chromosome duplication takes place in:** *(Recent Question 2014)*
    a. M phase
    b. GO phase Pattern
    c. S phase
    d. G2 phase

60. **True about protooncogene:** *(PGI May 2013)*
    a. Regulate cell growth and gene expression
    b. Found in normal cells
    c. Induced by virus
    d. Inactivated by virus
    e. May convert to oncogene

61. **Cyclin dependent kinase-2 (CDK-2) acts via:**
    a. Cyclin A
    b. Cyclin B *(PGI May 12)*
    c. Cyclin C
    d. Cyclin D
    e. Cyclin E

62. **Protein structure on chromatids where the spindle fibers attach during cell division is called?** *(DNB Aug 12 Pattern)*
    a. Nucleolus
    b. Satellite
    c. Kinetochore
    d. Centromere

63. **N-MYC amplification is associated with which tumor?**
    a. Burkitt lymphoma *(COMEDK 11)*
    b. Squamous cell carcinoma lung
    c. Astrocytoma
    d. Neuroblastoma

64. **Which among the following pairs of Oncogenes is activated by Translocation?** *(DNB Dec 10)*
    a. SIS and HST-l
    b. HGF and L-MYC
    c. TGF and CDK4
    d. ABL and C-MYC

65. **Which of the following genes is growth promoting marker for oncogenesis ?** *(MH 16)*
    a. Rb gene
    b. RAS gene
    c. p53 gene
    d. BRCA 1 gene

66. **Tumor suppressor gene is not involved in:**
    a. Breast cancers *(Recent Question 2014)*
    b. Neurofibromatosis
    c. Multiple endocrine neoplasia
    d. Retinoblastoma

67. **Cancers are usually associated with?** *(AIIMS Nov 2014)*
    a. Hypomethylation of oncogenes
    b. Methylation of tumor suppressor genes
    c. Loss of heterozygosity
    d. Mutation in introns

68. **RET gene mutation is associated with?**
    a. Pheochromocytoma *(Recent Question 2013)*
    b. Medullary carcinoma thyroid
    c. Lymphoma
    d. Renal cell carcinoma

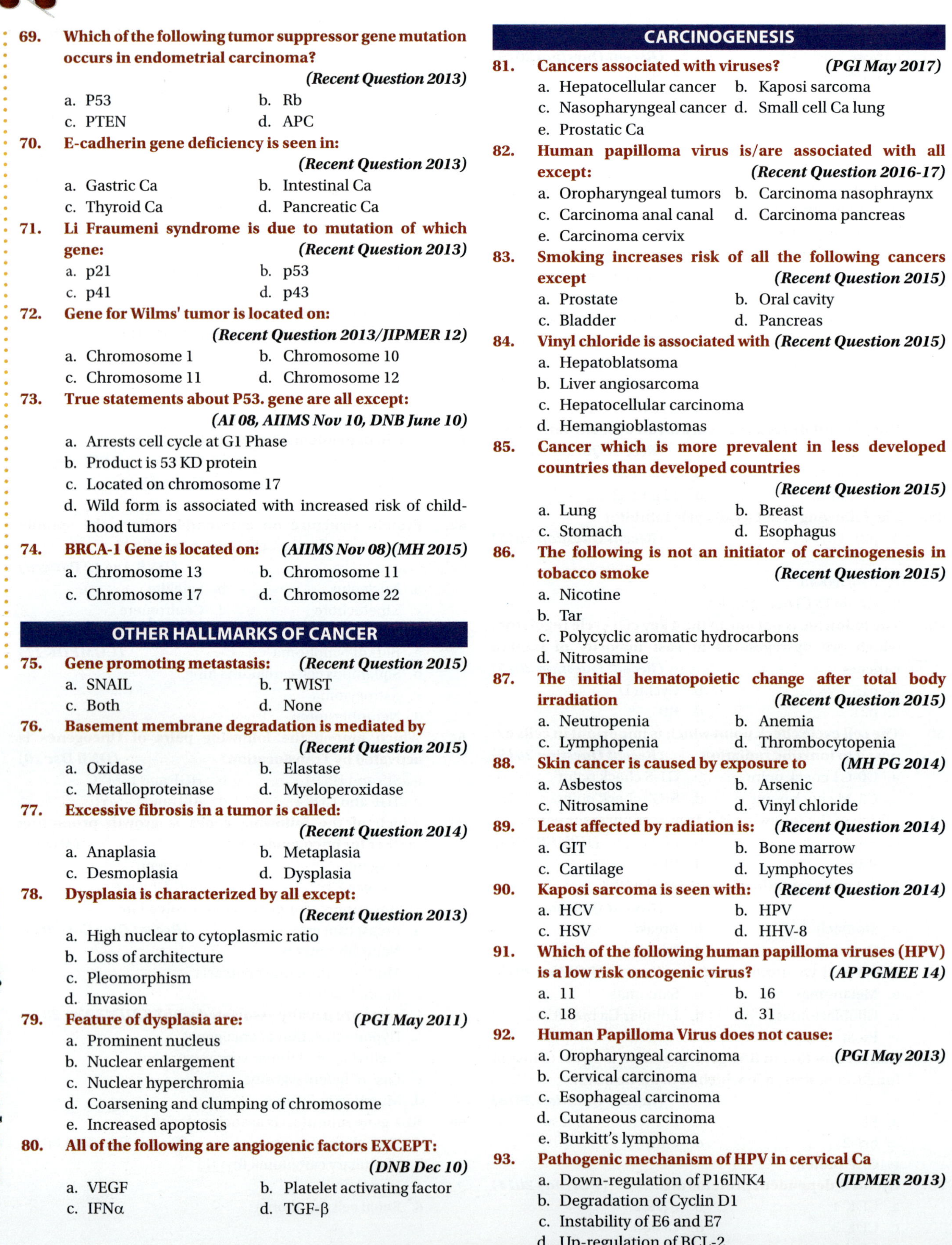

69. **Which of the following tumor suppressor gene mutation occurs in endometrial carcinoma?**
(Recent Question 2013)
   a. P53
   b. Rb
   c. PTEN
   d. APC

70. **E-cadherin gene deficiency is seen in:**
(Recent Question 2013)
   a. Gastric Ca
   b. Intestinal Ca
   c. Thyroid Ca
   d. Pancreatic Ca

71. **Li Fraumeni syndrome is due to mutation of which gene:**
(Recent Question 2013)
   a. p21
   b. p53
   c. p41
   d. p43

72. **Gene for Wilms' tumor is located on:**
(Recent Question 2013/JIPMER 12)
   a. Chromosome 1
   b. Chromosome 10
   c. Chromosome 11
   d. Chromosome 12

73. **True statements about P53. gene are all except:**
(AI 08, AIIMS Nov 10, DNB June 10)
   a. Arrests cell cycle at G1 Phase
   b. Product is 53 KD protein
   c. Located on chromosome 17
   d. Wild form is associated with increased risk of childhood tumors

74. **BRCA-1 Gene is located on:** *(AIIMS Nov 08)(MH 2015)*
   a. Chromosome 13
   b. Chromosome 11
   c. Chromosome 17
   d. Chromosome 22

OTHER HALLMARKS OF CANCER

75. **Gene promoting metastasis:** *(Recent Question 2015)*
   a. SNAIL
   b. TWIST
   c. Both
   d. None

76. **Basement membrane degradation is mediated by**
(Recent Question 2015)
   a. Oxidase
   b. Elastase
   c. Metalloproteinase
   d. Myeloperoxidase

77. **Excessive fibrosis in a tumor is called:**
(Recent Question 2014)
   a. Anaplasia
   b. Metaplasia
   c. Desmoplasia
   d. Dysplasia

78. **Dysplasia is characterized by all except:**
(Recent Question 2013)
   a. High nuclear to cytoplasmic ratio
   b. Loss of architecture
   c. Pleomorphism
   d. Invasion

79. **Feature of dysplasia are:** *(PGI May 2011)*
   a. Prominent nucleus
   b. Nuclear enlargement
   c. Nuclear hyperchromia
   d. Coarsening and clumping of chromosome
   e. Increased apoptosis

80. **All of the following are angiogenic factors EXCEPT:**
(DNB Dec 10)
   a. VEGF
   b. Platelet activating factor
   c. IFNα
   d. TGF-β

CARCINOGENESIS

81. **Cancers associated with viruses?** *(PGI May 2017)*
   a. Hepatocellular cancer
   b. Kaposi sarcoma
   c. Nasopharyngeal cancer
   d. Small cell Ca lung
   e. Prostatic Ca

82. **Human papilloma virus is/are associated with all except:** *(Recent Question 2016-17)*
   a. Oropharyngeal tumors
   b. Carcinoma nasophraynx
   c. Carcinoma anal canal
   d. Carcinoma pancreas
   e. Carcinoma cervix

83. **Smoking increases risk of all the following cancers except** *(Recent Question 2015)*
   a. Prostate
   b. Oral cavity
   c. Bladder
   d. Pancreas

84. **Vinyl chloride is associated with** *(Recent Question 2015)*
   a. Hepatoblatsoma
   b. Liver angiosarcoma
   c. Hepatocellular carcinoma
   d. Hemangioblastomas

85. **Cancer which is more prevalent in less developed countries than developed countries**
(Recent Question 2015)
   a. Lung
   b. Breast
   c. Stomach
   d. Esophagus

86. **The following is not an initiator of carcinogenesis in tobacco smoke** *(Recent Question 2015)*
   a. Nicotine
   b. Tar
   c. Polycyclic aromatic hydrocarbons
   d. Nitrosamine

87. **The initial hematopoietic change after total body irradiation** *(Recent Question 2015)*
   a. Neutropenia
   b. Anemia
   c. Lymphopenia
   d. Thrombocytopenia

88. **Skin cancer is caused by exposure to** *(MH PG 2014)*
   a. Asbestos
   b. Arsenic
   c. Nitrosamine
   d. Vinyl chloride

89. **Least affected by radiation is:** *(Recent Question 2014)*
   a. GIT
   b. Bone marrow
   c. Cartilage
   d. Lymphocytes

90. **Kaposi sarcoma is seen with:** *(Recent Question 2014)*
   a. HCV
   b. HPV
   c. HSV
   d. HHV-8

91. **Which of the following human papilloma viruses (HPV) is a low risk oncogenic virus?** *(AP PGMEE 14)*
   a. 11
   b. 16
   c. 18
   d. 31

92. **Human Papilloma Virus does not cause:**
   a. Oropharyngeal carcinoma *(PGI May 2013)*
   b. Cervical carcinoma
   c. Esophageal carcinoma
   d. Cutaneous carcinoma
   e. Burkitt's lymphoma

93. **Pathogenic mechanism of HPV in cervical Ca**
   a. Down-regulation of P16INK4 *(JIPMER 2013)*
   b. Degradation of Cyclin D1
   c. Instability of E6 and E7
   d. Up-regulation of BCL-2

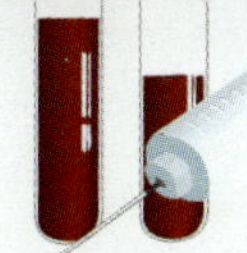

94. UV radiation: *(Recent Question 2013)*
- a. Prevents formation of Pyrimidine dimers
- b. Stimulates formation of Pyrimidine dimers
- c. Purine dimers
- d. Single gene deletion

95. The least radio sensitive tissue is: *(AI 10)*
- a. Nervous tissue
- b. Bone
- c. Kidney
- d. Thyroid

GENETIC BASIS OF CANCERS

96. All of the following are hereditary tumors except?
(Recent Question 2016-17)
- a. Retinoblastoma
- b. Ewings Sa
- c. Ca breast
- d. Nasopharyngeal Ca
- e. Ca pancreas

97. Tumors associated with AIDS? *(PGI Nov 2016)*
- a. DLBCL
- b. Ca breast
- c. Ca pancreas
- d. Kaposi Sarcoma
- e. Ca lung

98. Chromopthysis mechanism of carcinogenesis has been found to be associated with which of the following tumors? *(Recent Question 2016-17)*
- a. Sarcomas
- b. Osteosarcoma
- c. RCC
- d. ALL

99. True statement of Ataxia telangiectasia is?
- a. Seizure *(PGI Nov 2016)*
- b. IgA is low or absent
- c. Increased risk of Leukemia
- d. Hypoplasia of thymus
- e. Adaptive immune system is normal

100. Which of the following marker favours diagnosis of preinvasive and invasive cervical cancer:
- a. Ki67 *(Recent Question 2016-17)*
- b. Oncoprotein E6
- c. p16INK4, cyclin E, and Ki-67
- d. Oncoprotein E8

101. Which of the following marker/mutation is/are seen in papillary carcinoma of thyroid:
(Recent Question 2016-17)
- a. Synaptophysin
- b. RET/PTC
- c. P53
- d. NTRK1
- e. RAS

102. Chromothryps is false statement
(Recent Question 2015)
- a. Include simple deletions, inversions and translocations in chromosomes
- b. Found in higher frequencies in osteosarcomas and bone cancers
- c. Hundreds of chromosome breaks occur across single or several chromosomes
- d. DNA is repaired in a haphazard manner

103. BRAF mutation is seen in? *(Recent Question 2015)*
- a. Melanoma
- b. Squamous Cell Ca
- c. Papillary Ca thyroid
- d. Retinal hemangioblastoma

104. Most common translocation in Ewing's sarcoma is:
(Recent Question 2015)
- a. t (11;22)
- b. t (9;22)
- c. t (8;14)
- d. t (x;11)

PARANEOPLASTIC SYNDROMES

105. Paraneoplastic syndrome(s) associated with lymphoma? *(PGI Nov 2017)*
- a. SIADH
- b. Hypercalcemia
- c. Cushing's syndrome
- d. Acanthosis nigricans

106. All are signs of paraneoplastic syndrome in skin except?
- a. Tripe palm *(PGI Nov 2016)*
- b. Acanthosis nigricans
- c. Superficial thrombophlebitis
- d. Dermatomyositis
- e. Oslers node

107. Malignancy associated with hypercalcemia
(PGI Nov 2016)
- a. Breast cancer
- b. Prostate cancer
- c. Small cell lung cancer
- d. Nonsmall lung cancer

108. Migratory thrombophlebitis is seen in all except?
(JIPMER 2012, AI 08)
- a. Lung Ca
- b. Prostate Ca
- c. Colon Ca
- d. Pancreatic Ca

LABORATORY DIAGNOSIS OF CANCER

109. Tumour causing phosphaturia and osteomalacia is?
(AIIMS Nov 18)
- a. Peripheral nerve sheath
- b. Meningioma
- c. Fibrosarcoma
- d. Osteosarcoma

110. Sentinal lymph node biopsy is most significant for ?
(AIIMS Nov 18)
- a. CaVulva
- b. Ca Vagina
- c. Ca Endometrium
- d. Ca Cervix

111. Nobel Prize for 2018 was awarded for what contribution?
(AIIMS Nov 18)
- a. Negative immune regulation in treatment of cancer
- b. CAS9-CRISPER
- c. DNA repair syndromes
- d. Stem cell transplant

112. Gastrin is a marker of which carcinoma? *(JIPMER 18)*
- a. Medullary carcinoma of thyroid
- b. GIST
- c. Gastric carcinoma
- d. Pancreatic carcinoma/neuroectodermal tumour

113. Markers of carcinoma pancreas ? *(PGI Nov 2018)*
- a. Ca19-9
- b. Ca 125
- c. CEA
- d. AFP

114. Sarcoma on paraffin mount shows what markers?
(PGI Nov 2018)
- a. Desmin
- b. Vimentin
- c. PAX8
- d. WT1
- e. HMB 45

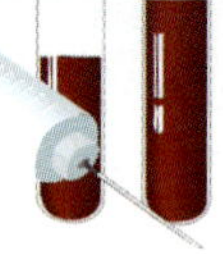

115. A 5-year-old child was presenting with proptosis. Microscopic examination has revealed round cell tumor and positive for desmin immunohistochemical marker. Most likely diagnosis is? *(AIIMS May 18)*
a. Leukemia
b. Embryonal rhabdomyosarcoma
c. Lymphoma
d. Primitive Neuroectodermal Tumor (PNET)

116. Biopsy from an eight-year-old child with leg swelling was showing small round blue tumor cells consistent with diagnosis of Ewing's sarcoma. What will be the best method to detect translocation t (11;22) in this malignancy? *(AIIMS May 18)*
a. Conventional karyotyping
b. Next generation sequencing
c. FISH
d. PCR

117. Which of the following immunohistochemical marker is positive in neuroendocrine tumor? *(Recent exam 2018)*
a. Cytokeratin
b. Synaptophysin
c. Calretinin
d. GFAP

118. Which of the following neoplasms shows ALK positivity? *(AIIMS May 2017)*
a. Ewing sarcoma
b. Inflammatory myofibroblastictumor
c. Synovial sarcoma
d. Fibromatosis

119. Fixative agent for PAP smear? *(AIIMS Nov 2017)*
a. Norma saline
b. Formalin
c. 95% ethanol
d. Air drying

120. Not seen in tumour lysis syndrome? *(AIIMS Nov 2017)*
a. Hyperphosphatemia
b. Hyperuricaemia
c. Hypercalcemia
d. Hyperkalaemia

121. In CA breast, based on Which stage/grade of IHC staining, FISH for gene amplification will be done?
a. Her2 neu 3+ *(AIIMS Nov 2017)*
b. Her2 Nu 2+
c. Her2 neu +
d. Will be done irrespective of above

122. ALK1 mutation seen mc with which hereditary hemorrhagic telangiectasia? *(JIPMER 2017)*
a. Type 1
b. Type 2
c. Type 3
d. Type 4

123. Carbohydrate marker of recurrent breast cancer is? *(JIPMER 2017)*
a. CA 15.3
b. CA 125
c. CEA
d. CA 19.9

124. For detection of carcinoma lip, stain used is? *(AIIMS Nov 2016)*
a. Giemsa
b. Crystal violet
c. Toulidine blue
d. Hematoxylin and eosin

125. AFP and CEA both rise in *(Recent Question 2016-17)*
a. Testicular ca
b. Hepatic ca
c. RCC
d. Germ cell tumor of ovary

126. A surgeon suspecting testicular carcinoma in a patient asks the intern to send the sample for histopathology, what is the fluid in which the intern should send the sample to the pathologist? *(AIIMS May 2016)*
a. Bouvin solution
b. 10% formalin
c. 95% ethanol
d. Alcohol

127. High level of β hCG is/are seen in all except:
a. Down syndrome *(Recent Question 2016-17)*
b. Neural tube defect
c. Germ cell tumor
d. Gestational trophoblastic disease
e. Multiple pregnancy

128. Neuroendocrine cell tumor markers are:
a. Chromogranin A *(Recent Question 2016-17)*
b. CD56
c. Neuron-specific enolase
d. Synaptophysin
e. Cytokeratin 7

129. Not true about cancer cachexia *(Recent Question 2015)*
a. Equal loss of both fat and lean muscle
b. Elevated basal metabolic rate
c. No evidence of systemic inflammation
d. TNFα (cachetin) plays an important role

130. Grading of cancers is does not depend on
a. Degree of differentiation *(Recent Question 2015)*
b. Number of mitoses
c. Architectural features
d. Size of primary lesion

131. Tumor markers and tumors –find the wrong match
a. Desmin–Carcinoma *(Recent Question 2015)*
b. Vimentin–sarcoma
c. Leucocyte specific antigen–lymphoma
d. S100–melanoma

132. Acid phosphatase is a tumor marker for
a. Pancreatic carcinoma *(Recent Question 2015)*
b. Prostatic carcinoma
c. Papillary carcinoma of thyroid
d. Renal cell carcinoma

133. Tumor marker for non-seminomatous testicular tumors *(Recent Question 2015)*
a. CEA
b. CA-125
c. CA-19-9
d. Alpha-fetoprotein

134. HMB-45 is positive in *(Recent Question 2015)*
a. Small cell carcinoma of lung
b. Adenocarcinoma of lung
c. Squamous cell carcinoma of lung
d. Angiomyolipoma of lung

135. CA-125 is used is the monitoring and treatment of *(Recent Question 2015)*
a. Ovarian cancer
b. Colon cancer
c. Breast cancer
d. Pancreatic cancer

136. An undifferentiated malignant tumor on immuno-histochemical stain shows cytoplasmic positivity of most of the tumor cells for cytokeratin. The most probable diagnosis of the tumor is: *(MH 16)*
a. Lymphoma
b. Carcinoma
c. Sarcoma
d. Malignant melanoma

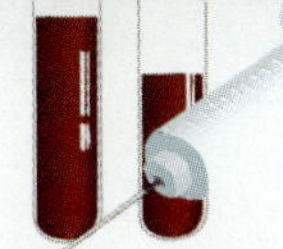

137. **Hypercalcemia as a paraneoplastic syndrome in lymphomas is due to elaboration of**
    a. PTHrP   *(Recent Question 2015)*
    b. PTH
    c. 1,25dihydroxy vitamin D
    d. PGE2

138. **Molecular profiling of cancer cells is obtained by**
                                (Recent Question 2015)
    a. Flow cytometry
    b. Immunohistochemistry
    c. DNA microarray analysis
    d. PCR

139. **Antibody not associated with paraneoplastic cerebellar degeneration**   *(Recent Question 2015)*
    a. Anti-Yo   b. Anti-Hu
    c. Anti-Ri   d. Anti-Tr

140. **Alpha feto protein is/are increased in:** *(PGI May 2015)*
    a. Yolk sac tumor   b. Seminoma
    c. Dysgerminoma   d. Non-seminoma
    e. Hepatocellular carcinoma

141. **Hypoglycemia occur as a paraneoplastic syndrome in:**
    a. Bronchogenic carcinoma   *(Recent Question 2015)*
    b. CA pancreas
    c. Fibrosarcoma
    d. RCC

142. **Test for carcinogenicity**   *(Recent Question 2015)*
    a. Kveim's test   b. Ame's test
    c. Schilling's test   d. Schick test

143. **Bortezomib, a proteasome inhibitor is used in the treatment of**   *(Recent Question 2015)*
    a. AML M3   b. CML
    c. Multiple myeloma   d. GIST

144. **Chemical carcinogen associated with cancer of renal pelvis**   *(Recent Question 2015)*
    a. Polycyclic hydrocarbons
    b. Cyclophosphamide
    c. Asbestos
    d. Cadmium

145. **Paraneoplastic neurologic syndrome not associated with antibodies**   *(Recent Question 2015)*
    a. Lambert-Eaton myasthenic syndrome
    b. Stiff pearson syndrome
    c. Limbic encephalopathy
    d. Necrotizing myelopathy

146. **The hallmark change in cell physiology that determines malignant phenotype**   *(Recent Question 2015)*
    a. Self sufficieny in growth signals
    b. Sustained angiogenesis
    c. Resistance to apoptosis
    d. Aerobic glycolysis

147. **Keratinization and pearl formation is seen in?**
                                (Recent Question 2015)
    a. Squamous cell Ca   b. Adenocarcinoma
    c. Small cell Ca   d. Basal cell Ca

148. **Which of the following is not correctly matched?**
    a. Melanoma - s100   *(AIIMS Nov 14)*
    b. Carcinoma - desmin
    c. Sarcoma - vimentin
    d. Lymphoma -leucocyte common antigen

149. **Calcitonin is a marker of:**   *(Recent Question 2014)*
    a. Prostate cancer
    b. Medullary carcinoma of thyroid
    c. Pheochromocytoma
    d. Pancreatic cancer

150. **MIC-2 is a marker of?**   *(DNB Aug 12 Pattern)*
    a. Ewing sarcoma
    b. Chronic lymphocytic leukemia
    c. Mantle cell lymphoma
    d. All of these

151. **Not a marker for muscle tumor:** *(Recent Question 2014)*
    a. Desmin   b. Actin
    c. Neurofilament   d. Intermediate filament

152. **The following is not a marker of melanoma:**
    a. S-100   b. MITF   *(JIPMER 2014)*
    c. CK-20   d. Vimentin

153. **Immunohistochemical marker for Rhabdomyosarcoma is:**   *(JIPMER 2014)*
    a. Desmin   b. Vimentin
    c. Cytokeratin   d. Neurofilament

154. **SS18 –SSX1 gene is associated with:**
                                (Recent Question 2013)
    a. Liposarcoma   b. Rhabdomyosarcoma
    c. Synovial sarcoma   d. Ewing's sarcoma

155. **Maternal serum AFP raised in:**   *(PGI May 2013)*
    a. Gestational Trophoblastic disease
    b. Down syndrome
    c. Omphalocoele
    d. Sacrococcygealtetatoma
    e. Neural tube defect

156. **True about Carcino embryonic antigen (CEA) is/are:**
                                (PGI May 2013)
    a. Used for monitoring of recurrence of colon cancer
    b. Specific for colon cancer
    c. Increased in smokers
    d. Increased in colon cancer
    e. Increased in Renal Carcinoma

157. **True about CA-125 is/are:**   *(PGI May 2013)*
    a. It is a Glycoprotein
    b. It is a specific marker
    c. It is Increased in colon carcinoma
    d. Normal range in pre-menopausal females is 200 U/ml
    e. May be elevated in Pelvic inflammatory disease

158. **Which amongst the following a marker of Carcinoma:**
    a. Cytokeratin   b. Vimentin   *(AI 12)*
    c. Calretinin   d. CD45

159. **Conventional cytogenetics are difficult in solid tumors especially in case of carcinoma cervix because of:**
                                (AIIMS Nov 10)
    a. High mitotic rate
    b. Bacterial contamination of the specimen
    c. Good metaphase activity
    d. Inadequate biopsy specimen

160. **Increased LDH helps in diagnosis of?**

(DNB Aug 12)

   a. Prostate carcinoma
   b. Hepatocellular carcinoma
   c. Pancreatic carcinoma
   d. Renal cell carcinoma

161. **AFP is elevated in:** *(PGI May 2011)*

   a. HCC
   b. Hepatoblastoma
   c. Infant hemangioendothelioma
   d. Amebic liver abscess
   e. Embryonic sarcoma

162. **Ames test in neoplasia is a test for:** *(AP 2013)*

   a. Teratogenicity   b. Mutagenicity
   c. Carcinogenicity   d. Clonality

163. **Elevated CA -125 are seen in:** *(PGI Nov 10)*

   a. Abdominal TB   b. Ca cervix
   c. Endometriosis   d. Ovarian Ca
   e. Endometrial Ca

164. **A 67-year male smoker presents with hemoptysis and cough. Bronchoscopic biopsy revealed undifferentiated tumor. The immunohistochemical marker that will be most helpful is:** *(DNB June 10, AIIMS Nov 09)*

   a. Calretinin   b. Vimentin
   c. Cytokeratin   d. TTF1

165. **Which of the following is not a tumor marker:**

   a. CEA   *(DNB Dec 10)*
   b. Tyrosinase
   c. Human leucocyte antigen
   d. AFP

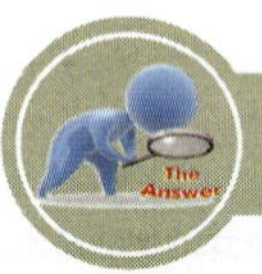

Answers with Explanations

1. **(b, c, d, e)** **b. Pleomorphism c. Loss of cell polarity d. Abnormal nuclear morphology; e. Abnormal mitosis**

2. **Ans. (a)** **Anaplasia** *(Ref: Robbins 9th ed p 269)*

Malignant neoplasms that are composed of poorly differentiated cells are said to be anaplastic. Lack of differ entiation, or anaplasia, is considered a hallmark of malignancy. The term anaplasia means "to form backward," implying a reversal of differentiation to a more primitive level.

3. **Ans. (b)** **Oropharyngeal carcinoma**

(Ref: Harrison's 19th ed/pg 467; table 99.1)

- Most common cancer all over the world (overall, considering both sexes together): **Lung cancer**
- Most common cancer all over the world: **Prostate cancer**
- Most common cancer (females) all over the world: **Breast cancer**
- Most common cause of cancer death in the world: **Lung cancer**
- 2nd most common cancer worldwide (overall): **Breast cancer**
- Causes of cancer death: lung > stomach > liver > colorectal > breast

4. **Ans. (a)** **Carcinoma breast, b. Carcinoma cervix**

(Ref: Park 23rd/ 382-83; Harshmohan 7th/198)

5. **Ans. (a)** **Gastrointestinal stromal tumors**

(Ref: Robbins 9th/pg 298; 8th/pg 295)

c-Kit
- It is a proto oncogene

- It is also known as Mast/stem cell growth factor receptor (SCFR), tyrosine-protein kinase Kit or CD117
- It is a receptor tyrosine kinase protein that in humans is encoded by the KIT gene.
- Activating mutations in this gene are associated with gastrointestinal stromal tumors, testicular seminoma, mast cell disease, melanoma, acute myeloid leukemia
- Inactivating mutations are associated with the genetic defect piebaldism.

6. **Ans. (a)** **Lung**

(Ref: Harrison's 19th ed/pg 467; table 99.1)

7. **Ans. (b)** **Breast**

(Ref: Harrison's 19th ed/pg 467; table 99.1)

8. **Ans. (b)** **Prostate**

(Ref: Harrison's 19th ed/pg 467; table 99.1)

9. **Ans. (c)** **Lung**

(Ref: Harrison's 19th ed/pg 467; table 99.1)

10. **Ans. (c)** **Development malformation**

(Ref: R 9th/pg 267)

Hamartoma:
- It is a **disorganized but benign-appearing mass** composed of cells **indigenous to that particular site**.
- Previously it was considered a **developmental malformation** but, hamartomas have been found to have **clonal recurrent translocations** involving genes encoding certain chromatin proteins

- So, hamrtomas are **considered neoplasms now**.
- E.g., Pulmonary chondroid hamartoma contains islands of disorganized, but histologically normal cartilage, bronchi, and vessels.

11. **Ans. (c) Normal tissue at abnormal site in the body**

(Ref: Robbins 9th/pg 267; 8th/pg 262)

12. **Ans. (d) Benign tumor of cartilaginous tissue**

(Ref: Robbins 9th/pg 267; 8th/pg 262)

13. **Ans. (c) Local invasion**

(Ref: Robbins 9th/pg 268; 8th/pg 263)

14. **Ans. (c) 10^9 cell**

(Ref: Robbins 9th/pg 267; 8th/pg 268)

15. **Ans. (a) Hamartoma** *(Ref: Robbins 9th/pg 267)*

Von Meyenburg Complexes (bile duct hamartomas) are small clusters of dilated bile ducts embedded in a fibrous, sometimes hyalinized, stroma located close to or within portal tracts.

16. **Ans. (c) Fibromatosis**

(Ref: Underwood's Pathology, by Simon Cross: Chapter 4)

Fibromatoses are apparently **autonomous proliferation** of **myofibroblasts,** occasionally forming **tumor like** masses. Eg Palmar Fibromatoses (Dupuytren's contractures), Desmoid tumor, Retroperitoneal fibromatosis and Peyronie's disease of penis.

17. **Ans. (c, e) c. Malformation; e. Neoplasms**

(Ref: Robbins 9th/pg 267; 8th/pg 262; Refer Ans 6)

18. **Ans. (c, e) c. Complex hyperplasia with atypia; e. Intraductal Carcinoma in situ**

(Ref: Robbins 9th/pg 270)

Discussing the options one by one:

Lesions	Relative Risk of malignancy	Description
A. Simple hyperplasia with atypia	1	Proliferation of ductal epithelium and/or stroma **without cytologic or architectural features suggestive of carcinoma in situ**
B. Simple hyperplasia without atypia	≤1	Epithelial hyperplasia i.e. presence of **> 2 cell layers**
C. Complex hyperplasia with atypia	4-5	Cellular proliferation **resembling carcinoma in situ** but lacking sufficient features for diagnosis as carcinoma
D. Complex hyperplasia without atypia	1.5-2	Individual cells may be **enlarged**, but, as in simple hyperplasia, the internal makeup of the cells is considered to be **normal**
E. Intraductal Carcinoma in-situ	8 -10	**Dysplastic changes are marked** and involve the **full thickness of the epithelium**, but **does not penetrate the basement membrane**

19. **Ans. (b) Metaplasia** *(Ref: Robbins 9th ed/pg 270)*

20. **Ans. (c) p53** *(Ref: Robbins 9th ed/pg 294)*

21. **Ans. (A→D→B→C)** *(Ref: Robbins 9th ed/pg 25)*

22. **Ans. (b) 1 and 3 are correct** *(Ref: Robbins 9th ed)*

23. **Ans. (a, b, c, d, e) a. Most common gene mutation found in human cancers; b. Causes cell cycle arrest at G1/S check point; c. Promote transcription of cell cycle inhibitors; d. Known as guardian of genome; e. Regulate cellular senescence** *(Ref: Robbins 9th ed/pg 294)*

24. **(a, c, d) a. One mutation is enough for causing tumors; c. Mutations of proto oncogenes is in somatic cells; d. Mutations can be transferred through germ line**

Oncogenes are produced from proto-oncogene by point mutations (single mutations) in both somatic cells or germ cells.

25. **Ans. (a) PTEN mutation**

(Ref: Robbins 9th ed p 298)

PTEN (phosphatase and tensin homologue) is a membrane-associated phosphatase encoded by a gene on chromosome 10q23 that is mutated in Cowden syndrome, an autosomal dominant disorder marked by frequent benign growths, such as skin appendage tumors, GI, and CNS growths; breast, endometrial, and thyroid carcinoma

26. **Ans. (b, c) b. CD 95; c. RAS**

27. **Ans. (a, e) a. G2-M; b. S phase** *(Ref: R 315)*

BRCA1 deficiency causes abnormalities in the S-phase checkpoint, the G_2/M checkpoint, the spindle checkpoint and centrosome duplication. Defects in this pathway leads to the activation of the salvage nonhomologous end joining pathway, formation of dicentric chromosomes, bridge-fusion-breakage cycles, and massive aneuploidy.

Contd...

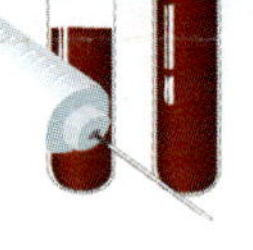

28. **Ans. (a, c, d, e) a. RB1-retinoblastoma; c. BRCA2-Breast cancer; d. n-MYC-Neuroblastoma; e. WT1 = Wilms' tumor** *(Ref: Robbins 291)*

PTEN (phosphatase and tensin homologue) mutated in Cowden syndrome, an autosomal dominant disorder marked by frequent benign growths, such as skin appendage tumors, GI, and CNS growths; breast, endometrial, and thyroid carcinoma.

29. **Ans. (b) Cell cycle will stop at G1** *(Ref: R9/ 290-292)*

- When hypophosphorylated, RB exerts antiproliferative effects by binding and inhibiting E2F transcription factors that regulate genes required for cells to pass through the G1-S phase cell cycle checkpoint. Normal growth factor signalling leads to RB hyperphosphorylation and inactivation, thus promoting cell cycle progression. Thus defective **phosphorylation will result in RB gene stopping the cell cycle at G1S transition**

30. **Ans. (d) Located on chr 13p14**

(Ref: Rb gene is located on Chr 13q14)

31. **Ans. (a, b, c) a. Has tyrosine kinase activity, b. Has pro-apoptotic activity present, c. A tumor suppressor protein**

(Ref: Robbins 9th/294)

32. **Ans. (a) Clear cell carcinomas**

(Ref: Robbins 9th/pg 721; 8th/pg 730)

33. **Ans. (a) PTEN** *(Ref: Robbins 9th/pg 721; 8th/pg 730)*

34. **Ans. (c) Hairy cell leukemia** *(Ref: Robbins 9th/1014)*

35. **Ans. (a) End of G1** *(Ref: Robbins 9th/pg 25; 8th/pg 285)*

G1-S is the primary point for regulation of cell growth

36. **Ans. (a) Colon cancer**

(Ref: Robbins 9th/pg 721; 8th/pg 730)

37. **Ans. (b) Medullary carcinoma of thyroid**

(Ref: Robbins 9th/pg 721; 8th/pg 730)

38. **Ans. (a) RB** *(Ref: Robbins 9th/pg 294; 8th/pg 291)*

RB gene (Chr 13q14) is the 'Governor of proliferation' and Key **negative regulator** of **G1/S** cell cycle transition

39. **Ans. (b) TP53** *(Ref: Robbins 9th/pg 294; 8th/pg 291)*

- HPV's genome consists of an early (E) gene region, a late (L) gene region, and a noncoding region that contains regulatory elements.
- E1, E2, E5, E6, and E7 proteins are expressed early in the growth cycle and are necessary for viral replication and cellular transformation.
- E6 and E7 proteins cause malignant transformation by targeting the human cell cycle regulatory molecules p53 and Rb (retinoblastoma protein), respectively, for degradation.

40. **Ans. (a) APC** *(Ref: Robbins 9th/pg 288; 8th/pg 284)*

Adenomatous polyposis coli (APC) gene

- On **Chr 5q21**[Q]
- **Gate-keeper of Colonic Neoplasia**[Q]
- Component of the **WNT signaling pathway**[Q]
- Controls cell fate, adhesion, and cell polarity during embryonic development.
- APC **controls** oncogenic effects of β-catenin so prevents carcinomas
- **Germline loss-of-function mutation → Familial adenomatous polyposis colon Cancer; (AD)**[Q]
- Other tumors induced: **Hepatoblastomas, Hepatocellular carcinomas**[Q]

41. **Ans. (a) Loss of heterozygosity** *(Ref: Robbins 9th/pg 288)*

42. **Ans. (a) KIT** *(Ref: Robbins 9th/pg 288; 8th/pg 285)*

43. **Ans. (c) E-cadherin** *(Ref: Robbins 9th/pg 288; 8th/pg 285)*

E-cadherin

- Loss-of-contact inhibition, by mutation of the E-cadherin/β-catenin axis is a key characteristic of carcinomas.
- Loss of E-cadherin contributes to the malignant phenotype by allowing easy disaggregation of cells, which can then invade locally or metastasize.
- Reduced cell surface expression of E-cadherin has been seen in Ca **esophagus, colon, breast, ovary, and prostate**.
- Germline loss- of-function mutations of the E-cadherin gene, known as CDH1, cause **familial gastric carcinoma**
- Some of the sporadic gastric carcinomas are also associated with loss of E-cadherin expression.

44. **Ans. (c) Endometrial carcinoma**

(Ref: Robbins 9th/pg 288)

45. **Ans. (a) Astrocytoma**

(Ref: Robbins 9th/pg 288; 8th/pg 285)

46. **Ans. (b) P16/INK4a**

(Ref: Robbins 9th/pg 288; 8th/pg 285)

Germline mutations of *p16* (*CDKN2A*) are present in 25% of melanoma-prone kindreds,
Somatically acquired deletion or inactivation of *p16* is seen in:

- 75% of pancreatic carcinomas, glioblastomas, esophageal cancers, and non–small-cell lung carcinomas.

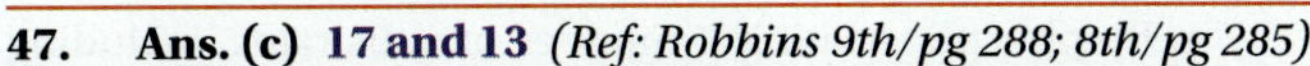

47. **Ans. (c)** **17 and 13** *(Ref: Robbins 9th/pg 288; 8th/pg 285)*

48. **Ans. (d)** **Cyclin D-CDK4 complex** *(Ref: R 9th/pg 25)*

49. **Ans. (c)** **p21** *(Ref: Robbins 9th/pg 288; 8th/pg 285)*

Loss of normal cell cycle control is central to malignant transformation and that at least one of four key regulators of the cell cycle (p16/INK4a, cyclin D, CDK4, RB) is dysregulated in the vast majority of human cancers.

50. **Ans. (c)** **G2-M check point** *(Ref: Robbins 9th/pg 25)*

Cells exposed to **ionizing radiation** → Cell cycle **arrested in G_2 and repair mechanisms activated.** Thus G2-M check point is important in cells exposed to ionizing radiation

51. **Ans. (a)** **RB** *(Ref: Robbins 9th/pg 292; 8th/pg 288)*

52. **Ans. (b)** **Breast** *(Ref: Robbins 9th/pg 292; 8th/pg 288)*

PTEN acts as a tumor suppressor by serving as a brake on the PI3K/AKT arm of the receptor tyrosine kinase pathway

PTEN (phosphatase and *ten*sin homologue) is a membrane-associated phosphatase, that is encoded by a gene on chromosome 10q23

It is mutated in Cowden syndrome, an autosomal dominant disorder marked by skin appendage tumors, and an increased incidence of epithelial cancers, particularly of the breast, endometrium, and thyroid

53. **Ans. (a, b, c);** **a. Melanomas; b. Sarcomas; c. Glioblastomas**

(Ref: Robbins 9th/pg 292; 8th/pg 288)

CDK4 activation by amplification or point mutation is seen in Glioblastoma, melanoma, sarcoma

54. **Ans. (e)** **GAP protein**

(Ref: Robbins 9th/pg 292; 8th/pg 288)

- RAS has an intrinsic GTPase activity that is accelerated by *GTPase-activating proteins (GAPs)*, which bind to the active RAS and augment its GTPase activity by more than 1000-fold, thereby terminating signal transduction.
- Thus, GAPs prevent uncontrolled RAS activity.
- Gain-of-function mutations in RAS proteins and loss-of-function mutations in GAPs lead to unchecked proliferation of cells.

55. **Ans. (d)** **CDK-4; e. CDK-6** *(Ref: Robbins 9th/pg 25)*

56. **Ans. (a)** **S phase**

(Ref: Robbins 9th/pg 25; 8th/pg 285; Cancer, By David Morris, 2003, Chapter 5)

Cells are **most radio-resistant in S phase** and **most radio-sensitive in M > G_2 phase.**

57. **Ans. (d)** **Transcription activator**

(Ref: Robbins 9th/pg 284)

MYC gene

- MYC is a **transcription factor** that acts to **reprogram somatic cells into pluripotent stem cells.**
- MYC translocations are seen in **Burkitt lymphoma** and is amplified in some **breast, colon, lung Carcinomas.**
- NMYC and LMYC genes are also amplified in **neuroblastomas** and **small cell cancers of lung**, respectively
- Notch signaling (T cell ALL), Wnt signaling (colon Ca) and Hedgehog signaling (medulloblastoma) pathways transform cells in part through upregulation of MYC gene.

58. **Ans. (d)** **M** *(Ref: Robbins 9th/pg 25; 8th/pg 285)*

59. **Ans. (c)** **S phase** *(Ref: Robbins 9th/pg 25; 8th/pg 285)*

S is the synthetic phase where **DNA replication** takes place

60. **Ans. (a, b, c, e); a. Regulate cell growth and gene expression; b. Found in normal cells; c. Induced by virus; e. May convert to oncogene** *(Ref: Robbins 9th/pg)*

Proto-Oncogenes

- **Unmutated counterparts** of genes found **normally in a cell** that promote **autonomous cell growth** in cancer
- **Function:** Regulate **Cell growth[Q], proliferation, inhibition of apoptosis[Q]** and **nuclear transcription[Q]**
- **Chromosomal translocation is the most common mechanism for activation of proto-oncogenes[Q]**
- **Proto-oncogenes** can also be **activated** by virus to **oncogenes**

61. **Ans. (a, e,);** **a. Cyclin A; e. Cyclin E**

(Ref: Robbins 9th/pg 25; 8th/pg 285; Refer to Ans 29 Above)

CDK2 forms a complex with **cyclin E** in late G1, which is involved in **G1/S transition.**

CDK2 also forms a complex with **cyclin A** at the S phase that facilitates **G2/M transition.**

62. **Ans. (c)** **Kinetochore**

(Ref: Emery's elements of Medical Genetics, 14th ed/pg 17)

- **Kinetochore** is a **protein structure on chromatids** where the spindle fibers attach during cell division to pull sister chromatids apart.
- **"Satellites:" Highly repetitive and abundant DNA sequences with sequence homogeneity,** that are easily separable from the main mass of DNA. **This satellite DNA includes tandem arrays—many copies, one right after another**
- **Centromere** region forms the **"pinched waist"** of **metaphase chromosomes, and is the site to which the spindle fibers attach, to separate daughter chromatids in mitosis.**

63. **Ans. (d)** **Neuroblastoma** *(Ref: Robbins 9th/pg 288)*

N-MYC causes, Neuroblastoma, small-cell Ca lung[Q]

64. **Ans. (d)** **ABL and C-MYC** *(Ref: Robbins 9th/pg 288)*

Answers with Explanations

Discussing the options one by one:

Oncogene	Method of activation
A. SIS and HST-I	Overexpression
B. HGF and L-MYC	Overexpression
C. TGF and CDK4	Overexpression
D. ABL and C-MYC	Translocation
E. RAS and BRAF	Point mutation

65.   **Ans. (b)**   **Ras gene**

(Ref: Robbins 9th/pg 288; 8th/pg 284)

66.   **Ans. (c)**   **Multiple endocrine neoplasia**

(Ref: R 9th/pg 291)

Multiple endocrine neoplasia (MEN) is caused by RET which is a Proto-oncogene

67.   **Ans. (b)**   **Methylation of tumor suppressor genes**

(Ref: Robbins 9th/pg 319)

Epigenetic alterations in cancers:
- **Abnormal DNA methylation**: hypomethylation or hypermethylation
- **Silencing of tumor suppressor genes** by **local hyper-methylation** of DNA is the **most common mechanism of cancers**
- Changes in histones near genes that **influence cellular behavior can also predispose to Cancers**

68.   **Ans. (b)**   **Medullary carcinoma thyroid**

(Ref: R 9th/pg 284)

The RET proto-oncogene
- A **receptor tyrosine kinase** that undergoes oncogenic conversion by **mutation and gene rearrangements**.
- RET protein is a **receptor for glial cell line–derived neurotrophic factor** and structurally related proteins that promote cell survival during neural development.
- Normally **expressed in neuroendocrine cells, such as parafollicular C cells of thyroid, adrenal medulla and parathyroid cell precursors.**
- In MEN-2A, mutations in RET extracellular domain → Medullary thyroid Ca, Adrenal and parathyroid tumors.
- In MEN-2B, mutations in cytoplasmic domain → Thyroid and adrenal tumors without parathyroid involvement
- In **familial** cases, **mutation is in germline** while in **sporadic** cases. **somatic rearrangements** are seen

69.   **Ans. (c)**   **PTEN** *(Ref: Robbins 9th/pg 291; 8th/pg 287)*

PTEN (Phosphatase and Tensin homologue)
- PTEN is a membrane-associated phosphatase encoded by a gene on **chromosome 10q23**
- Mutated in **Cowden syndrome** (an **autosomal dominant** disorder with **tumors of skin appendages** and an increased incidence of epithelial **cancers of breast, endometrium, and thyroid**).
- It acts as **a tumor suppressor** by serving as a brake on the pro-survival/pro-growth **PI3K/AKT pathway**.

- By phosphorylating a number of substrates, including BAD and MDM2, AKT **enhances cell survival.**
- **PI3K/AKT pathway is the most commonly mutated pathway in human cancer**s.

70.   **Ans. (a)**   **Gastric Ca** *(Ref: Robbins 9th/pg 291; 8th/pg 287)*

E-cadherin
- Loss-of-contact inhibition, by mutation of the E-cadherin/β-catenin axis is a key characteristic of carcinomas.
- Loss of E-cadherin contributes to the malignant phenotype by allowing easy disaggregation of cells, which can then invade locally or metastasize.
- Reduced cell surface expression of E-cadherin has been seen in Ca **esophagus, colon, breast, ovary, and prostate**.
- Germline loss- of-function mutations of the E-cadherin gene, known as CDH1, cause **familial gastric carcinoma**
- Some of the sporadic gastric carcinomas are also associated with loss of E-cadherin expression.

71.   **Ans. (b)**   **p53**

(Ref: Robbins 9th/pg 296; 8th/pg 290)

72.   **Ans. (c)**   **Chromosome 11**

(Ref: Robbins 9th/pg 298)

73.   **Ans. (d)**   **Wild form is associated with increased risk of child-hood tumors** *(Ref: Robbins 9th/pg 294)*

74.   **Ans. (c)**   **Chromosome 17** *(Ref: Robbins 9th/pg 291)*
- BRCA1 (chromosome 17q)
- BRCA2 (chromosome 13q)
- Wilms' tumor gene or WT1 gene (chromosome 11)
- NF2 gene (chromosome 22)

75.   **Ans. (c)**   **Both** *(Ref: Robbins 9th/pg 721)*

Genes that promote epithelial-mesenchymal transitions, like *TWIST* and *SNAIL*, may be important metastasis genes in epithelial tumors

76.   **Ans. (c)**   **Metalloproteinase** *(Ref: Robbins 9th/pg 721)*

Degradation of ECM (basement membrane) is carried out by **Metalloproteinases** (MMPs type **2 and 9**) also known as **Type IV collagenase[Q]**, cathepsin D, and urokinase plasminogen activator

77.   **Ans. (c)**   **Desmoplasia**

(Ref: Robbins 9th/pg 266; 8th/pg 260)

Basic components of tumors:
1. **Neoplastic cells**: constitute the tumor parenchyma
2. **Reactive stroma:** made up of connective tissue, blood vessels, cells of the immune system
- **Desmoplasia**-abundant **collagenous stroma** (fibrosis) in a tumor, stimulated by **parenchymal cells[Q]**

78.   **Ans. (d)**   **Invasion**

(Ref: Robbins 9th/pg 271; 8th/pg 265)

Dysplasia

- **Dysplasia** literally means **"disordered growth "**[Q]
- Epithelial dysplasia is a **premalignant lesion:** increased risk of cancer

Features of Dysplasia:

- **Pleomorphism**[Q] —variation in size and shape
- Abnormal **nuclear** morphology-**high N:C** ratio **(nuclear enlargement), hyperchromatic**[Q] nuclei
- Increased but typical **mitotic** figures[Q]
- **Loss of polarity**- disturbed orientation of cells

---

79. **Ans. (a, b, c); a. Prominent nucleus; b. Nuclear enlargement; c. Nuclear hyperchromia**

(Ref: R 9th/pg 271)

---

80. **Ans. (c) IFN a** *(Ref: Robbins 9th/pg 306; 8th/pg 298)*

Angiogenesis

- Tumor cannot enlarge beyond **1 to 2 mm**[Q] in diameter unless it has the capacity to induce angiogenesis.
- **Angiogenesis** is an important requirement for tumors to **undergo metastasis**

---

81. **Ans. (a, b, c) a. Hepatocellular cancer; b. Kaposi sarcoma; c. Nasopharyngeal cancer**

---

82. **(b) Carcinoma nasophraynx, d. Carcinoma pancreas**

(Ref: Robbins 9th/ 326-27])

---

83. **Ans. (a) Prostate** *(Ref: Robbins 9th/pg 276)*

- 90% of lung cancers occur in smokers.
- Smoking is also associated with an increased risk of cancers of the oral cavity, larynx, esophagus, stomach, bladder, and kidney, as well as some forms of leukemia.
- Cessation of smoking reduces the risk of lung cancer.

---

84. **Ans. (b) Liver Angiosarcoma** *(Ref: Robbins 9th/pg 428)*

---

85. **Ans. (d) Esophagus** *(Ref: Robbins 9th/pg 428; 8th/pg 423)*

- Liver (2-fold), cervical (2-fold), and esophageal (2- to 3-fold) cancers are more common in less developed countries.
- Stomach cancer incidence is similar in more and less developed countries but is much more common in Asia than North America or Africa.

---

86. **Ans. (a) Nicotine** *(Ref: Robbins 9th/pg 428; 8th/pg 423)*

---

87. **Ans. (c) Lymphopenia**

(Ref: Robbins 9th/pg 428; 8th/pg 423)

Radio-sensitive tissues

- Bone marrow cells and all stem cells
- Lymphocytes
- Immune response cells
- Mucosa lining of small intestines
- Breast tissue
- Gonads
- Sebaceous (fat) glands of skin

---

88. **Ans. (b) Arsenic** *(Ref: Robbins 9th/pg 721; 8th/pg 730)*

---

89. **Ans. (c) Cartilage** *(Ref: Robbins 9th/pg 428; 8th/pg 423)*

The main types of ionizing radiation are:

- X-rays and gamma rays (electromagnetic waves of very high frequencies),
- High-energy neutrons
- Alpha particles (composed of two protons and two neutrons)
- Beta particles (essentially electrons).

In the human body, the tissue most resistant to the effect of radiation is Cartilage > Bone

The body tissues can be divided into:

Radio-sensitive	Radio-resistant
• Bone marrow cells and all stem cells • Lymphocytes • Immune response cells • Mucosa lining of small intestines • Breast tissue • Gonads • Sebaceous (fat) glands of skin	• Brain and its Neurons • Kidney • Liver • Heart, large arteries and veins • Mature blood cells • Muscle cells • Cartilage

---

90. **Ans. (d) HHV-8** *(Ref: Robbins 9th/pg 325; Refer to pretexts)*

---

91. **Ans. (a) 11** *(Ref: Robbins 9th/pg 325; 8th/pg 314)*

HPV 6 and 11 are **low risk** oncogenic viruses, while HPV 16 and 18 are high risk oncogenic viruses.

---

92. **Ans. (e) Burkitt's lymphoma** *(Ref: Robbins 9th/pg 325)*

HPV causes Genital warts,[Q] Squamous cell Ca of cervix, anogenital region, head/neck[Q]

While Burkitt's lymphoma is caused by EBV

---

93. **Ans. (c) Instability of E6 and E7**

(Ref: Robbins 9th/pg 325)

---

94. **Ans. (b) Stimulates formation of Pyrimidine dimers**

(Ref: Robbins 9th/pg 428; 8th/pg 423)

Ultraviolet B Rays	Ionizing Radiation
• Leads to **formation of pyrimidine dimers in DNA**[Q] • Produces skin cancers like Squamous cell Ca, Basal cell Ca, and melanoma of skin	• **Particulate** radiation (α and β particles, protons, neutrons) are all carcinogenic • **Electromagnetic** (x-rays, γ rays) • X-ray causes DNA mutation by **Pyrimidine dimer breakdown**

---

95. **Ans. (b) Bone** *(Ref: Robbins 9th/pg 428; 8th/pg 423)*

---

96. **Ans. (b) Ewings Sa, e. Ca pancreas**

(Ref: Annexure 5; Harrisons 19th/ pg 595)

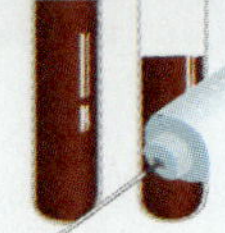

97. Ans. (a) DLBCL; d. Kaposi Sarcoma

(Ref: Robbins 9th/pg 316-318)

Most common mutations in type I endometrioid carcinomas act to increase signaling through the PI3K/AKT pathway, which is a hallmark of this particular tumor type.

Other genes involving PI3K/AKT pathway are:

- PTEN 30% to 80%
- PIK3CA, 40% of endometrioid carcinomas.
- KRAS, 25% of cases.
- ARID1A, 25-33% onethird of tumors.
- DNA mismatch repair genes 20%

98. Ans. (b) Osteosarcoma *(Ref: Robbins 9th/318)*

Chromothrypsis (A process in which in which a chromosome is "shattered" and then reassembled in a haphazard way.) has been observed in all 1-2% of cancers and 25% of osteosarcomas and then gliomas.

99. Ans. (b, c, d); b. IgA is low or absent, c. Increased risk of Leukemia, d. Hypoplasia of thymus

(Ref: Harrisons 19/2630)

Ataxia telangiectasia:

Immunodeficiency	Thymic hypoplasiaQ (most consistent defect) with cellular and humoral (IgA and IgG2)^Q immunodeficiency
Tumors seen	Lymphomas,^{Q} Hodgkin's disease,^{Q} T cell ALL and Breast cancer
Neuropathologic changes	• Loss of Purkinje, granule, and basket cells in the cerebellar cortex^Q (most striking change) and deep cerebellar nuclei.

100. Ans. (a, b, c) a. Ki67, b. Oncoprotein E6, c. p16INK4, cyclin E, and Ki-67

(Ref: Robbins 9th/1002-04; Harrison 19th/595; Harshmohan 7th/716)

101. Ans. (b) RET/PTC, d. NTRK1, e. RAS

(Ref: Robbins 9th/1095; Harrison 19th/2305; L and B 26th/764)

102. Ans. (a) Include simple deletions, inversions and translocations in chromosomes

(Ref: Robbins 9th/pg 428)

103. Ans. (a) Melanoma *(Ref: Robbins 9th/pg 286; 8th/pg 283)*

BRAF is a **serine/threonine protein kinase**, and is a member of the RAF family.

BRAF Mutations have been detected in: **Hairy cell leukemias, melanomas, benign nevi, colon carcinomas and dendritic cell tumors.**

104. Ans. (a) t (11;22) *(Ref: Robbins 9th/pg 317; 8th/pg 305)*

105. Ans. (b) Hypercalcemia

(Ref: Robbins 331)

Hypercalcemia is seen with Adult T-cell leukemia/lymphoma; Acanthosis nigricans is seen with Gastric carcinoma, Lung carcinoma, Uterine carcinoma

106. Ans. (a, e) a. Tripe palm, e. Oslers node

Dermatologic Disorders as paraneoplastic syndromes:

Acanthosis nigricans	Dermatomyositis
• Gastric carcinoma	• Bronchogenic carcinoma
• Lung carcinoma	• Breast carcinoma
• Uterine carcinoma	

107. Ans. (d) Nonsmall lung cancer *(Ref: Robbins 9th/719)*

Note that tumors that produce ACTH and ADH are predominantly small cell carcinomas, whereas those that produce hypercalcemia are mostly squamous cell carcinomas.

108. Ans. (b) Prostate Ca

(Ref: Robbins 9th/pg 332; 8th/pg 321)

Migratory thrombophlebitis

- Also called '**Trousseau sign**'
- Episodes of thrombophlebitis which are **recurrent** and appear in **different locations** over time
- It is seen in: **Pancreatic Ca, Bronchogenic Ca and Colon cancer**
- Not seen in Prostate Cancer

109. Ans. (c) Fibrosarcoma

Acquired hypophosphataemic osteomalacia is a rare tumour-associated disorder, first recognized in 1947. It is characterized by hypophosphataemia, phosphaturia, normocalcemia and osteomalacia in the absence of a nutritional or drug history suggestive of vitamin D deficiency or generalized renal tubular defects. Patients typically present with bone pain and proximal muscle weakness. Tumours associated with this disorder are generally of mesenchymal origin and benign. This condition has occasionally been associated with heamangiopericytoma, fibrous dysplasia, osteosarcoma, chondroblastoma, chondromyxoid fibroma, malignant fibrous histiocytoma, giant cell tumour, haemangioma, paraganglioma, prostate cancer and oat cell carcinoma of the lung

110. Ans. (a) Ca Vulva

The initial spread of vulval ca spreads to Inguinal, pelvic, ileal and periaotic lymph node. This allows the surgeon to assess the lymph node status by sentinel lymph node biopsy. Rest of the options mainly shows invasive property where they spread via hemtolymphoid pathway.

111. Ans. (a) Negative immune regulation in treatment of cancer

The 2018 Nobel Prize in Physiology or Medicine was awarded to James P. Allison and Tasuku Honjo "for their discovery of cancer therapy by inhibition of negative immune regulation". Their pioneering work on the CTLA4 and PD1 immune checkpoints revealed that these pathways act as so-called 'brakes' on the immune system. and showed that inhibition of these checkpoint pathways allow T cells to more effectively eradicate cancer cells. This research laid the foundation for the clinical development of immune checkpoint inhibitors, which have dramatically improved outcomes for many people with cancer.

112. Ans. (d) Pancreatic carcinoma/neuroectodermal tumour

113. Ans. (a, b) a. Ca19-9; b. Ca 125

114. Ans. (a) Desmin

115. Ans. (b) Embryonal rhabdomyosarcoma

116. Ans. (c) FISH

117. Ans. (b) Synaptophysin *(Ref: Robbins 9th ed p 717)*

The classic list of "NE markers" includes Synaptophysin (SYN), Chromogranin A (CHR), Neuron Specific Enolase (NSE), and CD56 (NCAM or Neural Cell Adhesion Molecule) and CD57 (Leu-7). We apply these marker by IHC method to identify the differentiation.

118. Ans. (b) Inflammatory myofibroblastictumor

(Ref: Robbins Basic Pathology, Chapter Neoplasia)

- Anaplastic lymphoma kinase (ALK) – Location: 2p23. It's also seen in Adenocarcinoma lung, Neuroblastoma, Inflammatory myofibroblastic tumor, Diffuse large B cell lymphoma. It's negative in Fibromatosis, one of the important thing to differentiate from difficult cases of inflammatory myofibroblastic tumor

119. Ans. (c) 95% ethanol

120. Ans. (c) Hypercalcemia

121. Ans. (b) Her2 neu 2+

122. Ans. (a) Type 1

ALK (2p23) gene mutation is seen in (hereditary hemorrhagic telangiectasia-1, Adenocarcinoma lung, Neuroblastoma, anaplastic large B cell lymphoma)

123. Ans. (a) CA 15.3

124. Ans. (c) Toulidine blue

(Ref: Early Diagnosis and Treatment of Cancer Series: Head and Neck Cancers, Wayne Koch Pg. 54)

- Toluidine blue stain is used as a marker to differentiate lesions at high risk of progression in order to improve early diagnosis of oropharyngeal carcinomas.

- Toluidine blue, an acidophilic metachromatic dye of thiazine group selectively stains acidic tissue components (sulfates, carboxylates and phosphate radicals), thus staining DNA and RNA.
- Toluidine blue has been established as a diagnostic adjunct in detecting oral lesions related to invasive carcinomas, carcinoma in situ or early asymptomatic oral carcinomas.

125. Ans. (b) Hepatic ca *(Ref: Robbins 9th /338, Henry 1392)*

Carcinoembryonic antigen (CEA) is raised in **ca colon, lung, liver, pancreas, stomach, and breast**, and alpha-fetoprotein (AFP), which is produced by **hepatocellular carcinomas, yolk sac remnants in the gonads, and occasionally teratocarcinomas and embryonal cell carcinomas.**

126. Ans. (b) 10% formalin

(Ref: Annexure 4; Bancrofts Stains)

This is a tricky Question!
- When you first see the term analysis for sperm, the answer is bouin's fluid. But what the examiner wants to know is whether you know that for histological diagnosis, the fixative is 10% formalin.

127. Ans. (b) Neural tube defect *(Ref: Robbins (SEA) 9th/337)*
- Beta hCG increased in: Gastric and pancreatic Ca, hepatoma, Ovarian Ca, germ cell tumor of testis, trophoblastic tumors, choriocarcinoma, and testicular tumors.

128. Ans. (a, b, c, d) a. Chromogranin A, b. CD56, c. Neuron-specific enolase, d. Synaptophysin

(Ref: Harrison 19th/558, 2337, 120e-2t)

129. Ans. (c) No evidence of systemic inflammation

(Ref: Robbins 9th/pg 331; 8th/pg 321)

Cancer Cachexia:

Progressive loss of body fat and lean body mass^Q with profound weakness, anorexia and anemia, seen in cancer. **TNF^Q** is the **major contributor** to cachexia with advanced cancer.
Equal loss of both **fat and lean muscle^Q**
Elevated basal metabolic rate
Evidence of **systemic inflammation** (e.g., an increase in acute phase reactants)

130. Ans. (d) Size of primary lesion *(Ref: Robbins 9th/pg 11)*

Grading of a tumor is based on its histopathological appearance, that includes Degree of differentiation, Number of mitoses, architectural features **and not on the size of primary lesion**

131. Ans. (a) Desmin–Carcinoma *(Ref: Robbins 9th/pg 11)*

Desmin is an IHC marker for **muscle tumors** and not Carcinoma

132. **Ans. (b)** **Prostatic carcinoma** *(Ref: Robbins 9th/pg 337)*

133. **Ans. (d)** **Alpha-fetoprotein** *(Ref: Robbins 9th/pg 337)*

134. **Ans. (d)** **Angiomyolipoma of lung** *(Ref: R 9th/pg 337)*

Lymphangiomyomatosis and **angiomyolipoma**: closely related entities characterized by hamartomatous proliferation of **HMB-45-positive** smooth muscle

135. **Ans. (a)** **Ovarian cancer** *(Ref: Robbins 9th/pg 337)*

136. **Ans. (b)** **Carcinoma** *(Ref: Robbins 9th/pg 11; 8th/pg 335)*

137. **Ans. (c)** **1,25dihydroxy vitamin D** *(Ref: R 9th/pg 337)*

138. **Ans. (c)** **DNA microarray analysis** *(Ref: R 9th/pg 337)*

Microarray can study several genes at a time. Hence it can be used in molecular profiling of cancer cells.

139. **Ans. (b)** **Anti-Hu** *(Ref: Robbins 9th/pg 337; 8th/pg 327)*

Antibodies to intracellular antigens, syndromes, and associated cancers

Antibody	Associated Neurologic Syndrome(s)	Tumors
Anti-Hu (ANNA1)	encephalomyelitis, subacute sensory neuronopathy	SCLC
Anti-Yo (PCA1)	Cerebellar degeneration	Ovary, breast
Anti-Rl (ANNA2)	Cerebellar degeneration, apsoclonus, bralnstem encephalitis	Breast, gynecologic, SCLC
Anti-Tr	Cerebellar degeneration	Hodgkin's lymphoma

140. **Ans. (a, d, e); a. Yolk sac tumor; d. Non-seminoma; e. Hepatocellular carcinoma** *(Ref: Robbins 9th/pg 337)*

141. **Ans. (c)** **Fibrosarcoma** *(Ref: Robbins 9th/pg 337)*

Hypoglycemia is seen as a paraneoplastic syndrome in fibrosrcoma and osteosarcoma

142. **Ans. (b)** **Ame's test** *(Ref: Robbins 9th/pg 337; 8th/pg 327)*

- The **Ames test** is a **biological assay** to **assess the mutagenic potential of chemical** compounds.
- Ames test **uses bacteria** (*Salmonella typhimurium* that carry mutations in genes involved in histidine synthesis) to test whether a given chemical can cause mutations in the DNA of test organism.
- **A positive test indicates** that the **chemical might act as a carcinogen**

It is a **quick and convenient** assay to estimate the carcinogenic potential of a compound because standard carcinogen assays on mice are time-consuming and expensive

143. **Ans. (c)** **Multiple myeloma** *(Ref: Robbins 9th/pg 337)*

Bortezomib, a proteasome inhibitor is used in the treatment of Multiple myeloma

144. **Ans. (a)** **Polycyclic hydrocarbons** *(Ref: R 9th/pg 337)*

145. **Ans. (d)** **Necrotizing myelopathy** *(Ref: R 9th/pg 337)*

146. **Ans. (d)** **Aerobic glycolysis** *(Ref: Robbins 9th/pg 337)*

- **Cancer cells** tend to **convert most glucose to lactate**[Q] even in presence of **ample oxygen (aerobic glycolysis)**[Q]

147. **Ans. (a)** **Squamous cell Ca** *(Ref: Robbins 9th/pg 1155)*

Malignant squamous epithelium with prominent central keratin pearls are seen in **Squamous cell Ca**

148. **Ans. (b)** **Carcinoma - desmin**

(Ref: Robbins 9th/pg 11; 8th/pg35; Refer table in Ans 158) *Desmin is an IHC marker for muscle tumors and not Carcinoma*

149. **Ans. (b)** **Medullary carcinoma of thyroid**

(Ref: Robbins 9th/pg 337; 8th/pg 327)

Calcitonin is a marker of **Medullary carcinoma of thyroid**; Hormones acting as tumor markers are-

150. **Ans. (a)** **Ewing sarcoma**

(Ref: Robbins 9th/pg 1203)

Mic2 is a **tumor marker** for **Ewing's sarcoma**
CD99 is a product of the MIC2 gene located on X and Y chromosomes.
It is seen in **Ewing's sarcoma/primitive neuro-ectodermal tumor (PNET) and lymphoblastic tumors.**

151. **Ans. (c)** **Neurofilament**

(Ref: Robbins 9th/pg 11; 8th/pg 35)

Markers for **muscle tumor** are: **Desmin, Actin, Intermediate filament, MYOD, myogenin**

152. **Ans. (c)** **CK-20**

(Ref: Robbins 9th/pg 11; 8th/pg 35)

The markers of **Melanoma** are **S-100, MITF (microphthalmia-associated transcription factor) and Vimentin**

153. **Ans. (a)** **Desmin**

(Ref: Robbins 9th/pg 11; 8th/pg 35)

154. **Ans. (c)** **Synovial sarcoma**

(Ref: Robbins 9th/pg 1223)

Synovial Sarcoma

- Immunohistochemistry yields positive reactions for **keratin and epithelial membrane antigen;**

- Most synovial sarcomas show a characteristic chromosomal translocation **t(x;18)(p11;q11)** producing *SS18-SSX1, SSX2, or SSX4* fusion genes that encode chimeric transcription factors

155. **Ans. (c, d, e); c. Omphalocoele; d. Sacrococcygeal tetatoma; e. Neural tube defect**

(Ref: Henry's 22nd/ pg 1392; Robbins 9th/pg 337; 8th/pg 327)

Alpha-fetoprotein

Structurally **related to Albumin**[Q]

In the fetus, AFP is **synthesized by yolk sac**[Q] **and fetal Hepatocytes**[Q]

Maternal serum AFP raised in **Omphalocele,**[Q] **Sacrococcygeal teratoma,**[Q] **Neural tube defect**[Q]

AFP can be used for **prenatal screening** for:

- **Neural tube defects**[Q] (**anencephaly** and **spina bifida**)
- **Down syndrome**[Q] (as part of triple test)
- **Omphalocele** and **gastroschisis** (**Acetylcholinesterase** levels may also be increased)
- **Sacrococcygeal teratoma**[Q]

Increased levels in Liver cancers[Q], **non-seminomatous**[Q] germ cell tumors of testis and non-neoplastic lesions like **Amebic liver abscess**[Q] **and Hepatitis**[Q] Sacrococcygeal teratoma (SCT) is the most frequent tumor in the neonatal period.

156. **Ans. (a, c, d); a. Used for monitoring of recurrence of colon cancer; c. Increased in smokers; d. Increased in colon cancer**

(Ref: Henry's 22nd/ pg 1392; Robbins 9th/pg 337; 8th/pg 327)

Carcino embryonic antigen (CEA)

- **Tumor marker** for **Carcinomas of colon, pancreas, lung, stomach and breast**.
- Can be used for **monitoring** of **recurrence of colon cancer**, but it is **not specific for colon cancer**.
- As **liver metabolizes CEA**, **liver damage** impairs CEA clearance and leads to **increased levels** in blood
- Also increased in **smokers, Alcoholic Cirrhosis, Ulcerative Colitis, Pancreatitis, hepatitis**

157. **Ans. (a, c, e); a. It is a Glycoprotein; c. It is Increased in colon carcinoma; e. May be elevated in Pelvic inflammatory disease**

(Ref: Robbins 9th/pg 337; 8th/pg 327; Ref: Henry's 22nd/ pg 1393)

CA-125:

- **Normal range** in pre-menopausal females is **0-35 U/mL**
- **Increased in Ovarian Ca**: non-mucinous epithelial (> 80%), serous, endometrioid and clear cell types
- Other Cancers with increased CA-125 levels are **Non-Hodgkin Lymphoma, Lung cancer, Endometrial Ca**
- Non-malignant diseases with increased CA-125: **Liver cirrhosis, Pelvic inflammatory disease including endometriosis and advanced abdominal or pelvic tuberculosis**

158. **Ans. (a) Cytokeratin** *(Ref: Robbins 9th/pg 11)*

159. **Ans. (b) Bacterial contamination of the specimen**

(Ref: Halder A, Halder S and Fauzdar A. A preliminary investigation of genomic screening in cervical carcinoma by comparative genomic hybridization. Indian J Med Res 122, November 2005, pp 434-446)

This question is a direct pick up from the above publication by our AIIMS faculty!

"Conventional cytogenetics are difficult in solid tumors especially in case of **carcinoma cervix** as **most biopsy sample is contaminated/infected** with microorganisms and **quality of metaphase preparation is poor."**

160. **Ans. (a) Prostate carcinoma**

(Ref: Robbins 9th/pg 337)

161. **Ans. (a, b, c, d); a. HCC; b. Hepatoblastoma; c. Infant hemangioendothelioma; d. Amebic liver abscess**

(Ref: Robbins 9th/pg 337; 8th/pg 327)

162. **Ans. (b) Mutagenicity**

(Ref: Robbins 9th/pg 337; 8th/pg 327)

163. **Ans. (a, b, c, d, e); a. Abdominal TB; b. Ca cervix; c. Endometriosis; d. Ovarian ca; e. Endometrial ca**

(Ref: Robbins 9th/pg 337; 8th/pg 327)

164. **Ans. (c) Cytokeratin**

(Ref: Robbins 9th/pg 337; 8th/pg 327)

An elderly smoker has a high risk of Small cell Ca and Squamous cell Ca lung; Of the given options, cytokeratin is a marker of squamous cell Carcinoma;

Discussing the options one by one,

Marker	Tumor
A. Calretinin	Malignant Mesothelioma
B. Vimentin	Mesenchymal tumors
C. Cytokeratin	Epithelial carcinomas (Squamous cell Ca and Adenocarcinoma)
D. TTF1	Adenocarcinoma

165. **Ans. (c) Human leucocyte antigen** *(Ref: R 9th/pg 337)*

CEA, Tyrosinase and AFP are tumor markers

- **Tyrosinase** has been demonstrated to be **a sensitive marker for melanoma**
- Human leucocyte antigen is not a tumor marker.

Note

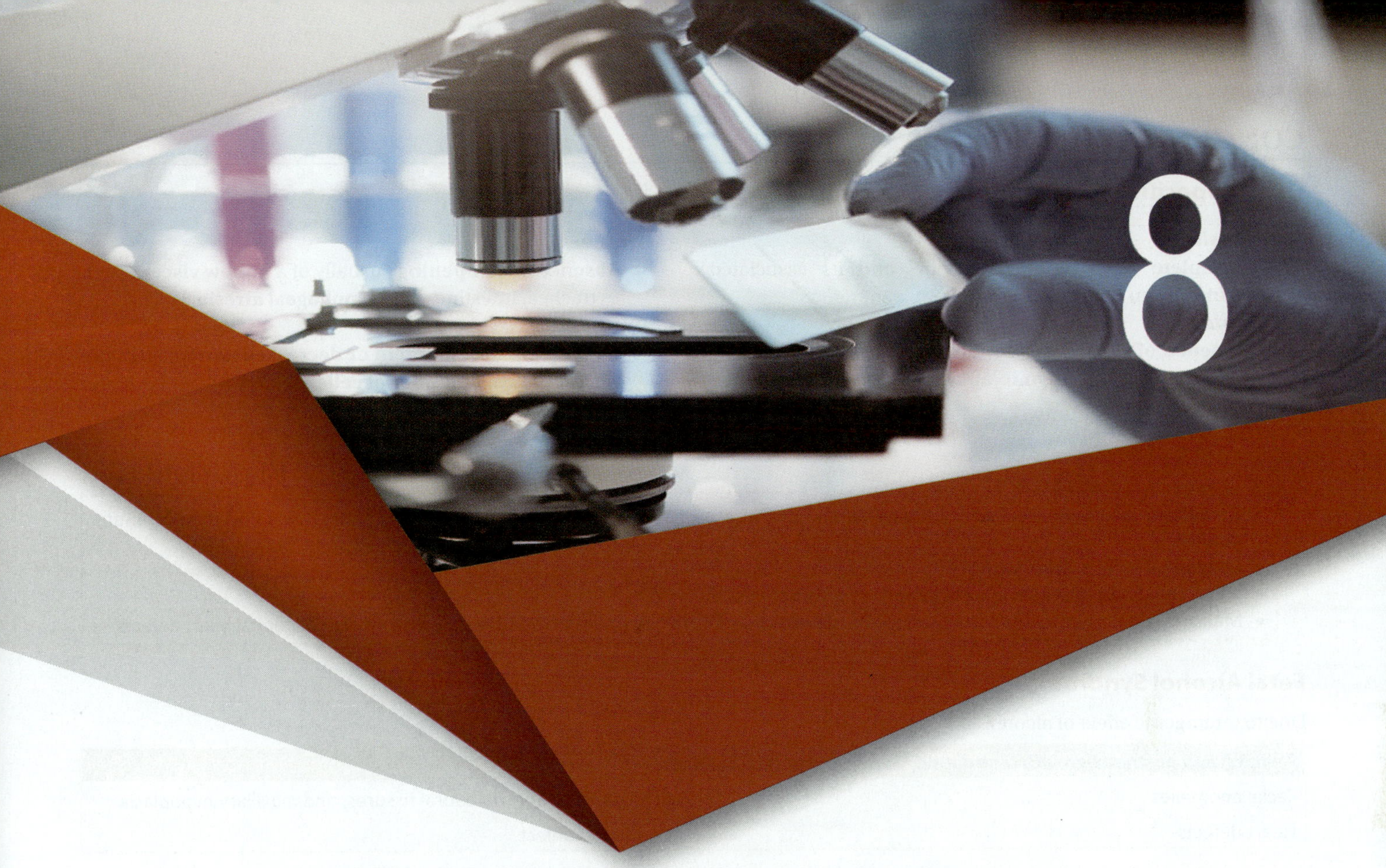

8

Diseases of Infancy and Childhood

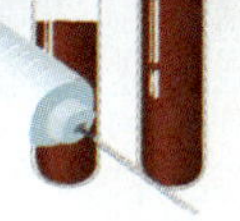

CONGENITAL ANOMALIES

Organ-Specific Disorders of Development

- *Agenesis:*
  - **Complete absence of an organ**[Q] and its associated **primodium. E.g., renal agenesis**[Q]
- *Aplasia:*
  - **Absence of organ**[Q] due to **failure of growth** of existing **primodium. E.g., thymic aplasia**[Q], found in **DiGeorge syndrome**

- *Atresia:*
  - **Absence of an opening**[Q] usually of a **hollow viscera** such as trachea, intestine. **E.g., esophageal atresia**
- *Hypoplasia:*
  - **Incomplete development or decreased size**[Q] of an organ with **decreased number of cells**

High Yield Facts

- **Hereditary disorders**: Derived from **parents** and are **transmitted in the germ line** through the generations and therefore, are familial.[Q]
- **Congenital** means **"born with"**[Q]
- **Some congenital diseases are not genetic**; e.g. Congenital syphilis[Q]
- **Malformations**: Due to **intrinsically abnormal** developmental process (multifactorial); e.g. Anencephaly, congenital heart defects[Q]

Fetal Alcohol Syndrome

Due to teratogenic effect of alcohol

Prenatal and postnatal growth retardation, psychomotor disturbances	
Facial anomalies	Microcephaly, short palpebral fissures, and maxillary hypoplasia
Heart defects	Atrial septal defect

High Yield Facts

- **Disruptions:** Secondary destruction (extrinsic disturbance in morphogenesis)[Q] of an organ that was **previously normal** in development. **Not heritable** and **no risk of recurrence**. E.g. Amniotic bands[Q]
- **Deformations:** Structural abnormalities (extrinsic disturbance in morphogenesis) due to **compression of growing fetus** by abnormal **biomechanical forces** like bicornuate uterus. **E.g., Clubfeet**[Q]. Most common underlying factor responsible for deformation is **uterine constraint**[Q]
- **Sequence:** Cascade of anomalies triggered by **one initiating aberration. E.g. Potter sequence (oligohydramnios sequence)**: Renal agenesis → Oligohydramnios → flattened facies, abnormalities of the hands and feet and pulmonary hypoplasia.
- **Malformation syndrome:** Constellation of **congenital anomalies** that *cannot* be explained on the basis of a single, localized, **initiating defect**. Usually caused by a specific chromosomal abnormality. E.g. **Down's syndrome**[Q]

CYSTIC FIBROSIS (MUCOVISCIDOSIS)

- Most common **lethal genetic disease**[Q] that affects Caucasian populations
- **Autosomal recessive,** inherited disorder of **ion transport channel.**

Chiefly Affects

- **Fluid secretion** from **exocrine glands**[Q]
- **Epithelial lining of the respiratory tract**[Q]: Chr lung disease due to recurrent infections,
- **Gastrointestinal**: **Pancreatic insufficiency, steatorrhea,** malnutrition, hepatic cirrhosis, intestinal obstruction

- **Reproductive tracts:** Male infertility[Q]

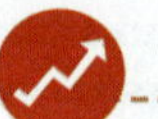

High Yield Facts

Cystic fibrosis
- *Haemophilus influenzae*[Q] and *S. aureus*[Q] are the **first organisms recovered** from lung secretions
- Antibiotic-resistant and **mucoid *P. aeruginosa***[Q] colonizes next.
- *Burkholderia cepacia* is pathognomonic organism

Primary Defect

- Abnormal function of an **epithelial chloride channel protein**[Q] encoded by the **Cystic Fibrosis Transmembrane conductance Regulator (CFTR) gene on chr7q31.2**[Q]

Other Defects Lie in

- Outwardly rectified **chloride channels**[Q]
- Inwardly rectified **potassium channels (Kir 6.1)**[Q]
- **Epithelial sodium channel (ENaC)**[Q]

Of these, the **interaction of CFTR** with **ENaC**[Q] is the most important step

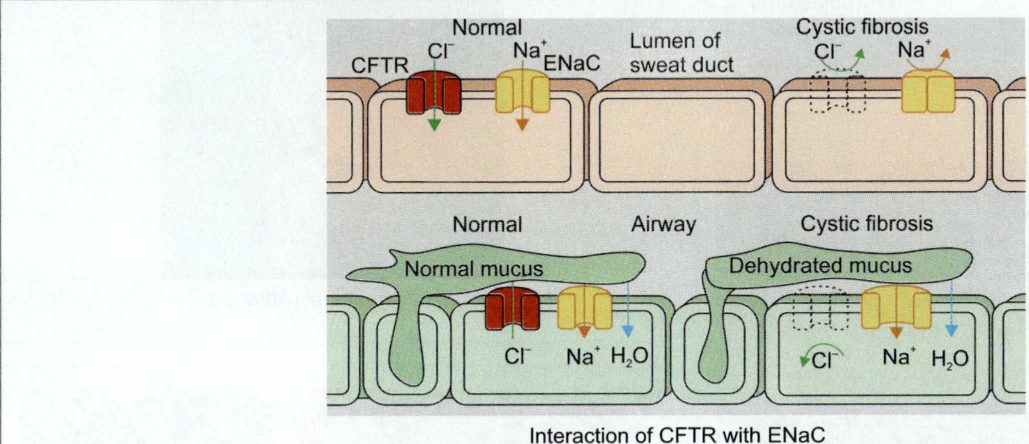

Interaction of CFTR with ENaC

Mechanism: Effect of CFTR Gene Mutation

ENaC (Epithelial sodium channel)

Site	Normal Function	In cystic fibrosis	Effect seen in CF
Apical exocrine glands of airway and GIT	Na uptake from luminal fluid	Increased Na and H_2O uptake from lumen	Thick, viscid secretions[Q]
Sweat ducts	Absorb luminal Na^+	Decreased reabsorption of Na and Cl	Salty sweat (high Na and Cl)[Q] (Hallmark of CF)

- Most common mutation: **class II mutation (ΔF508)**[Q]
- Leads to **defective processing**[Q] of the protein from the E.R to the Golgi apparatus

Systemic Involvement

Respiratory Tract

- **Upper respiratory tract disease** is almost **universal** in patients with CF[Q]
- **Chronic cough**[Q] and **sputum**[Q] production
- **Bronchiectasis**[Q], **atelectasis**[Q], infiltrates, hyperinflation, **Nasal polyps**[Q]

Genitourinary System

- **Azoospermia and infertility**[Q]
- Congenital **bilateral absence or obliteration**[Q] of the **vas deferens**[Q], due to defective liquid secretion may be seen

Gastrointestinal and Nutritional Abnormalities

- **Intestinal:** Meconium ileus[Q], distal intestinal obstruction syndrome (DIOS)[Q], rectal prolapse.
- **Pancreatic:** Pancreatic **exocrine in sufficiency**[Q], recurrent acute/chronic **pancreatitis**[Q]
- **Hepatic:** Focal **biliary cirrhosis**, or multilobular cirrhosis, prolonged **neonatal jaundice.**
- **Nutritional: Failure to thrive (protein-calorie malnutrition)**, hypoproteinemia, edema, fat-soluble vitamin deficiency
- **Salt-loss syndromes:** acute salt depletion, chronic **metabolic alkalosis**[Q]

Diagnosis

Criteria for Diagnosis of Cystic Fibrosis

- One or more characteristic **phenotypic features**[Q]
- **OR** a **history**[Q] of cystic fibrosis in a sibling
- **OR** a positive **newborn screening test** result (Serum Immunoreactive trypsinogen)

AND

- **Increased sweat chloride (>70 meq/L)**[Q] concentration on **two or more occasions**
- **OR** identification of **two cystic fibrosis mutations**[Q]
- **OR** demonstration of **abnormal epithelial an ion transport (transepithelial potential difference is raised)**[Q]

Sequencing the CFTR gene is the **gold standard** for diagnosis of cystic fibrosis[Q]

MALIGNANT TUMORS

Mnemonic

Small Round Blue Cell Tumors[Q]
Tumors with similar histology of small round cell include:

"Low NEW MRP"

- Lymphoma
- Ewing's Sarcoma
- Medulloblastoma
- Primitive Neuroectodermal tumor
- **N**euroblastoma
- **W**ilms' Tumor
- **R**etinoblastoma

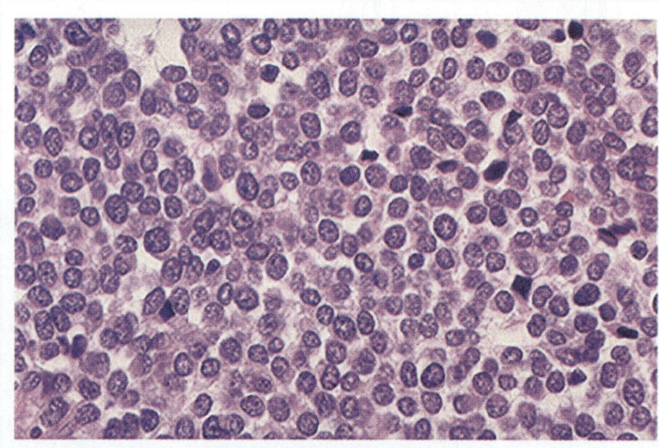
Small round blue cell tumor

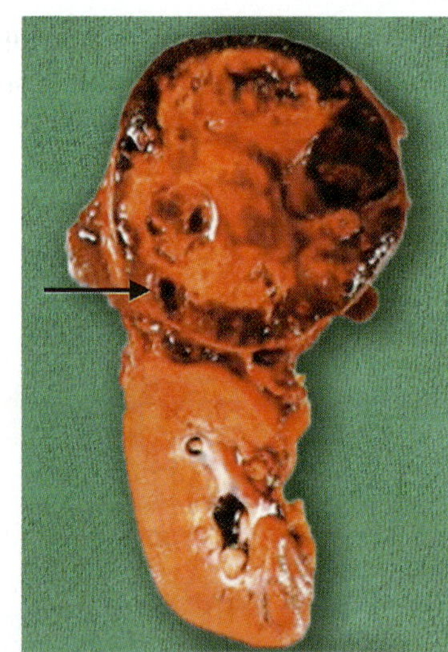
Neuroblastoma (Adrenal)

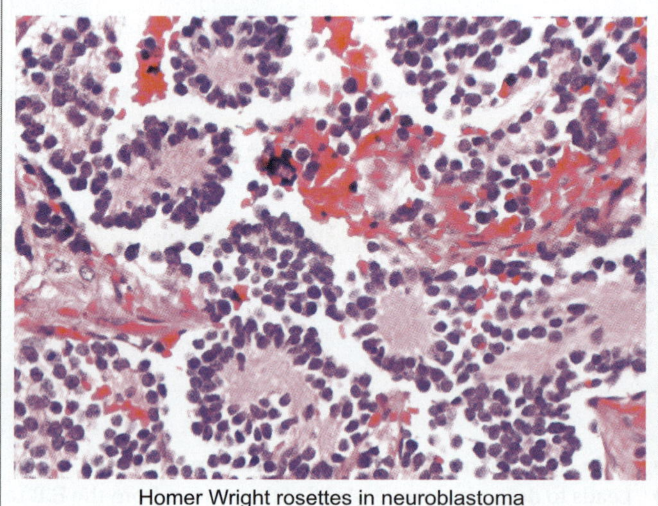
Homer Wright rosettes in neuroblastoma

High Yield Facts

The most frequent childhood cancers are:
(in order of decreasing frequency)[Q]
Leukemia (Most common is ALL)[Q] > Neuroblastoma > Wilms' tumor > Hepatoblastoma > Retinoblastoma

- **Hemangiomas[Q]** are the **most common tumors of infancy**
- **Characteristic** chromosomal translocation, **t(12;15)[Q]**, has been described in **congenital-infantile fibrosarcomas, (ETV6-NTRK3 fusion transcript)**
- **Sacrococcygeal teratomas** are the **most common teratomas of childhood[Q]**

NEUROBLASTIC TUMORS

Tumors of the **sympathetic ganglia** and **adrenal medulla** that are **derived** from **primordial neural crest cells.**

Neuroblastoma

Sites of Tumor

- **Adrenal medulla[Q] (MC site),** along the **sympathetic chain** in the **paravertebral region[Q]** of the abdomen (25%) and **posterior mediastinum[Q]** (15%) > **pelvis[Q]**, **neck**, and **brain** (cerebral neuroblastomas)

Morphology

- **Gross:** Often sharply demarcated by a **fibrous pseudo-capsule**
- **Microscopic:** Foci of **punctate intratumoral calcification**
- **Homer-Wright pseudorosettes[Q]** with **central space filled** with **neuropil (eosinophilic fibrillar material)[Q]**
- **Accompanied with:** Primitive neuroblasts **(ganglioneuroblastoma)[Q]**
- Stains +ve with **Neuron-specific enolase (NSE)**
- **E.M: central dense cores** (containing catecholamines) surrounded by a peripheral halo.

Metastasis

- **Hematogenous[Q] and lymphatic[Q]** route to **liver, lungs, bones, and bone marrow. Proptosis** and **ecchymosis** (spread to the **periorbital region)[Q]** is common.
- Disseminated neuroblastomas may present with **multiple cutaneous metastases ("blueberry muffin baby")[Q]**

- **Stage 4S("S"=special): Localized primary tumor** (as defined for stages 1,2A, or 2B) with dissemination limited to **skin, liver, and/or bone marrow; stage 4S is limited to infants younger than 1 year**

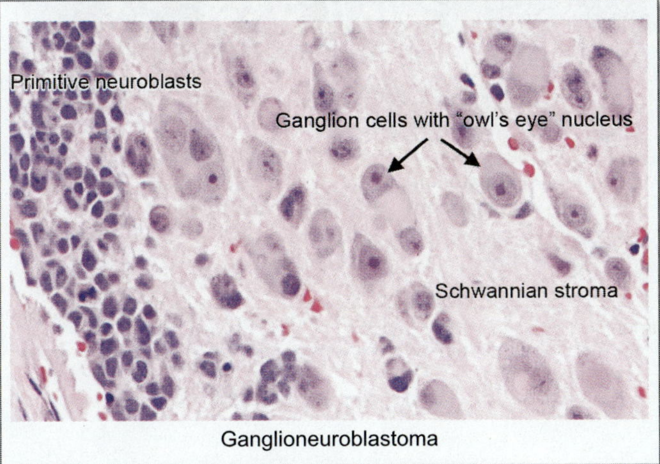

Prognostic Factors in Neuroblastoma

Variable	Favorable	Unfavorable
Stage	Stage 1, 2A, 2B, 4S[Q]	Stage 3, 4
Age	<18 months[Q]	>18 months
Schwannianstroma	Present	Absent
Mitosis-karyorrhexis index	< 200/5000 cells	> 200/5000 cells
DNA ploidy	Hyperdiploid[Q]	Near-diploid
N/myc	Not amplified	Amplified
Chromosome 11q loss	Absent	Present
TRKA expression	Present[Q]	Absent
TRKB expression	Absent	Present

High Yield Facts

Neuroblastoma
- Most common **extracranial solid tumor** of **childhood**[Q]
- Most common **abdominal tumor of childhood**[Q]
- Most **frequently diagnosed** tumor of **infancy (<1 year of age)**[Q]
- Median age at diagnosis is **18 months**[Q]
- **Mature ganglion cells (ganglioneuroma;** accompanied by the appearance of Schwann cells) on histology → signifies favorable outcome[Q]
- 98% cases are sporadic[Q]
- **2%** cases are **familial**[Q] (Germline mutations in the **anaplastic lymphoma kinase (ALK gene)**[Q]
- 90% of neuroblastomas, regardless of location, produce catecholamines: **vanillylmandelic acid (VMA) and homovanillic acid**

WILMS' TUMOR

- Most common **primary renal tumor of childhood**[Q]
- Peak incidence for Wilms' tumor is between **2 and 5 years**[Q]

Can be present as:
- **Synchronous:** Both kidneys involved **simultaneously**[Q]
- **Metachronous:** Kidney affected **one after the other**[Q]

Groups of congenital malformations with increased risk of Wilm's tumor:

WAGR syndrome (33% risk)[Q]	Denys-Drash syndrome (90% risk, Max)[Q]	Beckwith-Wiedemann syndrome (BWS)
• **WT1 gene: Chr 11p13**[Q] • **W**ilms' tumor, **A**niridia, **G**enital anomalies, and mental **R**etardation	• **Gonadal dysgenesis**[Q] (male pseudohermaphroditism) • Early-onset nephropathy **(diffuse mesangial sclerosis)**[Q] • Increased risk of **gonadoblastomas**[Q]	• **WT2 gene: 11p15.5** • Organomegaly: **Macroglossia**[Q], **hemihypertrophy**[Q], omphalocele, (adrenal cytomegaly)[Q] • **Genomic imprinting**[Q]

β-*catenin mutations is seen in 10% of sporadic Wilms' tumor.*
Nephrogenic rests[Q]: Putative **precursor lesions** of Wilms' tumors.
- **100%**[Q] in cases of **bilateral Wilms' tumor**
- **Increased risk** of developing Wilms' tumors in the **contralateral kidney**[Q]

Morphology
Triphasic combination:
- **Blastemal**-small blue tumor cells
- **Stromal**-fibrocytic or myxoid
- **Epithelial cell** -tubules or glomeruli

Anaplasia
- **Characteristic: Large, hyperchromatic, pleomorphic nuclei** and **abnormal mitoses.**
  - Loss of 11q and 16q, and gain in 1q
- **Signifies:** Presence of **TP53 mutations**[Q] and the **emergence of resistance**[Q] to chemotherapy
- **Increased risk** of recurrence and death-**adverse prognosis**[Q]

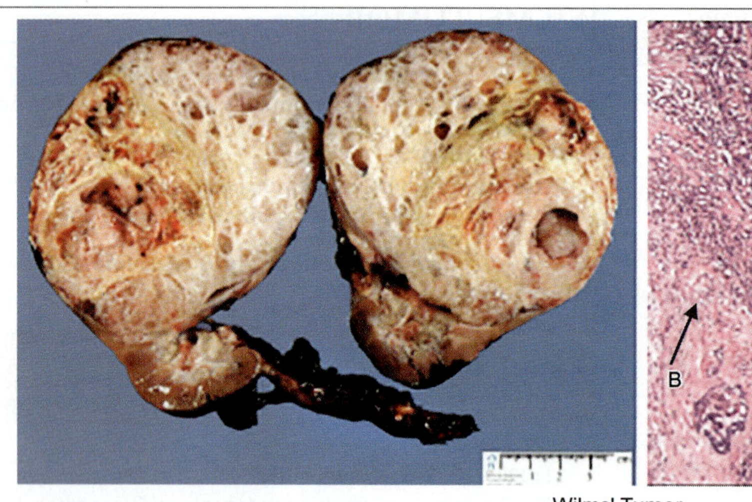

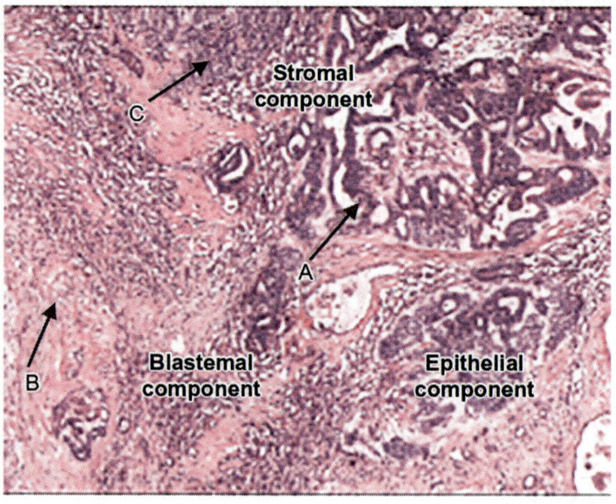

Wilms' Tumor

Image-Based Questions

1. **5 m Infant present with Abdominal mass in AIIMS Peds OPD along with dark pigmentation around eyes. CT scan suggested abdominal mass with punctate calcification. Biopsy of the same was done which has been shown below. What is your diagnosis?**

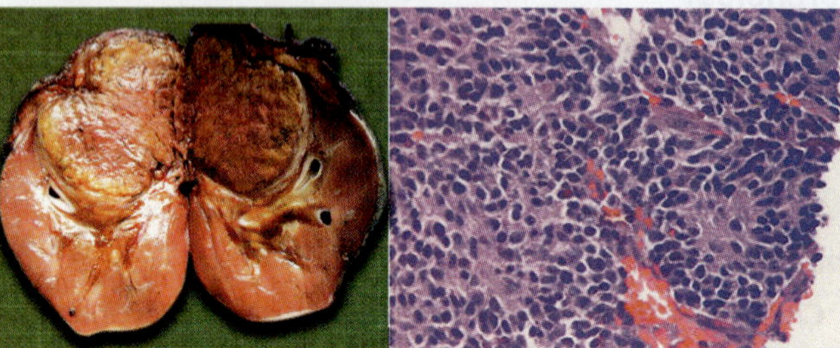

   a. Wilms' tumor with nephrogenic nests
   b. Neuroblastoma with rosettes
   c. Renal cell Ca with Papillary pattern
   d. Hepatoblastoma with rosettes

2. **2/male presented with abdominal mass. On CT scan intra-renal mass was seen, the biopsy of which has been shown below. What is your diagnosis?**

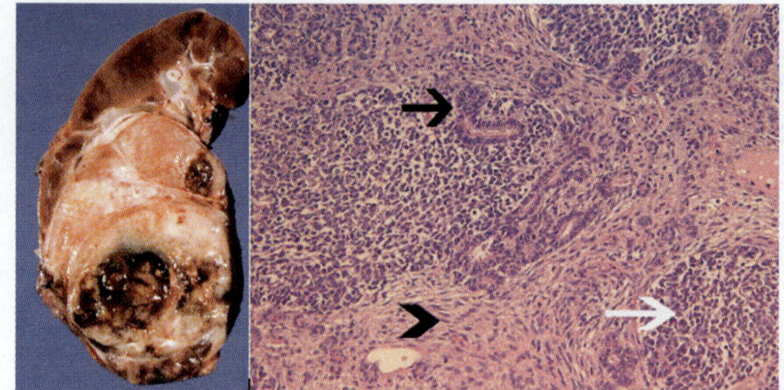

   a. Wilms' tumor with triphasic pattern
   b. Neuroblastoma with rosettes
   c. Renal cell Ca with Papillary pattern
   d. Hepatoblastoma with rosettes

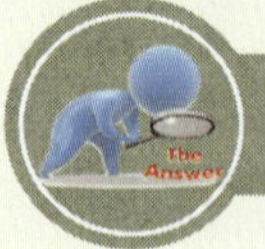

Answers of Image-Based Questions

1. **Ans. (b)** Neuroblastoma with rosettes
   - Abdominal mass along with dark pigmentation around eyes (Racoon eyes) with CT scan showing punctate calcification. Biopsy from the same shows homer wright rosette.
2. **Ans. (a)** Wilms' tumor showing intrarenal mass with triphasic pattern in biopsy.

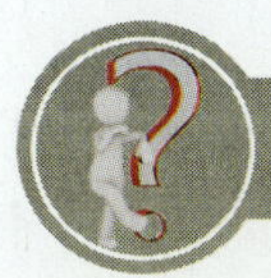

Multiple Choice Questions

1. **Feature(s) of Familial Mediterranean fever:**
   (PGI May 2019)
   a. Caused by mutations of the MEFV gene
   b. First fever attack occur only after 20 years of age
   c. Presentation include episodic bouts of acute peritonitis
   d. Amyloidosis occur as a complication
   e. Colchicine is used for treatment

2. **Which of the following is true about Wilms' tumor?**
   (PGI Nov 2018)
   a. Associated with aniridia b. Small unipolar cysts
   c. Presents in neonates d. Has pseudocapsule

3. **Which are primitive neuroectodermal tumors?**
   (PGI Nov 2018)
   a. Medulloblastoma b. Craniopharyngioma
   c. Meningioma d. Rhabdomyosarcoma

4. **Wilms' tumor has the following markers positive except?**
   (JIPMER 2017)
   a. Desmin b. Vimentin
   c. TTF-1 d. Cytokeratin

5. **All are good prognostic factors in neuroblastoma except:** *(Recent Question 2015)*
   a. Stage 4S b. Trk A expression
   c. Trk B expression d. Age <18 months

6. **For diagnosing cystic fibrosis sweat chloride level should be more than:** *(Recent Question 2015)*
   a. 20 mEq/L b. 40 mEq/L
   c. 60 mEq/L d. 70 mEq/L

7. **Most common cancer in children less than 10 years**
   (Recent Question 2015)
   a. Leukemia b. Neuroblastoma
   c. Brain tumor d. Wilms' tumor

8. **False statement about cystic fibrosis**
   (Recent Question 2015)
   a. Sweat chloride level >70 mEq/L is diagnostic
   b. ENAC activity of the sweat ducts increases
   c. Mycobacterium tuberculosis infection in rare
   d. Distal intestinal obstruction syndrome occurs in children

9. **The following is not a category A agent of bioterrorism**
   (Recent Question 2015)
   a. Anthrax b. Botulism
   c. Plague d. Brucellosis

10. **Most common site of metastases in neuroblastoma**
    (Recent Question 2015)
    a. Lung b Skull
    c. Liver d. Vertebrae

11. **All are true about Wilms' tumor except**
    a. Triphasic morphology *(Recent Question 2015)*
    b. MC renal malignancy in children
    c. Associated with cysts in liver
    d. Does not respond to chemotherapy and radiotherapy

12. **Find the false statement about cystic fibrosis**
    (Recent Question 2015)
    a. A normal sweat chloride test does not exclude the diagnosis
    b. Inhaled recombinant human deoxyribonuclease reduces the risk of acute exacerbations
    c. Ivacaftor, a potentiator of the CFTR channel is used to for patients with (ΔF508) mutation
    d. All the above

13. **The following is not one of the core prognostic factor of neuroblastoma:** *(Recent Question 2015)*
    a. Age at diagnosis
    b. Morphology
    c. Amplification of MYCN gene
    d. TRKA expression

14. **The genetic–abnormality associated with Beckwith-wiedeman syndrome** *(Recent Question 2015)*
    a. Negative missense mutation
    b. Genomic imprinting
    c. Deletion
    d. Balanced translocation

15. **Most common tumor of infancy:** *(Recent Question 2015)*
    a. Hemangioma b. Brain tumor
    c. Leukemia d. Neuroblastoma

16. **Passive smoke inhalation in non-smokers can be estimated by measuring the blood levels of**
    (Recent Question 2015)
    a. Cotinine b. Nicotine
    c. Hydrocarbons d. Carbon monoxide

17. **The following tumor is not common in the first decade**
    (Recent Question 2015)
    a. Ameloblastoma b. Retinoblastoma
    c. Neuroblastoma d. Rhabdomyosarcoma

18. **The following are small round blue cell tumors A/E**
    (Recent Question 2015)
    a. Lymphomas b. Osteosarcoma
    c. Neuroblastoma d. Rhabdomyosarcoma

19. **True regarding stge IV-S of neuroblastoma A/E**
    (Recent Question 2015)
    a. Limited to infants < 1 year
    b. Primary localize tumor
    c. Dissemination to bone
    d. Good prognosis

20. **A mother brings her 10 months old baby with the complaint that the swat is very salty. Past history revealed revealed meconium ileus in the new born period. Diagnosis** *(Recent Question 2015)*
    a. Hirschprung's disease
    b. Hyaline membrane disease
    c. Necrotizing enterocolitis
    d. Cystic fibrosis

21. **Most common cause of non-immune hydrops**
    a. Chromosomal abnormalities *(Recent Question 2015)*
    b. Fetal anemia
    c. Intrauterine infections
    d. Cardiovascular causes

22. **Cystic fibrosis gene is located in chromosome**
    (PGI Nov 2015/Recent Question 2015)
    a. 7p b. 7q
    c. 13p d. 22q

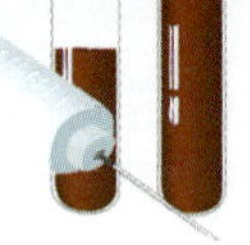

23. **Most common cause of death in Cystic fibrosis**
(Recent Question 2015)
a. Lower respiratory tract infections
b. Cardiovascular defects
c. Pancreatitis
d. Malnutrition and malabsorption

24. **The following tumor is not common in the first decade**
(Recent Question 2015)
a. Ameloblastoma   b. Retinoblastoma
c. Neuroblastoma   d. Rhabdomyosarcoma

25. **The following are small round blue cell tumors A/E**
(Recent Question 2015)
a. Lymphoma   b. Osteosarcoma
c. Neuroblastoma   d. Rhabdomyosarcoma

26. **Stippled calcification is seen in** *(Recent Question 2015)*
a. Wilms' tumor   b. Pheochromocytoma
c. Teratoma   d. Neuroblastoma

27. **Most common abdominal mass in children**
(Recent Question 2015)
a. Hydronnephrosis   b. Wilms' tumor
c. Neuroblastoma   d. Rhabdomyosarcoma

28. **Tumor with triphasic combination of blastmal, stromal and epithelial cell types** *(Recent Question 2015)*
a. Wilms' tumor   b. Teratoma
c. Melanoma   d. Neuroblastoma

29. **The following factor is associated with good prognosis in neuroblastoma** *(Recent Question 2015)*
a. TRLB expression   b. TRKA expression
c. MRP expression   d. Telomerase expression

30. **A mother brings hear 10-month-old baby with the complaint that the sweat is very salty-past history reveled meconium ileus in the new born period. What is your diagnosis ?** *(Recent Question 2015)*
a. Hirschsprung's disease
b. Hyaline membrane disease
c. Necrotizing enterocolitis
d. Cystic fibrosis

31. **Which is not associated with bilateral renal agenesis?**
(Recent Question 2015)
a. Potter facies   b. Renal agenesis
c. Polyhydramnios   d. Oligohydramnios

32. **Most common malignancy in children?**
(Recent Question 2015)
a. Leukemia   b. Brain tumors
c. Neuroblastoma   d. Retinoblastoma

33. **WAGR syndrome includes all except?**
(Recent Question 2015)
a. Wilms' tumor   b. Aniridia
c. Growth retardation d. Mental retardation

34. **Most common cause of extracranial solid tumor in children:** *(Recent Question 2015)*
a. Neuroblastoma   b. Wilms'tumor
c. Thymoma   d. Osteosarcoma

35. **Most important prognosticfactor of Wilms' tumor:**
(Recent Question 2015)
a. Histopathology   b. Ploidyof cells
c. Age < 1 yr   d. Mutation of 12p gene

36. **Small round cell tumors include:** *(Recent Question 2014)*
a. Wilms' tumor   b. Retinoblastoma
c. Rhabdomyosarcoma   d. All

37. **Sweat chloride in cystic fibrosis:** *(Recent Question 2014)*
a. Decreased   b. Increased
c. No change   d. May increase or decrease

38. **All are good prognostic factors for neuroblastoma except -** *(Recent Question 2014)*
a. Trk-A expression absent b. Absence of 1 p loss
c. Absence of 17 p gain   d. Absence of 11q loss

39. **Not a childhood tumor is?** *(Recent Question 2014)*
a. Neuroblastoma   b. Wilms' tumor
c. Small cell carcinoma d. Retinoblastoma

40. **Cystic fibrosis causes all except?** *(Recent Question 2014)*
a. Decreased chloride in sweat
b. Infertility
c. Increased infection   d. Pancreas involvement

41. **Children with germline retinoblastoma are more likely to develop other primary malignancies in their later lifetime course. Which of the following can occur in such patients?** *(AIIMS Nov 13)*
a. Osteosarcoma of lower limbs and soft tissue sarcoma
b. Thyroid carcinoma
c. Seminoma
d. Squamous cell carcinoma

42. **Bilateral proptosis is characteristically present in**
(AIIMS Nov 13)
a. Retinoblastoma   b. Rhabdomyosarcoma
c. Neuroblastoma   d. PNET

43. **Which histological finding in resected kidney indicated Bilateral Wilms' tumor?** *(JIPMER 2013)*
a. Blastemal component b. Nephrogenic rests
c. Skeletal muscle differentiation
d. Abnormal mitotic figures

44. **In cystic fibrosis mutation occurs at?**
(DNB Aug 12 Pattern)
a. One gene   b. Two gene
c. Three gene   d. Four gene

45. **All are true about cystic fibrosis except?** *(JIPMER 2012)*
a. Recurrent respiratory infections
b. Majority of males are infertile
c. Fasting hyperglycemia is a feature of early disease
d. Sweat chloride is >70 meq/l

46. **Which of the following congenital lesion is a deformity?**
(PGI Nov 2011)
a. Potter sequence   b. CTEV
c. Congenital heart disease d. Cleft lip
e. Imperforate anus

47. **Anaplasia in Wilms' tumor is evident by** *(PGI Nov 10)*
a. Increased mitosis   b. Pleomorphic nuclei
c. Large nucleus   d. p53 mutation
e. Increased response to chemotherapy

48. **True about nephrogenic rest:** *(PGI Nov 10)*
a. Associated with Wilms' tumor
b. Increased risk of Wilms' tumor in contralateral kidney
c. No association with Wilms' tumor
d. Abnormal embryonal renal tissue
e. High risk of Neuroblastoma

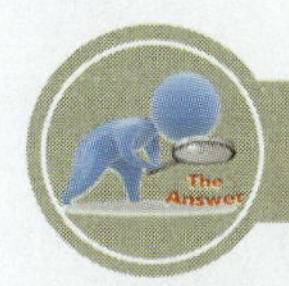 ## Answers with Explanations

1. **Ans. (a, c, d, e); a. Caused by mutations of the MEFV gene; c. Presentation include episodic bouts of acute peritonitis; d. Amyloidosis occur as a complication; e. Colchicine is used for treatment** (*Ref: R 9th/pg 259-260*)

2. **Ans. (a, d) a. Associated with aniridia; d. Has pseudocapsule**

Wilms' tumor is associated with WAGR syndrome which includes Aniridia, grossly have multilocular cysts, mostly well circumscribed and surrounded by a pseudocapsule. It is a pediatric tumor and can present in neonates.

3. **Ans. (a) Medulloblastoma**

4. **Ans. (c) TTF-1**

Wilms' tumor being mixed tumor has Desmin, Vimentin and Cytokeratin positive. Thyroid transcription factor-1 (TTF-1) is a sensitive marker for pulmonary and thyroid adenocarcinomas

5. **Ans. (c) Trk B expression** (*Ref: Robbins 9th/pg 475-479*)

6. **Ans. (d) 70 mEq/L** (*Ref: Robbins 9th/pg 466-470*)

7. **Ans. (a) Leukemia** (*Ref: Robbins 9th/pg 473-475*)

8. **Ans. (b) ENAC activity of the sweat ducts increases**

(*Ref: Robbins 9th/pg 466-470; 8th 465-470*)

In cystic fibrosis, there is decreased reabsorption of Na & Cl from sweat glands.

9. **Ans. (d) Brucellosis** (*Ref: Harrison 19th ed*)

Category A agents are the highest-priority pathogens. Greatest risk to national security because they (1) be easily disseminated (2) result in high mortality rates (3) might cause public panic (4) require special action for public health. **Category B** agents are the second highest priority pathogens and include those that are moderately easy to disseminate. **Category C** agents are the third highest priority.

10. **Ans. (b) Skull** (*Ref: Robbins 9th/pg 473-479*)

11. **Ans. (d) Does not respond to chemotherapy and radiotherapy** (*Ref: Robbins 9th/pg 479-481*)

12. **Ans. (c) Ivacaftor, a potentiator of the CFTR channel is used to for patients with (ΔF508) mutation**

(*Ref: Robbins 9th/pg 466-470; 8th/pg 465-470*)

13. **Ans. (d) TRKA expression** (*Ref: Robbins 9th/pg 479-481*)

14. **Ans. (b) Genomic imprinting** (*Ref: R 9th/pg 479-481*)

15. **Ans. (a) Hemangioma** (*Ref: Robbins 9th/pg 475*)

16. **Ans. (a) Cotinine** (*Ref: Robbins 9th/pg 475*)

17. **Ans. (a) Ameloblastoma** (*Ref: Robbins 9th/pg 474-475*)

18. **Ans. (b) Osteosarcoma** (*Ref: Robbins 9th/pg 474-475*)

19. **Ans. (c) Dissemination to bone** (*Ref: R 9th/pg 475-479*)

20. **Ans. (d) Cystic fibrosis** (*Ref: Robbins 9th/pg 466-470*)

21. **Ans. (d) Cardiovascular causes** (*Ref: R 9th/pg 475*)

22. **Ans. (b) 7q** (*Ref: Robbins 9th/pg 466-470*)

23. **Ans. (a) Lower respiratory tract infections**

(*Ref: Robbins 9th/pg 466-470; 8th/pg 475*)

24. **Ans. (a) Ameloblastoma** (*Ref: Robbins 9th/pg 475-479*)

25. **Ans. (b) Osteosarcoma** (*Ref: Robbins 9th/pg 475-479*)

26. **Ans. (d) Neuroblastoma** (*Ref: Robbins 9th/pg 475-479*)

27. **Ans. (c) Neuroblastoma** (*Ref: Robbins 9th/pg 475-479*)

28. **Ans. (a) Wilms' tumor** (*Ref: Robbins 9th/pg 479-481*)

29. **Ans. (b) TRKA expression** (*Ref: Robbins 9th/pg 475-479*)

30. **Ans. (d) Cystic fibrosis** (*Ref: Robbins 9th/pg 466-470*)

31. **Ans. (c) Polyhydramnios**

(*Ref: Robbins 9th/pg 452; 8th/pg 448N19: 1827*)

Potter sequence (oligohydramnios sequence)

- Bilateral Renal agenesis → Oligohydramnios → flattened facies, abnormalities of hands and feet and pulmonary hypoplasia.
- Neonates with bilateral renal agenesis die of pulmonary insufficiency from pulmonary hypoplasia rather than renal failure.

32. **Ans. (a) Leukemia** (*Ref: Robbins 9th/pg 473-475*)

The most frequent childhood cancers are: (in order of decreasing frequency)[Q]

- **Leukemia (Most common is ALL),[Q]** Neuroblastoma,[Q] Wilms' tumor, Hepatoblastoma, Retinoblastoma

33. **Ans. (c) Growth retardation** (*Ref: R 9th/pg 479-481*)

34. **Ans. (a) Neuroblastoma** (*Ref: Robbins 9th/pg 475-479*)

Neuroblastoma is the:

- Most common **extracranial solid tumor** of **childhood**[Q]
- Most common **abdominal tumor** of **childhood**[Q]
- Most **frequently diagnosed** tumor of **infancy (<1 year of age)**[Q]

35. Ans. (a) Histopathology

(Ref: Robbins 9th/pg 479-481; 8th/pg 479-481N19: 1759)

- **Histology** plays a major role in **risk stratification of Wilms'** tumor.
- **Absence of anaplasia** is considered a favorable histologic finding.
- Other prognostic factors for Wilms' tumor are: **age, stage, tumor weight, and loss of heterozygosity** at chromosomes 1p & 16q.

36. Ans. (d) All *(Ref: Robbins 9th/pg 475; 8th/pg 475)*

Small round blue cell tumors are Tumors with **similar histology of small round cell.**

"Low NEW MRP"	
• Lymphoma	• Neuroblastoma
• EwingSarcoma	• Wilms' Tumor
• Medulloblastoma	• Retinoblastoma
• Primitive Neuroectodermal Tumor	

37. Ans. (b) Increased *(Ref: Robbins 9th/pg 466-470)*

38. Ans. (a) Trk-A expression absent *(Ref: R 9th/pg 475-479)*

39. Ans. (c) Small cell carcinoma *(Ref: Robbins 9th/pg 475)*

Small cell Carcinoma of lungs is a tumor of adults.

40. Ans. (a) Decreased chloride in sweat

(Ref: R 9th/pg 466-470)

41. Ans. (a) Osteosarcoma of lower limbs and soft tissue sarcoma *(Ref: Robbins 9th/pg 475, 1339; 8th/pg 475, 1365)*

Clinical features of Neuroblastoma: reflect the tumor site and Extent of disease

Extent of disease	Clinical features
Localized disease	**Asymptomatic mass or as mass-related symptoms**; E.g. spinal cord compression, bowel obstruction and superior vena cava syndrome.
Metastatic disease	Fever, irritability, failure to thrive, bone pain, cytopenias, bluish subcutaneous nodules, **bilateral orbital proptosis, and periorbitalecchymoses (raccoon eyes)**
Neurologic involvement	Horner syndrome, nerve root compression
Paraneoplastic syndrome	Opsoclonus-myoclonus-ataxia syndrome
If catecholamines produced	Increased sweating, hypertension, secretory diarrhea (due to release of VIP)
Extensive tumors	Tumor lysis syndrome and DIC
Infants with stage 4S	Subcutaneous tumor nodules, massive liver involvement, limited bone marrow disease &a small primary tumor without bone involvement or other metastases.

42. Ans. (a) Retinoblastoma

(Ref: Robbins 9th/pg 475-479; 8th/pg 475-478)

Children with **germline retinoblastoma** are more likely to develop other primary malignancies like **Osteosarcoma** of **lower limbs** and **soft tissue sarcoma**, in their later lifetime course.

43. Ans. (b) Nephrogenic rests *(Ref: Robbins 9th/pg 479-481)*

Nephrogenic rests

- They are putative **precursor lesions of Wilms'** tumors
- Patients with presence of **nephrogenic rests in the resected specimen, are at an increased risk of developing Wilms' tumors in the contralateral kidney** and require frequent and regular surveillance.

44. Ans. (a) One gene *(Ref: Robbins 9th/pg 466-470)*

Cystic Fibrosisis an Autosomal recessive disease, caused by mutation in Cystic Fibrosis Transmembrane conductance Regulator (CFTR) gene on chr7q31.2, which leads to abnormal function of **ion transport channel.**

45. Ans. (c) Fasting hyperglycemia is a feature of early disease

(Ref: Refer Ans 7 & 10; Nelson 19th/pg 1996; Robbins 9th/pg 466-470; 8th/pg 465-470)

Cystic fibrosis-related diabetes (CFRD)

- **No diabetes is seen in CF patients younger than 10 yr while 40-50% show diabetes at $\geq$ 20 yr age;**
- **So diabetes is a late feature of CF, seen only in individuals who survive to adolescence & beyond.**
- Patients with CFRD have features of both **T1DM and T2DM.**
- There is pancreatic damage leading to slowly progressive insulin deficiency, along with insulin resistance

46. Ans. (b) CTEV *(Ref: Robbins 9th/pg 452; 8th/pg 448)*

Deformations or deformities are structural abnormalities (extrinsic disturbance in morphogenesis) due to **compression of growing fetus** by abnormal **biomechanical forces** like bicornuate uterus. **Eg: Clubfeet**[Q]

47. Ans. (a, b, c, d) a. Increased mitosis; b. Pleomorphic nuclei; c. Large nucleus; d. p53 mutation

(Ref: Robbins 9th/pg 481)

Anaplasia in Wilms' tumor (seen in **5%** of cases) is defined as the presence of cells with:
- Large, hyperchromatic, **pleomorphic nuclei**
- **Abnormalmitoses**

Anaplasia also correlates with the **presence of TP53 mutations; loss of p53** function makes anaplastic cells relatively **unresponsive to cytotoxic chemotherapy.**

48. Ans. (a, b, d) a. Associated with Wilms' tumor; b. Increased risk of Wilms' tumor in contralateral kidney; d. Abnormal embryonal renal tissue

(Ref: R 9th/pg 479-481)

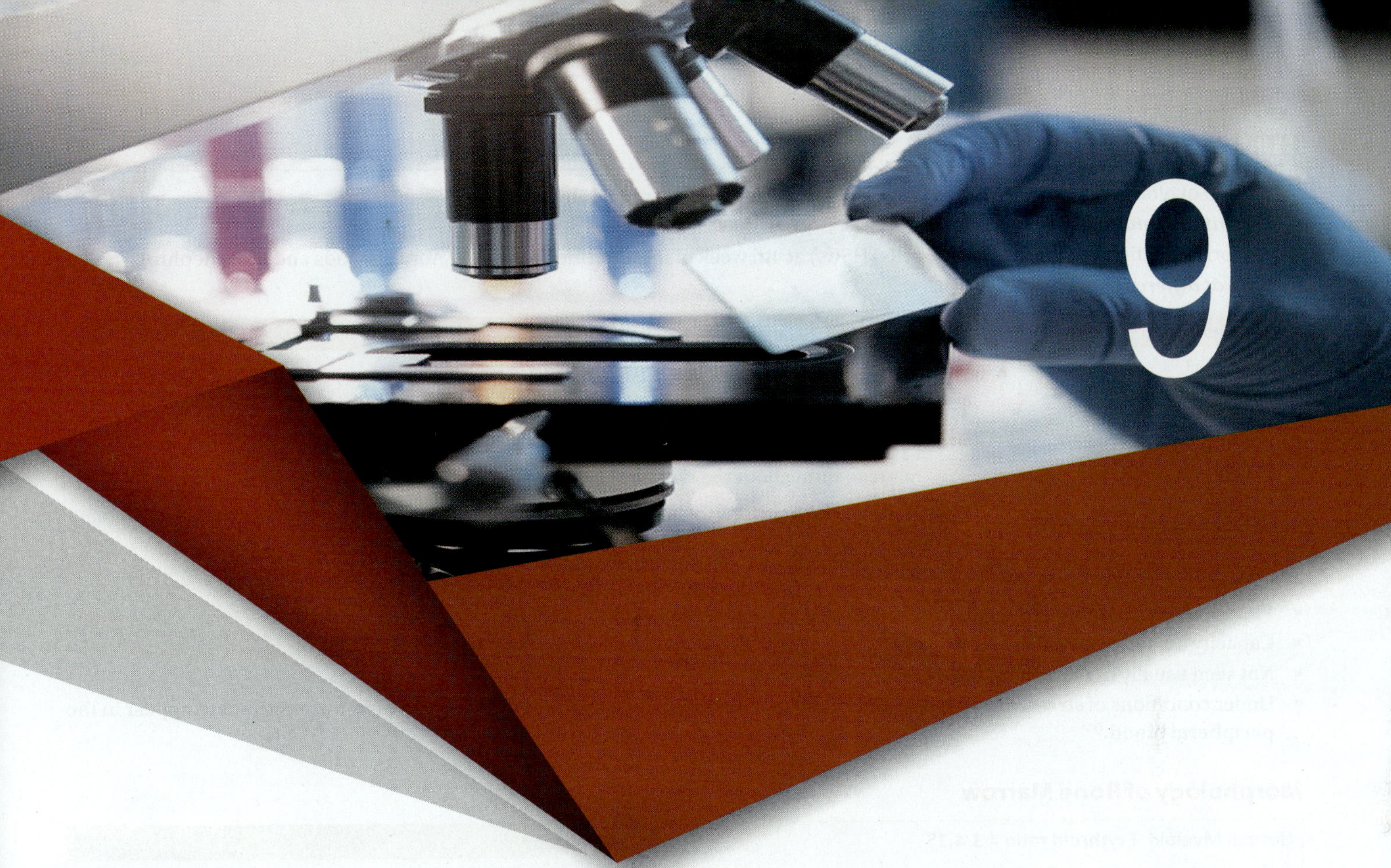

White Blood Cells and its Disorders

Key Points

- Hematopoiesis starts between 3-4th wk of Intrauterine life in yolk sac
- Leukopenia is abnormally **low WBC (TLC <4000/uL) while Leukocytosis is increase in the count of WBCs (>11,000/uL)**
- **Leukemia** refers to hematological neoplasms with involvement of **bone marrow & peripheral blood Lymphoma** refers to **discrete tissue masses**[Q] usually involving Lymph node, Spleen and Liver
- ALL is the **most common cancer of children.**
- **The most common leukemia** of adults in the **Western world is CLL.**
- The most common site for extranodal lymphoma is stomach
- **Follicular lymphoma is the most common** form of **indolent (low grade) NHL** in the West.
- **DLBCL, is the most common** form of **NHL in India**
- Burkitts lymphoma shows **"starry sky" pattern**
- Diagnostic Hallmark of Hodgkins lymphoma are Reed-Sternberg cells
- Cut off for blast counts in AML is <20% if AML is associated with cytogenetic abnormalities like t(15;17), t(8;21), inv(16)
- **BCR-ABL gene**[Q] (210 kDa in size) is hallmark of CML

Key Recent Updates

- CSF3R mutation is seen in CNL
- Provisional response to TKI is added in accelerated phase of CML.

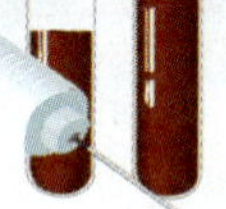

HEMATOPOIESIS

Formation of blood components during embryonic stage and throughout adult life

- *Definitive hematopoiesis:*
  - ○ Forms multipotent hematopoietic cells (HSCs) at 4th week of intrauterine life around Aorta, gonads and mesonephros
- *Sites at different ages:*

Age group	Site of Hematopoiesis
Embryo[Q]	Till the 3rd wk in Yolk sac;[Q] Up to 3rd month in Liver[Q]
Fetus	4th month onwards: Bone marrow[Q]
Birth	Bone marrow[Q]
Child	Bone marrow: throughout the skeleton[Q]
Adult	Bone marrow: Flat bone (Vertebra, ribs, sternum, pelvis)[Q] & proximal epiphysis of humerus & femur

Properties of Hematopoietic Stem Cells

- **Pluripotency**[Q] - Ability of a single HSC to generate all mature blood cells
- Capacity for **self-renewal**[Q]
- **Not** seen usually in **peripheral blood**[Q]
- Under conditions of **stress**, e.g. severe anemia or acute inflammation, HSCs are **mobilized from bone marrow** and appear in the **peripheral blood.**[Q]

Morphology of Bone Marrow

	Light Microscopy
Normal **Myeloid: Erythroid ratio = 3-4:1**[Q]	• Thin-walled **sinusoids**[Q] lined by **single layer of endothelial cells**
Normal ratio of **marrow cells: fat cells=1:1**[Q]	• Clusters of **hematopoietic & fat cells** within the interstitium
Normal Cellularity (%) = **100 − Age**[Q] • Decreases with age • At 10 yrs = 100-10 = 90% cellularity • At 30 yrs = 100-30 = 70% cellularity	• **Megakaryocytes** lie **next to sinusoids**[Q] where they release platelets • Red cell precursors (**Erythroblasts**) surround macrophages (so-called **nurse cells**)[Q]

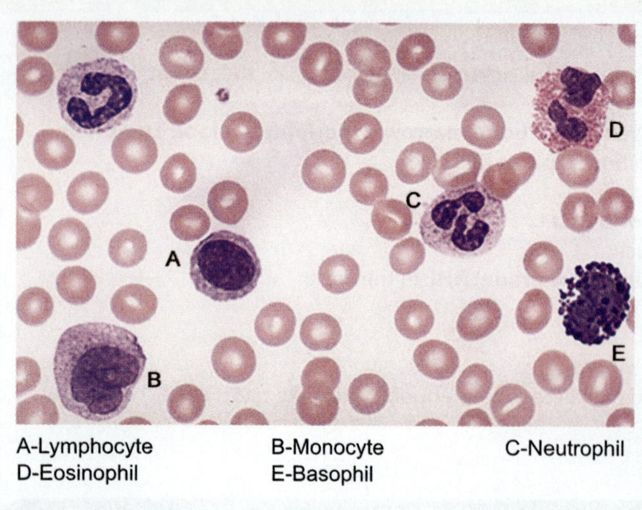

A-Lymphocyte   B-Monocyte   C-Neutrophil
D-Eosinophil   E-Basophil

High Yield Facts

- **Agranulocytosis: Clinically significant reduction in neutrophils** making one susceptible to bacterial & fungal infections.[Q]
- **Drugs are** the most common cause of **agranulocytosis**[Q]
- Serious infection increases when ANC < 500/mm³

DISORDERS OF WHITE BLOOD CELLS

- Quantitative defects
  - ○ Leucopenia
  - ○ Leucocytosis
- Qualitative defects

Leukopenia

- *Definition:*
  - ○ An abnormally **low white cell count** (leukopenia; **TLC <4000/μL)**[Q]

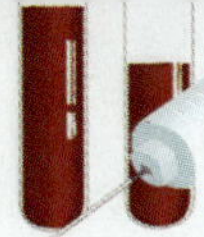

Lymphopenia

- **Definition**
  - Reduction in number of **lymphocytes** in blood
- **Etiology:**
  - **Congenital immunodeficiency diseases, e.g. SCID[Q]**
  - **Human immunodeficiency virus (HIV) infection[Q]**
  - **Glucocorticoids[Q]** or cytotoxic drugs
  - Autoimmune disorders
  - Malnutrition
  - **Acute viral infections[Q]**

Neutropenia

- **Definition**
  - **Reduction in the number** of neutrophils (<1500/µL) in the blood[Q]
- **Etiology**
  - **A. Drug Induced Neutropenia**
    - **Anti-bacterials – Chloramphenicol,[Q]** Cotrimoxazole, Ciprofloxacin, Nitrofurantoin
    - **Anti-inflammatory- Ibuprofen[Q]**
    - **Antithyroid-** Carbimazole, Propylthiouracil
    - **Anticonvulsants-** Valproate, Phenytoin
  - **B. Inadequate or ineffective granulopoiesis:[Q]**
    - **Aplastic anemia[Q]**
    - Infiltrative marrow disorders (e.g., tumors, granulomatous disease)
    - Infections: **Viral- Parvo B19[Q], HIV**, EBV
    - Ineffective hematopoiesis: **Megaloblastic anemias[Q]** & Myelodysplastic syndromes
    - **Kostmann syndrome[Q]:** Autosomal recessive congenital neutropenia
    - Cyclic Neutropenia
  - **C. Accelerated destruction or sequestration of neutrophils**
    - Immunological injury to neutrophils, e.g. **SLE[Q]**
    - **Splenomegaly[Q]**
    - Increased peripheral utilization: **bacterial, fungal, or rickettsial infections**

Leukocytosis

Increase in the number of WBCs (>11,000/µL)[Q]

Causes of Leukocytosis[Q]

Type of Leukocytosis	Causes
Neutrophilia (>75%)	• **Infection (bacterial)[Q]** & **Inflammation** including **MI[Q]** • Acute **stress** states (burns, post-surgery) • **Myeloproliferative** disorders: CML, **Polycythemia vera** • Others: **steroid[Q]** therapy, **Renal failure[Q]**
Eosinophilia (>400/µL)	• **Allergies: Asthma[Q], hay fever[Q], urticaria** • **Skin** diseases: Eczema, **dermatitis herpetiformis[Q]** • **Parasitic:** Ascariasis, **Hookworm[Q]**, Filariasis, Trichinosis • Others: **Tropical eosinophilia[Q], Hypereosinophilic syndrome, Hodgkin's disease**
Basophillia (>1%)	CML[Q], PCV, Ulcerative colitis[Q], Mastocytosis[Q], Myxedema
Monocytosis	• **Infections: TB[Q],** Kala azar, malaria, Syphilis • **Malignancies: AML-M4/5[Q]**, CMML, Hodgkin's • **Inflammatory** diseases: Ulcerative colitis[Q], Crohn's, SLE, Sarcoidosis
Lymphocytosis	• **Bacterial:** TB, **brucellosis**, Syphilis, *pertussis*, **Diphtheria[Q]** • **Viral infections: Infectious mononucleosis[Q]**, Mumps, **Malignancies: CLL[Q]**, NHL, **Hairy Cell Leukemia[Q]**

Qualitative defects in WBCs

Anomaly	Inheritance	Characteristic	Other features
May Hegglin anomaly	AD	**Basophilic inclusions** in WBCs	**Giant platelets & thrombocytopenia**
Alder-Reilly anomaly	AR	**Lilac inclusions** in Neutrophils	Stains with **Toluidine Blue**
Pegler Huet anomaly	AD	**Hypo-segmented** Neutrophils	**Distinct from Pseudo Pegler-Huet anomaly**
Döhle bodies		Patches of dilated endoplasmic reticulum that appear as sky-blue cytoplasmic "puddles."	
Toxic granules		Which are coarser and darker than the normal neutrophilic granules, represent abnormal azurophilic (primary) granules.	

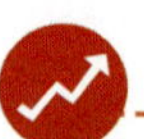

- Infection of **B lymphocytes** by EBV occurs in **Infectious Mononucleosis**
- Atypical lymphocytes that are characteristic of infectious mononucleosis are **CD8+ T** lymphocytes called **DOWNY cells**, that develop in response to the infected B lymphocytes.
- Reed Sternberg like cell are seen in **Infectious mononucleosis, Adult T cell lymphoma, Diffuse large B cell lymphoma**

- **Kikuchi disease** or 'histiocytic necrotizing lymphadenitis' is benign, recurrent necrotizing lymphadenitis
- Eosinophilic abscess in lymph node is characteristically seen in - **Kimura's disease**
- **Typhoid** (Enteric fever) presents with **lymphopenia** and not leukocytosis

NEOPLASTIC PROLIFERATIONS OF WHITE CELLS

- **Leukemia**: Hematological Neoplasms with involvement of **bone marrow and peripheral blood**[Q]
- **Lymphoma**: Hematological Neoplasms where proliferations arise as **discrete tissue masses**[Q] usually involving Lymph node, Spleen, Liver[Q]

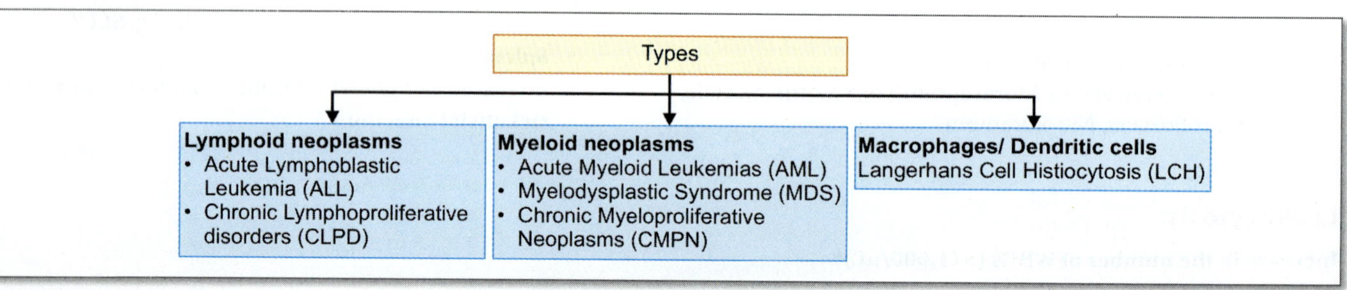

Lymphoid Neoplasms

World Health Organization (WHO) 2008 Classification of Lymphoid Neoplasms

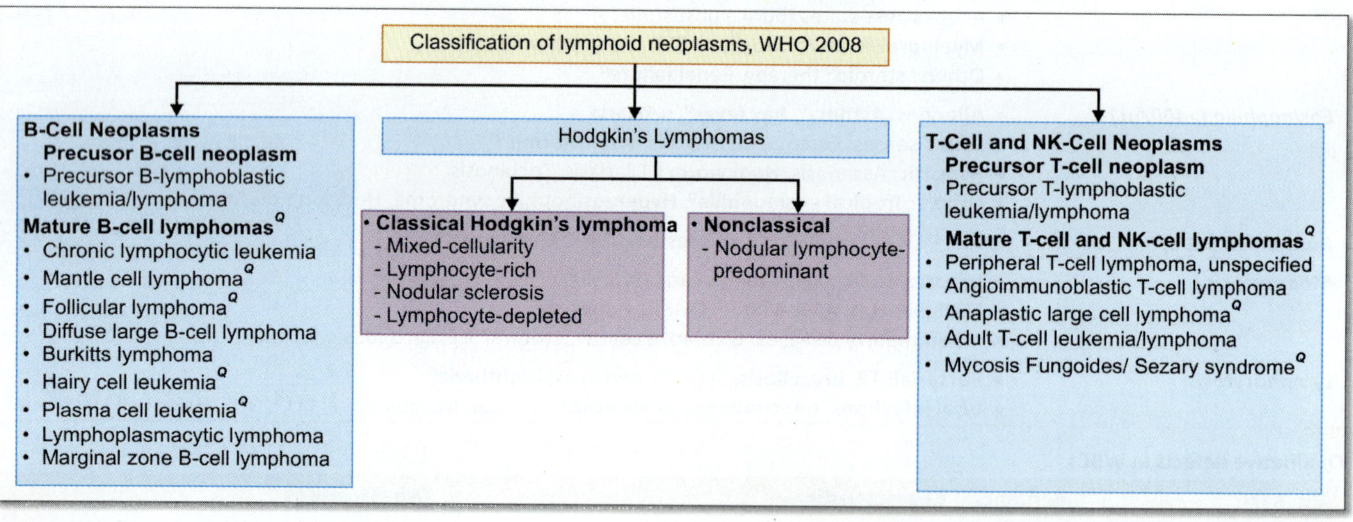

- **CD19** is the earliest recognizable marker of B cells & is lost when B cell becomes a plasma cell
- **CD 34** is the surface glycoproteins that is most often expressed in human hematopoietic stem cell

- Outside the hematopoietic system, **CD34** is expressed on **endothelial cells**.
- **CD 45** is found in **all hematopoietic cells except erythrocytes**
- **CD 46** is a receptor of pathogen like HHV-6, Streptococci
- PAX9 – Marker of B cells

Acute Lymphoblastic Leukemia (ALL)

- **Definition:**
  - **Neoplasms** of **immature B (pre-B)** or **T (pre-T) cells** which are referred to as **lymphoblasts**

- **Epidemiology:**
  - ALL is the **most common cancer of children**[Q], Peak Incidence: **3rd yr**[Q]
  - **Hispanics** have the highest incidence of any ethnic group.

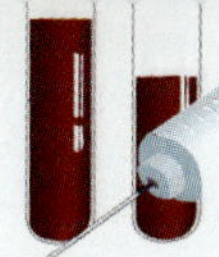

- *Pathogenesis:*
  - **T-ALLs** have **gain**-of-function mutations in **NOTCH1**[Q]
  - **B-ALLs** have **loss**-of-function mutations **PAX5**[Q], **E2A**[Q] & **EBF**[Q], or **t(12;21)**[Q] involving the genes **ETV6 and RUNX1**, 2 genes that are needed in very early hematopoietic precursor.
- *Clinical features:*
  - Abrupt **stormy onset**
  - Symptoms related to depression of marrow function:
    - **Fatigue** due to anemia;
    - **Fever** due to neutropenia; and
    - **Bleeding** due to thrombocytopenia
  - **Marrow expansion** and infiltration of the **sub-periosteum: sternal tenderness**[Q]
  - Generalized lymphadenopathy, Hepatosplenomegaly; **testicular enlargement**
  - **T-ALL:** Mediastinal mass **(Superior Mediastinal Syndrome)**[Q]
  - **CNS features:** headache, vomiting, and nerve palsies
- *Morphology:*
  - Hypercellular Bone Marrow; **> 20% lymphoblasts**[Q]
  - Compared with myeloblasts, **lymphoblasts** have **more condensed chromatin**, less conspicuous nucleoli & scanty agranular cytoplasm
  - Cytochemistry: Myeloperoxidase **(MPO) -ve**, Sudan Black B **(SBB): -ve**[Q]
  - **Diagnosis of choice**
  - Flow cytometry

Classification of ALL

FAB (French American British) Classification

ALL-subtype	L1	L2	L3 (Mature B-cells)Q
Morphology of Blasts	• Small Homogenous Blasts • Little Cytoplasm • Regular Nucleus, • Small indistinct nucleoli	• Large heterogeneous blasts • One or more nucleoli	• Large homogenous blasts • Abundant basophilic cytoplasm • Prominent **cytoplasmic vacuolation**[Q] • Resemble **Burkitt**[Q] **lymphoma**
Age group	Children	Adults	Adults
Prognosis	Good[Q]	Intermediate[Q]	Poor[Q]
Cytochemistry	PAS +	PAS +	PAS-, SBB+[Q]

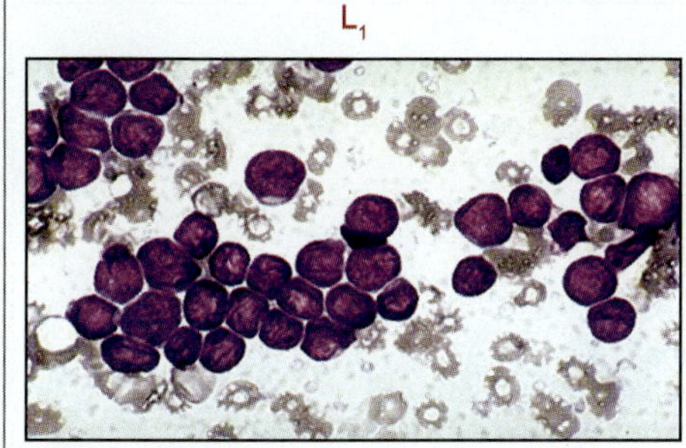

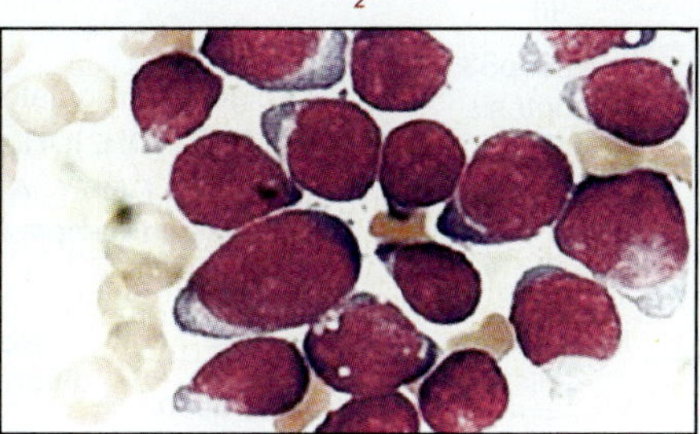

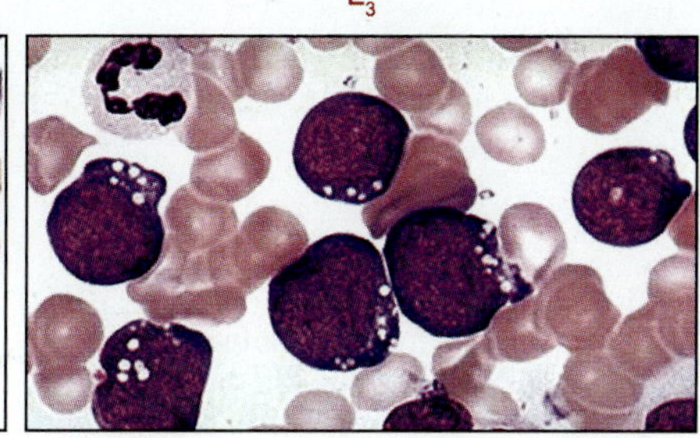

High Yield Facts

- **Mature B-cell ALL** is an uncommon type of **ALL**[Q] (1-2% of ALL cases) in children.
- Both **B-cell ALL** and **Burkitt lymphoma** are characterized by FAB **L3**[Q] morphology,
- Mature **B-cell ALL is** associated with **t(8;14)** & overexpression of the **c-myc** oncogene
- **T-ALL** commonly presents with Mediastinal mass **(Superior Mediastinal Syndrome)**[Q]
- **T-ALL** are **aggressive lymphomas.**[Q]
- In **T-ALL**, cells are positive for markers of blasts like- **Tdt,**[Q] **CD34** & T cell markers **CD1, CD2, CD5, CD7**[Q]
- **Response to treatment is the best prognostic marker in ALL**

WHO 2018: Classification of ALL

- B-Lymphoblastic leukemia, Not otherwise specified (NOS)
- B-Lymphoblastic leukemia with recurrent cytogenetic abnormality

1. t(12;21)ETV6–RUNXI	3. t (9;22) BCR–ABL1	5. B cell ALL with hyperdiploidy	7. BCR-ABL 1 like ALL (Provisional entitiy in 2018 WHO)
2. t (v,11)(KMT2A–MLL)	4. t(5;14) IgH-IL3	6. B cell ALL t(1, 19)–TCF3 –PBX1	8. iAMP 21 ALL.

- T-Lymphoblastic leukemia

Prognostic Factors in Acute Lymphoblastic Leukemia

Determinants	Favorable	Unfavorable
WBC/uL	<10,000	>2,00,000[Q]
Age	2–9 yr	<1 y, >10 y[Q]
Gender	Female	Male[Q]
Ethnicity	White	Black[Q]
L. node, liver, spleen enlargement	Absent	Massive
Testicular enlargement	Absent[Q]	Present[Q]
Central nervous system leukemia	Absent	Present[Q]
FAB morphologic features	L1[Q] Early pre–B-cell ALL	L2[Q] Pre–B-cell ALL Mature B-cell
Ploidy	Hyperdiploidy	Hypodiploidy<45
Cytogenetic markers	Trisomy 4, 10, 17[Q] t(12;21)	t(9;22) t(4;11)
Remission states	< 14 days	> 14 days

Acute Myeloid Leukemias (AML)

- *Definition:*
  - ○ **Neoplasms** of **myeloid cells** which are referred to **as myeloblasts**[Q]
- *Clinical features:*
  - ○ Same as ALL but in addition certain types of AML show:
    - **Chloromas (AML M2 > 5 > 4)**[Q]
    - **Gingival hyperplasia (AML M5 > 4)**[Q]
    - **DIC (AML M3)**[Q]
- *Predisposing Conditions:*

Genetic factors	Congenital bone marrow failure syndromes	Drugs
• **Down's syndrome**	• Kostmann syndrome	• Benzene
• **Fanconi's anemia**	• Diamond – Blackfan anemia	• Alkylating agents
• **Bloom's syndrome**		• Epipodophyl-lotoxins
• **Neurofibromatosis type 1**		• Ionizing radiation
• Klinefelter syndrome		
• Turner syndrome		

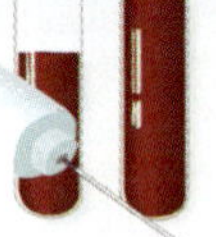

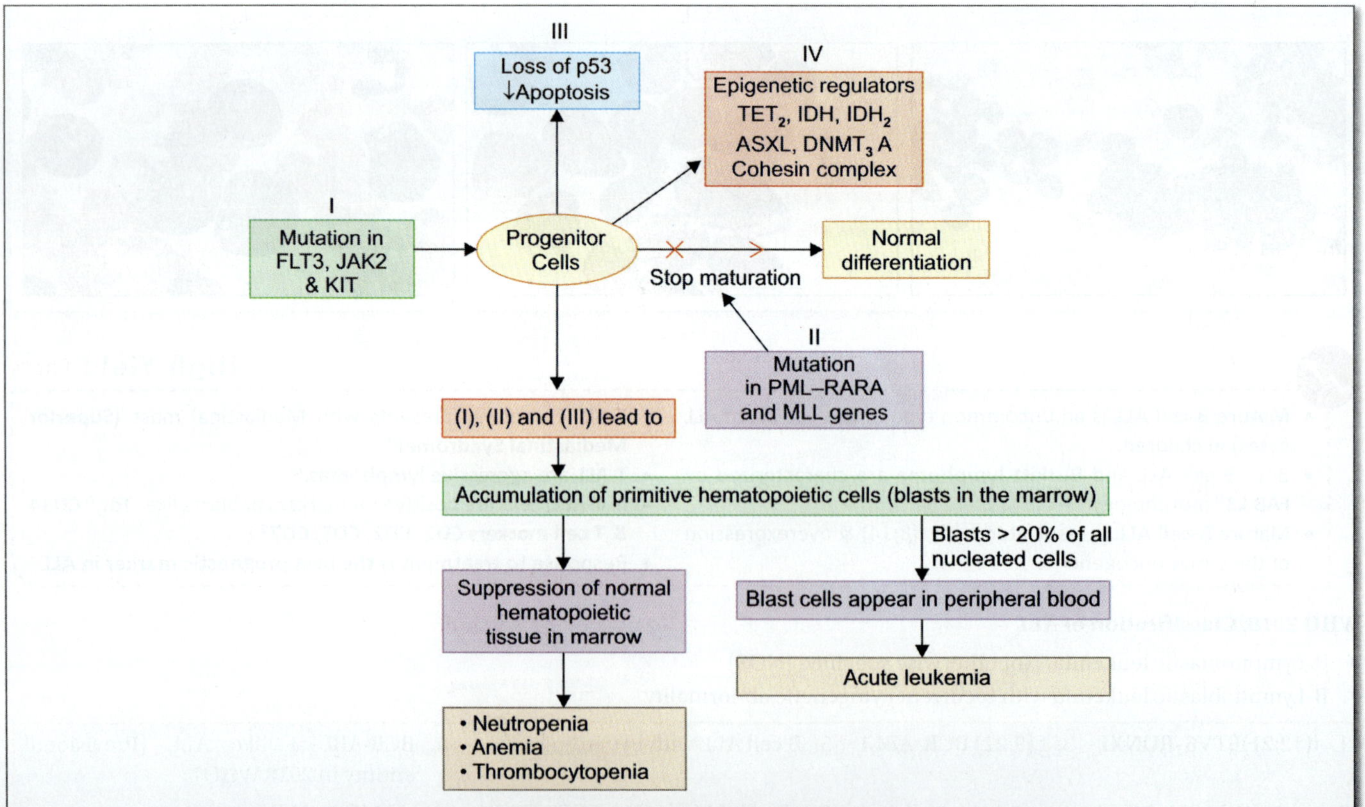

Pathogenesis of acute myeloid leukemia

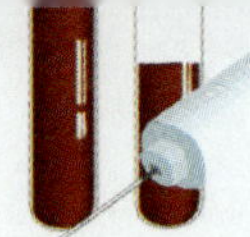

Major Subtypes of AML in the WHO Classification 2018

Class	Prognosis	FAB Subtype	Morphology/Comments
I. AML WITH RECURRENT GENETIC ABERRATIONS			
a. AML with balanced translocations			
AML with t(8;21)[Q] RUNX$_1$ – RUNX$_1$T$_1$	**Favorable**	M2[Q]	**Auer rods++;** abnormal cytoplasmic granules
AML with inv (16)[Q] CBFB-MYH II	**Favorable**	M4	abnormal eosinophilic precursors[Q]
AML with t(15;17) PML-RARA	**Intermediate**	M3	**Auer rods +++, high incidence of DIC[Q]**
AML with t(9,11) KMT$_{2A}$-MLL	**Poor**	Variable	
AML with BCR–ABL$_1$ mutation			Responds to R$_x$
b. AML with gene mutations AML with mutated NPM$_1$ AML with Biallelic mutation of CEBPA	Favorable Favorable		
II. AML WITH MDS-LIKE FEATURES			
AML with MDS-like cytogenetic aberrations	**Poor**	Variable	Associated with **5q-, 7q-, Monosomy 5 and 7[Q]**
III. AML, THERAPY-RELATED			
1. Post alkylating agents	**Very poor**	Variable	5–10 years after exposure • Unbalanced loss of chr. 5 & 7 & loss of p53
2. Post DNA topoisomerase II			1–5 years after exposure • Balanced chromosomal translocations
IV. AML, NOT OTHERWISE SPECIFIED (previously FAB)			
AML, minimally differentiated	Poor[Q]	M0	MPO –VE
AML without maturation	Intermediate	M1	MPO +ve in >3% of blasts
AML with myelocytic maturation	Intermediate	M2	myelocytic maturation, Auer Rods ++
AML with myelomonocytic maturation	Intermediate	M4	Myelocytic and monocytic differentiation **MPO +, NSE +[Q]**
AML with monocytic maturation	Intermediate	M5	Monoblasts and pro-monocytes predominate, **Non-specific esterase (NSE)+[Q]**
AML with erythroid maturation	Poor[Q]	M6	**>80% erythroid precursors**
AML with megakaryocytic maturation	Poor[Q]	M7	>50% megakaryocytic blasts **Most common Acute Leukemia in Down syndrome**

Diagnosis of AML

- *Bone marrow Morphology:*
  - ○ **> 20% myeloid blasts** in the **bone marrow[Q]**
  - ○ Myeloblasts have **delicate nuclear chromatin**, 2-4 nucleoli, and moderate cytoplasm with or without Auer rods
  - ○ **Auer rods: Most reliable** morphological feature of AML[Q]
    - Needle-like azurophilic fusiform inclusions in cytoplasm of myeloblasts
    - Stain +ve with **MPO and Sudan Black B[Q]**
    - Seen in AML **M2, M3** (also seen in **CML blast crisis** and **MDS**)[Q]
    - **Faggots:** bundles of Auer Rods in crisscross pattern[Q]
  - ○ **Phi Body**: round or oval inclusions in blasts[Q]
- *Cytochemistry:*
  - ○ Blasts stain positive for:
    - **Myeloid stain**: Myeloperoxidase **(MPO)**, Sudan Black B **(SBB)**-M2/3
    - **Monocytic stain**: Non-specific esterase (NSE) **M5[Q]**
    - Both **MPO/SBB** & **NSE**: **M4[Q]**
- **Diagnosis of choice**
  - Flow cytometry

High Yield Facts

Cytochemical stains	Cells stained
Myeloperoxidase (MPO)	Myeloid[Q]
Sudan Black B (SBB)	Myeloid[Q]
Periodic acid Schiff (PAS)	Lymphoid (Block positivity)[Q]
Non-specfic esterase (NSE)	Monocytes[Q] >>Myeloid
Acid phosphatase	T-lymphocyte[Q]
Tartarate resistant acid phosphatase (TRAP)	Hairy cell leukemia[Q]

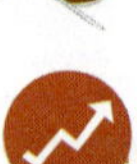

- **Pan B-** marker is **CD 19**^{Q}
- **Pan T-** marker is **CD3**^{Q}
- **Memory cells** have **CD45RO**^{Q}
- **CD 71:** Transferrin receptors
- **CD95**^{Q} is the major receptor for **apoptosis**
- Cut off for blast counts in AML is < 20% if AML is associated with cytogenetic abnormalities like t(15;17), t(8;21), inv(16)^Q
- AML causing **gum hypertrophy/infiltration** are **AML-M5, M4**^{Q}
- AML causing **extramedullary blast proliferations (Chloroms)** are AML **M2, M4, M5**^{Q}
- AML causing blast infiltrations in skin (**leukemia cutis**) are **AML M5, M4**^{Q}
- **Disseminated intravascular coagulation (DIC)**^{Q} can be seen in Acute promyelocytic leukemic (**APML, M3**)

Differences between Myeloblast and lymphoblast in Acute Leukemia

Parametres	Myeloblast	Lymhoblast
Size	Larger (18-20 μ)	Smaller (10-18 μ)
Cytoplasm	Moderate and granular	Scant and agranular
N/C ratio	High	Very high
Nuclear chromatin	Fine and stippled	Coarser
Nucleoli	2–5 prominent	0–2 Inconspicuous
Auer rods	Present	Absent
Accompanying cells	Myelocytes, metamyelocytes, stab and neutrophils	Lymphocytes

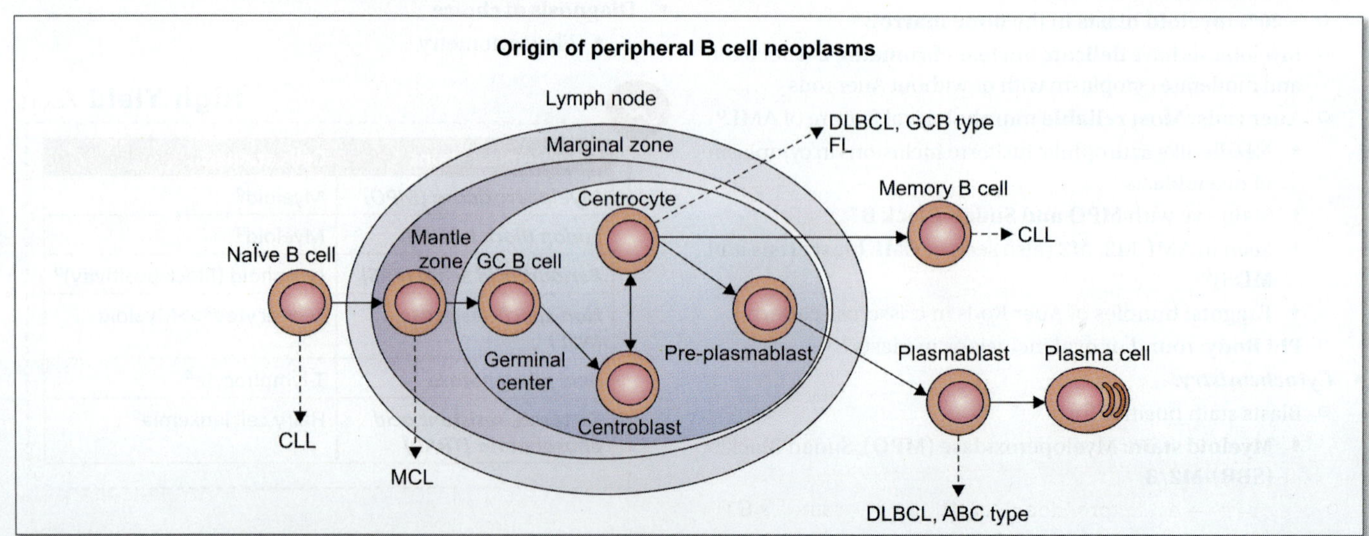

Peripheral B-Cell Neoplasms

Chronic Lymphocytic Leukemia (CLL)/ Small Lymphocytic Lymphoma (SLL)

- *Clinical criteria:*
  - Absolute **clonal lymphocytes >5000/uL**[Q]
  - **MC leukemia** of adults in the **Western world**.
  - Median age at diagnosis is **60 years; M:F = 2 : 1**
- MC mutation–Del 13q.
- Cell of origin–Naive B cell.
- *Peripheral Smear:*
  - **Small round lymphocytes** with scant cytoplasm (**CONVENT girl appearance**)[Q]
  - Occasional cells have distorted outline called **smudge cells**[Q]
  - Rarely **Warm type AIHA** may develop showing Spherocytes[Q]
- *Morphology of Lymph nodes:*
  - **Diffusely effaced**[Q] by an infiltrate of predominantly small lymphocytes (6- 12μm) between which lies larger activated lymphocytes- **proliferation centers**[Q] (**pathognomonic for CLL/SLL**), which contain **mitotically active cells.**
  - Overall CLL has **low mitotic rate**[Q] exc in proliferative center
- **Diagnosis of choice**
  - *Immunophenotyping*
  - **Dim Surface Ig** (usually IgM or IgM and IgD)[Q]
  - **Pan B-cell markers** CD19 + and CD20+[Q]
  - **CD23+ and CD5+**[Q]

- *Poor prognosis markers:*
  - Rai (stage 3 /4) and Binnet (stage C)
  - High β2 microglobulin
  - **Diffuse marrow** involvement
  - Lymphocyte doubling time (<1 yr)
  - **High LDH**
  - Increased Serum **CD23**[Q]
  - **Lack** of somatic IghVh **hypermutation**[Q]
  - **ZAP-70 +ve**
  - **CD38 +ve**
  - Presence of **NOTCH1 mutations**[Q]
- *Transformations of CLL (poor prognosis):*
  - Diffuse large B-cell lymphoma - **Richter syndrome** (5% – 10%)[Q]
  - Large-cell transformation to **prolymphocytic leukemia (PLL)**[Q]
  - **Acute Leukemia**
  - 2nd malignancy- **Melanoma and CNS tumors**[Q]

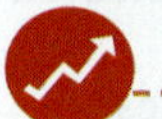

High Yield Facts

- Rai and Binnet staging system was used for CLL
- Almost never develops after radiation
- M.C genetic anomalies in CLL are **del 13q14.3**[Q], 11q, and 17p, and trisomy 12q.[Q]
- Micro-RNAs: **miR-15a and miR-16-1** (tumor suppressor genes): **good prognosis in CLL**[Q]
- CLL with Somatically **hypermutated** Ig genes have **indolent course**[Q]
- CLL with **Unmutated** Ig genes (naive B-cell origin) have **aggressive course**[Q]

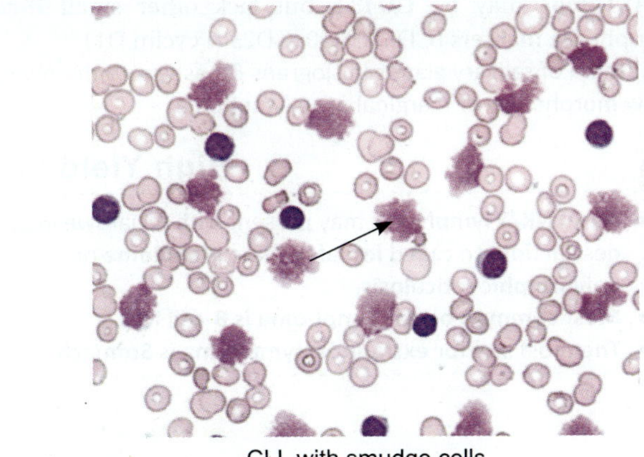

CLL with smudge cells

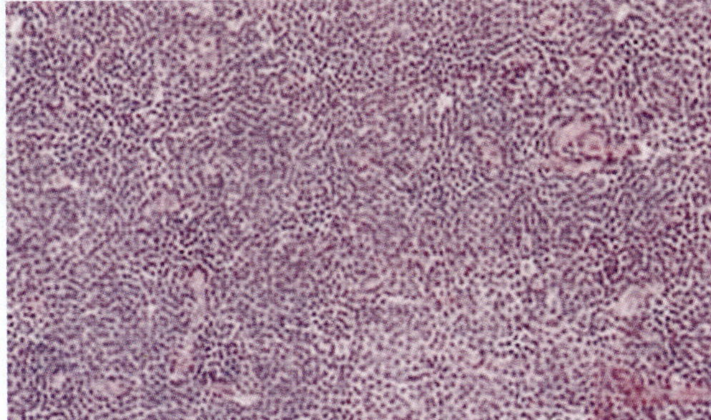

Lymph node biopsy showing effacement by small lymphocytes

Mantle Cell Lymphoma

- *Definition:*
  - Tumor arising from **mantle zone**[Q] which surrounds germinal centers
- *Seen in:*
  - **M>F;** Most common age: **5th-6th decade**
- *Pathogenesis:*
  - **t(11;14)**[Q] → overexpression of **cyclin D1** → promotes **G1-to S-phase** progression during the cell cycle.

- *Presentation:*
  - Usual presentation: **Lymphadenopathy** (with occasional spill to peripheral blood)[Q]
  - Unusual presentation: **Lymphomatoid polyposis**[Q]- mucosal involvement of the **small bowel or colon** producing **polyp-like** lesions
- *Morphology of lymph node:*
  - A **homogeneous population of small lymphocytes** with deeply **clefted (cleaved) nuclear** contours

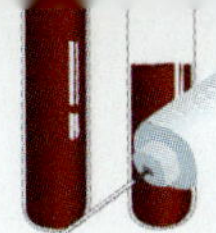

233

- *Immunophenotype:*
  - Express high levels of **cyclin D1, CD19, CD20, CD45 and surface Ig**[Q].
  - **CD5+ve**[Q] and **CD23–ve** which help to distinguish it from CLL/SLL.
  - **Most sensitive marker is SOX II**
- *Prognosis:*
  - Poor; Median survival of **3 - 4 years**.

Follicular Lymphoma

Most common form of **indolent (low grade) NHL** in the West.[Q]

- *Clinical feature*
  - Presents with painless, generalized **lymphadenopathy**.
- *Pathogenesis*
  - Arises from **germinal center of B** cells[Q]
  - Hallmark translocation **t(14;18)**[Q]
  - Mutations in **MLL gene**[Q] (histone-methyl transferase) that regulates **gene expression (90%)**
- *Morphology*
  - **Lymph node:** Predominantly **nodular** or **nodular & diffuse** growth pattern with **centrocytes** (small cleaved cells) along with **centroblasts**[Q]
  - **Bone marrow: paratrabecular** lymphoid aggregates[Q]
- *Immunophenotype*
  - Resemble **germinal center B cells CD19, CD20, CD10, surface Ig, and BCL6**[Q]
  - **CD5 –ve**[Q]
  - **BCL2** is expressed in more than 90% of cases[Q]
- *Histologic transformation occurs to:*
  - Diffuse large B-cell lymphoma **(DLBCL)**
  - Burkitt's lymphoma **(BL)**

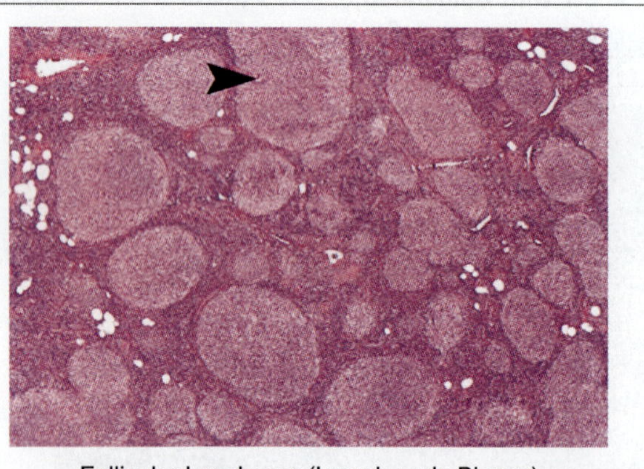

Follicular lymphoma (Lymph node Biopsy)

Burkitt's Lymphoma

Diffuse Large B-Cell Lymphoma (DLBCL)

Most common form of **NHL in India**[Q]

- *Epidemiology:*
  - **M>F,** Median age =**60 yrs**[Q]
- *Pathogenesis:*
  - Pathogenic event is dysregulation of **BCL6**[Q]
  - **10% – 20% have t(14;18)**[Q]
- *Morphology:*
  - Tumor cells have **large cell size** (4-5 times size of small lymphocyte) & **diffuse pattern** of growth. B4 is involved late
- *Immunophenotype:*
  - CD19+ and CD20+, CD10+ and **BCL6+, surface Ig+**[Q]
- *Special Subtypes:*

Immunodeficiency-associated large B-cell lymphoma	Primary effusion lymphoma
• Severe T-cell immunodeficiency • (HIV, allogeneic bone marrow transplantation) • Co-infection with **EBV**[Q]	• Malignant pleural effusion or ascites in advanced **HIV**[Q] infected patients • Co-infection with **KSHV/HHV-8**[Q] • IHC : CD38, CD30+, CD20 –

- *Prognosis:*
  - **Poor prognosis with aggressive course**

Malt Lymphoma (MALToma)

- **MALT lymphomas** express **B-cell antigens (CD19 and CD20)** & **monotypic surface Ig (IgM** without IgD).
- **MALTomas** may be **CD43+** but lack other small B-cell lymphoma markers (CD5, CD10, CD23 & cyclin D1)
- **MALToma** of salivary glands in sjogrens & hashimoto thyroiditis show morphology of marginal zone lymphoma

High Yield Facts

- **Nasal NK/T lymphoma** may present with facial swelling/destruction, so called **lethal midline granuloma** or **polymorphic reticulosis**.
- **Most common ocular lymphoma is B-cell NHL**
- **The most site for extranodal lymphoma is Stomach**

Pathogenesis	**MYC gene**[Q] **(chr 8)** (transcriptional regulator)-**characteristic** but not specific		
Hallmark translocations:	• **t(8;14)** myc; IgH – most characteristic[Q] • t(2;8) myc ; Ig κ • t(8;22) myc ; λ		
Subtypes/Varieties	**African (endemic)**	**Sporadic (Non-endemic)**	**Immunodeficiency associated (HIV)**
Site of involvement	• **Mandible (M.C)**[Q] • **Abdominal viscera**; E.g. kidneys, ovaries, adrenals	• **Ileocecal region(M.C)**[Q] • Peritoneum	• Lymph nodes • Bone marrow
EBV infection	**100%**[Q]	20-30%	25-40%

Contd...

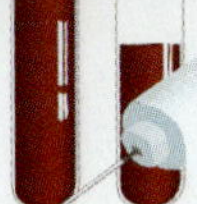

Morphology:	**Tumor: High mitotic index**[Q], **numerous apoptotic cells**, combined with **benign macrophages**. • Macrophages have abundant clear cytoplasm: characteristic **"starry sky" pattern.**[Q] **Bone Marrow:** • **Clumped nuclear chromatin** with distinct nucleoli, and royal blue cytoplasm containing clear cytoplasmic vacuoles.
Immunophenotype	Surface IgM+, CD19+, CD20+, **CD10+, and BCL6+**[Q]
Prognosis	Burkitt lymphoma is **very aggressive** but **responds well** to intensive **chemotherapy**

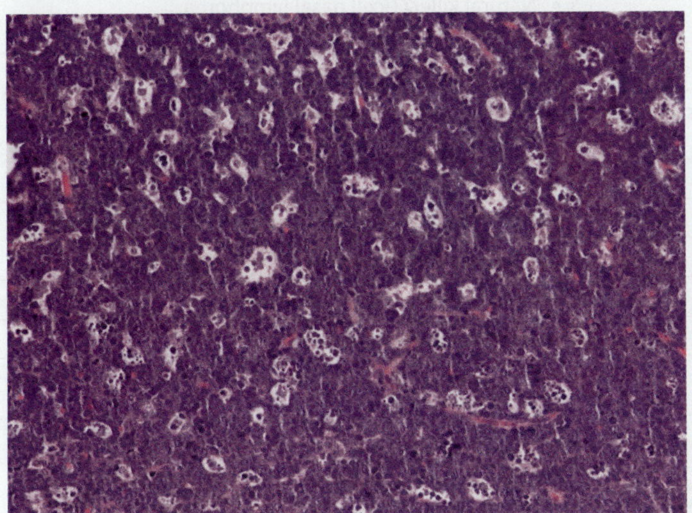

Burkitt lymphoma with starry sky pattern

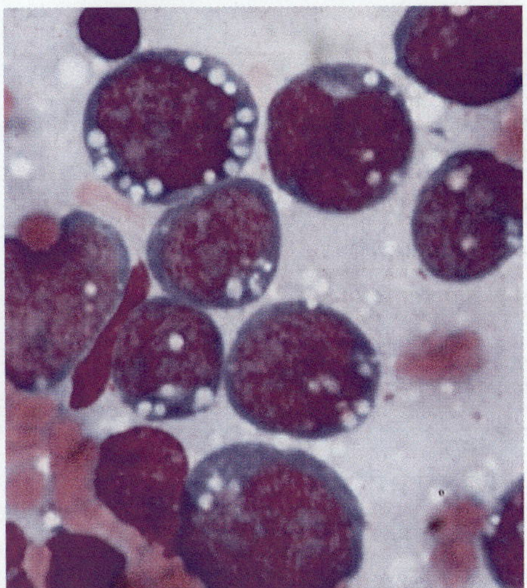

Cells showing cytoplasmic vacuoles

Hairy Cell Leukemia

Chronic B-cell leukemia characterized by **hairy cells, pancytopenia and splenomegaly**[Q]

- **Epidemiology:**
  - Median age: **55 years;** M:F ratio of **4-5 : 1.**

- **Pathogenesis:**
  - 90% of cases with activating point mutations in the **serine/threonine kinase BRAF v600E**[Q] (also +ve in **melanoma,** LCH and papillary lung Ca)[Q]

- **Morphology:**
  - **Peripheral smear:** Pancytopenia with **monocytopenia;** **'Hairy' tumor cells**- Tumor cells with Fine hair like projections, best recognized under the **phase-contrast microscope.**[Q]
  - On Electron microscopy: Hairy cells show **ribosomal-lamellar complexes**[Q]
  - Bone Marrow Aspirate: **Dry Tap (due to fibrosis in marrow)**[Q]
  - Bone Marrow Biopsy: Tumor nuclei surrounded by zone of clear cytoplasm giving rise to **"honeycomb"**[Q]**, "fried egg**[Q]**/chicken wire mesh"**[Q] appearance

- **Immunophenotype:**
  - CD19+ and CD20+, **surface Ig +**
  - **Characteristic marker: CD103**[Q] along with **CD11c, CD25**

- **Cytochemical markers:**
  - Tartrate resistant acid phosphatase **(TRAP), DBA 44** and **Annexin A1.**[Q]

- **Clinical Features:**
  - Infiltration of the bone marrow, liver, and spleen- **massive splenomegaly.**[Q]
  - **Pancytopenia** resulting from marrow involvement and splenic sequestration.
  - **Atypical mycobacterial** infections due to monocytopenia.

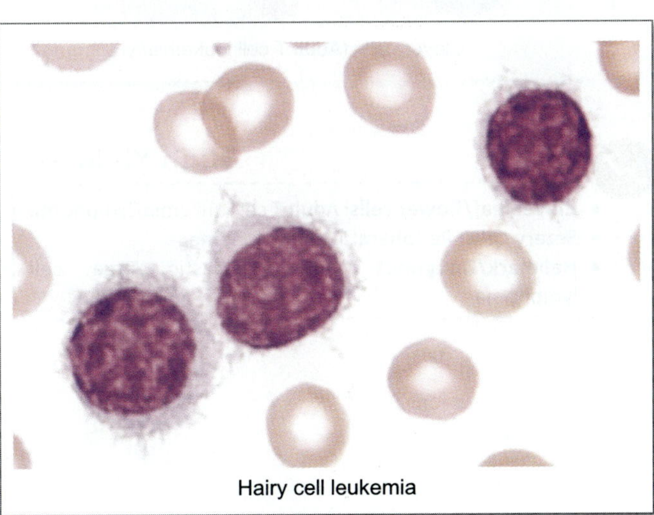

Hairy cell leukemia

Infections and Associations with Lymphoma	
Agent	Type of Lymphoma
Epstein Barr virus (EBV)	• Burkitt lymphoma (Africa) • Post Transplant Lymphoproliferative Disorders • AIDS–related lymphoma (central nervous system, others) • Natural killer/T-cell nasal lymphoma • Hodgkin lymphoma
Human T-lymphotropic virus I (HTLV-1)	Adult T-cell leukemia/lymphoma
Human herpes virus 8 (HHV8) or Kaposi sarcoma–associated herpes virus (KSHV)	• **Primary effusion lymphoma** • **Plasmablastic** lymphoma
Helicobacter pylori	Gastric MALToma
Hepatitis C virus	Splenic marginal zone lymphoma; other B-cell lymphomas
Campylobacter jejuni	Immunoproliferative small intestinal disease
Borrelia burgdorferi	Primary cutaneous B-cell lymphoma
Chlamydia psittaci	Ocular adnexal lymphoma

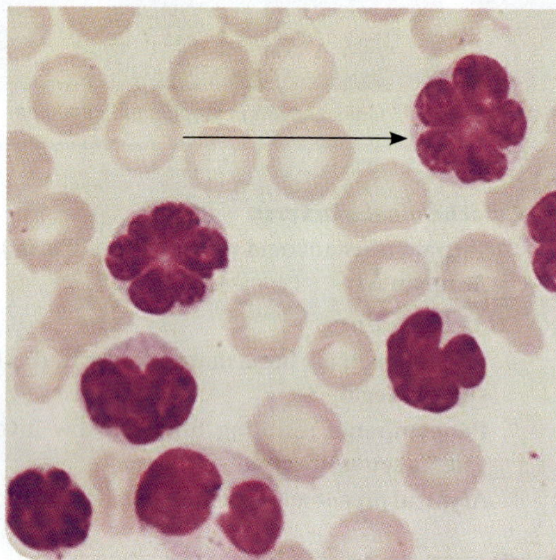

Clover cells (Adult T cell leukemia/lymphoma)

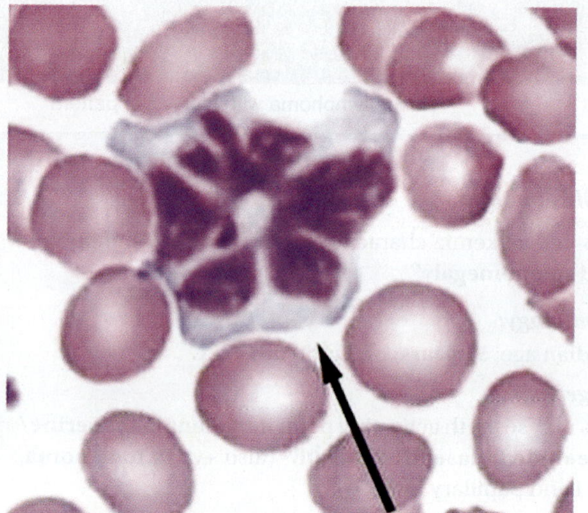

Sezary cell (Peripheral T cell lymphoma)

- **Clover leaf/flower cells:** Adult T cell leukemia/lymphoma
- **Sezary cells:** Peripheral T cell lymphoma
- **Hallmark/Doughnut cells:** Anaplastic large cell lymphoma

Plasma Cell Neoplasms and Related Disorders

Multiple Myeloma

- *Definition:* **Malignant proliferation of plasma cells** derived from a **single clone**.
- Classification and Diagnostic Criteria of Plasma cell neoplasms

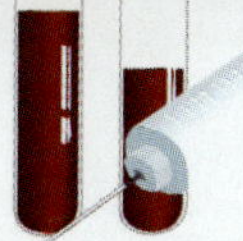

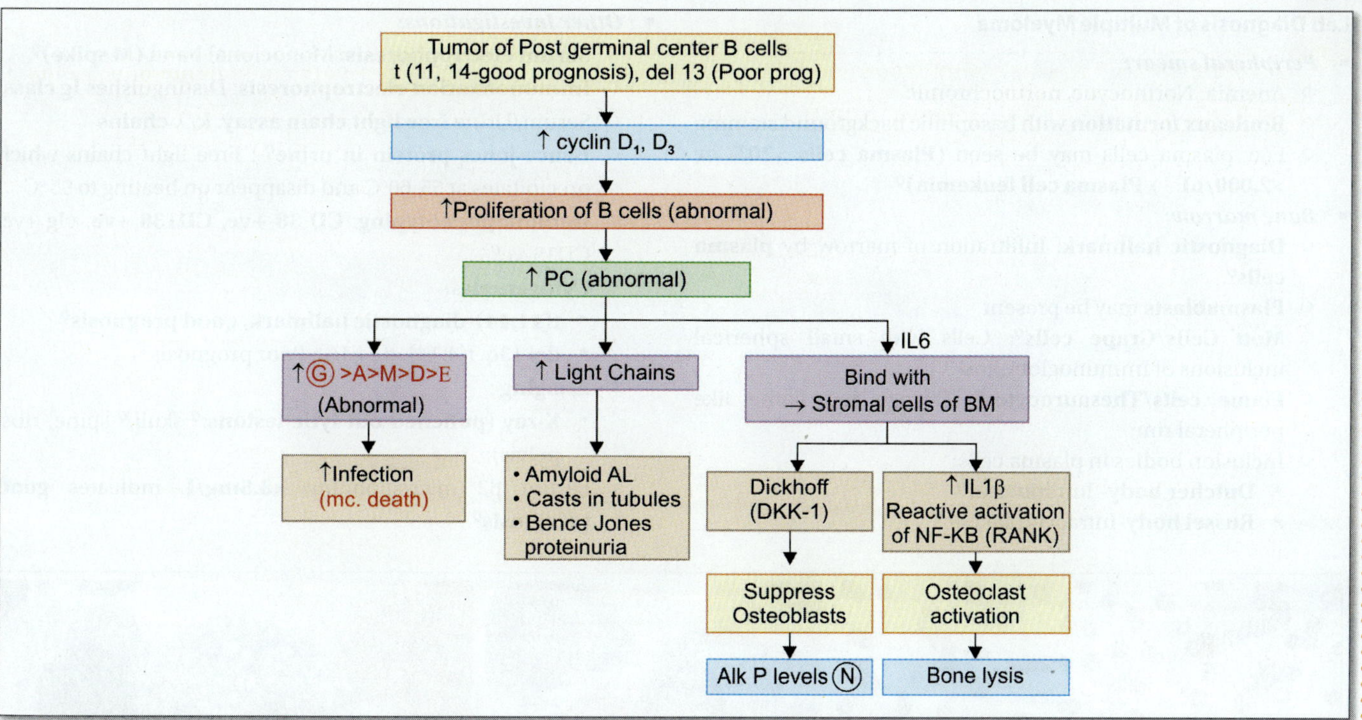

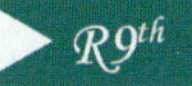

R9th Latest Update

Myeloma Defining Events (any 1 is sufficient for diagnosing multiple myeloma)
- ≥ 60% clonal plasma cells
- Involved/uninvolved free light chain ratio (>100)
- ≥ focal lesions of > 5 mm in size on (MRI)

Classification of Plasma Cell Neoplasma (WHO 2017)

MGUS	Smoldering Myeloma	Multiple Myeloma
IgG/A/M MGUS [All criteria must be met] • Serum monoclonal protein (IgG or IgA or IgM <3 g/dL AND • Clonal BM plasma cells <10% AND • No myeloma defining events (see below)	• Serum monoclonal protein (IgG or IgA) ≥3 g/dL or • Urinary monoclonal protein ≥500 mg/24 h and/or • Clonal BM plasma cells 10% – 60%	• Clonal BM plasma cells of ≥10% or • Biopsy-proven bony or extramedullary plasmacytoma
	AND	**AND**
	• No myeloma defining events or amyloidosis (no CRAB and no SLIM) as details below	• 1 or more myeloma defining events as details below ≥1 CRAB feature(s) OR ≥1SLiM feature(s)

Myeloma defining events are evidence of end organ damage that can be attributed to the underlying plasma cell proliferative disorder, especially
C: Calcium elevation (>11 mg/dL or >1 mg/dL higher than ULN)
R: Renal insufficiency (creatinine clearance < 40 mL/min or serum creatinine >2 mg/dL)
A: Anemia (Hb <10 g/dL or 2 g/dL < normal)
B: Bone disease (≥1 lytic lesions on skeletal radiography, CT, or PET-CT).
OR, in the absence of **CRAB**, any one or more of the following biomarkers or malignancy, referred to here as the
SLiM criteria: SLiM: **S** = ≥Sixty-percent (≥60%) clonal BM plasma cells; **Li**=Serum free Light chain ratio involved:
uninvolved ≥100; **M** = >1 focal lesions (≥5 mm each) detected by MRI studies

Lab Diagnosis of Multiple Myeloma

- *Peripheral smear:*
  - Anemia: Normocytic, normochromic
  - **Rouleaux formation** with basophilic background staining
  - Few plasma cells may be seen **(Plasma cells >20% or >2,000/uL → Plasma cell leukemia)[Q]**
- *Bone marrow:*
  - **Diagnostic hallmark**: Infiltration of marrow by **plasma cells[Q]**
  - **Plasmablasts** may be present
  - **Mott Cells/Grape cells[Q]:** Cells with small spherical inclusions of Immunoglobulins
  - **Flame cells/Thesaurocytes[Q]:** Orange red flame like peripheral rim
  - Inclusion bodies in plasma cells:
    - **Dutcher body**- Intranuclear[Q]
    - **Russel body**-Intracytoplasmic[Q]

- *Other Investigations:*
  - **Serum electrophoresis:** Monoclonal band **(M spike)[Q]**
  - **Immunofixation electrophoresis**: Distinguishes **Ig class**
  - Serum/Urine **free light chain assay: k/λ chains**
  - **Bence jones protein in urine[Q]** : Free light chains which precipitates at 55-60°C and disappear on heating to 95 °C
  - **Immunophenotyping: CD 38 +ve, CD138 +ve**, cIg +ve, CD19-ve[Q]
  - **Cytogenetics:**
    - **t(11;14)-diagnostic hallmark, good prognosis[Q]**
    - del 13q, t(4;14), t(14;16): Poor prognosis
  - **Imaging** :
    - **X-ray (punched out lytic lesions:[Q]** skull,[Q] spine, ribs, pelvis);
  - Serum β2 microglobulin: **<3.5mg/L** indicates **good prognosis[Q]**

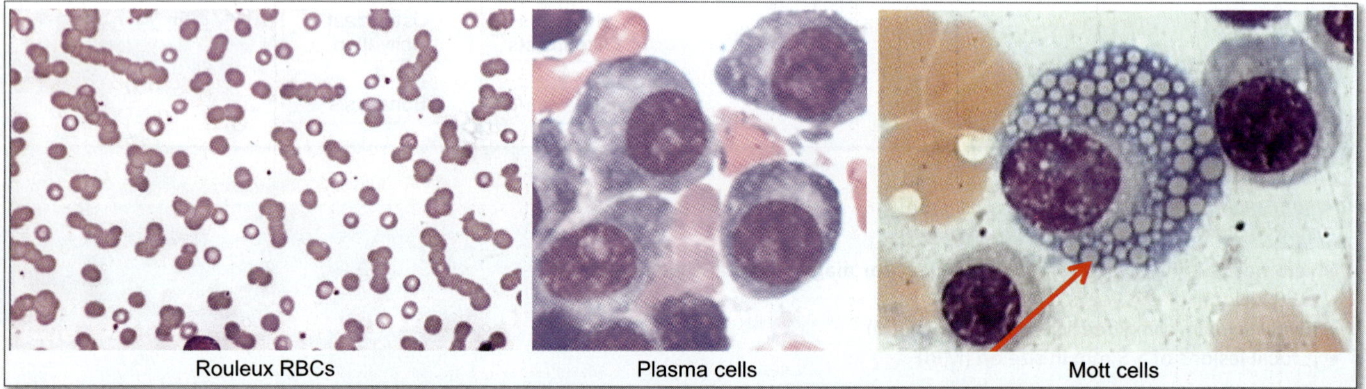

Rouleux RBCs   Plasma cells   Mott cells

High Yield Facts

- M spike : **IgG(most common)[Q]** >A>M>D>E
- Free light chains are called Bence-Jones proteins- **not detected** by **urine protein dipsticks[Q]**
- **IL-6[Q]** helps in **survival and proliferation** of myeloma cell proliferation.
- Other growth factors for myeloma cells-**IL1 β[Q] and VEGF[Q]**
- **Most common** cytogenetic abnormality in myeloma is 13q->t (11,14)
- **Osteolytic lesions[Q]** in bone are due to involvement of **RANK-L[Q]** (receptor activator of nuclear factor kappa B ligand) → **activates osteoclasts**
- **POEMS[Q]:** Polyneuropathy, Organomegaly, Endocrinopathy, Multiple Myeloma & Skin Changes
- **Alkaline Phosphatase levels in multiple myeloma is normal** and not raised, as there is no bone formation and only bone lysis.

- Mc mutation: **MYD88**
- *Clinical features:*
  - Anemia, lymphadenopathy, Hepatosplenomegaly & hyperviscosity
- *Immunophenotyping:*
  - CD 138 +, cy IgM+, CD19 +

HODGKIN LYMPHOMA (HL)

- *Characteristics:*
  - Arises in lymph nodes (**M.C cervical region**)[Q] & spreads to anatomically **contiguous lymphoid tissues[Q]**
- *Clinical features:*
  - **Pel Ebstein fever (Intermittent fever every alternate week)[Q]**
  - **Lymphadenopathy;** Affected lymph nodes nodes become painful with alcohol ingestion[Q]
- *Pathogenesis:* Mc mutation: Rel transcription activators
  - Activation of the **transcription factor NF-κB** is a common event in **classical HL.**
  - Cytokines (e.g., **IL-5, IL-10, M-CSF**), chemokines (e.g, **eotaxin**), & other factors (e.g., **immunomodulatory factor galectin-1**) that are secreted by Reed-Sternberg cells

Waldenstrom Macroglobulinemia

- *Definition:*
  - Indolent **lymphoproliferative disorder** characterized by Lymphoplasmacytic cell proliferation in marrow with secretion of **IgM**

- *Morphology:*
  ○ Reed-Sternberg cells **(R.S cells)** surrounded by **T lympho-cytes** in a rosette-like manner[Q]
  ○ **Diagnostic Hallmark: Reed-Sternberg cells**: **(45 μm)** binucleate cell or single nucleus with multiple nuclear lobes.[Q]

- *Poor prognostic markers:*
  ○ Albumin <4.0 g/dL, Hemoglobin <10.5 g/dL, Male sex, 45 years of age or more, Stage IV disease, Leukocytosis at or above 15,000/mm³, Lymphocytopenia

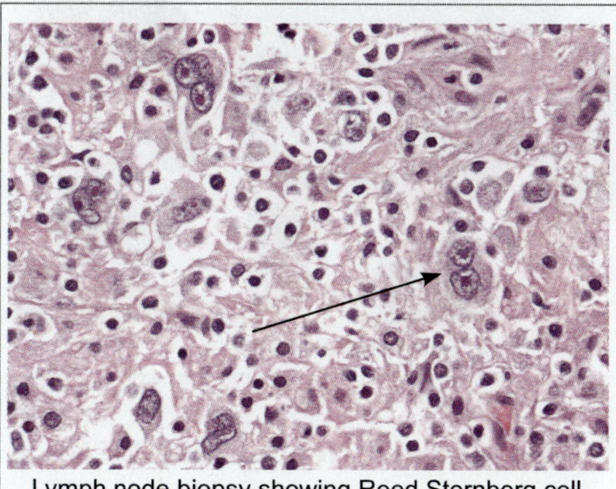

Lymph node biopsy showing Reed Sternberg cell

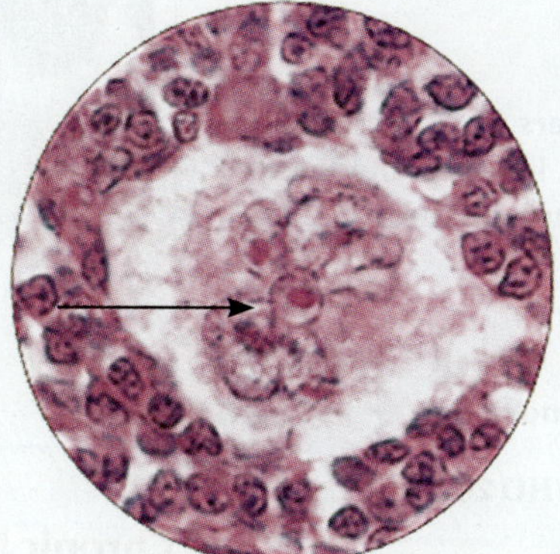

Lacunar cell

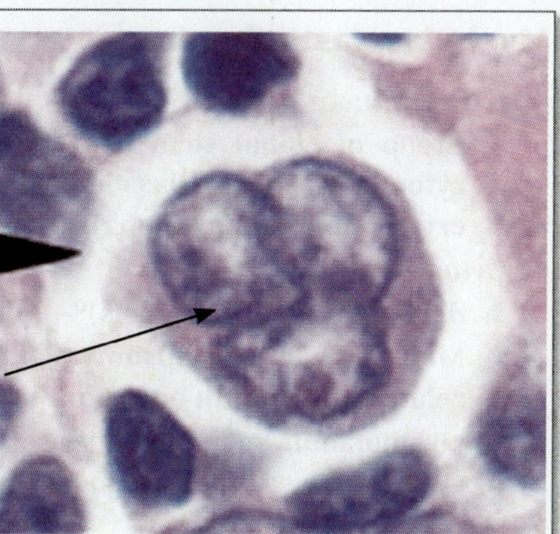

Popcorn cells

Description of different Subtypes of Hodgkin Lymphoma

Subtype	Morphology	Immunophenotype	Association with EBV	Typical Clinical Features
Nodular sclerosis	Lacunar cells **(clear space around nucleus)**[Q] **Fibrous strands**[Q] & **plasma cells**[Q]	CD15+, CD30+;	usually **EBV-**	**MC in World**[Q]; **M=F;** usually stage I or II; frequent **mediastinal** involvement; **Good prognosis**[Q]
Mixed cellularity	Mononuclear cells	CD15+, CD30+;	**70% EBV+**	**MC in India**[Q], stage III or IV; M > F; biphasic incidence; **Good prognosis**[Q]
Lymphocyte rich	Mononuclear cells	CD15+, CD30+;	**40% EBV+**	Uncommon; M > F, **Good prognosis**[Q]
Lymphocyte depletion	Reticular variant:	CD15+, CD30+;	**90% EBV+ (Maximum)**[Q]	Uncommon; M>F; **HIV infected**[Q] **Poorest Prognosis**[Q]
Lymphocyte predominance	Lymphocytic & Histiocytic (popcorn cell)[Q]	**CD20+,** CD15-, C30-;	EBV-	Uncommon; young males with cervical or axillary L. nodes, **Best Prognosis**[Q]

Clinical Staging of Hodgkin's and Non-Hodgkin's Lymphomas (Ann Arbor Classification)

Stage	Distribution of Disease
I	Involvement of a **single lymph node region** (I) or a single extra-lymphatic organ or site (IE).
II	Involvement of **two or more lymph node** regions on the **same side of diaphragm** alone (II) or localized involvement of an extra-lymphatic organ or site (IIE).
III	Involvement of lymph node regions on **both sides of the diaphragm** without (III) or with (IIIE) localized involvement of an extra-lymphatic organ or site.
IV	Diffuse involvement of **one or more extra-lymphatic organs** or sites with or without lymphatic involvement.

All stages are further divided on the basis of: **Absence (A)** or **Presence of (B)** symptoms:[Q], Unexplained fever, Drenching night sweats, and/or, Unexplained weight loss > 10%

Treatment

ABVD (Adriamycin, Bleomycine, Vineblastine & Dacarbazine) regimen is standard line of treatment[Q]

MYELOID NEOPLASMS

Three broad categories of myeloid neoplasia exist:

- Acute myeloid leukemias (AML): discussed previously
- Myelodysplastic syndromes (MDS)
- Chronic Myeloproliferative Neoplasms (CMPN)

Myelodysplastic Syndromes

- ***Definition:***
  - Group of **clonal stem cell disorders** characterized by **cytopenias, dysplasias** in either lineage, **ineffective erythropoiesis** and a **high risk of transformation to AML.**[Q]
- ***Cytogenetics***
  - **del 5q (MC best prognosis)**[Q]—**Adults**
  - Monosomy 5[Q], **Monosomy 7, del 7q (MC treatment related MDS;[Q] both have poor prognosis)**[Q]
  - p53 mutation–aggressive disease ⎤ **WHO 2017**
  - –y, del 11q–very good prognosis ⎦

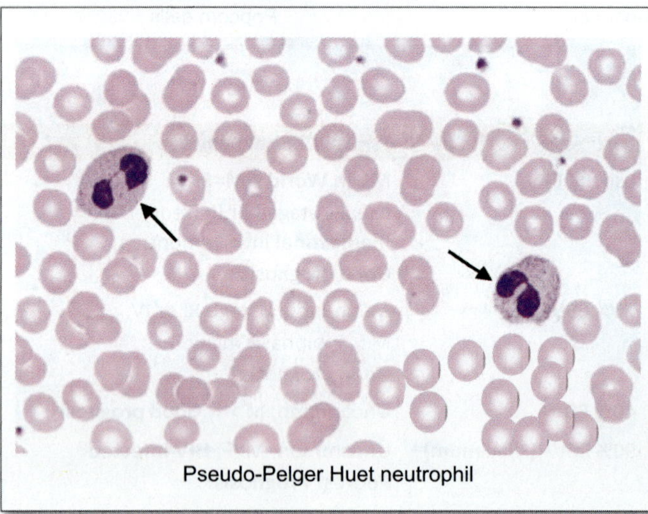

Pseudo-Pelger Huet neutrophil

- ***Bone marrow Morphology:***
  - Cytopenias with features of dysplasia can be seen in either of the series like:

Erythroid series	Myeloid series	Megakaryocytic series
• **Ring sideroblasts**[Q] • Megaloblastic maturation • Nuclear budding • Nuclear bridging	• Hypo or defective granulation • Toxic granulations • **Döhle bodies** • **Pseudo-Pelger-Hüet**[Q] **neutrophils**	• Micromega-karyocytes • Single nuclear lobes • Multiple separate nuclei **(Pawn ball Megakaryocytes)**[Q]

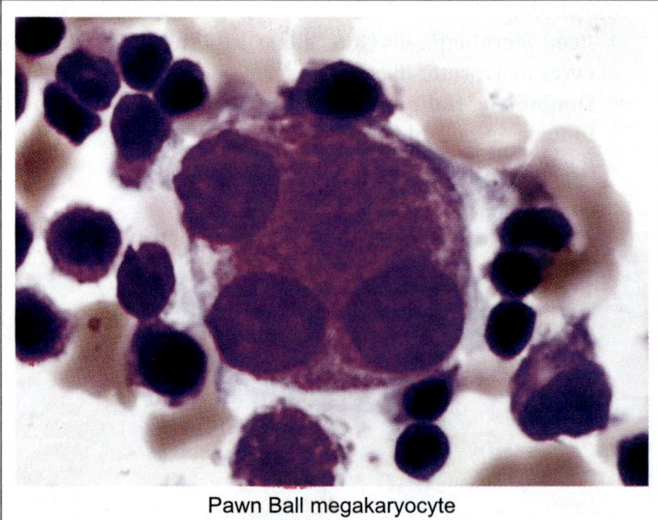

Pawn Ball megakaryocyte

Chronic Myeloproliferative Neoplasms (CMPN)

- ***Definition:***
  - Presence of **mutated tyrosine kinases**[Q] or **other acquired aberrations** in signaling pathways that lead to growth factor independence leading to:
    - Increased proliferation of bone marrow
    - Extra-medullary hematopoiesis
    - **Marrow fibrosis** and peripheral blood cytopenias
    - **Transformation to acute leukemia**

We will now discuss the types of CMPN:

Chronic Myelogenous Leukemia (CML)

- ***Characterized by:***
  - **BCR-ABL gene**[Q] (210 kDa in size)
  - **ABL gene on chr 9q translocates to BCR gene on chr 22q** which **activates tyrosine kinase**[Q]
- ***Cell of origin:***
  - **Pluripotent hematopoietic stem cell**[Q]
- ***Etiology:***
  - Radiation exposure, No genetic predisposition
- ***Epidemiology:***
  - M> F; **Median age-5ᵗʰ -6ᵗʰ decade**
- ***Clinical features:***
  - Presents with **massive splenomegaly**, hepatomegaly and lymphadenopathy.[Q]
- ***Peripheral smear:***
  - Increased TLC (30,000/uL – 10,00,000/uL), **myeloid bulge**[Q] (myelocytes and metamyelocytes) and **basophilia.**[Q]
- ***LAP score:***
  - **Low**[Q]

- ***Bone marrow Morphology:***
  - ○ Hypercellular marrow (Not required for diagnosis but **for staging**)[Q]
  - ○ Increased small, **dysplastic forms of megakaryocytes**.
    - • Scattered macrophages with abundant wrinkled, green-blue cytoplasm so-called **sea-blue histiocytes/ Pseudo-Gaucher cells**[Q]
- **Diagnosis of choice**
  - • Cytogenetics -FISH/PCR

The Philadelphia Chromosome

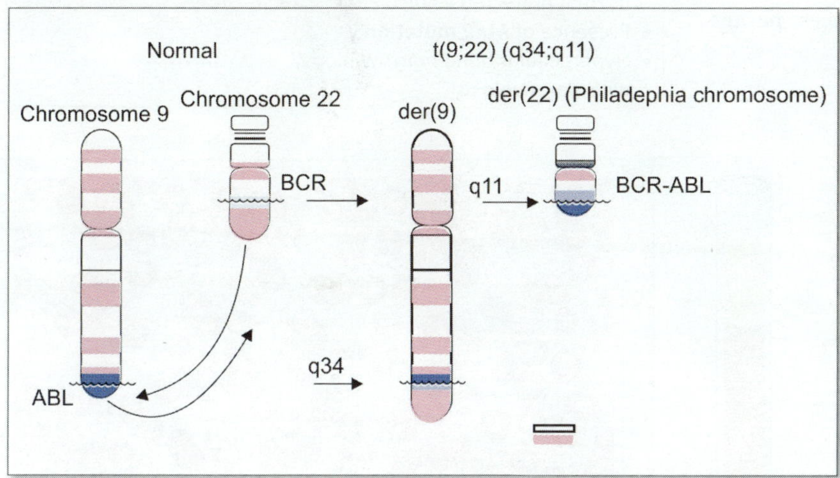

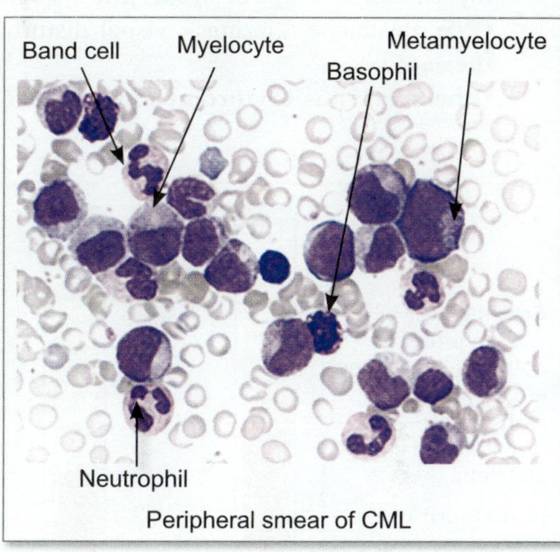

WHO Diagnostic Criteria for Different Phases of CML (WHO 2017)

Accelerated Phase	Blast phase/ blast crisis
• **Blasts 10–19%** in blood or marrow[Q] • Peripheral blood **basophilia ≥ 20%**[Q] • Newer Cytogenetic clonal evolution • Persistent thrombocytopenia ($<100 \times 10^9$/L) • Persistent thrombocytosis ($>1{,}000 \times 10^9$/L) unresponsive to therapy • Increasing splenomegaly & WBC count unresponsive to therapy • Provisional response to TKI-Tyrosine kinase inhibitors • **Provisional" response-to-TKI (tyrosine kinase inhibitors) criteria is added- Occurrence of 2 or more mutations or resistance to therapy are added**	• **>20%** blasts[Q] (*Wintrobe's latest 13th ed: >30%) • Clusters of blasts on BM biopsy • Extramedullary myeloid tumors (granulocytic sarcomas, **chloromas**)[Q] • Lymphoblasts in any number should be reported as they signify poor prognosis

High Yield Facts

Conditions Associated with Abnormal Leukocyte Alkaline Phosphatase (LAP) Scores	
High LAP score (>130)	**Low LAP Score (<15)**
• **Infections (Leukemoid reaction)**[Q] • **Growth factor therapy** • **Myeloproliferative disorders other than CML (ET, PCV, Myelofibrosis)**[Q] • **AML**[Q] • **Hodgkin's disease**[Q] • **Inflammatory disorders** • **Pregnancy,**[Q] **oral contraceptives** • **Stress** • **Drugs (lithium, corticosteroids, estrogen)**	• **CML**[Q] • **Paroxysmal nocturnal hemoglobinuria**[Q] • **Hereditary Hypophosphatemic Rickets** • **Myelodysplastic syndromes** • **Rare infections or toxic exposures**

Polycythemia Vera

- ***Epidemiology:***
  - Mean age = 60yrs; M:F=1-2:1
- ***Genetic abnormality:***
  - Most frequent genetic abnormality in PCV is **JAK2 V617F**[Q]
- ***Clinical Features:***
  - **CVS: Hypertension**[Q], venous or arterial **thrombosis**, myocardial ischemia or stroke, pruritus after bath
  - **CNS:** Headache, dizziness. visual disturbances, **paraesthesias**
  - **Others:** Pruritus, **erythromelalgia,**[Q] **gout**[Q]

- **Diagnosis:** *Requires all 3 major criteria or first 2 major + minor criteria*

Major Criteria	Minor Criteria
• **Hemoglobin >16.5 g/dl**[Q] **in men, >16 g/dL in women** or HCT >49% in men or >48% is woman. Increased red cell mass >25% above mean normal predicted value. • Presence of ***JAK2* mutation**[Q] • Hypercellular bone marrow biopsy with **panmyelosis**[Q]	• **Low serum erythropoietin level**[Q]

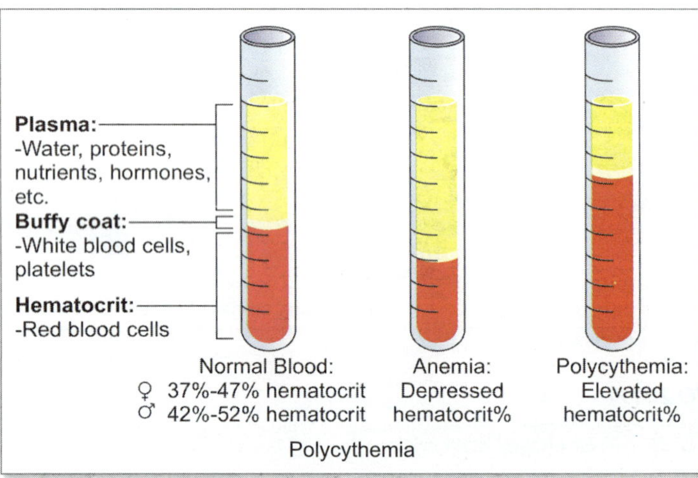

Polycythemia

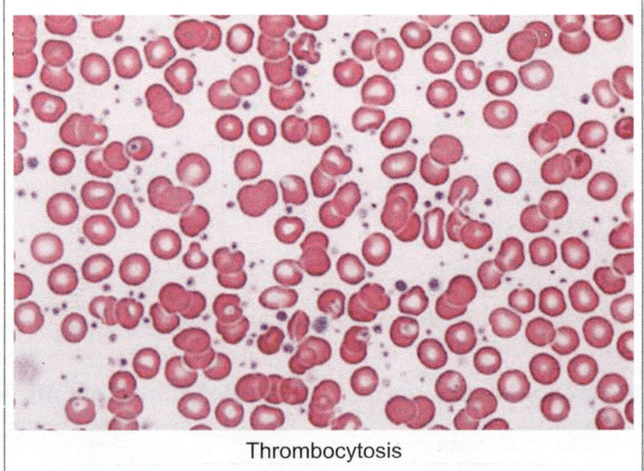

Thrombocytosis

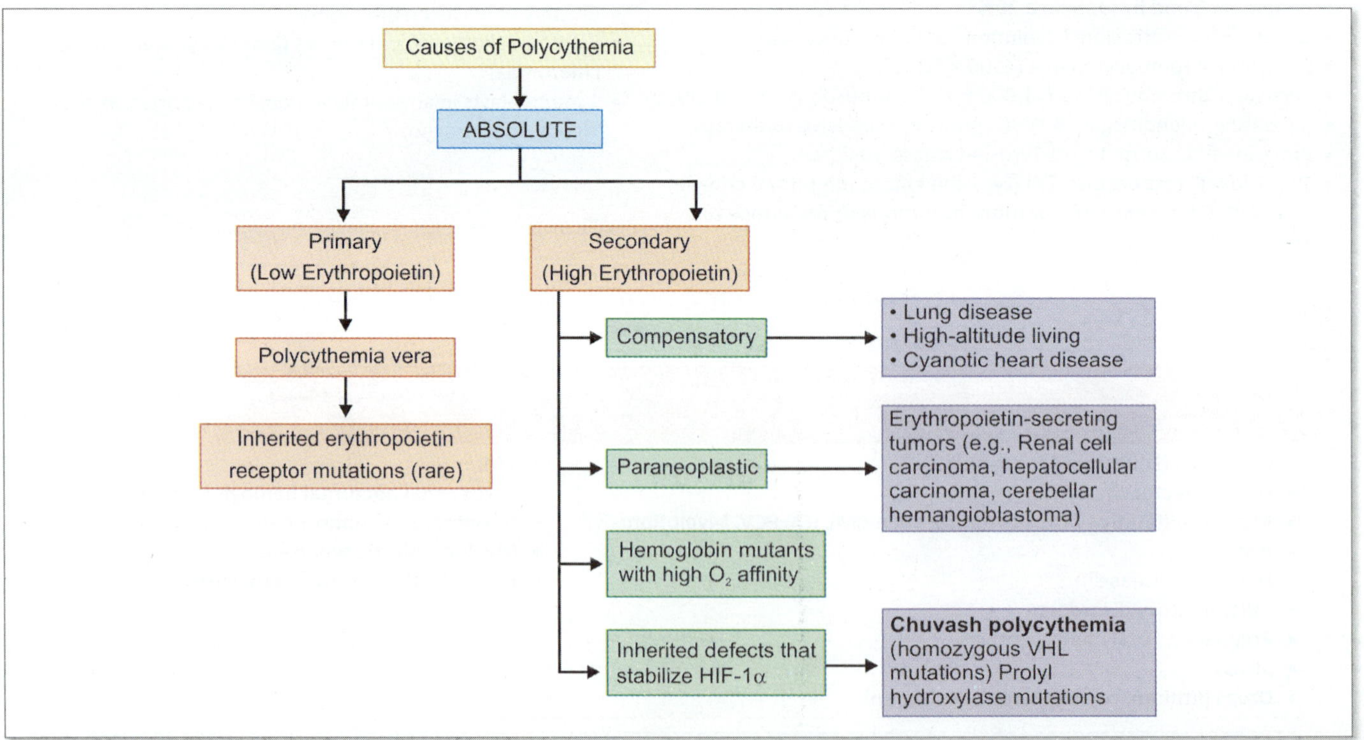

Essential Thrombocythemia/Primary Thrombocytosis

- *Epidemiology*
  - Mean age = **50-60 yrs; M=F**
- *Clinical Feature*
  - **Microvascular occlusion** may lead to **transient ischemic attacks**[Q], digital ischemia with **paraesthesia** & gangrene. **Bleeding**[Q] may also be seen, due to platelet function defects
- *Peripheral smear*
  - **Thrombocytosis** with **abnormalities in size, shape & granularity** of platelets
- *Diagnosis:*
  - All 4 or first 3 major + 1 minor criteria

Major criteria	Minor criteria
• Sustained platelet count **≥4.5 Lakhs/uL**[Q] • Bone marrow biopsy showing proliferation of megakaryocytes, • **Exclusion** of WHO criteria for PV, PMF, CML, MDS • *JAK2* mutation[Q], CALR or MPL mutations	• Absence of evidence of reactive thrombocytosis

Chronic Idiopathic Myelofibrosis/Agnogenic Myeloid Metaplasia (AMM)

- *Epidemiology:*
  - Mean age: 6th–7th decade; M=F
- *Hallmark:*
  - Hallmark of primary myelofibrosis is: **obliterative marrow fibrosis**[Q]
- *Peripheral smear:*
  - Marrow distortion due to fibrosis leads to the premature release of nucleated erythroid and early granulocyte progenitors **(leukoerythroblastosis)**[Q]
  - Erythroids damaged in fibrotic marrow results in :Tear drop-shaped RBCs **(dacrocytes)**[Q]
- *Diagnosis requires: All 3 Major + at least 1 minor criteria*

Major Criteria	Minor Criteria
• Atypical megakaryocytic hyperplasia, with **collagen fibrosis**[Q] • Exclusion of WHO criteria for PV, CML, MDS, or other MPDs • *JAK2*V617F mutation[Q], CALR, MPL	• Leukoerythroblastosis[Q] • ↑ LDH • Anemia • Palpable splenomegaly • Leucocytosis >11,000

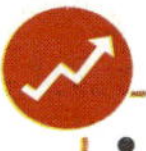

High Yield Facts

- **Ph chr** discovered by Nowell & Hungerford in 1960
- **Ring sideroblasts are** erythroblasts with **iron-laden mitochondria**[Q] visible as **perinuclear granules** in **Iron/ Prussian blue/Perl's**[Q] staining
- **Pseudo-Pelger-Hüet neutrophils**[Q]: bilobed hypogranular dysplastic neutrophils[Q]

MYELODYSPLASTIC/ MYELOPROLIFERATIVE (MDS/MPN) NEOPLASMS

- **Definition:**
  - Group of disorders with features of **both myeloproliferative and myelodysplastic syndromes**[Q]
- *Includes:*
  - Chronic myelomonocytic leukemia (CMML)
  - Atypical CML (a-CML)
  - Juvenile myelomonocytic leukemia (JMML)

Other

Newer Myeloproliferative Neoplasms (MPNs)	
MPN	**Mutation seen**
• Systemic mastocytosis	• Constitutive **c-KIT** kinase activation
• Chronic eosinophilic leukemia	• Constitutive **PDGFRα/β** kinase activation
• Stem cell leukemia	• Constitutive **FGFR1** kinase activation

JUVENILE MYELOMONOCYTIC LEUKEMIA (JMML)

- *Definition*
  - It is a **childhood mixed MDS/MPD** that includes childhood leukemias previously classified as CMML, juvenile CML, and infantile monosomy 7 syndrome.
- *Diagnostic Criteria:*

Genetic Criteria (Any 1 is sufficient)	Required Criteria (All 4 needed)	Other criteria
• NFI mutation • CBL mutation (germ line) • Somatic mutation of KRAS/NRAS/ PTPN11	• Peripheral blood monocytes > 1.0×10^9/L • Blasts + promonocytes <20% in blood and marrow • Absence of Philadelphia chromosome or BCR/ABL fusion gene • Splenomegaly	• Increased hemoglobin F for age • Immature granulocytes in peripheral blood • Clonal chromosomal abnormality (i.e., includes monosomy 7) • GM-CSF hypersensitivity of myeloid progenitors in vitro • Hypophosphorylation od STAT 5 or Monosomy 7

High Yield Facts

- **JMML is the most common MDS/MPD of children**
- Increased hemoglobin F is seen in JMML
- JMML is associated with NF1

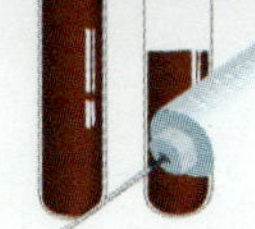

Theory

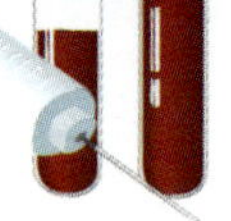

LANGERHANS CELL HISTIOCYTOSIS (LCH) HISTIOCYTOSIS X[Q]

- ***Current classification:***
  - **Unifocal** (i.e., single-system, single-site disease)
  - **Multifocal** (i.e., single-system, multiple-site disease)
  - **Disseminated** histiocytosis (i.e., multisystem disease)
- ***Diagnosis: Light microscopy***
  - Basic histologic lesion: **granulomas,** containing histiocytes or Langerhans cells, mature eosinophils, lymphocytes, giant cells, neutrophils & plasma cells
  - The **Langerhans cell**[Q] (large mononuclear cells with few cytoplasmic vacuoles) is the '**sine qua non' (essential)** of the diagnostic lesion
- ***Electron microscopy***
  - **Birbeck granules (tennis racket appearance)**[Q]
- ***Immunohistochemistry***
  - **CD1a**[Q]**, S-100**[Q] **or Langerin (CD 207)**[Q] demonstration on the surface of LCH cells
- ***Prognosis***
  - LCH may be a **self-limiting** disease, which may resolve spontaneously[Q]
  - For most patients with LCH, the prognosis is **excellent**
  - Patients with **multisystem** disease may experience fatal **organ failure**

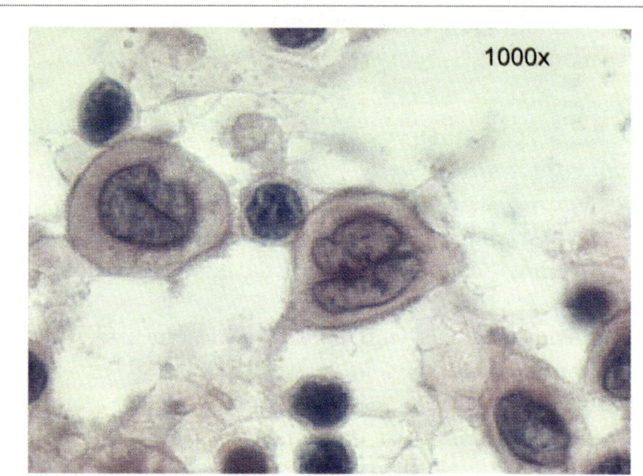

Langerhans cells with convoluted nuclei with longitudinal grooves ("coffee-bean" shaped)

High Yield Facts

- **Bone** is the **most commonly involved** organ[Q]
- **Skull** is the most commonly involved **site in both children and adults**[Q]
- Unifocal eosinophilic granuloma of bone is the most common form of the disease[Q]
- **"Punched out"** appearance of skeletal lesions is typically seen in LCH[Q]
- **Pulmonary LCH** occurs more commonly in **males** & is **associated with smoking**
- **Pneumothorax** is seen in **25--40%** cases of **pulmonary LCH**
- **Eosinophilic granuloma:**[Q] bone lesions, with no visceral involvement
- **Letterer-Siwe disease:**[Q] When granulomas involve multiple viscera
- **Hand-Schüller-Christian disease**[Q]: Triad of multiple bone lesions, exophthalmos and diabetes insipidus (DI)

Thymoma

- ***Definition:***
  - Tumors of **thymic epithelial cells**
- ***Epidemiology:***
  - Usually seen in adults **older than 40 years** of age; rare in children; Males = females
- ***Location:***
  - **Anterior superior mediastinum**, neck, thyroid
- ***Gross Morphology:***
  - **Lobulated**, firm, gray-white masses of **up to 15 to 20 cm in size.**
  - Sometimes have areas of cystic **necrosis and calcification**.
  - Most are **encapsulated**, but 25% of the tumors penetrate the capsule & **infiltrate perithymic structures**
- ***Histology:***
  - **Sheets of epithelial cells** giving **arborizing pattern** of reactivity along with interspersed **lymphoid cells.**
  - **IHC** –CK + CD45

High Yield Facts

Post Transplant Lymphoproliferative Disorder (PTLD)

- Post-transplant lymphoma occurs due to **proliferation of B cells**
- 90% of **early** (<1 year post-transplant) PTLDs are **EBV positive**, when EBV-CTL immunity is lowest
- **Late** (>2 years post-transplant) PTLDs are **frequently EBV negative**, can be of T-cell origin, and may have a poorer prognosis.
- Majority of **PTLDs are CD20+**, but not all PTLDs are of B-cell phenotype and not all are EBV positive.
- **T-cell PTLD tends** to occur **late**, often more than 10 years after transplantation.

2018 Revision to the World Health Organization Classification of Leukemia & Lymphoma

Category	Latest modification	Category	Latest modification
New Acute Myeloid Leukemia Subtypes 2016	AML with RUNX1mutation AML with BCR-ABL 1 mutation AML with biallelic CEBPA mutations Familial AML/MDSmultiple types- EBPA,RUNX,GATA	*ALL*	Early precursor T-ALL –CD7,CD2, CD3 , Myeloid markers+
Myeloid neoplasms *CML*	*Refer* to CML in text	*Essential thrombocythemia and Primary myelofibrosis*	CALR and MPL mutation is needed in addition to JAK-2 mutation
CNL (chronic neutrophilic leukemia)	CSF3R mutations added	*Polycythemia Vera*	Hb cut off reduced to 16.5 gm% in males and 16 gm% in females or Hematocrit >49% (m) and 48% (f)
MDS	Del9q is an MDS related entity only in the absence of NPM1 mutations SF3B1 mutation is strongly associated with ringed sideroblast	*Systemic mastocytosis*	Removed from Chronic myeloproliferative neoplasms

WHO 2018 Update

The Cancer Genome Atlas (TCGA) project showing 9 classes of AML

Class 1: Transcription factor fusions
e.g. t(8;21), inv(16), and t(15;17)

Class 2: Nucleophosmin 1
NPM1 mutations

Class 3: Tumor suppressor genes
e.g. *TP53* and *PHF6* mutations

Class 4: DNA methylation-related genes
DNA hydroxymethylation e.g. *TET2* , *IDH1* and *IDH2*
DNA methyltransferases

Class 5: Activated signalling genes
e.g. *FLT3*, *KIT RAS* mutation..

Class 6: Chromatin-modifying, genes
e.g. *ASXL1* and *EZH2* mutations., fusions, KMT2A-PTD

Class 7: Myeloid transcription factor genes
e.g. *CEBPA*, *RUNX1* mutations

Class 8: Cohesin complex genes
e.g. STAG2, RAD21, SMC1, SMC2 mutations

Class 9: Spliceosome-complex genes
e.g. *SRSF2*, *U2AF1*, *ZRSR2* mutations

Image-Based Questions

1. A 4-year-old male presents with fever, bleeding gums and fatigue for 4 days. CBC shows Hb of 8 gm%, TLC 86,000/UL, Platelet count of 25,000/ul. DLC shows Neutrophils 20%, Lymphocyte 40%, Eosinophils 10%, Basophils 0%, Monocytes 5%, Abnormal cells 25%. Bone marrow aspiration shows cells as shown in figure 60%. What is your diagnosis?

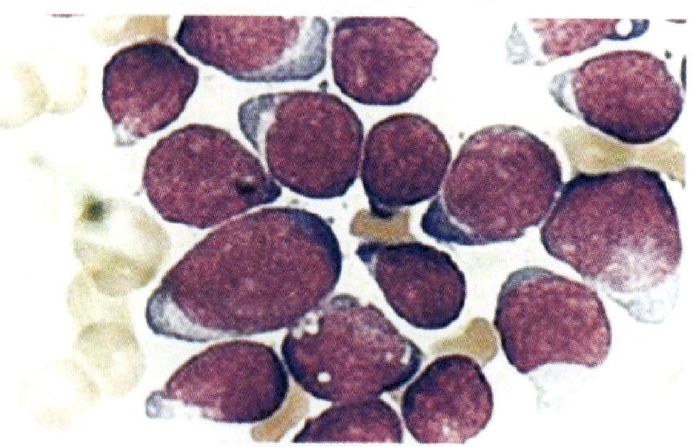

a. Chronic myeloid leukemia
b. Chronic lymphoid leukemia
c. Acute leukemia
d. Myelofibrosis

2. A 10-year-old boy presents to AIIMS OPD with mass in the abdomen. On imaging the paraaortic LN is enlarged. Biopsy from the lymph node suggests a pattern as shown in the figure. What is the underlying abnormality?

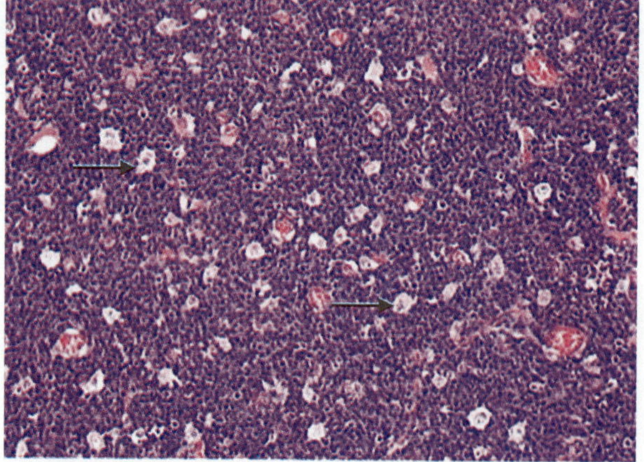

a. p53 gene mutation
b. RB gene mutation
c. Translocation involving BCR-ABL genes
d. Translocation involving MYC gene

3. Peripheral smear showing the given figure is likely to be seen in all except:

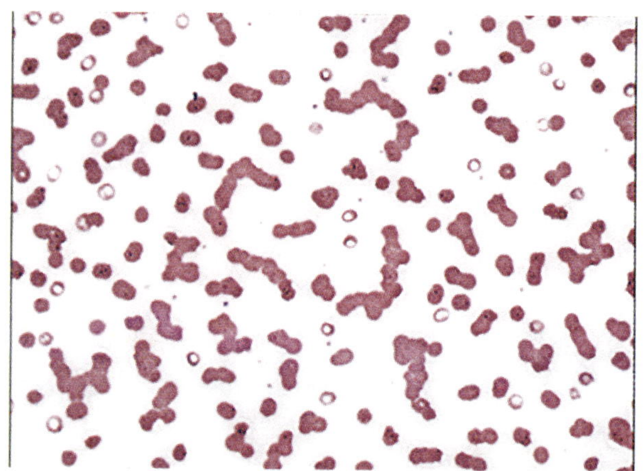

a. Hypergammaglobinemia
b. Severe anemia
c. Multiple myeloma
d. Hemolytic anemia

4. For which procedure it is used?

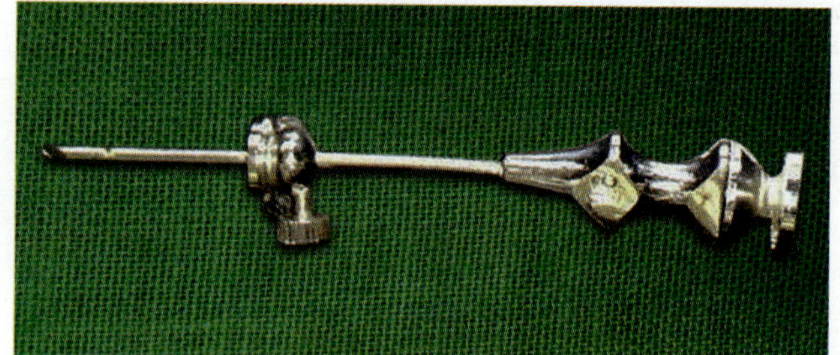

a. Bone marrow examination
b. Liver biopsy
c. Pleural biopsy
d. Lumbar puncture

5. 40/F presented to Medicine OPD with fever and mucosal bleeding of 3 days. CBC shows Hb-9.8 gm%, TLC = 15,700/cumm, Platelet count = 15,000/cumm. Peripheral smear showed findings as shown in figure. His cytogenetics revealed t(8;21). What is your diagnosis?

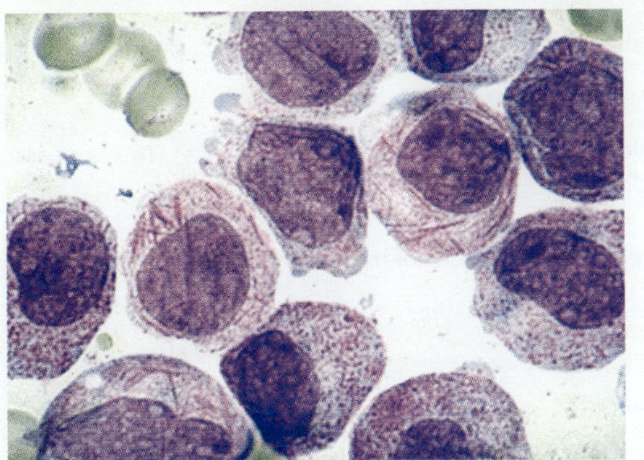

a. AML
b. CML
c. MDS
d. ALL

6. The most important investigation in the given case to diagnose if the condition is a neoplasm?

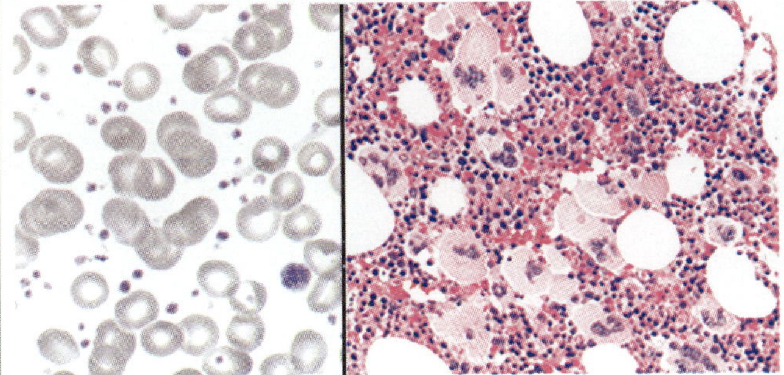

a. JAK-2
b. EPO level
c. PaO_2
d. Bone marrow aspiration and biopsy

7. 55/M presented with fatigue and dragging sensation in the abdomen to AIIMS OPD. He send the patients sample to a pathologist initially performed hemogram which revealed Hb = 8 gm%, TLC = 1500/cumm, platelet count = 79,000/cumm. He also reported some bizzare looking cells which are shown below. Which stain will the pathologist like to do to diagnose the condition?

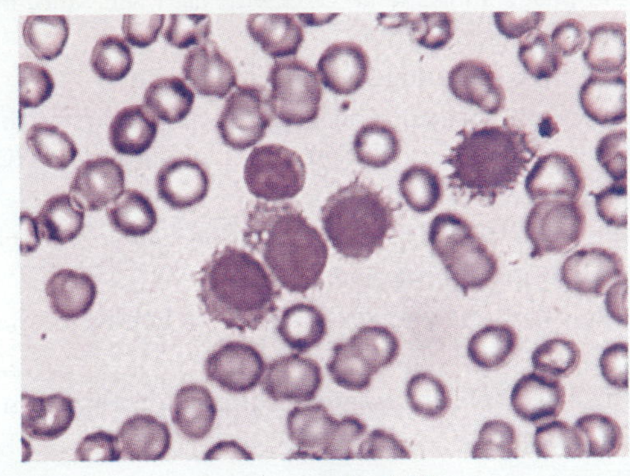

a. PAS
b. NSE
c. MPO
d. TRAP

8. A 10-year-chid with bilateral cervical lymphadenopathy. Lymph node biopsy was performed, which showed cells as given in the figure. Which of the following is true regarding this condition?

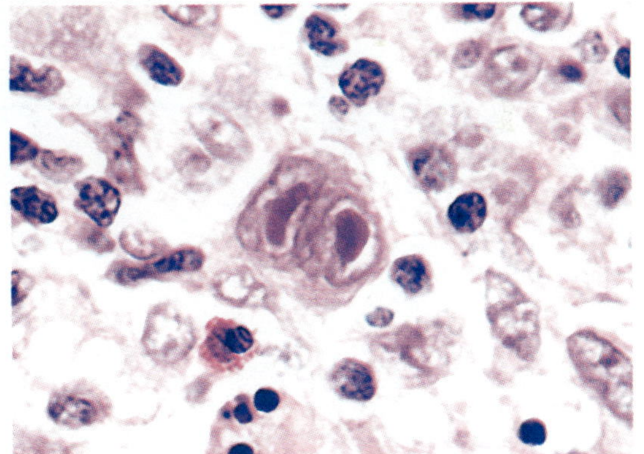

a. Hodgkin lymphoma: EBV and embryo cell
b. Non-Hodgkin lymphoma HIV and Giant B cell
c. TB, Mycobacteria and tiny granuloma
d. Hodgkin lymphoma: EBV and Reed Sternberg cell

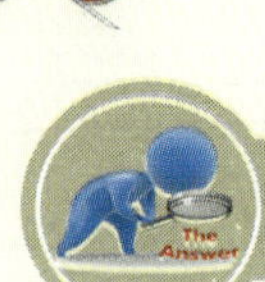

Answers of Image-Based Questions

1. **Ans. (c) Acute leukemia**
   - The image shows large cells with high N:C ratio, immature chromatin which are blasts. With >20% blasts, the diagnosis is acute leukemia.

2. **Ans. (d) Translocation involving MYC gene**
   - The arrow marked shows cleared area (stars as macrophages) amidst hugely proliferating tumor cells (sky). This appearance of starry sky is seen in Burkitts lymphoma having MYC gene translocation.

3. **Ans. (d) Hemolytic anemia**
   - The smear shows rouleux formation seen in multiple myeloma, severe anemia & cases of hypergammaglobinemia.

4. **Ans. (a) Bone marrow examination**
   - This is Klima bone marrow aspiration needle for marrow aspiration and biopsy

5. **Ans. (a) AML**
   - The blasts cells shows Auer rods inside them which are a hallmark of AML.

6. **Ans. (a) JAK-2**
   - The figure shows increased platelets in smear and increased megakaryocytes in bone marrow. To diagnose this as essential thrombocythemia (neoplasm); JAK-2 mutation analysis should be done.

7. **Ans. (d) TRAP**
   - The peripheral smear in the question shows hairy cells which can be diagnosed with TRAP stain.

8. **Ans. (d) Hodgkin lymphoma: EBV and Reed Sternberg cell**
   - Figure shows Reed Sternberg cells in Hodgkins lymphoma which are EBV infected.

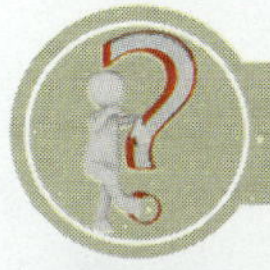

Multiple Choice Questions

NON-NEOPLASTIC WBC DISORDERS

1. A patient presented with intermittent fever, no wt loss, no anorexia, retroperitoneal mass. Peripheral smear finding were normal. Gross and microscopy of the mass is given. What is the most likely diagnosis?

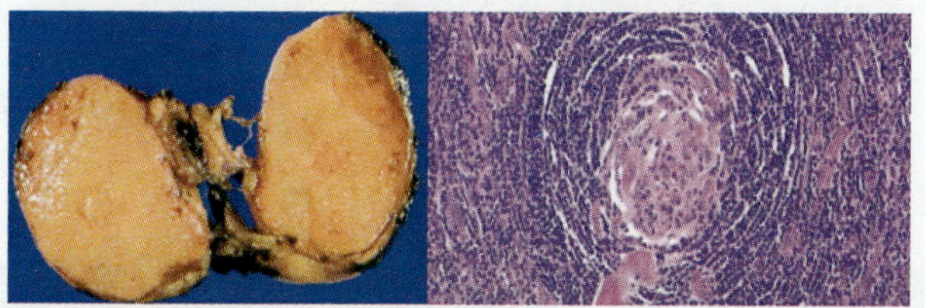

   a. Non-Hodgkin's lymphoma   *(AIIMS Nov 18)*
   b. Castleman disease
   c. Angiolymphoid hyperplasia

2. HHV-8 is related to all except: *(AIIMS May 18)*
   a. Primary effusion lymphoma
   b. Kaposi sarcoma
   c. Castleman disease
   d. Adult T cell lymphoma

3. Which of the following represents the marked area in the histology of lymph node?   *(AIIMS May 2017)*

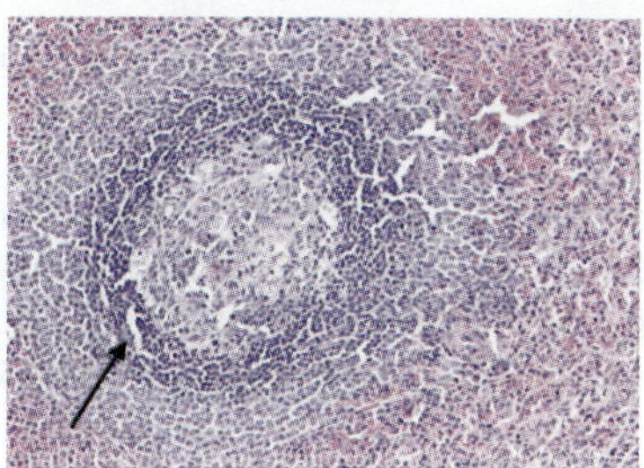

   a. Mantle zone   b. Marginal zone
   c. Paracortical area   d. Germinal centre

4. Dohle bodies with giant platelets are seen in:
   a. May heggalin anomaly   *(JIPMER 2017)*
   b. Pelger huet anomaly
   c. Chediak higashi syndrome
   d. Bernard solier syndrome

5. Which of the following cells will increase in case of parasite infection?   *(AIIMS Nov 2016)*

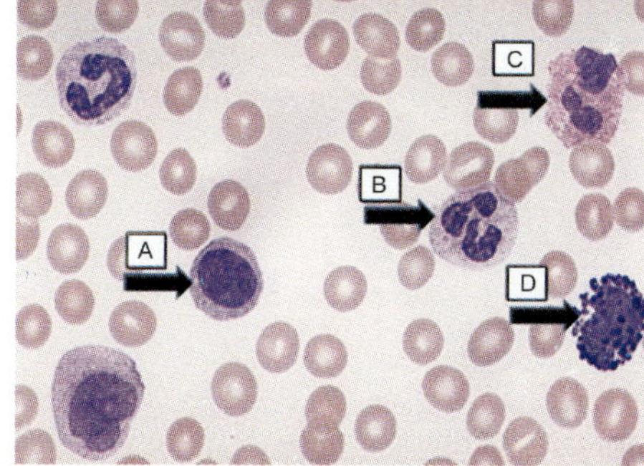

   a. A   b. B
   c. C   d. D

6. Identify the arrow marked cell in the given condition below?   *(AIIMS May 2016)*

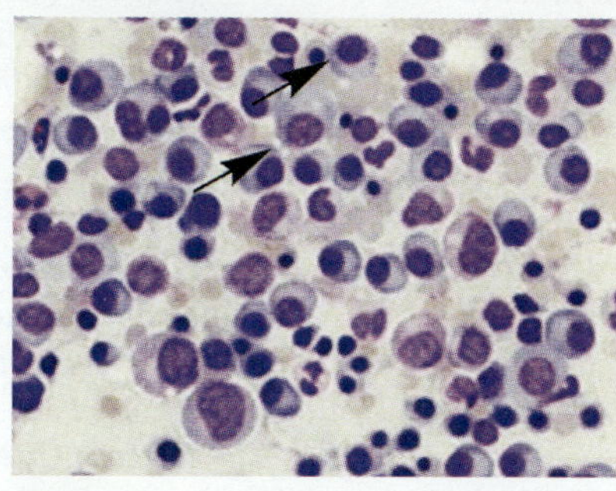

   a. Macrophage   b. Lymphocyte
   c. Plasma cell   d. Eosinophil

7. About the given instrument below all of the following statements are true except?   *(AIIMS May 2016)*

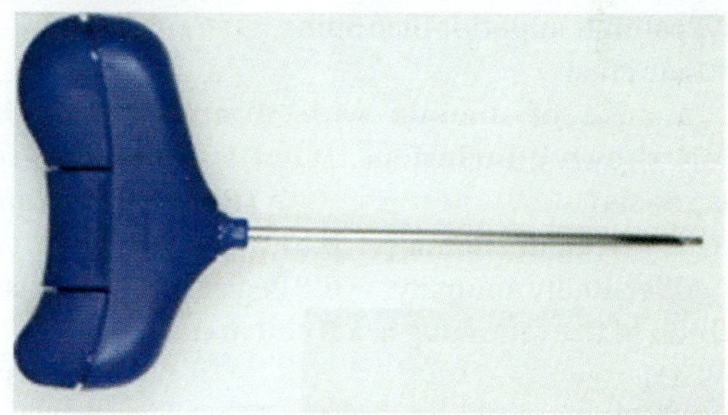

   a. Done for diagnosis of infiltrative and granulomatous diseases
   b. No need of breath holding during the procedure
   c. Can be done in prone or lateral position
   d. Platelet count of <40000/ul is contraindication

8. A Warthin–Finkeldey cell is a type of giant multinucleate cell found in hyperplastic lymph nodes early in the course of: *(Recent Question 2016-17)*
   a. Measles   b. Hodgkins
   c. Kala azar   d. Syphilis

9. For which procedure is the following instrument used?

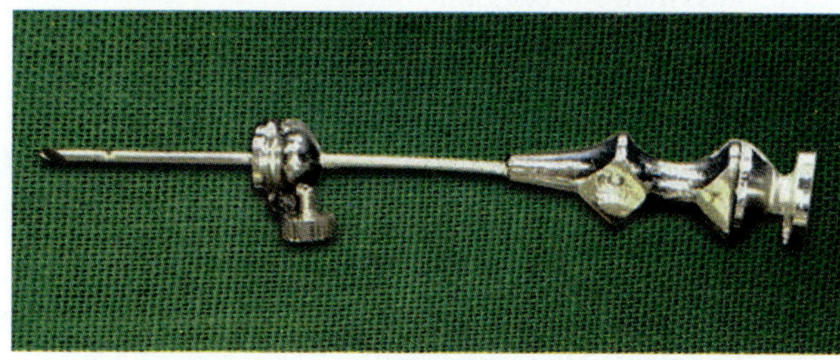

   a. Bone marrow examination   *(AIIMS Nov 2015)*
   b. Liver biopsy
   c. Pleural biopsy
   d. Lumbar puncture

10. Marker of T -lymphocyte is: *(Recent Question 2016)*
   a. CD8   b. CD20
   c. CD19   d. CD45

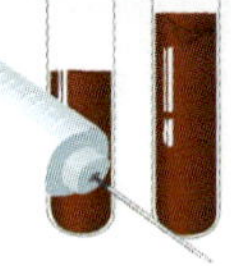

11. **Host receptor for streptococcus pyogenes is?**
    (Recent Question 2015)
    a. CD4   b. CD21
    c. CD44   d. CD46

12. **Serious infections can occur when absolute neutrophil count decreases below?** *(Recent Question 2016)*
    a. Less than 500/ul   b. Less than 800/ul
    c. Less than 1000/u   d. less than 2000/ul

13. **Eosinophillia is found in?** *(Recent Question 2016)*
    a. Cryptococcus   b. HPV
    c. Stronglyloides   d. Typhoid

14. **1st cell of RBC development** *(Recent Question 2016)*
    a. Pro erythroblast   b. Intermediatenormoblast
    c. Reticulocyte   d. Basophilic erythroblast

15. **Dilated endoplasmic reticulum is called as?**
    (Recent Question 2015)
    a. Asteroid bodies   b. Bamboo bodies
    c. Hirano bodies   d. Dohle bodies

16. **In infant, Bone Marrow biopsy is done from?**
    a. Tibia   *(Recent Question 2015)*
    b. Sternum
    c. Posterior superior Iliac Spine
    d. Iliac crest

17. **In a case of anemia with thrombocytopenia and PMN showing inclusions. What is the most probable diagnosis?** *(Recent Question 2015)*
    a. May Hegglin anomaly   b. Evan syndrome
    c. Alder-Reilly anomaly   d. Pegler Huet Anomaly

18. **Which of the following is a B cell marker?**
    a. CD1   *(PGI May 2014)*
    b. CD 10   c. CD1a
    d. CD19   e. CD20

19. **Pan B cell marker:** *(WB PG 2014)*
    a. CD 19p   b. CD 19q
    c. CD 16   d. CD 21

20. **Infectious mononucleosis affects?** *(JIPMER 2014)*
    a. B-cells   b. T-cells
    c. NK cells   d. Macrophages

21. **The peripheral blood eosinophil count in Eosinophilia-myalagia syndrome is usually** *(Bihar PG 2014)*
    a. Between 500 to 2000 cells/ microilter
    b. 2000 to 5000 cells/microliter
    c. Less than 500 cells/microliter
    d. More than 5000 cells/microliter

22. **In an ablated animal, myeloid series cells are injected. Which of following is seen after incubation period -**
    (AIIMS May 12)
    a. RBC   b. Fibroblast
    c. T lymphocytes   d. Hematopoetic stem cell

23. **All of the following stem cell populations are found within the bone marrow, except -** *(AI 12)*
    a. Endothelial Progenitor cells
    b. Myoblast Progenitor cells
    c. Mesenchymal stem cells
    d. Hematopoietic stem cells

24. **Leukocyte common antigen is:** *(WB PG 2012)*
    a. CD 45   b. CD 20
    c. CD 19   d. CD 41

25. **Generalized necrotising lymphadenopathy is -** *(AI 11)*
    a. Kimura disease
    b. Kikuchi disease
    c. Non-Hodgkin's lymphoma
    d. Castleman's disease

26. **Eosinophilic abscess in lymph node is characteristically seen in -** *(DPG 11)*
    a. Kimura's disease   b. Hodgkin's lymphoma
    c. Tuberculosis   d. Sarcoidosis

27. **Which of the following surface glycoproteins is most often expressed in human hematopoietic stem cell?**
    (DPG 10)
    a. CD22   b. CD45
    c. CD15   d. CD34

ACUTE LEUKEMIA

28. **Which of the following is not a provisional entity according to Revised WHO-2016 classification of Acute leukemia?** *(AIIMS May 18)*
    a. AML with BCR-ABL
    b. ALL with hyperploidy
    c. AML with $RUNX_1$
    d. Early T cell precursor leukemia

29. **How will you differentiate mediastenal mass from thymoma differentiating it from ALL?** *(AIIMS Nov 18)*
    a. Cytokeratin   b. CD1a
    c. CD3   d. Tdt

30. **A patient presented with painless b/l proptosis. What is the next investigation to diagnose it as chloroma?**
    (AIIMS Nov 2017)
    a. Blood haemoglobin   b. Peripheral smear
    c. Platelets   d. Bone marrow (reticulin)

31. **All of the following are seen in the development of T lymphocyte at a point except?** *(AIIMS May 2017)*
    a. Tdt   b. CD34
    c. PAX5   d. Cd1a

32. **A 7 year old presents with fever, weight loss. On examination he was pale and had significant lymphadenopathy. Bone marrow histology is as given below. What is the most probable diagnosis?** *(AIIMS May 2017)*

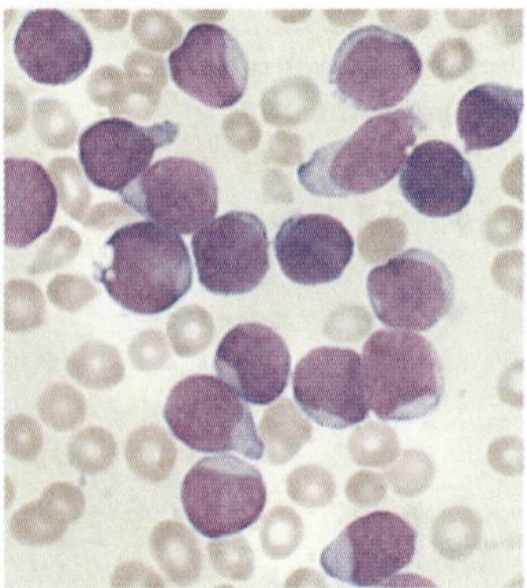

    a. ALL
    b. AML
    c. Aplastic anaemia
    d. Juvenile myelomonocyticleukemia

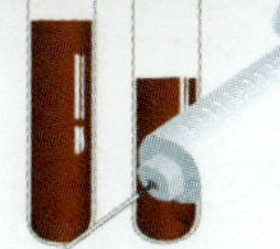

33. Good prognosis for ALL is? *(JIPMER 2017)*
a. Age > 10 yrs
b. Hyperdiploidy
c. T cell variant
d. TLC >1,00,000/ul

34. Best candidate for Autologus bone marrow transplant?
a. Multiple myeloma *(JIPMER 2017)*
b. Leukemia
c. Thalassemia
d. Congenital Immunodeficiency

35. Most commom translocation in acute promyelocytic leukemia? *(PGI May 2017)*
a. t(8:14)
b. t(15:17)
c. t(9:22)
d. t(8:11)
e. t(11:14)

36. Which one is best prognostic factor for ALL?
a. Hyperploidy *(AIIMS Nov 2015)*
b. Orgnomegaly
c. TLC more than 50,000/ul
d. Response to treatment

37. Auer rods are specific for *(Recent Question 2015)*
a. Acute myeloid leukemia
b. Acute lymphocytic leukemia
c. Chronic lymphocytic leukemia
d. Hodgkin's lymphoma

38. True about ALL *(Recent Question 2015)*
a. tdT positive
b. Gamma globulins
c. t(8,14)
d. Insidious onset

39. Dohle bodies are seen in *(Recent Question 2015)*
a. Neutrophils
b. Macrophages
c. Plasma cells
d. Histiocytes

40. All are true regarding hemophagocytic lymphohistiocytosis (HLH) except? *(Recent Question 2015)*
a. Activation of macrophages and CD 8+ T cells
b. Cytopenias due to phagocytosis of progenitors in bone marrow
c. HTLV-1 is a cause in immunodeficient patients
d. Abnormal liver function tests

41. Stain used for diagnosis of granulocytic sarcoma
a. Myeloperoxidase *(Recent Question 2015)*
b. Leukocyte alkaline phosphatase
c. Nonspecific esterase
d. Neuron specific enolase

42. Most common type of AML in Down's syndrome
(Recent Question 2015)
a. M2
b. M3
c. M6
d. M7

43. The following parameter in ALL indicates poor prognosis *(Recent Question 2015)*
a. Age >10 years
b. WBC count <50000/mm³ at diagnosis
c. Hyperdiploidy
d. Early pre-B phenotype

44. Drug that is not used in the treatment of ALL
(Recent Question 2015)
a. Rituximab
b. Methotrexate
c. Vincristine
d. Daunorubicin

45. Most common type of all in children
(Recent Question 2015)
a. Pre-B cell ALL
b. Mature B cell ALL
c. Pre-T cell ALL
d. Mature T cell ALL

46. Chloroma is a *(Recent Question 2015)*
a. Lymphoma
b. Leukemia
c. Sarcoma
d. Carcinoma

47. A 35 year old male presented with complaints of bleeding gums. There is history of recurrent infections in the past 1 year. On examination, pallor present. Peripheral smear of the same patient is shown below. Identify the arrow marked structure? *(Recent Question 2015)*
a. Dohle body
b. Normoblast
c. Auer Rod
d. Heinz bodies

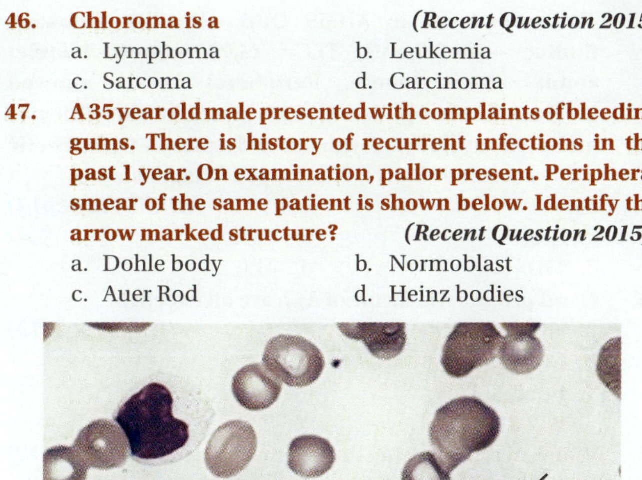

48. In Acute lymphoblastic leukaemia favourable prognostic factors includes all except? *(MH PG 2014)*
a. Age of 2 to 10 yrs
b. Low white cell count
c. Presence of t (12; 21)
d. Presence of t (9; 22)

49. Which one of the following is the likely diagnosis based on the smear given above: *(AP PGMEE 2015)*
a. Acute myelogenous leukemia
b. Acute lymphoblastic leukemia
c. Hairy cell leukemia
d. Chronic lymphocytic leukemia

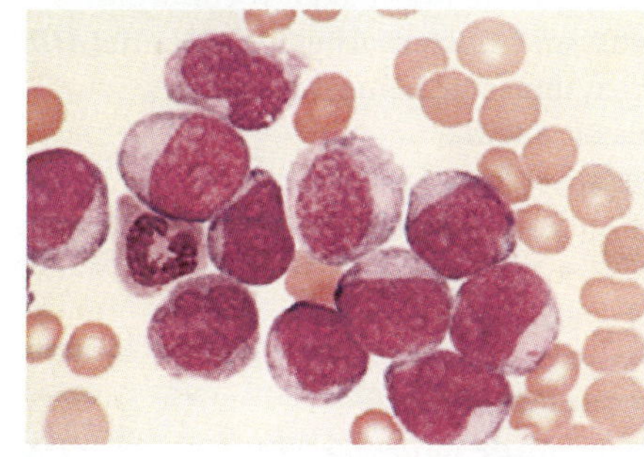

50. Good prognosis of AML are all except?
(Recent Question 2015)
a. t(15;17)
b. t(8;21)
c. inv 16
d. t(12;21)

51. Most common malignancy of blood is?
(Recent Question 2016)
a. ALL
b. CLL
c. AML
d. CML

52. AML causing Gum hypertrophy- *(Recent Question 2014)*
a. M1
b. M2
c. M3
d. M4

53. DIC is common in which AML- *(Recent Question 2014)*
a. Monocytic (M5)
b. Promyelocytic (M3)
c. Erythrocytic (M6)
d. Megakaryocytic (M7)

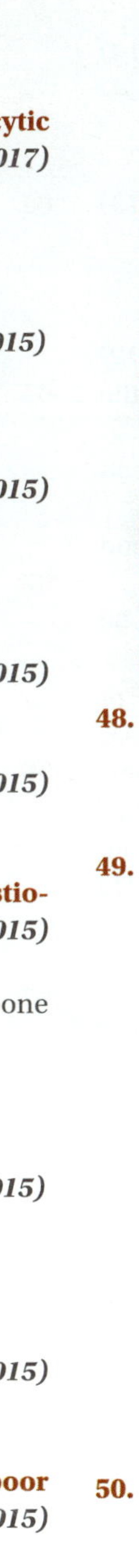

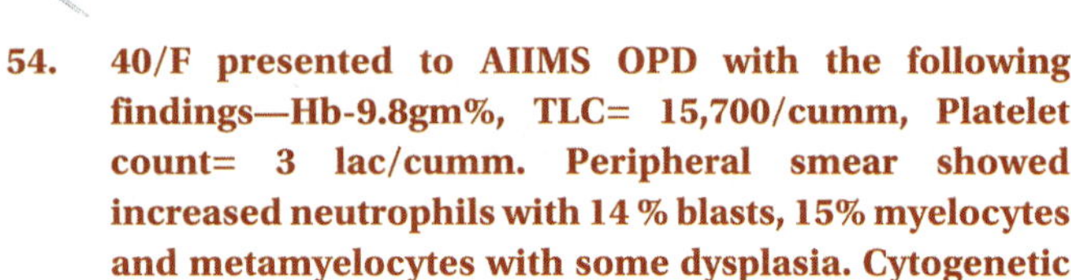

54. 40/F presented to AIIMS OPD with the following findings—Hb-9.8gm%, TLC= 15,700/cumm, Platelet count= 3 lac/cumm. Peripheral smear showed increased neutrophils with 14 % blasts, 15% myelocytes and metamyelocytes with some dysplasia. Cytogenetic study revealed t(8;21). What is your diagnosis?

(AIIMS May 2014)

a. AML b. CML

d. MDS d. ALL

55. Good prognostic factor of ALL are all except?

a. Hyperdiploidy *(JIPMER 2013)*

b. Female

c. Pre B ALL

d. t(12;21)

56. Which of the following statements is true- *(AIIMS May 12)*

a. Peak incidence of Chronic myeloid leukemia is in the fifth to sixth decades of life

b. Hairy cell leukemia in more than 50 years has a good prognosis

c. Acute lymphoid leukemia in less than 1 year has good prognosis

d. Chronic lymphocytic leukemia occurs in less than 50 years of age

57. A 10 year old child presents with pallor & history of blood transfusion 2 months back. On investigation, Hb –4.5gm/dl, total count 60,000/cu mm and blasts. platelet count- 2 lacs/cumm and CD 10(+)ve, CD 19 (+) ve, CD 117 (+) ve, MPO (+) ve& CD 33(-)ve. What is the most likely diagnosis? *(AIIMS Nov 11)*

a. ALL

b. AML

c. Undifferentiated leukemia

d. Mixed phenotypic acute leukemia

58. Least likely to be Pre-leukemic condition is:

a. Paroxysmal nocturnal hemoglobinuria *(AIIMS Nov 11)*

b. Paroxysmal cold hemoglobinuria

c. Aplastic anemia

d. Myelodysplastic syndrome

59. Most Common extranodal site of Lymphoma in HIV is?

a. CNS *(DNB Dec 10)*

b. GIT

c. Retroperitoneum

d. Mediastinum

60. Poor prognostic indicator in ALL- *(DNB June 10)*

a. Age < 2 year

b. TLC 4,000-10,000/mm3

c. Presence of testicular involvement at presentation

d. Presence of blasts in peripheral smear

HODGKIN'S LYMPHOMA

61. Lymphohistocytic variant of Reed Sternberg seen in which subtype of Hodgkin lymphoma?

a. Nodular sclerosis *(Recent exam 2018)*

b. Lymphocyte rich

c. Lymphocyte predominant

d. Lymphocyte depleted

62. A 20 year old male presented with cervical lymphadenopathy. Histology of lymph node shows RS cell with vague nodule formation and background T reactive lymphocytes. The cells were positive for CD20, LCA, EMA and negative for CD 15 and CD30. Diagnosis is? *(AIIMS May 2017)*

a. NLPHL

b. T cell rich B cell lymphoma

c. Nodular sclerosis Hodgkin

d. CLL

63. True about lymphoma? *(PGI Nov 2016)*

a. Mantle cell origin is in germinal centre

b. DLBCL is most common in India

c. CD5/3/8 are markers of B cell lymphoma

d. Burkitts lymphoma arises from Germinal centre

64. True about CML is? *(PGI Nov 2016)*

a. If Imatinib not working then Dasatinib can be used

b. BCR-ABL activates tyrosine kinase

c. BM biopsy is essential for diagnosis

d. Blast crisishas > 10% blasts

65. EBV is not associated with? *(AIIMS May 2016)*

a. Lymphocyte predominant HD

b. Plasmablastic lymphoma

c. Nasopharyngeal Ca

d. Mixed cellularity HD

66. True about Hodgkin's lymphoma: *(PGI May 2016)*

a. Often localized to single axial group of lymph node

b. Hepatomegaly is always present

c. Contiguous spread of lymph node

d. Can be cured by chemotherapy & radiotherapy

e. Commonly presents with painless lymphadenopathy

67. CD 30 is/are marker for: *(Recent Question 2016-17)*

a. Anaplastic large cell lymphoma

b. Embryonal cell carcinoma

c. Squamous Cell Carcinoma

d. Seminoma

e. Hodgkin's lymphoma

68. Bimodal distribution is seen in? *(Recent Question 2016-17)*

a. Hodgkins lymphoma

b. DLBCL

c. ALL

d. CML

69. RS cell having same immunophenotyping are present in which subtypes of Hodgkin's lymphoma:

a. Nodular sclerosis *(Recent Question 2016-17)*

b. Lymphocyte predominant

c. Lymphocyte rich

d. Mixed cellularity

e. Lymphocyte depletion

70. In which following subtypes of Hodgkin lymphoma, the diagnostic R-S giant cells are usually negative for CD 15 and CD 30? *(AP PGMEE 2013)*

a. Mixed cellularity

b. Lymphocyte rich

c. Lymphocyte depletion

d. Lymphocyte predominance

71. **A 10 year child presented with bilateral cervical lymphadenopathy. Lymph node biopsy was performed, which showed cells as given in the figure. Which of the following is true regarding this condition?** *(AIIMS Nov 2015)*

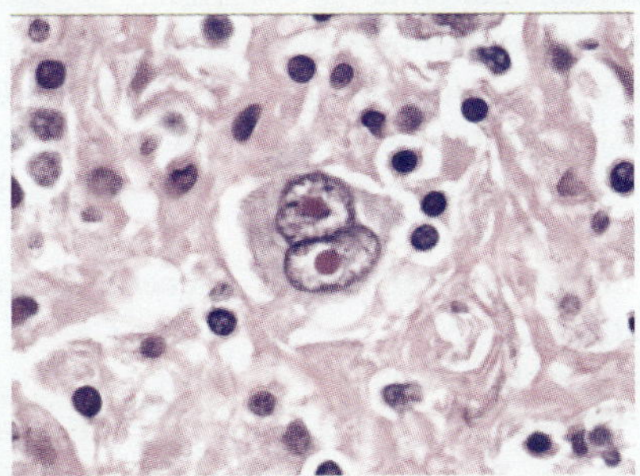

   a. Hodgkin lymphoma; EBV and embryo cell
   b. Non Hodgkin lymphoma; HIV and Giant B cell
   c. TB, Mycobacteria and tiny granuloma
   d. Hodgkin lymphoma: EBV and Reed Sternberg cell

72. **All are true regarding Reed Sternburg cell immunophenotype in classical Hodgkin lymphoma**
   a. Positive for CD15 and CD30 *(Recent Question 2015)*
   b. Negative for other B-cell markers, T-cell markers, and CD45
   c. Positive for PAX 5
   d. Overexpression of BCL-6

73. **Hodgkin lymphoma type that more commonly presents as fever of unknown origin**
   a. Nodular sclerosis *(Recent Question 2015)*
   b. Mixed cellularity
   c. Lymphocyte predominance
   d. Lymphocyte depletion

74. **Hodgkins lymphoma type not associated with EBV** *(Recent Question 2015)*
   a. Nodular sclerosis   b. Lymphocyte rich
   c. Lymphocyte depleted   d. Mixed cellularity

75. **Sea blue histiocytes are seen in** *(Recent Question 2015)*
   a. Chronic lymphoblastic leukemia
   b. Chronic myeloid leukemia
   c. Langerhan cell histiocytosis
   d. Burkitt lymphoma

76. **Which of the following types of Hodgkin's lymphomas is not associated with Epstein Barr virus?**
   a. Lymphocyte depletion *(Recent Question 2015)*
   b. Mixed cellularity
   c. Lymphocye rich
   d. Lymphocyte predominance

77. **A 35 year old female presents with cervical and axillary lymphadenopathy. There is history of fever and drenching night sweats. She is diagnosed to have hodgkin's lymphoma. What is the stage of the disease?** *(Recent Question 2015)*
   a. II-A   b. II-B
   c. IIE-A   d. IIE-B

78. **True about Hodgkin's lymphoma is/are?**
   a. Axial lymphnadenopathy *(PGI Nov 2015)*
   b. hepatomegaly is common
   c. Contiguous spread of lymph node
   d. Can be cured by chemotherapy
   e. An arbor classification is useful

79. **Reticular variant of Reed Sternberg found in which subtype of hodgkin's?** *(Recent Question 2015)*
   a. Lymphocyte rich Hodgkins lymphoma
   b. Lymphocyte poor Hodgkins lymphoma
   c. Lymphocyte predominant Hodgkins lymphoma
   d. Nodular Sclerosis

80. **Popcorn cell is seen with which Hodgkins lymphoma?** *(Recent Question 2015)*
   a. Lymphocyte rich Hodgkins lymphoma
   b. Lymphocyte poor Hodgkins lymphoma
   c. Lymphocyte predominant Hodgkins lymphoma
   d. Nodular Sclerosis

81. **CD 15+/ CD30+ lymphoma among the following are?**
   a. Mixed cellularity Hodgkin lymphoma *(PGI May 2014)*
   b. Mantle cell lymphoma
   c. Diffuse T- cell lymphoma
   d. NLPHL
   e. Acute lymphoblastic leukemia

82. **Choose the FALSE statement regarding Hodgkin's lymphoma** *(APPGMEE 14)*
   a. Affected lymph nodes become painful with alcohol ingestion
   b. Ann Arbor Stage II is involvement of two or more lymph node groups on both sides of the diaphragm
   c. 'B symptoms' are fever, night sweats and ≥ 10% weight loss in 6 months
   d. ABVD regimen is standard line of treatment

83. **A person is having painless lymphadenopathy. On biopsy, binucleated owl shaped nuclei with clear vacuolated area is seen. On IHC CD 15 and CD 30 were positive. What is the most probable diagnosis?**
   a. Nodular sclerosis *(AIIMS Nov 2013)*
   b. Large granular lymphocytic lymphoma
   c. Lymphocyte depletion type
   d. Lymphocyte predominant HD

84. **Most common Non Hodgkins lymphoma is**
   a. Diffuse large B cell lymphoma *(AIIMS Nov 2013)*
   b. Follicular lymphoma
   c. Anaplastic large cell lymphoma
   d. Large T-cell leukemia/lymphoma

85. **Flow cytometry is done on:** *(AIIMS May 2013)*
   a. Polycythemia
   b. Thrombocytosis
   c. Basophil
   d. Lymphocytes

86. **Reed Sternberg like cell are seen in:**
   a. Adult T cell lymphoma *(PGI May 2013)*
   b. Extranodal NK-Cell Lymphoma
   c. Marginal zone lymphoma
   d. Diffuse large B cell lymphoma
   e. Infectious mononucleosis

87. **All are poor prognostic factors for Hodgkin's lymphoma except:** *(PGI Nov 2011)*
   a. Young age
   b. Involvement of stomach
   c. Lymphocyte depletion
   d. Extranodal metastasis
   e. Large mediastinal mass

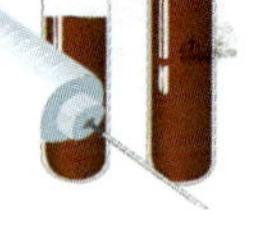

88. Which of the following malignancy is associated with underlying progression and spreads characteristically in a stepwise fashion and hence staging the disease is an important prognostic factor?
a. Hodgkin's lymphoma *(MH 11, DNB Dec 08)*
b. Multiple myeloma
c. Mature T cell NHL
d. Mature B cell NHL

89. True about nodular lymphocytic predominant Hodgkin's lymphoma- *(PGI Nov 10)*
a. Consists predominantly of classical RS cells
b. CD 15 & CD 30 positive
c. Made up of T lymphocytes
d. EBV positive
e. Has good prognosis

90. L & H variants of the Reed-Sternberg cells are positive for *(MH 16)*
a. CD 20   b. CD 15
c. CD 30   d. EBV

NON-HODGKIN LYMPHOMA

91. In Alibert bazin syndrome, origin of lymphoma is from? *(JIPMER 18)*
a. Eosinophill   b. B lymphocyte
c. Monocyte   d. T lymphocyte

92. CLL/SLL arises from which cell? *(AIIMS Nov 2017)*
a. Mature B cell
b. Naive B cell
c. Centrocytes of germinal center
d. Progenitor B-cell

93. Which of the following Immunohisto chemistry marker is used in Cyclin D1 negative Mantle cell lymphoma?
a. SOX11   b. ITRA 1 *(AIIMS May 2017)*
c. MYD88   d. Annexin V

94. A 35 year old presented with fever. On examination he had enlarged and ulcerated tonsils. His peripheral blood smear showed lymphocytosis. Monospot test was negative. Tonsillectomy was done. The biopsy of the same showed large cells mixed with lymphocytes. The cells were positive for CD20, EBVLMP1, MUM1, CD 79a. Background cells were positive for CD3. The cells are negative for CD15. Your most probable diagnosis?

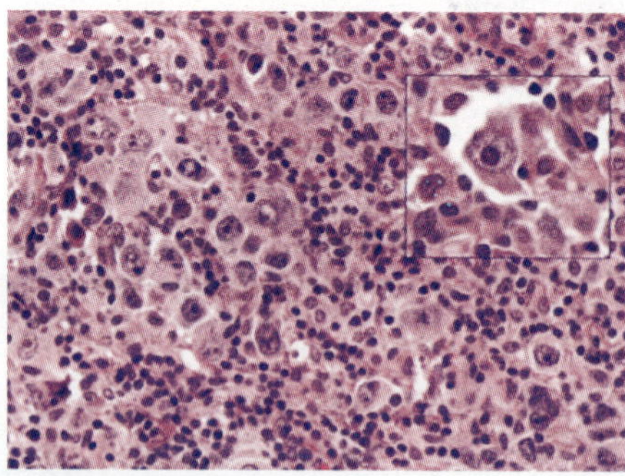

a. Infectious mono-nucleosis *(AIIMS May 2017)*
b. Hodgkin lymphoma
c. EBV positive – DLBL
d. EBV positive mucocutaneous ulcer

95. PAX-5 is a marker for? *(AIIMS May 2017)*
a. Diffuse large B-cell lymphoma
b. Hodgkins lymphoma
c. Anaplastic lymphoma
d. Lymphoblastic lymphoma
e. AML

96. TRAP positivity is seen in? *(JIPMER 2017)*
a. Hairy cell leukemia   b. ALL
c. Burkitts lymphoma   d. T-cell leukemia

97. Primary extranodal neoplasms is/are? *(PGI Nov 2017)*
a. Burkitt lymphoma   b. Waldeyer's ring lymphoma
c. Gastric lymphoma   d. Thyroid lymphoma
e. Mycosis fungoides

98. BRAF mutation is seen in? *(Recent Question 2016-17)*
a. LCH   b. Colon Ca
c. Hairy cell leukemia   d. AML M7

99. A 10 yr old boy with mass in the abdomen. On imaging the paraaortic LN is enlarged. On biopsy starry sky appearance is seen. What is the underlying abnormality? *(AIIMS May 2015)*
a. p53 gene mutation
b. RB gene mutation
c. Translocation involving BCR-ABL genes
d. Translocation involving MYC gene

100. All are true about CLL except? *(PGI Nov 2015)*
a. Most common leukemia of adults in west
b. Diagnosed incidentally
c. Not treated in stage A
d. CD38 is poor prognostic marker
e. Most common age group is pediatric

101. CD5 is expressed in *(Recent Question 2015)*
a. Mantle cell lymphoma
b. Chronic myeloid lymphoma
c. Follicular lymphoma
d. Burkitt lymphoma

102. CD 30 positivity and t(2;5) is characteristic of *(Recent Question 2015)*
a. Langerhans cell histiocytosis
b. Lymphoplasmacytic lymphoma
c. Null cell lymphoma
d. Follicular lymphoma

103. Cyclin D1 is expressed in *(Recent Question 2015)*
a. Follicular lymphoma
b. Chronic lymphoid lymphoma
c. Mantle cell lymphoma
d. Splenic marginal zone lymphoma

104. CD20 is positive in all the following lymphomas except
a. Mantle cell lymphoma *(Recent Question 2015)*
b. Lymphocyte rich HL
c. Follicular lymphoma
d. Butkitt lymphoma

105. Find the false statement about diffuse large B cell lymphoma *(Recent Question 2015)*
a. Most common form of NHL
b. Waldeyer ring is involved commonly
c. Extranodal sites are also involved
d. Bone-marrow involvement in early phase

106. True about endemic Burkitt lymphoma:
(Recent Question 2015)
a. All are associated with EBV infection
b. Abdominal amass involving ileocaecum and peritoneum and peritoneum
c. Most aggressive form
d. Bone marrow is commonly involved

107. Not true about anaplastic large T cell lymphoma
a. t(2;5) translocation *(Recent Question 2015)*
b. CD30 (ki-1) positive
c. Large anaplastic cells containing horseshoe-shaped nuclei and voluminous cytoplasm
d. ALK positive tumors carry worst prognosis

108. Neoplastic cells with multilobated nuclei (cloverleaf or flower cells) are seen in *(Recent Question 2015)*
a. Diffuse large B cell lymphoma
b. Adult T cell leukemia
c. Anaplstic large T cell lymphoma
d. Mycosis fungoides

109. Hallmark cells are seen in: *(Recent Question 2015)*
a. Anaplastic large cell lymphoma
b. Burkitt's lymphoma
c. Hairy cell leukaemia
d. Mantle cell lymphoma

110. Clover leaf cells are seen in: *(Recent Question 2015)*
a. Burkitt's lymphoma
b. Adult T cell leukemia-lymphoma
c. Hairy cell lymphoma
d. Mantle cell lymphoma

111. Gastric MALTomas may express all of the following except: *(Recent Question 2015)*
a. CD5
b. CD19
c. CD20
d. CD43

112. IgA lymphoma is seen in? *(Recent Question 2016)*
a. Spleen
b. Lymph nodes
c. Small Intestine
d. Large Intestine

113. Spleniculi means *(Recent Question 2015)*
a. Splenic calculi
b. Splenic atrophy
c. Splenic malignancy
d. Accessory spleen

114. A 60 year old male presents with generalized lymphadenopathy and hepatosplenomegaly. Immunophenotype: CD5 and CD19 are positive and CD10 negative. Diagnosis *(Recent Question 2015)*
a. Follicular lymphoma
b. Burkitt lymphoma
c. Hairy cell leukemia
d. CLL

115. Translocation t(8;14) of c-MYC gene is seen in
a. Follicular lymphoma *(Recent Question 2015)*
b. Burkitt lymphoma
c. Mantle cell lymphoma
d. Diffuse large B cell lymphoma

116. Characteristic translocation in mantle cell lymphoma *(Recent Question 2015)*
a. t(11;14)
b. t(15;17)
c. t(9;22)
d. t(8;14)

117. True about follicular lymphoma: *(PGI May 2015)*
a. Lymphadenopathy is the most common presentation
b. BCL-1 positive
c. CD5 positive
d. More common in males than females

118. True about Chronic Lymphocytic Leukemia:
a. Most common leukemia in adult *(PGI May 2015)*
b. Proliferation center is pathognomonic
c. Massive splenomegaly
d. Radiotherapy & chemotherapy are given in treatment

119. EBV is associated with? *(Recent Question 2015)*
a. Burkitts Lymphoma
b. Adamintinoma
c. Follicular lymphoma
d. CLL

120. CD 30 marker for
a. Anaplastic large cell lymphoma
b. Seminoma
c. Embroyonal cell ca
d. Hodgkins lymphoma

121. An elderly male presents with anemia and fatigue. O/E splenomegaly-2 cm palpable below costal margin. Hemogram showed Pancytopenia. Which is the most common etiology?
(Recent Question 2014, DNB July 2014)
a. Hairy cell leukemia
b. CML
c. Thalassemia
d. Follicular lymphoma

122. Mantle cell lymphomas are positive for all of the following, except - *(Recent Question 2014)*
a. CD23
b. CD20
c. CD5
d. CD45

123. Lethal midline granuloma is - *(Recent Question 2014)*
a. T cell lymphoma
b. B-celllymphoma
c. NK/T cell lymphoma
d. LCH

124. Most common ocular lymphoma-
(Recent Question 2014)
a. T-cell lymphoma
b. Hodgkin's lymphoma
c. B-cell NHL
d. Pre T-cell lymphoma

125. Cyclin-D & IGH fusion gene is associated with?
(Recent Question 2014)
a. Mantle cell Lymphoma
b. Follicular carcinoma
c. Melanomas
d. Burkitt lymphoma

126. Commonest site for extranodal lymphoma is
a. Liver
b. Stomach *(APPGMEE 14)*
c. Small intestine
d. Large intestine

127. Following gene when mutated, protects tumor cells from Apoptosis *(APPGMEE 14)*
a. BCL – 2
b. BRCA
c. RB
d. TGF – β

128. One of the following leukemia almost never develops after radiation *(APPGMEE 14)*
a. Acute myeloid leukemia
b. Chronic myeloid leukemia
c. Acute lymphoblastic leukemia
d. Chronic lymphocytic leukemia

129. Histological presence of "Hallmark Cells" with horse shoe-like or embryoid like nuclei and voluminous cytoplasm are seen in *(APPGMEE 14)*
a. Anaplastic large celllymphoma (ALKpositive)
b. Familial Medullary Carcinoma
c. Familial Neuroblastoma
d. LymphocytepredominancetypeHodgkin's lymphoma

130. "Smudge cells" in the peripheral smear are characteristic of *(APPGMEE 14)*
a. Chronic myelogenous leukemia
b. Chronic lymphocytic leukemia
c. Acute myelogenous leukemia
d. Acute lymphoblastic leukemia

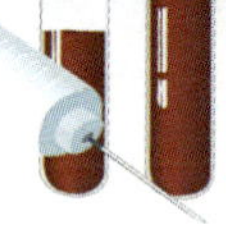

131. Burkitt's lymphoma is positive for?
a. CD5 *(Recent Question 2013)*
b. CD 15
c. CD20
d. CD25

132. A patient of 70 years, presented with generalized lymphadenopathy. WBC count was 20,000/mm³ and blood film showed >70% mature looking lymphocytes. Next investigation that should be done:
a. LN biopsy *(AIIMS May 2013)*
b. Peripheral blood Immunophenotyping
c. Bone marrow aspiration
d. Peripheral blood cytogenetics

133. Marker for Lymphoma is: *(AIIMS May 2013)*
a. S-100
b. HMB-45
c. Leukocyte common antigen
d. Cytokeratin

134. All are true about Mantle cell lymphoma except:
a. Associated with (11;14) translocation *(PGI May 2013)*
b. Overexpression of the BCL protein
c. CD 5 positive
d. CD 23 positive
e. Centroblasts frequently seen

135. Lymphoma associated with translocation of c-myc is?
a. Follicular Lymphoma *(JIPMER 2013)*
b. Mantle cell Lymphoma
c. Burkitts Lymphoma
d. Anaplastic large cell lymphoma

136. Most common Non-Hodgkin's lymphoma of orbit:
a. B cell   b. T cell *(AIIMS May 2012)*
c. NK cell   d. Plasma cell

137. International prognostic index for lymphomas includes the following prognostic factors, except:
a. Stage of disease *(AIIMS May 11)*
b. Number of extralymphatic sites involved
c. LDH
d. Hemoglobin and albumin

138. True about abdominal lymphoma: *(PGI Nov 2011)*
a. GIT lymphoma most commonly has polypoid appearance
b. Primary small intestinal lymphoma are most commonly located in ileum
c. Lymphoma is most common primary malignant neoplasm of spleen
d. Stomach is most common site for extranodal lymphoma
e. MALT lymphoma is associated with H. pylori infection

139. Features of hairy cell leukemia are all except:
a. Splenomegaly *(PGI May 2011)*
b. Hepatomegaly
c. Vasculitic syndromes
d. Pancytopenia
e. Erythema multiforme

140. Massive splenomegaly is found in: *(PGI May 2011)*
a. Hairy cell leukemia
b. CML
c. Typhoid
d. Sickle cell anemia
e. ITP

141. Compared to the other leukemias, hairy cell leukemia is associated with which of the following infections -
a. Parvovirus D 19 *(MH 10)*
b. Mycoplasma
c. Atypical mycobacteria
d. Salmonella

PLASMA CELL NEOPLASMS

142. All of the following are feature of waldenstorm macroglobulinemia except:? *(PGI May 18)*
a. Hyperviscosity
b. Polycythemia
c. Treated with alkylating agents
d. Low grade lymphoplasmacytoid lymphoma
e. IgG paraprotein

143. Myeloma associated with good prognosis? *(JIPMER 18)*
a. t (11 : 14)   b. t (14 : 18)
c. del 17   d. t (14, 16)

144. Origin of lymphoplasmacytic lymphoma (Waldenstorm Macroglobulinemia) is from? *(JIPMER 18)*
a. Germinal centre T cell
b. Germinal centre B cell
c. Post germinal centre B cell
d. Pre germinal centre B cell

145. Which of the following hematological condition is depicted below? *(Recent exam 2018)*

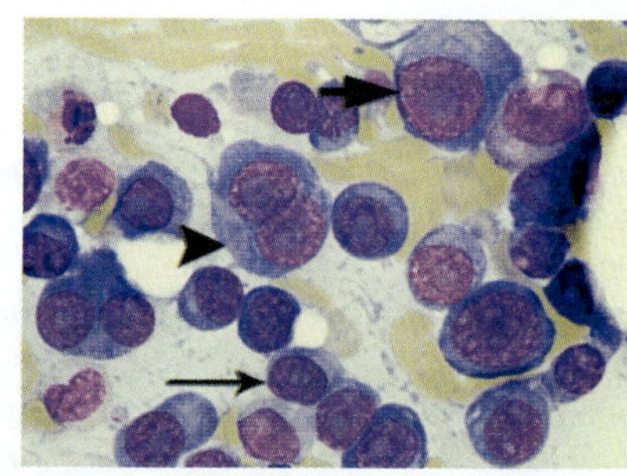

a. Multiple myeloma
b. Megaloblastic anemia
c. Chronic myeloid leukemia
d. Metastasis

146. Multiple myeloma causes? *(AIIMS May 2017)*
a. Cast nephropathy   b. Amyloidosis
c. Cryoglobinemia   d. Interstitial nephritis
e. Nephrocalcinosis

147. An elderly male presented with history of intractable diarrhea. His bone marrow and renal biopsy as shown below. Which of the following is the most appropriate diagnosis? *(AIIMS May 2017)*

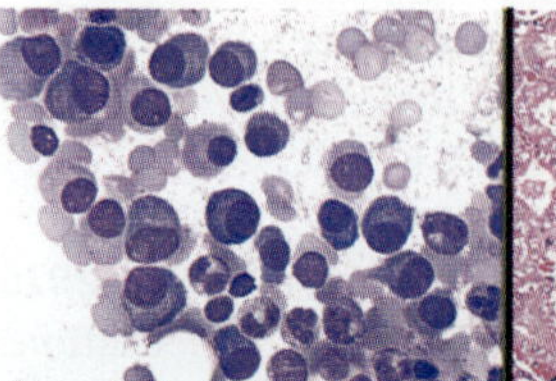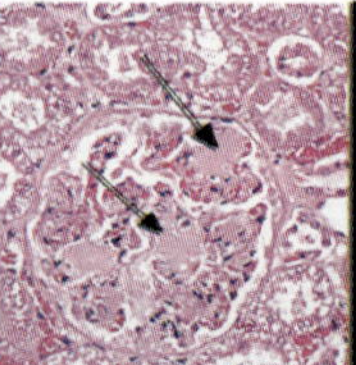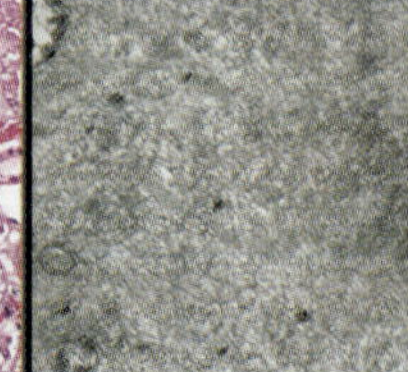

a. Leishmaniasis   b. Multiple myeloma
c. Lymphoma   d. Urate nephropathy

148. MYD88 L265P mutation is seen in? *(JIPMER 2017)*
a. Hairy cell leukemia
b. Waldenstrom Macroglobulinemia
c. Multiple Myeloma
d. AML

149. Large homogenous eosinophilic inclusions in plasma cells are called *(Recent Question 2015)*
a. Dutcher bodies   b. Councilman bodies
c. Russell bodies   d. Mallory hyaline bodies

150. Russell bodies are seen in *(Recent Question 2015)*
a. Mast cells   b. Plasma cells
c. Histiocytes   d. Langerhan cells

151. The single most important predictor of survival in multiple myeloma *(Recent Question 2015)*
a. IL-6 levels
b. Bence jones proteinuria
c. CD 138 positivity
d. Serum β_2-microglobulin

152. In multiple myeloma treatment, the following drug is avoided during induction therapy for transplant candidates *(Recent Question 2015)*
a. Thalidomide   b. Bortezomib
c. Melphalan   d. Dexamethasone

153. False statement about monoclonal gammopathy of unknown significance *(Recent Question 2015)*
a. <3g/dL of monoclonal protein
b. No bence jones proteinuria
c. Bone marrow plasma cells < 10%
d. Does not progress to multiple myeloma

154. M splike in waldenstorm macroglobulinemia is due to *(Recent Question 2015)*
a. IgM   b. IgG
c. IgA   d. IgD

155. False statement about MGUS *(Recent Question 2015)*
a. Few progress to multiple myeloma
b. Asymptomatic
c. Secrete M protein
d. Bence jones proteinuria

156. POEM syndrome. E stands for: *(Recent Question 2016)*
a. Endocrinopathy   b. Edema
c. Eosinophilia   d. Erythema

157. Life span of plasma cell *(Recent Question 2016)*
a. 12 hr   b. 24 hrs
c. 48 hrs   d. Days to weeks

158. Multiple myeloma is a tumor of? *(Recent Question 2015)*
a. B-lymphocyte   b. T-lymphocyte
c. Lymph nodes   d. Plasma cell

159. A patient presents with bone pain. X-ray reveals destructive lesions. Lab investigations show shypercalcemia. Serum electrophoresis shows M spike, while Bone marrow shows 35% plasma cells. What is your diagnosis? *(JIPMER 2014)*
a. MGUS   b. Smoldering myeloma
c. Multiple myeloma   d. Plasma cell leukemia

160. Beta-2 –microglobulin is a tumor marker for *(Bihar PG 2014)*
a. Multiple myeloma   b. Lung cancer
c. Colonic neoplasm   d. Choriocarcinoma

161. Proliferation and survival of myeloma cells are dependent on which of the following cytokines?
a. IL-1   b. IL-6   *(APPGMEE 14)*
c. IL-2   d. IL-5

162. Multiple myeloma-all are true except? *(JIPMER 2013)*
a. Proteinuria   b. Visual disturbance
c. Bleeding   d. Dystrophic calcification

163. Bence jones proteinuria is derived from? *(JIPMER 2013)*
a. Alpha globulins   b. Light chain globulins
c. Gamma globulins   d. Delta globulins

164. Malignancy associated with Waldenstrommacroglobulinemia? *(JIPMER 2013)*
a. Mycosis fungoides
b. Smoldering myeloma
c. Primary effusion lymphoma
d. Lymphoplasmacytic lymphoma

165. Which of the metabolic abnormality is seen in multiple myeloma? *(DNB 08/ DPG 11)*
a. Hyponatremia
b. Hypokalemia
c. Hypercalcemia
d. Hyperphosphatemia

166. Multiple myeloma is diagnosed by - *(JIPMER 11)*
a. 24 hours urine protein
b. Kidney biopsy
c. > 10% plasmocytosis
d. Rouleaux formation in blood

167. Lymphoplasmacytoid lymphomas may be associated with *(AIPGMEE 10)*
a. IgG   b. IgM
c. IgA   d. IgE

168. Which of the following is not a minor diagnostic criteria for multiple myeloma? *(AIIMS Nov 10, 08)*
a. Lytic bone lesions
b. Plasmacytosis greater than 20%
c. Plasmacytoma on biopsy
d. Monoclonal globulin spike on serum electrophoresis of> 2.5 *g/dl* for IgG, > 1.5 g/dl for IgA

169. Not a feature of multiple myeloma *(AIIMS May 05)* *(WB PG 2016)*
a. Hypercalcemia
b. Anemia
c. Hyperviscosity
d. Elevated alkaline phosphatase

CHRONIC MYELOPROLIFERATIVE NEOPLASMS

170. True about BCR-ABL 'traits' are all except? *(JIPMER 18)*
a. P190 has an indolent course
b. P190 is a bad prognostic factor
c. P230 is positive in chronic neutrophilc leukemia
d. P230 has an indolent course

171. A 40-year-old woman is on treatment for CLL. Over the past few months she noticed swellings in the neck and axilla which was rapidly increasing in size. She complains of feeling feverish and experiences weight loss. Which of the following is responsible? *(JIPMER 18)*
a. Richter transformation
b. Progression of CLL
c. EBV infection
d. Immunodeficient hemolytic anemia
e. MHC non-expression

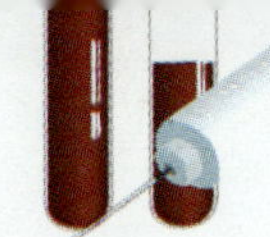

172. A 60-year-old male living in hilly area has Hb of 16 gm% ,TC 21000/ul. DLC showed metamyelocytes and myelocytes 40%, N25% L40%, E5%. Platelet count 3.25 lakh/u. He presented with hypertension and on examination, spleen was just palpable below costal margin. What is the next step?   *(AIIMS Nov 2017)*
   a. Bone marrow with reticulin stain
   b. JAK STAT mutation assessment
   c. Philadelphia chromosome
   d. Erythropoietin levels

173. 45/m presented with leuko-erythroblastic blood picture with dacrocytes. What is bone marrow finding?
   a. Fatty degeneration with erythroid cell hyperplasia with megakaryocytes   *(JIPMER 2017)*
   b. Abundant fat cells
   c. Focal cellular marrow with hypocellular areas and atypical megakaryocytes.
   d. Hypercellular marrow with prominent blasts

174. Which of the following statements is true regarding juvenile chronic myeloid leukemia?
          (Recent Question 2016-17)
   a. Philadelphia chromosome is negative.
   b. Thrombocytopaenia is uncommon.
   c. The prognosis is better than the adult form of chronic myeloid leukemia.
   d. Single agent chemotherapy with busulfan or hydroxyurea can achieve remission.

175. Robertsonian translocation is seen in?
          (Recent Question 2016)
   a. AML   b. CML
   c. ALL   d. CLL

176. True about Robertsonian translocation is?
          (Recent Question 2016)
   a. Acrocentric chromosome involved
   b. Balanced translocation
   c. Large part is lost   d. Poor prognosis

177. Which of the following is not a characteristic feature of Myelodysplastic syndrome?   *(Recent Question 2015)*
   a. Leucoerythroblastic blood picture
   b. Pawn ball megakaryocytes
   c. Pseudo pelger heut cells
   d. Transformation to AML

178. The following is true regarding polycythermia vera ?
   a. Raised ESR   *(Recent Question 2015)*
   b. Decrease LAP score
   c. Thrombocytopenia   d. Leukocytosis

179. Best investigation for BCR-ABL *(Recent Question 2015)*
   a. Flow cytometry
   b. Fluorescent in situ hybridization
   c. EISA
   d. Polymerase chain reaction

180. Hyposegmented neutrophils are seen in
   a. Megaloblastic anemia   *(Recent Question 2015)*
   b. Sideroblastic anemia
   c. Accelerated phase of CML
   d. Blast crisis phase of CML

181. Erythromelalgia is polycythemia vera is a complication of   *(Recent Question 2015)*
   a. Erythrocytosis   b. Thrombocytosis
   c. Granulocytosis   d. Lymphocytosis

182. Treatment of choice for CML   *(Recent Question 2015)*
   a. Sorafenib   b. Imatinib mesylate
   c. Sunitinib   d. Erlotinib

183. Not seen in polycythemia vera   *(Recent Question 2015)*
   a. Platelet function abnormalities
   b. Normal red cell morphology
   c. Abnormal oxygen saturation
   d. Low ESR

184. Which of the following is NOT commonly seen in poly-cythemia vera ?   *(MH 16)*
   a. Thrombosis
   b. Hyperuricemia
   c. Prone for Acute Leukemia
   d. Spontaneous severe infection

185. Not seen in essential thrombocytosis
          (Recent Question 2015)
   a. Activating mutation in JAK2 gene
   b. Abnormally large platelets
   c. Erythromelagia   d. Marrow fibrosis

186. Triad of leukoerythroblastosis, tear drop erythrocytes and large platelets is seen in   *(Recent Question 2015)*
   a. Essential thrombocytosis
   b. Primary myelofibrosis
   c. Myelodysplastic syndrome
   d. Langerhan cell histiocytosis

187. False regarding myelodysplastic syndromes
          (Recent Question 2015)
   a. Hypercellular bone marrow
   b. Increased neutrophil alkaline phosphastase
   c. Ringed sideroblasts
   d. Pawn ball megakaryocytes

188. Mutation seen in systemic mastocytosis
          (Recent Question 2015)
   a. FGFR1 fusion genes   b. BCR-ABL fusion gene
   c. JAK 2 point mutation   d. c-kit point mutation

189. Leukocyte alkaline phosphatase score is decreased in
   a. Pregnancy   *(Recent Question 2015)*
   b. Polycythemia vera
   c. Infections
   d. Myelodysplastic syndrome

190. Highest LAP score is seen in?   *(Recent Question 2015)*
   a. Acute Myeloid Leukemia
   b. Polycythemia Vera
   c. Chronic myeloid Leukemia
   d. Paroxysmal Nocturnal Hemoglobinuria

191. Dwarf megakaryocytes with unilobed nucleus is char-acteristic of   *(Recent Question 2015)*
   a. Myelodysplastic syndrome
   b. Essential thrombocytosis
   c. Chronic myeloid leukemia
   d. Polycythemia vera

192. 45/m presents with leukoerythroblastic blood picture in PBS with drytap, What is your diagnosis?
          (Recent Question 2015)
   a. AML   b. CML
   c. ALL   d. Myelofibrosis

193. BCR-ABL fusion gene is detected by?
          (Recent Question 2015)
   a. Flow cytometry   b. FISH
   c. Karyotyping   d. RT-PCR

194. **All are true about Polycythemia vera except-**
(Recent Question 2014, AIIMS 01)
a. Increased vit B$_{12}$
b. Decreased LAP score
c. Leucocytosis
d. Increased platelets

195. **Bone marrow finding in myelofibrosis-**
(Recent Question 2014)
a. Dry tap (hypocellular)
b. Megaloblastic cells
c. Microcytic cells
d. Thrombocytosis

196. **Pseudo-Pelger-Huet cells are seen in-**
a. Hairy cell leukemia   *(Recent Question 2014, 2013)*
b. Multiple myeloma
c. Myelodysplastic syndrome
d. Hodgkin's lymphoma

197. **Polycythemia is not caused by-**   *(Recent Question 2014)*
a. Renal carcinoma
b. Liver carcinoma
c. Cerebellar hemangioma
d. Lung carcinoma

198. **Which of the following is not a myeloproliferative disease**   *(Recent Question 2014)*
a. Polycythemia vers
b. Acute myeloid leukemia
c. Chronic myeloid leukemia
d. Essential thrombocytosis

199. **In patients with Chronic Myeloid Leukemia**
(AP PGMEE 14)
a. ABL gene on Chr. 22 is trans-located to BCR gene on Chr.9
b. The fusion gene bcr-abl forms a protein with tyrosine kinase activity
c. Splenomegaly is unusual
d. Philadelphia chromosome positive patients respond poorly to Imatinib

200. **Which of the following is not a chronic myeloproliferative disorder?**   *(AP PGMEE 14)*
a. Polycythemia vera
b. Myeloid metaplasia
c. CML
d. Essential thrombocytopenia

201. **About CML in children true is:**   *(AIIMS Nov 2013)*
a. Translocation between long arm of chr 9 and short arm of chr 22
b. Protein tyrosine kinase inhibitor are the drug of choice
c. Most commonly presents in blast crisis
d. 2nd most common malignancy

202. **Myelofibrosis leading to a dry tap on bone marrow aspiration is seen with which of the following condition?**
a. Burkitt's lymphoma   *(AIIMS May 2013)*
b. Acute erythroleukemia
c. Acute Megakaryocytic Leukemia
d. Acute Myelomonocytic Leukemia

203. **In myelodysplastic syndrome, ring sideroblast is seen in:**   *(WB PG 2011)*
a. Mitochondria
b. Golgi body
c. Nuclear membrane
d. ER

HEAVY CHAIN DISEASES

204. **Palatal edema is significant for?**   *(JIPMER 18)*
a. Alpha heavy chain disease
b. Gamma heavy chain disease
c. Mu chain disease
d. Beta heavy chain disease

LCH

205. **Which of the following cell is seen in LCH?**
a. Eosinophil   *(Recent Question 2016-17)*
b. Basophils
c. Neutrophil
d. Langerhans cell

206. **In Langerhans Cell Histiocytosis, the characteristic abnormality seen is**   *(AIIMS May 2015)*
a. Birbecks granules
b. Macrophages
c. Plasma cell
d. Giant cell

207. **Langerhans cell shows which of these?**
(Recent Question 2015)
a. Badminton racquet appearance
b. CD 100a
c. MPO +
d. Birbeck's granules

208. **Localised langerhans cells histiocytosis affecting head & neck is -**   *(Recent Question 2014)*
a. Letterer-siwe disease
b. Pulmonary langerhans cell histiocytosis
c. Hand-schuller-christian disease
d. Eosinophilic granuloma

209. **CD marker for Langerhans cell histiocytosis is?**
(Recent Question 2013, DNB Aug 12)
a. CD 17
b. CD 23
c. CD la
d. CD 117

210. **About Pulmonary Langerhans cell histiocytosis, all are true EXCEPT:**   *(WB PG 2012)*
a. Associated with smoking
b. Pneumothorax in 10% cases
c. 20-40 years male predominance
d. Corticosteroids have role in treatment

Answers with Explanations

1.   Ans. (b)   Castleman disease

Based on clinical presentation, Castleman disease has been divided into a solitary and a multicentric form. The solitary form presents as a mass located most commonly in the mediastinum, neck, lung, axilla, mesentery, broad ligament, retroperitoneum, and several other sites. Grossly, it is round, well circumscribed, with a solid gray cut surface and can measure 15 cm or more in diameter. The follicles show marked vascular proliferation and hyalinization of their abnormal or atrophic germinal centers, surrounded by concentrically arranged small lymphocytes imparting an 'onion-skin' pattern .

Remember angiolymphoid hyperplasia shows thick walled blood vessels with prominent endothelial cells and inflammatory eosinophilia infiltrates.

2.   Ans. (d)   Adult T cell leukemia

HHV 8 is associated with
- Castleman disease
- Primary effusion lymphoma
- Kaposi sarcoma

3.   Ans. (a)   Mantle zone *(Ref: R 9/p 583)*

A normal lymph node has 2 areas: Cortex → Lymphoid follicles and paracortical areas, Medulla → predominantly blood vessels

Structures in a Follicle

- **Germinal center:** Round/oval zone containing pale staining cells, surrounded by darker cells
- **Mantle zone:** Small dark coloured unchallenged B cells surrounding pale staining germinal centers
- **Marginal zone:** Light zone surrounding follicles; contains postfollicular memory B cells derived after stimulation of recirculating cells from T cell dependent antigen; named "marginal cells" due to location

4.   Ans. (a)   May heggalin anomaly

May-Hegglin anomaly (MHA) is an autosomal dominant disorder characterized by thrombocytopenia, giant platelets containing few granules; and large, well-defined, basophilic, cytoplasmic inclusion bodies in granulocytes that resemble Döhle bodies

5.   Ans. (c)   C

(Ref: Wintrobes 13th ed. Pg. 303; Wintrobes Atlas)

Key to the figure:
- A: Lymphocyte
- B: Neutrophil
- C: Eosinophil
- D: Basophil

Eosinophils are increased in parasitic infection

6.   Ans. (c)   Plasma cell *(Ref: Wintrobes 13th ed. Pg. 303; Wintrobes Atlas)*

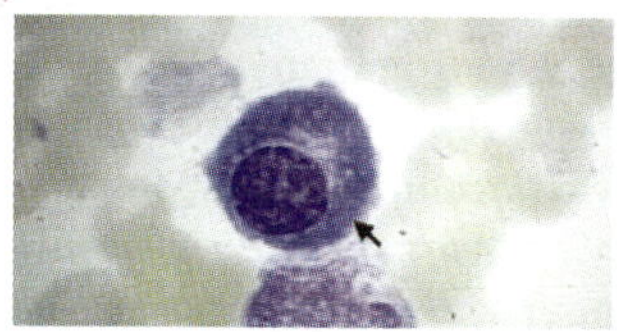

Plasma cells are spherical or ellipsoid and range from 5 to 30 μm in size. The cytoplasm is abundant & basophilic (deep blue); with a well-defined perinuclear clear zone that contains Golgi apparatus.

7.   Ans. (d)   Platelet count of <40000/ul is contraindication

(Ref: Dacie Practical Hematology 10th ed/ pg 163)

The given image is of **Jamshedi Bone marrow biopsy needle.** Most are **14 to 18 gauge;**

In most of the situations where bone marrow aspiration is indicated (eg suspected Acute Leukemia, thrombocytopenia is usually present; So, platelet count of < 40,000/uL is not a contraindication to bone marrow aspiration

8.   Ans. (a)   Measles

9.   Ans. (a)   Bone marrow examination

(Ref: Dacie Practical Hematology, 10thed/163; Complete review of Pathology 1st/761)

This is a Sahli's bone marrow aspiration needle. (Sahli's needle has a Screw on the side; S for S)

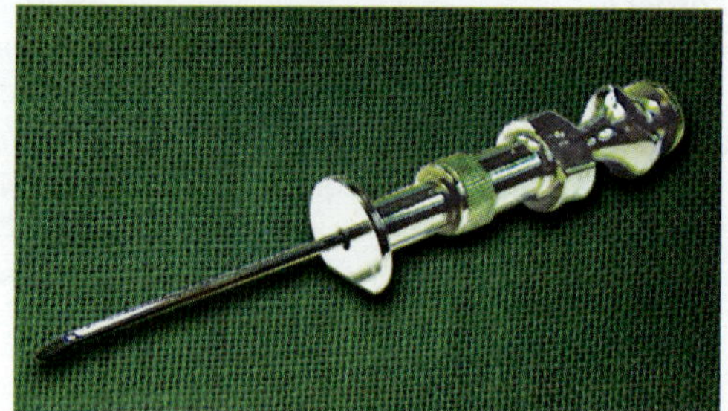

Klima's bone marrow aspiration needle (no side screw)

10.   Ans. (a)   CD8 *(Ref: Robbins 9th/pg 590; 8th/pg 600)*

11.   Ans. (d)   CD46 *(Ref: Wintrobes 12th/pg 2523)*

CD46 (Complement Membrane Cofactor Protein): It is a receptor to a number of pathogens, such as herpes virus 6, M protein of group A streptococci, Neisseria gonorrhoeae, and Escherichia coli.

12.   Ans. (a)   Less than 500/ul *(Ref: Robbins 9th/pg 583)*

Serious infections are most likely when the neutrophil count falls below 500 per mm3.

13.   Ans. (c)   Stronglyoides

(Ref: Robbins 9th/pg 583 8th/pg 593)

Parasitic infestations: Ascariasis, **Hookworm, Strongyloides,** Filariasis, Trichinosis can cause eosinophillia

| 14. | Ans. (a) **Pro erythroblast** (*Ref: Robbins 9th/pg 580-581*) |

| 15. | Ans. (d) **Dohle bodies** |

(*Ref: Robbins 9th/pg 583 9th/pg 593*)

In sepsis or severe inflammatory disorders, there can be morphologic changes in the neutrophils:

- Cytoplasmic vacuoles
- *Toxic granules*
- *Döhle bodies*

| 16. | Ans. (a) **Tibia** (*Ref: Wintrobe's 12th/pg 10*) |

Iliac crest[Q] is the **most common** site for **bone marrow sampling overall in adults**, while in children it is Anterior medial **tibial**[Q] area, below tibial tuberosity

| 17. | Ans. (a) **May Hegglin anomaly** |

(*Ref: Wintrobe's 12th/pg 1549*)

- Anemia with thrombocytopenia & inclusions in neutrophils is suggestive of May Hegglin anomaly
- **Evan syndrome:** Autoimmune hemolytic Anemia with thrombocytopenia

| 18. | Ans. (b, d, e); b. CD 10; d. CD19; e. CD20 |

(*Ref: Robbins 9th/pg 590; 8th/pg 600*)

| 19. | Ans. (a) **CD 19p** |

(*Ref: Robbins 9th/pg 590; 8th/pg 600; Wintrobe's 12th/pg 2504*)

CD19 is the pan B cell marker; Since it is present on Chr 16p, so the best suitable answer here is CD 19p

| 20. | Ans. (a) **B-cells** (*Ref: Wintrobe's 12th/pg 1589-1593*) |

Pathogenesis of Infectious Mononucleosis: Caused by Ebstein Barr Virus (**EBV**)[Q] **infection**

- **Entry** of EBV in the **oral cavity**[Q]
- EBV initially **infects oral epithelial cells** à symptoms of **pharyngitis.**[Q]
- **Intracellular**[Q] **viral replication** and cell lysis with **release of new virions**
- Virus **spreads to contiguous structures** such as the **salivary glands**[Q]
- Eventual **viremia** & **infection of B lymphocytes**[Q] in the peripheral blood & entire lymphoreticular system, including **liver & spleen**.
- **DOWNY cells** are **atypical CD8+ T lymphocytes** that are characteristic of infectious mononucleosis[Q]
- DOWNY cells exhibit **both suppressor & cytotoxic**[Q] functions that develop **in response to the infected B lymphocytes.**

| 21. | Ans. (b) **2000 to 5000 cells/microliter** |

(*Ref: Medscape (http://emedicine.medscape.com/article/329614-overview)*)

The peripheral blood eosinophil count in Eosinophilia-myalgia syndrome is usually **2000 to 5000 cells/microliter**

CDC definition of 'Eosinophilia-myalagia syndrome'

- Incapacitating myalgias,
- Blood **eosinophil count greater than 1000** cells/µl, and
- **No evidence of infection** (eg, trichinosis) **or neoplastic** conditions that could account for these findings.

| 22. | Ans. (a) **RBC** (*Ref: Robbins 9th/pg 580-581*) |

- **Myeloid cells** are WBCs like **neutrophils, monocytes, Basophils, RBCs and Platelets**.
- **Lymphoid cells** include **B-Lymphocyte, T-lymphocyte and NK cells**.

So following injection of myeloid series cells, RBCs will be released into peripheral blood.

| 23. | Ans. (b) **Myoblast Progenitor cells** |

(*Ref: Robbins 9th/pg 580-581*)

- Endothelial Progenitor cells, Mesenchymal stem cells and Hematopoetic stem cells are found in the bone marrow.
- Mesenchymal stem cells are multipotent stromal cells constituting 0.001-0.01% of bone marrow cells.

| 24. | Ans. (a) **CD 45** |

(*Ref: Robbins 9th/pg 590; 8th/pg 600; Wintrobe's 12th/pg 2522*)

CD 45

- Found in all hematopoietic cells except erythrocytes.
- CD45 plays an essential role in lymphocyte activation.
- Peripheral blood naïve T cells are CD45RA, whereas memory (activated) T cells are CD45RO+

| 25. | Ans. (b) **Kikuchi disease** |

(*Ref: Rheumatology: Diagnosis and Therapeutics; Edited by John J. Cush, Arthur Kavanaugh, Charles Michael Stein; Lippincott Williams & Wilkins, 2005; pg 228*)

Kikuchi Disease

- **Kikuchi-Fujimoto disease or histiocytic necrotizing lymphadenitis** is a **benign**, rare disorder that affects young women (more so than men) with **recurrent necrotizing lymphadenitis.**
- MC involves **cervical region, Histology:** Zone of **necrosis** surrounded by blast-like plasmacytoid lymphocytes

| 26. | Ans. (a) **Kimura's disease** |

(*Ref: Ioachim's Lymph Node Pathology. Harry L. Ioachim, L. Jeffrey Medeiros; Lippincott Williams & Wilkins, 2009. Pg 190*)

Kimura's Disease

- **Eosinophilic abscess in lymph node is seen**
- A chronic inflammatory disorder involving subcutaneous tissue & lymph nodes predominantly in the head & neck region & is characterized by **angiolymphoid proliferation & eosinophilia**
- **in Kimura disease, salivary gland involvement, Glomerulonephritis, Nephrotic syndrome, Eosinophilia & increased IgE are more common than in Kikuchi disease**

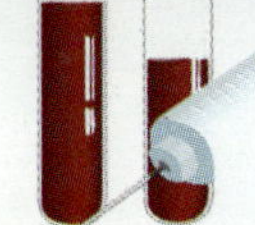

- Angiolymphoid hyperplasia with eosinophilia (ALHE), owing to some histologic similarities, can be confused with or mistaken for an early stage of *Kimura disease*.

27. **Ans. (d) CD34** *(Ref: Robbins 9th/pg 590; 8th/pg 600)*

28. **Ans. (b) ALL with hyperploidy**

All with hyperploidy is known terminology
Provisional entities in new WHO classification

Leukemia	Provisional entities
AML	AML with BCR-ABL-1 AML with mutated RUNX$_1$
ALL	Early T cell precursor ALL

29. **Ans. (a) Cytokeratin**

A mediastenal mass has a differential of thymoma and T cell ALL. T –ALL will have the markers TDT (Lymphoblast), CD 1a & CD3. Thymoma has 2 components epithelial and lymphoid component so is positive for EMA, **cytokeratin 7 & 20**, CD57 CD5, bcl-2, calretinin, vimentin, **CD3**, CD1a, CD20, CD99 and Ki67 & **TdT**.

30. **Ans. (b) Peripheral smear**

Myeloid (granulocytic) sarcoma, or myeloblastoma are extramedullary blast proliferation.These tumors are called chloromas because some appear green or turn green in dilute acid secondary to expression of MPO. The tumors are usually localized; they often involve bone, periosteum, soft tissues, lymph nodes, or skin. Common sites are the orbit and the paranasal sinuses.

The diagnosis can be made if Auer rods are detected on blasts in peripheral smear or if myeloid origin is confirmed by cytochemical or immunohistochemical methods . The diagnosis should be suspected if eosinophilic myelocytes are present in hematoxylin and eosin–stained biopsy sections. Imprint preparations can be helpful.

31. **Ans. (c) PAX5** *(Ref: R 9/ p 590)*

PAX-5 is a B Cell marker.

32. **Ans. (a) ALL** *(Ref: R 9/ 611)*

- The picture is that of a lymphoblast. Lymphoblasts will be 3-4x larger than a mature RBC, High nuclear to cytoplasmic ratio, Round Nucleus with immature chromatin (not clumped), Prominent nucleoli, Cytoplasm is scant, light blue and lacks granules

33. **Ans. (b) Hyperdiploidy**

34. **Ans. (b) Leukemia**

(Ref: Wintrobes 13/p 734)

Autologous stem cell support after myeloablative therapy has been successful for treatment of acute myelogenous leukemia (AML), non-Hodgkin lymphoma, and Hodgkin disease

35. **Ans. (b) t(15:17)**

36. **Ans. (a, d) a. Hyperploidy; d. Response to treatment**

(Ref: Robbin's 9th/ 590-592; Complete review of Pathology 1ˢᵗ/280)

Discussing options one by one:

- Hyperploidy	**Intermediate prognosis; can be considered good**
- **Organomegaly**	L. Node, liver, spleen enlargement, Testicular enlargement → poor prognosis
- **TLC more than 50000/ul**	Poor prognosis; TLC <10,000/ul has good prognosis
- **Response to treatment**	Early response to treatment is a good prognostic factor but non responsive is a poor prognostic factor

The best answer suited here is Response to treatment > *hyperploidy as remission status at 14 days is the best guide to prognosis; and so the best prognostic factor.*

37. **Ans. (a) Acute Myeloid Leukemia**

(Ref: Robbins 9th/pg 612 8th/622)

38. **Ans. (a) tdT positive** *(Ref: Robbins 9th/pg 590)*

39. **Ans. (a) Neutrophils** *(Ref: Robbins 9th/pg 583/ 8th/593)*

40. **Ans. (c) HTLV is a cause in immunodeficient patients**

(Ref: Robbins 9th/pg 239-242)

EBV rather than HTLV-1 is implicated in HLH

41. **Ans. (a) Myeloperoxidase** *(Ref: Robbins 9th/pg 612; 8th/622)*

CD117 is a Myeloid series marker
- *Granulocytic(Myeloid) sarcoma, or Myeloblastoma, is an extramedullary tumor*
- Also called **chloromas** because some appear/turn green in dilute acid secondary to expression of MPO
- Usually localized; often involve bone, periosteum, soft tissues, lymph nodes, or skin.
- Common sites are the **orbit ¶nasal sinuses;**
- Can involve GIT, genitourinary tract, breast, cervix, salivary glands, mediastinum, pleura, peritoneum & bile duct

42. **Ans. (d) M7** *(Ref: Robbins 9th/pg 612; 8th/622)*

43. **Ans. (a) Age >10 years** *(Ref: Robbins 9th/pg 590-592)*

44. **Ans. (a) Rituximab** *(Ref: Robbins 9th/pg 590-592)*

45. **Ans. (a) Pre-B cell ALL** *(Ref: Robbins 9th/pg 590-592)*

46. **Ans. (b) Leukemia** *(Ref: Robbins 9th/pg 612; 8th/622)*

47. **Ans. (c) Auer Rod** *(Ref: Robbins 9th/pg 590-592)*

48. **Ans. (d)** **Presence of t (9;22)**

(Ref: Robbins 9th/pg 590-592)

49. **Ans. (a)** **Acute myelogenous leukemia**

(Ref: Robbins 9th/pg 590-592)

The peripheral smear shows myeloblasts having **delicate nuclear chromatin**, 2-4 nucleoli, and moderate cytoplasm. One of them shows Auer rods. So it is a case of AML.

50. **Ans. (d)** **t(12;21)** *(Ref: Robbins 9th/pg 612; 8th/pg 622)*

AML with $t(8;21)^Q$ in V 16 and t(15, 17) have Favorable Prognosis

51. **Ans. (a)** **ALL**

(Ref: Robbins 9th/pg 590-592)

52. **Ans. (d)** **M4** *(Ref: Robbins 9th/pg 612; 8th/pg 622)*

- AML causing **gum hypertrophy** are AML-**M5,M4**
- AML causing **extramedullary blast proliferations (Chloromas)** are AML **M2, M4, M5**
- AML causing blast infiltrations in skin (leukemia cutis) are AML **M5, M4**

53. **Ans. (b)** **Promyelocytic (M3)**

(Ref: Robbins 9th/pg 612; 8th/pg 622)

Acute Promyelocytic Leukemic (APML, M3) cells can induce **Disseminated intravascular coagulation (DIC)**

54. **Ans. (a)** **AML** *(Ref: Robbins 9th/pg 612; 8th/pg 622)*

This **40 yr old** female is presenting with **leukocytosis and increased blast counts** in the peripheral smear. The cytogenetic study done here shows **t(8;21)**. This finding is **suggestive of Acute myeloid leukemia even if there are <20% blast counts.**

- It cytogenetic abnormalities like **t(15;17), t(8;21), inv(16)** are encountered in a patient with symptomatic myeloid disease, **AML should be diagnosed despite the lower blast percent.**

55. **Ans. (c)** **Pre B ALL** *(Ref: Robbins 9th/pg 590-592)*

56. **Ans. (a)** **Peak incidence of Chronic myeloid leukemia is in the fifth to sixth decades of life**

(Ref: Robbins 9th/pg 590-592, 616-618

Discussing the options one by one,

a.	True
b.	False; **Prognosis** is **worse for those > 50 yrs** age & those with **a Hb level <10 g/dL** & white cell counts $<2 \times 10^9$/L
c.	False; ALL in children < 1 yr & >10 yrs has poor prognosis
d.	False; **Median age at diagnosis of CLL is 60 years**

57. **Ans. (d)** **Mixed phenotypic acute leukemia**

(Ref: WHO Classification of Hemato-Lymphoid Tumors, 4th edition, 2008, pg 150)

The child has severe Anemia & Leukocytosis with blasts on peripheral smear. So this is a case of leukemia.

Immunophenotyping suggests:

Immunophenotype	Lineage
CD 10(+)ve,	B-Cell marker
CD 19 (+)ve,	B-Cell marker (most specific)
CD 117 (+) ve,	Myeloid Cell marker
MPO (+) ve	Myeloid Cell marker (most specific)
CD 33(-)ve	Myeloid Cell marker

As both B-cell and myeloid lineages are positive, this is a case of Mixed phenotypic acute leukemia (MPAL).

58. **Ans. (b)** **Paroxysmal cold hemoglobinuria**

(Ref: Wintrobe's 12th/pg chap 78)

- Paroxysmal nocturnal hemoglobinuria (PNH), Aplastic anemia & Myelodysplastic syndrome predispose to Leukemia

59. **Ans. (a)** **CNS** *(Ref: Harrison 18th/pg Chapter 189)*

Lymphoma in HIV

- **90% of lymphomas in HIV** are **B cell** in phenotype; more than half contain **EBV DNA**.
- *Immunoblastic lymphomas* account for **60% of the cases** of lymphoma in patients with AIDS.
- *Primary CNS lymphoma* accounts for **20%** of the cases of lymphoma in patients with HIV infection.
- **Most common extranodal site involved in Lymphoma in HIV is the CNS**, which is involved in one-third of all patients with lymphoma.

60. **Ans. (c)** **Presence of testicular involvement at presentation**

(Ref: Robbins 9th/pg 590-592;8th/pg600-603)

61. **Ans. (c)** **Lymphocyte predominant**

(Ref: Robbins 9th ed p 608)

Lymphohistiocytic variants (L&H cells) with polypoid nuclei, inconspicuous nucleoli, and moderately abundant cytoplasm are characteristic of the lymphocyte predominance subtype Hodgkin lymphoma.

62. **Ans. (a)** **NLPHL** *(Ref: R 9/p 606)*

This is classical description of NLPHL. (Nodular lymphocyte predominant Hodgkin lymphoma)

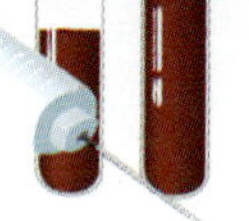

63. Ans. (b, d) **b. DLBCL is most common in India; d. Burkitts lymphoma arises from Germinal centre**

(Ref: Robbins 9th/pg 602-603)

About other options,

a. Mantle cell lymphoma arises from mantle layer & not germinal centre

c. CD 5, CD 3 & CD 8 are T cell markers

64. Ans. (a) **a. If Imatinib not working then Dasatinib can be used; b. BCR-ABL activates tyrosine kinase**

(Ref: Dacie Practical Hematology, 10th ed/163; Robbins 9th/pg 616-618)

Note: Bone marrow aspirate/biopsy is used for staging of CML & is not an essential criteria for diagnosis; Blast crisis has > 20% blasts in bone marrow/peripheral smear

65. Ans. (a) **a. Lymphocyte predominant HD**

(Ref: Robbins 9th/pg 325)

EBV is associated with Plasmablastic lymphoma, Nasopharyngeal carcinoma & Mixed cellularity Hodgkin disease

66. Ans. (a, c, d, e) **a. Often localized to single axial group of lymph node; c. Contiguous spread of lymph node d. Can be cured by chemotherapy & radiotherapy e. Commonly presents with painless lymphadenopathy**

(Ref: Harrison 19th/708-09; Robbins(SAE) 9th/607,610-11; Oxford Textbook of Haematology 2nd/211; CMDT 2016/ 530-31; Ref: Harrisons 19e/ pg 700

In stage E of Hodgkin Lymphoma (Ann Arbor staging), localized, solitary involvement of extralymphatic tissue, excluding liver and bone marrow is seen; So hepatomegaly may not be always present in Hodgkin disease.

67. Ans. (a, b, e) **a. Anaplastic large cell lymphoma; b. Embryonal cell carcinoma; e. Hodgkin's lymphoma**

(Ref: Robbins (SAE) 9th/590,605)

68. Ans. (a) **Hodgkins lymphoma**

(Ref: Robbins 9th/pg 606-611)

69. Ans. (a, c, d, e) **a. Nodular sclerosis; c. Lymphocyte rich; d. Mixed cellularity; e. Lymphocyte depletion**

70. Ans. (d) **Lymphocyte predominance**

(Ref: Robbins 9th/pg 606-611/ 8th pg 616-621)

Lymphocyte predominance is CD20+, CD15-, CD30-;

71. Ans. (d) **Hodgkin Lymphona: EBV and Ree Sternberg cell** *(Ref: Robbins 9th/pg 606-611/ 8th pg 616-621)*

Figure show binucleated R-S cell seen in hodgkin lymphona

72. Ans. (d) **Overexpression of BCl-6** *(Ref: R 9th/pg 606-611)*

73. Ans. (b) **Mixed cellularity** *(Ref: Robbins 9th/pg 606-611)*

74. Ans. (a) **Nodular sclerosis** *(Ref: R 9th/pg 606-611)*

75. Ans. (b) **Chronic myeloid leukemia**

(Ref: Robbins 9th/pg)

Sea-blue–colored histiocytes: Results from increased cell death and subsequent deposition of phospholipids in the macrophages in bone marrow.

Seen in: High rates of intramedullary cell death due to: *lipid storage diseases, myelodysplastic syndromes, lymphomas, chronic myelogenous leukemia, idiopathic thrombocytopenic purpura, autoimmune neutropenia, and β-thalassemia major.*

76. Ans. (d) **Lymphocyte predominance**

(Ref: Robbins 9th/pg 606-611)

77. Ans. (b) **II-B**

(Ref: Robbins 9th/pg 606-611/ 8th pg 616-621)

Involvement of **two or more lymph node** regions on the **same side of diaphragm** alone (II) or localized involvement of an extra-lymphatic organ or site (IIE).

Presence of (B) symptoms:[Q]

- Unexplained fever,
- Drenching night sweats, and/or
- Unexplained weight loss > 10%

78. Ans. (a, b, c, d, e); **a. Axial lymphnadenopathy; b. hepatomegaly is common; c. Contiguous spread of lymph node; d. Can be cured by chemotherapy; e. An arbor classification is useful**

(Ref: Robbins 9th/pg 606-611)

79. Ans. (b) **Lymphocyte poor Hodgkins lymphoma**

(Ref: Robbins 9th/pg 606-611; 8th/pg 616-621)

Reticular variant of Reed Sternberg cell is found in Lymphocyte depletion of hodgkin's disease

80. Ans. (c) **Lymphocyte predominant Hodgkins lymphoma** *(Ref: Robbins 9th/pg 606-611)*

81. Ans. (a) **Mixed cellularity Hodgkin lymphoma**

(Ref: Robbins 9th/pg 606-611; 8th/pg 616-621)

In Mixed cellularity type, which is a **Classical Variety** of Hodgkin lymphoma, CD 15+/ CD30+

82. Ans. (b) **Ann Arbor Stage II is involvement of two or more lymph node groups on both sides of the diaphragm**

(Ref: Robbins 9th/pg 606-611; 8th/pg 616-621; Harrison 18th/ Chapter 110)

- Affected lymph nodes become painful with alcohol ingestion: TRUE

- Ann Arbor Stage II is involvement of two or more lymph node groups on both sides of the diaphragm: FALSE, as it is involvement of **two or more lymph node** regions on the **same side of diaphragm.**
- 'B symptoms' are fever, night sweats and ≥ 10% weight loss in 6 months: TRUE
- ABVD regimen is standard line of treatment for Hodgkin disease: True

83. Ans. (a) Nodular sclerosis *(Ref: Robbins 9th/pg 606-611)*

- Binucleated owl shaped nuclei with clear vacuolated area refers to Lacunar cells.
- **Lacunar cells** are seen in the **nodular sclerosis** subtype of Hodgkin's disease
- Lacunar cells have delicate, folded, or multilobate nuclei and abundant pale cytoplasm that is often disrupted during the cutting of sections, leaving the nucleus sitting in an empty space (lacuna)

84. Ans. (a) Diffuse large B cell lymphoma

(Ref: Robbins 9th/pg 595-596; 8th/pg 606-607)

Most common Non Hodgkins lymphoma is Diffuse large B cell lymphoma

Diffuse large B cell lymphoma (DLBCL)

85. Ans. (d) Lymphocytes *(Ref: Robbins 9th/pg 592)*

Flow cytometry is done to detect surface molecules like CD markers on:

- **Lymphocytes** for the diagnosis of **chronic lymphoproliferative disorders**
- **Blasts** for diagnosis of **Acute Leukemias**

86. Ans. (a, d, e); a. Adult T cell lymphoma; d. Diffuse large B cell lymphoma; e. Infectious mononucleosis

(Ref: Wintrobe's 12th/pg 2312)

Reed-Sternberg cells are **not absolutely specific for HL** Reed Sternberg like cell are seen in

- Adult T cell lymphoma,
- Diffuse large B cell lymphoma &
- Infectious mononucleosis

EBV-infected B cells resembling Reed Sternberg cells are found in the lymph nodes of individuals with **infectious mononucleosis,** strongly suggesting that EBV-encoded proteins play a part in the remarkable metamorphosis of B cells into Reed-Sternberg cells.

87. Ans. (a) Young age *(Ref: Wintrobe's 12th/pg 2319)*

Involvement of stomach (stage IV disease), Lymphocyte depletion, Extranodal metastasis (stage IV disease), Large mediastinal mass & old age are some of the poor prognostic factors in HD

Poor prognostic factors for Hodgkin's lymphoma

- Albumin <4.0 g/dl, Hemoglobin <10.5 g/dl, Male sex, 45 years of age or more, Stage IV disease
- Leukocytosis at or above 15,000/mm³, Lymphocytopenia (lymphocytes ≤600/mm³ and/or <8% of TLC).

88. Ans. (a) Hodgkin's lymphoma *(Ref: R 9th/pg 606-611)*

Ann Arbor staging is used for Hodgkin's lymphoma staging;

89. Ans. (e) Has good prognosis

(Ref: Robbins 9th/pg 606-611; 8th/pg 616-621)

a. False, popcorn cells are present
b. False, it is CD 15 & CD 30 negative
c. False, because both B & T lymphocytes, plasma cells & eosinophils are present;
d. False, because it is EBV negative
e. True;

90. Ans. (a) CD 20 *(Ref: Robbins 9th/pg 606-611)*

91. Ans. (d) T lymphocyte

Mycosis fungoides, also known as **Alibert-Bazin syndrome** or granuloma fungoides, is the most common form of cutaneous T-cell lymphoma. It generally affects the skin, but may progress internally over time. Symptoms include rash, tumors, skin lesions, and itchy skin.

92. Ans. (b) Naive B cell *(Ref: Robbins 9e pg 593)*

93. Ans. (a) SOX11

WHO 2016 Hematolymphoid textbook.

Mantle Zone Lymphoma

- Positive stains - CD5, CD19 (strong), CD20 (strong), cyclin D1/BCL1 (variable nuclear staining since cells are at different stages of cell cycle) also CD22, CD43, CD79a, FMC7, surface IgM or IgD, kappa or lambda, BCL2
- SOX 11 positive in cyclin D1 negative mantle lymphoma.
- Negative stains - CD23, usually CD10; also BCL6, CD11c, TdT, T cell antigens

94. Ans. (c) EBV positive – DLBL

(Ref: Hematological malignancies, WHO. Page No. 223)

EBV positive DLBL	EBV positive muco-cutaneous ulcer (WHO 2016 entity
Immunocompetent	Immuno-compromised
Patients > 50 years old	30-50 years old
The cells are positive for CD20, CD79a, IRF4/MUM1 positive, EBV LMP1 and EBNA negative, CD15 negative. Background are predominantly T lymphocytes	B-cell immunophenotype with uniform expression of CD30, MUM1, PAX5, and OCT-2, and variable CD20, CD45, CD15, CD79a, and BCL-6 expression

We can rule out infectious mononucleosis as monospot test is positive and Hodgkins lymphoma as CD 15 is negative.

95. Ans. (a, b) a. Diffuse large B-cell lymphoma; b. Hodgkins lymphoma

PAX-5 is a B-cell differentiation including lymphoblasts (used as a novel pan B-cell marker); also seen in R-S cells in NLPHL (+) vs. classic HL (weak).

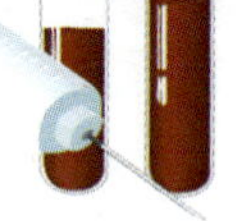

96. Ans. (a) **Hairy cell leukemia**

97. Ans. (c, d, e) c. **Gastric lymphoma; d. Thyroid lymphoma; e. Mycosis fungoides**

At least one quarter of non-Hodgkin's lymphomas (NHL) arise from tissue other than lymph nodes and even from sites which normally contain no lymphoid tissue. These forms are referred to as primary extranodal lymphomas. Gastrointestinal localizations, CNS, skin (Mycosis fungoidosis), thyroid, testis. Primary nodal NHL have presentation in lymph node, Waldeyer's ring, spleen or bone marrow

98. Ans. (c) **Hairy cell leukemia**

99. Ans. (d) **Translocation involving MYC gene**

(Ref: Robbins 9th/pg 597; 8th/607)

- Macrophages with abundant clear cytoplasm showing: characteristic **"starry sky" pattern** are seen in Burkitt lymphoma

100. Ans. (e) **Most common age group is pediatric**

(Ref: Robbins 9th/pg 593; 8th/pg 603)

Indications to treat in CLL are as follows:

- Rai stage 0–II disease in patients who are symptomatic, have progressive anemia/thrombocytopenia or lymphocytosis
- Rai stages III/IV
- Bulky or progressive lymphadenopathy or splenomegaly
- AIHA/ITP

101. Ans. (a) **Mantle cell lymphoma** *(Ref: R 9th/pg 602-603)*

102. Ans. (c) **Null cell lymphoma**

(Ref: Wintrobe's 12thed/pg 2169)

Features of Anaplastic large cell lymphoma (ALCL):

- ALK rearrangements present
- CD30+
- t(2;5) seen but t(1;2) is most common.
- Because the variants are of **T- or null-cell origin** and occur in a similar age group as the t(2;5): they are also called ALKoma

103. Ans. (c) **Mantle cell lymphoma** *(Ref: R 9th/pg 602-603)*

104. Ans. (b) **Lymphocyte rich HL** *(Ref: R 9th/pg 597)*

105. Ans. (d) **Bone - marrow involvement in early phase**

(Ref: Robbins 9th/pg 608)

106. Ans. (a) **All are associated with EBV infection**

(Ref: Robbins 9th/pg 591; 8th/pg 691)

107. Ans. (d) **ALK positive tumors carry worst prognosis**

(Ref: Robbins 9th/pg 605; 8th/615)

Anaplastic Large-Cell Lymphoma (ALK Positive)

- **Defined by the presence of rearrangements in the ALK gene on chromosome 2p23**→ break the *ALK* locus → formation of chimeric genes encoding ALK fusion proteins à Activate tyrosine kinases à trigger **JAK/STAT pathway**
- Typically composed of **large anaplastic cells**, with **horseshoe-shaped nuclei & voluminous cytoplasm (so-called hallmark cells)**
- Tumor cells cluster about venules& infiltrate lymphoid sinuses, **mimicking a metastatic carcinoma**.
- **Detection of ALK protein in tumor cells is a reliable indicator of an *ALK* gene rearrangement** as ALK is not expressed in normal lymphocytes or other lymphomas
- **Have good prognosis**

108. Ans. (b) **Adult T cell leukemia** *(Ref: Robbins 9th/pg 605)*

109. Ans. (a) **Anaplastic large cell lymphoma**

(Ref: Robbins 9th/pg 591)

110. Ans. (b) **Adult T cell leukemia lymphoma**

(Ref: Robbins 9th/pg 591; 8th/pg 691)

111. Ans. (a) **CD5** *(Ref: Robbins 9th/pg 603; 8th/pg 613)*

- **MALT lymphomas** express **B-cell antigens (CD19 and CD20)&monotypic surface Ig (IgM** without IgD).
- **MALTomas** may be **CD43+** but lack other small B-cell lymphoma markers (CD5, CD10, CD23 &cyclin D1)

112. Ans. (c) **Small intestine**

(Ref: WHO Hemato-lymphoid Tumors 4thed 2008 pg 197-199)

Heavy chain disease (HCD) comprises of 3 rare B-cell neoplasms that produces monoclonal heavy chains (IgG, IgA, IgM) and no light chains.

Alpha HCD/IgA lymphoma

- Most common HCD
- Variant of extranodal marginal zone lymphoma
- Also called immunoproliferative small intestine disease (IPSID); Caused by **C. jejuni** infection
- **Site:** GIT: **small intestine (MC)** and mesenteric lymphnodes, gastric and colonic mucosa

113. Ans. (d) **Accessory spleen** *(Ref: Robbins 9th/pg)*

Accessory spleens or spleniculi are seen in

- Gastrosplenic ligament
- Lienorenal ligament
- Gastrophrenic ligament
- Greater omentum
- Broad ligament of uterus
- Spermatic cord.

114. Ans. (d) **CLL** *(Ref: Robbins 9th/pg 593; 8th/pg 603)*

CD5 +tumors are CLL and Mantle zone lymphoma.

115. Ans. (b) **Burkitt lymphoma** *(Ref: Robbins 9th/pg 597)*

116. Ans. (a) **t (11;14)** *(Ref: Robbins 9th/pg 597; 8th/pg 607)*

117. Ans. (a) Lymphadenopathy is the most common presentation *(Ref: Robbins 9th/pg 594; 8th/pg 604)*

118. Ans. (a, b, c) a. Most common leukemia in adult; b. Proliferation center is pathognomonic; c. massive splenomegaly *(Ref: Robbins 9th/pg 593)*

119. Ans. (a) Burkitts Lymphoma

(Ref: 9th/pg 597; 8th/pg 607)

120. Ans. (a) Anaplastic large cell lymphoma

(Ref: Robbins 9th/pg 605; 8th/pg 615)

121. Ans. (a) Hairy cell leukemia *(Ref: R 9th/pg 603-604)*

In the given scenario an elderly male presents with Anemia, Splenomegaly & Pancytopenia.

Discussing the options one by one:

- **Hairy cell Leukemia:** Chronic B-cell leukemia characterized by **hairy cells, pancytopenia and splenomegaly**[Q]
- **CML:** Massive splenomegaly with Basophilic Leukocytosis seen
- **Thalassemia:** Jaundice, severe anemia (requiring transfusion), hepatosplenomegaly with leukoerythroblastosis, usually presents in childhood
- **Follicular lymphoma:** Lymphadenopathy ± Leukocytosis

122. Ans. (a) CD23 *(Ref: Robbins 9th/pg 602-603)*

- CLL is positive for CD23;

123. Ans. (c) NK/T cell lymphoma

(Ref: Wintrobe's 12th/pg 2169)

Nasal NK/T lymphoma may present with facial swelling/destruction, so called **lethal midline granuloma** or **polymorphic reticulosis**. Occurs more commonly in **males**, with a median age of **50 to 55 years**.

124. Ans. (c) B-cell NHL *(Ref: Wintrobe's 12th/pg 2154)*

- Most common ocular lymphoma is B-cell NHL
- Most **orbital lymphomas** are of **B-cell origin** and are **low-grade**, particularly in the conjunctiva or eyelids, but can be a large B-cell lymphoma in the lacrimal gland or retrobulbar area.

125. Ans. (a) Mantle cell lymphoma

(Ref: Robbins 9th/pg 602-603; 8th/pg 612-613)

126. Ans. (b) Stomach *(Ref: Wintrobe's 12th/pg 2177)*

- Commonest site for **extranodal lymphoma is Stomach**
- **Gastrointestinal tract** is the **most common site for extranodal NHL (10 to 15%** of all NHL).
- **Stomach** accounts for 50% **of gastrointestinal lymphomas**

127. Ans. (a) BCL – 2 *(Ref: Robbins 9th/pg 594-595)*

- **BCL2 antagonizes apoptosis** and **promotes survival of follicular lymphoma cells.**
- **BCL stands for 'B Cell Lymphoma'**

128. Ans. (d) Chronic lymphocytic leukemia

(Ref: Robbins 9th/pg 593; 8th/pg 603; Wintrobe's 12th/pg 2214)

- **Unlike other leukemias, there is no firm evidence linking an occupational exposure or radiation with an increased incidence of CLL**

129. Ans. (a) Anaplastic large cell lymphoma (ALK positive)

(Ref: Robbins 9th/pg 605; 8th/pg 615)

Histological presence of "**Hallmark Cells**" with horse shoe-like or embryoid like nuclei and voluminous cytoplasm are seen in Anaplastic large cell lymphoma (ALK positive)

130. Ans. (b) Chronic lymphocytic leukemia

(Ref: Robbins 9th/pg 593; 8th/pg 603)

"Smudge cells"

- Also called '**Basket cells**', '**shadow cells of Gumprecht**'
- Caused by **decrease in Vimentin**
- May predict **good prognosis**
- Seen mainly in **CLL**; Also have been reported in **AML, CML, ALL** & in normal peripheral smear, but rare;

131. Ans. (c) CD20

(Ref: Robbins 9th/pg 597; 8th/pg 607)

132. Ans. (b) Peripheral blood Immunophenotyping

(Ref: Robbins 9th/pg 593-604; 8th/pg 613-614)

Most likely this is a case of **Non-Hodgkin Lymphoma with spill over in the peripheral blood.**
Hence, next investigation that should be done is **Immunophenotyping of Peripheral blood Lymphocytes**

133. Ans. (c) Leukocyte common antigen

(Ref: R 9th/pg 590)

Since Lymphoma arises from mature leukocytes, so **Lymphoma cells are positive for Leukocyte common antigen (CD45).**

134. Ans. (d, e) d. CD 23 positive; e. Centroblasts frequently seen

(Ref: Robbins 9th/pg 602-603; 8th/pg 612-613)

Discussing the options about Mantle cell lymphoma, one by one,

- Associated with t(11;14) translocation: TRUE, t(cyclin D1;Ig heavy chain)
- Overexpression of the BCL protein: TRUE, as Bcl2 is overexpressed
- CD 5 positive: TRUE
- **CD 23 positive: FALSE, It is CD 23 -ve**
- **Centroblasts frequently seen: FALSE, Centroblasts & centrocytes are seen in Follicular lymphoma**

135. Ans. (c) Burkitts Lymphoma *(Ref: Robbins 9th/pg 597)*

Lymphoma associated with **translocation of c-myc** is **Burkitt's Lymphoma**

136. Ans. (a) B cell *(Ref: Wintrobe's 12th/pg 2154)*

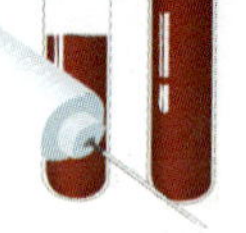

137. Ans. (d) Hemoglobin and albumin

(Ref: Wintrobe's 12th/pg 2154)

International prognostic index for lymphomas does not include Hemoglobin and albumin

Adverse Factor	Risk Group
Performance status ≥ 2	Low
LDH > normal	Low-intermediate
Extra-nodal sites ≥ 2	High-intermediate
Stage III / IV disease	High
Age > 60 years	High

138. Ans. (b, c, d, e) b. Primary small intestinal lymphoma are most commonly located in ileum; c. Lymphoma is most common primary malignant neoplasm of spleen; d. Stomach is most common site for extranodal lymphoma; e. MALT lymphoma is associated with H. pylori infection

(Ref: Wintrobe's 12th/pgs 12th ed -2152, Sternburg 1462-1464)

GIT involvement in NHL

- **Gastrointestinal tract** is the **most common extranodal site** of Lymphoma, at presentation
- Involved **in 10 to 15% of adults with NHL**.
- **Stomach** is most frequently involved (option D), followed by the **small intestine, the colon, and esophagus**.
- **H. pylori** play a role in the development of most **MALT lymphomas (option E)**
- **Abdominal pain** is the most common presenting symptom.
- Dyspepsia, nausea & early satiety, suggest stomach involvement.
- Gross appearance of low-grade lymphoma resemble **peptic ulcers**; others have **enlarged mucosal folds; flat and either hyperemic or normal mucosa may also be seen.**
- Patients with rectal involvement usually present with hematochezia or a change in bowel habits
- **Obstruction, intussusception, or perforation** are associated with **aggressive small bowel lymphomas**, particularly Burkitt lymphoma and intestinal T-cell lymphoma.
- **Ileum is the most common site (60%-65%) (option B)** involving **small intestine lymphoma** followed by jejunum (20%-25%), duodenum (6%-8%)
- **Mantle cell lymphoma** presents with **GI symptoms in 20 to 30%** of patients & **multiple polyposis**
- Lymphomatous polyposis of GIT is not restricted to MCL & is also seen in follicular lymphoma (FL) & MALToma (But this is a rare presentation)
- Abnormal histology in the gastrointestinal tract is found in >80% of MCL patients

For option C:

- Most common benign tumors of spleen: **Cavernous hemangioma**
- Most common malignant tumor of spleen: **lymphoma**

139. Ans. (c, e); c. Vasculitic syndromes; e. Erythema multiforme *(Ref: Robbins 9th/pg 603-604; 8th/pg 613-614)*

Features of hairy cell leukemia include splenomegaly, Hepatomegaly & Pancytopenia.

140. Ans. (a, b) a. Hairy cell leukemia; b. CML

(Ref: Harrison 18th/Chapter 59)

Diseases Associated with Massive Splenomegaly

- **Chronic myeloid leukemia**
- Lymphomas
- **Hairy cell leukemia**
- Myelofibrosis with myeloid metaplasia
- **Polycythemia vera**
- Gaucher's disease
- Chronic lymphocytic leukemia
- Sarcoidosis
- Autoimmune hemolytic anemia
- Diffuse splenic hemangiomatosis

141. Ans. (c) Atypical mycobacteria

(Ref: Robbins 9th/pg 603-604; 8th/pg 613-614)

Hairy cell leukemia is associated with Atypical Mycobacteria.

142. Ans. (b, e) b. Polycythemia; e. IgG paraprotein

143. Ans. (a) t (11 : 14)

144. Ans. (c) Post germinal centre B cell

145. Ans. (a) Multiple myeloma *(Ref: Robbins 9th ed p 599)*

Normal plasma cell ha e characteristic eccentrically placed nucleus. Malignant plasma cells have a perinuclear clearing due to a prominent Golgi apparatus and an eccentrically placed nucleus. Relatively normal-appearing plasma cells, plasma-blasts with vesicular nuclear chromatin and a prominent single nucleolus, or bizarre, multinucleated cells may predominate. Other cytologic variants stem from the dysregulated synthesis and secretion of Ig, which often leads to intracellular accumulation of intact or partially degraded protein. Such variants include flame cells with fiery red cytoplasm

146. Ans. (a, b, c, d, e) a. Cast nephropathy; b. amyloidosis; c. Cryoglobinemia; d. Interstitial nephritis; e. nephrocalcinosis *(Ref: Wintrobe 13/p 2377)*

Approximately 5% of myeloma gammaglobulins show reversible precipitation in the cold, so-called cryoglobulins, forming either a flocculent precipitate or a gel-like coagulum when the serum is cooled. The most common findings on autopsy include tubular atrophy and fibrosis (77%), tubular hyaline casts (62%), tubular epithelial giant cell reaction (48%), and nephrocalcinosis. Acute and chronic pyelonephritis can also be seen.

147. Ans. (b) Multiple myeloma *(Ref: R 9/ 595)*

Key to the image:1 → Increase in plasma cells in marrow, 2 → Kidney biopsy with pink deposits in glomerulus, 3 → Fibrils in electron microscope. So the diagnosis is **Multiple myeloma, probably AL amyloidosis of kidney**

148. Ans. (b) Waldenstrom Macroglobulinemia

MYD88 (L265P) mutation is detectable in all patients with Waldenström's macroglobulinemia, therefore representing a hallmark of the disease.

149. Ans. (c) Russell bodies (*Ref: Robbins 9th/pg 598-602*)

The globular inclusions in the plasma cells are referred to as **Russell bodies** (if cytoplasmic) or **Dutcher bodies** (if nuclear).

150. Ans. (b) Plasma Cells (*Ref: 9th/pg 598-602/8th 608-612*)

151. Ans. (d) Serum b2-microglobulin

(*Ref: Robbins 9th/pg 598-602/8th 608-612*)

β2-M concentration is the strongest and most reliable prognostic factor for multiple myeloma. It depends not only on tumor burden but also on renal function. Elevated β2-M values predict early death

152. Ans. (d) Dexamethasone

(*Ref: Robbins 9th/pg 598-602*)

153. Ans. (d) Does not progress to mutiple myeloma

(*Ref: Robbins 9th/pg 598-602/8th 608-612*)

1% monoclonal gammopathy of unknown significance progress to multiple myeloma /year

154. Ans. (a) IgM (*Ref: Robbins 9th/pg 598-602*)

155. Ans. (d) Bence jones proteinuria (*Ref: R 9th/pg 598-602*)

156. Ans. (a) Endocrinopathy (*Ref: Robbins 9th/pg 598-602*)

157. Ans. (d) Days to week (*Ref: Robbins 9th/pg 598-602*)

Life span of plasma cells is almost same as that of Memory lymphocytes (days to months or even years)

158. Ans. (d) Plasma cell (*Ref: Robbins 9th/pg 598-602*)

Multiple myeloma is a **malignant proliferation of plasma cells** derived from a **single clone**.

159. Ans. (c) Multiple myeloma (*Ref: Robbins 9th/pg 598-602*)

In the given scenario, patient has **bone pain, destructive bony lesions** on X Ray, **hypercalcemia, M spike** and **35% plasma cells in Bone marrow** à Diagnostic of **Multiple Myeloma**

160. Ans. (a) Multiple myeloma (*Ref: Robbins 9th/pg 598-602*)

Serum β2 microglobulin level <3.5mg/L indicates **good prognosis, in multiple myeloma.**

161. Ans. (b) IL-6 (*Ref: Robbins 9th/pg 598-602*)

IL-6 helps in **survival and proliferation** of **myeloma cells**

162. Ans. (d) Dystrophic calcification (*Ref: R 9th/pg 598-602*)

Calcification in multiple myeloma is due to hypercalcemia (**metastatic calcification**) and **not dystrophic calcification.**

163. Ans. (b) Light chain globulins

(*Ref: R 9th/pg 598-602*)

Excretion of **light chains** in the **urine** has been referred to as **Bence Jones proteinuria**.
Light chains includes κ and λ **(kappa and lambda)**

164. Ans. (d) Lymphoplasmacytic lymphoma

(*Ref: Robbins 9th/pg 598-602; 8th/pg 608-612*)

Waldenstrom Macroglobulinemia

Indolent lymphoproliferative disorder characterized by:
- Lymphoplasmacytic cell proliferation in marrow (**Lymphoplasmacytic lymphoma**) with secretion of **IgM**
- **Clinical Features** Anemia, lymphadenopathy, Hepato-splenomegaly and hyperviscosity
- CD138+, cyIgM+, CD19+

165. Ans. (c) Hypercalcemia

(*Ref: Robbins 9th/pg 598-602; 8th/pg 608-612*)

166. Ans. (c) > 10% plasmocytosis

(*Ref: Robbins 9th/pg 598-602; 8th/pg 608-612*)

Multiple myeloma is diagnosed by > 10% plasmacytosis

167. Ans. (b) IgM

(*Ref: Robbins 9th/pg 598-602*)

Lymphoplasmacytic cell proliferation in marrow (**Lymphoplasmacytic lymphoma**) with secretion of **IgM**

168. Ans. (c) Plasmacytoma on biopsy

(*Ref: Wintrobe's 12th/pg 2377*)

Durie and Salmon criteria for diagnosis of Multiple myeloma.
A minimum of 1 major and 1 minor criterion needed, although (1) + (a) is not sufficient, or 3 minor criteria that must include (a) and (b).

However, **International myeloma working group 2011 has revised** the criteria as mentioned in pretexts.

169. Ans. (d) Elevated alkaline phosphatase

(*Ref: Robbins 9th/pg 598-602; 8th/pg 608-612*)

Alkaline Phosphatase levels in multiple myeloma is normal and not raised, as there is no bone formation and only bone lysis.

170. Ans. (a) P190 has aggressive course

CML can have 3 types of transcripts.
- P190–Poor prognosis Seen in ALL
- P210–Seen in CML
- P230–Seen in CNL good prognosis

171. Ans. (a, d) a. Richter transformation; d. MHC non-expression is way to escape immunity but of to mark one a > d.

172.   Ans. (d)   Erythropoietin levels

In this case the d/d of the clinical details given is polycythemia. Since he is from hilly area, it may be due to secondary causes. To rule out primary (low epo) vs secondary cause (high epo), erythropoietin must be the next logical step.

173.   Ans. (c)   Focal cellular marrow with hypocellular areas and atypical megakaryocytes.

(Ref: WHO Textbook of hematolymphoid tissues 2016/ p 47)

174.   Ans. (a)   Philadelphia chromosome is negative

(Ref: Robbins 9th/pg 616-617)

175.   Ans. (b)   CML

(Ref: Robbins 9th/pg 616- 618; 8th 626-628)

176.   Ans. (a)   Acrocentric chromosome involved

(Ref: Robbins 9th/pg 160, Refer Genetics chapter)

177.   Ans. (a)   Leucoerythroblastic blood picture

(Ref: Robbins 9th/pg 614- 615; 8th 624-625)

Myelodysplastic syndrome usually results in pancytopenia rather than leukoerythroblastic blood picture.

178.   Ans. (d)   Leukocytosis *(Ref: Robbins 9th/pg 618- 619)*

Polycythermia vera results in Panmyelosis (increase in all myeloid components including leukocytes)

179.   Ans. (b)   Florescent in situ hybrdization

(Ref: Robbins 9th/pg 170)

In PCV: Reddening, swelling, and pain in the digits (erythromelalgia) may occur and are typically associated with extreme platelet elevations.

180.   Ans. (d)   Blast crisis phase of CML

(Ref: Robbins 9th/pg 616- 618)

181.   Ans. (b)   Thrombocytosis

(Ref: Robbins 9th/pg 618)

182.   Ans. (b)   Imatinib mesyiate

(Ref: Robbins 9th/pg 617)

183.   Ans. (c)   Abnormal oxygen saturation

(Ref: Robbins 9th/pg 618)

184.   Ans. (d)   Spontaneous severe infection

(Ref: Robbins 9th/pg 618)

185.   Ans. (d)   Marrow fibrosis *(Ref: Robbins 9th/pg 620/630)*

186.   Ans. (b)   Primary myelofibrosis

(Ref: Robbins 9th/pg 620/630)
The most characteristic peripheral blood finding in **PMF** is myelophthisis, defined by the presence of **leukoerythroblastosis** (presence of nucleated red blood cells, metamyelocytes, myelocytes, myeloblasts, and megakaryocytes) and dacryocytosis (**Tear drop RBCs**)

187.   Ans. (b)   Increased neutophil alkaline phosphatase

(Ref: Robbins 9th/pg 617)

188.   Ans. (d)   c-kit point mutation *(Ref: R 9th/pg 616-620)*

Myeloproliferative disorders include:

Disease	Tyrosine kinase involvement
Chronic myeloid leukemia	ABL1
Myeloid and lymphoid neoplasms with eosinophilia	PDGFRA/Bor FGFRA
Polycythemia vera	JAK2 V61 7F, JAK EXON 12
Primary myelofibrosis	JAK2 V 6174 , MPL W515 K/L
Essential thrombocythemia	JAK2 V617 F , MPL W 515 K/L

189.   Ans. (d)   Myelodyplastic syndrome

(Ref: R 9th/pg 614)

190.   Ans. (b)   Polycythemia Vera

(Ref: Wintrobe's 12th/pg 180-190)

191.   Ans. (a)   Myelodysplastic Syndrome

(Ref: Robbins 9th/pg 614- 615)

192.   Ans. (d)   Myelofibrosis *(Ref: Robbins 9th/pg 620)*

193.   Ans. (b)   FISH *(Ref: Robbins 9th/pg 616-618)*

- **Flow cytometry:** is used for **immunophenotyping** in Leukemias & Lymphomas
- **FISH- used for detecting submicroscopic chromosomal aberrations of BCR-ABL fusion**
- **Karyotyping**: Used for detecting **chromosomal defects of at least 5 mb size** (low sensitivity)
- **RT-PCR**: used for **quantitative DNA estimation**

194.   Ans. (b)   Decrease LAP score *(Ref: R 9th/pg 618-619)*

Increased vit B12- is seen in all myeloproliferative neoplasms including polycythemia vera due to increased levels of transcobalamin II

195.   Ans. (a)   Dry tap (hypocellular) *(Ref: Robbins 9th/pg 620)*
In Myelofibrosis bone marrow is replaced by fibrosis, giving a dry tap on bone marrow aspiration

196.   Ans. (c)   Myelodysplastic syndrome

(Ref: R 9th/pg 614-615)

Pseudo-Pelger-Hüet neutrophils: bilobed hypogranular dysplastic neutrophils[Q] seen in Myelodysplastic syndromes.

197. Ans. (d) Lung carcinoma

(Ref: Robbins 9th/pg 618-619)

Polycythemia is not caused by Lung Carcinoma.

198. Ans. (b) Acute myeloid leukemia

(Ref: Robbins 9th/pg 616; 8th/pg 626)

AML is not a myeloproliferative disease

199. Ans. (b) The fusion gene bcr-abl forms a protein with tyrosine kinase activity *(Ref: Robbins 9th/pg 616-618)*

a. FALSE, as **ABL gene is on chr 9q** while BCR is on chr 22q
b. The **fusion gene bcr-abl forms a protein with tyrosine kinase activity**: TRUE
c. FALSE; **Massive splenomegaly is a feature of CML**
d. FALSE; as **response to Imatinib is good in patients with Philadelphia chromosome +ve**

200. Ans. (d) Essential thrombocytopenia

(Ref: Robbins 9th/pg 616-618; 8th/pg 626-628)

- Myeloid metaplasia is other name of myelofibrosis.
- Essential thrombocytosis is CMPD (not thrombocytopenia)

201. Ans. (b) Protein tyrosine kinase inhibitor are the drug of choice *(Ref: Robbins 9th/pg 616-618)*

a. FALSE; as translocation **is between long arms of chr 9 & 22**
b. TRUE; **Imatinib- a tyrosine kinase inhibitor is the drug of choice**
c. FALSE; **Most commonly presents in the chronic phase**
d. FALSE; **Commonest tumor in children is ALL, followed by CNS tumors.**

202. Ans. (d) Acute Megakaryocytic Leukemia

(Ref: Robbins 9th/pg 620; 8th/pg 630)

Myelofibrosis leading to a dry tap on bone marrow aspiration is seen with **Acute Megakaryocytic Leukemia**.

Conditions in which Myelofibrosis is seen are:

- Primary Myelofibrosis (PMF)
- **Secondary Myelofibrosis:**
- Myeloproliferative Neoplasms- CML, PCV, ET
- Myeloid Neoplasms- AML M7, MDS
- Hairy cell Leukemia, Hodgkin's, Multiple Myeloma
- Metastasis
- Granulomatous diseases- TB, Sarcoidosis
- Autoimmune disease- SLE, Systemic sclerosis

- Others-Paget's disease, Renal osteodystrophy, Radiation, HyperPTH

203. Ans. (a) Mitochondria

(Ref: Robbins 9th/pg 614-615)

In **myelodysplastic syndrome, ring sideroblast is seen in Mitochondria**

204. Ans. (b) Gamma heavy chain disease

Franklin's disease **(gamma heavy chain disease)** It is a very rare B-cell lymphoplasma cell proliferative **disorder** which may be associated with autoimmune **diseases** and infection is a common characteristic of the **disease**. It is characterized by lymphadenopathy, fever, anemia, palatal edema, malaise, hepatosplenomegaly, and weakness.

205. Ans. (d) Langerhans cell

(Ref: Robbins 9th/pg 631-632)

206. Ans. (a) Birbecks granules

(Ref: Robbins 9th/pg 531)

Birbeck granules

- Also known as Langerhans bodies or **X granules**
- Seen on Electron microscopy
- Rod-shaped organelles with a central striation and terminal vesicular dilation, giving them a 'tennis racket' appearance.

207. Ans. (d) Birbeck's granules

(Ref: Wintrobe's 12th/pg 1573)

208. Ans. (d) Eosinophilic granuloma

(Ref: 9th/pg 621-622)

Localised langerhans cells histiocytosis affecting head & neck is **Eosinophilic granuloma**

209. Ans. (c) CD la

(Ref: Robbins 9th/pg 621-622)

CD marker for Langerhans cell histiocytosis is CD 1a

210. Ans. (b) Pneumothorax in 10% cases

(Ref: Wintrobe's 12th/pg pg 1577)

- **Pneumothorax is seen in 25-40% cases of pulmonary LCH**

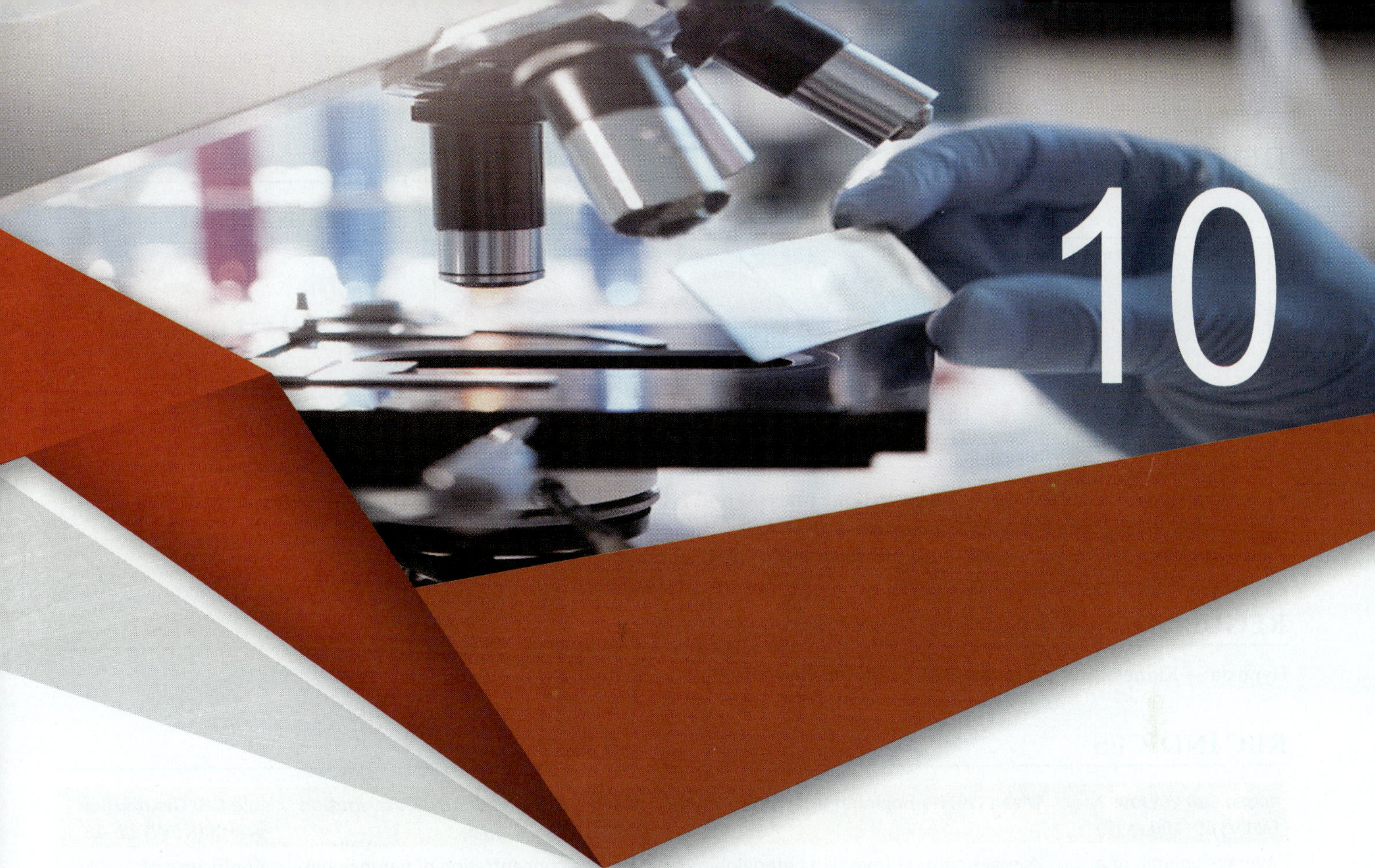

10

Red Blood Cells and its Disorders

Key Points

- » **Hemoglobin** can be first visualized at **polychromatic (Intermediate) erythroblast^Q** stage
- » **Early recovery in acute blood loss is marked by thrombocytosis**
- » Decreased free serum haptoglobin, Hemoglobinuria, Methemoglobinuria, Hemosiderinuria are hallmark of intravascular hemolysis
- » **Most common** mutation in Hereditary spherocytosis are **Ankyrin^Q > band 3 >Spectrin and band 4.2**
- » Both **intravascular and extravascula** repisodic hemolysis is seen in^Q in G6PD-deficient individuals
- » **Sickle cell anemia results from point mutation in 6th codon of β-globin^Q** $\rightarrow$ replacement of a **glutamate** residue with a **valine** residue
- » α **and** β **Thalassemia results from decreased production of** α **and** β **chains respectively**
- » PNH results from acquired somatic clonal mutation of **PIG-A gene^Q** resulting in loss of **GPI**
- » **Divalent metal transporter type 1 (DMT-1) helps in absoption of Iron from Intestine but is not specific for Iron absorption**
- » **Hypersegmented neutrophils is the earliest abnormality to appear in macrocytic anemia**
- » **Aplastic anemia** refers to a **marrow hypoplasia** and **pancytopenia**

Key Recent Updates

- » Eosin 5-maleimide (EMA) binding test is recent screening test for diagnosis of HS
- » FLAER is an Alexa488-labeled inactive variant of aerolysin to diagnose and monitor patients with PNH.

DEVELOPMENT OF RBCs

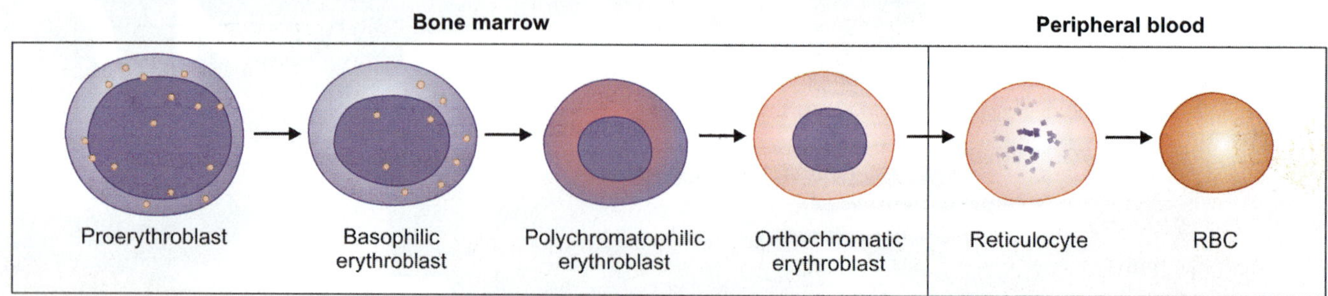

- Reticulocytes takes **4–5 days (1–3 days in bone marrow and 1–2 days in peripheral circulation)**[Q] to **mature** into RBCs
- **Ferritin** molecules can be seen at **proerythroblast stage**[Q] by **electron microscopy**
- **Hemoglobin** can be first visualized at **polychromatic (Intermediate) erythroblast**[Q] stage

REGULATION OF ERYTHROPOIESIS

Hypoxia → Kidney → Erythropoietin → Bone marrow → Manufactures and releases RBCs

RBC INDICES

Mean Cell Volume (MCV) 80–100 m (fl)	Mean Cell Hemoglobin (MCH) 30 ± 3 (pg)	Mean Cell Hemoglobin Concentration (MCHC) 34 ± 2 (g/d)	Red Cell Distribution Width (RDW) 12–16
Average volume of a red cell	Average content (mass) of hemoglobin per red cell, MCH = Hb/RBC count[Q]	Average concentration of hemoglobin in a given volume of packed red cells, MCHC = Hb/MCV[Q]	**Coefficient of variation** of red cell volume[Q]

- **Hematocrit** or **Packed cell volume:** ratio of the volume of RBCs to total volume of blood
- **Hct or PCV = MCV × RBC concentration**

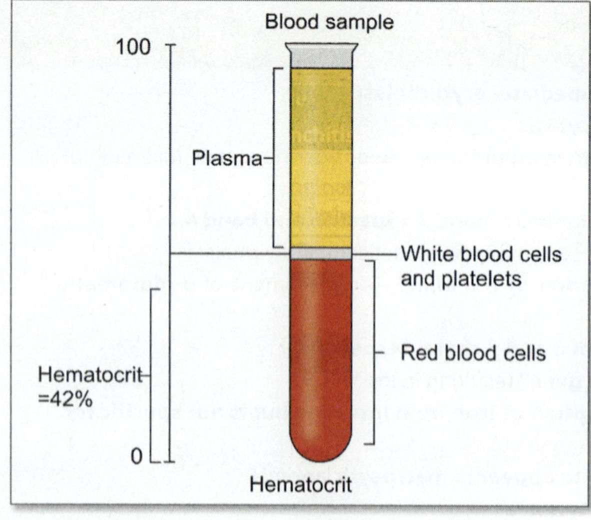

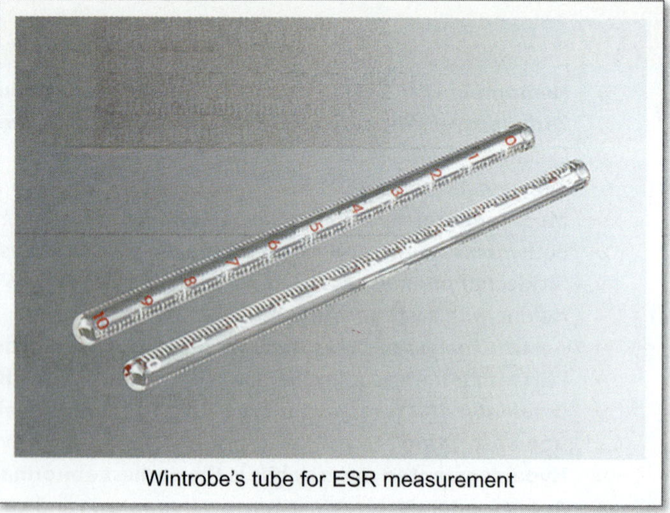
Wintrobe's tube for ESR measurement

ESR

- *Definition:*
  - Measurement of **sedimentation of RBCs** in diluted blood (EDTA or Citrate) after standing for **1 hr** in an open-ended glass tube of 30 cm length mounted vertically on a stand.

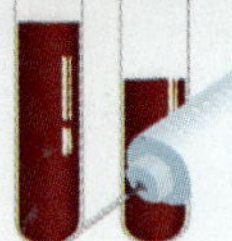

- **Characteristics:**
  - It is **slower to respond** to acute disease activity
  - **It is insensitive to small changes** in disease activity.
  - It is **less specific than CRP** because it is influenced by immunoglobulins & Anemia.
- **Stages of sedimentation:**
  - Formation of **rouleaux**
  - Period of **fast settling**
  - Period of **packing of the rouleaux** at the bottom of the tube
- **Normal value:**
  - Men: < 15 mm/hr
- **Very low ESR:**
  (0–1 mm)
  - Polycythemia, hypo- or afibrinogenemia, congestive cardiac failure & abnormalities of red cells such as poikilocytosis, spherocytosis, or sickle cells.
- **Very high ESR**
  (>100 mm)
  - Tuberculosis, Hodgkin's disease, multiple myeloma, chronic infective or inflammatory conditions
- **Factors influencing ESR**

Increased ESR	Lower ESR
• Old age	• Extreme leucocytosis
• Female	• **Polycythemia**
• **Pregnancy**	• **Spherocytosis**, microcytosis
• **Anemia**	• Hyperviscosity
• Paraprotein (Multiple Myeloma)	• Low Protein; fibrinogen, gammaglobulins
• Hypergammaglobulinemia	• Technical factors; dilution, clotted sample
• Macrocytosis	• **Afibrinogenemia**
• Elevated fibrinogen (infection, inflammation malignancy)	**No effect**
• Technical factors: dilution, high temperature	• Obesity
	• Body temperature
	• Recent meal
	• Aspirin, NSAIDs

Erythrocyte Sedimentation Rate is zero in Afibrinogenemia

ANEMIA

Definition: Functionally defined as **an insufficient RBC mass** to adequately **deliver oxygen** to peripheral tissues

WHO Criteria

Category	Hb (g/d)^Q cut-off for Anemia	Mean Normal Hb (g/d)
Adult male	< 13	14.5
Adult female	< 12	13.5
Pregnant female	< 11	12.5
Child < 6 yr	< 11	12

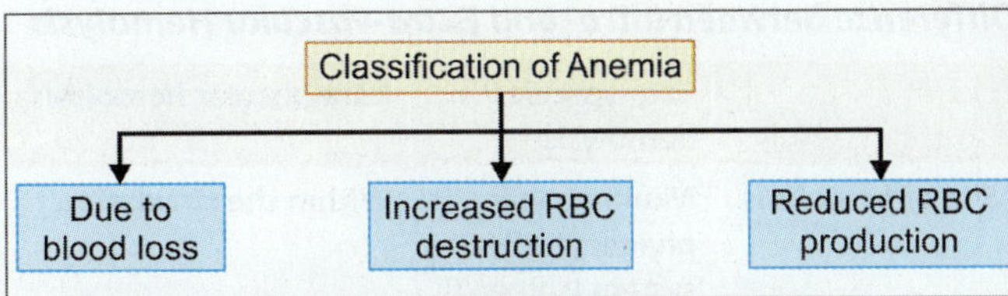

Anemia Due to Blood Loss

Acute Blood loss

- **Etiology:**
  - **External** (trauma, or obstetric hemorrhage)
  - **Internal** (e.g., from bleeding in the gastrointestinal tract, rupture of the spleen, rupture of an ectopic pregnancy, subarachnoid hemorrhage)
- **Pathophysiology:**
  - Loss of intravascular volume → Intravascular shift of water from the interstitial fluid compartment → *Hemodilution* → *Lowering of hematocrit*
- **Features:**
  - *Early recovery is marked by thrombocytosis^Q*
  - On **day 5- reticulocytosis starts^Q**
  - **Massive** bleeding- **granulocytosis** (leukocytosis)^Q
  - Day 7: reticulocytosis (10–15%)^Q
  - **MCV increases^Q** as newly produced RBC's are larger

Chronic Blood Loss

Anemia is the only manifestation

Hemolytic Anemias: Due to increased RBC Destruction

Characterized by:

- **Shortened** RBC life **span^Q** (normal = 120 days)^Q
- **Increase** in **erythropoiesis^Q**
- Accumulation of **hemoglobin degradation^Q** products

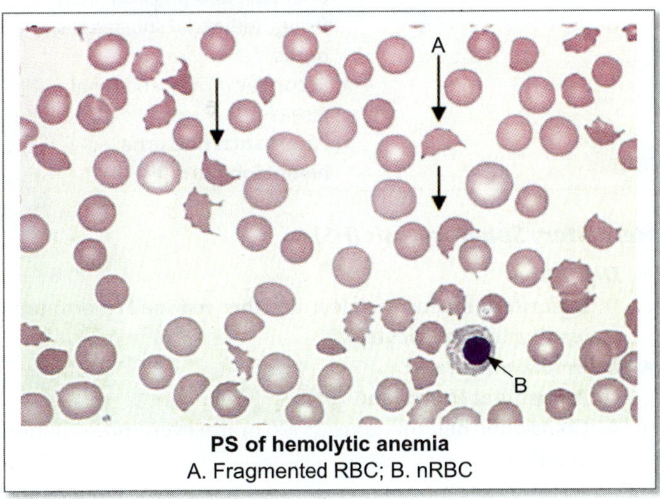

PS of hemolytic anemia
A. Fragmented RBC; B. nRBC

Difference between Intra- and Extra-vascular Hemolysis

	Extravascular hemolysis	Intravascular hemolysis
Site of hemolysis	Mononuclear phagocytes[Q] RE system (**spleen[Q]**)	Within the circulation[Q]
Diseases causing hemolysis	Thalassemia,[Q] sickle cell anemia[Q]	PNH,[Q] G6PD deficiency[Q] angiophatic
Serum haptoglobin	Normal	Decreased[Q]
Hemoglobinuria	Not seen	Positive[Q]
Methemoglobinuria	Not seen	Positive[Q]
Hemosiderinuria	Not seen	Positive[Q]
Serum unconjugated bilirubin	Moderately elevated	Mildly elevated
Splenomegaly	**Usual[Q]**	Uncommon

Classification of Hemolytic Anemias

Hereditary	Acquired
Membrane defects	**Immune**
• Hereditary spherocytosis	• *Autoimmune:* Warm or Cold antibody type
• Hereditary elliptocytosis	• *Alloimmune*
Enzyme defects	▪ Hemolytic transfusion reaction
• G6PD deficiency	▪ Hemolytic disease of the newborn
• Pyruvate kinase deficiency	▪ Allografts, especially stem cell transplantation
Hemoglobin	• Drug associated
Genetic abnormalities (HbS, HBc, unstable)	• **Red cell fragmentation syndromes**
	• **March hemoglobinuria**
	• **Infections:** Malaria, Clostridia
	• **Chemical and physical agents:** Drugs, industrial substances, burns
	• **Secondary:** Liver and renal disease
	• **Paroxysmal nocturnal hemoglobinuria**

Hereditary Spherocytosis (HS)

- *Definition:*
  - **Inherited** intrinsic defect in the red cell membrane leading to **spherocytes**[Q]
- *Inheritance pattern:*
  - **Autosomal Dominant-75%**[Q]
  - Compound heterozygous-25%[Q] (more severe, presentation at birth)

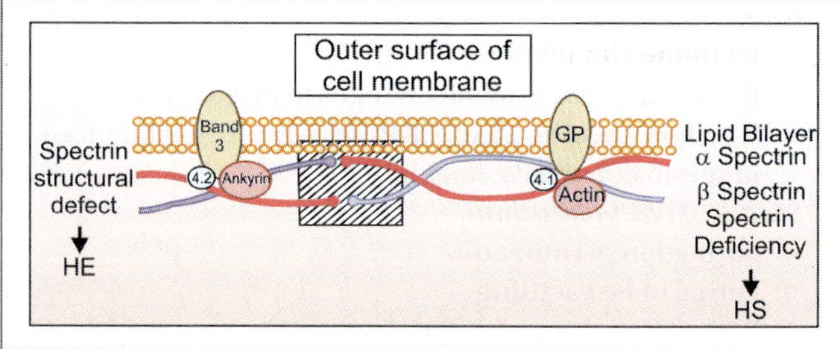

- ○ **Spectrin** (α/β)-major protein forming tetramers[Q]
- ○ **Actin**-binds spectrin tetramers[Q]
- ○ **Protein 4.1**- binds **spectrin** to inner surface of RBC membrane
- ○ **Band 3**- RBC 's transmembrane ion transporter[Q]
- ○ **Ankyrin**-bridge between Spectrin and Band 3 helped by **Pallidin (band 4.2)**[Q]

- *Pathogenesis*

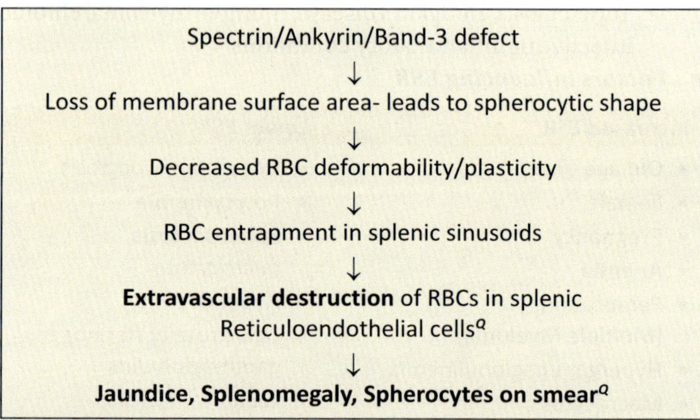

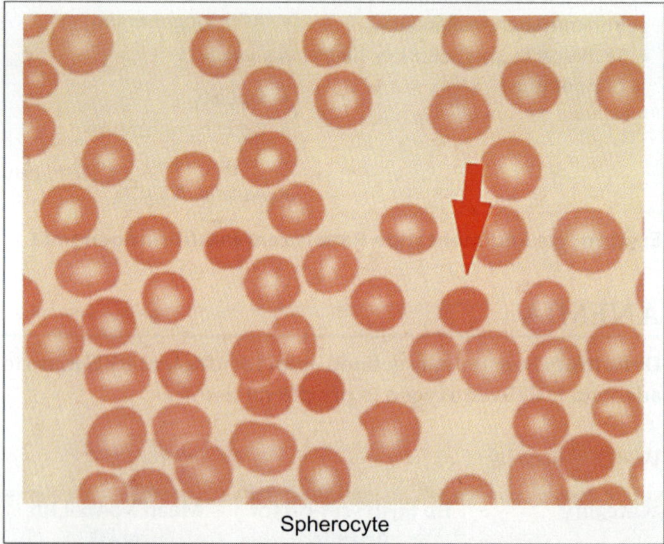

Spherocyte

- *Clinical feature*
  - **Triad of** Jaundice + hemolytic anemia + splenomegaly (with a f**amily history of gall stones**)
  - **Pigment type**[Q] of gall stones are common

- *Diagnosis*
  - **PS**: Micro-spherocytosis of uniform size (**variable size**^{Q} in Immune Hemolytic Anemia).
  - **Decreased MCV, Increased MCHC**^{Q}, **Increased 'glycerol lysis test'**^{Q}
  - **Increased fragility** on Osmotic fragility testing (**OFT**): shift of curve to **right**^{Q}
    - **24-hr incubated OFT** is the **most sensitive** test to diagnose HS^Q
    - Diagnosis of choice -eosin-5-maleimide flow cytometric test

High Yield Facts

- **Life span** of RBC in HS is **20 days**^{Q} against a normal of 120 days
- **Most common** mutation in HS: **Ankyrin**^{Q}**> band 3> Spectrin and band 4.2**^{Q}
- **α-spectrin** mutations (Autosomal recessive) leads to **most severe** phenotypes^Q
- In **Spectrin** mutations, the most common RBC abnormality is **Hereditary Elliptocytosis > spherocytosis**^{Q}

Hemolytic Disease Due to Red Cell Enzyme Defects

Four Types

- Glucose-6-Phosphate Dehydrogenase (**G6PD**) deficiency (**most common**)^Q, Pyruvate Kinase deficiency, Pyrimidine-5' nucleotidase deficiency, Hereditary methemoglobinemia

Glucose-6-Phosphate Dehydrogenase (G6PD) Deficiency

- *Inheritance:*
  - **X-linked recessive** trait (Chr Xq28)^Q
- *Epidemiology:*
  - **Highest prevalence** in Kurdish **Jews**> African
- *Pathogenesis:*
  - **Mechanism**: **Hemolysis** occur due to **oxidative stress**^{Q} due to **deficient G6PD** activity
  - **Defective pathway:** hexose monophosphate (**HMP**) shunt → leads to **deficient NADPH**^{Q}
  - Normally NADPH reduces **oxidized glutathione (GSSG)** to **reduced glutathione (GSH), which neutralizes H_2O_2**

Increased H_2O_2 cross-links reactive sulfhydryl groups on globin chains

↓

Forms membrane bound precipitates known as **Heinz bodies.**^{Q}

↓

Heinz bodies **damage the RBC membrane** to cause **intravascular hemolysis**^{Q}

↓

Splenic macrophages pluck out the Heinz bodies

↓

Extravascular hemolysis forming **bite cells** and **Spherocytes**^{Q}

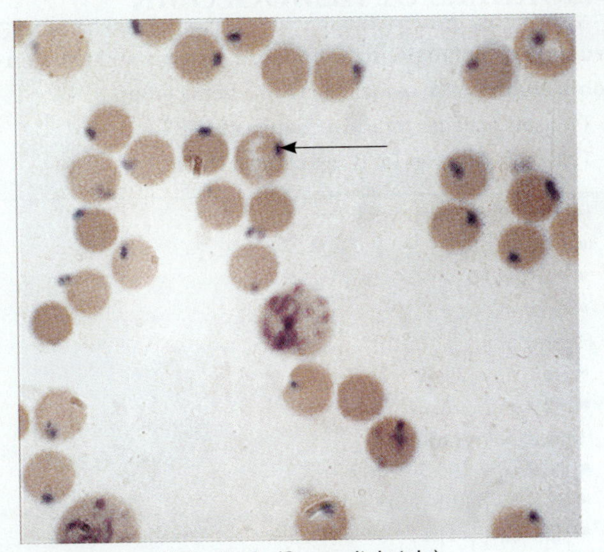

Heinz body (Supra vital stain)

- *Variants of G6PD*
  - Most common **normal variant**, G6PD B+^{Q}
  - **Most severe variants**: G6PD A- and G6PD **Mediterranean, Canton**^{Q}
- *Inciting events*
  - Refer Ans
- *Lab Diagnosis*

Peripheral smear:	Screening assay:^{Q}
- **Heinz body on supravital staining**^{Q} - **Anisopoikilocytosis** with polychromasia^Q - **"Bite cells"**^{Q} - **Microspherocytes** - Increased Reticulocyte %^{Q}	- Methemoglobin reduction test Fluorescent spot test **Diagnostic assay:**^{Q} - Quantitative G-6-PD enzyme assay by **electrophoresis** - DNA analysis by PCR

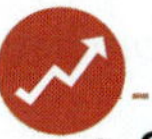

High Yield Facts

- **G6PD deficiency causes self-limited hemolysis**, which stops with release of younger G6PD abundant RBC's (**even in presence of offending drug**)^Q
- Both **intravascular and extravascular** hemolysis^Q in G6PD-deficient individuals.
- G6PD deficient individuals are **protected** against **malaria**^{Q}
- Most frequently implicated food is the **fava bean**, which generates oxidants when metabolized called **"Favism"**^{Q}
- WHO classification of G6PD is **Class I (most severe)** to **Class V (least severe)**^{Q}

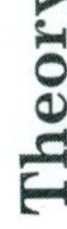

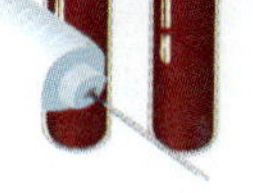

DISORDERS OF HEMOGLOBIN

Structure of Hemoglobin: Composed of **two α-and two non–α-globin chains**, each associated with a heme group

- Two sets of genes for the α chains: **chr 16[Q]**
- Two pairs of genes for β, γ, δ chains: **chr 11[Q]**

- Hemoglobins (embryonic)
  - Gower 1 ($\varsigma_2\varepsilon_2$)
  - Portland ($\varsigma_2\gamma_2$)
  - Gower 2 ($\alpha_2\varepsilon_2$)
- Hemoglobins (at Birth)
  - Hb F $\alpha_2\gamma_2$ (75)%
  - Hb A $\alpha_2\beta_2$ (25)%
- Hemoglobins (adults)
  - Hb A $\alpha_2\gamma_2$ (96.5-97.5)%
  - Hb A$_2$ $\alpha_2\delta_2$ (2.5-3.5)%
  - Hb F $\alpha_2\gamma_2$ (<1)%

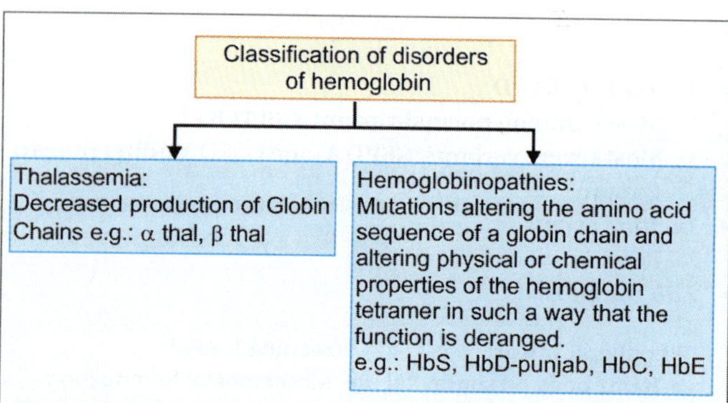

Sickle Cell Anemia

- **Defect:**
  - **Point mutation in 6th codon of β-globin[Q]** $\rightarrow$ replacement of a **glutamate** residue with a **valine** residue.[Q]
  - Production of **HbS** with abnormal physiochemical properties that promotes the **polymerization** of deoxygenated hemoglobin.

- **Pathogenesis:**

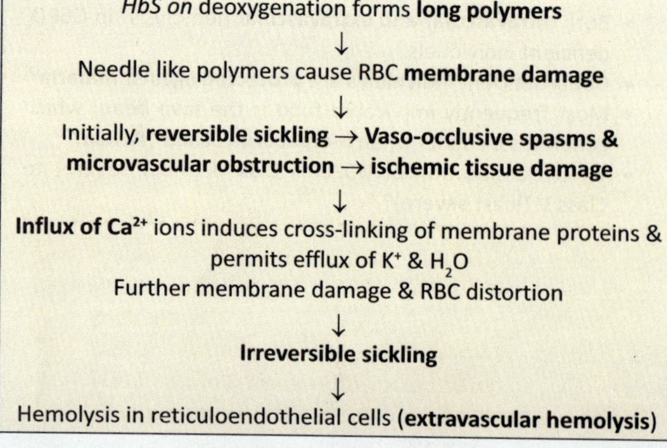

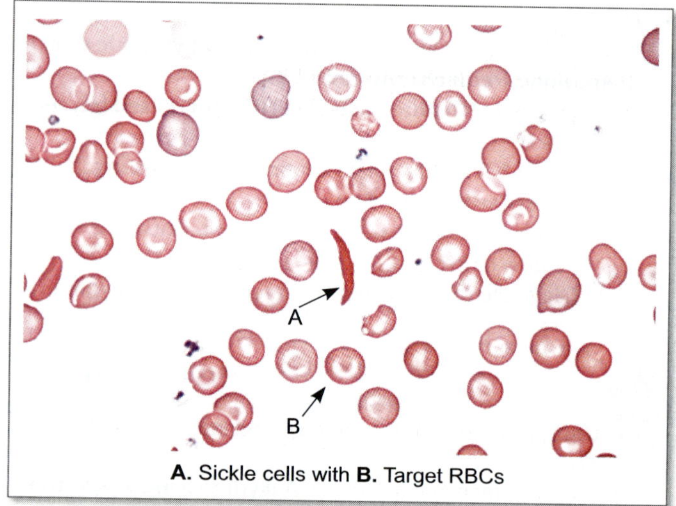

A. Sickle cells with **B.** Target RBCs

- *Factors affecting Sickling:*

Factors INCREASING Sickling	Factors DECREASING Sickling
- **Dehydration[Q]** - Increase in MCHC[Q] - Decrease in pH[Q], Increase in ionic strength - De-oxygenation Inflammation	- Other Hemoglobins like: HbA, HbF*[Q] - **Concomitant alpha thalassemia[Q]** - Re-oxygenation

- *Clinical features*
  - **Hand-foot syndrome or dactylitis[Q]**
  - **Priapism** and **erectile dysfunction.[Q]**
  - **Stroke and retinopathy[Q]**
  - **Cardiomegaly is a feature**
  - **Autosplenectomy[Q]**: multiple infarcts in splenic artery causes spleen to be reduced to fibrous tissue (splenic atrophy → **spleen may become nonpalpable**)[Q]
  - **Chronic hemolysis:** impaired growth and development.
  - **Renal involvement**: Papillary necrosis & **hyposthenuria[Q]** (inability to concentrate urine)
  - Infection
  - Vaso-occlusive crises/Acute painful crises
  - Acute chest syndrome[Q]
  - Sequestration crises
  - Aplastic crises
- *Diagnosis*
  - **PS:** Irreversibly **sickle RBCs** and **target cells** (increased after autosplenectomy). **Howell-Jolly bodies** if asplenia.[Q]
  - **Sickling test:** Mixing a blood sample with an oxygen consuming reagent, such as **metabisulfite or dithionate** induces sickling of RBCs, if HbS is present.[Q]
  - **Spleen biopsy: Gamma gandy bodies[Q]**
  - **X-ray:** "Crew-cut" appearance of skull, **fish-mouth vertebra[Q]**
  - **Hemoglobin electrophoresis**
  - **Hb-HPLC** (High Performance Liquid Chromatography): **investigation of choice[Q]**
  - **Prenatal diagnosis:** by analysis of fetal DNA obtained by amniocentesis or chorionic biopsy.

High Yield Facts

Hemoglobins with abnormal solubility

Abnormal Hb	Residue	Mutation	Molecular pathology
HbS	β6	Glu→ Val	Polymenzation
HbC	β6	Glu → Lys	Crystallization
HbD-Punjab	β121	Glu → Gln	Increases poymer is S/D heterozygote

Severity of the hemolysis[Q] correlates with the percentage of **irreversibly** sickled cells

- Sickle RBCs are **mechanically fragile**, leading to some **intravascular hemolysis[Q]**
- **Sickle cell anemia, G6PD deficiency, Thalassemias, absence of Duffy antigen on RBCs protect against malaria[Q]**
- **HbSC disease is milder** than sickle cell disease
- Sickle cell anemia usually **presents after first 6 months** of life
- **Splenomegaly** is first noted **after 6 months** of age
- **Gamma Gandy bodies** contains fibrous tissue, foci of fibrosis with Iron or Calcium salts
- **Gamma Gandy bodies seen in portal hypertension, Sickle cell anemia, Splenic congestion, CML** and some cases of leukemia and lymphoma

Thalassemia

- *Definition*
  - A heterogeneous group of disorders caused by **inherited mutations** that **decrease the synthesis** of **globin** chains.
- *Distribution*
  - Worldwide: **Mediterranean**, Africa, South east Asia.
  - In India- **Sindh[Q], Punjab, Gujrat and Bengal**
- *Classification (PS)*
  - α Thalassemia: **decreased production of α chains**
  - β Thalassemia: **decreased production of β chains**
  - Others: δβ-Thalassemias, γδβ-thalassemias, αβ-thalassemias
- *Diagnosis*
  - Moderate to severe **microcytic hypochromic anemia with aniso-poikilocytosis**
  - **Polychromasia, Target RBCs, Basophilic stippling,[Q] Howell jolly bodies[Q]**
  - **Reticulocyte** count is **increased but <5%[Q] due to ineffective erythropoiesis**
- **NESTROFT: Naked Eye Single Tube Red cell Osmotic Fragility Test[Q]**

- Assesses osmotic fragility of RBCs at a single concentration of buffered saline **(0.36% in single tube)[Q]**

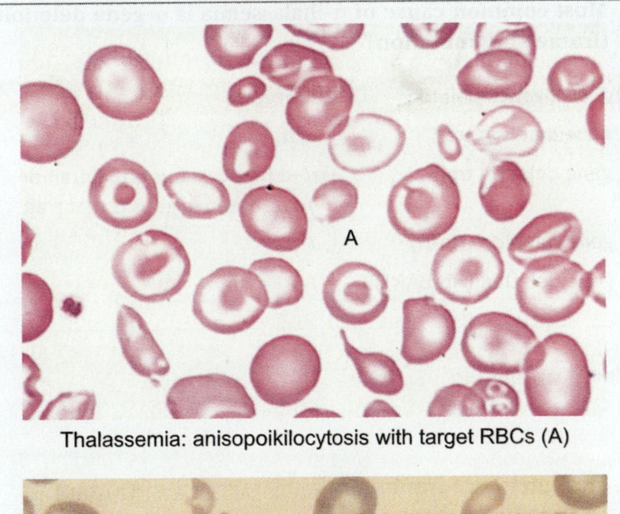

Thalassemia: anisopoikilocytosis with target RBCs (A)

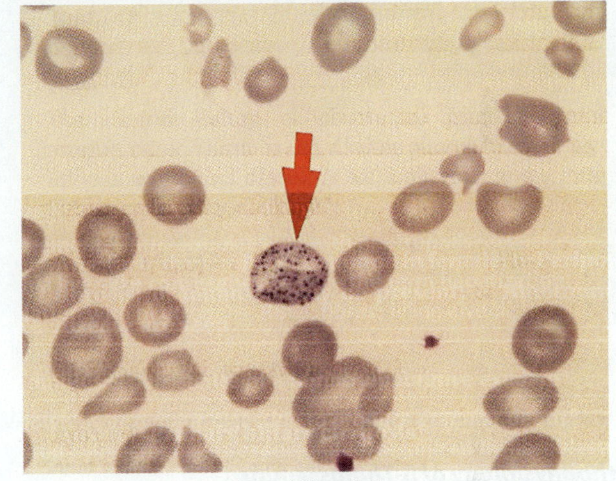

Basophillic stipling

Screening test

Mentzer Index[Q] = Mean corpuscular volume (MCV)/RBC count This test helps in differentiating iron deficiency from thalassemia

In Thalassemia trait	In Iron deficiency Anemia
Mentzer's index<13[Q] (RBC count is normal with a low MCV)	Mentzer's index > 13[Q] as (RBC count as well as MCV is low)

- *Diagnosis of choice:* HPLC; High performance liquid, and chromatography/Electrophoresis

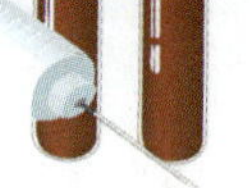

α-Thalassemia

- **Normally 4 α-genes[Q] synthesize 2 α chains:** α, α/α, α
- **Most common cause of** α-thalassemia is **α-gene deletion[Q] (frame-shift mutation)[Q]**

No. of α genes deleted	Genotype
1 gene deletion trait	-, α/α, α[Q]
2 gene deletion trait	−α/−α homozygous α thal trait or —/α, α heterozygous α thal trait
3 gene deletion (Hb-H)[Q]	-,-/-, α
4 gene deletion (Hb-BART)[Q]	-,-/-,-

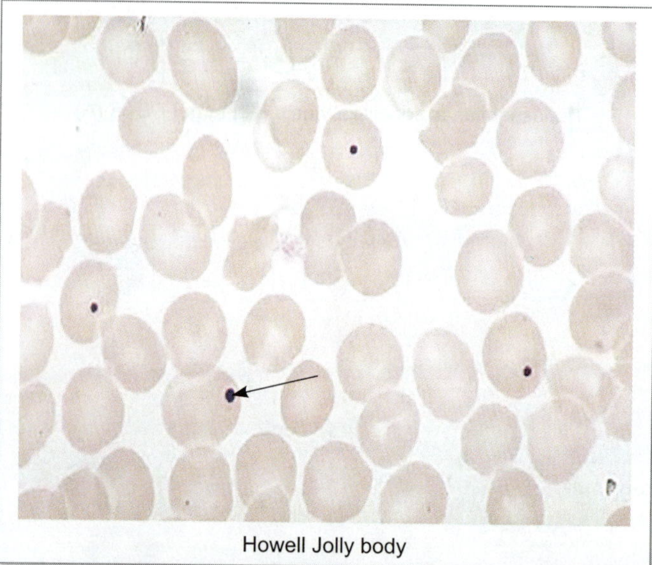

Howell Jolly body

β-Thalassemias

Types of Mutations in β-Thalassemias

- **Splicing mutations: Most common cause** of β(+) thalassemia.[Q]
- **Promoter region mutations:** β(+) thalassemia[Q]
- **Terminator mutations:** Most common cause of β(0) thalassemia[Q]

High Yield Facts

Most common mutation in β thalassemia in India:
- **IVS-1, position 5 (G → C) (most common mutation)[Q]**
- 619-bp deletion[Q]
- Codons 8/9, frameshift mutation
- Codons 41/42, frameshift mutation
- IVS-1, position 1 (G → T)

β-Thalassemias:

Clinical classification	Manifestations	Globin genotype (normal= β/β)
Thalassemia trait (minor)	• Asymptomatic • May have mild anemia	β/β_0 $\beta/\beta+$
Thalassemia intermedia	• Mild to moderate anemia • Variable need of blood transfusions	$\beta+/\beta+$[Q]
Thalassemia major	• Severe anemia & Jaundice • Presents in childhood • Requires multiple transfusion Hemolytic facies • Hepatosplenomegaly	$\beta+/\beta+$ $\beta+/\beta_0$ β_0/β_0[Q]

Pathophysiology of β-Thalassemias

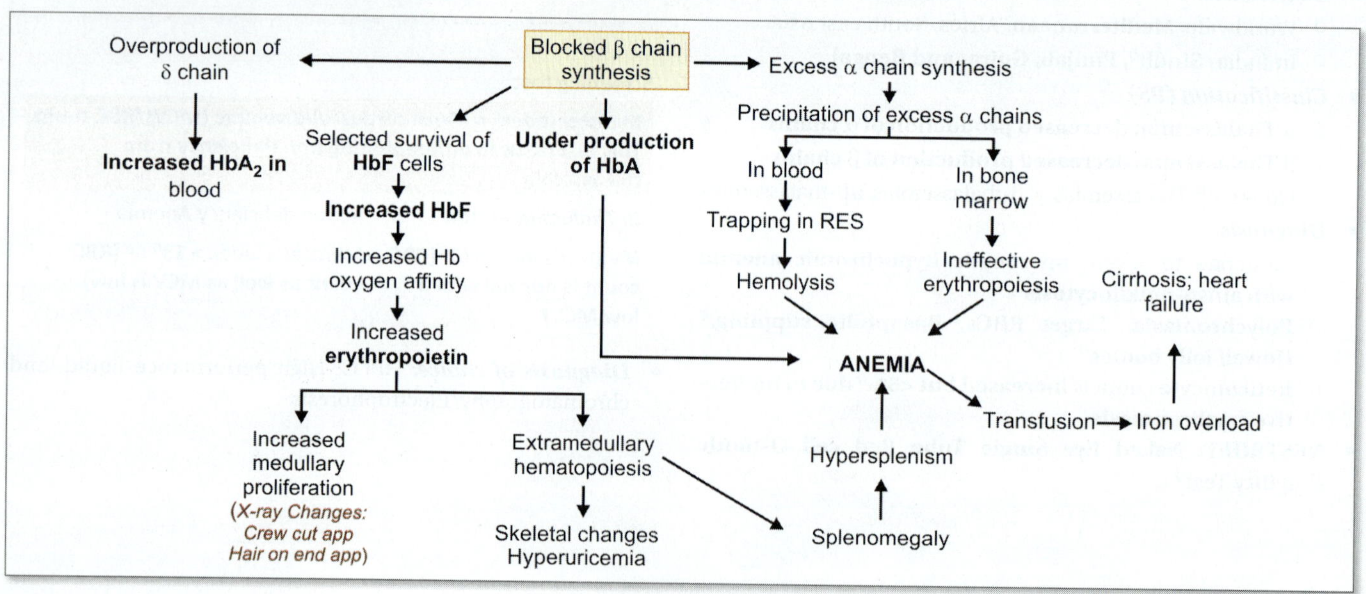

Paroxysmal Nocturnal Hemoglobinuria (PNH)

- *Definition*
  - A triad of Intravascular hemolysis, Thrombosis & Pancytopenia

- *Underlying defect*
  - Acquired somatic clonal mutation of **PIG-A gene[Q]** resulting in **loss of GPI (Glycosyl phospahtidyl inositol)** linked proteins like CD55, CD59

- *Pathophysiology*
  - Deficiency of **Regulators of complement activity** → **Inappropriate complement activation** → **Intravascular hemolysis** & destruction of WBCs & platelets causing **pancytopenia.**[Q]

- *Diagnosis*
  - **Acidified serum hemolysis test (HAM's test):**[Q]
  - Patient's RBC gets lysed in acidic pH in presence of complements
  - **Alkaline phosphatase: Low LAP** score[Q] in PNH patients
  - **Gold standard: Flow cytometry**: **absence of GPI-linked proteins such as CD59/CD55**[Q]
  - **FLAER (Fluorescent aerolysin)**- Most recently introduced test to diagnose PNH[Q] – **Diagnosis of choice**

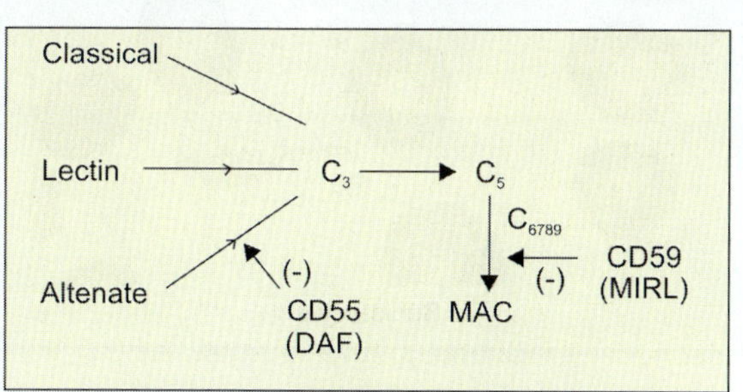

PNH pathophysiology

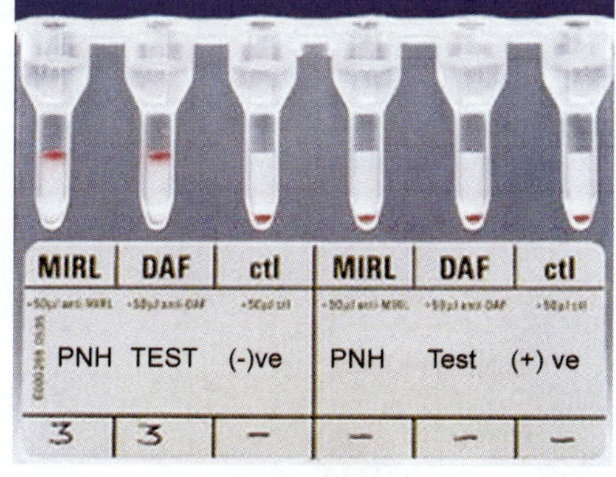

PNH Card test

- PIG-A gene is **X-linked** which **encodes Glycosyl phospahtidyl inositol(GPI)** anchor protein.
- 5% to 10% of PNH patients develop **AML or MDS**[Q]
- PNH has high association with **aplastic anemia**[Q]
- **Thrombosis is the leading cause of disease-related death in PNH**[Q]
- In PNH, hemolysis occurs at night due to slight decrease in blood pH during sleep, which increases the activity of complement

Immunohemolytic Anemias

- *Definition*
  - Hemolytic anemias caused by antibodies that bind to red cells, leading to their premature destruction.

- *Classification*
  - Autoimmune (*see below*)
  - Alloimmune Eg: Hemolytic disease of New born, Rh Incompatibility

- *Etiology*

Warm Antibody Type (IgG Ab Active at 37°C)[Q]	Cold Antibody Type (IgM Ab Active Below 37°C)[Q]
Primary (idiopathic) **Secondary** • Autoimmune (SLE, Evans syndrome) • Lymphoid neoplasms eg: CLL[Q] • Drugs: ■ **Antigenic type**[Q]: Penicillin, Cephalosporins ■ **Innocent bystander type** (Immune complex): Penicillin ■ **Tolerance-breaking:** Alpha methyl dopa[Q]	**Primary (idiopathic)** **Secondary:** • **Acute:**[Q] Mycoplasma pneumoniae, EBV, CMV, Influenza and HIV • **Chronic:** Lymphoid neoplasms **Cold Hemolysin Type (Ab Active Below 37°C)** Viral infections.

- *Diagnosis:*
  - **PS:** Anisopoikiocytosis, Polychromasia, **Spherocytes**[Q]
  - **Increased Reticulocyte %**
  - **Coomb's test** is **positive** in **Immune hemolytic anemia**[Q]
    - **Direct** Coomb's test- Detects **Antibody on RBC Surface**[Q]
    - **Indirect** Coomb's test- Detects **Antibody in Serum**[Q]

- **Evans Syndrome:** Auto Immune Hemolytic Anemia (AIHA) + thrombocytopenia
- **Paroxysmal cold hemoglobinuria is** seen in children following viral infections.
- **In Paroxysmal cold hemoglobinuria, intravascular hemolysis** and **hemoglobinuria seen**
- **Paroxysmal cold hemoglobinuria is due to Donath Landsteiner Antibodies (IgG)[Q]** that bind to **P blood group[Q]** antigen on RBC at 4°C → **Complement-mediated lysis of RBCs at** 37°C

- **In Cold agglutinin disease,** chronic **intravascular hemolysis** occur on **exposure to cold (0-5 C)[Q]**
- **Cold agglutinin disease is due to** binding of **IgM** to "i" **Ag** on RBC's at 32°C[Q] → activates complements at **37°C**
- Both intravascular & extravascular hemolysis is seen in **Cold agglutinin disease**

Red Cell Fragmentation Syndromes

Macroangiopathic Hemolytic Anemia	Microangiopathic Hemolytic Anemia[Q]
Cardiac hemolysis • Prosthetic heart valves • Perivalvular leaks **Arteriovenous malformations**	• **Hemolytic Uremic Syndrome (HUS)[Q]** • **Thrombotic Thrombocytopenic Purpura (TTP)[Q]** • **Disseminated intravascular coagulation (DIC)[Q]** • **Malignant hypertension[Q]** • Pre-eclampsia/HELLP • March hemoglobinuria • Vasculitis • Connective tissue disorders Eg. SLE,[Q] Scleroderma • Giant hemangioma (Kasabach-Merritt syndrome)[Q]

Microangiopathic Hemolytic Anemia (MAHA) For detail Discussion, refer Bleeding Disorders

- **Characterized by:** Hemolytic anemia due to RBC fragmentation.
- **Pathophysiology:** Microvascular lesion → luminal narrowing, due to **deposition of fibrin and platelets** → traumatic **damage** → red cell fragmentation → Appearance of *schistocytes,[Q] burrcells, helmet cells, triangle cells* in blood smears.
- **Schistocytes:** Fragmented RBC's with 1-3 sharp spicules; (>3/5000)

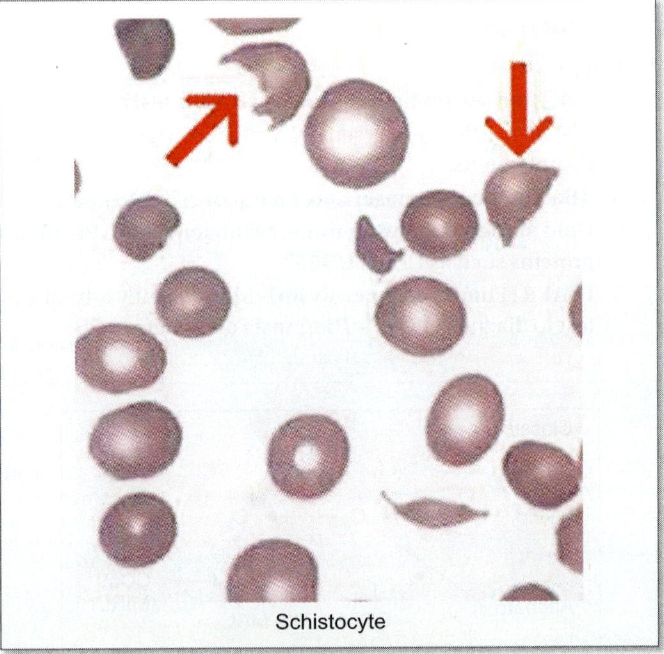

Schistocyte

Anemias of Decreased Erythropoiesis

NUTRITIONAL-DEFICIENCY ANEMIA: Important examples are:
- Iron-deficiency anemia
- Folic acid and B_{12} deficiency anemia
- Vit C, Copper and Zinc deficiency

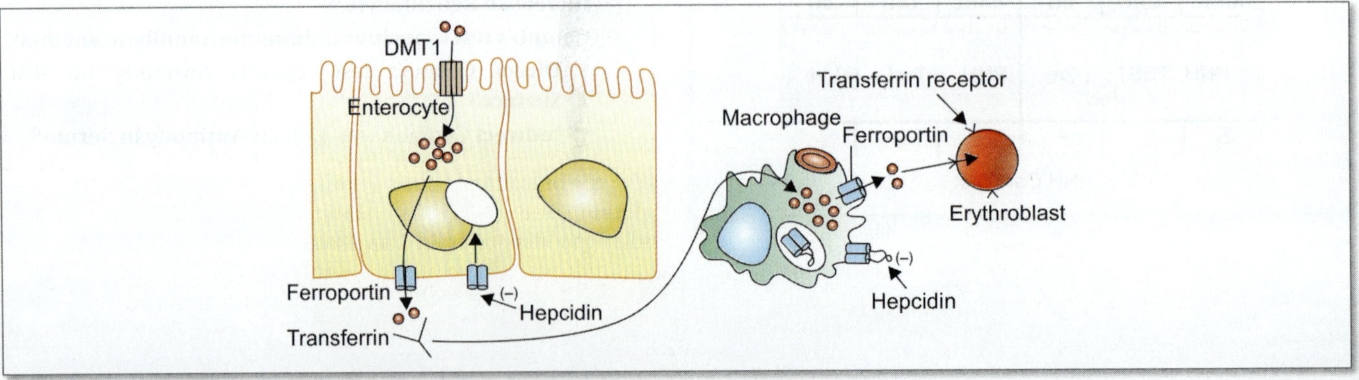

Iron Deficiency Anemia

Iron Metabolism

Site of Iron absorption: Mainly occurs in **proximal small intestine (duodenum and jejunum)**[Q]

At the brush border of the absorptive cell,
$Fe^{3+} \rightarrow Fe^{2+}$ by a ferrireductase: **Duodenum cytochrome B**
↓
Transport across the membrane by DMT-1*
↓
In gut cell, Iron may be stored as mucosal **ferritin** or transported by **ferroportin** at basolateral surface
↓
In the process of release from basolateral surface,
$Fe^{2+} \rightarrow Fe^{3+}$ by hephaestin**
↓
Fe^{3+} is taken up by **transferring in blood** to storage **tissue ferritin**

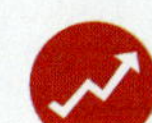

High Yield Facts

- **Amount of iron** needed to replace RBC's lost through senescence amounts to **20 mg/day**
- Normally, an adult male absorbs **1 mg** of elemental iron daily to meet needs[Q]
- Iron-deficiency anemia is the **most common anemia prevalent in India**[Q]
- Iron-deficiency anemia has higher incidence in females, particularly **pregnant females**[Q]
- **Hepcidin** is the **principal iron regulatory hormone**; it is **negatively** regulated by **ferroportin**[Q]

*__Divalent metal transporter type 1 (DMT-1)__: also known as natural resistance macrophage-associated protein type 2 (Nramp 2) or DCT-1[Q]
__Hephaestin__ is similar to **ceruloplasmin, the copper-carrying protein.[Q]

Iron Deficiency Anemia

Etiology	Increased Demand for Iron	Increased Iron Loss	Decreased Iron Intake or Absorption
	• Rapid growth in infancy or adolescence • Pregnancy[Q] • Erythropoietin therapy	• Acute or Chronic blood loss (Hookworm,[Q] Carcinoma colon[Q]) • Menstruation • Phlebotomy as treatment for polycythemia vera	Inadequate diet Malabsorption (Celiac ds,[Q] Crohn's ds) Malabsorption due to surgery (postgastrectomy,[Q] Bilroth II[Q]) Acute or chronic inflammation Chronic Renal Failure[Q]
Clinical features	• Depend on the severity & chronicity of anemia • **Fatigue, pallor, reduced exercise capacity, cheilosis**[Q] (fissures at the corners of the mouth)		• **Koilonychia**[Q](spooning of the fingernails); **Platynychia**[Q]: flattening of the fingernails • Pharyngeal webs: **Plummer Vinson syndrome**[Q]

Stages of Iron Deficiency

Features	Stage 1 (Prelatent)	Stage 2 (Latent)	Stage 3 (Anemia)
Symptoms	None	Fatigue, malaise	Pallor ± pica
Hemoglobin	Normal	**Normal**[Q]	**Reduced**[Q]
MCV	Normal	Normal	Reduced
Serum ferritin	**Reduced**[Q]	**<12 µg/L**[Q]	**<12 µg/L**[Q]
Transferrin saturation	Normal	<16%[Q]	<16%
Free erythrocyte protoporphyrin	Normal	↑[Q]	↑[Q]
Serum transferrin receptor	**Normal**[Q]	↑	↑
Bone marrow iron	Reduced	Absent	Absent

Lab diagnosis		
Lab diagnosis	**Peripheral smear:** • Anisocytosis, microcytic hypochromic RBCs • **Pencil RBCs/cigar**[Q] shaped RBCs are seen • **Target RBCs** in severe cases • **Reticulocyte %**[Q]**-not raised** • **Platelets-often increased**[Q]	**RBC Indices:** • **MCV < 80fl** • **MCH < 25pg** • **MCHC< 27g/dl** • **Increased RDW (>14)**[Q] • **Serum Iron studies:** Refer to table below
Response to therapy	• **Rapid subjective improvement**, with decrease in fatigue, **before any improvement in anemia** • **Earliest hematologic evidence: increase in reticulocyte % & their hemoglobin content.** • **Reticulocytes attain maximal value (5 to 10%) on 5th to 10th day** of therapy	

Serum Iron Studies: (to Distinguish the Differential Diagnosis)

Differential Diagnosis of Microcytic Anemia

Tests	Normal Values	Iron Deficiency	Anemia of chronic disease	Thalassemia	Sideroblastic Anemia
Peripheral Smear	N/N	Micro/hypo	N/N or micro/hypo	Micro/hypo with target RBCs	Micro/hypo or Dimorphic
S. Iron (ug/dl)	50-150	<30	<50	Normal to high	Normal to high
(TIBC) (ug/dl)	30-300	>360	<300	Normal	Normal
Transferrin saturation %	33%	<10	10–20	30–80	30–80
Ferritin (µg/L; ng/ml)	50-300	<15	30–200	50–300	50–300
Hb electrophoresis	–	Normal	Normal	Abnormal	Normal

*TIBC: Total Iron Binding Capacity

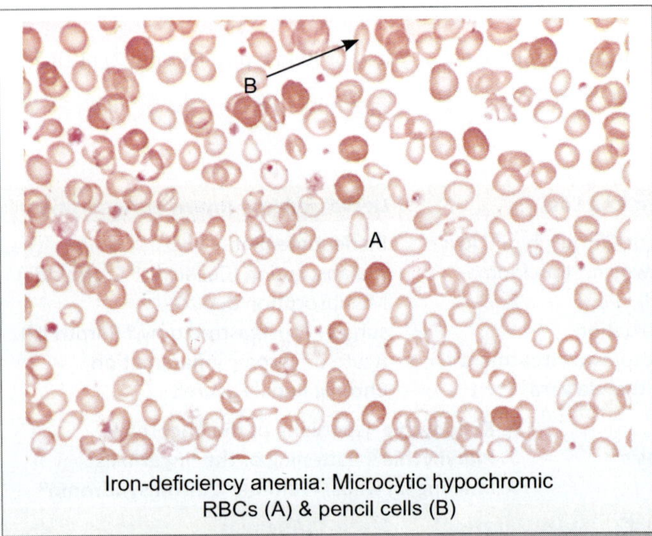

Iron-deficiency anemia: Microcytic hypochromic RBCs (A) & pencil cells (B)

ANEMIA OF CHRONIC DISEASE

Hypoferremia in presence of Adequate Reticuloendothelial Stores

Etiology (for > 1–2 months)

- **Chronic Inflammation**: Rheumatoid Arthritis, Systemic Lupus Erythematosus
- **Chronic Infections**: TB, Chronic osteomyelitis, HIV
- **Malignancy**: Hodgkin's disease and Non-Hodgkin Lymphoma
- Miscellaneous: Alcoholic liver disease

SIDEROBLASTIC ANEMIA

- *Definition*
  - A heterogeneous group of disorders characterized by **amorphos iron deposits** in **erythroblast mitochondria**

- *Classification*

Hereditary	X-linked (XLSA): (Pearson syndrome)
Acquired	Refractory anemia with ring sideroblasts **(RARS)/Pure SA (PSA)**
Reversible	Alcoholism Lead poisoning Drugs (isoniazid, pyrazinamide, chloramphenicol) Copper deficiency (zinc ingestion, copper chelation Hypothermia

- Sideroblasts can be seen in Iron overload

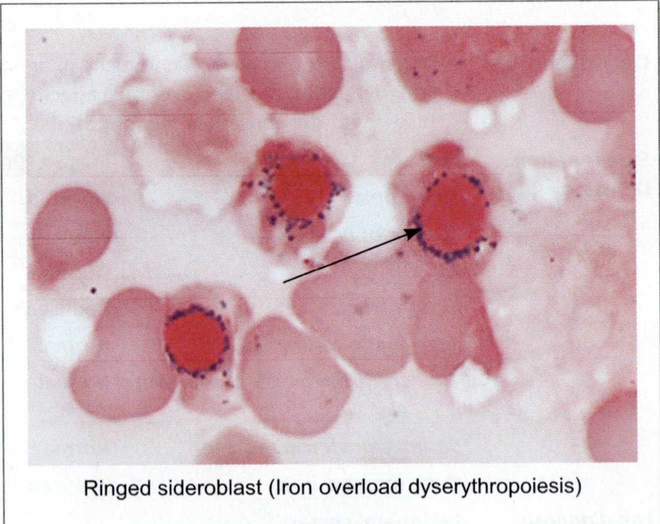

Ringed sideroblast (Iron overload dyserythropoiesis)

MEGALOBLASTIC ANEMIA

- *Definition:*
  - **Impairment of DNA synthesis** that leads to **ineffective hematopoiesis** & distinctive **morphologic changes,**

including **abnormally large erythroid precursors** in bone marrow & RBCs in peripheral smear

- *Etiology*
  - **Cobalamin Deficiency**
    - **Dietary deficiency**
    - **Malabsorbtion:** Ileal resection, Fish tapeworm infection
    - **Intrinsic factor Deficiency:** Pernicious anemia
    - **Increased requirements**: Pregnancy
  - **Folic acid deficiency**
    - **Dietary deficiency:** Malnutrition, **Alcoholics**[Q]
    - **Impaired absorption: Celiac Sprue**[Q], Small bowel resection/disease, **Anticonvulsants/ OCPs**
    - **Increased requirements:** Infancy, **Pregnancy**[Q], **Hemolytic anemias**
  - **Drug-induced suppression of DNA synthesis**
    - **Folate antagonists,** Alkylating agents
    - Metabolic inhibitors of synthesis of:
    - Purine: **hydroxyurea,**[Q] **6-MP, azathioprine**
    - Pyrimidine: **5-fluorouracil; cytosine** arabinoside
  - **Inborn errors**
    - Defective folate metabolism
    - Defective vitamin B_{12} metabolism
    - Hereditary orotic aciduria[Q]
    - Lesch-Nyhan syndrome[Q]
- *Peripheral smear*
  - **Anisopoikilocytosis, macrocytic** RBCs; **Macro-ovalocytosis** are highly **characteristic.**[Q]
  - Tear drop RBCs, Howel Jolly bodies, Cabot ring & Basophilic stippling may be seen
  - **Macrocytes** appear "hyperchromic," but the **MCHC is not elevated**.
  - Even though there is **mild hemolysis, reticulocyte count is low**
  - Neutrophils are also larger than normal **(macropolymor-phonuclear)**[Q] and show **nuclear hypersegmentation**[Q] **(>=5 lobes in >5% neutrophils) Earliest abnormality to appear**[Q]
- *Bone marrow*
  - Markedly **hypercellular** with **megaloblastic changes**[Q] at all stages of erythroid development
  - Derangement in **DNA synthesis** → **apoptosis of** precursors of all 3 lineages in marrow **(ineffective hematopoiesis)** → **pancytopenia.**[Q]
  - **Hallmark: nuclear cytoplasmic maturation asynchrony**[Q]
  - **Megaloblast with sieve like chromatin**[Q]
- *Other tests*
  - In vit B12 deficiency, serum **MMA (Methyl malonic acid) level is raised.**[Q]
  - **Serum homocysteine is raised** in both early **cobalamin and folate deficiency**[Q]
  - **Increased LDH levels**[Q]

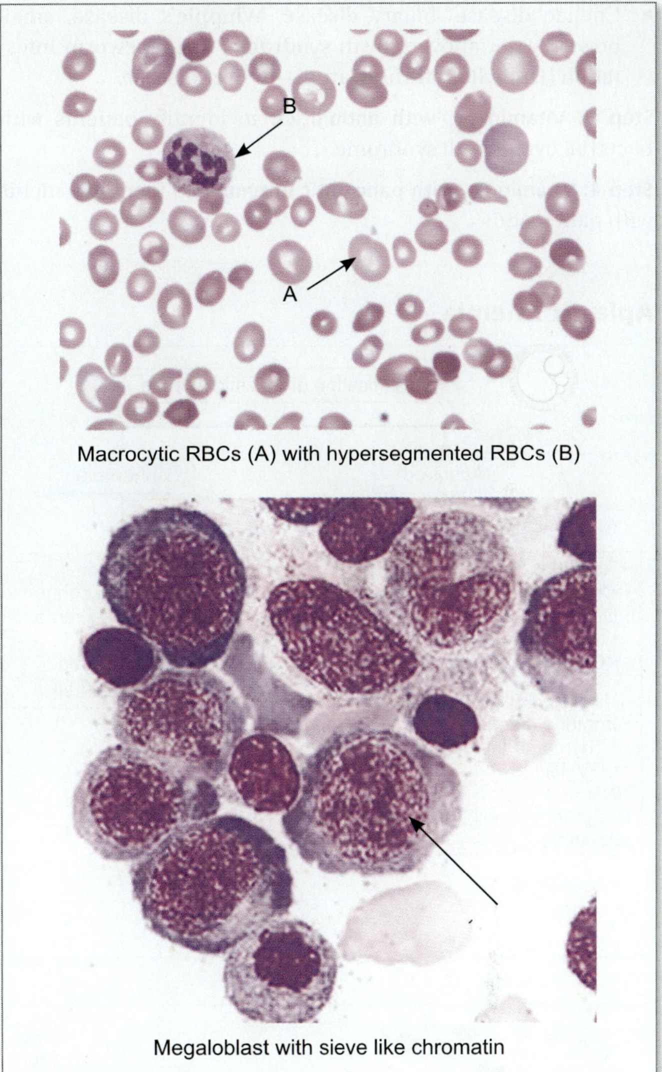

Macrocytic RBCs (A) with hypersegmented RBCs (B)

Megaloblast with sieve like chromatin

Schilling test

Step 1: oral vitamin B_{12} plus intramuscular vitamin B_{12}

- Patient is given radiolabeled vit B_{12} followed by i.m injection of unlabeled vit B_{12} an hour later to temporarily saturate B_{12} receptors in the liver.
- The patient's urine is then collected over the next 24 hours to assess the absorption.
- Normally, the ingested radiolabeled vitamin B_{12} will be absorbed into the body and get excreted in the urine.
- Normal result: **> 10% of radiolabeled vit B_{12}** in the **urine** over the first 24 hours.
- In patients with pernicious anemia or with deficiency due to impaired absorption, less than 10% of the radiolabeled vitamin B_{12} is detected → we proceed to step 2

Step 2: Vitamin B[12] with oral intrinsic factor

- Normal excretion indicates lack of intrinsic factor production, or pernicious anemia.
- Low value on the second test implies **abnormal intestinal absorption** (malabsorption):

- Coeliac disease, biliary disease, Whipple's disease, small bowel bacterial overgrowth syndrome, fish tapeworm infestation (Diphyllobothrium latum), or liver disease.

Step 3: Vitamin B$_{12}$ with antibiotics: to identify patients with bacterial overgrowth syndrome.

Step 4: Vitamin B$_{12}$ with pancreatic enzymes: to identify patients with pancreatitis

Aplastic Anemia

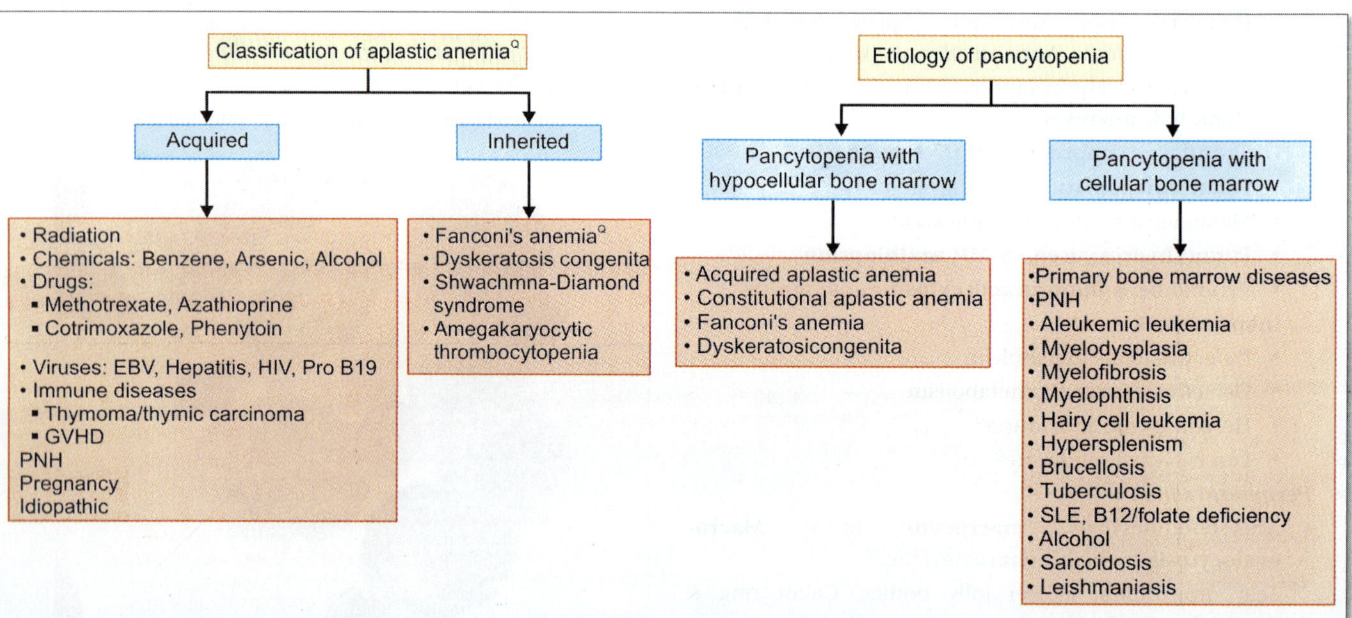

HYPOPROLIFERATIVE ANEMIAS

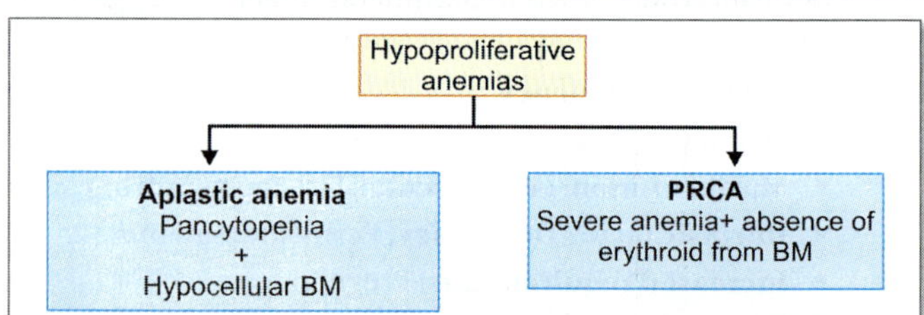

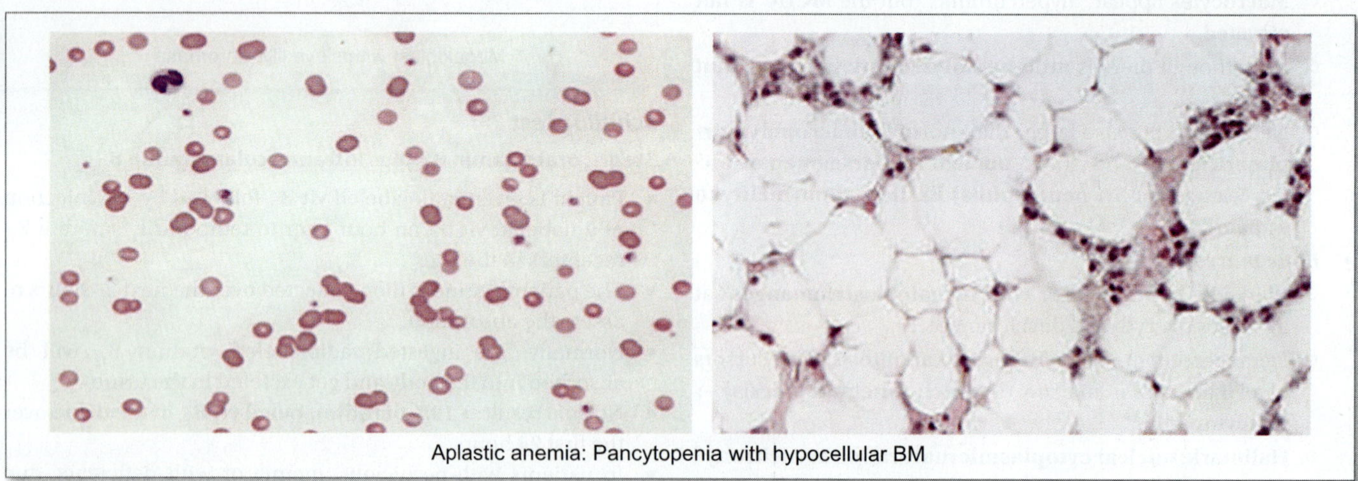

Aplastic anemia: Pancytopenia with hypocellular BM

Pure Red Cell Aplasia (PRCA)

Pure red cell aplasia is a primary marrow disorder in which only **erythroid progenitors are suppressed.**

Classification of Pure Red Cell Aplasia

Self-limited: Transient erythroblastopenia of childhood

Hereditary: Congenital pure red cell aplasia (**Diamond-Black-fan syndrome**)[Q]

Acquired

- **Thymoma**
- **Lymphoma**s: CLL, Large granular lymphoma,[Q] Hodgkin's,[Q] Non Hodgkin's
- **Paraneoplastic** to solid tumors
- Connective tissue disorders: **SLE, JRA, RA**
- **Virus:** Parvovirus B19[Q], hepatitis, HTLV, EBV
- **Pregnancy**[Q]

- **Drugs:** Phenytoin, azathioprine, chloramphenicol, procainamide, isoniazid[Q]
- **Post ABO incompatible transplant**[Q]

MYELOPHTHISIC ANEMIA

- **Definition**
  - A form of marrow failure in which space-occupying lesions replace normal marrow elements.
- **Etiology**
  - **Metastasis** from breast, lung, and prostate Carcinoma
  - **Infiltrative process** (e.g., granulomatous disease)
  - Spent phase of **myeloproliferative** disorders
  - Storage disorders: Eg. Gaucher's disease

- **Peripheral Smear**
  - **Leukoerythroblastosis:** Abnormal release of nucleated RBC's and immature granulocytic forms into peripheral smears.
  - Tear drop-shaped red cells (**Dacrocytes**)

High Yield Facts

Diagnostic Criteria for Severe Aplastic Anemia[Q]
Bone marrow cellularity of <25% along with 2 of the following:
- Neutrophil count<500/μl[Q]
- Platelet count<20,000/μl[Q]
- Absolute reticulocyte count of <60,000/μl[Q]

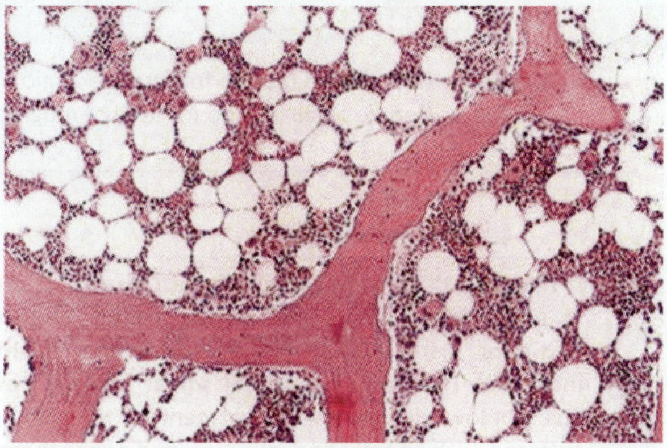

Normal marrow

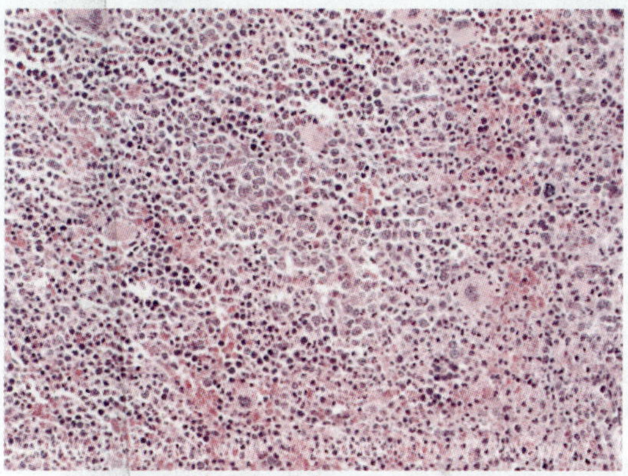

Hypercellular marrow

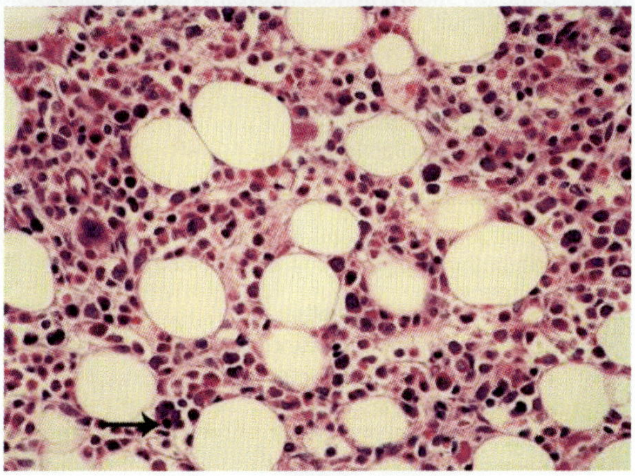

PRCA

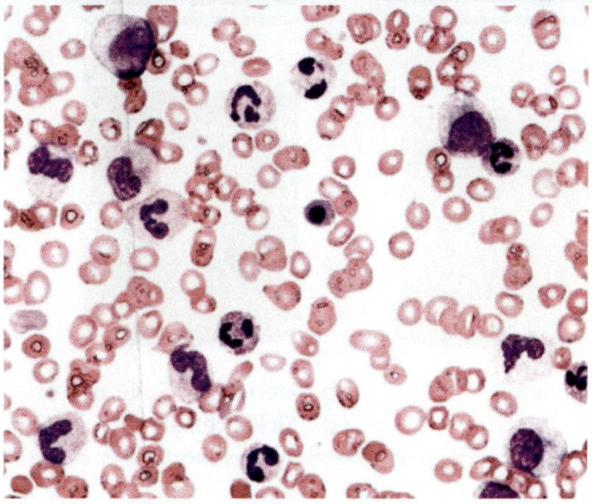

Leukoerythroblastosis

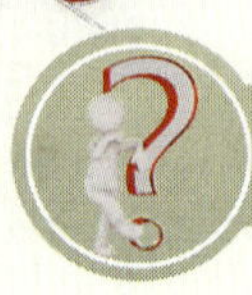

Image-Based Questions

1. The given figure shows a special stain on RBCs. Which of the following stains cannot be used for this?

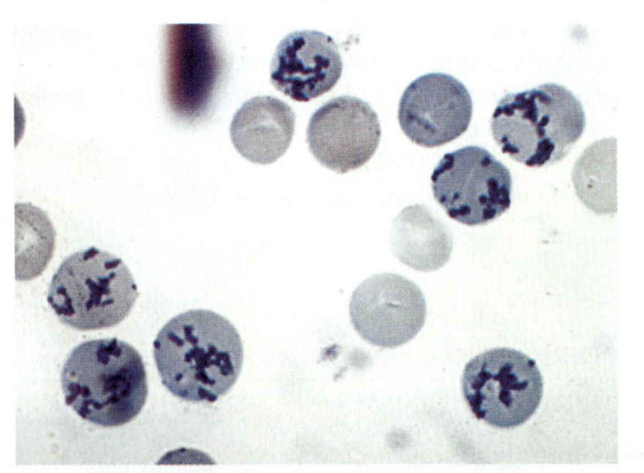

   a. New Methylene blue
   b. Crystal violet
   c. Brilliant cresyl blue
   d. Methyl violet

3. In the above case, the following investigation was done. Identify the test ?

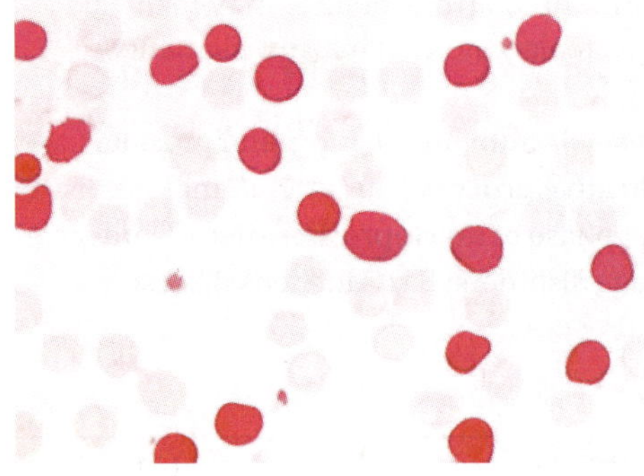

   a. APT test
   b. Kleihauer-Bethke acid elution for fetal hemoglobin
   c. Kleihauer-Bethke alkali elution for fetal hemoglobin
   d. Rossetting

2. The given figure shows urine sample from a patient who presented with anemia and Jaundice. (compare with normal sample on left). In which of the following condition this can be seen?

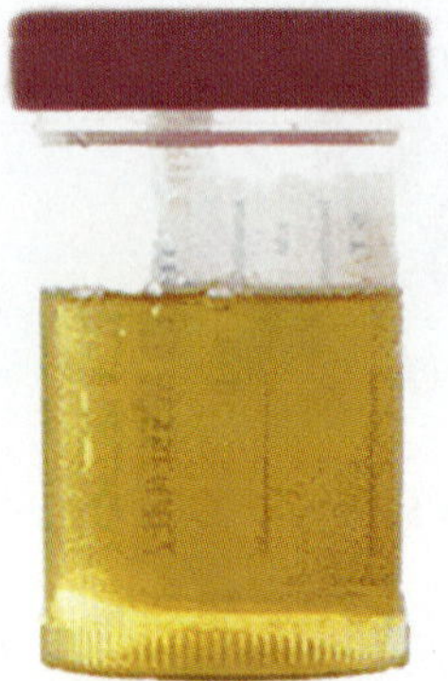
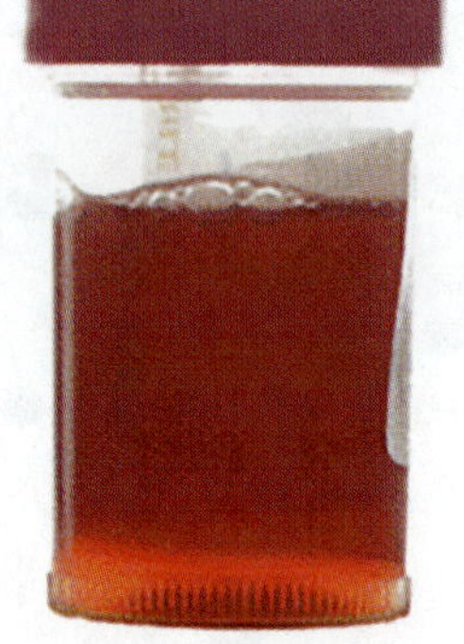

   a. Thalassemia
   b. Hereditary Spherocytosis
   c. PNH
   d. Sickle cell anemia

4. A male aged 20 years, native from Orissa had presented to AIIMS Medicine OPD with high grade fever with chills and rigor. His routine CBC revealed mild neutrophillia and increased TLC while Peripheral smear findings have been given below. He was given treatment for the same after he suffered with anemia and jaundice, and a repeat smear was done (as shown in next figure). What is your diagnosis?

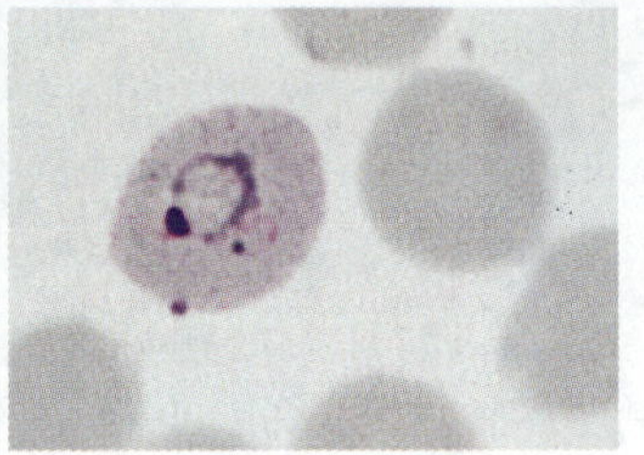
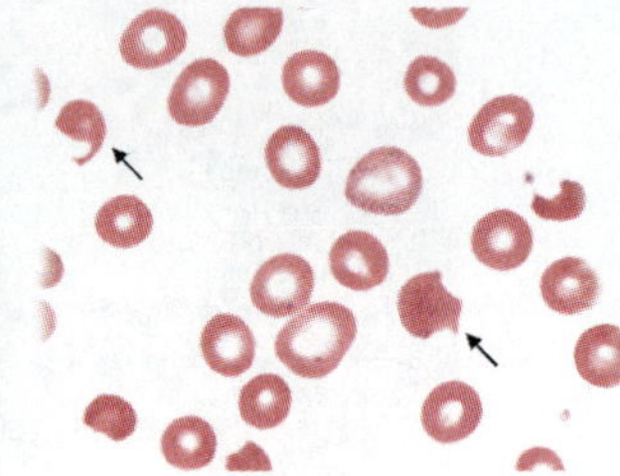

   a. *P. vivax* and bite cells
   b. *P. falciparum* and bite cells
   c. Babesia and schistocytes
   d. *P. vivax* and scistocytes

5. **A 5-year-old male child presented to AIIMS pediatrics OPD with severe transfusion requiring anemia and Jaundice. On examination Liver and spleen were palpable 5 cm below the costal margin. Peripheral smear analysis showed the following? What is your diagnosis?**

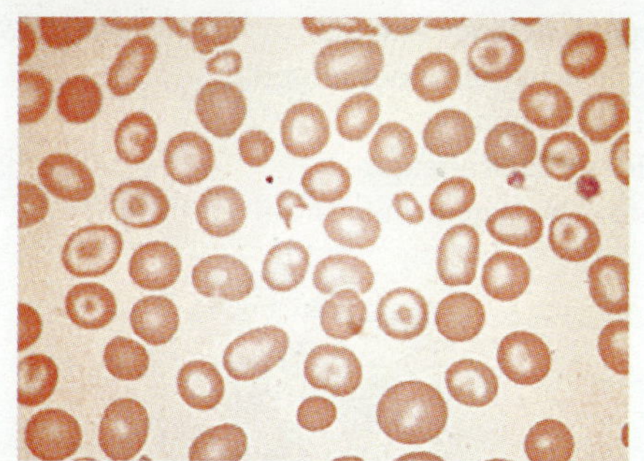

a. Nutritional anemia
b. Aplastic anemia
c. Autoimmune hemolytic anemia
d. Thalassemia

6. **A 45-year-old male presented to OPD with severe fatigue. On examination he was found to have severe anemia, and petechial spots. Given below is the picture of Peripheral smear and bone marrow biopsy. What is your diagnosis?**

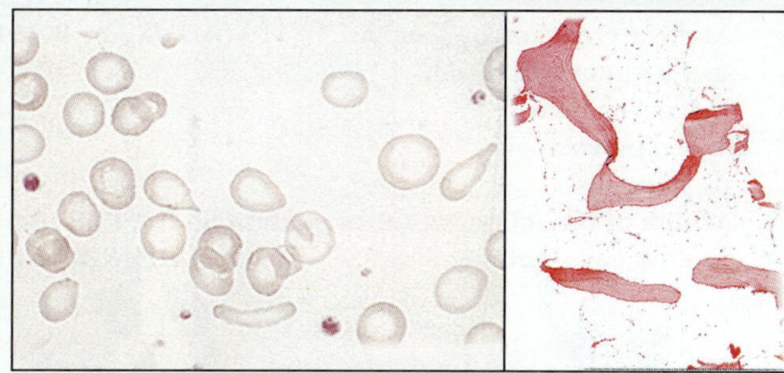

a. Iron deficiency anemia
b. Megaloblastic anemia
c. Aplastic anemia
d. Pure red cell aplasia

Answers of Image-Based Questions

1. **Ans. (d) Methyl violet**
   - This is staining of reticulocyte with supravital stains which includes New Methylene blue, Crystal violet, Brilliant cresyl blue

2. **Ans. (c) PNH**
   - **A case of anemia and Jaundice suggests hemolytic anemia.** Red coloured urine suggests hemoglobinuria seen in a case of intravascular hemolysis like PNH.

3. **Ans. (b) Kleihauer-Bethke acid elution for fetal hemoglobin**
   - In this figure the dark red colored cells are RBC which have resisted acid elution and have HbF, while ghost RBCs (light colored) lack HbF and so denatured with alkali and eluted with adding acid. **Kleihauer-Betke acid elution method to quantify the magnitude of feto-maternal bleed.**

4. **Ans. (a) *P. vivax* and bite cells**
   - **The given condition is malaria and shows trophozoite stage of *Plasmodium vivax*.** On giving anti malarials like Primaquine, hemolysis may be precipitated showing bite cells in peripheral smear.

5. **Ans. (d) Thalassemia**
   - Severe transfusion requiring anemia and Jaundice with smear showing Anisopoikilocytosis and targets on smear suggests Thalassemia.

6. **Ans. (c) Aplastic anemia**
   - The given peripheral smear shows pancytopenia while bone marrow biopsy shows hypocellular marrow seen in a case of Aplastic anemia.

Multiple Choice Questions

RBCs AND ANEMIA

1. Maltese cross can be seen in: *(AIIMS Nov 2019)*
a. Pneumocystis carinii
b. Leishmaniasis
c. Cryptococcosis
d. Babesiosis

2. Which of the following tubes contain Sodium fluoride as anticoagulant? *(AIIMS Nov 18)*

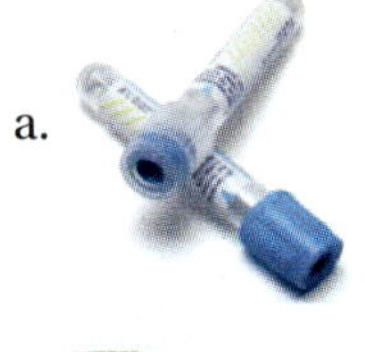

a.

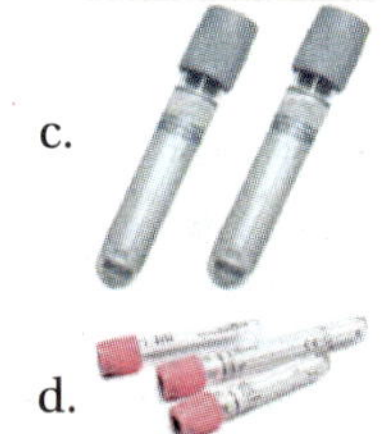

c.

b.

d.

3. Formula for calculating reticulocyte production index: *(JIPMER Nov 2019)*
a. Retic × hct/ normal hct
b. Corrected ret × hct /45 | maturation index
c. Reticulocyte percentage × RBC count
d. Reticulocyte counted × 100/number of red cells

4. Ring sidroblast in myelodysplastic syndrome is associated with which gene mutation? *(JIPMER 18)*
a. ASXL 1
b. EZH2
c. TET2
d. SF3B1

5. What should be the sequence of events during collection of blood sample? *(AIIMS Nov 2017)*
a. Ask the patient his name verify from file Label the sample at bedside → collect blood
b. Look at the file → Collect sample → Label the sample at bedside
c. Prelabel the sample vials → Check the file patient details → Collect sample
d. Collect sample → Confirm name from file → Label the sample vial

6. Which vacutainer is used for electrolyte estimation?
a. Na Citrate
b. EDTA *(AIIMS Nov 2017)*
c. Fluoride
d. Lithium heparin

7. What does the red cell distribution width (RDW) deal with? *(AIIMS May 2017)*
a. Hypochromia
b. Anisocytosis
c. Poikilocytosis
d. Anisochromia

8. A 25 year old female came to OPD 1 year after postpartum. She was treated for iron deficiency anemia while pregnancy. Now she is pale and her Hb was 5% and reticulocyte count was 9%. Her corrected retic count is? *(AIIMS May 2017)*
a. 6
b. 4.5
c. 3
d. 1

9. Acetone free methanol in leishman stain does which of the following? *(AIIMS May 2017)*
a. Fixes cells to slide
b. Colour of cell
c. Causes metabolic and enzymatic activity to stop
d. Washes the slide

10. A 26-year-old patient having RBC count 2 lakhs/mm³, PCV 30% and haemoglobin 9.3, what is the type of anemia?
a. Iron deficiency anemia *(AIIMS Nov 2016)*
b. Folic acid deficiency anemia
c. Thalassemia
d. Sideroblatic anemia

11. Identify the organism in the given Image?

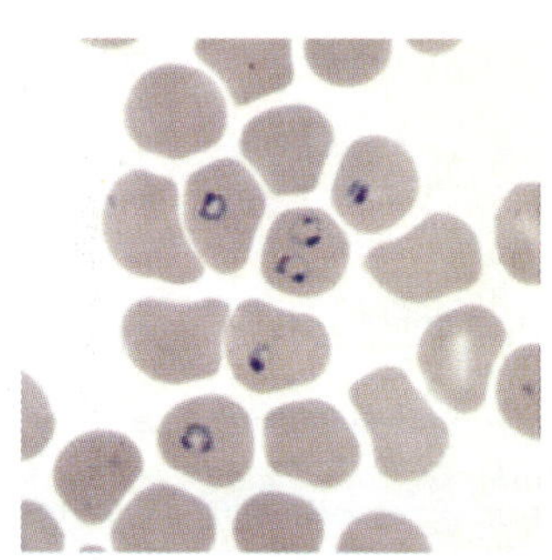

a. P. vivax
b. P. ovale *(AIIMS Nov 2016)*
c. P. falciparum
d. P. malariae

12. The rate of production of red blood cells by the human bone marrow is? *(Recent Question 2016)*
a. 1.5×10^6 cells/second
b. 1.5×10^3 cells/second
c. 7.5×10^6 cells/second
d. 7.5×10^3 cells/second

13. Identify the predominant abnormally shaped red cell type seen in the peripheral smear given below: *(Recent Question 2016)*

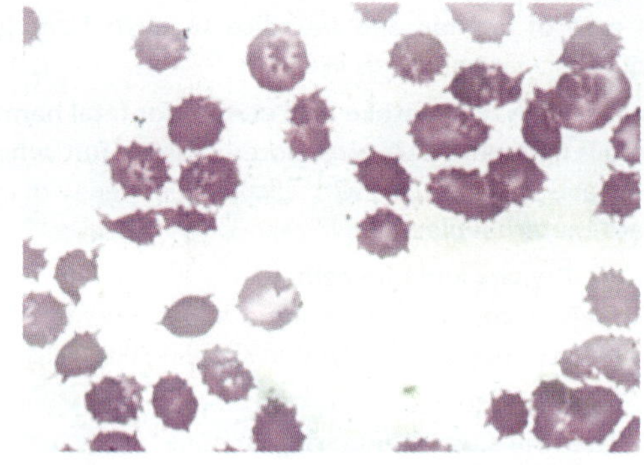

a. Macrocyte
b. Acanthocyte
c. Dacrocyte
d. Elliptocyte

14. Erythropoetin in fetus is secreted by? *(Recent Question 2016)*
a. Liver
b. Marrow
c. Spleen
d. Kidney

15. Most mature normoblast is: *(JIPMER Nov 2019)*
a. Orthochromic normoblast
b. Pronormoblast
c. Polychromatic normoblast
d. Basophilic normoblast

16. 1st stage of RBC development is? *(Recent Question 2016)*
a. Pro erythroblast
b. Intermediate normoblast
c. Reticulocyte
d. nRBC

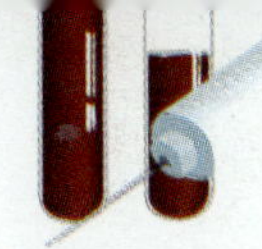

17. **Spur cells are seen in** *(Recent Question 2015)*
 a. Hereditary spherocytosis b. G6PD deficiency
 c. Liver disease d. Sideroblastic anemia

18. **Spiculated RBCs with evenly spaced spikes are called**
 (Recent Question 2015)
 a. Acanthocytes b. Stomatocytes
 c. Echinocytes d. Dacryocytes

19. **Most common cause of splenic rupture is:**
 (Recent Question 2015)
 a. Malaria b. ITP
 c. Thalassemia d. Cirrhosis

20. **Supravital staining is used for?** *(Recent Question 2015)*
 a. Nucleated RBCs b. Reticulocytes
 c. Basophils d. Myeloblasts

21. **When osmotic fragility is normal, RBCs begin to hemolyse when suspended in saline:**
 (Recent Question 2015, DNB 99)
 a. 0.33% b. 0.48%
 c. 0.9% d. 1.2%

22. **True about reticulocyte is?** *(Recent Question 2014)*
 a. Stained by supravital staining
 b. Myeloid cell
 c. Romanowsky stains are used
 d. 5% is normal

23. **Ratio of fat cells and blood cells in bone marrow is-**
 (Recent Question 2014, 2013)
 a. 1 : 4 b. 1 : 2
 c. 1 : 1 d. 2 : I

24. **Howel-Jolly bodies may be seen after-**
 (Recent Question 2014, AI 99)
 a. Hepatectomy b. Splenectomy
 c. Pancreatectomy d. Cholecystectomy

25. **Cabot's ring is seen in?** *(Recent Question 2014)*
 a. Megaloblastic anemia
 b. Sickle cell disease
 c. Iron deficiency anemia
 d. Autoimmune anemia

26. **Cyanosis is not seen in severe anemia because:**
 (AIIMS May 2012)
 a. Anemic hemoglobin has greater oxygen carrying capacity per unit gram of hemoglobin
 b. A critical concentration of reduced hemoglobin is required
 c. Increased RBC number counterbalances the oxygen shortage
 d. Blood flow through the skin is decreased in anemia

27. **ESR is a very critical investigation in the diagnosis of TB. Which of the following is true about ESR in TB?**
 a. No change in ESR *(AIIMS May 2012)*
 b. Confirms recovery from TB
 c. ESR is raised because of increased RBC aggregate
 d. ESR is raised due to decreased RBC size

28. **All are true about polycythemia vera except?**
 a. Increased ESR *(DNB Aug. 12 Pattern)*
 b. Decreased erythropoietin
 c. Increased LAP score
 d. Increased blood volume

29. **Cabot's ring in RBC is seen in?** *(DNB Aug 12, Dec 09)*
 a. Acquired hemolytic anemia
 b. Hemochromatosis
 c. Thalassemia
 d. After splenectomy

30. **If you are in PHC, which anticoagulant is used to sent the blood sample for blood glucose estimation'?**
 a. EDTA *(AIIMS Nov 11)*
 b. Heparin
 c. Potassium oxalate
 d. Potassium oxalate + sodium fluoride

31. **True about RBC and anemia:** *(PGI Nov 2011)*
 a. In female of reproductive age 12.5% is cut of value for anemia
 b. In newborn Hb level is 15 gm%
 c. Microcytosis occurs in folic acid deficiency
 d. Macrocytosis may occur in Celiac disease
 e. Normocytic normochromic anemia is found in chronic diseases

32. **Which of the following indicates hemolysis?**
 (JIPMER 11)
 a. Target cells b. Schistocytes
 c. Acanthocytes d. Basophilic stippling

33. **Pappenheimer bodies are composed of ?**
 a. Copper b. Zinc *(DNB June 10)*
 c. Iron d. Lead

ESR

34. **In which of the following condition(s) erythrocyte sedimentation rate is increased:** *(PGI May 2019)*
 a. Increased serum immunoglobulin level
 b. Spherocytosis
 c. Increased plasma viscosity
 d. Sickle cell anemia
 e. Increased level of C-reactive protein

35. **ESR is decreased in all the following conditions except**
 a. Polycythemia *(Recent Question 2015)*
 b. Sickle cell anemia
 c. Congestive cardiac failure
 d. Multiple myeloma

36. **Decreased ESR is seen in** *(Recent Question 2016)*
 a. Sickle cell Anemia
 b. Increased fibrinogen
 c. Anemia
 d. Hypoviscosity

HEMOLYTIC ANEMIAS

37. **In hereditary spherocytosis, which of the following is/ are increased?**
 (PGI May 18)
 a. Haptoglobin b. Spleen size
 c. MCHC d. MCV
 e. LDH

38. **Secondary hemolytic anemia is seen in all except?**
 (JIPMER 18)
 a. CML b. CLL
 c. CRRT d. ECMO

39. **Eosin-5-Maleamide flow cytometry is used for diagnosis of?** *(JIPMER 18)*
a. G6PD
b. Hereditary spherocytosis
c. Sickle cell anemia
d. Alpha thalassemia

40. **Schistocytes seen in which of the following?**
a. HUS *(PGI Nov 2018)*
b. TTP
c. Prosthetic heart valves
d. Alpha thalassemia

41. **Acanthocytes are seen in?** *(PGI MAY 18)*
a. Hallervorden-Spatz disease
b. Abetalipoproteinemia
c. Severe liver disease
d. Ataxia telangiectasia
e. McLeod syndrome

42. **Blister cells seen in which condition?** *(JIPMER 2017)*
a. G6PD deficiency   b. Thalassemia
c. Sickle cell anemia   d. AIHA

43. **Cold agglutinins are directly against which of the following RBC antigens?** *(JIPMER Nov 2019)*
a. I
b. P
c. Le
d. Rh

44. **A 25-year-old female presented in December month with chronic fatigue and cyanosis with bluish lips and arthralgia. Peripheral blood film is shown below. What is the likely cause?** *(AIIMS Nov 2016)*

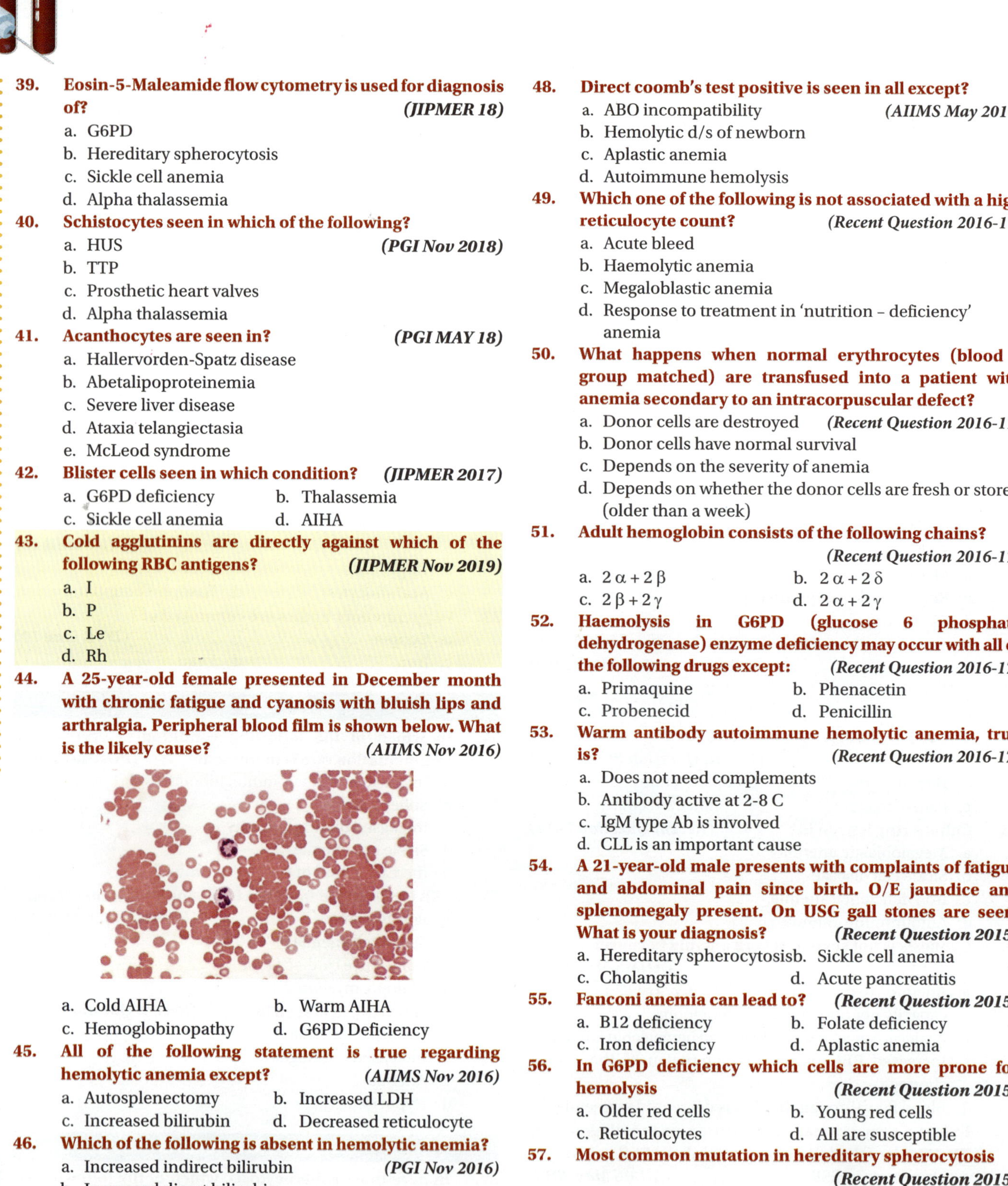

a. Cold AIHA   b. Warm AIHA
c. Hemoglobinopathy   d. G6PD Deficiency

45. **All of the following statement is true regarding hemolytic anemia except?** *(AIIMS Nov 2016)*
a. Autosplenectomy   b. Increased LDH
c. Increased bilirubin   d. Decreased reticulocyte

46. **Which of the following is absent in hemolytic anemia?**
a. Increased indirect bilirubin *(PGI Nov 2016)*
b. Increased direct bilirubin
c. Increased reticulocyte count
d. Jaundice
e. Increased LDH

47. **True about sickle cell anemia is?** *(JIPMER 2016)*
a. More susceptible to infections especially by Pneumococcus
b. Sickling is irreversible
c. Bone pain is common in small bones
d. HbA2 is increased

48. **Direct coomb's test positive is seen in all except?**
a. ABO incompatibility *(AIIMS May 2016)*
b. Hemolytic d/s of newborn
c. Aplastic anemia
d. Autoimmune hemolysis

49. **Which one of the following is not associated with a high reticulocyte count?** *(Recent Question 2016-17)*
a. Acute bleed
b. Haemolytic anemia
c. Megaloblastic anemia
d. Response to treatment in 'nutrition – deficiency' anemia

50. **What happens when normal erythrocytes (blood – group matched) are transfused into a patient with anemia secondary to an intracorpuscular defect?**
a. Donor cells are destroyed *(Recent Question 2016-17)*
b. Donor cells have normal survival
c. Depends on the severity of anemia
d. Depends on whether the donor cells are fresh or stored (older than a week)

51. **Adult hemoglobin consists of the following chains?** *(Recent Question 2016-17)*
a. $2\alpha + 2\beta$ b. $2\alpha + 2\delta$
c. $2\beta + 2\gamma$ d. $2\alpha + 2\gamma$

52. **Haemolysis in G6PD (glucose 6 phosphate dehydrogenase) enzyme deficiency may occur with all of the following drugs except:** *(Recent Question 2016-17)*
a. Primaquine   b. Phenacetin
c. Probenecid   d. Penicillin

53. **Warm antibody autoimmune hemolytic anemia, true is?** *(Recent Question 2016-17)*
a. Does not need complements
b. Antibody active at 2-8 C
c. IgM type Ab is involved
d. CLL is an important cause

54. **A 21-year-old male presents with complaints of fatigue and abdominal pain since birth. O/E jaundice and splenomegaly present. On USG gall stones are seen. What is your diagnosis?** *(Recent Question 2015)*
a. Hereditary spherocytosis b. Sickle cell anemia
c. Cholangitis   d. Acute pancreatitis

55. **Fanconi anemia can lead to?** *(Recent Question 2015)*
a. B12 deficiency   b. Folate deficiency
c. Iron deficiency   d. Aplastic anemia

56. **In G6PD deficiency which cells are more prone for hemolysis** *(Recent Question 2015)*
a. Older red cells   b. Young red cells
c. Reticulocytes   d. All are susceptible

57. **Most common mutation in hereditary spherocytosis** *(Recent Question 2015)*
a. Spectrin   b. Ankyrin
c. Glycophorin A   d. Band 3

58. **Most common mutation in hereditary elliptocytosis** *(Recent Question 2015)*
a. Spectrin   b. Ankyrin
c. Glycophorin A   d. Band 4.2

59. **Drug that is safe in G6PD deficiency** *(Recent Question 2015)*
a. Primaquine   b. Acetanilid
c. Quinidine   d. Dapsone

60. **Duffy antigen is associates with:** *(Recent Question 2016)*
    a. Plasmodium vivax
    b. Falciparum
    c. Ovale
    d. Malariae

61. **In hereditary spherocytosis, which gene is altered?** *(Recent Question 2016)*
    a. Spectrin
    b. Laminin
    c. Desmin
    d. Vimentin

62. **Warm Antibodies are?** *(Recent Question 2016)*
    a. Complete Antibody
    b. Incomplete Antibody
    c. Heterophillic antibody
    d. IgM

63. **Best treatment of atypical HUS is?** *(Recent Question 2016)*
    a. Plasmapheresis
    b. Antibiotics
    c. IvIG
    d. Dialysis

64. **Direct coomb's test is positive in hemolytic anemia due to** *(Recent Question 2015)*
    a. Paraxysmal cold hemoglobinuria
    b. Paroxysmal nocturnal hemoglobinuria
    c. Idiopathic thrombocytopenic purpura
    d. Hemolytic uremic syndrome

65. **Not used in the treatment of PNH**
    a. Cyclosporine *(Recent Question 2015)*
    b. Eculizumab
    c. Bone marrow transplantation
    d. Leucocyte depleted blood transfusion

66. **Hemolytic crisis in hereditary spherocytosis is precipitated by** *(Recent Question 2015)*
    a. Parvovirus B19 infection
    b. Infectious mononucleosis
    c. Human T-cell leukemia virus
    d. Cytomegalo virus

67. **A 25 year old patient presents with the history of dyspnea on exertion for 3 weeks. Investigations revealed Hb–7g/dl, reticulocyte count 18% and positive coomb's test. Diagnosis** *(Recent Question 2015)*
    a. Autoimmune hemolytic anemia
    b. Paroxysmal nocturnal hemoglobimuria
    c. Sickle cell anemia
    d. Hereditary spherocytosis

68. **Kleiheur Bethke test is done for?** *(APPGMEE 2015)*
    a. Cephalopelvic disproportion
    b. Fetomaternal haemorrhage
    c. Determining karyotype of normal fetus
    d. Diagnosing fetal infections

69. **Features of hemolytic anemia are all except?** *(Recent Question 2015)*
    a. Hemoglobinemia
    b. Bilirubinemia
    c. Reticulocytosis
    d. Haptoglobin increased

70. **Direct globulin test is positive in?**
    a. PNH *(Recent Question 2014)*
    b. Sickle cell anemia
    c. Thalassemia
    d. Paroxysmal cold hemoglobinuria

71. **Intracorpuscular hemolytic anemia is seen in-** *(Recent Question 2014)*
    a. Autoimmune hemolytic anemia
    b. TTP
    c. Thalassemia
    d. Infection

72. **Not true about hereditary spherocytosis-** *(Recent Question 2014)*
    a. Defect in ankyrin
    b. Decreased MCV
    c. Decreased MCHC
    d. Reticulocytosis

73. **In sickle cell anemia all are true except:** *(Recent Question 2014)*
    a. Sickle cells
    b. Target cells
    c. Howell jolly bodies
    d. Ringed sideroblast

74. **Person having heterozygous sickle cell trait is protected from infection of –** *(Recent Question 2014)*
    a. Plasmodium falciparum
    b. P. vivax
    c. Pneumococcus
    d. Salmonella

75. **All are features of haemolytic uremic syndrome, except-** *(Recent Question 2014)*
    a. Hyperkalemia
    b. Anemia
    c. Renal microthrombi
    d. Neuro psychiatric disturbances

76. **Thalassemia gives protection against-** *(Recent Question 2014)*
    a. Filaria
    b. Kala-azar
    c. Malaria
    d. Leptospirosis

77. **Donath Landsteiner antibody is seen in-**
    a. PNH *(Recent Question 2014)*
    b. Waldenstrom's macroglobulinemia
    c. Paroxysmal cold hemoglobinuria
    d. Malaria

78. **HUS is differentiated from TTP by?** *(JIPMER 2014)*
    a. Presence of Microangipathic hemolytic anemia
    b. Renal failure
    c. Neurological symptoms
    d. Absence of fever

79. **Maternal blood from fetal blood can be differentiated by?** *(JIPMER 2014)*
    a. Osmotic fragility test
    b. Kleihaurbethke test
    c. APT test
    d. Bubble test

80. **Reagent used in APT test?** *(JIPMER 2014)*
    a. Sodium hydroxide
    b. Sodium chloride
    c. Sodium acetate
    d. Sodium bicarbonate

81. **Severe Hereditary spherocytosis can be seen due to defect of the following protein?** *(JIPMER 2014)*
    a. α-Spectrin
    b. Ankyrin
    c. Band 3
    d. Band 4.2

82. **KleihauerBetke test is used to detect** *(APPGMEE 14)*
    a. Ferning pattern in follicular phase
    b. Cephalopelvic disproportion
    c. Fetomaternal blood leak
    d. Sperm–cervical mucus interaction

83. **A 16-year-old Afro-American boy presenting with non-healing ulcer of foot with recurrent pneumonia, chronic hemolytic anemia. The peripheral blood erythrocytes showed some RBCs with peculiar appearance. Most likely cause is:** *(AIIMS Nov 14/ Nov 2013)*
    a. Single amino acid base substitution
    b. Trinucleotide repeat
    c. Antibody to RBC membrane
    d. Genomic imprinting

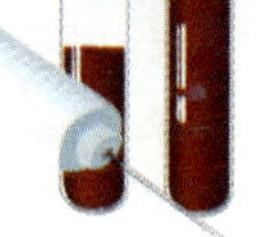

84. Person having heterozygous sickle cell trait is protected from infection of: *(AIIMS May 2013/Nov 12)*
- a. P. falciparum
- b. P. vivax
- c. Pneumococcus
- d. Salmonella

85. True about β-thalassemia: *(PGI May 2013)*
- a. Common in India
- b. Change in β-globin gene
- c. Microcytosis
- d. Increased HbF
- e. Secondary hemochromatosis may occur

86. Autosplenectomy is seen in? *(DNB Aug 12 Pattern, DNB June 10)*
- a. Hereditary spherocytosis
- b. G6 PD deficiency
- c. Sickle cell anemia
- d. Thalassemia major

87. False about Sickle cell anemia is? *(JIPMER 2012)*
- a. Fetal Hb persists at high conc in adult life as it is protective
- b. Co existant alpha thal is milder disease
- c. Aplastic crisis is related to spleen
- d. Sequestration crisis is related to spleen

88. Which is false about hemolytic anemia?
- a. Decreased LDH *(JIPMER 2012)*
- b. Decreased Haptoglobin
- c. Decreased RBC survival
- d. Increased Uncongugated Bilirubin

89. Which of the following is not true about HS?
- a. Extravascular hemolysis *(JIPMER 2012)*
- b. Mutation in protein of RBC membrane
- c. Young RBCs are normal in shape
- d. After splenectomy, Spherocytes disappear

90. Which is false about G6PD deficiency?
- a. X linked recessive *(JIPMER 2012)*
- b. Young RBCs are more prone to hemolysis
- c. Episodic hemolysis
- d. Both intravascular & extravascular hemolysis is seen

91. A 23-year-old female presented with jaundice and pallor for 2 months. Her peripheral blood smear shows the presence of spherocytes. The most relevant investigation to arrive at a diagnosis is *(AIIMS May 11)*
- a. Reticulocyte count
- b. Osmotic fragility test
- c. Coombs test
- d. Tests for PNH

92. Reticulocyte index ≥2.5 is/are seen in: *(PGI Nov 2011)*
- a. Hemolysis
- b. Blood loss
- c. Hemoglobinopathy
- d. Iron deficiency anemia
- e. Macrocytic anemia

93. Drugs that do not carry risk of hemolysis in persons with G-6-PD deficiency: *(PGI May 2011)*
- a. Primaquine
- b. Paracetamol
- c. Ceftriaxone
- d. Nitrofurantoin
- e. Vitamin K analogues

94. Schistocytes are found in: *(PGI May 2011)*
- a. Microangiopathichemolytic anemia
- b. HUS
- c. Hereditary schistocytosis
- d. Thrombotic thrombocytopenic purpura
- e. DIC

95. Most common cause of hereditary spherocytosis? *(DNB Dec 11)*
- a. Spectrin
- b. Glycophorin
- c. Ankyrin
- d. Band 4

96. Heinz bodies are seen in: *(MAHA 11)*
- a. Thalassemia
- b. G6PD deficiency
- c. Hereditary spherocytosis
- d. Paroxysmal nocturnal hemoglobinuria

97. Unconjugated hyperbilirubinemia with increased urobilinogen is seen in: *(AI 10)*
- a. Hemolytic anemia
- b. Liver cirrhosis
- c. Bile duct obstruction
- d. Sclerosing cholangitis

98. In hereditary spherocytosis mutation not seen is? *(DNB Dec 10)*
- a. Ankyrin
- b. Spectrin
- c. Band-3
- d. Na+ Cl- channel protein

99. A Newborn with ABO incompatibility will characteristically show the presence of following on peripheral smear: *(AIIMS Nov 10)*
- a. Schistocytes
- b. Elliptocytes
- c. Microspherocytes
- d. Polychromasia

100. A 5 year old male child presents with episodic jaundice and anemia since birth. Which of the following is least likely diagnosis?
- a. Hereditary spherocytosis
- b. Sickle cell disease
- c. PNH
- d. G6PD deficiency

ABNORMALITIES OF HEMOGLOBIN

101. A 6-year-old patient with anemia, on electrophoresis shows HbF 90%, Hb A2/=3%. Which of the following will be seen on peripheral smear? *(AIIMS Nov 2017)*

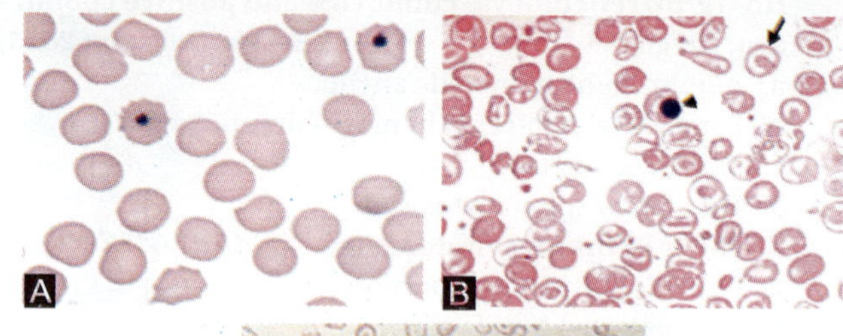

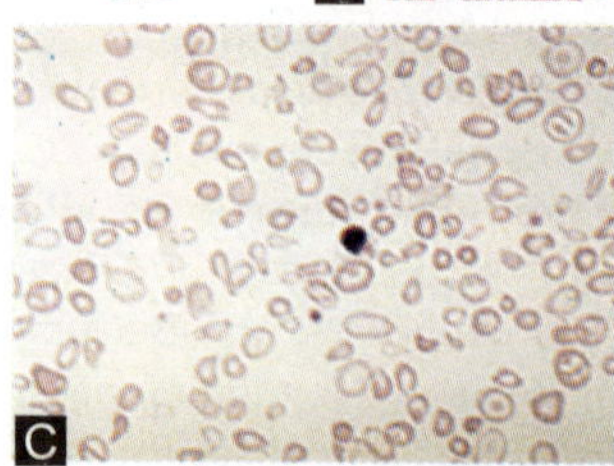

- a. A, B
- b. A, C
- c. ABC
- d. B, C

102. CBC done on a patient who had come for blood transfusion revealed MCV 56fl, Hb 13 gm%, MCHC 32 gm/dl & RDW 14, RBC count 6million/ul
- a. Sideroblastic anaemia
- b. b-Thalassemia disease
- c. b-Thalassemia trait
- d. Iron deficiency anemia

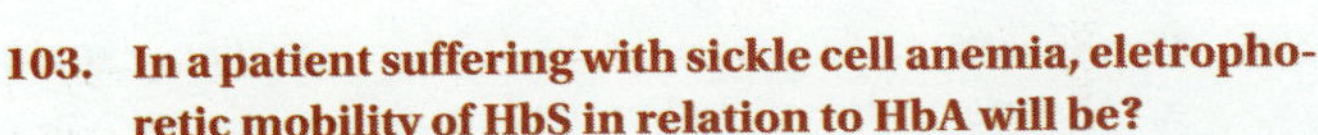

103. In a patient suffering with sickle cell anemia, eletrophoretic mobility of HbS in relation to HbA will be?

(AIIMS Nov 2015)

a. Retarded
b. Accelerated
c. Same
d. Will depend upon concentretation of HbS

104. Screening test for thalassemia   *(Recent Question 2015)*

a. Alkali denaturation test
b. Kleihauer test
c. Hb electrophoresis
d. NESTROFT

105. Bart hemoglobin is tetramer of   *(Recent Question 2015)*

a. α chain
b. β chain
c. γ chain
d. δ chain

106. Hemoglobin H disease is caused by deletion

a. Single α globin chain   *(Recent Question 2015)*
b. Two α globin chains
c. Three α globin chains
d. All α globin chain

107. All the following features precipitate sickling of HBS except   *(Recent Question 2015)*

a. Hypoxia
b. Dehydration
c. Infections
d. Alkalosis

108. Autosplenectomy is seen in

(WB PG 2016) (Recent Question 2015)

a. Hereditary spherocytosis
b. Sickle cell anemia
c. Thalassemia
d. G6PD deficiency

109. Sickle cell disease is less severe in

(Recent Question 2015)

a. HbSC
b. Females
c. Thalassemia
d. All the above

110. A young adult presents with history of bone pains, recurrent chest infections and dyspnea. Peripheral blood smear shows. (refer Q149) what is you diagnosis?

(Recent Question 2015)

a. Megaloblastic anemia
b. Hereditary spherocytosis
c. Sickle cell anemia
d. Thalassemia

111. In HbM the position of point mutation

(Recent Question 2015)

a. β chain, 87th codon, Histidine → Tyrosine
b. α chain, 87th codon, Histidine → Tyrosine
c. β chain, 6th codon, Glutamine → Valine
d. β chain, 6th codon, Glutamine → Lysine

112. Mutation in sickle cells disease is an example of

a. Silence mutation   *(Recent Question 2015)*
b. Missense mutation
c. Nonsense mutation
d. Frameshift mutation

113. In α-thalassemia, HbBarts is said when number of gene loci affected is: *(PGI May 2015)*

a. 1
b. 2
c. 3
d. 4
e. None

114. 25/f came to OPD with anemia, jaundice and joint pain. Which of the following statements is not true about the condition?   *(APPGMEE 2015)*

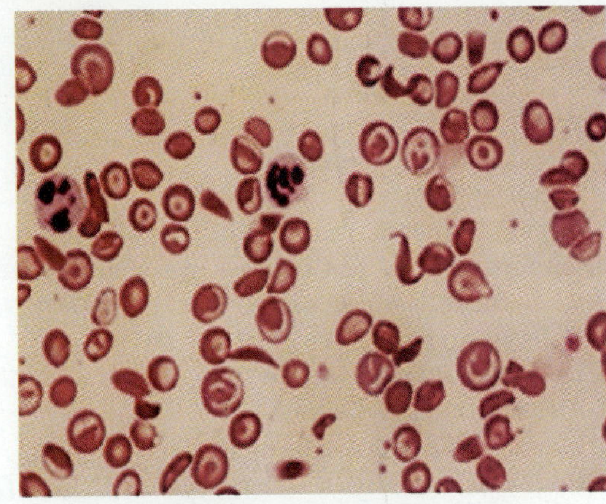

a. She can have pulmonary syndrome
b. She can have retinopathy
c. Hydroxyurea can help her
d. HbF and HbA2 will be undetectable

115. Boy born to mother who is O-ve has blood group B+ve. He developed jaundice on day 1, Peripheral blood smear is given, which cell is absent?

(Recent Question 2015)

a. Sickle cell
b. Aniocytosis
c. Target cell
d. Schistocytes

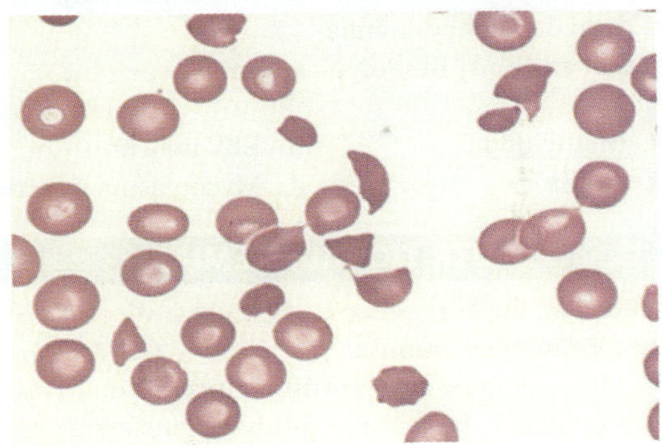

116. All are seen in sickle cell anemia EXCEPT?

a. Target cells
b. Jaundice   *(DNB June 11)*
c. Reticulocytosis
d. High hematocrit

117. Heterozygous sickle cell anemia gives protection against: *(AI 10)*

a. G6PD
b. Malaria
c. Thalassemia
d. Dengue fever

118. HbH is associated with: *(AI 11)*

a. Deletion of 3 alpha genes
b. Deletion of 4 alpha genes
c. Deletion of 2 beta genes
d. Deletion of 1 beta genes

119. NESTROFT test is used in screening of -

a. Thalassemia   *(AIIMS Nov 11)*
b. Autoimmune hemolytic anemia
c. Spherocytosis
d. G6PD deficiency

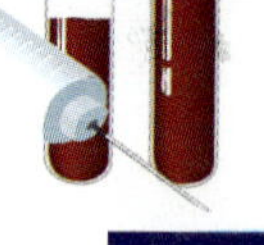

OTHER HEMOLYTIC ANEMIAS

120. **Which of the following tests is gold standard to diagnose a case of PNH?** *(Recent exam 2018)*
    a. HAMS test
    b. Sucrose lysine test
    c. Flow cytometry
    d. Bone marrow

121. **CD59 deficiency leads to:**
    a. PNH
    b. Chédiak–Higashi disease
    c. Hairy cell leukemia
    d. Hemolytic uremic syndrome

122. **An abnormal Ham test is most likely associated with which of the following?** *(AIIMS Nov 11)*
    a. Defect in spectrin
    b. Defective GPI anchor
    c. Defect in complement
    d. Mannose-binding residue defect

123. **PNH is associated with a deficiency of:** *(AI 10)*
    a. DAF
    b. MIRL
    c. GPI anchored protein
    d. All of the above

124. **Mutation of which of the following gene is most important in paroxysmal nocturnal hemoglobinuria**
    a. Decay accelerating factor (DAF) *(AI 10)*
    b. Membrane inhibitor of reactive lysis (MIRL)
    c. Glycosylphosphatidyl inositol (GPI)
    d. CD8 binding protein

125. **Schistocyte is/are found in:** *(PGI May 10)*
    a. TTP
    b. DIC
    c. Severe iron deficiency
    d. March hemoglobinuria
    e. Iron deficiency anemia

126. **Warm antibody hemolytic anemia is seen in?** *(DNB June 10)*
    a. Methyldopa
    b. EBV infection
    c. Quinine
    d. Mycoplasma infection

NUTRITIONAL ANEMIAS

127. **Which of the following is the best indicator to assess iron deficiency anemia:** *(AIIMS Nov 2019)*
    a. TIBC increased, Ferritin increased, Transferrin saturation increased, Serum transferrin receptors increased
    b. TIBC reduced, Ferritin reduced, Transferrin saturation reduced, Serum transferrin receptors decreased
    c. TIBC increased, Ferritin reduced, Transferrin saturation reduced, Serum transferrin receptors decreased
    d. TIBC increased, Ferritin reduced, Transferrin saturation reduced, Serum transferrin receptors increased

128. **Hepcidin inhibits the function of which of the following?**
    a. DMT-1 *(AIIMS Nov 2019)*
    b. Hephaestin
    c. Ceruloplasmin
    d. Ferroportin

129. **Iron enters enterocyte by:** *(AIIMS Nov 2019)*
    a. DMT-1
    b. Ferroportin
    c. Ferritin
    d. Hephaestin

130. **Hypoproliferative anemia(s) is/are:** *(PGI May 2019)*
    a. Anemia of chronic inflammation
    b. Anemia due to chronic renal disease
    c. Iron deficiency anemia
    d. Myelodysplastic syndrome
    e. Sickle cell anemia

131. **Which of the following is/are lower in anaemia of chronic diseases as compared to iron deficiency anaemia?** *(PGI May 18)*
    a. TIBC (Total iron binding capacity)
    b. Serum ferritin
    c. Serum iron
    d. Transferrin saturation
    e. Iron stores

132. **Microcytosis on peripheral blood smear is/are seen in?**
    a. Iron deficiency anemia *(PGI May 18)*
    b. Thalassaemia
    c. Sideroblastic anemia
    d. Vit. B12 deficiency
    e. Folate deficiency

133. **Differential diagnosis for microcytic anemia is?** *(PGI Nov 2018)*
    a. Lead poisoning
    b. Sideroblastic anemia
    c. Occult blood loss
    d. Atransferrenemia

134. **All decrease in iron deficiency anemia except?** *(AIIMS Nov 2017)*
    a. Ferritin
    b. TIBC
    c. Iron
    d. Transferrin

135. **Which of these is not involved in iron metabolism?** *(AIIMS Nov 2017)*
    a. Hepcidin
    b. Ferroportin
    c. Transthyretin
    d. Ceruloplasmin

136. **Which of the following would be the findings of sideroblastic anemia?** *(AIIMS May 2017)*
    a. Coarse basophilic stippling in lead poisoning
    b. erythroid hypoplasia in marrow
    c. Dimorphic anaemia
    d. Increase transferrin saturation
    e. Increase MCHC

137. **Which of the following is accurate regarding the internal iron homeostasis in iron deficiency anemia** *(JIPMER 2018)*
    a. Transferrin receptor 1 - iron responding elements increases transferrin receptor mRNA concentration and synthesis
    b. Ferritin mRNA concentration – iron response element increases and ferritin synthesis decreases
    c. Ferritin mRNA concentration – iron response element decreases and Ferritin synthesis increases
    d. Transferrin receptor 1 - iron responding elements decreases transferrin receptor mRNA concentration and increases synthesis

138. **Which of the following are true regarding a child with iron deficiency anaemia** *(JIPMER 2017)*
    a. Raised MCV
    b. Raised transferrin saturation
    c. Increased TIBC
    d. Increased ferritin

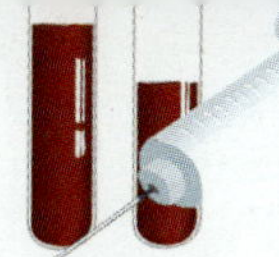

139. **Following are causes of megaloblastic anemia except?**
   a. Defect in DNA synthesis   *(PGI Nov 2016)*
   b. Folic acid deficiency
   c. Lead toxicity   d. Vit B12 deficiency

140. **Match List-I with List-II and select the correct answer using the code given below the Lists?**
                (Recent Question 2016-17)

List-I (Blood picture)	List-II (Type of Anemia)
A. Microcytic, hypochromic red cells	1. Vitamin B12 deficiency anemia
B. Macrocytic, hypochromic red cells	2. Thalassemia major
C. Large number of early, intermediate and late erythroblasts	3. Aplastic anemia
D. Low reticulocyte count	4. Iron-deficiency anemia

  Code:

	A	B	C	D
a.	1	4	2	3
b.	2	3	4	1
c.	4	1	2	3
d.	3	1	2	4

141. **Which of the following conditions does not cause pancytopenia?**   *(Recent Question 2016)*
   a. Hypersplenism
   b. Aplastic anemia
   c. Cancer infiltrating the bone-marrow
   d. Hemolysis from G6PD enzyme deficiency

142. **Which of the following is least likely?**
   a. Celiac disease   *(Recent Question 2016-17)*
   b. Thalassemia major
   c. Nutritional anemia
   d. Paroxysmal nocturnal haemoglobinuria

143. **Iron metabolism and regulation are important for RBC precursor cell. Which of the following helps in regulation of iron metabolism but is not specific for iron?**
   a. Hepcidin   b. DMT-1 *(AIIMS Nov 2015)*
   c. Ferroportin   d. Ferritin

144. **Transfer of Iron from enterocyte to plasma is inhibited by?**   *(Recent Question 2016-17)*
   a. Hepsidin   b. DMT-1
   c. Ferroportin   d. Hepestin

145. **Iron stores are best indicated by?**
             (Recent Question 2016)
   a. S. ferritin   b. S. Iron
   c. S. transferrin   d. TIBC

146. **Release ferroportin store is controlled by?**
             (Recent Question 2016)
   a. Hepsidin   b. Transferrin
   c. Ferritin   d. Hepoxin

147. **Which of the following correctly describes principle of Prussian blue stain?**   *(Recent Question 2016)*
   a. Ferrocyanide to ferricyanide
   b. Ferrocyanide to ferroferric cyanide
   c. Ferroferric cyanide to ferrocyanide
   d. Ferrocyanide to ferricferro cyanide

148. **True about Hereditary Hemochromatosis a/e:**
   a. Mutations in the HFE gene   *(Recent Question 2016)*
   b. Autosomal recessive disorder
   c. Excess iron affects organ function
   d. Diagnosed by serum ferritin

149. **Pappenheimer body is seen in:** *(Recent Question 2016)*
   a. Sideroblast   b. Siderocyte
   c. Reticulocyte   d. Bite cells

150. **Calculate iron deficit for a 50 kg person, with Hb-5g/dL. Add 1000 mg for stores.**   *(Recent Question 2015)*
   a. 2150 mg   b. 1650 mg
   c. 1150 mg   d. 1575 mg

151. **A 50 year old male has Hb 9.2g/dL and MCV112fL. Next step:**   *(Recent Question 2015)*
   a. Iron supplement   b. Folate supplement
   c. Transusion   d. Check B12 and folate level

152. **A 40 year old female presents with signs of heart failure. Hb-6 g/dL, MCV-112. Next step** *(Recent Question 2015)*
   a. Check B12 and folate levels
   b. Blood transfusion
   c. Start iron tablets
   d. Start folate supplementation

153. **MCV is increased in the following anemia**
   a. Iron deficiency anemia   *(Recent Question 2015)*
   b. Sideroblastic anemia
   c. Anemia of chronic disease
   d. Folate deficiency anemia

154. **Find the false statement regarding megaloblastic anemia**   *(Recent Question 2015)*
   a. Hypersegmented neutrophils are the earliest manifestation
   b. Reticulocyte count decreased
   c. Hypercellular bone marrow
   d. MCHC is increased

155. **20-year-old female present with features of anemia. Blood tests: Hb-5g/dL, MCV – 52 fL, MCHC–20 g/dL, PCV – 32%. Diagnosis**   *(Recent Question 2015)*
   a. Phenytoin toxicity
   b. Fish tape worm infection
   c. Hook worm infection
   d. Blind loop syndrome

156. **Most sensitive indicator of iron deficiency anemia**
             (Recent Question 2015)
   a. Packed cell volume   b. Hemoglobin
   c. Serum ferritin   d. Serum iron

157. **Macrocytic anemia with MCV> 110 fL is seen in**
             (Recent Question 2015)
   a. Thiamine deficiency   b. B12 deficiency
   c. Hypothyroidism   d. Phenytoin tocixity

158. **Iron deficiency anemia and anemia of chronic disease can be differentiated by the following parameter**
             (Recent Question 2015)
   a. Microcytic, hypochromic anemia
   b. Serum iron
   c. TIBC
   d. Transferrin saturation

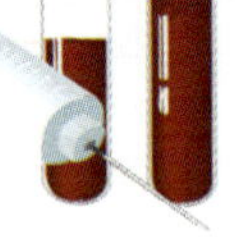

159. In a patient with thalassemia major, who had received multiple blood transfusions, the serum iron overload can be detected by *(Recent Question 2015)*

a. Serum ferritin level
b. Blood iron level
c. Total iron binding capacity
d. Blood hemoglobin level

160. Iron absorption is increased by *(Recent Question 2015)*

a. Phytates
b. Tannates
c. Plant food
d. Ascorbic acid

161. Microcytic anemia is not seen in the following condition *(Recent Question 2015)*

a. Osteomyelitis
b. Leukopenia
c. Papilliary necrosis
d. Stroke

162. True statement about anemia of chronic disease

a. Increased serum ferritin *(Recent Question 2015)*
b. Increased serum iron
c. Increased TIBC
d. Increased transferring saturation

163. Average serum ferritin value in males *(Recent Question 2015)*

a. 50 mg/dL
b. 100 mg/dL
c. 200 mg/dL
d. 500 mg/dL

164. Most important inflammatory mediator, involved in anemia of chronic disease? *(Recent Question 2015)*

a. IL-1
b. IL-6
c. TNFa
d. IFN-Y

165. True about iron deficiency anemia *(JIPMER 2015)*

a. Parenteral iron is indicated when anemia response slowly to oral iron
b. Ferrous sulphate 200mg has less elemental iron then the same dose of ferrous gluconate
c. Sustained release iron is a useful way of giving larger doses
d. Absorption of iron is increased by ascorbic acid

166. This patient came with anemia. This peripheral smear shows. *(APPGMEE 2015)*

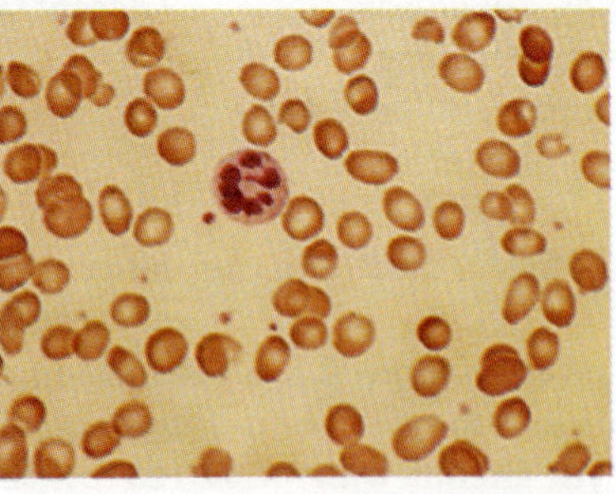

a. Microcytic hypochromic anemia due to iron deficiency
b. Macrocytic anemia
c. Target cells of thalassemia
d. Spherocytes of autoimmune hemolytic anemia

167. Which of the following is not associated with microcytic hypochromic anemia? *(APPGMEE 2015)*

a. Chronic Lead poisoning
b. Thalassemia
c. Hereditary spherocytosis
d. Iron deficiency

168. Red cells containing granules of non-heme iron, which gives positive Prussian blue reaction with Perl's stain as well as stain with Romanowsky dyes (referred to as pappenheimer bodies) are known as: *(AP 2012)*

a. Schistocytes
b. Spherocytes
c. Sideroblasts
d. Siderocytes

169. A 5-year-old child presents with pallor and constipation with Hb-6 gm%. Which is the most appropriate therapy? *(Recent Question 2015)*

a. Packed cell RBC's
b. Oral iron therapy
c. Parenteral iron
d. Hematologist referral

170. Most sensitive marker in iron deficiency anemia:

a. TIBC *(Recent Question 2014)*
b. Serum ferritin
c. Serum Iron
d. Serum transferrin saturation

171. Normal transferrin saturated with iron is ? *(Recent Question 2014)*

a. 20%
b. 35%
c. 50%
d. 70%

172. Response to iron in iron deficiency anemia is denoted by? *(Recent Question 2014, DNB 09)*

a. Restoration of enzymes
b. Reticulocytosis
c. Increase in iron binding capacity
d. Increase in hemoglobin

173. Iron deficiency causes *(Recent Question 2014)*

a. Megaloblastic anemia
b. Microcytic hypochromic anemia
c. Macrocytic hypochromic anemia
d. Microcytic hypochromic anemia

174. Bone marrow in lead poisoning contains?

a. Ringed siderocytes *(JIPMER 2014)*
b. Giant metamyelocytes
c. Dwarf megakaryocytes
d. Fibrotic changes

175. All of the following statements about iron deficiency anemia are true except? *(AIIMS Nov 2013)*

a. Latent iron deficiency is most common presentation in India
b. Transferrin saturation is less than 16%
c. Serum ferritin is the earliest marker
d. It can present without detectable abnormalities

176. Leptocyte in blood smears seen in? *(Recent Question 2013)*

a. Sickle cell anemia
b. Thalassemia
c. Post splenectomy
d. Uremia

177. First sign of improvement in oral iron therapy is? *(DNB Aug. 12 Pattern) (WBPG 2015)*

a. Reticulocytosis
b. Raise of hemoglobin
c. Raise in RBC count
d. Increase in ESR

178. Parameter increased in IDA? *(JIPMER 2012)*

a. RBC protoporphyrin
b. Serum Iron level
c. Serum ferritin
d. Transferrin saturation

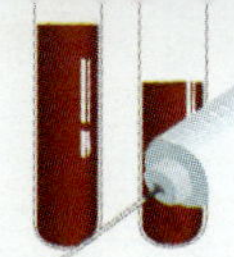

179. A 35-year-old lady on treatment for rheumatoid arthritis has following lab findings: Hb-9 gm/dl, MCV- 55 fl, serum iron-30 ug/dl, ferritin- 200 ng/ml, TIBC- 298 ug/dl. What is the most probable diagnosis? *(AIIMS Nov 11)*
   a. Thalassemia minor   b. Thalassemia major
   c. Anemia of chronic disease
   d. Iron deficiency anemia

180. 33-years-old alcoholicon ATT presents with increased serum iron and increased transferrin saturation. Diagnosis? *(JIPMER 11)*
   a. Iron deficiency anemia   b. Sideroblastic anemia
   c. Megaloblastic anemia   d. Anemia of chronic disease

181. A patient with microcytic hypochromic anemia. Hb-9 g%, serum iron-20 microg/dl, ferritin level-800 ng/ml, transferrin percentage saturation is 64%. What is possible diagnosis? *(AIIMS Nov 10)*
   a. Atransferrinemia
   b. Iron deficiency anemia
   c. DMT 1 mutation
   d. Anemia of chronic disorder

182. A 60-years-old female presents with history of 8 blood transfusions in 2 yrs. Her Hb-6.0gm/dl, TLC-5800/cumm, platelet- 3.4 lakhs/cumm, MCV-60 fl, RBC-2.1 lakhs/mm³. She is having hypochromic microcytic anemia. Which investigation is not needed?

   (AIIMS Nov 10)
   a. Evaluation for pulmonary hemosiderosis
   b. Urinary hemosiderin
   c. Bone marrow examination
   d. G1 endoscopy

183. A man presents with fatigue. Hemogram analysis done suggested low Hb, high MCV. The next investigation is?
   (Recent Question 2015)
   a. Vit B_{12}/folatelevels   b. Bone Marrow
   c. S. Iron studies   d. Reticulocyte count

184. Which of the following does not indicate Megaloblastic anemia? *(AIIMS May 2013/ Nov 2012)*
   a. Increased reticulocyte count
   b. Raised Bilirubin
   c. Mild splenomegaly
   d. Nucleated RBC

185. Symptoms of folate deficiency occur in association with which of the following? *(PGI May 2011)*
   a. Nitrous oxide   b. Pyrimethamine
   c. Sodium nitroprusside   d. Sodium valproate
   e. 5-FU

186. Macrocytic anemia is seen in all EXCEPT·
   a. Vitamin B_{12} deficiency   *(DNB June 10)*
   b. Hemolytic anemia
   c. Post hemorrhagic anemia
   d. Anemia of chronic disease

HYPOPROLIFERATIVE ANEMIAS

187. Criteria for severe aplastic anemia are all except?
   a. BM cellularity <25%   *(JIPMER 2017)*
   b. Reticulocyte <60,000/ul
   c. Platelet <20,000/ul
   d. Absolute neutrophil count <1500/ul

188. Bone marrow failure with neutropenia and exocrine pancreatic deficiency is a feature of ? *(JIPMER 2017)*
   a. Fanconi anemia
   b. Dyskeratosis congenita
   c. Diamond Blackfan syndrome
   d. Diamond Schwachman syndrome

189. Parvovirus preferentially involves in which of the following cells:
   a. Erythroid progenitors   b. Myeloid precursors
   c. Megakaryocytes   d. Both a & c

190. All of the following are causes of increased reticulocyte count except?
   a. Treatment of megaloblastic anaemia with Vit B12
   b. Congenital dyserythropoetic anaemia
   c. Hereditary spherocytosis
   d. Aplastic anaemia

191. The following drug is not associated with pure red cell aplasia: *(Recent Question 2015)*
   a. Phenytoin   b. Isoniazid
   c. Erythropoietin   d. None of the above

192. Pancytopenia with hypocellular bone marrow seen in:
   a. Fanconi's anemia   *(Recent Question 2015)*
   b. Paroxysmal nocturnal hemoglobinuria
   c. Hairy cell leukemia
   d. Myelopthisis

193. 2-year-old child presents with short stature and café-au-lait spots. Bone marrow aspiration yields a little material and mostly containing fat. What is your diagnosis: *(Recent Question 2015)*
   a. Fanconi anemia
   b. Dyskeratosis congenita
   c. Tuberous sclerosis
   d. Osteogenesis imperfecta

194. Dry tap is a feature: *(Recent Question 2015)*
   a. Anemia of chronic disease
   b. Megaloblastic anemia
   c. Aplastic anemia
   d. Sickle cell anemia

195. MC tumor associated with pure red cell aplasia:
   a. Hepatoma   *(Recent Question 2015)*
   b. Hodgkins lymphoma
   c. Thymoma
   d. Bronchogenic carcinoma

196. 2/F presented with maculopapular rash 24hrs after onset of mild fever. There was prominent erythema over the cheek. The causative organism also causes?
   a. CMV   b. ALL   *(JIPMER 2014)*
   c. DIC   d. PRCA

197. Pure red cell aplasia is associated with all except?
   (AIIMS Nov 2013)
   a. ABO incompatibility after renal transplant
   b. 5q- syndrome
   c. Drugs
   d. Large granular lymphocytic leukemia

198. Pancytopenia with cellular bone marrow is seen in all except: *(WBPG 2015)*
   a. Megaloblastic Anemia   b. MDS
   c. PNH   d. G6PD deficiency

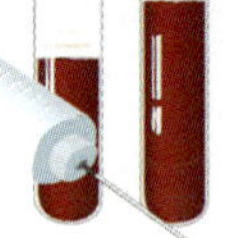

199. Prominent reticulocytosis is a feature of:

(WBPG 2015)

a. Aplastic Anemia   b. Hemolytic Anemia

c. Nutritional Anemia   d. Anemia of chronic disease

200. Aplastic anemia can progress to all except: *(DPG10)*

a. AML

b. Myelodysplastic anemia

c. Pure red cell aplasia

d. Paroxysmal nocturnal hemoglobinuria

201. True about Dyskeratosis congenita: *(PGI May 2011)*

a. Pancytopenia

b. Nail dystrophy

c. Hyperkeratosis

d. X-linked

e. Leukoplakia

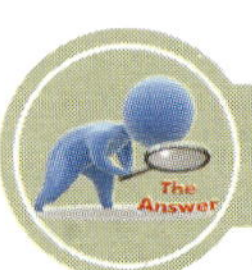

Answers with Explanations

---

1.   Ans. (d) Babesiosis

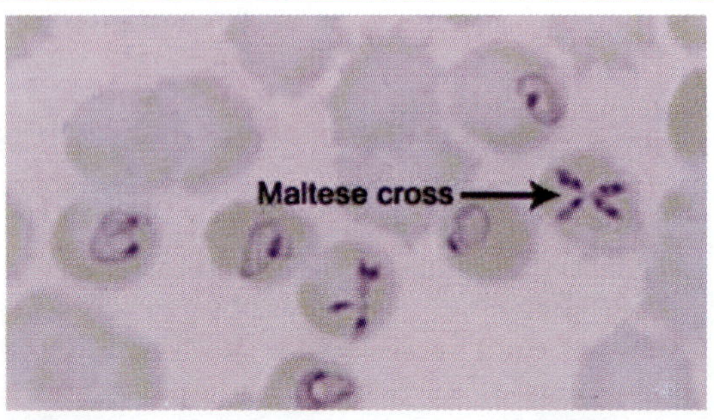

Babesia microti in a thin blood smear. Note the classic "Maltese Cross" tetrad-form in the infected RBC in the lower part of the image.

---

2.   Ans. (c) Gray

Hemoguard stopper	Tube content	Determination
	Serum separator tube (SST)	All biochemistry not mentioned elsewhere (1 tube), microbiology (1 tube)
	Heparin	Chromosome studies, lead, amino acids, troponin
	Fluoride/ oxalate	Glucose
	EDTA	Full blood count (FBC) and ESR, C3/C4, hemoglobin A1c, homocysteine, ACTH
	Plain (No additive)	LDH, Ca, drugs (Phenytoin, theophylline, lithium), endo-crine testing (except thyroid)
	Sodium citrate	Coagulation testing, PT, INR, APTT, D-Dimer, etc...
	ESR	Westergren Sedimentation Rate; requires full draw

---

3.   Ans. (b) Corrected ret × hct /45 | maturation index

(Ref: Harrison 19th ed/pg 396)

---

4.   Ans. (d) SF3B1

---

5.   Ans. (a) Ask the patient his name verify from file Label the sample at bedside → collect blood

---

6.   Ans. (d) Lithium heparin

(Ref: Henry Clinical chemistry)

Heparin, a mucoitin polysulfuric acid, is an effective anticoagulant available as lithium heparin (LiHep) and sodium heparin (NaHep) in green-top tubes. Heparin accelerates the action of antithrombin III, neutralizing thrombin and preventing the formation of fibrin. Heparin has an advantage over EDTA as an anticoagulant, as it does not affect levels of ions such as calcium. However, heparin can interfere with some immunoassays. Heparin should not be used for coagulation or hematology testing.

---

7.   Ans. (b) Anisocytosis

Red Cell Distribution width

- The RDW is an index of the variation in cell size and volume within the red cell population.

Normal Value

- RDW-SD 39-46 fL, RDW-CV 11.6-14.6% in adult

Condition with Increased RDW:

- Iron deficiency anaemia
- Folate/vit B12 deficiency anaemia

---

8.   Ans. (c) 3 *(Ref: Harrison 19th Edition. Page No. 396)*

Reticulocyte Count has two Corrections

- Correction for the degree of anaemia (Absolute reticulocyte count) and Correction for the prolonged duration of stay of reticulocyte in peripheral smear.

Corrected reticulocyte count → Reticulocyte count X Hb or

Hct of patient/Normal Hb or Hct

    = 9 X 5/15

    = 9/3 = 3

Corrected reticulocyte count = 3 %

---

9.   **Ans. (a)**   **Fixes cells to slide**

(Ref: Bancroft's Histochemical Techniques, Page 90-98)

Acetone Free Methanol is the Fixative in Leishmann Stain

- If acetone is there it will destroy the cell membrane

---

10.   **Ans. (b)**   **Folic acid deficiency anemia**

(Ref: Robbins 9th/pg 631)

- **Hematocrit** or **Packed cell volume:** ratio of the volume of RBCs to total volume of blood
- Hct or PCV = MCV × RBC concentration

Now coming back to the question:

- MCV =PCV/RBC count (in millions) = 30/0.2 = 150 (Increased)
- MCH= Hb/RBC count = 9.3/ 0.2= 46 (Increased)
- MCHC= Hb/ MCV= 31 (Normal)

The answer here is clearly macrocytic anemia (increased MCV as macrocytosis) so the correct option is b. Folic acid deficiency anemia

---

11.   **Ans. (c)**   **P. falciparum**

(Ref: Practical hematology, Dacie pg 110)

---

12.   **Ans. (a)**   **1.5 × 106 cells/second**

(Ref: Wintrobes 12th ed/pg 107-108)

- Bone marrow produces approximately **2.4 million new erythrocytes per second** (2.4×10^6/s) in human adults.
- They circulate for about 100–120 days
- The closest to this data is option A (hence the answer)

---

13.   **Ans. (b)**   **Acanthocyte** *(Ref: Dacie 11th/pg 85)*

---

14.   **Ans. (a)**   **Liver** *(Ref: Robbins 9th/pg 618; 8th/pg 628)*

Sources of erythropoietin:

Fetus: Liver

Adult:

- Interstitial cells in peritubular capillary bed of kidneys (85%)
- Perivenous hepatocytes in the liver (15%)
- Brain (protective effect against excitotoxic damage triggered by hypoxia)
- Uterus and oviducts (mediate estrogen-dependent angiogenesis).

---

15.   **Ans. (a)**   **Orthochromic normoblast** *(Ref: R 9th/pg 580)*

---

16.   **Ans. (a)**   **Pro erythroblast** *(Ref: Robbins 9th/pg 580)*

---

17.   **Ans. (c)**   **Liver disease** *(Ref: Dacie 11th/pg 85)*

---

18.   **Ans. (c)**   **Echinocytes** *(Ref: Dacie 11th/pg 85)*

---

19.   **Ans. (a)**   **Malaria** *(Ref: Robbins 9th/pg 625)*

- **Most common cause of splenic rupture is Trauma**
- **Most common cause of spontaneous splenic rupture in the world is Infectious Mononucleosis**
- **Most common cause of spontaneous splenic rupture in India is Malaria**

---

20.   **Ans. (b)**   **Reticulocytes** *(Ref: Dacie 11th/pg34)*

---

21.   **Ans. (b)**   **0.48 %** *(Ref: Dacie 11th/pg246)*

When osmotic fragility is normal, RBC's begin to hemolyse when suspended in 0.48 % saline

Osmotic Fragility Test

- Gives an indication of the **surface area/volume ratio** of erythrocytes.
- Normally RBCs start hemolysing at 0.5% NaCl and is completely hemolysed at 0.3% NaCl
- It is useful in the diagnosis of **hereditary spherocytosis** & screening for **thalassaemia.**
- Red cells that are **spherocytic** have **increased osmotic fragility** i.e. take up less water in a hypotonic solution before rupturing than do normal red cells.

Conditions associated with:

Increased osmotic fragility (OF)	Decreased (OF)
• Hereditary spherocytosis • Hereditary elliptocytosis (HE) • Hereditary stomatocytosis • Autoimmune hemolytic anemia	• Thalassaemia • Enzyme abnormalities • Hereditary xerocytosis • Iron deficiency

---

22.   **Ans (a)**   **Stained by supravital staining**

(Ref: Dacie 11th/pg34; Refer Ans 2 Above)

- Reticulocytes stained on Romanowsky stain (used for usual hematological staining) are called polychromatophils;
- However it is not a specific stain;

---

23.   **Ans. (c)**   **1: 1** *(Ref: Robbins 9th/pg 582; 8th/pg 592)*

Ratio of fat cells and blood cells in bone marrow is 1:1

---

24.   **Ans. (b)**   **Splenectomy**

(Ref: Dacie 11th/pg 85; Robbins 9th/pg 632; 8th/pg 643)

Howell–Jolly Bodies

- Howell–Jolly bodies are **nuclear remnants**.
- They are **small, round cytoplasmic inclusions** that **stain purple** on a Romanowsky stain.
- Seen after **splenectomy, in splenic atrophy, pernicious anemia, coeliac disease**

---

25.   **Ans. (a)**   **Megaloblastic anemia**

(Ref: Wintrobe's Atlas of Clinical Hematology, 1st Edition, 2007, chapter 1)

26. **Ans. (b)** **A critical concentration of reduced hemoglobin is required** (*Ref: Harrison 18th/pg Chapter 35*)

- Cyanosis becomes apparent when the concentration of **reduced hemoglobin in capillary blood > 4 g/dL**.
- It is the **absolute,** rather than the *relative*, **quantity of reduced Hb** that is **important in producing cyanosis**.
- In a patient with severe anemia, the *relative* quantity of reduced Hb in the venous blood may be very large, but the *absolute* quantity of reduced Hb is still small. Therefore, patients with **severe anemia & even *marked* arterial desaturation may not display cyanosis.**

27. **Ans. (c)** **ESR is raised because of increased RBC aggregate**

(*Ref: Dacie 11th/pg102*)

In **TB, ESR is raised** because of increased RBC aggregates ESR is increased by any cause or focus of inflammation

28. **Ans. (a)** **Increased ESR** (*Ref: Dacie 11th/pg105*)

In **polycythemia vera, ESR is decreased due to decrease in rouleaux formation or increase the RBC surface area to volume ratio.**

29. **Ans. (a)** **Acquired hemolytic anemia**

(*Ref: Wintrobe's 12th; Atlas of Clinical Hematology, 1st Edition, 2007 chapter 1*)

Cabot's ring in RBC is seen in **Acquired hemolytic anemia Pernicious Anemia > Hemolytic Anemias > Post Splenectomy; Lead poisoning**

30. **Ans. (d)** **Potassium oxalate + sodium fluoride**

(*Ref: Teitz clinical chemistry*)

Anticoagulant used to send blood sample for **glucose** estimation is **Potassium oxalate + sodium fluoride**

31. **Ans. (b, d, e); b. In newborn Hb level is 15 gm%; d. Macrocytosis may occur in Celiac disease and e. Normocytic normochromic anemia is found in chronic diseases**

(*Ref: Robbins 9th/pg 645-654; Wintrobe's 12th/pg 1221*)

32. **Ans. (b)** **Schistocytes**

(*Ref: Hematology: Basic principles and practice, 6th edition, 2013 chapter 32; Robbins 9th/pg 640; 8th/pg 650*)

Discussing the options one by one

a. **Target cells**: Seen in **Thalassemia, Liver disease, Abetalipoproteinemia, severe Iron deficiency anemia**
B. **Schistocytes**: Seen in **Microangiopathic hemolytic anemia**
C. Acanthocytes: See table below
D. Basophilic stippling: See table below

33. **Ans. (c)** **Iron** (*Ref: Wintrobe's Atlas of Clinical Hematology, 1st Edition, 2007 chapter 1*)

34. **Ans.** **(a) Increased serum immunoglobulin level; (e) Increased level of C-reactive protein** (*Ref: Dacie 11th pg 105*)

Erythrocyte Sedimentation Rate is zero in Afibrinogenemia

Increased ESR	Lower ESR
• Old age	• Extreme leukocytosis
• Female	• **Polycythemia**
• **Pregnancy**	• Spherocytosis, microcytosis
• **Anemia**	• Hyperviscosity
• Paraprotein (Multiple Myeloma)	• Low protein, fibrinogen, gammaglobulins
• **Hypergammaglobulinemia**	• Technical factors; dilution, clotted sample
• Macrocytosis	• Afibrinogenemia
• Elevated fibrinogen (infection, inflammation malignancy)	**No effect**
• **Technical factors:** Dilution, high temperature	• Obesity
	• Body temperature
	• Recent meal
	• Aspirin, NSAIDs

35. **Ans. (d)** **Multiple myeloma** (*Ref: Dacie 11th/pg 105*)

36. **Ans. (a)** **Sickle cell Anemia** (*Ref: Dacie 11th/pg 105*)

37. **Ans. (b, c, e)** **b. Spleen size; c. MCHC; e. LDH**

Decreased MCV, Increased MCHC, and ↑ LDH. It also causes splenomegaly.

38. **Ans. (a)** **CML**

CLL IS USUALLY ASSOCIATED WITH AIHA.

Extracorporeal membrane oxygenation (ECMO) is a treatment that uses a pump to circulate blood through an artificial lung back into the bloodstream of very ill baby. This system provides heart-lung bypass support outside the baby's body. This can be associated with hemolysis Continuous renal replacement therapy (CRRT) can also have secondary hemolysis

39. **Ans. (b)** **Hereditary spherocytosis**

A flow cytometry-based test using eosin-5-maleimide (EMA) dye is used for diagnosis of hereditary spherocytosis (HS). Eosin-5-maleimide (EMA) dye, which reacts covalently with lysine-430 on the first extracellular loop of band-3 protein helps detecting HS, as vertical bonds are usually broken in HS.

40. **Ans. (a, b, c)** **a. HUS; b. TTP; c. Prosthetic heart valves**

41. **Ans. (a, b, c, e)** **a. Hallervorden-Spatz disease; b. Abeta-lipoproteinemia; c. Severe liver disease; e. McLeod syndrome**

42. **Ans. (a)** **G6PD deficiency** (*Ref: Wintrobes 13/p 2089*)

The peripheral blood smear IN G6PD def contains spherocytes and eccentrocytes or "blister" cells.

43. **Ans. (a)** **I** *(Ref: Robbins 9th/pg 643)*

44. **Ans. (a)** **Cold AIHA**

The given figure is of RBC agglutination. The history is suggestive of agglutination occurring in the month of December that is cold induced. Cold Agglutinin Type. This form of immunohemolytic anemia is caused by IgM antibodies that bind red cells avidly at low temperatures (0°–4°C).

45. **Ans. (d)** **Decreased reticulocyte**

46. **Ans. (b)** **Increased direct bilirubin**

Increased indirect bilirubin and not direct bilirubin are the findings in hemolytic anemia

	MCV	% S	% A	% A$_2$	% F
AS	N	35–38	62–65	< 3.5	<1
SS	N	88–93	0	<3.5	5–10
S/β° thalassaemia	L	88–93	0	>3.5	5–10

47. **Ans. (d)** **HbA2 is increased**

(Ref: Practical hematology by Dacie 11th ed/ pg 312)

In sickle cell anema, HbA2 is decreased and not increased.

48. **Ans. (c)** **Aplastic anemia**

(Ref: Wintrobe 13th ed / Page 576)

Coomb's test is **positive** in **Immune hemolytic anemia**
- They can be of 2 types:
  - **Direct Coomb's test**- Detects Antibody on RBC Surface[Q]
  - **Indirect Coomb's test**- Detects Antibody in Serum

Out of the given options: Aplastic anemia is not a hemolytic anemia and so is automatically the answer here.

49. **Ans. (c)** **Megaloblastic anemia**

Megaloblastic anemia has a low normal Retic % as it is a nutritional anemia.

50. **Ans. (b)** **Donor cells have normal survival.**

(Ref: Robbins 9th ed. Pg. 631-632)

This Question is based on the knowledge that in intracorpuscular defect of RBCs the defect lies in the RBCs itself and not in spleen or vessels and so any erythrocytes (blood – group matched) are transfused into a patient will not be destroyed. Hence the answer is **donor cells have normal survival.**

51. **Ans. (a)** **2 α + 2 β** *(Ref: Robbins 9th/pg 638-642)*

52. **Ans. (d)** **Penicillin** *(Ref: Robbins 9th/pg 644-645)*

Penicillin causes hemolysis by mechanism of autoimmune hemolytic anemia and not G6PD deficiency mediated.

53. **Ans. (d)** **CLL is an important cause**

54. **Ans. (a)** **Hereditary spherocytosis**

This is a case of anemia (fatigue), splenomegaly (abdominal pain) with jaundice and gall stones since birth. These findings suggest a inherited causes of extravascular hemolysis. The best option is Hereditary spherocytosis.

55. **Ans. (d)** **Aplastic anemia** *(Ref: Robbins 9th/pg 653)*

56. **Ans. (a)** **Older red cells** *(Ref: Robbins 9th/pg 634; 8th/ pg 644)*

Because mature red cells do not synthesize new proteins, G6PD– or G6PD Mediterranean enzyme activities fall quickly to levels inadequate to protect against oxidant stress as red cells age. Thus, older red cells are much more prone to hemolysis than younger ones.

57. **Ans. (b)** **Ankyrin** *(Ref: Robbins 9th/pg 632; 8th/pg 642)*

Most common mutation:
- Hereditary spherocytosis is Ankyrin>Band-3>spectrin
- Hereditary elliptocytosis is Spectrin

58. **Ans. (a)** **Spectrin** *(Ref: Robbins 9th/pg 632; 8th/pg 642)*

59. **Ans. (c)** **Quinidine** *(Ref: Robbins 9th/pg 634-635)*

Quinidine do not carry risk of hemolysis in persons with G-6-PD deficiency

60. **Ans. (a)** **Plasmodium vivax** *(Ref: Harrison 18th/pg 1014)*

Duffy antigen/chemokine receptor (**DARC**), also known as **Fy glycoprotein** (FY) or **CD234** (Cluster of **D**ifferentiation 234)
- Duffy antigen is located on the surface of RBCs, and is named after the patient in which it was discovered.
- glycosylated membrane protein and a non-specific receptor for several chemokines.
- The protein is also the receptor for the human malarial parasites Plasmodium vivax and Plasmodium knowlesi.
- Polymorphisms in this gene are the basis of the Duffy blood group system

61. **Ans. (a)** **Spectrin** *(Ref: Robbins 9th/pg 632; 8th/pg 642)*

62. **Ans. (b)** **Incomplete Antibody**

(Ref: Wintrobes 12th/ed pg 959)

IgM-coated RBCs may spontaneously agglutinate because the pentameric antibody can cross-link RBCs. The capability for **IgM antibodies** to agglutinate saline-suspended RBCs without additional reagents has led to the traditional terminology of **"complete" antibodies**. In contrast, **IgG antibodies** typically require antihuman globulin (AHG) to agglutinate saline-suspended RBCs and are thus termed **"incomplete" antibodies**.

Now as warm Antibodies are IgG, so they are "Incomplete antibodies"

63. Ans. (a) Plasmapheresis

(Ref: Robbins 9th/pg 941; 8th/pg 952; Harrison 19th/pg 740-745)

Treatment of Atypical HUS

- Fresh frozen plasma can induce remission.
- Plasma exchange may benefit patients with deficiency of **Complement Factor H or Factor I** by replenishing the missing protein or removing the antibodies.

64. Ans. (a) Paraxysmal cold hemoglobinuria

(Ref: Robbins 9th/pg 643; 8th/pg 653)

65. Ans. (a) Cyclosporine *(Ref: Wintrobes pg 1011)*

66. Ans. (a) Parvovirus B19 infection

(Ref: Harrison 18th/pg 1478)

- Aplastic/hypoplastic crises resulting from parvovirus B19 infection may occur in Hereditary spherocytosis just as is seen in individuals with other chronic hemolytic disorders.
- Parvovirus B_{19} selectively infects erythroid precursors and inhibits their growth.
- Erythropoietic arrest leads to a sudden decrease in hemoglobin concentration and reticulocytopenia.

67. Ans. (a) Autoimmune hemolytic anemia *(Ref: 9th/pg 643)*

68. Ans. (b) Fetomaternal haemorrhage

(Ref: Oski's Pediatrics: Principles & Practice, chapter 66; Dacie 11th/pg 307)

APT test for differentiation of fetal & adult (maternal) hemoglobin in stool or vomitus
- Mix 1 volume of sample with 5 volumes of water.
- Centrifuge mixture and remove clear-pink supernatant solution containing hemoglobin.
- Mix 1 ml of 1% sodium hydroxide with 4 ml supernatant and observe color change after 2 minutes.
  - Remains **pink: Hemoglobin F**
  - Turns **yellow-brown: Hemoglobin A** (maternal blood)

A common approach to evaluating FMH is the **rosette test to screen for the presence of fetal cells** followed by the **Kleihauer-Betke acid elution method to quantify the magnitude of feto-maternal bleed.**
The Kleihauer-Betke acid elution method:
- **Quantitative estimate of the volume of FMH** based on different solubility properties of HbF&HbA.
- On a peripheral smear **treated with an acidic solution** & counterstained, red cells containing acid-soluble **HbA appear as pale ghosts** compared to **deeply red stained red cells containing acid-resistant HbF**
- Can also be used to detect HbF containing cells in β-thalassemia, hereditary persistence of hemoglobin F, sickle cell disease &**myelodysplastic syndrome**.

- Increased HbF is also found in congenital red cell aplasia (Blackfan-Diamond syndrome) & congenital aplastic anemia (Fanconianemia), JMML, presence of erythropoietic stress (haemolysis, bleeding, recovery from acute bone marrow failure) and in pregnancy.

69. Ans. (d) Haptoglobin increased

(Ref: Robbins 9th/pg 631-632)

Haptoglobin

- A glycoprotein that is synthesized in the liver.
- It consists of two pairs of αchains and two pairs of β chains.
- With hemolysis, free Hb readily dissociates into dimers of α & β chains; the α chains bind avidly with the β chains of haptoglobin in plasma or serum to form a complex

70. Ans. (d) Paroxysmal cold hemoglobinuria

(Ref: Robbins 9th/pg 642; 8th/pg 654)

Direct globulin test is positive in Paroxysmal cold hemoglobinuria, as anti P antibody is formed.

71. Ans. (c) Thalassemia *(Ref: 9th/pg 631-632)*

Intra-corpuscular hemolytic anemia is seen in thalassemia

72. Ans. (c) Decreased MCHC *(Ref: 9th/pg 632-633)*

In hereditary spherocytosis, **increased** rather than decreased MCHC is seen

73. Ans. (d) Ringed sideroblast

(Ref: Robbins 9th/pg 635-636)

Ring sideroblasts are not seen in sickle cell anemia, but in Sideroblastic Anemia
Peripheral smear finding in sickle cell anemia:
- Ansiopoikilocytosis, polychromasia, Increased Retic %
- Irreversibly **sickle RBCs** and **target cells** (increased after autosplenectomy).
- **Howell-Jolly bodies** due to asplenia.[Q]

74. Ans. (a) Plasmodium falciparum

(Ref: Robbins 9th/pg 635-636; 8th/pg 645-646; Wintrobe's 12th/pg 1038)

Person having heterozygous sickle cell trait is protected from infection of Plasmodium falciparum
Mechanism by which patients with sickle cell trait are protected against Malaria:
- **Preferential sickling of parasitized cells** has been seen in the blood of children with sickle cell trait & malaria.
- **Selective removal of sickled cells** from the circulation probably reduces the degree of parasitemia and substantially limits the infectious process.

75. Ans. (d) Neuro psychiatric disturbances

(Ref: Robbins 9th/pg 941; 8th/pg 952-953)

Neuro-psychiatric disturbances are not a feature of hemolytic uremic syndrome, but may be seen in TTP

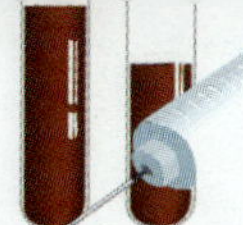

76. **Ans. (c) Malaria**

(Ref: Wintrobe's 12th/pg 1084)

RBCs with common Hemoglobinopathies (i.e. α- & β-thalassemias, HbS, HbC, HbE) & enzyme (**glucose-6-phosphate dehydrogenase [G6PD]) defects** have shown **a reduced parasite invasion/growth** and an **increased susceptibility to phagocytosis** of the infected RBC as a **malaria-protective effect.**

77. **Ans. (c) Paroxysmal cold hemoglobinuria**

(Ref: Robbins 9th/pg 642; 8th/pg 654)

Paroxysmal cold hemoglobinuria:
- Rare **intravascular hemolysis** and **hemoglobinuria.**
- **IgGs Abs[Q]** that bind to the **P blood group[Q]** antigen on RBC (direct antibody testing positive)are **called Donath Landsteiner Antibodies[Q]**
- Binds to RBC's at a low temperature (optimally at 4°C), but when the temperature is shifted to 37°C, lysis of red cells takes place in the presence of complement
- Seen in children following **viral infections.[Q]**

78. **Ans. (d) Absence of fever** *(Ref: Robbins 9th/pg 941)*
- In both HUS & TTP, there is Microangiopathic hemolytic anemia, Renal failure & Neurological symptoms.
- Fever & neurologic findings are seen in TTP, not in HUS

79. **Ans. (c) APT test**

(Ref: Oski's Pediatrics: Principles & Practice, chapter 66; Dacie 11th/pg 307)

80. **Ans. (a) Sodium hydroxide**

(Ref: Oski's Pediatrics: Principles & Practice, chapter 66; Dacie 11th/pg 307)

81. **Ans. (a) α-Spectrin**

(Ref: 9th/pg 632-633; 8th/pg 642-643)

82. **Ans. (c) Fetomaternal blood leak**

(Ref: Oski's Pediatrics: Principles & Practice, chapter 66; Dacie 11th/pg 307; Refer to Ans 81)

83. **Ans. (a) Single amino acid base substitution**

(Ref: Robbins 9th/pg 635-636; 8th/pg 645-647)

This is a case of 16 year old boy presenting with foot ulcer, recurrent pneumonia and chronic hemolytic anemia. This history of **non-healing ulcer** and **repeated infection** along with given peripheral smear finding is suggestive of **Sickle cell anemia. Point mutation in 6th codon of β-globin** that leads to **replacement of glutamate by valine** residue

84. **Ans. (a) P. falciparum** *(Ref: Robbins 9th/pg 635-636)*
- HbA/S heterozygotes (**Sickle cell trait**) have a **6-fold reduction** in risk of dying from **severe falciparum** malaria.

- Due to impaired parasite growth at **low oxygen tensions** and **reduced parasitized red cell cyto-adherence**.
- **Parasite multiplication** in HbA/E heterozygotes is **reduced** at high parasite densities.

85. **Ans. (a, b, c, d, e); a. Common in India; b. Change in β-globin gene; c. Microcytosis; d. Increased HbF; e. Secondary hemochromatosis may occur**

(Ref: Robbins 9th/pg 638-642)

a.	True	**Distribution:[Q]** of β thalassemia: • Mediterranean, Africa, middle-east, Pakistan, India and South east Asia. • In India- **Sindh[Q]**, Punjab, Gujrat and Bengal have higher prevalence
b.	True	**Decreased synthesis** of **β-globin** chains due to mutation of beta globin gene
c.	True	Marked **aniso-poikilocytosis, microcytic hypochromic** RBC's
d.	True	Selected survival of HbF cells in thalassemia causes increased level of HbF in blood
e.	True	**Repeated transfusion in thalassemia causes Iron overload** leading to Secondary hemochromatosis

86. **Ans. (c) Sickle cell anemia** *(Ref: Robbins 9th/pg 635-636)*

Patients of sickle cell anemia may undergo auto-splenectomy[Q] due multiple infarcts in splenic artery causes spleen to be reduced to fibrous tissue (splenic atrophy → **spleen may become non-palpable**)[Q]

87. **Ans. (c) Aplastic crisis is related to spleen**

(Ref: Robbins 9th/pg 635-636)

a. Fetal Hb persists at high conc in adult life as it is protective: TRUE; HbF has increased O_2 affinity, so decreases sickling;
b. Co-existant alpha thalassemia is milder disease: TRUE
c. Aplastic crisis is related to spleen: FALSE, as aplastic crisis is related to Parvovirus B19 infection
d. Sequestration crisis is related to spleen: TRUE, as it is due to hyperslenism

88. **Ans. (a) Decreased LDH** *(Ref: 9th/pg 631-632)*

In hemolytic anemia, there is decreased haptoglobin, decreased RBC survival, increased unconjugated bilirubin & Increased LDH.

89. **Ans. (d) After splenectomy, Spherocytes disappear**

(Ref: Robbins 9th/pg 632-633; 8th/pg 642-643)

Discussing options about HS one by one,
a. TRUE, as hemolysis occurs in spleen
b. TRUE, as Spectrin/Ankyrin/Band-3 defect is seen in HS
c. TRUE, as RBCs get damaged & deformed in circulation
d. FALSE; **After splenectomy, Spherocytes are still present, but hemolysis of these spherocytes in spleen is prevented**

90.   **Ans. (b)**   **Young RBCs are more prone to hemolysis**

(Ref: Robbins 9th/pg 634-635; 8th/pg 644-645)

Discussing the options about G6PD deficiency one by one,

a. TRUE; It has X linked recessive: inheritance

b. Young RBCs are more prone to hemolysis: FALSE, rather **younger RBCs are more resistant to hemolysis** - *Wintrobe's 12th/pg 935-937*

- As red cells age, the activity of G6PD declines.
- The normal enzyme (G6PD B) has an in vivo half-life of 62 days
- In contrast, the **G6PD variants associated with hemolysis are unstable** and have **much shorter half-lives**.
- The **anemia is self-limited** because the old susceptible population of erythrocytes is replaced by **younger RBC with sufficient G6PD activity to withstand an oxidative assault.**

c. Episodic hemolysis: TRUE, as it occurs only when exposed to inciting factors like infection & certain drugs;

d. Both intravascular & extravascular hemolysis is seen: TRUE

91.   **Ans. (c)**   **Coombs test**

(Ref: 9th/pg 643-644; 8th/pg 653-654)

A 23-year-old female presented with jaundice and pallor for 2 months. Her peripheral blood smear shows the presence of spherocytes. This scenario is suggestive of Autoimmune hemolytic Anemia

The most relevant investigation to arrive at a diagnosis is Coombs test

92.   **Ans. (a, b, c); a. Hemolysis; b. Blood loss; c. Hemoglobinopathy** *(Ref: Robbins 9th/pg 631-632)*

93.   **Ans. (b, c); b. Paracetamol; c. Ceftriaxone**

(Ref: Robbins 9th/pg 634-635; 8th/pg 644-645)

Paracetamol & Ceftriaxone do not carry risk of hemolysis in persons with G-6-PD deficiency

94.   **Ans. (a, b, c, d, e); a. Microangiopathic hemolytic anemia; b. HUS; c. Hereditary schistocytosis; d. Thrombotic thrombocytopenic purpura; e. DIC**

(Ref: Robbins 9th/pg 941)

Schistocytes are found in Microangiopathic hemolytic anemia, HUS, Hereditary schistocytosis, TTP, DIC

95.   **Ans. (c)**   **Ankyrin**

(Ref: Robbins 9th/pg 632-633)

96.   **Ans. (b)**   **G6PD deficiency** *(Ref: Robbins 9th/pg 634-635)*

Heinz bodies are seen in G6PD deficiency

97.   **Ans. (a)**   **Hemolytic anemia**

(Ref: Robbins 9th/pg 631-632)

Unconjugated hyperbilirubinemia with increased urobilinogen is seen in Hemolytic anemia

98.   **Ans. (d)**   **Na+ Cl– channel protein (Ref: R 9th/pg 632-633)**

99.   **Ans. (c)**   **Microspherocytes** *(Ref: Robbins 9th/pg 631-632)*

ABO incompatibility causes immune hemolytic anemia which is characterized by Spherocytes on peripheral smear

100.   **Ans. (c)**   **PNH** *(Ref: Robbins 9th/pg 631-632)*

- The given scenario is suggestive of episodes of hemolysis since birth, so it is probably due to a hereditary cause.
- Out of the given options, **hereditary spherocytosis, Sickle cell disease & G6PD deficiency** are **inherited causes** of hemolytic anemia, so they usually present in early childhood.
- **PNH is due to an acquired somatic mutation in PIG A gene, which usually presents in adults. So, PNH is the** least likely diagnosis in this cause.
- Remember that, **Sickle cell disease usually presents beyond 6 months age, due to high HbF concentration before that**, which prevents sickling

101.   **Ans. (c)**   **ABC**

Looking at the history and HPLC finding, it looks Thalassemia major which will have severe anisopoikilocytosis, (slide C) nRBC (slide B) and Howell jolly body (slide A)

102.   **Ans. (c)**   **b-Thalassemia trait**

This patient has a normal Hb but low MCV. So if you calculate the Mentzer index= MCV/RBC count, it comes to 9.3, which is less than 13 which is indicative of Thalassemia trait.

103.   **Ans. (a)**   **Retarded**

(Ref: Complete review of Pathology 1st /343)

Pathogenesis of Sickle cell anemia:

Sequence of codon 6 of the Beta-chain changed from GAG in the normal gene to GTG in the sickle cell gene, resulting in substitution of **valine for glutamic** acid

Concept:

So if you see, the charge of amino acid is changing from **charged (glutamic acid, more negative) to neutral amino acid (valine),** *so when we do an electrophoresis, the* **mobility of HbS will be lesser than HbA towards Anode (i.e retarded) (which is positively charged).**

<table>
<tr><td rowspan="2">At alkaline pH;
Cathode(–)</td><td>HbA2 → HbC → HbS → HbF → HbA</td></tr>
<tr><td align="right">Anode (+)</td></tr>
</table>

104.   **Ans. (d)**   **NESTROFT**

(Ref: Robbins 9th/pg 638; 8th/pg 648)

Screening tests for Thalassemia trait: NESTROFT (Naked Eye Single Tube Red cell Osmotic Fragility Test)[Q] *assesses osmotic fragility of red cells at a single concentration of buffered saline* **(0.36% in single tube)**[Q]

105. Ans. (c) γ **chain** *(Ref: Robbins 9th/pg 638; 8th/pg 648)*

106. Ans. (c) Three α **globin chains** *(Ref: Robbins 9th/pg 638)*

Classification of α-thalassemia:
- Normally 4 α-genes synthesize: **2** α **chains** → α,α/α,α
- Most common cause of α-thalassemia is α-**gene deletion (frame-shift mutation)**[Q]

107. Ans. (d) Alkalosis *(Ref: Robbins 9th/pg 635; 8th/pg 645)*

108. Ans. (b) Sickle cell anemia *(Ref: Robbins 9th/pg 635)*

Multiple infarcts in splenic artery causes spleen to be reduced to fibrous tissue referred to autospnectomy (splenic atrophy → **spleen may become non-palpable)**

109. Ans. (d) All the above

(Ref: Robbins 9th/pg 635; 8th/pg 645)

110. Ans. (c) Sickle cell anemia *(Ref: Robbins 9th/pg 635)*

111. Ans. (b) α **chain, 87th codon, Histidine → Tyrosine**

(Ref: Wintrobes 12th ed 1060-1070)
- M (met) hemoglobins are characterized by heme-iron oxidation and result in cyanosis.
- HbM Iwate (HBA 87th position his → tyr)

112. Ans. (b) Missense mutation *(Ref: Robbins 9th/pg 635)*

113. Ans. (d) 4 *(Ref: Robbins 9th/pg 638; 8th/pg 648)*

114. Ans. (d) HbF and HbA2 will be undetectable

(Ref: Wintrobes 12th ed p 1062)

The given peripheral blood picture shows sickle cells. Pulmonary syndrome & retinopathy are complications of Vaso-occlusive crises. Hydroxyurea increases HbF levels and so is used for treatment. HPLC diagnosis suggests **increase in HbS, HbA2, and HbF** while Hb A is decreased.

115. Ans. (a) Sickle cell *(Ref: Robbins 9th/pg 635; 8th/pg 645)*

The given scenario is of Rh incompatibility resulting in Hemolytic disease of newborn. The RBC morphology shows anisopoikilocytosis, polychromasia, target RBCs and Schistocytes.

116. Ans. (d) High hematocrit *(Ref: Robbins 9th/pg 635-636)*

In sickle cell anemia: Target cells, Jaundice & Reticulocytosis are seen
But hematocrit is low (not high), as it is an anemia

117. Ans. (b) Malaria *(Ref: 9th/pg 635-636; 8th/pg 645-647)*

118. Ans. (a) Deletion of 3 alpha genes *(Ref: 9th/pg 638-642)*

119. Ans. (a) Thalassemia

(Ref: Robbins 9th/pg 638-642; 8th/pg 648-652)

120. Ans. (c) Flow cytometry

(Ref: Robbins 9th/pg 643)
PNH is diagnosed by flow cytometry, which provides a sensitive means for detecting red cells that are deficient in GPI-linked proteins such as CD59 & CD55

121. Ans. (a) PNH

(Ref: Robbins 9th/pg 642)

122. Ans. (b) Defective GPI anchor

(Ref: R 9th/pg 642-643)

An abnormal Ham test is seen in PNH, which is due to defective GPI anchor

123. Ans. (d) All of the above

(Ref: Robbins 9th/pg 642-643)

PNH is associated with a deficiency of DAF (CD55), MIRL (CD59) & GPI anchored protein

124. Ans. (c) Glycosyl phosphatidyl inositol

(Ref: Robbins 9th/pg 642-643; 8th/pg 652-653)

125. Ans. (a, b, d); a. TTP; b. DIC; d. March Hemoglobinuria
(Ref: Robbins 9th/pg 631-632)

126. Ans. (a) Methyldopa *(Ref: Robbins 9th/pg 643-644)*

Drugs causing warm Ab type Autoimmnue Hemolytic Anemia:
- **Antigenic type**[Q]: penicillin and cephalosporins
- **Innocent bystander type** (Immune complex type): Penicillin
- **Tolerance-breaking**: Alpha methyl dopa[Q]

127. Ans. (d) TIBC increased, Ferritin reduced, Transferrin saturation reduced, Serum transferrin receptors increased *(Ref: Robbins 9th/pg 659)*

128. Ans. (d) Ferroportin *(Ref: Robbins 9th/pg 659)*

Hepcidin is a regulator of iron metabolism. **Hepcidin** inhibits iron transport by binding to the iron export channel ferroportin which is located on the basolateral surface of gut enterocytes and the plasma membrane of reticuloendothelial cells (macrophages).

129. Ans. (a) DMT-1 *(Ref: Robbins 9th/pg 659)*

The DMT1 protein, also known as Nramp2, SLC11A2, and DCT1, conducts iron transport at two distinct compartments of the cell: (1) It facilitates iron uptake at the apical cell membrane in for instance duodenal enterocytes (2) It transports iron across erythroid precursors in the bone marrow

130. Ans. (a) Anemia of chronic inflammation; (b) Anemia due to chronic renal disease; (c) Iron deficiency anemia; (d) Myelodysplastic syndrome *(Ref: Robbins 9th/pg 659)*

Anemias of Decreased Erythropoiesis: Important Examples are:
- Iron deficiency anemia, Folic acid and B_{12} deficiency anemia, vitamin C, Copper and Zinc deficiency. ACD, MDS, Aplastic and pre red cell aplasia

131. Ans. (a) TIBC (Total iron binding capacity)

132. Ans. (a, b, c) a. Iron deficiency anemia; b. Thalassaemia; c. Sideroblastic anemia

133. Ans. (a) Lead poisoning (b)Sideroblastic anemia (c)Occult blood loss (d) Atransferrenemia

All 4 will cause microcytic anemia hypochromic

134. Ans. (b) TIBC

Transferrin is quantified in terms of the amount of iron it will bind, a measure called the total iron-binding capacity (TIBC; In the average subject, the plasma iron concentration is ~(100 μg/dl), and the TIBC is ~(300 μg/dl).
Serum iron concentration is reduced in iron deficiency, and the TIBC is often increased

135. Ans. (c) Transthyretin *(Ref: Wintrobes 14th/p 813)*

Ceruloplasmin acts as an oxidase for a variety of substrates, one of which is ferrous iron . There is evidence that ceruloplasmin is required for the optimal mobilization of iron from cells to plasma.

136. Ans. (a, c, d) a. Coarse basophilic stippling in lead poisoning; c. Dimorphic anaemia; d. Increase transferrin saturation

Findings in sideroblastic anemia: Serum Iron: High; Increased ferritin levels; Normal total iron-binding capacity; High transferrin saturation, MCV is usually normal or low. lead poisoning will show coarse basophilic stippling of red blood cells on peripheral blood smear. Specific test: Prussian blue stain of RBC Erythroid hyperplasia is found on bone marrow examination

137. Ans. (a) Transferrin receptor 1 - iron responding elements increases transferrin receptor mRNA concentration and synthesis

138. Ans. (c) Increased TIBC

139. Ans. (c) Lead toxicity

In megaloblastic anemia there is defect in DNA synthesis lead toxicity causes iron deficiency anemia

140. Ans. (c) 4 1 2 3 *(Ref: Robbins 9th/pg 643)*

141. Ans. (d) Haemolysis from G6PD enzyme deficiency

(Ref: Robbins 9th/pg 643)

G6PD deficiency causes anemia and not pancytopenia

142. Ans. (b) Thalassemia major *(Ref: Robbins 9th/pg 631)*

Though all the options mentioned can cause Iron deficiency resulting in microcytic hypochromic RBCs. Thalassemia will result in raised ferritin (due to increased GIT absorption & multiple transfusions) and not low ferritin.

143. Ans. (b) DMT-1

(Ref: Wintrobe 13ed /pg 811; Robbin's 9th/649; Complete review of Pathology 1st/314)

About DMT-1:
- Mucosal uptake of **non-heme iron** begins at **brush border** of mucosal cell, mediated by divalent metal ion transporter 1 **(DMT1, also known as Nramp2, SLC11A2).**
- Levels of DMT1 are markedly increased in iron-deficient animals.
- *In addition to iron, DMT1 has been shown to transport a variety of divalent metal ions, including Mn^{2+}, Co^{2+}, Cu^{2+}, Zn^{2+}, Cd^{2+}, and Pb^{2+}. (Hence non -specific)*
- It acts as a proton symporter; protons accompany metal ions into the cell.

Hepcidin: principal iron regulatory hormone; and is **negatively** regulates **ferroportin on basolateral surface of enterocyte**[Q]

144. Ans. (a) Hepsidin *(Ref: Robbins 9th/pg 649; 8th/pg 659)*

145. Ans. (a) S.ferritin *(Ref: Robbins 9th/pg 649; 8th/pg 659)*

146. Ans. (a) Hepsidin *(Ref: Robbins 9th/pg 649; 8th/pg 659)*

Ferroportin which regulates the Iron release from tissue store house is regulated by hepsidin hormone released by liver.

147. Ans. (d) Ferrocyanide to ferricferrocyanide

(Ref: T. Singh 3rd ed/pg 21)

Prussian Blue Stain:
Purpose: To demonstrate ferric iron in tissue sections.
Principle: The reaction occurs with the treatment of sections in acid solutions of ferrocyanides. Any **ferric ion (+3)** in the tissue combines with the **ferrocyanide** and results in the formation of a bright blue pigment called 'Prussian blue" or **ferric ferrocyanide.**

148. Ans. (d) Diagnosed by serum ferritin

(Ref: Robbins 9th/pg 649; 8th/pg 659)

Hereditary hemochromatosis (Autosomal recessive)is caused due to mutations of HFE gene on chr6p21.3.

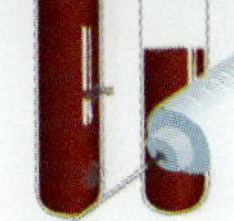

149. Ans. (b) Siderocyte *(Ref: Robbins 9th/pg 649)*

Pappenheimer bodies: Siderotic mitochondria of the developing cell may be retained in some circulating erythrocytes (Pathognomonic siderocytes)

150. Ans. (a) 2150 mg *(Ref: Wintrobes 12ed/814)*

Treatment of anemia due to iron deficiency.

The total dose is calculated from the amount of iron needed to restore the hemoglobin deficit plus an additional amount to replenish stores.

> **Total iron deficit [mg]** = body weight [kg] × (target Hb (15)-actual Hb) [g/dl] × 2.4 + **Iron for iron stores** (depot iron) [mg]

In this question: 50 × (15-5) × 2.4 + 1000 = 2200 mg
Nearest correct option is A i.e 2150 mg

151. Ans. (b) Folate supplement *(Ref: Robbins 9th/pg 645)*

152. Ans. (d) Start folate supplementation

(Ref: Robbins 9th/pg 645)

153. Ans. (d) Folate deficiency anemia *(Ref: R 9th/pg 645)*

154. Ans. (d) MCHC is increased *(Ref: Robbins 9th/pg 645)*

MCHC: Mean Corpuscular Hemoglobin Concentration
- Low in iron deficiency anemia and thalassemia.
- Increased in spherocytosis

155. Ans. (c) Hook worm infection *(Ref: Robbins 9th/pg 649)*

The findings in the question are suggestive are Iron deficiency anemia. Hookworm infection can cause this among the given options.

156. Ans. (c) Serum ferritin *(Ref: Robbins 9th/pg 649-652)*

Among the options provided, **most sensitive marker in iron deficiency anemia is Serum ferritin**.
Serum ferritin reflects the **storage of Iron** which is **decreased** even in the **pre-latent stage** of Iron deficiency Anemia and is the **most sensitive** marker.

157. Ans. (b) B12 deficiency *(Ref: Robbins 9th/pg 645)*

158. Ans. (c) TIBC *(Ref: Robbins 9th/pg 649)*

Total Iron Binding Capacity (TIBC) is increased in IDA while it is decreased in ACD.

159. Ans. (a) Serum ferritin level *(Ref: Robbins 9th/pg 649)*

Serum ferritin level is the best marker of Iron store levels.

160. Ans. (d) Ascorbic acid *(Ref: Robbins 9th/pg 649-652)*

Iron Absorption

- **Site of iron absorption: duodenum and upper jejunum (proximal small intestine)[Q].**
- **Ferrous form (Fe²⁺) of Iron is absorbed[Q].**
- Transport of Fe^{2+} into enterocyte occurs **via DMT1[Q].**

Increased by	Decreased by
• **Acids[Q]**	• Alkalies
• **Ascorbic acid (Vitamin C)[Q]**	• **Phosphates[Q]**
	• **Phytates[Q]**
• Amino acid containing SH-group	• Tetracycline
• **Meat (these reduce Fe^{3+} to Fe^{2+})**	• Presence of other food in stomach

161. Ans. (b) Leukopenia *(Ref: Robbins 9th/pg 649)*

162. Ans. (a) Increased serum ferritin *(Ref: R 9th/pg 649)*

163. Ans. (b) 100 µg/dL *(Ref: Robbins 9th/pg 649)*

164. Ans. (b) IL-6 *(Ref: Wintrobes 13th ed/pg 1223)*

Cytokines most often implicated in the pathogenesis of ACD are TNF, IL-1, IL-6, and the interferons. However, **IL-6 is the potent inducer of hepcidin**, proposed as a **major mediator of the iron abnormalities of ACD.**

165. Ans. (d) Absorption of iron is increased by ascorbic acid

(Ref: Robbins 9th/pg 649; 8th/pg 659; Wintrobes 12th ed/827)

a. False Parenteral Iron is given in severe iron deficiency anemia or if patient is unable to tolerate oral iron.
b. False as ferrous sulphate (65mg/325mg) has more Iron than gluconate (37.5mg/325mg)
c. False as parenteral iron is best
d. True, refer to table above

166. Ans. (b) Macrocytic anemia *(Ref: Robbins 9th/pg 645)*

The peripheral smear here shows hypersegmental neutrophil and macro-ovalocytes, suggestive of macrocytic anemia.

167. Ans. (c) Hereditary spherocytosis *(Ref: R 9th/pg 632)*

168. Ans. (d) Siderocytes *(Ref: Wintrobes 12th ed/ 848)*

169. Ans. (b) Oral iron therapy *(Ref: Robbins 9th/pg 649-652)*

The history provided is suggestive of Iron deficiency (nutritional) Anemia. Oral Iron therapy is the treatment of choice.

170. Ans. (b) Serum ferritin *(Ref: Robbins 9th/pg 649-652)*

171. Ans. (b) 35% *(Ref: Robbins 9th/pg 649-652)*

172. Ans. (b) Reticulocytosis

(Ref: Robbins 9th/pg 649-652; 8th/pg 659-662; Wintrobe's 12th/ pg 829)

Response to iron therapy:

- **Rapid subjective improvement**, with disappearance or marked diminution of fatigue, lassitude, and other

Contd...

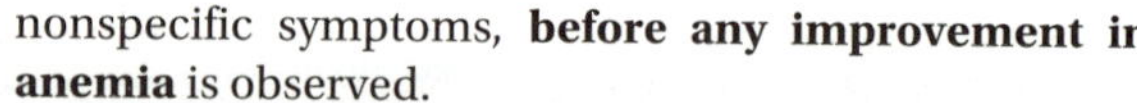

nonspecific symptoms, **before any improvement in anemia** is observed.

- **Earliest hematologic evidence** of response to treatment is an **increase in reticulocytes % & Hb content.**
- **Maximal reticulocytes % is on 5th to 10thday** after institution of therapy & thereafter returns to normal.
- Maximum value usually ranges from 5 to 10% and is inversely related to the level of hemoglobin.
- **Hemoglobin level** is the **most accurate** measure of the **degree of anemia** in iron deficiency

173. Ans. (b) **Microcytic hypochromic anemia**

(Ref: Robbins 9th/pg 649-652; 8th/pg 659-662)

Iron deficiency causes Microcytic hypochromic anemia

Differential diagnosis of microcytic hypochromic RBC's[Q]:

- Iron Deficiency Anemia
- Anemia of Inflammation/chronic disease
- Thalassemia
- Sideroblastic Anemia

174. Ans. (a) **Ringed siderocytes**

(Ref: Wintrobe's 12th/pg 848)

Bone marrow in lead poisoning contains Ringed siderocytes.

Hematologic findings in **Lead poisoning** include:

- Anisocytosis with microcytic Hypochromic Anemia
- Basophilic stippling
- Ringed sideroblasts in bone marrow may be seen

175. Ans. (a) **Latent iron deficiency is most common presentation in India**

(Ref: Robbins 9th/pg 649-652; 8th/pg 659-662)

a. False- Manifest (Anemia), not Latent (pre-anemia) iron deficiency is most common presentation in India

b. True- Saturation of transferrin is always reduced to <16%. At this level of saturation, iron delivery to erythroid precursors is limited.

c. True-Most sensitive marker in iron deficiency anemia is Serum ferritin

d. True-The onset of iron deficiency anemia is usually insidious & progression of symptoms is gradual. As a result, patients accommodate remarkably well to advancing anemia & may not present with clinical features

176. Ans. (b) **Thalassemia** *(Ref: Robbins 9th/pg 649-652)*

Leptocytes are **flattened red cells** in which the **volume-to-surface area ratio is decreased.** Seen in **iron deficiency anemia and thalassemia** in which the red cells with a low mean cell hemoglobin (MCH) and mean cell volume (MCV) are unusually resistant to osmotic lysis.

177. Ans. (a) **Reticulocytosis** *(Ref: Robbins 9th/pg 649-652)*

178. Ans. (a) **RBC protoporphyrin** *(Ref: R 9th/pg 649-652)*

Heme in Hb consists of Iron & Porphyrin.

In **Iron deficiency anemia, free erythrocyte protoporphyrin increases**, which is due to excess of protoporphyrin over

iron in heme synthesis. Each RBC contains less hemoglobin, resulting in microcytosis & hypochromia.

Stages in the Development of Iron Deficiency; Refer to pretexts of this chpater

179. Ans. (c) **Anemia of chronic disease**

(Ref: Robbins 9th/pg 649-652; 8th/pg 659-662)

This is a case of 35 year, female presenting with microcytic anemia. (Hb-9gm/dL, MCV- 55 fL).

Serum Iron studies reveal:

- Serum iron-30 ug/dL → Low
- Ferritin- 200 ng/mL and TIBC- 298 ug/dl levels are suggestive of Anemia of chronic disease.

180. Ans. (b) **Sideroblastic anemia**

(Ref: Wintrobe's 12th/pg 847-848)

This is an Alcoholic patient on Anti TB drugs (isoniazid, pyrazinamide) who presents with features of iron overload on iron studies (increased serum iron & increased transferrin saturation). These features are suggestive of sideroblastic anemia.

181. Ans. (a) **Atransferrinemia** *(Ref: Wintrobe's 12th/pg 814)*

This patient with **microcytic hypochromic** anemia, has **high ferritin level** (800 ng/ml) & **increased transferrin percentage saturation** (64%). The most possible diagnosis is Atransferrinemia.

Atransferrinemia

- It is a rare **congenital autosomal recessive** condition with low transferrin level in the body.
- So whatever transferrin is left, is saturated.
- It presents with hypochromic microcytic anemia, decreased serum levels of iron, TIBC, and increased serum level of ferritin (as iron absorption is markedly increased but iron transfer to eryrthropoetic tissues are reduced)

High transferrin saturation (64% in this case) & high ferritin level, excludes Iron deficiency Anemia *(option B excluded)*

In DMT 1 mutation, transferrin saturation is low (hence *option C* **excluded)**

High transferrin saturation excludes Anemia of chronic disease *(option D)*

182. Ans. (c) **Bone marrow examination**

This is a 60 yr old female presents with history of 8 blood transfusions in 2 yrs presenting with severe degree of hypochromic microcytic anemia. The most probable diagnosis is **Iron deficiency anemia, for which one of the underlying causes can be chronic blood loss.**

The investigations required for assessing the patients conditions are:

- **Evaluation for pulmonary hemosiderosis**: to exclude bleeding from alveolus;
- **Urinary hemosiderin**: to assess iron overload (due to repeated blood transfusions)
- **G1 endoscopy**: to assess GI bleeds which may cause such severe iron deficiency over a period of time.

Idiopathic pulmonary hemosiderosis:
- **Recurrent alveolar bleeding** may eventually produce **pulmonary hemosiderosis and fibrosis**.
- Presents with **hemoptysis, dyspnea, alveolar opacities** on chest Xray & **anemia**.
- Iron in the shed blood is converted to hemosiderin by pulmonary macrophages, but it cannot be used for Hb synthesis.
- Thus, **repeated hemorrhages can lead to iron deficiency** despite a normal total amount of body iron.

Bone marrow examination is not required to investigate for Iron deficiency anemia, hence the answer

---

183. Ans. (d) Reticulocyte count

(Ref: Robbins 9th/pg 645-648)

- This is a tricky question as the initial investigation looks like B_{12}/ folate levels, as the patient has macrocytosis.
- But remember, Macrocytosis can also be seen in hemolytic anemia, as newer RBC precursors released are larger in size.
- So the initial investigation should be reticulocyte count
- If reticulocyte % is low it can be macrocytic anemia & if there is reticulocytosis, then it can be a case of hemolytic anemia.

---

184. Ans. (a) Increased reticulocyte count

(Ref: Robbins 9th/pg645-648; 8th/pg 654-658)

Reticulocyte count does not increase in Megaloblastic anemia

---

185. Ans. (e) 5-FU *(Ref: Robbins 9th/pg 645-648)*

Drug induced causes of macrocytic anemia: by drugs that suppress DNA synthesis
- Folate antagonists
- Alkylating agents
- Metabolic inhibitors of:
  - Purine synthesis: Hydroxyurea, 6-mercatopurine, azathioprine
  - Pyrimidine synthesis: 5-fluorouracil; cytosine arabinoside

---

186. Ans. (d) Anemia of chronic disease *(Ref: 9th/pg 652-653)*

Anemia of chronic disease leads to microcytic anemia and not macrocytic anemia

---

187. Ans. (d) Absolute neutrophil count <1500/ul

(Ref: Wintrobes 13/p 1189)

A bone marrow cellularity of <25% and markedly decreased values of at least two of three hematopoietic lineages (neutrophil count <500/µl, platelet count <20,000/µl, and absolute reticulocyte count of <60,000/µl) define SAA

---

188. Ans. (d) Diamond Schwachman syndrome

(Ref: Wintrobes 13/p 1523-1533)

Shwachman-Diamond syndrome (SDS) is an autosomal recessive disorder characterized by exocrine pancreatic insufficiency and persistent or intermittent neutropenia

and an increased susceptibility to infections. Hematologic problems also can include anemia, thrombocytopenia, and pancytopenia

---

189. Ans. (a) Erythroid progenitors

(Ref: Robbins 9th ed p 655)

A special form of red cell aplasia occurs in individuals infected with parvovirus B19, which preferentially infects and destroys red cell progenitors. Normal individuals clear parvovirus infections within 1 to 2 weeks; as a result, the aplasia is transient and clinically unimportant. However, in persons with moderate to severe hemolytic anemias, even a brief cessation of erythropoiesis results in rapid worsening of the anemia, producing an aplastic crisis.

---

190. Ans. (b, d) b. Congenital dyserythropoetic anaemia; d. Aplastic anaemia

---

191. Ans. (d) None of the above

(Ref: Robbins 9th/pg 653-655)

- **Drugs:** associated with PRCA are Phenytoin, azathioprine, chloramphenicol, procainamide, isoniazid[Q]

---

192. Ans. (a) Fanconi's anemia

(Ref: Harrison 18th/Chapter 107)

---

193. Ans. (a) Fanconi anemia *(Ref: Robbins 9th/pg 653)*

---

194. Ans. (c) Aplastic anemia *(Ref: Robbins 9th/pg 653)*

---

195. Ans. (c) Thymoma *(Ref: Robbins 9th/pg 653)*

---

196. Ans. (d) PRCA *(Ref: Robbins 9th/pg 635-636)*

In the case provided, the child develops maculopapular rash 24hrs after onset of mild fever. There was prominent erythema over the cheek. It suggests **Erythema infectiosum caused by parvovirus B19 infection. Parvovirus also causes aplastic crisis in any hemolytic anemia** due to suppression of early erythroblasts by acting on P receptors.

---

197. Ans. (b) 5q- syndrome *(Ref: 9th/pg 653-655)*

Pure red cell aplasia is not associated with 5q- syndrome Pure red cell aplasia is a primary marrow disorder in which only erythroid progenitors are suppressed.

---

198. Ans. (d) G6PD deficiency

(Ref: Harrison 18th/pg Chapter 107)

Pancytopenia with cellular bone marrow is not seen in G6PD deficiency, which is a type of hemolytic anemia

---

199. Ans. (b) Hemolytic Anemia

(Ref: Robbins 9th/pg 631-632)

Prominent reticulocytosis is a feature of Hemolytic Anemia, while all others in the options have normal/ low reticulocyte count

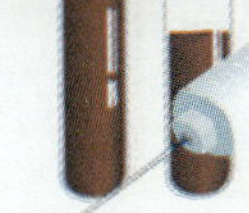

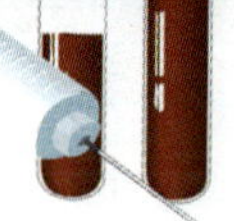

200. Ans. (c) Pure red cell aplasia *(Ref: Robbins 9th/pg 653-655)*

Aplastic anemia can progress to
- AML
- Myelodysplastic anemia
- Paroxysmal nocturnal hemoglobinuria

Aplastic anemia cannot progress to Pure red cell aplasia

201. Ans. (a, b, c); a. Pancytopenia; b. Nail dystrophy; c. Hyperkeratosis

(Ref: Robbins 9th/pg 653-655; 8th/pg 662-664)

In Dyskeratosis congenita, there is Pancytopenia, Nail dystrophy & Hyperkeratosis.

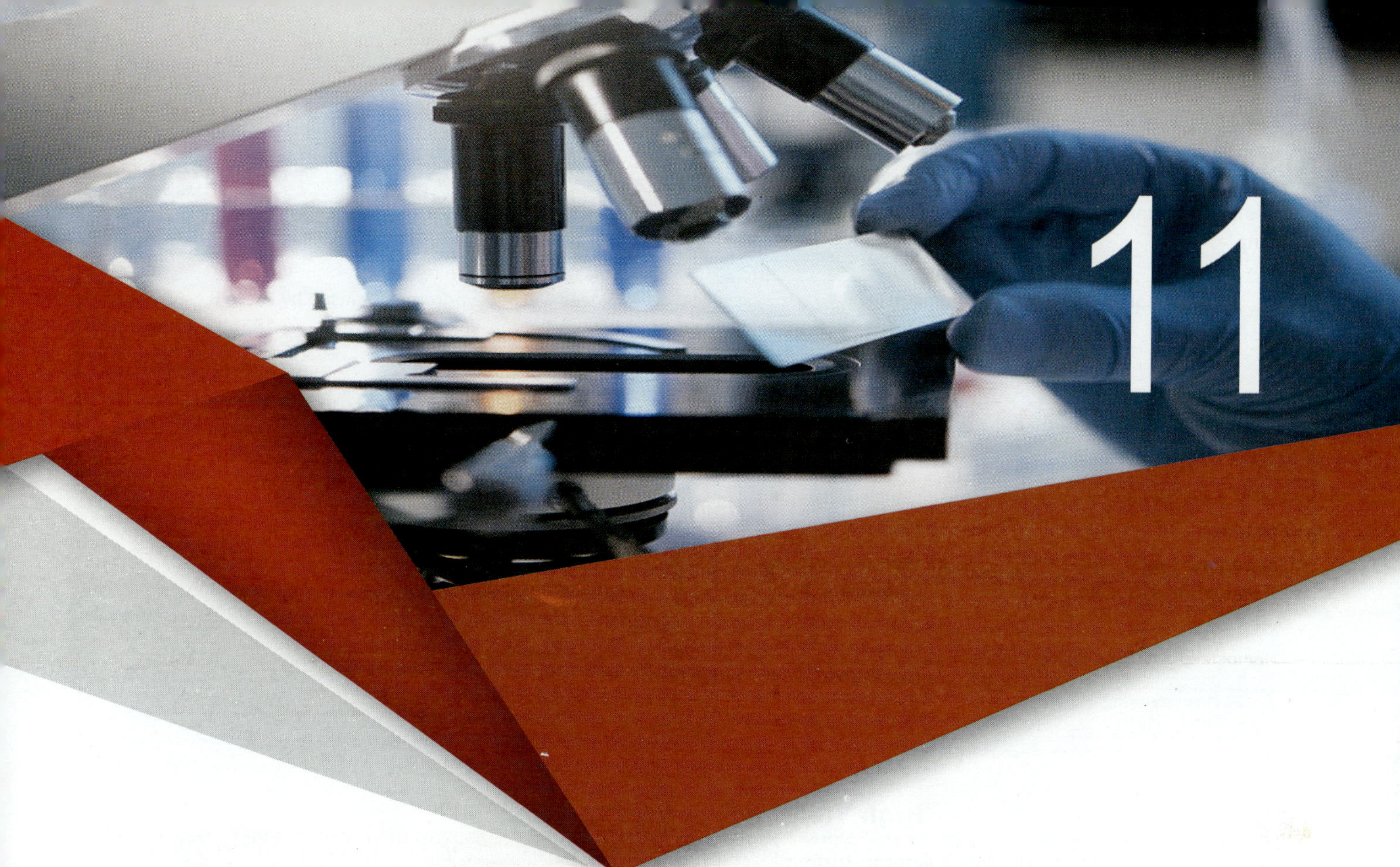

Bleeding and Coagulation Disorders

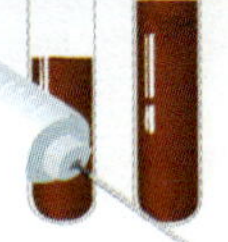

HEMOSTASIS

Process of formation of a **blood clot**[Q], which **prevents or limits** bleeding.

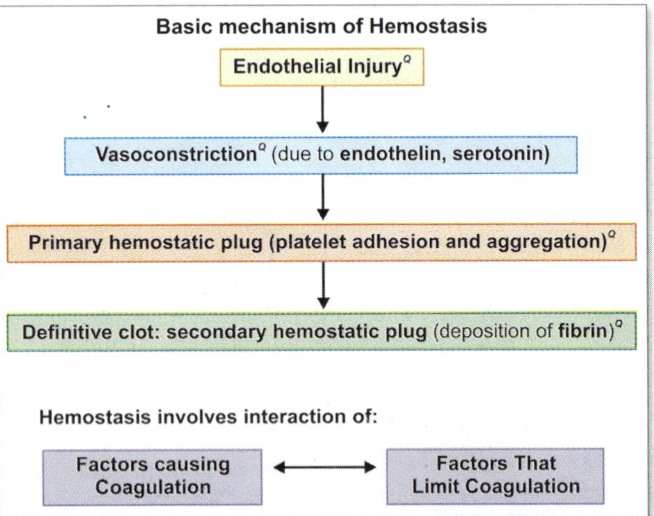

Basic mechanism of Hemostasis

Endothelial Injury[Q]

↓

Vasoconstriction[Q] (due to **endothelin, serotonin**)

↓

Primary hemostatic plug (platelet adhesion and aggregation)[Q]

↓

Definitive clot: secondary hemostatic plug (deposition of **fibrin**)[Q]

Hemostasis involves interaction of:

Factors causing Coagulation	←→	Factors That Limit Coagulation

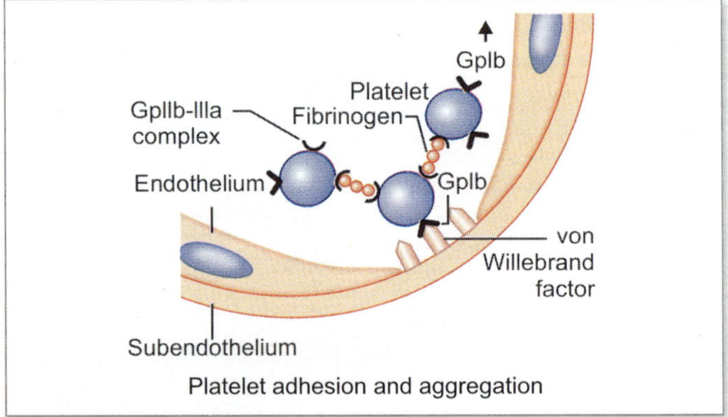

Platelet adhesion and aggregation

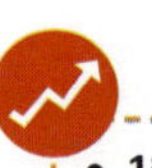

High Yield Facts

- **1st response** to endothelial injury is **vasoconstriction**
- Endothelial injury **activates extrinsic pathway** by releasing **tissue factor**

Formation of Primary Hemostatic Plug

Platelet Plug Formation: 2 Processes

- *Platelet adhesion:*
  - vWF on **endothelium**[Q] with Gp Ib/IX on **platelets**[Q]
- *Platelet aggregation:*
  - Gp IIb/IIIa on **platelets**[Q] that bridges adjacent platelets[Q]

PLATELET: Disc shaped anucleate[Q] cell fragments shed from megakaryocytes

α-Granules contains:	Dense (or δ) granules contain: ("DENSE")
• **P-selectin (adhesion molecule)**	• aDENosine diphosphate (ADP)[Q]
• **Fibrinogen**[Q]	• Serotonin[Q]
• **Coagulation factors: V[Q], VIII[Q], vWF[Q]**	• Epinephrine[Q]
• **Platelet factor 4[Q]** (a heparin binding chemokine)	• Ionized calcium[Q]
• Platelet derived growth factor (**PDGF**)	
• Transforming growth factorβ (**TGF-β**)	

Mnemonic

"B comes before G & Ib comes before IIb"	
Disease	**Deficient Gp**
Bernard Soulier syndrome	**Ib** / IX
Glanzmann thrombasthenia	**IIb** / IIIa

Formation of Secondary Hemostatic Plug

Coagulation Cascade

Series of **amplifying**[Q] **enzymatic reactions** that leads to the deposition of an **insoluble fibrin clot**.[Q]

Each Reaction Step Involves

- **Enzyme** (an **activated coagulation factor**)
- **Substrate** (an **inactive proenzyme** form of a coagulation factor)
- **Cofactor** (a reaction accelerator)

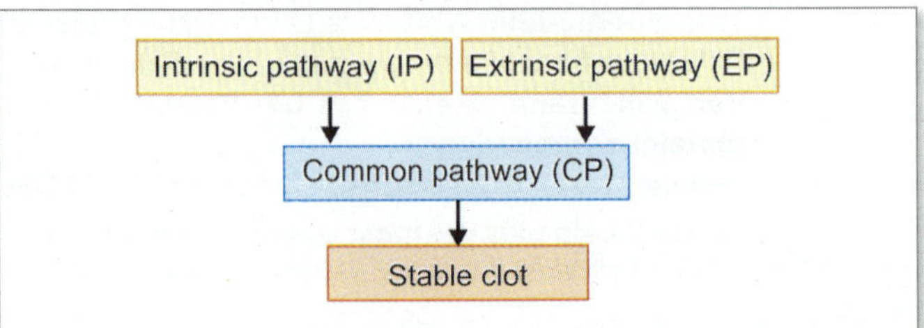

Role of Coagulation Factors

- **Clotting factors** normally circulate in plasma in their **inactive forms**[Q]
- Components are assembled on a **negatively charged phospholipid surface**[Q], provided by **activated platelets**[Q]
- Based on laboratory assays: Coagulation cascade can be of **extrinsic and intrinsic pathways**[Q]

High Yield Facts

- All clotting factors are synthesized by **LIVER,**[Q] except **factor VIII, from endothelium**[Q]
- Factor **VIIa/tissue factor** complex is the most important activator of **factor X**[Q]
- Factor **IXa/ VIIIa** complex is the most important activator of **factor X**[Q]
- **Factor Xa** converts **prothrombin to thrombin** which requires factor **Va**[Q] as cofactor
- **Factor Va** is the **'fundamental protease of the coagulation system'**[Q]
- **Thrombin** is called **'Master regulator of clotting pathway'**[Q]
- **F VIII dose** = VIII levels (Target – bleeding) × 0.5 IU/kg

Overview of Coagulation Pathway

Three Pathways that make the Classical Blood Coagulation Pathway

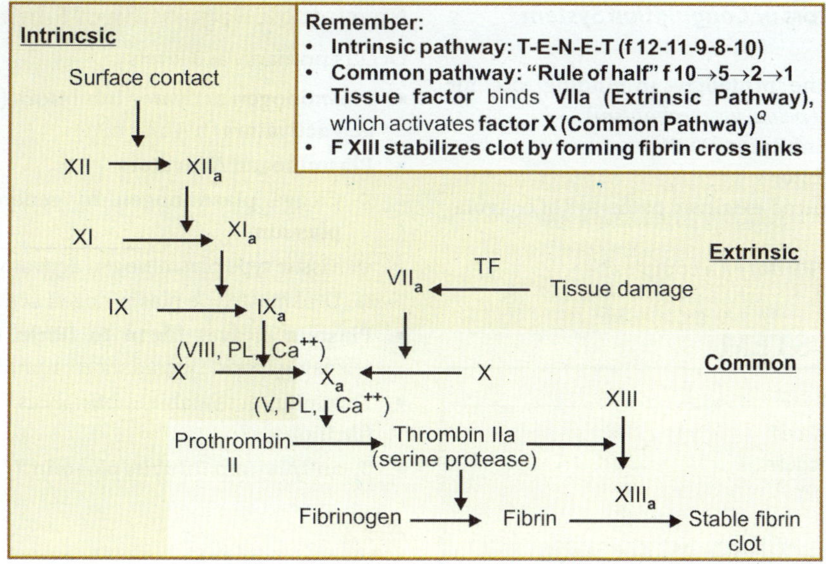

Functions of Thrombin

- It converts soluble plasma **fibrinogen to insoluble fibrin**[Q]
- Activates factor **XIII (fibrin-stabilizing factor)** to factor **XIIIa**, which covalently cross-links & thereby **stabilizes the fibrin clot.**[Q]
- **Thrombin** is the **most potent activator of platelets**[Q]
- **Pro-inflammatory** effects-contribute to tissue **repair and angiogenesis**[Q]
- Some **anticoagulant** effects

Factors that Limit Coagulation

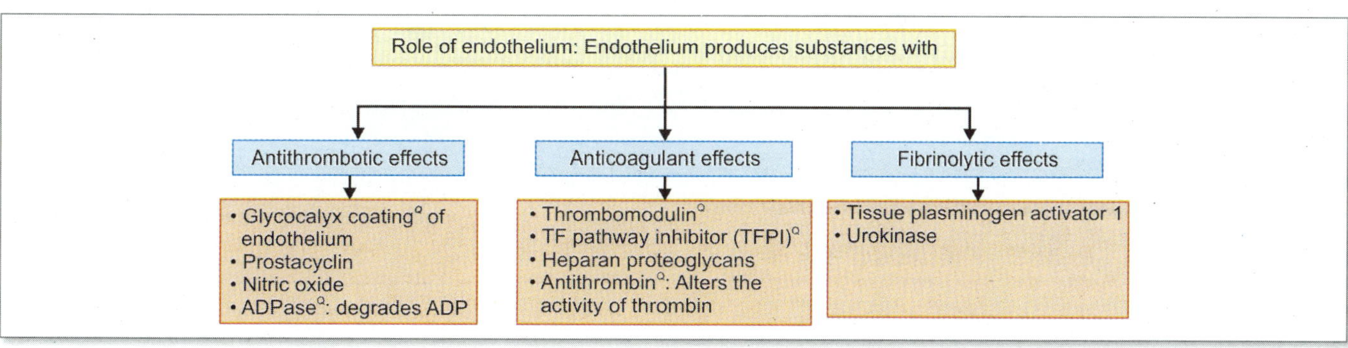

Vitamin K–Dependent Coagulation Factors

- **Vitamin K, a fat-soluble vitamin** is a **cofactor for carboxylation** of the Y-carbon of the glutamic acid residues of vitamin K-dependent factors
- Vitamin K-dependent factors are F- **II, VII, IX, and X**[Q] and anticoagulant **proteins C, S and Z**[Q]
- A critical step for **calcium and phospholipid binding**[Q] of these proteins
- The enzymes Y glutamyl carboxylase and **epoxide reductase** are critical for the **regeneration of vitamin K.**[Q]
- **Earliest** coagulation factor affected due to **Vit K def.** is **factor VII**[Q] (shortest $t_{1/2}$)
- **Warfarin blocks** the action of **epoxide reductase** and **competitively inhibits** the effects **of vitamin K.**[Q]
- **Abnormal plasma proteins** produced in **Vit K def.** are called PIVKA
- **Abnormal prothrombin produced in Vit K def.** are called des Y-carboxy prothrombin (DCP)
- **Mutations** in the genes encoding the **gamma-carboxylase (GGCX)**[Q] or **vitamin K epoxide reductase complex 1 (VKORC1)**[Q] result in **defective enzymes (1 to 30% of normal activity)**[Q]
- Vit K deficiency bleeding can be treated by **high doses of vitamin K**[Q], replacement therapy with **FFP** or **Plasma concentrate**[Q]

Some Important Regulators of Coagulation System

- **Thrombomodulin**
  - Has a transmembrane **proteoglycan-binding site for thrombin**[Q] (*See figure below for mechanism*).
- **Tissue Factor Pathway Inhibitor (TFPI)**
  - Plasma protease inhibitor
  - Regulates the TF–induced **extrinsic pathway**[Q] of coagulation.
  - TFPI **inhibits** the **TF/FVIIa/FXa complex**[Q]

FIBRINOLYTIC SYSTEM

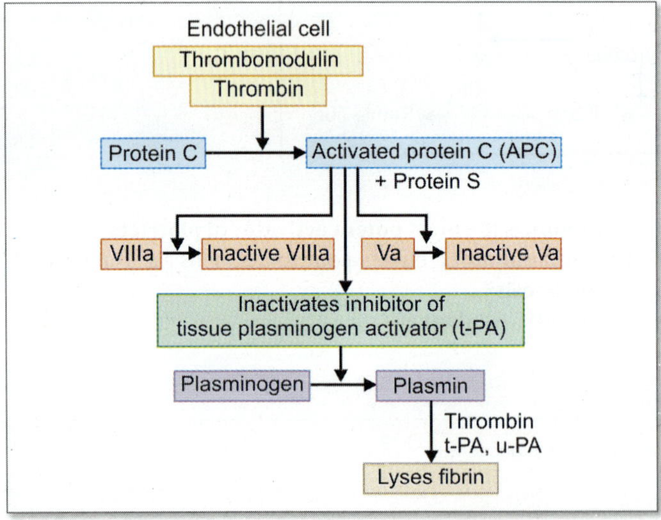

Physiologic Regulation of Fibrinolysis

Occurs primarily at 3 levels

- **Plasminogen activator inhibitors** (PAIs) **inhibit plasminogen activators** (tPA and uPA)
- **Plasminogen Activators**
  - Cleave **plasminogen** to generate the active enzyme **plasmin**
  - Tissue type plasminogen activator **(tPA)**[Q]
  - Urokinase type plasminogen activator **(uPA)**[Q]
- **Plasmin** cleaves **fibrin to fibrin fragments** (fibrinolysis) releasing Fibrin Degradation products (FDP) and D-dimers
- Thrombin-activatable fibrinolysis inhibitor (**TAFI**) **limits fibrinolysis**[Q]
- β_2-**antiplasmin inhibits plasmin.**[Q]

- **Protein S** is the **cofactor for Protein C**[Q]
- **Thrombomodulin, Protein C and Protein S** are synthesized from **liver**[Q]
- **Thrombomodulin inhibits** activation of **factor V and factor VIII**[Q]
- **D-dimer** is used to diagnose **deep-venous thrombosis (DVT)** and **pulmonary embolism.**[Q]

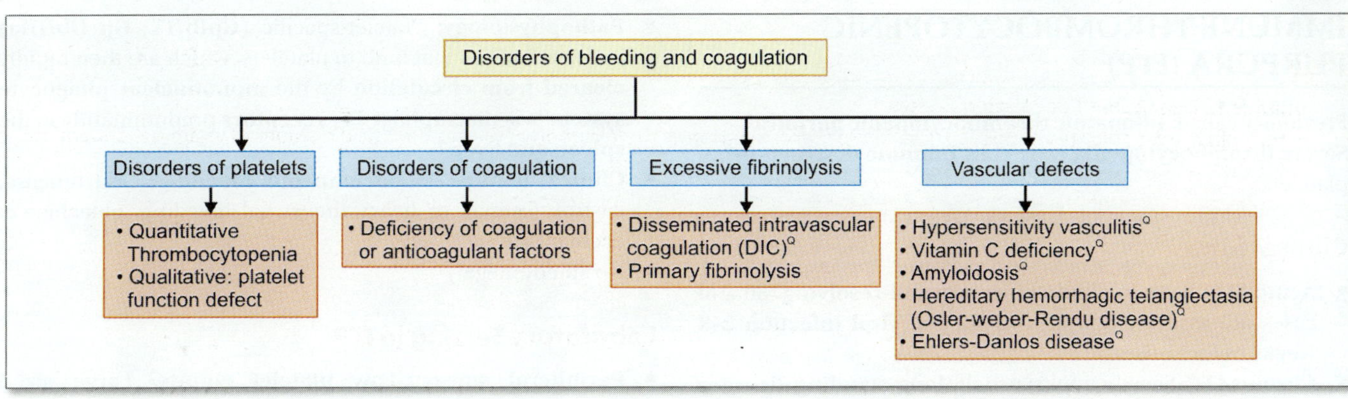

POINTS TO REMEMBER

- TAFI is Thrombin activated fibrinolysis inhibition
- Thrombin bound to thrombomodulin activates TAFI
- Removes lysine residues from fibrin & prevents fibrinolysis

CLINICAL DIFFERENCES BETWEEN DISORDERS OF PLATELETS/VESSELS AND COAGULATION

Characteristics	Disorders of Platelets/ Vessels	Disorders of Coagulation
Petechiae^Q	Common	Rare
Hematomas^Q	Rare	Common
Ecchymoses^Q	Characteristic: small and multiple	Common: large and solitary
Hemarthrosis^Q	Rare	Characteristic
Sex of patient	F>>M	M>>F
Family history	Rare (except vWD)	Common

THROMBOCYTOPENIA

Definition < **1.5 lac/cu mm**^{Q}

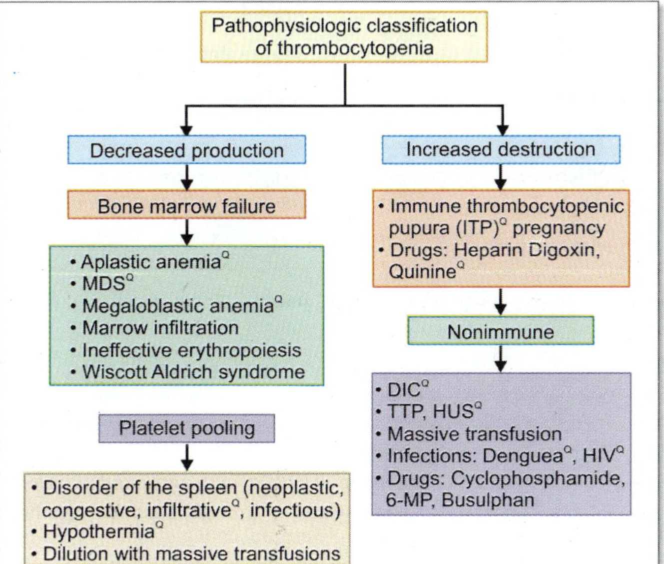

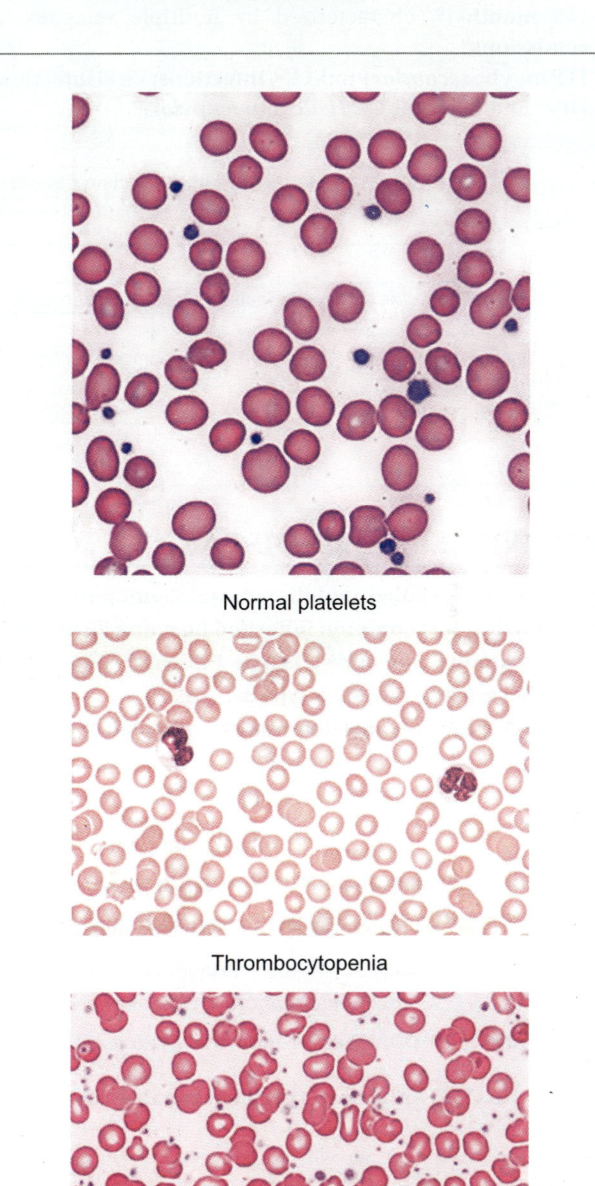

Normal platelets

Thrombocytopenia

Thrombocytosis

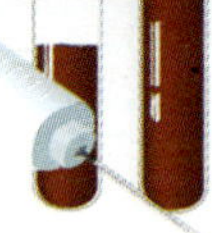

IMMUNE THROMBOCYTOPENIC PURPURA (ITP)

Previously called: **Idiopathic thrombocytopenic purpura**[Q]

Severe **thrombocytopenia** caused by **immune destruction**[Q] of platelets.

Clinical forms:

- **Acute ITP:** Seen in children; usually **self-resolving.** 50% of cases are associated with a **history of viral infection 2–3 weeks before onset.**[Q]
- **Chronic ITP:** Seen in adults; usually **long-standing disorder (>6 months)**[Q], characterized by **multiple relapses and remissions**[Q]
- **ITP** may be *secondary* to: SLE[Q], Infections: Viral infections[Q], HIV[Q] and hepatitis C[Q], *Helicobacter pylori*[Q]

- **Pathophysiology:** Platelet-specific (**GpIb/IX; Gp IIb/IIIa**) **autoantibodies** that bind to platelets, which are then rapidly **cleared from circulation** by the **mononuclear phagocyte system**[Q] via macrophage **Fcγ receptors** predominantly in the **spleen and liver.**[Q]
- **Clinical feature: Mucocutaneous bleeding:** Oral mucosa, gastrointestinal, or heavy menstrual bleeding, petechiae & ecchymoses
- No splenomegaly

Laboratory Testing in ITP

- **Peripheral smear:** Low **platelet counts**, **Large sized platelets,**[Q]
- **BM shows (not required otherwise):** Increased young form of **megakaryocytes,**[Q] **Clot retraction**, which depends on platelets, is **defective.**[Q]

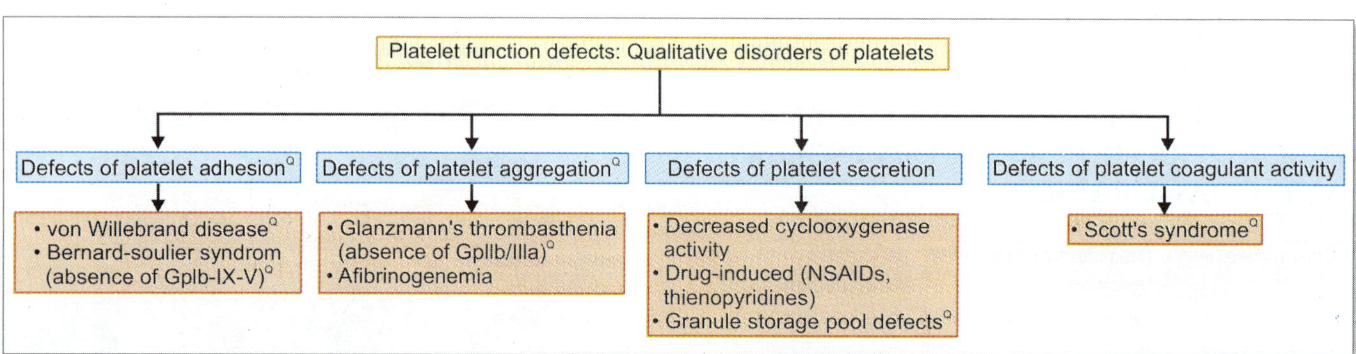

VON WILLEBRAND DISEASE

Also known as **Angiohemophilia**[Q], **pseudohemophilia**[Q]

- vWD is the **most common inherited bleeding disorder.**[Q]
- Most **common type** of vWD is **type 1** disease[Q]
- Most **severe** type of vWD is **type 3** disease[Q]
- All **vWD are Autosomal dominant except type 3**[Q]

3 types	Types	Type 1	Type 2	Type 3
	Defect	**Partial deficiency**[Q] of vWF	**Qualitative** vWF defects	**Severe deficiency** of vWF[Q]
	Inheritance	**Autosomal Dominant**[Q]	**Autosomal Dominant**[Q]	Autosomal Recessive[Q]
C/F	• "Platelet-like" superficial bleeding Except in severe VWD-type 3			
Investigations	• Coagulation tests: **Prolonged apTT**[Q], Normal PT and TT; **Ristocetin induced platelet aggregation**[Q] defective			
	• Serum electrophoresis: **Decreased vWF multimers in type 1 and 3**[Q]			
Treatment	• **DDAVP or Desmopressin**, causes a **transient rise in FVIII & VWF; FFP**			

Functions of vWF: Adhesion of **platelets to sub-endothelium**[Q], Binding protein for **FVIII** (**Increases FVIII half-life in circulation**).[Q]

High Yield Facts

- **Primary hemostatic plug** consists of: **Platelets, Fibrinogen, Entrapped RBCs & WBCs**[Q]
- **Primary plug is reversible**[Q]
- **Platelet aggregation** is followed by **platelet contraction**[Q]
- **Large platelets**[Q] are seen in **Bernard Soulier syndrome**
- Bernard Soulier syndrome & Glanzmann thrombasthenia are **Autosomal recessive**[Q]

- Bleeding in **Glanzmann thrombesthenia** is **more severe**[Q] than Bernard Soulier syndrome
- **P-selectin** causes **adherence of WBCs**[Q] with **activated platelets**
- **Primary hemostatic plug is loose** → Stronger secondary hemostatic plug required
- Weibel Palade bodies on vWF is synthesized by endothelial cells and α granules on platelets

Platelet Aggregation Studies

Disease	Platelet Aggregation studies			Other Features
	Collagen	ADP	Ristocetin	
Bernard–Soulier disease	N	N	Absent	Giant platelets[Q]
Glanzmann's thrombasthenia	Absent[Q]	Absent[Q]	N/Reduced[Q]	Absent clot retraction
Von Willebrand's disease	N	N	Absent[Q]	Corrected by factor VIII:vWF
Storage pool disease	Absent	Absent	N	Absent dense bodies[Q]

HEPARIN INDUCED THROMBOCYTOPENIA AND THROMBOSIS (HITT)

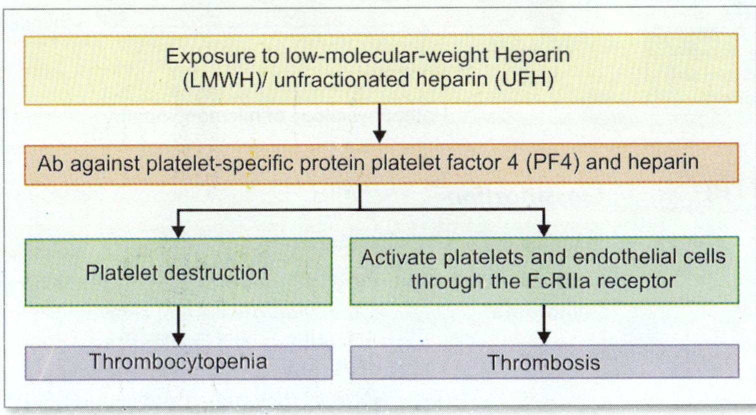

Mnemonic

4 T's in the diagnostic of HITT

- *T*hrombocytopenia (decrease of ≥ 50% platelet count)
- *T*iming of : HIT develops after exposure to **heparin for 5–14 days**[Q]
- *T*hrombosis in **50%**[Q]
- o*T*her causes of thrombocytopenia not evident.

THROMBOTIC MICROANGIOPATHIES

- Hemolytic-uremic syndrome (HUS)
- Thrombotic thrombocytopenic purpura (TTP)

Hemolytic-Uremic Syndrome (HUS)

Characterized by Triad of:

- Acute onset of **microangiopathic hemolytic anemia**[Q] (**schistocytes**[Q], **burr cells**[Q], **or helmet cells**[Q] on peripheral blood smear) (**Hallmark of HUS**)[Q]
- **Renal Failure**[Q]
- **Thrombocytopenia**[Q]

Classification

Points	Typical HUS	Atypical HUS
Also Called	**Epidemic**[Q]**, diarrhea-positive, D+ HUS**[Q]	**Non-epidemic**[Q]**, diarrhea-negative, D- HUS**[Q]
Etiology	• **E. coli**[Q] **(O157:H7)-Shiga-like toxins**[Q] • **Shigella dysenteriae**[Q]	• Inherited **mutations** of complement-regulatory proteins: **Factor I, H and CD46**[Q] causing **hyperactivation of complement** • **APLA: (lupus anticoagulant)**[Q]**,** Complications of **pregnancy**[Q] or the postpartum period. • **Systemic sclerosis**[Q] **& malignant hypertension.**[Q] • **Drugs: e.g., cyclosporine**[Q]**, FK-506**[Q]**, OKT3, mitomycin C,**[Q] **Ganciclovir, OCP'**

Pathogenesis

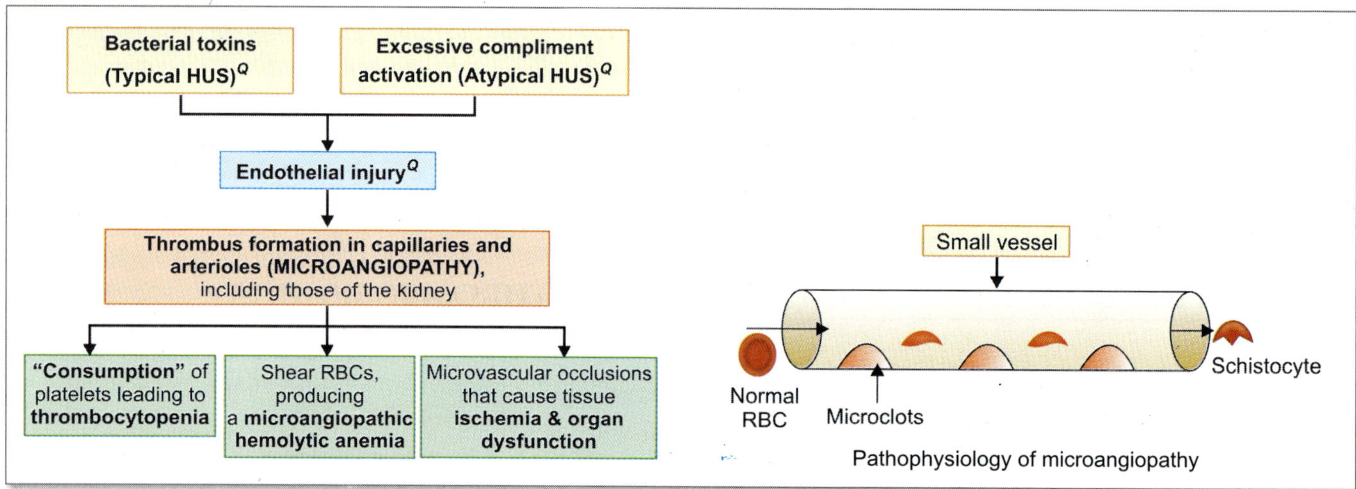

Thrombotic Thrombocytopenic Purpura (TTP)

Pentad of findings:

- Microangiopathic hemolytic anemia
- **Thrombocytopenia**^{Q}
- **Neurologic findings**^{Q}
- **Renal failure**^{Q}
- **Fever**^{Q}

Classification

Inherited	Acquired
Upshaw-Schulman syndrome^Q	• **Deficiencies of ADAMTS13**^{Q}, a plasma **metalloprotease** that **cleaves vWF** multimers into smaller sizes. • ↑ in **HIV**^{Q} and in **pregnant** women • Drugs (**ticlopidine** and **clopidogrel**)^Q

TESTS USED TO EVALUATE BLEEDING AND COAGULATION DISORDERS

Test	Description and Significance	Abnormal values in: platelet Abnormalities
Bleeding time (BT) (normal: 3–8 min)^Q	• Time taken for a standardized skin puncture to stop bleeding. • Tests the ability of vessels to vasoconstrict & platelets to form a hemostatic plug.	
Tourniquet test (Hess test)^Q	• BP cuff inflated to above diastolic pressure for 5 minutes • Appearance of ≥ **20 petechiae**^{Q} in 1 sq inch area of forearm indicates **capillary fragility, thrombocytopenia**, or platelet **abnormalities**.	
Prothrombin time (PT)^Q (12-15 sec)	Time taken for clotting to occur when **tissue thromboplastin**^{Q} (brain extract) and **calcium** are added to the patient's plasma to **activate extrinsic pathway**^{Q}	• **Deficiencies or inhibitors of factors VII, X, and V; II and I;**^{Q} • Lupus inhibitors; heparin; **warfarin**^{Q} • Liver disease
Activated Partial thrombo-plastin time (aPTT)^Q (26-37 sec)	Time taken for clotting when **Kaolin/Silica** is added to **activate intrinsic pathway**^{Q}	• Deficiencies or inhibitors of: • Prekallikrein, high-molecular-weight kininogen • Factors XII, XI, IX, VIII, X^Q, V^Q, II^Q and I; • **Lupus inhibitors; heparin**^{Q}**; warfarin therapy**^{Q}
Thrombin time (TT) (14-19 sec)	Time taken for clotting when **thrombin is added** to the patient's plasma to test for **conversion of fibrinogen to fibrin (depends on fibrinogen levels)**^{Q}	• **Afibrinogenemia**^{Q} • **Dysfibrinogenemia**^{Q} • **Hypofibrinogenemia,**^{Q}

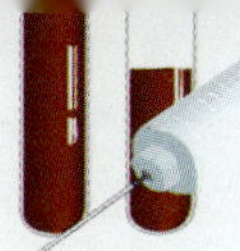

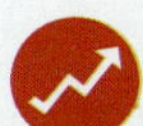

- Clot retraction time & Prothrombin consumption index are used to asses platelet function
- Clot retraction failure of clot retraction in 1–4 hours indicates **thrombocytopenia** or **abnormal platelet function**[Q].
- **Ratio** of anticoagulant (**Trisodium citrate**): Blood = **1:9**[Q]
- Sample required: **Platelet poor plasma** (PPP)[Q]
- Storage: **Room temperature**[Q]
- Test should ideally be performed **within 2 hours**[Q] of sample collection

- **Prothrombin time (PT)** assay screens **extrinsic + common pathway**[Q] (factors VII, X, V, II, and fibrinogen).
- **Partial thromboplastin time (PTT)** assay screens **intrinsic pathway + common pathway**[Q] (factors XII, XI, IX, VIII, X, V, II, and fibrinogen).
- Clotting time (CT) (normal: 5–10 min)[Q] time taken for the patient's blood to **clot in a test tube**, very **insensitive test**; Not used now a days.

DISSEMINATED INTRAVASCULAR COAGULATION (DIC)

DIC is an **acute, subacute, or chronic thrombo-hemorrhagic** disorder characterized by the **excessive activation of coagulation**[Q] and the **formation of thrombi** in the **microvasculature of the body**[Q].

Etiology of DIC

Sepsis: • **Bacterial: Staphylococci**[Q], **meningococci**[Q], **gram-negative bacilli, Anerobic**[Q] • **Mycotic: Histoplasmosis & Aspergillosis, Parasitic, Viral**	**Immunologic disorders:** • Acute hemolytic transfusion reaction • Transplant rejection • **GVHD**[Q]
Trauma and tissue injury: Brain injury (gunshot), **Rhabdomyolysis**[Q]	**Drugs: Warfarin (especially in neonates with protein C deficiency)**[Q]
Vascular disorders: Giant hemangiomas **(Kasabach-Merritt syndrome)**[Q]	**Envenomation:** Snake, Insect bites
Obstetrical complications: Abruptio placentae[Q], Amniotic-fluid embolism, Dead fetus syndrome, **Septic abortion**[Q]	**Liver disease: Fulminant hepatic failure**[Q] Cirrhosis, **Fatty liver of pregnancy**[Q]
Cancer ("SLAP"): Stomach Ca, **L**ung Ca, **A**cute promyelocytic leukemia (APML)[Q] **P**ancreas (most common) & **P**rostate Adenocarcinoma[Q]	**Miscellaneous: Shock**[Q], ARDS, **Massive transfusion**[Q]

- **Most sensitive** test for DIC is elevated **Fibrin Degraded Products (FDPs) level**[Q]
- **DIC is unlikely diagnosis** in the **presence of normal levels of FDP (High negative predictive value)**[Q]
- **D-dimer test** is **more specific**[Q] for detection of FDPs; Indicates that the **cross-linked fibrin**[Q] has been **digested by plasmin.**[Q]
- **Decreased Fibrinogen level is seen in DIC**[Q]
- **High-grade DIC: Increased** levels of **antithrombin III** or **plasminogen activity <60% of normal.**[Q]
- The reference concentration of D-dimer is less than 0.5 µg/mL fibrinogen-equivalent units (FEU)
- Sample collected in - plasma (with sodium citrate anticoagulant, 3.2%)

Two Major Mechanisms Trigger DIC

- Release of **tissue factor**[Q] & other **pro-coagulants**, into the circulation, and
- **Widespread injury** to the **endothelial cells**[Q]

Lab Diagnosis

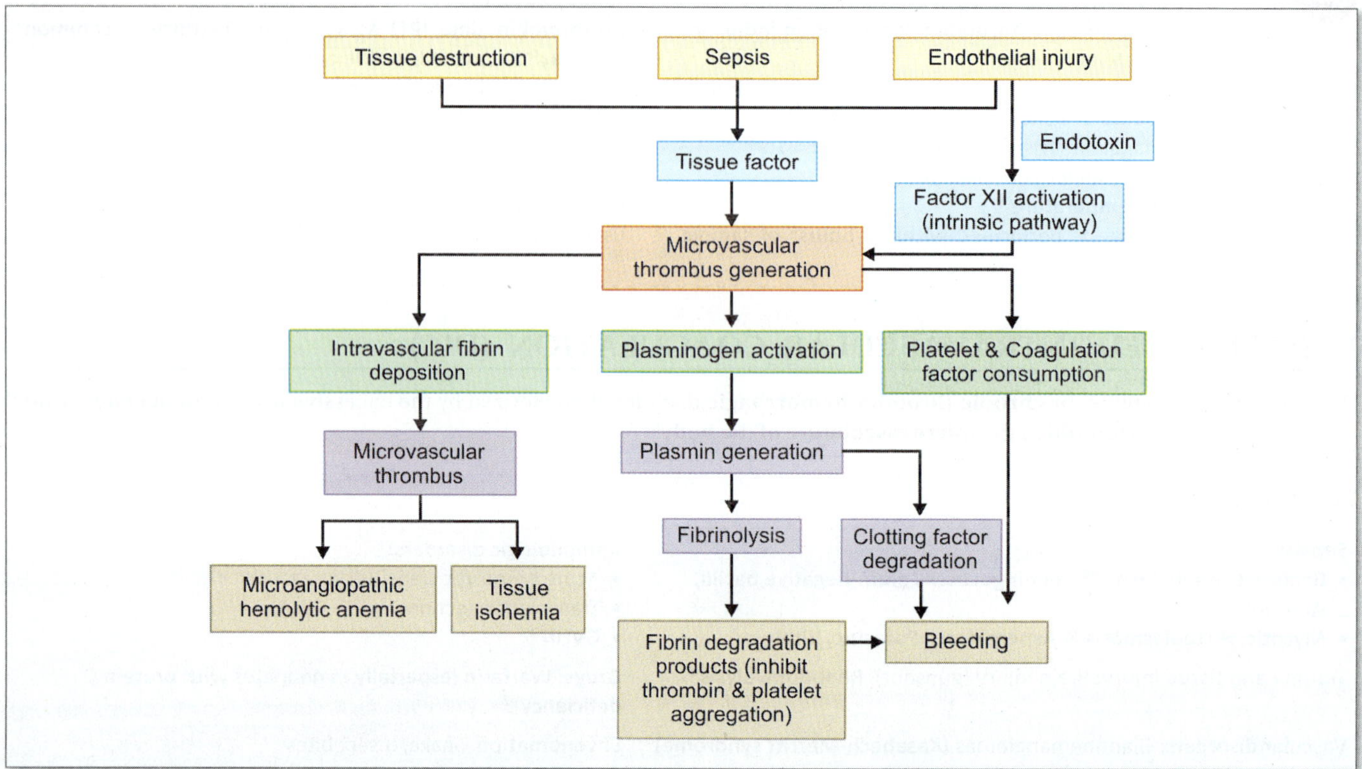

- *Hemogram:*
  - Reduced **platelet counts < 100,000/uL**[Q]
- *Peripheral smear:*
  - Presence of **schistocytes (fragmented red cells)**[Q] in peripheral blood smear
- *Coagulation tests:*
  - Prolongation of **PT, aPTT and/or TT**[Q]
- *Other investigations:*
  - **Most sensitive** test for DIC is elevated **FDP (Fibrin Degraded Products) level**[Q]
  - **DIC** is **unlikely diagnosis** in the **presence of normal levels of FDP (High negative predictive value)**[Q]
  - **D-dimer test** is **more specific**[Q] for detection of fibrin degradation products; indicates that the **cross-linked fibrin**[Q] has been **digested by plasmin.**[Q]
  - **Decreased Fibrinogen level is also seen in DIC**[Q]
  - **High-grade DIC: Increased** levels of **antithrombin III** or **plasminogen activity <60% of normal.**[Q]

THROMBOSIS

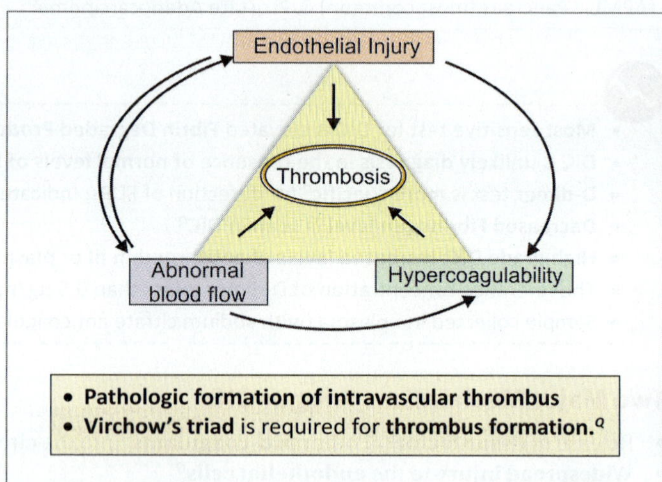

- **Pathologic formation of intravascular thrombus**
- **Virchow's triad** is required for **thrombus formation.**[Q]

Endothelial Injury

- **Most important factor**[Q] causing thrombosis in **arterial and cardiac** circulation
- Endothelial injury → platelet activation → thrombus formation in **high stress circulation like arteries**[Q]
- **Endothelial dysfunction**- shifts pattern of gene expression in endothelium to "**prothrombotic.**" state

Stasis or Turbulent Blood Flow

- Turbulence causes arterial,[Q] whereas stasis causes venous thrombosis.[Q]

- Aortic and arterial dilations called **aneurysms**[Q] result in local stasis[Q]
- A dilated atrium in Rheumatic mitral valve stenosis is a site of profound stasis[Q] and a prime location for thrombosis[Q]
- Hyperviscosity syndromes like polycythemia[Q] and with deformed red cells as in sickle cell anemia.[Q]

Blood Hypercoagulability

- It can either be primary (inherited) or secondary (acquired) hypercoagulable state.

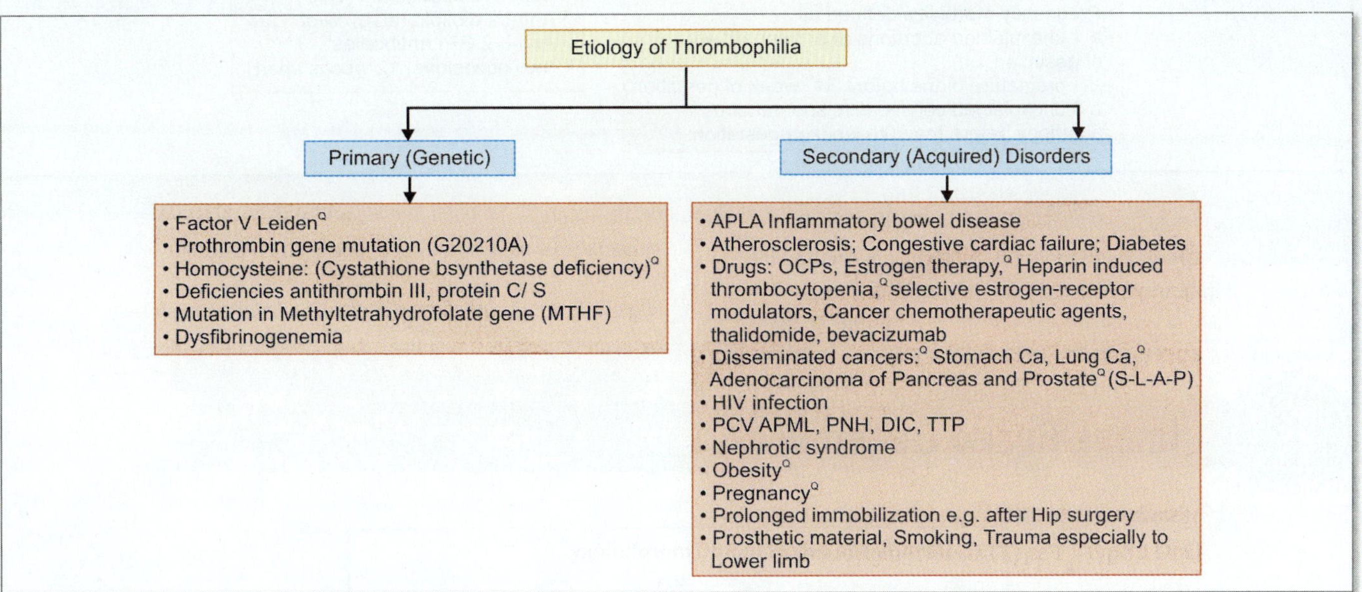

Investigations for Thrombophilia

- **Kaolin Clotting Time (KCT)**[Q]
- **Dilute Russel Viper Venom Test (DRVVT)**[Q]
- **Platelet neutralisation test**[Q]

High Yield Facts

- Glutamine → arginine substitution at amino acid residue 506 that renders **factor V resistant** to cleavage and inactivation by protein C (also called **Activated Protein C resistance**)
- Factor V Leiden[Q] is the most common inherited cause of hypercoagulability
- **Antithrombin III, Protein C or Protein S deficiency** causes **venous thrombosis only**[Q]
- **Factor V Leiden** causes most commonly **venous thrombosis**[Q] but also **arterial thrombosis**
- Hyperhomocystinemia, APLA, DIC, HIT, PNH, Polycythemia Vera and dysfibrinogenemia cause both-arterial and venous thrombus[Q]
- Thrombomodulin is produced by all endothelial cells except those of cerebral microcirculation[Q]
- Thrombocytopenia (decrease of ≥ 50% platelet count), **T**iming of : HIT develops after exposure to **heparin for 5–14 days**[Q], Thrombosis in **50%**[Q], **OT**her causes of thrombocytopenia not evident.

ANTIPHOSPHOLIPID ANTIBODY (APLA) SYNDROME

Autoantibody[Q]-mediated **acquired**[Q] thrombophilia characterized by **recurrent**[Q] **arterial or venous thrombosis**[Q] and/or **pregnancy morbidity** in the presence of **autoantibodies against phospholipid (PL)**-binding **plasma proteins (β-2 GPI)**[Q]

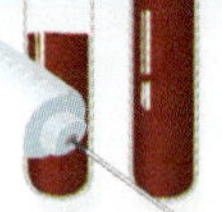

Pathophysiology

Diagnostic Criteria

One clinical event and at least one laboratory abnormality.

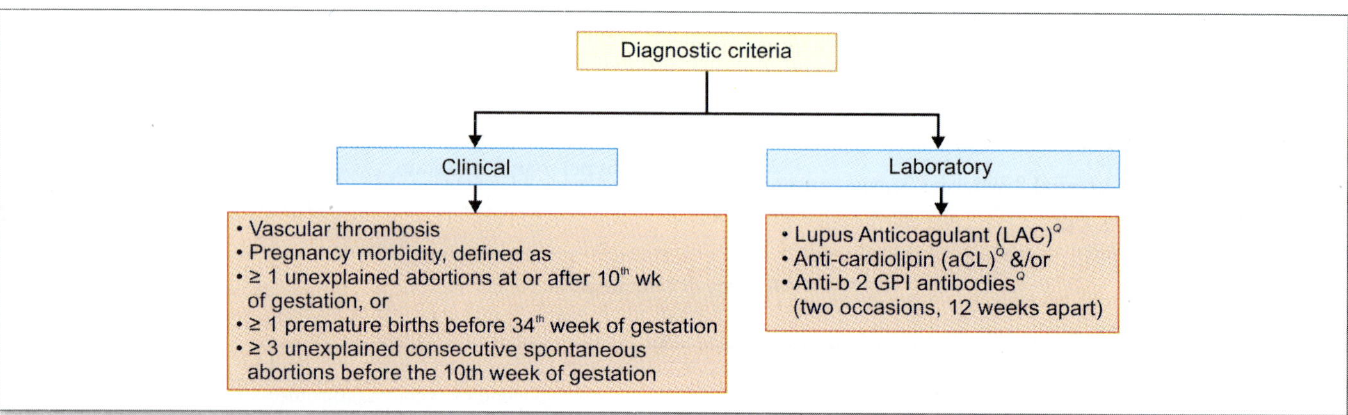

Image-Based Question

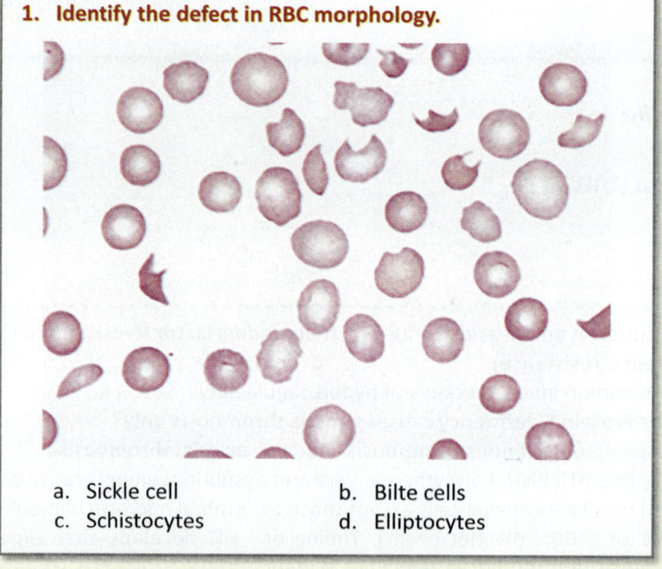

Answer of Image-Based Question

1. **Ans. (c) Schistocytes**
   - The given smear shows helmet cells with spiculated ends in a case of microangiopathic hemolytic anemia.

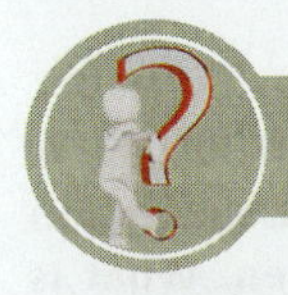

Multiple Choice Questions

DISORDERS OF PRIMARY HEMOSTASIS

1. **Glanzmann thrombasthenia is due to defect in**
   (Recent Question 2019)
   a. Gp IIb/IIIa
   b. Gp Ib-IX
   c. CD68
   d. Von Willebrand factor

2. **Bleeding time increased in which of the following conditions?** *(Recent Question 2018)*
   a. Von Willebrand disease
   b. Hemophilia A
   c. DIC
   d. Both a & c

3. **Which of the following is true regarding Bernard-Soulier syndrome?** *(Recent Question 2018)*
   a. It is due to defect in platelet adhesion
   b. It is due to defect in platelet aggregation
   c. It is due to defect in platelet receptor GpIb-IX
   d. Both a and c

4. **Which of the following is/are released from dense granules of platelets?** *(PGI Nov 2017)*
   a. Serotonin
   b. Histamine
   c. PDGF
   d. ATP
   e. Lysosome

5. **Platelet adhesion to vessel wall is due to?**
   (AIIMS May 2015)
   a. Factor IX
   b. Fibrinogen
   c. vWF
   d. Fibronectin

6. **Which of the following is not a component of the dense granules of platelets?** *(Recent Question 2015)*
   a. ADP
   b. Calcium
   c. Epinephrine
   d. Platelet factor 4

7. **Earliest event of vascular trauma is?**
   (Recent Question 2016)
   a. Vasoconstriction
   b. Platelet adhesion
   c. Platelet aggregation
   d. Vasodilatation

8. **Which of the following is a qualitative defect of platelet?** *(Recent Question 2016)*
   a. VWD
   b. Hemophillia A
   c. Hemophillia C
   d. Glanzman thrombasthenia

9. **PDGF is present in which granules of platelets?**
   (Recent Question 2016)
   a. Alpha
   b. Beta
   c. Delta
   d. None

10. **In von Willebrand disease, what is true ?**
    (Recent Question 2016)
    a. Ristocetin aggregation test is decreased
    b. Ristocetinaggregation is Increased
    c. No effect
    d. May be increased or decreased

11. **An adolescent female presents with palpable purpura. Her hemogram suggested only anemia. What is your diagnosis?** *(Recent Question 2015)*
    a. ITP
    b. TTP
    c. HUS
    d. HSP

12. **Bernard Soulier syndrome is a defect in?**
    (Recent Question 2015)
    a. Platelet Aggregation
    b. Platelet Adhesion
    c. Platelet activation
    d. Platelet agglutination

13. **A 7 years old boy presented with sudden onset petechiae and purpura. There was a history of URTI 2 weeks back. On examination, there was no hepatosplenomegaly. He is most probably suffering from:** *(Recent Question 2015)*
    a. ALL
    b. Acute viral infection
    c. ITP
    d. Aplastic Anemia

14. **Platelet aggregation is caused by?**
    (Recent Question 2014)
    a. Nitrous oxide
    b. Thromboxone A2
    c. Aspirin
    d. PGE2

15. **Glanzmanns disease is-** *(Recent Question 2014)*
    a. Congenital defect of platelets
    b. Congential defect of RBCs
    c. Defect of neutrophils
    d. Clotting factor deficiency

16. **Vasoconstricting mediator is-** *(Recent Question 2014)*
    a. Prostacyclin
    b. Thromboxane-A$_2$
    c. PGG2
    d. Lipoxins

17. **All the following conditions cause thrombocytopenia except** *(Recent Question 2014)*
    a. Giant hemangioma
    b. Infectious mononucleosis
    c. HIV infection
    d. Iron deficiency anemia

18. **vWF is useful in:** *(Recent Question 2014)*
    a. Platelet adhesion
    b. Platelet aggregation
    c. Clot formation
    d. Fibrinolysis

19. **Fever, fluctuating neurological symptoms, renal failure and severe thrombocytopenia are characteristic of**
    (Recent Question 2015)
    a. Hemolytic uremic syndrome
    b. Thrombotic thrombocytopenic purpura
    c. Idiopathic thrombocytopenic purpura
    d. Disseminated intravascular coagulation

20. **All the following are associated with HUS except**
    a. E coli O157:H7 *(Recent Question 2015)*
    b. Shigelladysentriae type 1
    c. Staphylococcus aureus
    d. Streptococcus pneumoniae

21. **A 4-year-old boy with sudden onset of petechial rashes. History of viral illness 2 weeks ago present. Investigations reveal thrombocytopenia and anti-platelets antibodies. What is your diagnosis?**
    (Recent Question 2015)
    a. Immune thrombocytopenic purpura
    b. Henochschonleinpurpura
    c. Thrombotic thrombocytopenic purpura
    d. Haemolytic uremic syndrome

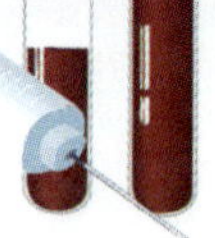

22. After tonsillectomy, a 9 year old child is having continuous bleeding. Bleeding time and PTT are prolonged. Platelet count and PT are normal. What is your diagnosis *(Recent Question 2015)*
a. Von willebrand disease
b. Vitamin K deficiency
c. Immune thrombocytopenic purpura
d. Hemophilia A

23. Find the false statement about TTP
a. Renal failure *(Recent Question 2015)*
b. Negative direct anti-globulin test
c. Antibodies to ADAMTS 13
d. PT and aPTT are prolonged

24. True regarding heparin induced thrombocytopenia *(Recent Question 2015)*
a. Platelet counts usually <10,000/uL
b. Increased risk of thrombosis
c. Associated with severe bleeding
d. HIT antibodies disappear in 5-14 days

25. Anticoagulant used for complete blood count? *(Recent Question 2015)*
a. Trisodium citrate   b. Heparin
c. EDTA   d. Potassium oxalate

26. Increased PT indicates *(Recent Question 2015)*
a. Platelet function defect
b. Intrinsic pathway defect
c. Extrinsic pathway defect
d. Common pathway defect

27. The following feature differentiates TTP and DIC
a. Elevated D-dimers *(Recent Question 2015)*
b. Schistocytes in peripheral smear
c. Thrombocytopenia
d. Increased thrombin time/Decreased fibrinogen

28. Glanzmann thrombasthenia is due to: *(Recent Question 2015)*
a. Abnomal platelet granule formation
b. Deficiency of von willebrand factor
c. Dysfunction of GpIIb-IIIa
d. Dysfunction of GpIb-IX

29. Spontaneous bleeding usually occurs when the platelet counts fall below *(Recent Question 2015)*
a. 20000/uL   b. 50000/uL
c. 100000/uL   d. 120000/uL

30. Disorder of platelet aggregation: *(Recent Question 2015)*
a. Bernard soulier syndrome
b. Glanzmann's thrombasthenia
c. Idiopathic thrombocytopenic purpura
d. Gray platelet syndrome

31. All are true about chronic ITP except:
a. Common in females *(Recent Question 2015)*
b. Anti platelet antibodies
c. Splenomegaly
d. I.V. immunoglobulin used in treatment

32. Evans syndrome is: *(Recent Question 2015)*
a. Autoimmune hemolytic anemia + ITP
b. Autoimmune hemolytic anemia + TTP
c. Autoimmune hemolytic anemia + HUS
d. Autoimmune hemolytic anemia + vWD

33. Five years old child presents with oliguria. There is history of bloody diarrhea 2 weeks ago. Coagulation tests are normal. Peripheral smear is given. What is your diagnosis: *(Recent Question 2015)*

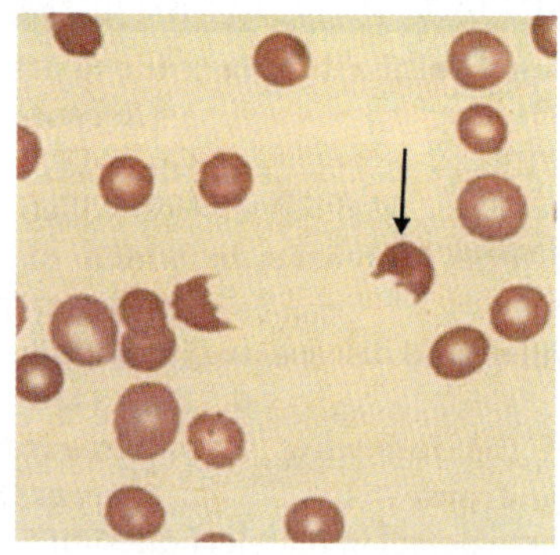

a. Thrombotic thrombocytopenic purpura
b. Idioppathic thrombocytopenic purpura
c. G6PD deficiency
d. Hemolytic uremic syndrome

34. The following is not a platelet function test
a. Bleeding time *(Recent Question 2015)*
b. Prothrombin time
c. Clot retraction time
d. Prothrombin consumption index

35. Giant platelets, thrombocytopenia and cytoplasmic inclusions in the neutrophils is characteristic of
a. May hegglin anomaly *(Recent Question 2015)*
b. Pelgerheut anomaly
c. Wiskott Aldrich syndrome
d. Gray platelet syndrome

36. Which plasma protein is necessary for adhesion of platelets to subendothelialfibres? *(APPGMEE 14)*
a. Glycoprotein IIb   b. Von Willebrand factor
c. Platelet factor 3   d. Factor X

37. Select the FALSE statement among the following: *(APPGMEE 14)*
a. Anti-D is used in Immune Thrombocytopenic purpura
b. DDAVP is used in von Willebrand disease type 3
c. DDAVP is used in severe form of Hemophilia A
d. EACA is used in Factor XI deficiency for minor bleeds

38. HUS is differentiated from TTP by? *(JIPMER 2014)*
a. Presence of MAHA
b. Renal failure
c. Neurological symptoms
d. Absence of fever

39. Platelet is attached to collagen in endothelium via: *(AIIMS Nov 2013)*
a. Factor 8   b. Factor 9
c. vWF   d. Fibronectin

40. Not true about von Willebrand disease:
a. aPTT is normal *(PGI May 2013)*
b. Bleeding time is normal
c. Most common pattern of inheritance is autosomal recessive
d. Bleeding from mucosa in oral cavity may present
e. Normal platelet count

41. **A newborn baby presented with profuse bleeding from the umbilical stump after birth. Rest of the examination and PT, APTT are within normal limits. Most probable diagnosis is-** *(AIIMS May 12)*
   a. Factor X deficiency
   b. Glanzmann thrombasthenia
   c. Von willebrand disease
   d. Bernard soulier disease

42. **What abnormalities will be present in a patient is having deficiency of Von Willebrand factor?** *(DNB Aug 12 Pattern, DNB Dec 09)*
   a. Increased apTT, Increased- PT
   b. Decreased.PT, Increased apTT
   c. Normal PT, Normal apTT
   d. Normal PT, IncreasedaPTT

43. **Which is not true regarding Bernard Soulier syndrome**
   a. Ristocetin aggregation is normal *(AI 11)*
   b. Aggregation with collagen and ADP is normal
   c. Large platelets
   d. Thrombocytopenia

44. **Which of the following statements about platelet function defects is true?** *(AI 11)*
   a. Normal platelet count with prolonged bleeding time
   b. Thrombocytopenia with prolonged bleeding time
   c. Thrombobocytosis with prolonged bleeding time
   d. Normal platelet count with normal bleeding time

45. **Increased bleeding time is seen in:** *(PGI May 2011)*
   a. Coumarin derivative administration
   b. Thrombocytopenia
   c. Congenital afibrinogenemia
   d. DIC
   e. Hemophilia A

46. **Normal platelet count is/are seen in -** *(PGI Nov 10)*
   a. DIC
   b. Shaken baby syndrome
   c. Microangiopathic hemolytic anemia
   d. Splenomegaly
   e. Kaasabach- Merritt syndrome

47. **A 25-year-old asymptomatic female underwent pre-op coagulation testing. Her BT was 3 minutes, PT was 15/14 seconds, aPTT 45/35 seconds. Platelet counts were 2.5 lac/uL, factor VIII levels 60 IU/dl. Most likely diagnosis is:** *(AIIMS Nov 11)*
   a. Factor IX deficiency
   b. vWD type 3
   c. Factor VIII inhibitor
   d. Lupus anticoagulant

48. **Which test is NOT used to assess the Platelet function?**
   a. Clot retraction time *(Recent Question 2013)*
   b. Bleeding time
   c. Ristocetin induced assay
   d. Clot lysis time

DISORDERS OF SECONDARY HEMOSTASIS

49. **Which of the following is required for the function of heparin ?** *(AIIMS May 18)*
   a. Protein C
   b. Protein S
   c. Antithrombin III
   d. Thrombomodulin

50. **True about Hemophillia B are?** *(PGI Nov 2018)*
   a. Autosomal recessive
   b. Cryoprecipitate for treatment
   c. Haemophila B had factor 8 <5%
   d. X linked
   e. PT is raised

51. **Increase PT is seen with?** *(PGI May 18)*
   a. Vitamin K deficiency
   b. Factor V deficiency
   c. Factor VIII deficiency
   d. Factor IX deficiency
   e. Warfarin administration

52. **Which of the following is true regarding Von willebrand disease?** *(Recent exam 2018)*
   a. Type 1&3 are associated with quantitative defects in vWF
   b. Normal platelet count
   c. Desmopressin stimulates release of VWF
   d. All of the above

53. **Which of the following is the most common manifestation of hemophilia?** *(Recent exam 2018)*
   a. Hemoptysis
   b. Hemarthrosis
   c. Hematemesis
   d. Mucosal bleeding

54. **In PT test, the addition of Ca^{2+} & tissue thromboplastin activates which pathway?** *(AIIMS Nov 2017)*
   a. Extrinsic
   b. Intrinsic
   c. Fibrinolytic
   d. Common

55. **Which coagulation factor is not in circulating form in blood?** *(JIPMER 2017)*
   a. F Xl
   b. F X
   c. F III
   d. F XIII

56. **Which of the following is not associated with prolonged prothrombin time?** *(PGI Nov 2017)*
   a. Haemophilia A
   b. Von-Willebrand disease
   c. Factor VII deficiency
   d. Disseminated intravascular coagulation(DIC)

57. **Both PT and aPTT will be increased in deficiency of?**
   a. Factor 2
   b. Factor 5 *(PGI May 2017)*
   c. Factor 8
   d. Factor 10
   e. Factor 12

58. **Feature(s) of XIII factor deficiency is/are:**
   a. Delayed wound closure *(PGI May 2016)*
   b. Clot solubility tests are abnormal
   c. ↑aPTT
   d. ↑PT
   e. ↑ BT

59. **Which of the following statement(s) is/are correct except:** *(PGI May 2016)*
   a. Increased PT in extrinsic pathways
   b. Increased aPTT in instrinsic pathways
   c. If platelet count is > 1.5 lac/microL, then normal homeostasis present
   d. BT is decreased in platelet abnormality

60. **Endotoxin first damages ?** *(Recent Question 2016-17)*
   a. Endothelium
   b. RBC
   c. Platelets
   d. WBC

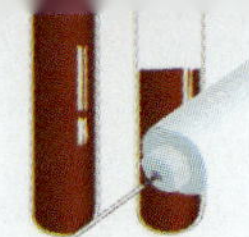

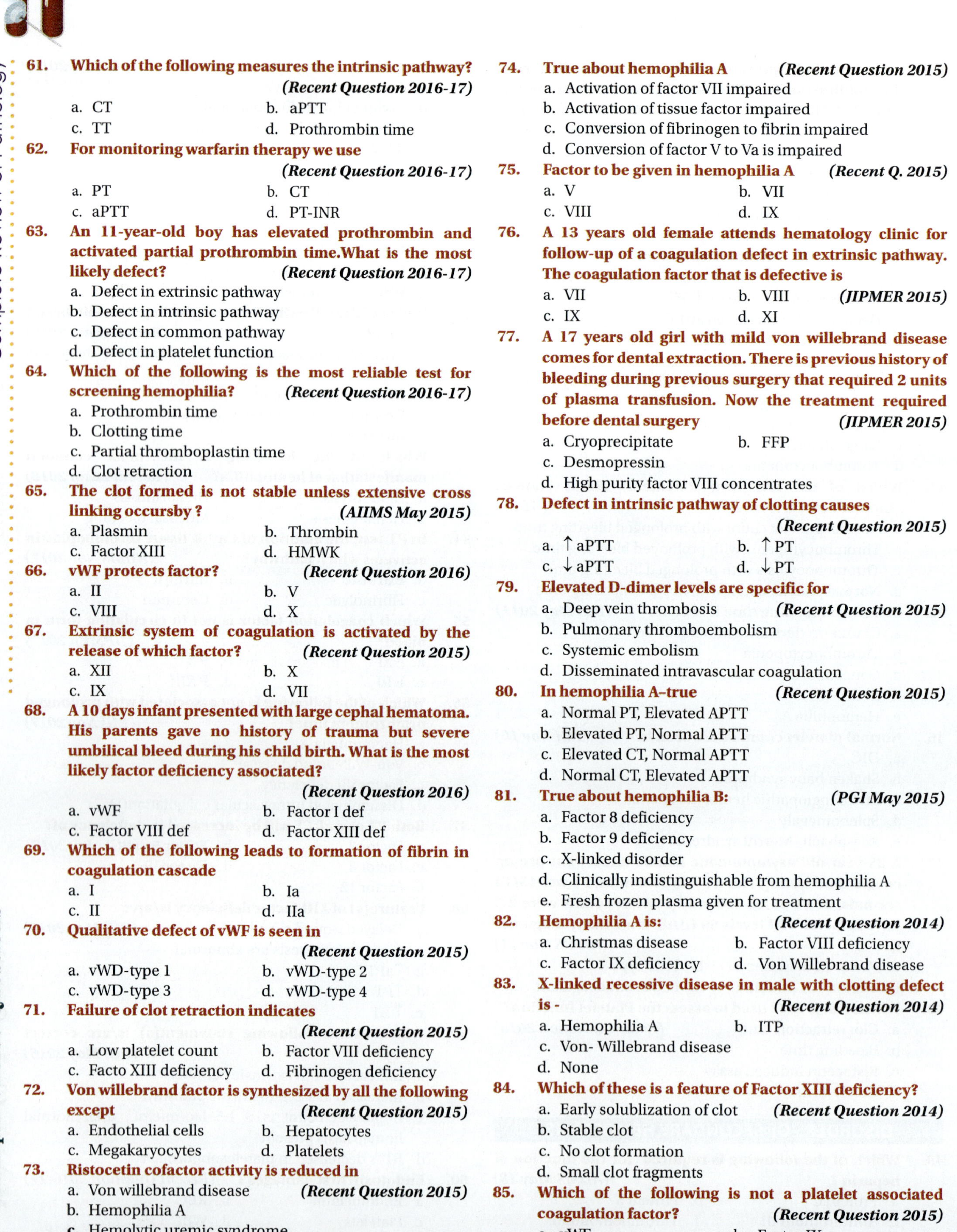

61. Which of the following measures the intrinsic pathway?
(Recent Question 2016-17)
a. CT
b. aPTT
c. TT
d. Prothrombin time

62. For monitoring warfarin therapy we use
(Recent Question 2016-17)
a. PT
b. CT
c. aPTT
d. PT-INR

63. An 11-year-old boy has elevated prothrombin and activated partial prothrombin time.What is the most likely defect? *(Recent Question 2016-17)*
a. Defect in extrinsic pathway
b. Defect in intrinsic pathway
c. Defect in common pathway
d. Defect in platelet function

64. Which of the following is the most reliable test for screening hemophilia? *(Recent Question 2016-17)*
a. Prothrombin time
b. Clotting time
c. Partial thromboplastin time
d. Clot retraction

65. The clot formed is not stable unless extensive cross linking occursby ? *(AIIMS May 2015)*
a. Plasmin
b. Thrombin
c. Factor XIII
d. HMWK

66. vWF protects factor? *(Recent Question 2016)*
a. II
b. V
c. VIII
d. X

67. Extrinsic system of coagulation is activated by the release of which factor? *(Recent Question 2015)*
a. XII
b. X
c. IX
d. VII

68. A 10 days infant presented with large cephal hematoma. His parents gave no history of trauma but severe umbilical bleed during his child birth. What is the most likely factor deficiency associated?
(Recent Question 2016)
a. vWF
b. Factor I def
c. Factor VIII def
d. Factor XIII def

69. Which of the following leads to formation of fibrin in coagulation cascade
a. I
b. Ia
c. II
d. IIa

70. Qualitative defect of vWF is seen in
(Recent Question 2015)
a. vWD-type 1
b. vWD-type 2
c. vWD-type 3
d. vWD-type 4

71. Failure of clot retraction indicates
(Recent Question 2015)
a. Low platelet count
b. Factor VIII deficiency
c. Facto XIII deficiency
d. Fibrinogen deficiency

72. Von willebrand factor is synthesized by all the following except
(Recent Question 2015)
a. Endothelial cells
b. Hepatocytes
c. Megakaryocytes
d. Platelets

73. Ristocetin cofactor activity is reduced in
a. Von willebrand disease *(Recent Question 2015)*
b. Hemophilia A
c. Hemolytic uremic syndrome
d. Thrombotic thrombocytopenic purpura

74. True about hemophilia A *(Recent Question 2015)*
a. Activation of factor VII impaired
b. Activation of tissue factor impaired
c. Conversion of fibrinogen to fibrin impaired
d. Conversion of factor V to Va is impaired

75. Factor to be given in hemophilia A *(Recent Q. 2015)*
a. V
b. VII
c. VIII
d. IX

76. A 13 years old female attends hematology clinic for follow-up of a coagulation defect in extrinsic pathway. The coagulation factor that is defective is
a. VII
b. VIII *(JIPMER 2015)*
c. IX
d. XI

77. A 17 years old girl with mild von willebrand disease comes for dental extraction. There is previous history of bleeding during previous surgery that required 2 units of plasma transfusion. Now the treatment required before dental surgery *(JIPMER 2015)*
a. Cryoprecipitate
b. FFP
c. Desmopressin
d. High purity factor VIII concentrates

78. Defect in intrinsic pathway of clotting causes
(Recent Question 2015)
a. ↑ aPTT
b. ↑ PT
c. ↓ aPTT
d. ↓ PT

79. Elevated D-dimer levels are specific for
a. Deep vein thrombosis *(Recent Question 2015)*
b. Pulmonary thromboembolism
c. Systemic embolism
d. Disseminated intravascular coagulation

80. In hemophilia A–true *(Recent Question 2015)*
a. Normal PT, Elevated APTT
b. Elevated PT, Normal APTT
c. Elevated CT, Normal APTT
d. Normal CT, Elevated APTT

81. True about hemophilia B: *(PGI May 2015)*
a. Factor 8 deficiency
b. Factor 9 deficiency
c. X-linked disorder
d. Clinically indistinguishable from hemophilia A
e. Fresh frozen plasma given for treatment

82. Hemophilia A is: *(Recent Question 2014)*
a. Christmas disease
b. Factor VIII deficiency
c. Factor IX deficiency
d. Von Willebrand disease

83. X-linked recessive disease in male with clotting defect is - *(Recent Question 2014)*
a. Hemophilia A
b. ITP
c. Von- Willebrand disease
d. None

84. Which of these is a feature of Factor XIII deficiency?
a. Early solublization of clot *(Recent Question 2014)*
b. Stable clot
c. No clot formation
d. Small clot fragments

85. Which of the following is not a platelet associated coagulation factor? *(Recent Question 2015)*
a. vWF
b. Factor IX
c. Factor XI
d. Factor XIII

86. Hemophilia C is deficiency of *(WBPG 2015)*
a. Factor VIII
b. Factor IX
c. Factor X
d. Factor XI

87. LakiLorand factor is *(Recent Question 2014)*
a. Factor X
b. Factor XI
c. Factor XII
d. Factor XIII

88. Levels of all coagulation factors are increased in pregnancy EXCEPT *(APPGMEE 14)*
a. Factor VIII
b. Factor IX
c. Factor X
d. Factor XI

89. Factor Xa is necessary for conversion of prothrombin to thrombin *(APPGMEE 14)*
a. Only in the extrinsic pathway
b. Only in the intrinsic pathway
c. As part of both extrinsic and intrinsic pathways
d. Only if the normal blood clotting cascade is inhibited

90. Isolated rise in aPTT is seen in? *(Recent Question 2013)*
a. Von Willebrand's disease
b. Factor 7 deficiency
c. Vitamin K deficiency
d. Anti phospholipid antibodies

91. Increased Prothrombin time is/are seen in:
a. Pt on oral anticoagulant *(PGI May 12)*
b. Pt with liver disease
c. Factor X deficiency
d. Factor VII deficiency
e. Vit. K deficiency

92. Prolonged apTT, but asymptomatic is seen in deficiency of factor *(JIPMER 2012)*
a. V
b. VII
c. X
d. XII

93. All of the following are true about blood coagulation, except: *(AI 11)*
a. Factor X is part or both intrinsic and extrinsic pathways
b. Extrinsic pathway is activated by contact with negatively charged surfaces
c. Intrinsic pathway can be activated in vitro
d. Calcium is required in several steps of coagulation

94. True regarding prothrombin time measurement?
a. Platelet rich plasma is required *(AIIMS Nov 11)*
b. Activate with kaolin
c. Should be measured within 2 hours
d. Immediate refrigeration to preserve coagulation factor viability

95. Increased PT and Normal PTT are found in? *(DNB Dec 11)*
a. Von Willebrand disease
b. Factor 7 deficiency
c. Factor 8 deficiency
d. Thrombin deficiency

96. The best screening test for hemophilia - *(DNB Dec 11)*
a. PT
b. CT
c. PTT
d. BT

97. Prolonged PT and Normal PTT may be seen in:
a. Thrombocytopenia
b. DIC *(DNB June 11)*
c. Vit. K deficiency
d. Aspirin toxicity

98. A 9 years old boy with elevation in both PT and aPTT. What is the diagnosis? *(AIIMS Nov 10)*
a. Defect in extrinsic pathway
b. Defect in intrinsic pathway
c. Platelet function defect
d. Defect in common pathway

DIC

99. Which among the following laboratory investigation is best to reveal about bleeding in Disseminated Intravascular Coagulation (DIC)? *(AIIMS May 18)*
a. Increased PT
b. Increased aPTT
c. Decreased fibrinogen
d. Increased FDPs

100. Most common cause of DIC *(Recent Question 2015)*
a. Obstetric complications
b. Cyanotic heart disease
c. Malignancies
d. Extensive burns

101. The most sensitive test for DIC is *(Recent Question 2015)*
a. Bleeding time
b. Clotting time
c. Prothrombin time
d. FDP level

102. The following is not a contraindication for heparin in DIC *(Recent Question 2015)*
a. If the platelet count cannot be maintained at $\geq$ 50,000/mcL
b. In cases of central nervous system/gastrointestinal bleeding
c. Placental abruption
d. DIC associated with malignancy

103. What is not associated with DIC *(Recent Question 2015)*
a. Thrombocytopenia
b. Increased PT
c. Hyperfibrinogenemia
d. Increased FDP

104. DIC causes all except? *(Recent Question 2014)*
a. Increased fibrinogen level
b. Increased d-dimer
c. Decreased platelet counts
d. Decreased clotting factors

105. In DIC, following are seen except *(Recent Question 2014)*
a. Fibrinogen decreased
b. Thrombocytopenia
c. Normal APTT
d. PT elevation

THROMBOPHILIAS

106. Which of the following is true regarding Factor V Leiden mutation? *(Recent exam 2018)*
a. Increased risk of deep vein thrombosis
b. Factor V becomes resistant to cleavage by protein C
c. Glutamine to Arginine substitution at 506
d. All of the above

107. True about hematological disorder? *(PGI May 2017)*
a. In Haemophilia B factor 8 is useful.
b. Both PT and aPTT are increased in DIC
c. IV Ig is useful in ITP
d. Cryoprecipitate is useful in hemophilia A

108. Most common inherited hyper coagulation defect?
a. Factor 5 mutation *(Recent Question 2016-17)*
b. Prothrombin mutation
c. Hyperhomocytenemia
d. Protein C deficiency

109. Tumors causing thrombosis are all except? *(Recent Question 2016-17)*
a. Stomach
b. Lung
c. Pancreas
d. Breast

110. Antithrombin is activated by? *(Recent Question 2016)*
a. Heparin
b. Factor I
c. Fctor V
d. Factor VIII

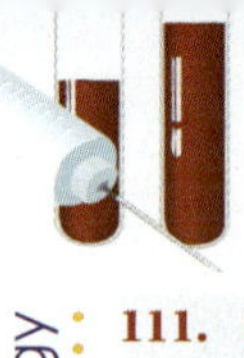

111. Which of the following is not a usual cause of DVT?
(Recent question 2016)
a. Injury
b. Hypothermia
c. Stasis
d. Hypercoagubility

112. Treatment of antiphospholipid antibody syndrome
(Recent Question 2015)
a. Warfarin for life
b. Warfarin for 1 year
c. IV immunoglobulin
d. Glucocorticoids

113. Not a feature of antiphospholipid antibody syndrome
a. Budd-Chiari syndrome   *(Recent Question 2015)*
b. Coomb's positive hemolytic anemia
c. Libman sacks endocarditis
d. Priaspism

114. Leiden mutation is related to?   *(Recent Question 2015)*
a. Factor V
b. Factor VIII
c. Antithrombin III
d. Severe inherited bleeding

115. All antibodies are seen in APLA except?
a. Anti-β2 glycoprotein   *(Recent Question 2015)*
b. Anti-Prothrombin
c. Anti-Phospholipid
d. Anti-Cardiolipin

116. All are true about Virchow's triad except-
(Recent Question 2014)
a. Concerns the risk of intravascular thrombus
b. Depends on endothelial injury
c. Depends on platelet activation
d. Depends on stasis

117. Leiden factor is -   *(Recent Question 2014)*
a. Factor VI
b. Factor VIII
c. Factor IV
d. Factor V

118. All endothelial cells produce thrombomodulin except those found in -   *(Recent Question 2013, AI 05)*
a. Hepatic circulation
b. Cutaneous circulation
c. Cerebral microcirculation
d. Renal circulation

119. Heparin treatment is monitored by:
(Recent Question 2013)
a. PT INR
b. aPTT
c. Vit K levels
d. PT

120. Presentation of antiphospholipid syndrome includes:
a. Recurrent abortion   *(PGI May 2013)*
b. Fetal death
c. Both arterial and venous thrombosis
d. Prolonged aPTT
e. Prolonged PT

121. Which of the following antibodies is most frequently seen in Antiphospholipid Syndrome?   *(AI 11)*
a. Beta 2 microglobulin antibody
b. Anti-nuclear antibody
c. Anti-centromere antibody
d. Anti- beta 2 glycoprotein antibody

122. Both arterial and venous thrombosis occur in:
a. Antiphospholipid antibodies   *(PGI Nov 2011)*
b. Antithrombin III deficiency
c. Hyperhomocysteinemia
d. Protein C deficiency
e. Mutation in factor V gene

123. Hypercoagulability due to defective factor V gene is called   *(AIIMS 10)*
a. Lisbon mutation
b. Leiden mutation
c. Aruiphospholipid syndrome
d. Inducible thrombocytopenia syndrome

124. Warfarin skin necrosis is caused by-
(Recent Question 2014)
a. Protein C / Protein S deficiency
b. APLA
c. Vitamin K deficiency
d. Fibrinogen deficiency

125. Tissue Factor Pathway Inhibitor (TFPI) inhibits?
(Recent Question 2013)
a. Factor V
b. Factor VII
c. Factor X
d. Factor IV

126. Screening test for patients suspected of having a hyper-coagulable State includes?   *(Recent Question 2013)*
a. Russell viper venom time
b. Prothrombin time
c. Heparin cofactor II
d. Clotting Factor levels

127. International Normalised Ratio (INR) is defined as?
a. (PT patient/ PT control)^{ISI}
b. (PT control/ PT patient)^{ISI}
c. (PT patient/ PT control)$^{1/ISI}$
d. (PT control/ PT patient)$^{1/ISI}$

128. Increased clotting time and decreased platelet count is associated with?   *(WBPG 10, 12)*
a. Vascular injury
b. Volume contraction
c. Decreased platelet clumping
d. Decreased platelet phospholipid

129. Warfarin therapy is monitored by:
(Recent Question 2013)
a. PT INR
b. apTT
c. Vit K levels
d. PT

Answers with Explanations

1.   **Ans. (a)**   Gp IIb/IIIa

2.   **Ans. (d)**   Both a & c

BT	↑
Deficiency of platelets	Functional defect of platelets
VWD is adhesion defect as platelets cannot bind with vessel wall. So primary hemostatic plug is not formed.	Dic is hyper coagulable to state so many clots are formed which consume all platelets.

3.   **Ans. (d)**   Both a and c

(Ref: Robbins 9th/pg 660)

Bernard-Soulier syndrome illustrates the consequences of defective adhesion of platelets to subendothelial matrix. Bernard-Soulier syndrome is caused by an inherited deficiency of the platelet membrane glyco protein complex Ib-IX. This glycoprotein is a receptor for vWF and is essential for normal platelet adhesion to the subendothelial extracellular matrix.

4.   **Ans. (a, b, d) a. Serotonin; b. Histamine; d. ATP**

The dense granules of platelets contain adenosine diphosphate (ADP), adenosine triphosphate (ATP), ionized calcium, serotonin and histamine. PDGF is a constituent of alpha granules.

5.   **Ans. (c)**   vWF *(Ref: Robbins 9th/pg 660; 8th/pg 670)*

Platelet adhesion to vessel wall is due to vWF on endothelium and GpIb/IX receptors on the surface of platelets.

6.   **Ans. (d)**   Platelet factor 4 *(Ref: Robbins 9th/pg 660)*

Dense (or δ) granules of platelets contain: (**"DENSE"**)
- a**DEN**osine diphosphate **(ADP)**[Q], Serotonin[Q], Epi-nephrine[Q], Ca

7.   **Ans. (a)**   Vasoconstriction *(Ref: Robbins 9th/pg 661)*

Endothelial Injury causes vasoconstriction[Q] (due to endothelin, serotonin) immediately and markedly reduces blood flow to the injured area.

8.   **Ans. (d)**   Glanzman thrombesthenia *(Ref: R 9th/pg 660)*

9.   **Ans. (a)**   Alpha *(Ref: Robbins 9th/pg 660; 8th/pg 670)*

α-Granules **of platelets contains**:
- **Pselectin, Fibrinogen[Q], V[Q], VIII[Q], and vWF[Q], Platelet factor 4[Q], (PDGF), TGF-β**

10.   **Ans. (a)**   Ristocetin aggregation test is decreased

(Ref: Wintrobe's 12th ed/1392)

Ristocetin cofactor assay[Q]/Ristocetin induced platelet aggregation is decreased or absent in vWD

11.   **Ans. (d)**   HSP *(Ref: Harrison 18th/Chapter 53)*

12.   **Ans. (b)**   Platelet Adhesion

(Ref: Robbins 9th/pg 660; 8th/pg 670)

13.   **Ans. (c)**   ITP *(Ref: 9th/pg 657-658; 8th/pg 667-668)*

A 7 year old boy presented with sudden onset petechiae and purpura with a history of URTI 2 weeks back and there is no hepatosplenomegaly. He is most probably suffering from ITP. For complete discussion on **ITP**; Refer to pretext of this chapter.

14.   **Ans. (b).**   Thromboxone A2

(Ref: Robbins 9th/pg 116-117)

Thromboxone A2 (TXA2)

- It is **produced by activated platelets** and has prothrombotic properties
- It is an **Arachidonic acid metabolite** of COX pathway
- Functions: It is a potent **platelet aggregator & vasocon-strictor**
- Its effect is **neutralized by prostacyclin (PGI2)**

15.   **Ans. (a)**   Congenital defect of platelets

(Ref: Robbins 9th/pg 660; 8th/pg 670)

Glanzmanns disease is a congenital defect of platelets; Refer Ans 4 above;

16.   **Ans. (b)**   Thromboxane-A2 *(Ref: Robbins 9th/pg 116-117)*

17.   **Ans. (d)**   Iron deficiency anemia

(Ref: Robbins 9th/pg 657-658; 8th/pg 667-668; Wintrobe's 12th/ pg 1595)

Thrombocytopenia refers to platelet count < **1.5 lac/cu mm**[Q]

Refer to pretext of this chapter for important causes of Thrombocytopenia

- **Thrombocytopenia** is seen in **50%** of patients with **Infectious Mononucleosis**
- **Thrombocytosis** is seen in **Iron deficiency Anemia**, platelet counts rise to twice the normal value and **return to normal with Iron therapy.** Exact cause unknown, but probably **due to ↑ level of Erythropoietin**

18.   **Ans. (a)**   Platelet adhesion *(Ref: Robbins 9th/pg 661)*

2 major **functions of vWF** are: Platelet adhesion via GpIb/ IX and Stabilizes factor VIII in circulation

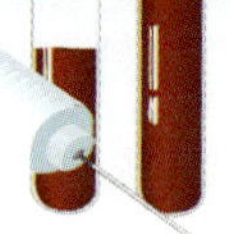

19. Ans. (b) Thrombotic thrombocytopenic purpura

(Ref: Robbins 9th/pg 659; 8th/pg 669)

- Features of hemolytic uremic syndrome include Hyperkalemia (due to deranged renal function), Anemia (due to hemolysis) & renal microthrombi
- But Neuro psychiatric disturbances are seen in TTP & not in HUS

20. Ans. (c) Staphulococcus aureus

(Ref: Robbins 9th/pg 659)

21. Ans. (c) Thrombotic thrombocytopenic purpura

(Ref: Robbins 9th/pg 659; 8th/pg 669)

Thrombocytopenia and anti-platelets antibodies in a child presenting with purpura after 2 weeks of viral illness is characteristic of ITP.

22. Ans. (a) Von Willebrand disease

(Ref: Robbins 9th/pg 661)

a. Von willebrand disease: True: Bleeding time and aPTT prolonged, PT and platelet count normal
b. Vitamin K deficiency: False: PT prolonged
c. Immune thrombocytopenic purpura: False aPTT is normal
d. Hemophilia A: Flase: Bleeding time normal

23. Ans. (d) PT and aPTT are prolonged *(Ref: R 9th/pg 662)*
PT and aPTT are normal and not prolonged.

24. Ans. (b) Increased risk of thrombosis *(Ref: R 9th/pg 657)*

Options:

a. Platelet counts usually <10,000/uL: **False:** *T*hrombocytopenia (decrease of >50%)
b. Increased risk of thrombosis: True: seen in 50%
c. Associated with severe bleeding: False: Bleeding is uncommon in HIT
d. HIT antibodies disappear in 5-14 days: False: they appear after 5-14 days.

25. Ans. (c) EDTA *(Ref: Robbins 9th/pg 656)*

K2 (Dipotassium)-EDTA is the common anticogualant for hemogram analysis.

26. Ans. (c) Extrinsic pathway defect

(Ref: Robbins 9th/pg 661)

27. Ans. (d) Increased thrombin time/Decreased fibrinogen

(Ref: Robbins 9th/pg 663; 8th/pg 673)

Increased thrombin time/Decreased fibrinogen is seen in DIC only not in TTP.

28. Ans. (c) Dysfunction of GpIIb-IIIa

(Ref: Wintrobe's 13th ed/pg 689)

29. Ans. (a) 20000/uL *(Ref: Robbins 9th/pg 662; 8th/pg 692)*

In general, the risk of significant spontaneous hemorrhage increases gradually as the platelet count drops to <50 $\times$ 10^9/L and is high at counts <5 $\times$ 10^9/L. So among the options the best answer is 10,000/ul.

30. Ans. (b) Glanzmann's thrombasthenia

(Ref: Robbins 9th/pg 662)

31. Ans. (c) Splenomegaly

(Ref: Robbins 9th/pg 657; 8th/pg 667)

Splenomegaly is very rare in ITP

32. Ans. (a) Autoimmune hemolytic anemia + ITP

(Ref: Wintrobe's 13th ed/pg 968)

Evans syndrome: Antiplatelet antibodies in patients with ITP do not usually cross-react with RBCs. However, RBC fragmentation because of weak complement activation, may occur. Such patients may also have a positive Coombs test and autoimmune hemolytic anemia. This is referred as Evans syndrome.

33. Ans. (d) Hemolytic uremic syndrome

(Ref: R 9th/pg 659)

Features of oliguria following an episode of diarrhea with peripheral smear finding of Schistocytes (Helmet cells) is suggestive of Hemolytic uremic syndrome.

34. Ans. (b) Prothrombin time

(Ref: Robbins 9th/pg 662)

a. **Bleeding time** assess ability of platelets to iorm platelet plug
b. **Prothrombin time asseses extrinsic pathway of coagulation**
c. **Clot retraction study** measures the time taken for a platelet plug to undergo last step of retraction, which indicates overall platelet function.
d. An abnormal **Prothrombin consumption index** indicates impaired availability of platelet membrane phospholipid for coagulation.

35. Ans. (a) May hegglin anomaly

(Ref: Wintrobe's 12th ed/pg 1549)

May-Hegglin anomaly is a rare, dominantly inherited disorder characterized by large (2 to 5 μm), well-defined, basophilic and pyroninophilic inclusions in granulocytes (neutrophils, eosinophils, basophils, monocytes) and accompanied by thrombocytopenia and giant platelets containing few granules.

36. Ans. (b) Von Willebrand factor

(Ref: Robbins 9th/pg 661)
Von Willebrand factor is necessary for adhesion of platelets to subendothelial fibres.

37.   Ans. (b)   DDAVP is used in von Willebrand disease type 3

(Ref: Wintrobe's 12th/pg 1392, 1410)

DDAVP is used in von Willebrand disease type 1 & 2a, but not in type 3

38.   Ans. (c)   Neurological symptoms

(Ref: Robbins 9th/pg 659)

HUS is differentiated from TTP by **Absence of neurological symptoms**

- **Neurologic findings (due to microthrombi formed in vessels of CNS) are present in TTP in addition to the triad seen in HUS (Microangiopathic hemolytic anemia, Thrombocytopenia & Renal failure)**

39.   Ans. (c)   vWF

(Ref: Robbins 9th/pg 661; 8th/pg 671)

Platelet is attached to collagen in endothelium via vWF

40.   Ans. (a, b, c); a. aPTT is normal; b. Bleeding time is normal; c. Most common pattern of inheritance is autosomal recessive

(Ref: Robbins 9th/pg 661; 8th/pg 671)

Discussing the options about von Willebrand disease, one by one-

A.	False	vWF stabilizes factor VIII, which takes part in Intrinsic pathway. So in vWD, when **vWF is deficient, apTT is prolonged**
B.	False	Because there is **defective platelet adhesion in vWD →↑ BT**
C.	False	Most common pattern of inheritance is **Autosomal dominant for vWD type I**
D.	True	Mucosal bleeding is seen in vWD.
E.	True	In vWD platelet count is normal

41.   Ans. (b)   Glanzmann thrombasthenia

(Ref: Robbins 9th/pg 660; 8th/pg 670)

A newborn baby presented with profuse bleeding from the umbilical stump after birth.

This is a case of severe inherited bleeding disorder. As **PT & apTT are normal, Glanzmann thrombasthenia** is the most probable cause, which can present with **profuse bleeding soon after birth;**

It can be **diagnosed by platelet aggregation studies,** which will be defective.

The other differential diagnosis in this scenario is **Factor XIII deficiency** (not given in the option)

42.   Ans. (d)   Normal PT, Increased a PTT

(Ref: R 9th/pg 662)

In vWD, **Normal PT, Increased a PTT**

vWF stabilizes factor VIII, which takes part in Intrinsic pathway. So in vWD, when vWF is deficient, **Intrinsic** pathway of coagulation is affected, giving rise to **prolonged apTT**; but as extrinsic pathway is not affected, PT remains normal

43.   Ans. (a)   Ristocetin aggregation is normal

(Ref: Robbins 9th/pg 660; 8th/pg 670)

44.   Ans. (a)   Normal platelet count with prolonged bleeding time *(Ref: Robbins 9th/pg 660; 8th/pg 670)*

In **platelet function defects**, there is **normal platelet count** with **prolonged bleeding time**

45.   Ans. (b, c, d); b. Thrombocytopenia; c. Congenital afibrinogenemia; d. DIC *(Ref: Robbins 9th/pg 656)*

↑ **bleeding time (BT) is seen in:**

A.	Coumarin derivative administration	No	PT (initially) followed by both PT & apTT will be abnormal
B.	Thrombocytopenia	Yes	Because of defective formation of primary hemostatic plug
C.	Congenital afibrinogenemia	No	PT, TT & apTT will be abnormal, as formation of stable clot is only affected
D.	DIC	Yes	Due to thrombocytopenia inDIC
E.	Hemophilia A	No	apTT abnormal, PT normal

46.   Ans. (b)   Shaken baby syndrome *(Ref: R 9th/pg 657-658)*

Normal platelet count is/are seen in Shaken baby syndrome.

47.   Ans. (c)   Factor VIII inhibitor

(Ref: Wintrobe's 12th/pg 1452)

This is the case of an asymptomaticfemale with normal BT, PT & platelet counts; aPTT is ↑, factor VIII levels (N=50-150 IU/dl) are near normal.

This is a **controversial** MCQ, as both factor VIII inhibitor & lupus anticoagulant are possible answers

Discussing the options one by one:

A.	Factor IX deficiency	Also called Hemophilia B, excluded because patient is asymptomatic; Factor IX deficiency leads to clinical bleeding
B.	vWD type 3	Excluded because patient is asymptomatic & BT is normal
C.	**Factor VIII inhibitor**	**Best possible answer as patient is asymptomatic with prolonged aPTT due to mild deficiency of factor VIII**
D.	Lupus anticoagulant	Second best answer, as isolated ↑aPTT in an asymptomatic female can be due to Lupus anticoagulant. However, **usually the patient presents with thrombocytopenia & prolonged PT also.**

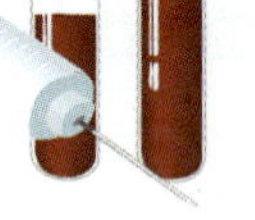

48.   **Ans. (d)**   **Clot lysis time**

(Ref: Wintrobe's 12th/pg 499)

Discussing the options one by one,

A. Clot retraction time	Used to assess the **global contractile function** of platelets; hence it is a test for platelet function
B. Bleeding time	First screening test to assay **platelet function defects**
C. Ristocetin induced assay	Ristocetin induced **platelet adhesion** and **aggregation study** is used to asses **vWF and gplb/IX deficency**
D. Clot lysis time	Used for assessing FXIII deficiency which is responsible for strength of clot

49.   **Ans. (c)**   **Antithrombin III**

50.   **Ans. (b)**   **Cryoprecipitate for treatment (c) Haemophila B had factor 8 <5%**

Hemophilia B is deficiency of factor 9.

51.   **Ans. (a, b, e)** **a. Vitamin K deficiency; b. Factor V deficiency; e. Warfarin administration**

52.   **Ans. (d)**   **All of the above**

53.   **Ans. (b)**   **Hemarthrosis**

(Ref: Robbins 9th/pg 663)

In all symptomatic haemophilia cases there is a tendency toward easy bruising and massive hemorrhage after trauma or operative procedures. In addition, "spontaneous" hemorrhages frequently occur in regions of the body that are susceptible to trauma, particularly the joints, where they are known as hemarthroses. Recurrent bleeding into the joints leads to progressive deformities that can be crippling. Petechiae are characteristically absent.

54.   **Ans. (a)**   **Extrinsic**

To PT we add of Ca^{2+} & tissue thromboplastin which activates extrinsic pathway, while to test for aPTT we add kaolin, silica which activates intrinsic pathway.

55.   **Ans. (c)**   **F III**

Tissue factor (factor III) is also called as platelet tissue factor. It is found on the outside of blood vessels and is not exposed to the bloodstream. It initiates the extrinsic pathway at the site of injury.

56.   **Ans. (a, b)** **a. Haemophilia A; b. Von-Willebrand disease**

Haemophilia A is a deficiency of FVIII & Von-Willebrand disease is a defect of vWF so both of them are associated with aPTT rather than PT.

57.   **Ans. (a, b, d) a.**   **Factor 2; b.**   **Factor 5; d.**   **Factor 10**

Both PT and aPTT will be increased in deficiency of factors of common pathway.

58.   **Ans. (a, b)**   **a. Delayed wound closure, b. Clot solubility tests are abnormal**

(Ref: Harrison 19th/ 733, 736; CMDT 2016/ 556-57)

59.   **Ans. (d)**   **BT is decreased in platelet abnormality**

(Ref: Robbins 9th/118-119)

60.   **Ans. (a)**   **Endothelium** *(Ref: Robbins 9th/pg 131-133)*

61.   **Ans. (b)**   **aPTT** *(Ref: Robbins 9th/pg 656-661)*

62.   **Ans. (d)**   **PT-INR** *(Ref: Wintrobe's 12th/pg 1489)*

63.   **Ans. (c)**   **Defect in common pathway**

(Ref: Robbins 9th/pg 118-119)

64.   **Ans. (c)**   **Partial thromboplastin time**

(Ref: Robbins 9th/pg 656)

65.   **Ans. (c)**   **Factor XIII** *(Ref: Robbins 9th/pg 662; 8th/pg 672)*

66.   **Ans. (c)**   **VIII** *(Ref: Wintrobe's 13th/pg 1389)*

vWF is required for normal platelet adhesion, and also acts as a carrier of factor VIII in the plasma

67.   **Ans. (d)**   **VII** *(Ref: Robbins 9th/pg 662; 8th/pg 672)*

68.   **Ans. (d)**   **Factor XIII def** *(Ref: Robbins 9th/pg 662)*

- Abnormal bleeding manifests shortly after birth, when bleeding from the healthy umbilical cord remnant occurs.
- Umbilical stump bleeding is an uncommon presentation for other congenital bleeding disorders. Rebleeding at circumcision is also common.
- The most life-threatening complication of factor XIII deficiency is spontaneous intracranial hemorrhage

69.   **Ans. (d)**   **IIa** *(Ref: Robbins 9th/pg 662; 8th/pg 672)*

70.   **Ans. (b)**   **vWD-type 2**

(Ref: Robbins 9th/pg 663; 8th/pg 673)

71.   **Ans. (a)**   **Low platelet count** *(Ref: Robbins 9th/pg 657)*

- This test measures the amount of time it takes for a blood clot to pull away from the walls of a test tube (Shrinking).
- The edges of the blood vessel wall at the point of injury are slowly brought together again to repair the damage.
- It is used to evaluate and manage blood platelet disorders, including Glanzmann's thrombasthenia
- So Clot retraction depends primarily on the number and activity of the blood platelets

72. **Ans. (b)** **Hepatocytes**

(Ref: Robbins 9th/pg 662; 8th/pg 672)

73. **Ans. (a)** **Von willebrand disease**

(Ref: Robbins 9th/pg 660)

74. **Ans. (c)** **Conversion of fibrinogen to fibrin impaired**

(Ref: Robbins 9th/pg 660; 8th/pg 670)

75. **Ans. (c)** **VIII** *(Ref: Robbins 9th/pg 660; 8th/pg 670)*

76. **Ans. (a)** **VII** *(Ref: Robbins 9th/pg 660; 8th/pg 670)*
Factor VII is involved in extrinsic pathway.

77. **Ans. (c)** **Desmopressin**

Endothelial stores of vWF can be released therapeutically with administration of desmopressin, So its administration can be helpful for treatment of mild vWD deficiency.

78. **Ans. (a)** ↑ **aPTT** *(Ref: Robbins 9th/pg 662; 8th/pg 672)*

79. **Ans. (d)** **Disseminated intravascular coagulation**

(Ref: Wintrobe's 12th/pg 1437)

- Levels of fibrin degradation products, including cross-linked fibrin degradation products (D-dimer), are usually increased in the presence of acute venous thromboembolism.
- Absence of an elevated level of D-dimer in patients undergoing an evaluation for acute DVT or PE has an excellent negative predictive value for thrombosis.

80. **Ans. (a)** **Normal PT, Elevated APTT**

(Ref: Robbins 9th/pg 662; 8th/pg 672)

81. **Ans. (b, c, d, e);** **b. Factor 9 deficiency; c. X-linked disorder; d. Clinically indistinguishable from hemophilia A; e. Fresh frozen plasma given for treatment**

(Ref: Robbins 9th/pg 662; 8th/pg 672)

About option E. The ideal treatment for hemophilia B is Factor IX concentrate or Prothrombin Complex. But FFP is an alternative when these are not available, hence we will take option E as true.

82. **Ans. (b)** **Factor VIII deficiency** *(Ref: R 9th/pg 662-663)*

- **Hemophilia A is Factor VIII deficiency**
- **Hemophilia B is Factor IX deficiency**
- **Hemophilia C is Factor XI deficiency**
- **Pseudo-Hemophiliais vWD**
- **Parahemophilia is factor V deficiency**

83. **Ans. (a)** **Hemophilia A** *(Ref: Robbins 9th/pg 662-663)*
X-linked recessive disease in male with clotting defect is Hemophilia A

84. **Ans. (a)** **Early solublization of clot**

(Ref: Wintrobe's 12th/pg)

Early solublization of clot is a feature of **Factor XIII deficiency**

85. **Ans. (b)** **Factor IX**

(Ref: Wintrobe's 12th/pg 499)

Platelet associated coagulation factors are:Fibrinogen, vWF, Factor V, XI, XIII & HMWK

86. **Ans. (d)** **Factor XI**

(Ref: Robbins 9th/pg 662-663)
Hemophilia C is Factor XI deficiency

87. **Ans. (d)** **Factor XIII** *(Ref: Wintrobe's 12th/pg 1452)*
LakiLorand factor is the other name for Factor XIII

88. **Ans. (d)** **Factor XI** *(Ref: Wintrobe's 12th/pg 1403)*

In pregnancy,

- **Factor II & V remain unchanged**
- **Factor XI & XIII are decreased**
- **Other coagulation factors ↑ making pregnancy a hypercoagulable state**

89. **Ans. (c)** **As part of both extrinsic and intrinsic pathways**

(Ref: Robbins 9th/pg 118-119; 8th/pg 119)

Activated factor IX along with factor VIIIa (Intrinsic pathway) & factor VIIa (extrinsic pathway), converge to activate Factor X to Xa is necessary for conversion of prothrombin to thrombin(common pathway)

90. **Ans. (a, d); a. Von Willibrand's disease; d. Anti phospholipid antibodies**

(Ref: Robbins 9th/pg 662)

Isolated rise in aPTT is seen in Von Willibrand's disease, as vWF deficiency causes factor VIII destabilization;
Even Anti phospholipid antibodies (option D). seen in APLA can cause ↑aPTT, but prolongation of PT & TT can also be seen; So the best answer is A.

91. **Ans. (a, b, c, d, e); a. Pt on oral anticoagulant; b. Pt with liver disease; c. Factor X deficiency; d. Factor VII deficiency; e. Vit. K deficiency**

(Refer to Pretext of this chapter)

92. **Ans. (d)** **XII**

(Ref: Wintrobe's 12th/pg 1403)

Factor XII deficiency usually is **not associated with hemorrhagic manifestations**. On the other hand, **myocardial infarction and thrombophlebitis** have been observed in patients with severe factor XII deficiency. However please note that the above theory is currently debated as other procoagulant factors have also been found to have a role.

93. Ans. (b) Extrinsic pathway is activated by contact with negatively charged surfaces

(Ref: Robbins 9th/pg 118-119; 8th/pg 119)

Discussing options about blood coagulation one by one-

A. Factor X is part of both intrinsic and extrinsic pathways: True, refer Ans 50 above

B. Extrinsic pathway is activated by contact with negatively charged surfaces: False, as negatively charged surfaces activate intrinsic pathway

C. Intrinsic pathway can be activated in vitro: True

D. Calcium is required in several steps of coagulation: True, Calcium acts as a cofactor for activation of coagulation factors

94. Ans. (c) Should be measured within 2 hours

(Ref: Dacie 11th/pg)

- **Ratio** of anticoagulant (**Trisodium citrate**): Blood= **1:9**[Q]
- Sample required: **Platelet poor plasma** (PPP)[Q]
- Storage: **Room temperature**[Q]
- Test should ideally be performed **within 2 hours**[Q] of sample collection
- **Prothrombin time (PT)** assay screens **extrinsic + common pathway**[Q] (factors VII, X, V, II, and fibrinogen).
- **Partial thromboplastin time (PTT)** assay screens **intrinsic pathway + common pathway**[Q] (factors XII, XI, IX, VIII, X, V, II, and fibrinogen).

95. Ans. (b) Factor 7 deficiency *(Ref: Robbins 9th/pg 656)*

Disease	PT	apTT
A. Von Willebrand disease	N	↑
B. Factor 7 deficiency	↑	N
C. Factor 8 deficiency	N	↑
D. Thrombin deficiency	↑	↑

96. Ans. (c) PTT

(Ref: Robbins 9th/pg 662-663)

Best screening test for hemophilia (both A & B) is apTT, which is ↑.

97. Ans. (c) Vit. K deficiency *(Ref: Robbins 9th/pg 656)*

Disease/ Condition	BT	PT	apTT
A. Thrombocytopenia	↑	N	N
B. DIC	↑	↑	↑
C. Vit. K deficiency	N	↑	↑ (late)
D. Aspirin toxicity	↑	N	N

98. Ans. (d) Defect in common pathway

(Ref: Robbins 9th/pg 656; 8th/pg 666)

Defect in common pathway leads to elevation of both PT & apTT.

99. Ans. (c) Decreased fibrinogen

(Ref: Wintrobe pg 684)

Though ↑ FDP is the most sensitive test for DIC bleeding occurs due to defective aggregation of platelets and decreased fibrinogen. (Remember aggregation also requires fibrinogen).

100. Ans. (a) Obstetric complications

(Ref: Harrison 18th ed/pg 1390)

The most common causes are bacterial sepsis, malignant disorders such as solid tumors or acute promyelocytic leukemia, and obstetric causes. DIC is diagnosed in almost one-half of pregnant women with abruptio placentae, or with amniotic fluid embolism

101. Ans. (d) FDP level *(Ref: Robbins 9th/pg 663-664)*

102. Ans. (d) DIC associated with malignancy

(Ref: Robbins 9th/pg 662; 8th/pg 672)

About use of Heparin in DIC:

- Low doses of continuous infusion heparin (5–10 U/ kg per h) may be effective in patients with low-grade DIC associated with *solid tumor, acute promyelocytic leukemia, or in a setting with recognized thrombosis.*
- Heparin is also indicated for the **treatment of purpura fulminans** during the **surgical resection of giant hemangiomas and during removal of a dead fetus.**
- In **acute DIC,** the use of heparin is likely to **aggravate bleeding**.
- To date, the use of heparin in patients with severe DIC has no proven survival benefit.

103. Ans. (c) Hyperfibrinogenemia

(Ref: R 9th/pg 663-664)

104. Ans. (a) ↑ fibrinogen level

(Ref: Robbins 9th/pg 663-664)

105. Ans. (c) Normal APTT

(Ref: Robbins 9th/pg 663-664)

106. Ans. (d) All of the above

(Ref: Robbins 9th/pg 123)

Factor V Leiden mutation results in glutamine to arginine substitution at amino acid residue 506 that renders factor V resistant to cleavage and inactivation by protein C. As a result, an important antithrombotic counterregulatory pathway is lost and chances of thrombosis are highly raised.

107. Ans. (b, c, d) b. Both PT and aPTT are increased in DIC; c. IV Ig is useful in ITP; d. Cryoprecipitate is useful in hemophilia A

108. Ans. (a) Factor 5 mutation

Factor V leiden is MC

109. Ans. (d) Breast (*Ref: Robbins 9th/pg 663-664*)

Thrombosis is breast carcinoma is least common among given options

110. Ans. (a) Heparin (*Ref: Harrison 18th/pg 1403*)

- Antithrombin, a serine protease inhibitor, regulates coagulation by inactivating thrombin and other procoagulant enzymes, including factors Xa, IXa, XIa, and XIIa.
- Once bound to Heparin, the natural anticoagulant effect of Antithrombin is potentiated, resulting in the accelerated binding and inactivation of serine proteases, and factor Xa and thrombin in particular.
- The inhibition of these factors affects the common pathway of coagulation, resulting in decreased formation of thrombin and fibrin.

111. Ans. (b) Hypothermia

(*Ref: Robbins 9th/pg 663; 8th/pg 673*)

112. Ans. (a) Warfarin for life (*Ref: Harrison 19th/pg 2135*)

- After the first thrombotic event, APS patients should be placed on **warfarin for life**, aiming to achieve an international normalized ratio (INR) ranging from **2.5 to 3.5**, alone or in combination with **80 mg of aspirin daily**.
- Pregnancy morbidity is prevented by a combination of **heparin with aspirin 80 mg daily. IV immunoglobulin (IVIg)** 400 mg/ kg every day for 5 days may also prevent abortions, whereas glucocorticoids are ineffective

113. Ans. (d) Priaspism (*Ref: Robbins 9th/pg 123-124*)

Hypercoagulability due to defective factor V gene is called Leiden mutation

- **Factor V Leiden[Q]:** glutamine → arginine substitution at amino acid residue 506 that renders **factor V resistant** to cleavage and inactivation by protein C.

114. Ans. (a) Factor V (*Ref: Robbins 9th/pg 123; 8th/pg 123*)

115. Ans. (b) Anti-Prothrombin (*Ref: Robbins 9th/pg 124*)

116. Ans. (c) Depends on platelet activation

(*Ref: Robbins 9th/pg 122; 8th/pg 122*)

117. Ans. (d) Factor V (*Ref: Robbins 9th/pg 123-124*)

Leiden factor is factor V.

118. Ans. (c) Cerebral microcirculation

(*Ref: Robbins 9th/pg 663*)

Thrombomodulin is produced by all endothelial cells except those of cerebral microcirculation

119. Ans. (b) aPTT (*Ref: Dacie 11th pg 472*)

Therapeutic treatment with UFH is given by continuous intravenous infusion and is usually monitored using the APTT, which is repeated 6 h after every dose change.

120. Ans. (a, b, c, d); a. Recurrent abortion; b. Fetal death; c. Both arterial and venous thrombosis; d. Prolonged aPTT

(*Ref: Robbins 9th/pg 124; 8th/pg 123*)

Autoantibody[Q]-mediated **acquired[Q] thrombophilia** characterized by **recurrent[Q] arterial or venous thrombosis[Q]** and/or **pregnancy morbidity** in the presence of **autoantibodies against phospholipid (PL)**-binding **plasma proteins (β-2 GPI)[Q]**

APLA can result in ↑ phospholipid based assays like PT, aPTT, TT.

But isolated Increase in aPTT is most commonly seen

121. Ans. (d) Anti- beta 2 glycoprotein antibody

(*Ref: Robbins 9th/pg 124; 8th/pg 123*)

Anti- beta 2 glycoprotein antibody is most frequently seen in Antiphospholipid Syndrome

122. Ans. (a, c, e); a. Antiphospholipid antibodies; c. Hyperhomocysteinemia; e. Mutation in factor V gene

(*Ref: Wintrobe's 12th/pg 1465*)

Both arterial and venous thrombosis occur in:

• APLA syndrome	• Heparin induced Thrombocytopenia (HIT)
• Hyperhomocystinemia	
• Factor V leiden	• (PNH)
• DIC	• Polycythemia Vera (PCV)
	• Dysfibrinogenemia

123. Ans. (b) Leiden mutation

(*Ref: Robbins 9th/pg 123-124*)

124. Ans. (a) Protein C/Protein S deficiency

(*Ref: Wintrobe's 12th/pg 1490*)

Warfarin skin necrosis

- Due to **warfarin-induced rapid reduction in protein C levels** in patients with a **pre-existing inherited protein C deficiency** that results in a **hypercoagulable state and thrombosis.**
- Not all heterozygous protein C–deficient patients receiving warfarin experience this complication, and not all patients with this complication have protein C deficiency.

125. Ans. (c) Factor X (*Ref: Robbins 9th/pg 121; 8th/pg 116*)

TFPI is a major anticoagulant, present in plasma and associated with vascular endothelium. TFPI binds to and neutralizes factor Xa to inhibit coagulation.

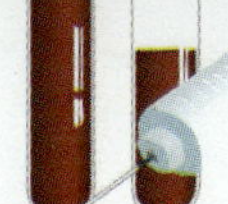

126. Ans. (a) Russell viper venom time

(Ref: R 9th/pg 123-124)

Screening Laboratory Evaluation for Patients Suspected of Having a Hypercoagulable State

- **Activated protein C resistance** (diluting patient plasma with factor V–deficient plasma)
- **Prothrombin G20210A mutation** testing by polymerase chain reaction
- Activity assays for **antithrombin, protein C, and protein S**
- Activated partial thromboplastin time, mixing studies, and **dilute Russell viper venom time**
- Fasting total plasma **homocysteine level**
- **Anticardiolipin & β_2-glycoprotein 1 antibody testing** by enzyme-linked immunosorbent assays
- **Factor VIII activity**

127. Ans. (a) (PT patient/ PT control)ISI

(Ref: Wintrobe's 12th/pg 1489)

128. Ans. (a) Vascular injury

(Ref: Robbins 9th/pg 663-664)

- DIC shows ↑ CT and low Platelet counts
- DIC begins with factors that causes endothelial (vascular) injury (refer to pretext of this chapter)

129. Ans. (a) PT INR

(Ref: Wintrobe's 12th ed/pg 1489)

Patients with recurrent thrombosis should receive **long-term warfarin therapy** at a dosage to maintain an international normalized ratio **(INR) value of 2.0 to 3.0.**

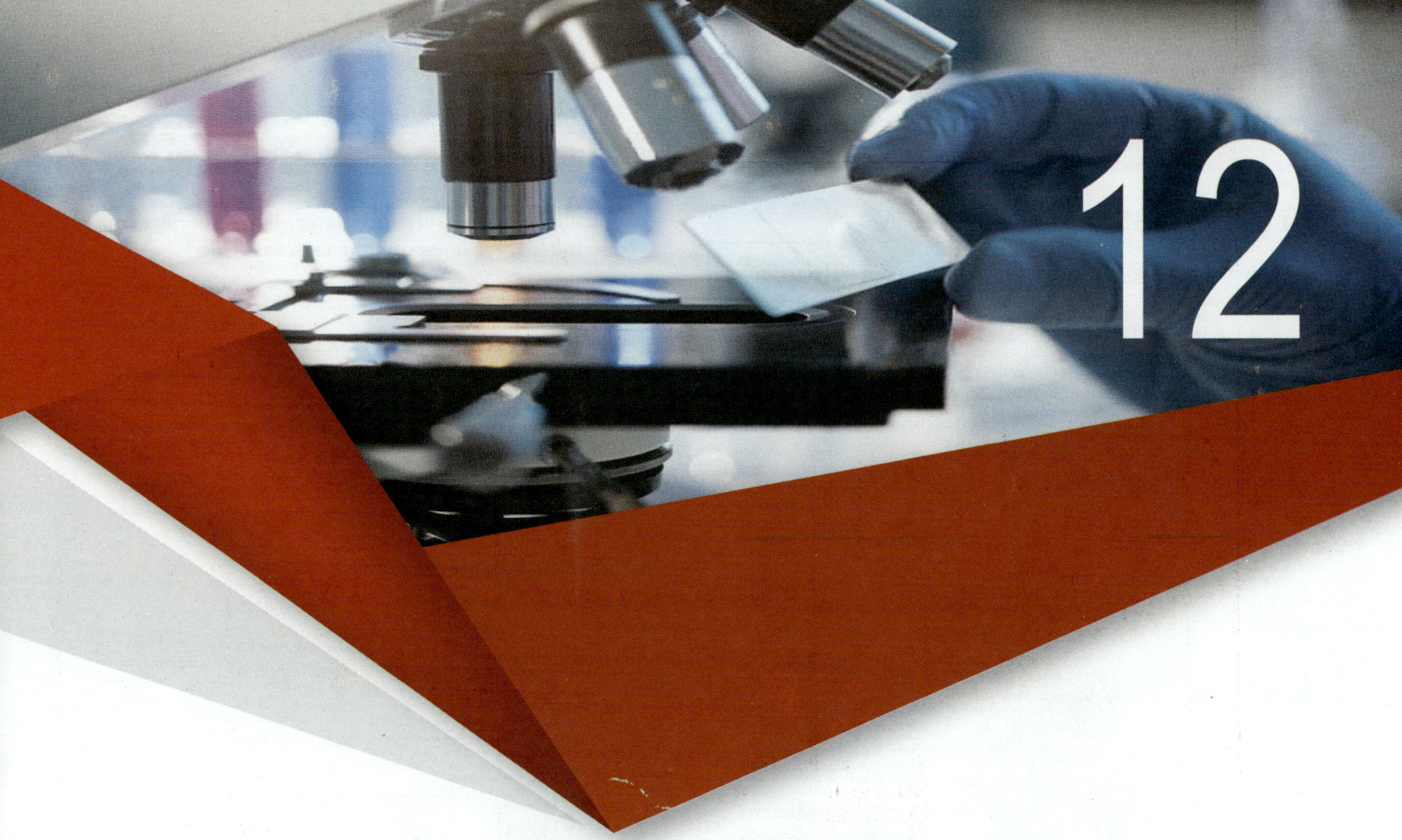

12

Cardiovascular System and its Disorders

Key Points

- **Fatty streak is seen in Aortas of infants,** virtually all adolescents, even those without known risk factors
- **Most common**[Q] vessel involved & Most common **site**[Q] of atherosclerotic aneurysm is *Lower abdominal aorta*
- **Hyperplastic arteriolosclerosis is seen** in Malignant hypertension
- **Hyaline arteriolosclerosis is seen in** Benign hypertension and Diabetes mellitus (DM)
- Most important cause of true **aortic aneurysms are atherosclerosis**
- **Most common cause of dissection is hypertension**
- **Anti-endothelial** cell antibodies are seen in **Kawasaki's disease**
- **Strawberry tongue is seen in Kawasaki disease**
- **Microscopic hallmark** of HSP is the deposition of **IgA in the walls** of involved blood vessels.
- **Most common** vascular tumor: **Capillary hemangioma**
- **Time for reversible injury in heart is 30 mins**
- **Intravenous drug abusers: Right side** of heart is affected
- Dilated cardiomyopathy is **most common**
- **HOCM** is the **leading cause of** unexplained left ventricular hypertrophy
- **Native cardiac valve endocarditis-Staphylococcus aureus**
- The most common cardiac tumor is the **secondaries or metastasis**
- The most common primary cardiac tumor in the adults is **the myxoma**
- The most common cardiac tumor in the children is the **rhabdomyoma**.

Key Recent Updates

- Most common vascular tumor is hemangioma
- Aschoff's nodule is hallmark of Rheumatic heart disease.

BLOOD VESSELS: OVERVIEW

The basic histological layers of the blood vessels (particularly arteries) are:

- Tunica intima (Innermost layer)-single layer of **endothelial cells** [Q]
- Internal elastic lamina
- Tunica media (Middle layer)- constituents depends on the type of artery as explained below
- External elastic lamina
- Tunica adventitia (Outermost layer)-loose connective tissue containing nerve fibers and the **vasa vasorum** [Q]

High Yield Facts

- All vessels **except capillaries** [Q] have three-layered architecture consisting of an **intima, media, and adventitia**.
- There are 3 types of capillaries-**continuous, fenestrated & sinusoidal**

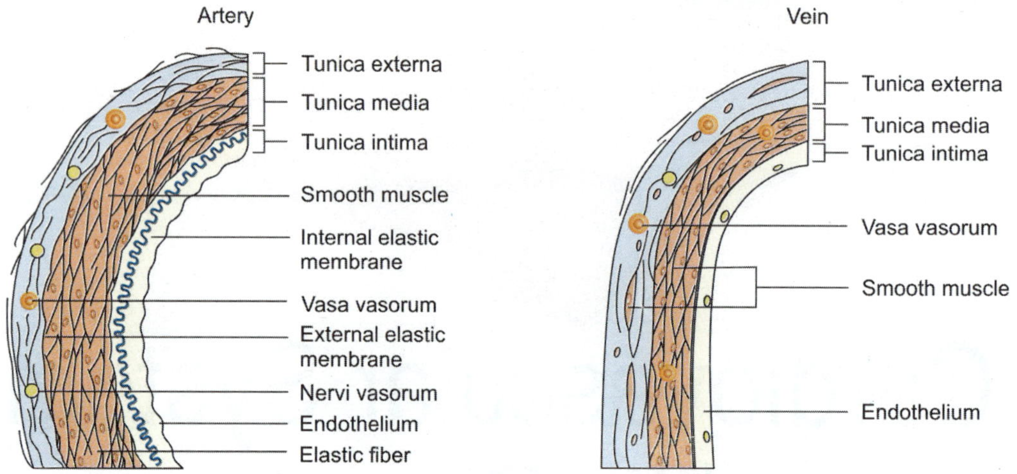

Arteries are divided into three types			
	Large or Elastic Arteries	**Medium or Muscular Arteries**	**Small Arteries (0.2 mm) Arterioles (20-100 µm)**
Type of vessel	Aorta & major branches **Pulmonary arteries**	Smaller branches of aorta (coronary & renal)	• Within tissues and organs.
Characteristic feature	Tunica media is **rich in elastin fibers** [Q]	Tunica media is rich in **smooth muscle cells** [Q]	**Resistance vessels** is other name of arterioles

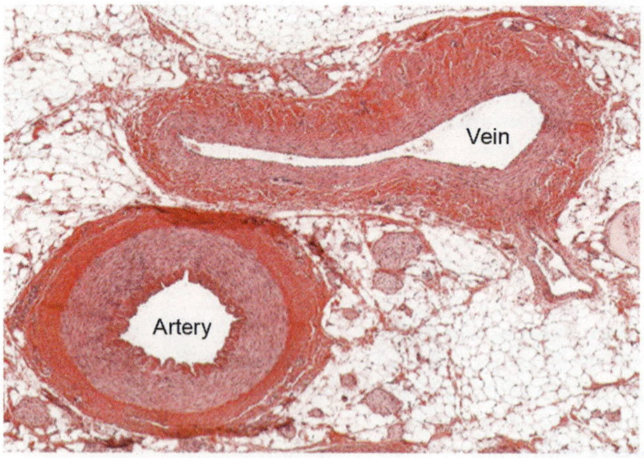

Vascular anomalies

Developmental/ Berry/ Saccular Aneurysms

Cause
- Structural abnormality of the involved vessel
- Absence of smooth muscle and intimal elastic lamina[Q]

Features
- 90%- found **near major arterial branch points**[Q] in the anterior circulation of brain

Arteriovenous Fistulas

Cause
- Direct connections between arteries and veins

Features
- **Bypass the intervening capillary bed.**[Q]

Fibromuscular Dysplasia (FMD)

Cause
- Focally thickened segments of vessel wall
- Medial and intimal hyperplasia and fibrosis

Features
- Most frequent in **young women**[Q]
- Immediately adjacent vessel segments have **markedly attenuated media**[Q] **-leading to aneurysms**[Q]

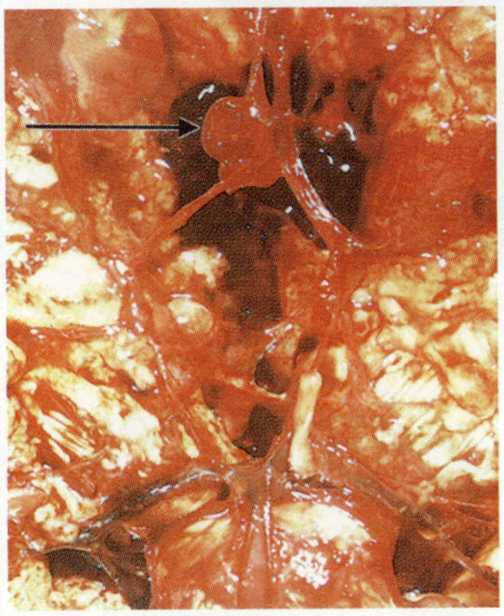

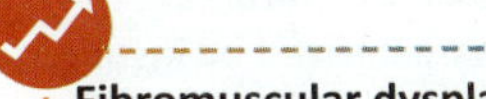

Berry aneurysm

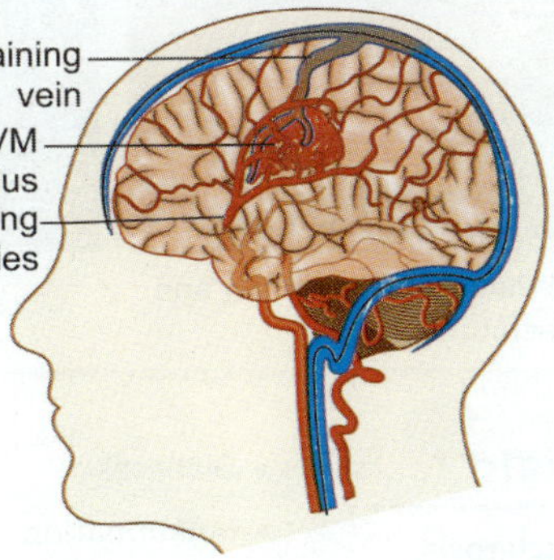

A-V fistula

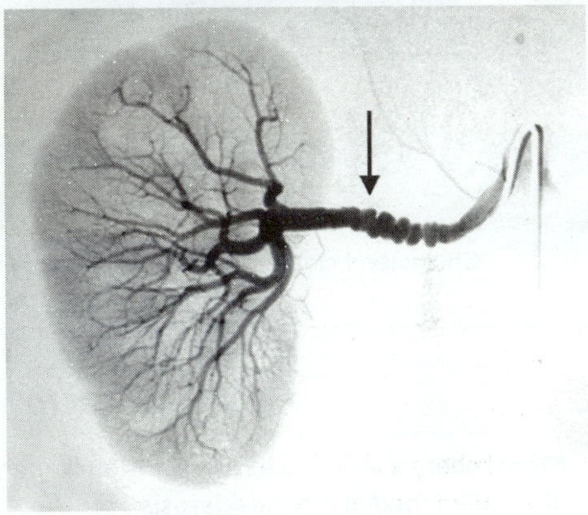

MRA or arteriography: string or beads appearance S/o FMD

High Yield Facts

Fibromuscular dysplasia
- Cause of **renovascular hypertension** in **young females** [Q]
- **No association with oral contraceptives or increased estrogen expression.**[Q]
- On angiography, the vessels have a "**string of beads**"[Q] appearance (due to **markedly attenuated media**[Q])

VESSEL SCLEROSIS

Denotes **arterial wall thickening** and **loss of elasticity**

Type of vessel sclerosis

Arteriosclerosis (vessel lumen becomes narrow)

Hyaline
- Homogeneous pink hyaline arteriolar wall thickening
- Plasma protein leakage with increased smooth muscle cell synthesis.
- Seen in: Benignhypertension (HT)
  : Diabtes mellitus (DM)

Hyperplastic
- Smooth muscle proliferation leads to concentric laminated arteriolar thickening **(Onion skinning)**
- Associated with **fibrinoid necrosis** & **necrotizing arteriolitis** (Vessel wall necrosis)
- Seen in: Malignant HT.

Monckeberg medial sclerosis (vessel lumen is normal)
- Calcification of media of blood vessels typically involving internal elastic membrane.
- Do not encroach on vessel lumen.
- Age > 50 yrs
- Not clinically significant

Atherosclerosis (vessel lumen becomes narrow)
- Most frequent
- Clinically important
- Characterized by atheroma/ plaque consisting of raised focal lesion

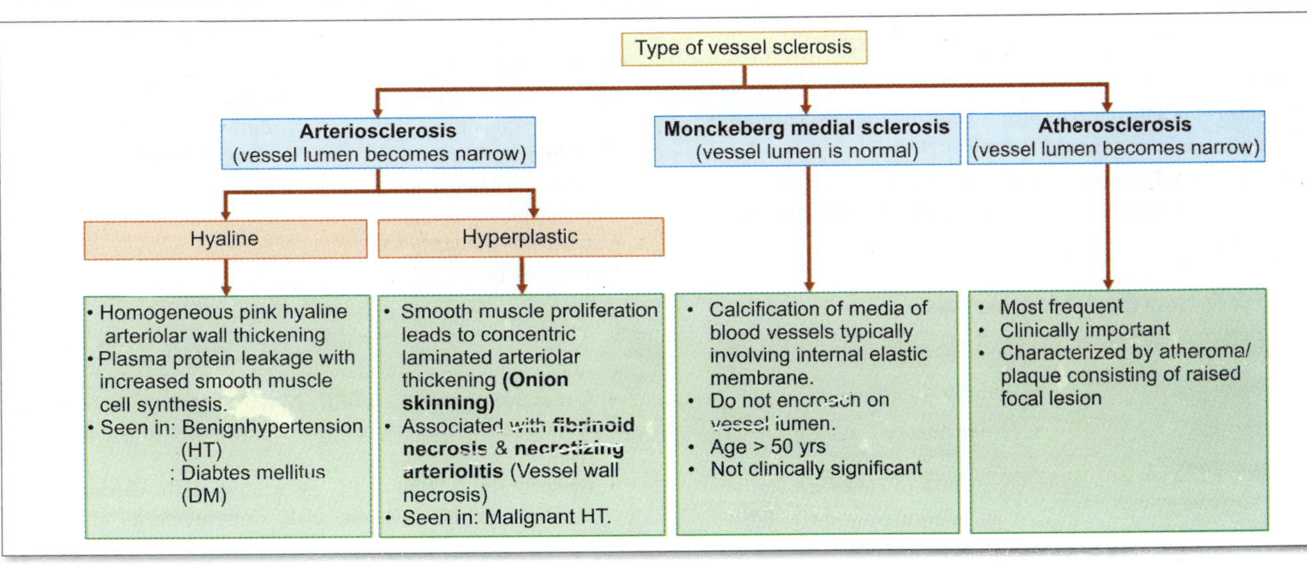

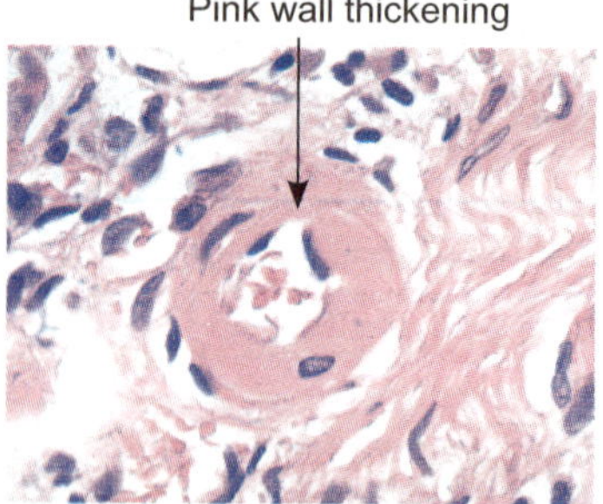

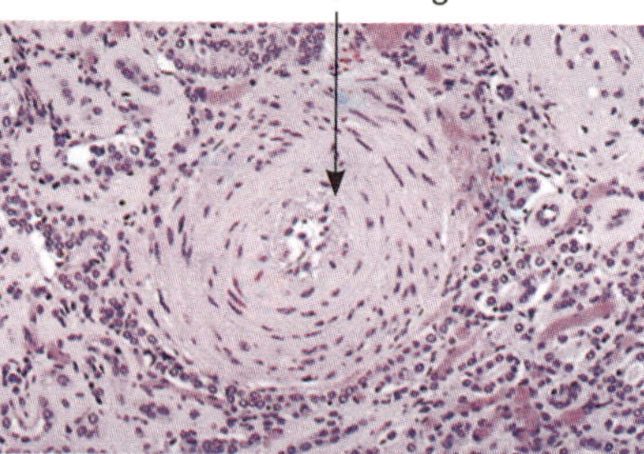

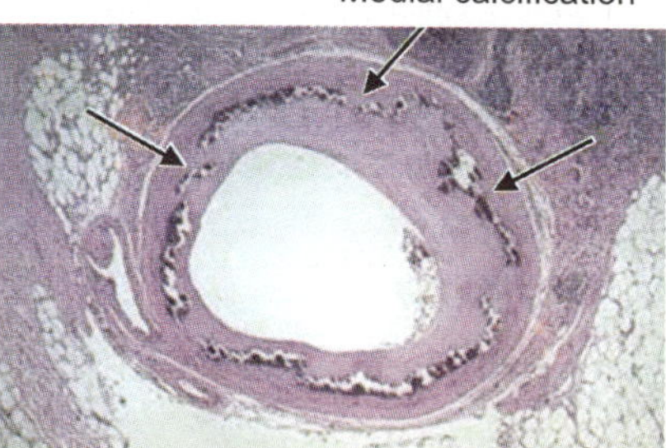

Hyaline Arteriolosclerosis

Hyperplastic Arteriolosclerosis

Mönckeberg Medial Sclerosis

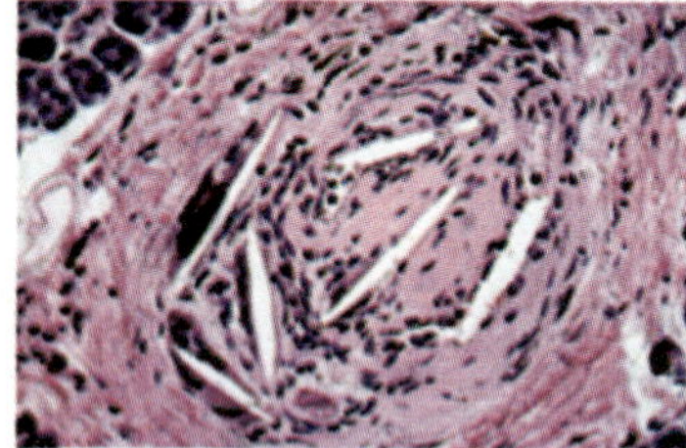

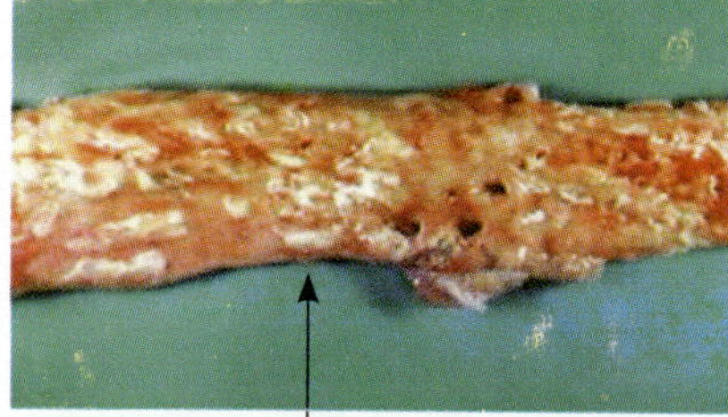

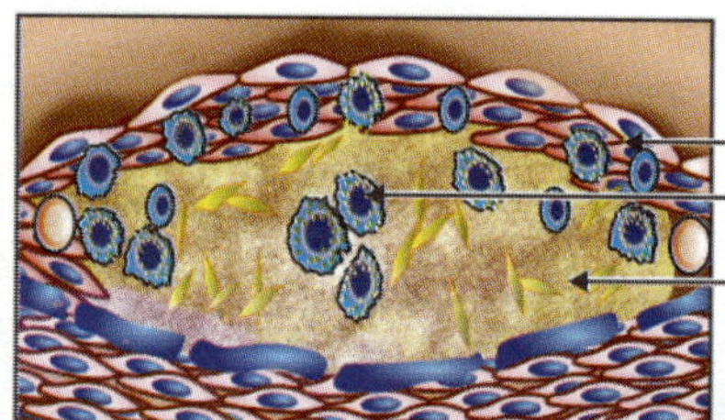

Cholesterol clefts

Atherosclerotic Plaque: white-yellow and encroach on the lumen

Schematic diagram of Atherosclerotic Plaque

High Yield Facts

Mönckeberg's arteriosclerosis, or Mönckeberg's sclerosis, also called medial calcific sclerosis

- Example of **dystrophic calcification**[Q]
- Prevalence **increases with age**[Q]
- More frequent in **diabetes mellitus**[Q], chronic kidney disease, and systemic lupus erythematosus
- **Non obstructive lesion**[Q]
  Hyperplastic arteriolosclerosis is pathological change seen in malignant hypertension
  - Arterioles of all organs of body are affected but **favored sites** are:
    Kidney[Q], **Small intestine**[Q], **Gall bladder**[Q], **Peri pancreatic fat**[Q], **Periadrenal fat**[Q]

Atherosclerosis plaque is **present within the intima**[Q], has a **core of lipid (cholesterol & its esters) & a covering of fibrous cap.**

Histopathology of Atherosclerotic Plaque

- **Fibrous cap**[Q] – Consists of **smooth muscle cells, collagen.**
- **'Shoulder'**[Q] – **Cellular area** around cap having **macrophages, smooth muscle cells and T lymphocytes.**
- **Necrotic core**–Debris of **dead cells, foam cells**, lipid (cholesterol, **cholesterol clefts.**[Q]) **fibrin and variably organized thrombus.**

Major Risk Factors for Atherosclerosis

Modifiable	Nonmodifiable (Constitutional)
• Hyperlipidemia	• Genetic abnormalities
• Hypertension	• Family history
• Cigarette smoking	• Increasing age

Contd...

• Diabetes	• Male gender
• Inflammation	• Stress (Type A personality)
• Physical inactivity	

Additional Risk Factors for Atherosclerosis

a. Inflammation: ▪ Present during **all stages of atherosclerosis**[Q], **linked with atherosclerotic plaque formation and rupture**[Q] ▪ Marker-CRP	**d. Metabolic syndrome:** ▪ Characterized by **insulin resistance, hypertension, dyslipidemia (↑ LDL & ↓ HDL), hypercoagulability, proinflammatory state**[Q]
b. Hyperhomocysteinemia	**e. Factors Affecting Hemostasis:** ▪ Elevated plasminogen activator inhibitor 1 and thrombinase
c. Lipoprotein a [Lp(a)]: ▪ Altered form of LDL that contains the **apolipoprotein B-100** portion of LDL linked to apolipoprotein A (apo A) ▪ Structural similarity to **plasminogen.**[Q]	**f. Infection:** ▪ *Herpesvirus, Cytomegalovirus & Chlamydophila pneumoni*

High Yield Facts

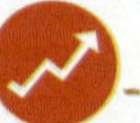

- **C-reactive protein (CRP): Most sensitive** marker of inflammation that correlate with **ischemic heart disease risk**[Q]
- **Lipoprotein a [Lp(a)]** is associated with **coronary & cerebrovascular disease risk, independent of total cholesterol or LDL levels**[Q]

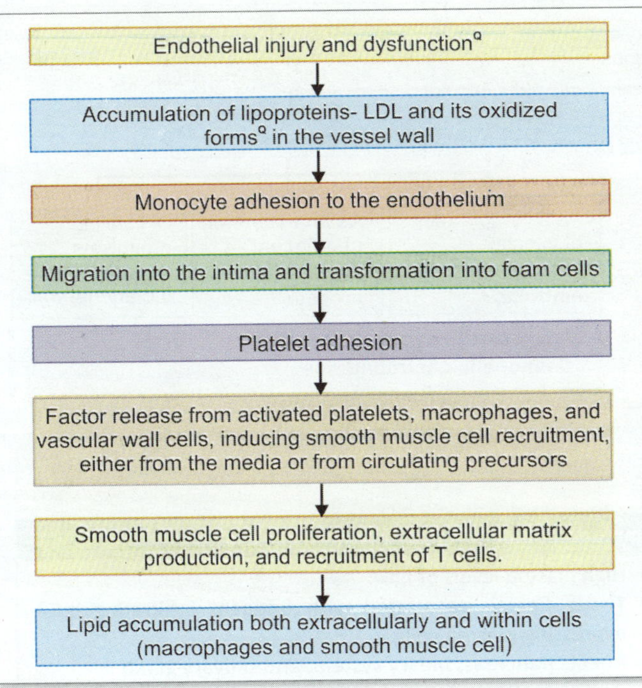

High Yield Facts

- **Endothelial injury and dysfunction** is the cornerstone of the **response-to-injury hypothesis**[Q]
- **Non-denuding endothelial dysfunction underlies most human atherosclerosis**[Q]
- Most important causes of endothelial dysfunction are hemodynamic disturbances[Q] & hypercholesterolemia[Q]
- Foam cells **are lipid laden smooth muscles cells/tissue macrophages or Blood monocytes**[Q]
- In foam cells **oxidized LDL** is ingested by the **scavenger receptors**[Q] present on macrophages & smooth muscle cells[Q]

Morphology of Atherosclerosis

- Fatty steak
  - **Earliest lesion** of atherosclerosis is composed of **lipid filled foam cells.**[Q]
  - Begin as yellow flat spots **less than 1 mm**[Q]
  - **Donot**[Q] cause flow disturbances.
  - **Seen in Aortas of infants, virtually all adolescents, even those without known risk factors.**[Q]
- Atherosclerotic Plaque
  - Characterized by **intimal thickening and lipid accumulation**[Q], which together form plaques
  - White-yellow and **encroach on the lumen**[Q] of the artery

In descending order[Q], the most extensively involved vessels in Atherosclerosis are:	
Lower abdominal aorta	**Most common**[Q] vessel involved & Most common **site**[Q] of atherosclerotic aneurysm
Coronary arteries	**Left Anterior Descending is Most common**[Q] coronary artery involved → causes MI

Contd...

Popliteal arteries	**Most common peripheral vessel**[Q] with aneurysm formation → ischemic gangrene of lower limbs
Internal carotid arteries	Cause stroke
Vessels of circle of Willis	Cause stroke

- Vessels spared in Atherosclerosis are upper extremities vessels,[Q] mesenteric & renal arteries except at their ostia[Q]

Type of Plaques

Characteristics	Stable Plaques	Vulnerable/ Unstable Plaques
Fibrous cap	Dense	Thin
Lipid cores	Minimal	Large
Inflammation	Minimal	Marked
Clinical Manifestations	Due to **chronic ischemia**	**Fatal ischemic complications**

Acute plaque change is described as:

- Rupture, ulceration, or erosion, Hemorrhage into a plaque, Atheroembolism, Aneurysm formation

ANEURYSM

- *Definition:*
  - Localized abnormal dilation of a blood vessel or the wall of the heart
- *Types:*
  - **True aneurysm**
  - **False/Pseudoaneurysm**
- *Characteristics:*
  - Involves **attenuated intact arterial wall** or **thinned ventricular wall** of the heart
  - Vascular wall defect leading **to extravascular hematoma that freely** communicates with intravascular space[Q]
- *Associated Conditions:*
  - **Atherosclerosis**[Q]
  - **Syphilis**[Q]
  - **Congenital vascular aneurysms**[Q]
  - **Post MI ventricular aneurysms.**[Q]
  - **Post MI rupture contained by pericardial adhesion**[Q]
  - **Leakage at the suture junction of vascular anastomosis**[Q]
- *Etiology:*
  - Most important cause of true **aortic aneurysms** are **atherosclerosis**[Q] > hypertension

The inherited causes of aneurysm are: M-L-E	
Marfan syndrome	Defective synthesis of the protein **fibrillin**[Q]
Loeys Dietz syndrome	Defect in **elastin & collagen type I & III** due to mutation in **TGF-B receptor**[Q]
Ehlers-Danlos syndrome	Defect in **collagen type III**[Q]

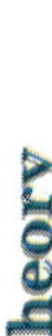

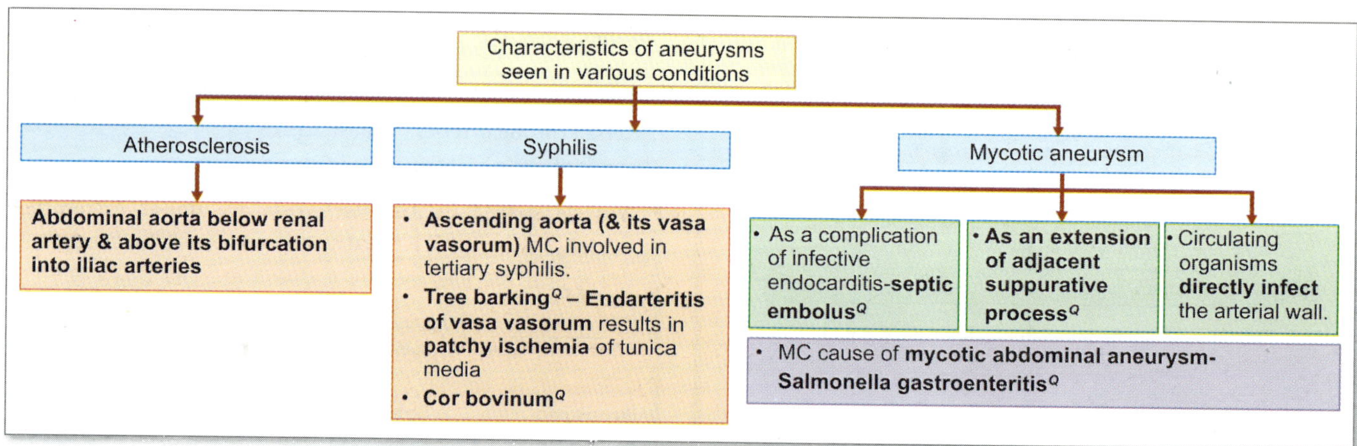

R9th Latest Update

Inflammatory aneurysms	Immunoglobulin G4 (IgG4)-related disease
Younger patients;[Q] Present with back pain • Elevated inflammatory markers (e.g., elevation of **C-reactive protein**[Q]) • **Abundant lymphoplasmacytic inflammation**[Q] with many macrophages & sometimes giant cells • Associated with **dense periaortic scarring that can extend into the anterior retroperitoneum**[Q] • Cause: **Localized**[Q] immune response to the abdominal aortic wall	• High plasma levels of IgG4 • **Tissue fibrosis associated with frequent infiltrating IgG4-expressing plasma cells.**[Q] • Affects **pancreas, biliary system, and salivary gland.**[Q] • **Cause aortitis and periaortitis → aneurysms.**[Q] • Responds well to **steroid therapy.**

AORTIC DISSECTION

- **Definiton:**
  - Blood separates the laminar planes of the **media** to form a blood-filled channel within the aortic wall
- **Epidemiology:**
  - 40-60 years; at younger age in Marfan's syndrome
- **Etiology:**
  - **Most common cause of dissection is hypertension**[Q]
- **Types depending on level of aorta affected:**

Type A	Type B
• Involves **ascending** aorta or **both**[Q] ascending & descending aorta	• **Does not involves ascending aorta**[Q] but lesion begins **distal to subclavian artery.**[Q]

De Bakey   Type I   Type II   Type III

Stanford   Type A .   Type A   Type B

- **Histology:**
  - **The most frequent preexisting histologically detectable lesion is cystic medial degeneration**[Q]
  - **Inflammation is characteristically absent.**

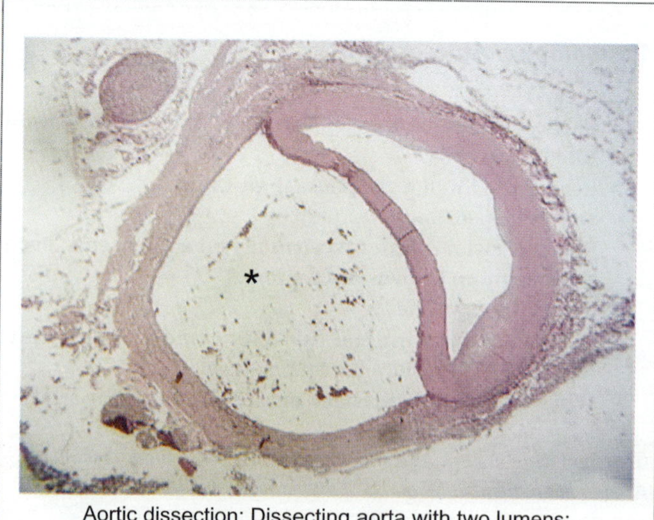

Aortic dissection: Dissecting aorta with two lumens: true lumen in the right, while false lumen in the left*

- **Double-barreled aorta**-Formed when the dissecting hematoma re-enters the lumen of the aorta through a **second distal intimal tear**[Q], creating a new false vascular channel
- **Chronic dissection**: When false channels are **endothelialized**[Q]
- **Cystic medial necrosis (CMN) involves large arteries, in particular the aorta,** [Q]
- In CMN, there is accumulation of **basophilic ground substance in the media**[Q] with cyst-like lesions

Diseases causing CMN
- **Marfan's syndrome**[Q], **Chronic aortic dissection**[Q], **Bicuspid aortic valve**[Q], **Scurvy**[Q], **Aortic aneurysm**[Q], **Atheroslerotic disease**[Q], **Hypertension**[Q], **Ehler danlos syndrome (type IV)**[Q]

VASCULITIS

Vasculitis is the **inflammation** of **vessel wall.**

Classification

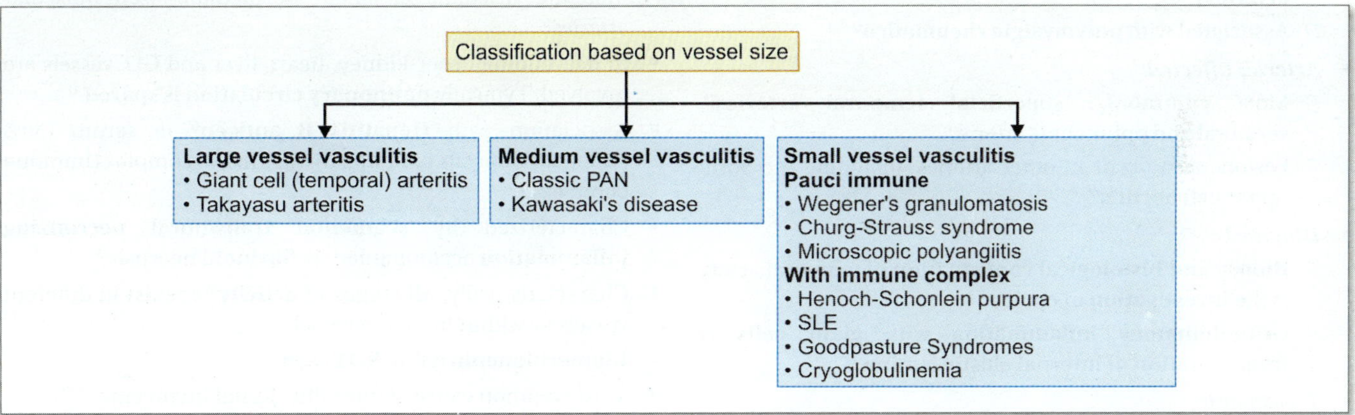

Antibodies in Vasculitis

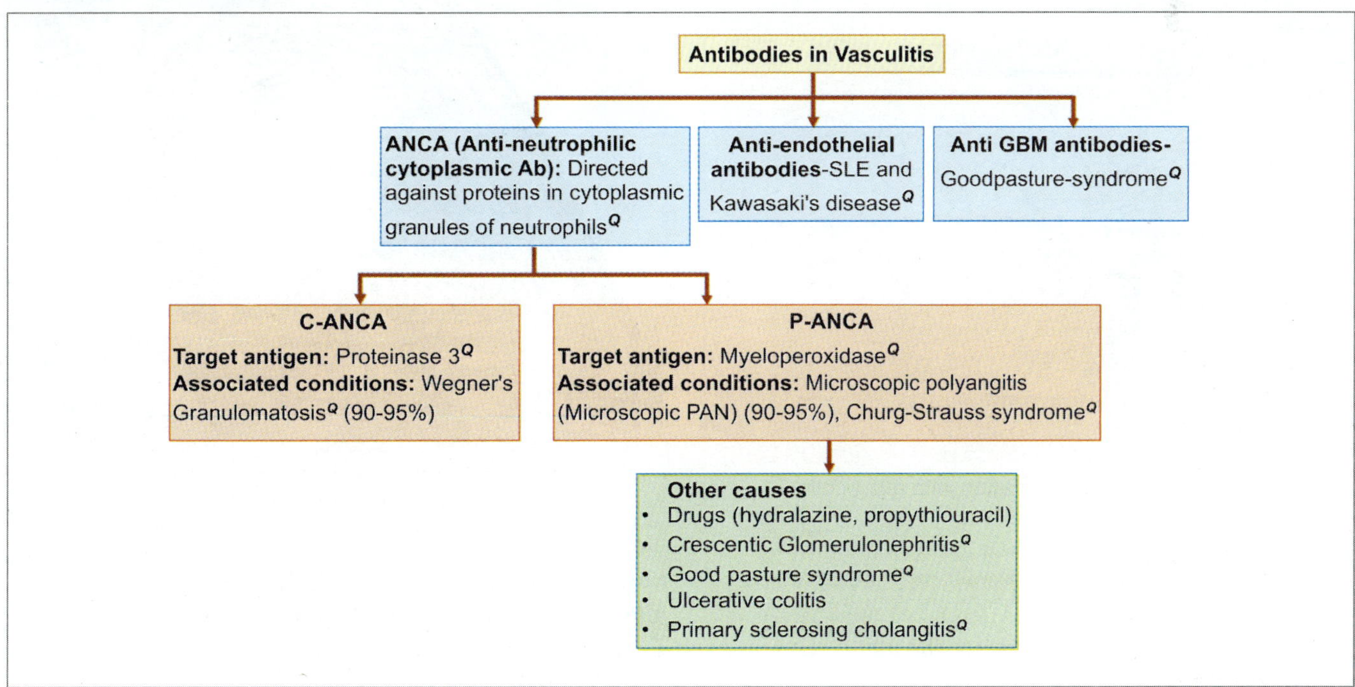

Large Vessel Vasculitis

Giant Cell (Temporal) Arteritis/Cranial Arteritis

- *Epidemiology:*
  - **Most common type of vasculitis in adults** (usually >50 years)
- *Pathophysiology:*
  - **T-cell mediated immune response**[Q] against **vessel wall antigens**[Q] that releases proinflammatory cytokines (**particularly TNF**[Q])
- *Clinical features:*
  - **Fever, anemia (normocytic normochromic)**[Q]**, high ESR, and headaches (most common)**
  - **Most specific symptom- jaw claudication**[Q]
  - **Sudden blindness** (due to involvement of **ophthalmic arteries**)
  - Associated with **polymyalgia rheumatica**[Q]
- *Arteries affected:*
  - **Most commonly: superficial temporal arteries**[Q], vertebral and ophthalmic arteries.
  - Lesions also occur in other arteries, including the aorta (**giant cell aortitis**[Q])
- *Diagnosis:*
  - **Biopsy and histological confirmation** of temporal artery is the **investigation of choice**.
  - **Granulomatous inflammation with giant cells & fragmentation of internal elastic lamina.**[Q]
- *Treatment:*
  - Corticosteroids & anti-TNF therapies are the **drug of choice**

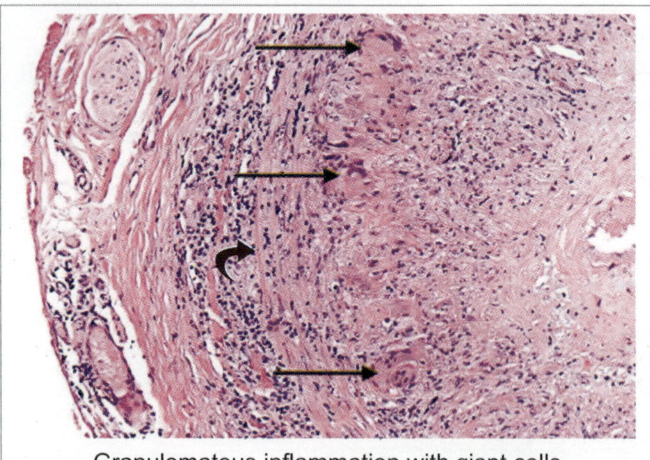
Granulomatous inflammation with giant cells

Takayasu's Arteritis

- *Epidemiology:*
  - Seen in **adult female**[Q]<50 years of age.
- *Characteristic:*
  - **Granulomatous vasculitis of medium and larger arteries**[Q]

- *Clinical features:*
  - Ocular disturbances & marked **weakening of the pulses in the upper extremities** (hence the name **pulseless disease**[Q])
- *Vessels involved:*
  - **Most common vessel involved - subclavian artery**[Q]
  - **Least common vessel involved- coronary vessels**[Q]
  - Aortic arch & its branches involved, so also called **Aortoarteritis or Aortic Arch syndrome**[Q]
  - Pulmonary artery involvement in half the cases can cause pulmonary hypertension[Q]

Medium Vessel Vasculitis

Polyarteritis Nodosa (PAN)

- Systemic vasculitis of small- or medium-sized muscular arteries[Q]
- In descending order-kidney, heart, liver and GIT vessels are involved. Typically **pulmonary circulation is spared**.[Q]
- Association with **Hepatitis B antigen**[Q] in serum (30% patients)-Deposits contain HBsAg-HBsAb complex (immune complex)[Q]
- Characterized by **segmental transmural necrotizing inflammation** accompanied by **fibrinoid necrosis**[Q]
- Characteristically, **all stages of activity**[Q] **coexist** in different vessels or within the same vessel
- **Glomerulonephrits**[Q] is **NOT** seen.
- Most common cause of mortality: **Renal involvement**[Q]

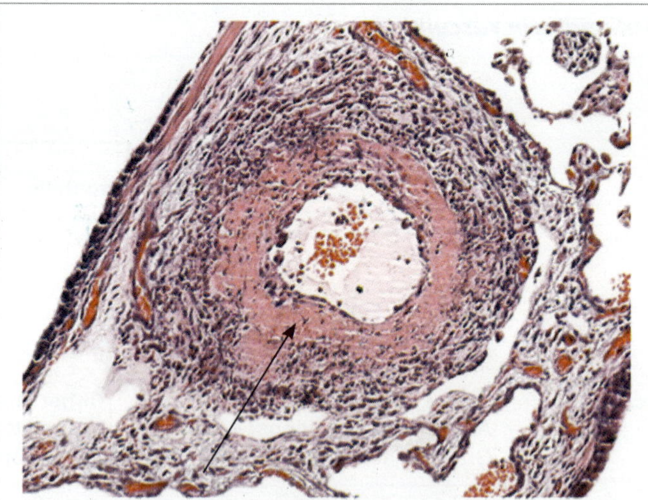
Fibrinoid necrosis: accumulation of amorphous, proteinaceous material in the tissue matrix

Kawasaki's Disease (Infantile Polyarteritis, Mucocutaneous Lymph Node Syndrome)

- **Acute febrile**[Q], usually self-limited illness of **infancy and childhood**[Q] (80% patients are ≤ 4 years)
- It is associated with an **arteritis** affecting **large to medium-sized, and even small vessels**

- **Diagnostic criteria:**
  - **Anti-endothelial** cell antibodies[Q].
  - Leading cause of **acquired heart disease**[Q] in children.
  - **Coronary artery** involvement[Q] → aneurysms that rupture or thrombose → **Acute Myocardial Infarction**[Q]

> Fever for > 5 days
> +
> 4 from conjunctivitis, adenopathy, rash, erythema of hands/feet & mucosa involvement. (CARE – M)

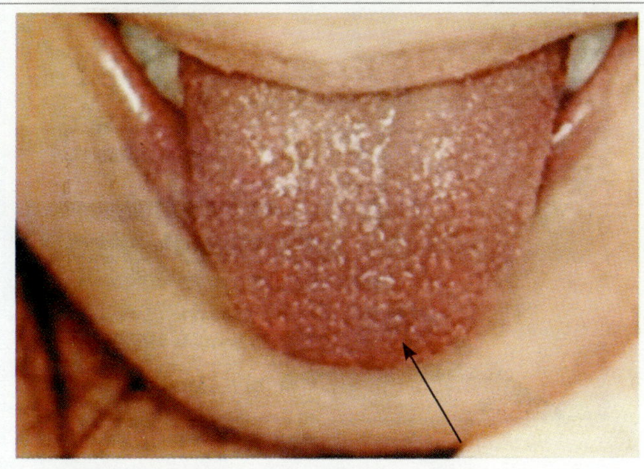
Kawasaki's disease: Shows typical strawberry tongue

Mnemonic

Kawasaki's disease (CREAM)
- **C**-Conjunctivitis (non-exudative); non purulent conjuncivits
- **R**-Rash (Polymorphous non-vesicular)
- **E**-Edema (or erythema of hands or feet)
- **A**-Adenopathy (cervical, often unilateral and non suppurative)
- **M**-Mucosal involvement (erythema or fissures or crusting at times referred as **strawberry tongue**[Q])
- **F**-Fever (**most important constitutional symptom**[Q])

Small Vessel Vasculitis

Microscopic Polyangiitis/Leukocytoclastic Vasculitis/Hypersensitivity Vasculitis

- **Necrotizing vasculitis**[Q] that generally affects capillaries, as well as small arterioles and venules
- All lesions are of **same age**[Q] in any given patient and are **distributed more widely**[Q].
- **Necrotizing glomerulonephritis** (90% of patients) and **pulmonary capillaritis** are **common**.
- Typically **spare medium-sized and larger arteries**[Q]; consequently, **infarcts are uncommon**[Q]
- Granulomatous inflammation is **absent**[Q]
- **P-ANCA**[Q] is present is majority of the patients.
- **Leukocytoclastic vasculitis**[Q] -vessel wall infiltrated with **intact and apoptotic neutrophils**[Q]

- **Clinical features**-palpable cutaneous purpura[Q], hemoptysis, hematuria and proteinuria

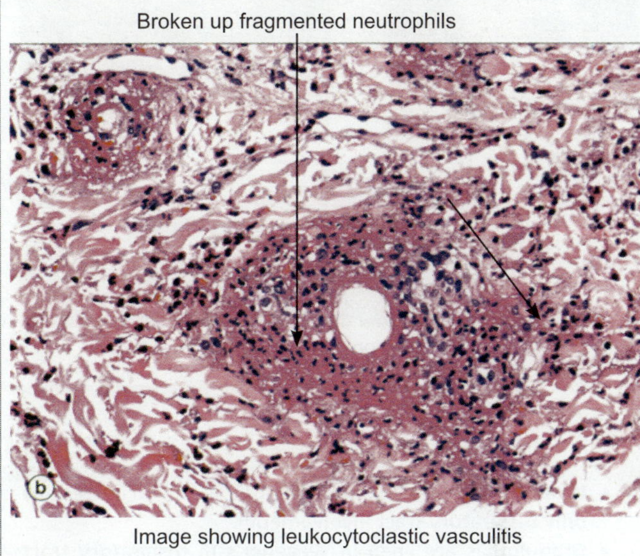

Image showing leukocytoclastic vasculitis

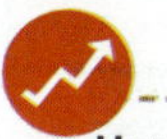
High Yield Facts

Hypersensitivity Vasculitis
- Seen most commonly in **Post capillary venules**[Q]
- Mic- **leukocytoclastic vasculitis**[Q]

Churg-Strauss Syndrome (Allergic Granulomatosis and Angiitis)

- Small-vessel necrotizing vasculitis classically associated with **asthma, allergic rhinitis**[Q]
- **Lung infiltrates, peripheral hypereosinophilia**, and **extravascular necrotizing granulomata**[Q]
- **P-ANCA**[Q] present in less than 50% of patients
- Multisystem diseases with cutaneous involvement (**palpable purpura**[Q]), gastrointestinal tract bleeding, and renal disease (primarily as **focal and segmental glomerulosclerosis**)[Q]
- The heart is involved in 60% of patients and accounts for almost **half of the deaths** in the syndrome[Q]
- New name suggested is–**EGPA**-Eosinophilic granulomatosis with polyangiitis

Granulomatosis with Polyangiitis

- Previously called as **Wegener's granulomas**

Necrotizing vasculitis which is characterized by **triad of**

- Acute necrotizing granulomas of either **upper (more commonly) or lower respiratory tract**[Q] or both.
- **Necrotizing or granulomatous vasculitis**[Q] affecting small to medium-sized vessels (e.g., capillaries, venules, arterioles, and arteries), most prominent in the lungs and upper airways.
- **Focal necrotizing, often crescentic, glomerulonephritis.**[Q]

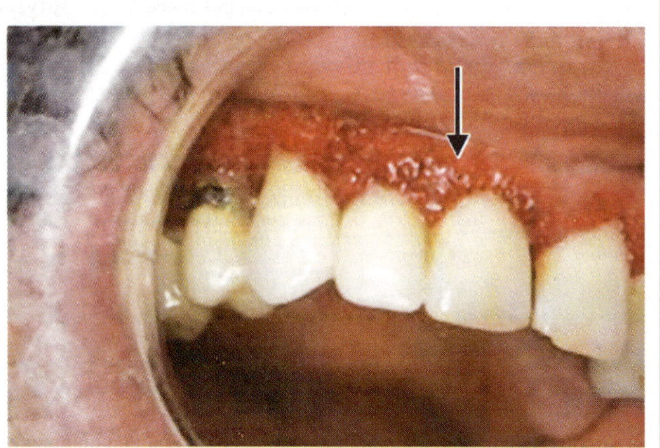

Wegener's granulomatosis: Strawberry gums

High Yield Facts

- Limited Wegener's granulomatosis[Q] is characterized by only respiratory tract involvement[Q]
- Granulomas are seen in Wegener's in respiratory tract but not in renal parenchyma[Q]
- Patients with classical PAN[Q] are ANCA negative
- PAN is the commonest cause of mononeuritis multiplex.[Q]

Henoch-Schonlein Purpura (HSP)/Anaphylactoid Purpura/Purpura Rheumatica

- **Definition:**
  - **Systemic vasculitis** syndrome involving **small size vessels.**[Q]

- **Epidemiology:**
  - **Most common small vessel** vasculitis in children
  - Usually **follows an upper respiratory tract infection**[Q] *(in 2/3rd cases)*

- **Pathophysiology:**
  - Vasculitis is caused by **immune complex deposition**
  - Most common antibody seen in these immune complexes is **IgA** (elevated)

- **Clinical features (tetrad)**
  - **Palpable purpura (Most common sites**[Q]**-buttocks and exterior surface of legs and arms),**
  - **Arthritis or arthralgia**
  - **Renal involvement (proteinuria,**[Q] Microscopic hematuria with RBC casts in urine),
  - **Colicky Abdominal pain and/or upper GI bleed**

- **Diagnosis:**
  - Platelet count is normal or elevated (as Purpura **does not occurs due to a low platelet** count but due to **vasculitis)**
  - Serum complement levels are **normal**
  - **M**icroscopic hallmark of HSP is the deposition of **IgA in the walls**[Q] of involved blood vessels.
  - **Morphology of vasculitis-leukocytoclastic vasculitis**[Q]

- **Treatment:**
  - Administration of **glucocorticoids** (Prednisolone)
- **Prognosis:**
  - **Excellent** and disease is **self limiting.**
  - **Incidence of renal involvement in adults is 45–85%, while it is 20–50% in children**

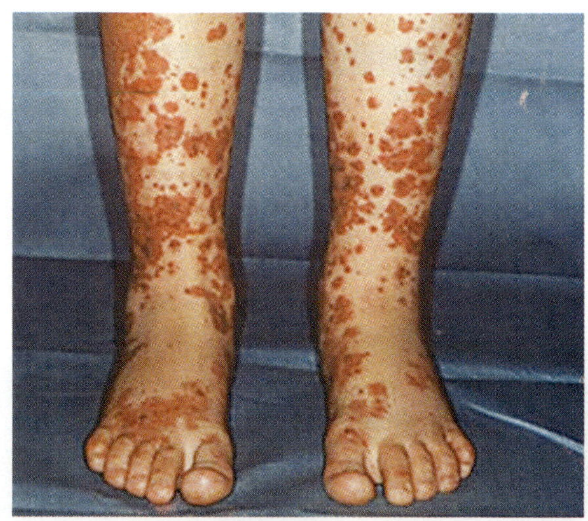

Palpable Purpura

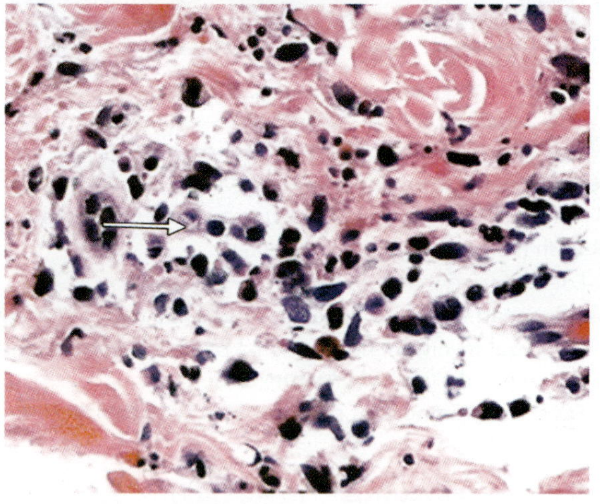

Leukocystoclastic vasculitis

Behçet's Disease

- Small-to-medium vessel **neutrophilic vasculitis**[Q]
- Clinical triad of **recurrent oral aphthous ulcers, genital ulcers, and uveitis**[Q]
- **Sin qua non** for diagnosis- **Oral ulceration (hallmark)**[Q]
- **Positive pathergy test**[Q]- if a papule or **pustule >2 mm, 24-48 hours** after needle prick, depth of 5 mm
- **HLA-B51**[Q] associated
- Microscopic findings are nonspecific- neutrophils are seen infiltrating vessels walls
- Immunosuppression with steroids or TNF-antagonist therapies is generally effective.

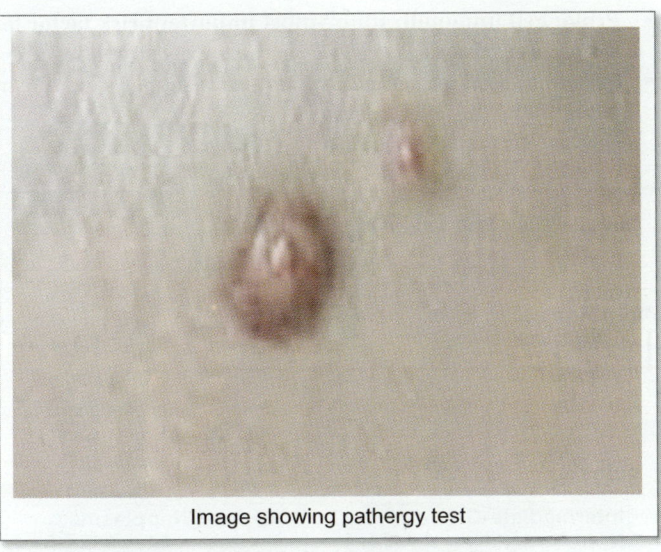

Image showing pathergy test

Buerger's Disease (Thromboangitis Obliterans)

- **Segmental, thrombosing**, acute and chronic inflammation[Q] of **medium-sized and small**[Q] arteries,
- **Tibial and radial arteries**[Q], with secondary extension into the **veins and nerves** of the extremities.
- Seen in **heavy cigarette smokers;**[Q] Onset is **before 35 years of age**[Q]
- Associated with **HLA B5 and HLA A9**[Q].
- Associated with **hypersensitivity to intradermal injections of tobacco extracts.**[Q]
- Mic-**segmental thrombosing vasculitis extending into contiguous veins & nerves, encasing all in fibrous tissue.**[Q]
- Thrombus contains **microabscess** with **granulomatous inflammation.**[Q]

Clinically

• **Intermittent claudication**[Q]-leg pain induced by exercise that is relieved on rest	• **Instep claudication**[Q]- Instep foot pain induced by exercise	• Superficial nodular phlebitis and cold induced Raynaud's phenomenon

- Treatment includes smoking cessation.

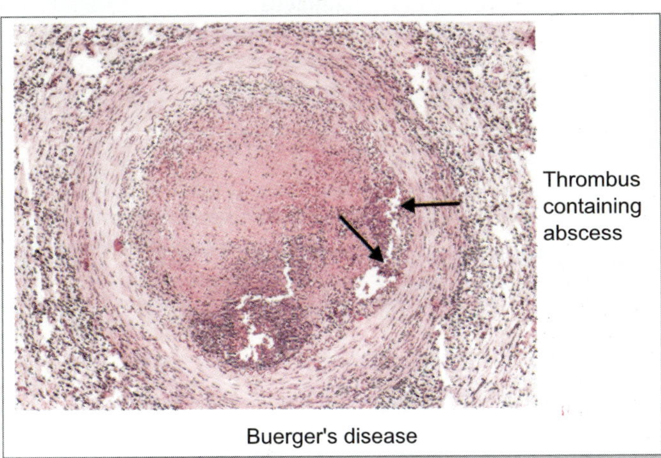

Thrombus containing abscess

Buerger's disease

Infectious Vasculitis

Caused by vascular infections that can weaken arterial walls and culminate in mycotic aneurysms

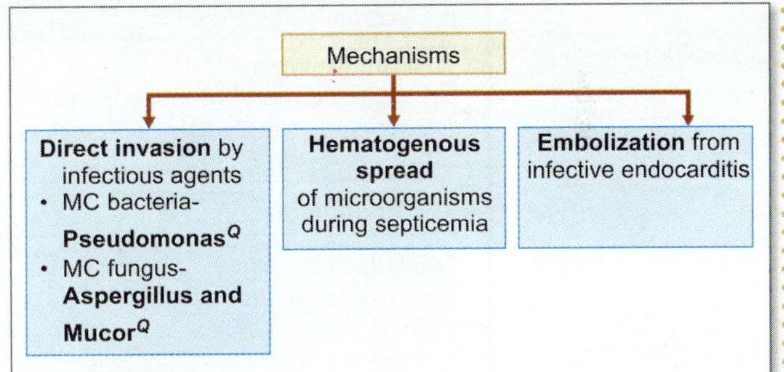

Mnemonic

Granulomatous vasculitis

WTC has TB

W – **W**egener's

T – **T**akayasu

C – **C**hurg- Strauss

T – **T**emporal arteritis

B – **B**uerger's disease.

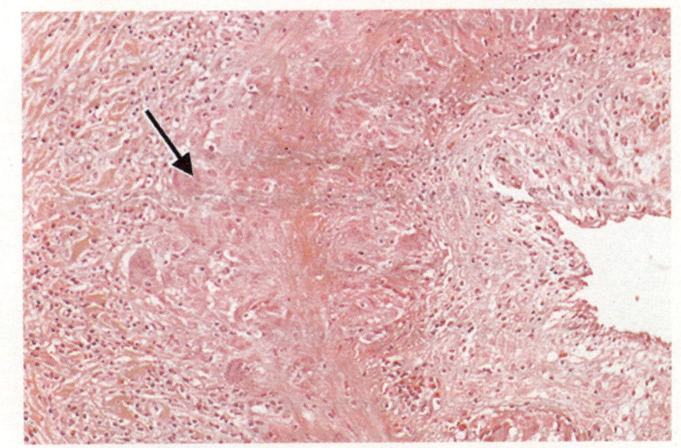

Granulomatous vasculitis: we can see epithelioid cells and giant cells s/o granulomatous vasculitis

VEINS AND LYMPHATICS

Varicose veins and phlebothrombosis/thrombophlebitis together account for at least 90% of clinical venous disease.

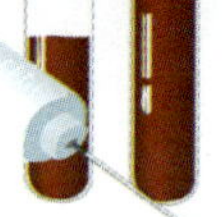

Thrombophlebitis and Phlebothrombosis

- Involvement of **deep leg veins**[Q] accounts for more than 90% of cases.

- **Prolonged immobilization**[Q]-**most important risk factor** for deep venous thrombosis (DVT) in the lower extremities.
- **Systemic hypercoagulability**[Q]: often also plays a role in potentiating thrombophlebitis.

VASCULAR TUMORS

Classification of Vascular Tumors and Tumor-Like Conditions

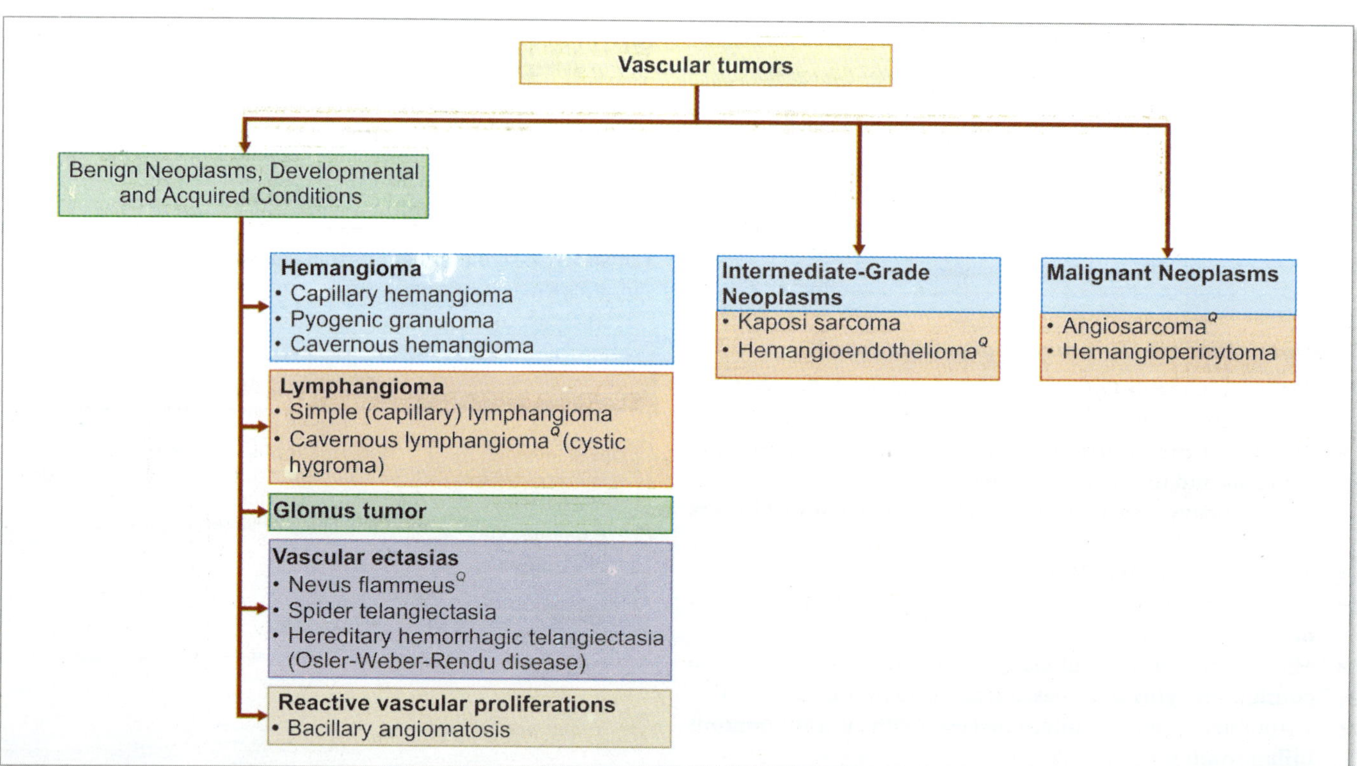

Benign Tumors

Hemangioma

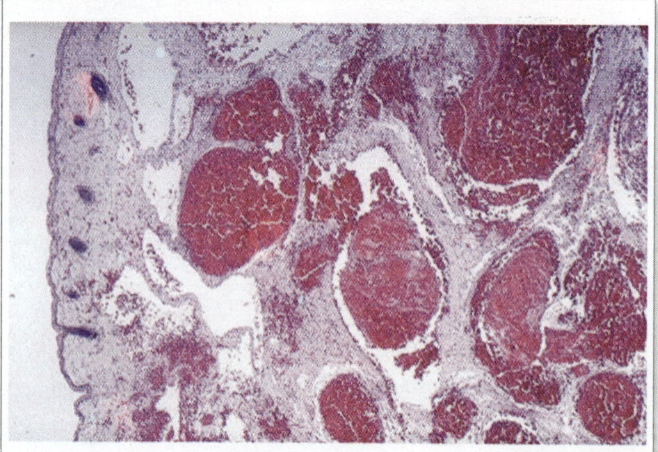

A proliferation of vascular channels filled with red blood cells, consistent with a hemangioma

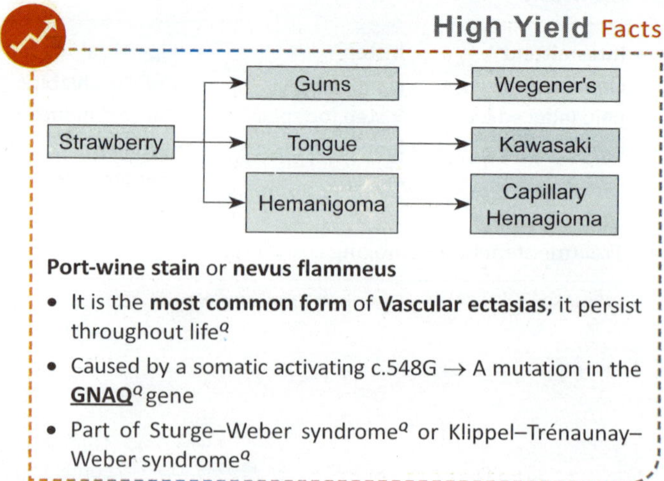

Port-wine stain or **nevus flammeus**

- It is the **most common form** of **Vascular ectasias;** it persist throughout life[Q]
- Caused by a somatic activating c.548G → A mutation in the **GNAQ**[Q] gene
- Part of Sturge–Weber syndrome[Q] or Klippel–Trénaunay–Weber syndrome[Q]

Capillary Hemangioma

Most common vascular tumor, occurs in skin, mucus membrane & viscera.

Strawberry[Q] or Juvenile Hemangioma	Pyogenic Granulomas
• Very common • Occurs in **new borns**[Q] • **Completely regress**[Q] by age 7	Red pedunculated lesions on skin, gingival, or oral mucosa (resembling **granulation tissue**[Q]) **Pregnancy tumor** (granuloma gravidarum) • Occurs in < 1% of patients; **Usually regresses**[Q] after delivery • Pyogenic granuloma in the gingiva of pregnant women[Q]

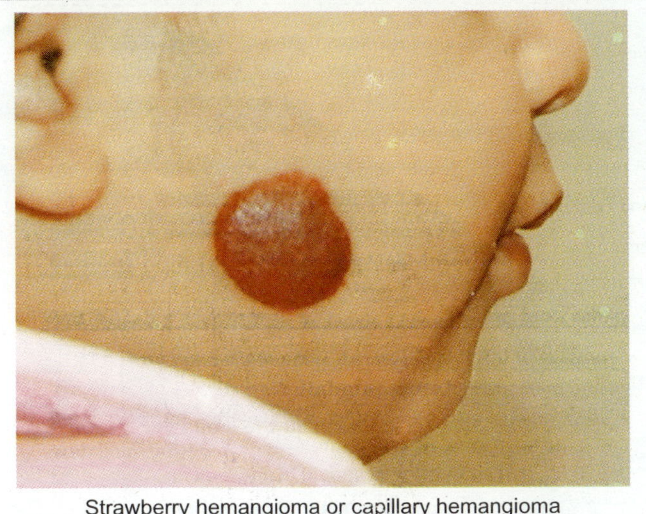

Strawberry hemangioma or capillary hemangioma

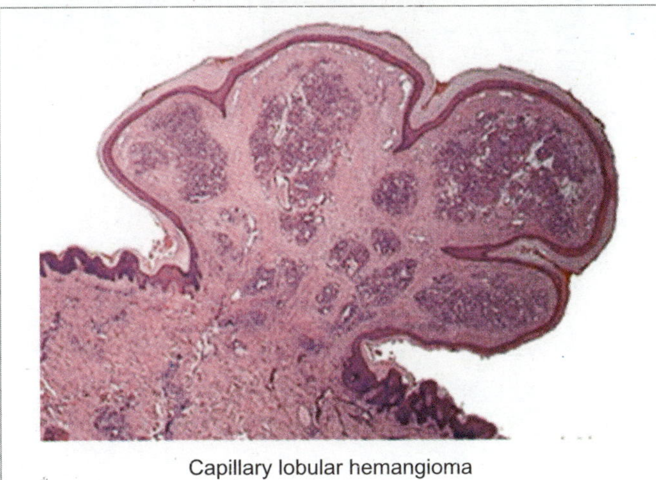

Capillary lobular hemangioma

Cavernous Hemangiomas

- Are more infiltrative, frequently involve deep structures
- **Do not**[Q] spontaneously regress.
- Intravascular thrombosis and associated dystrophic calcification are **common**[Q].
- Component of **von Hippel-Lindau disease**[Q], with vascular lesions in cerebellum, brain stem, retina, pancreas, and liver.

Lymphangioma

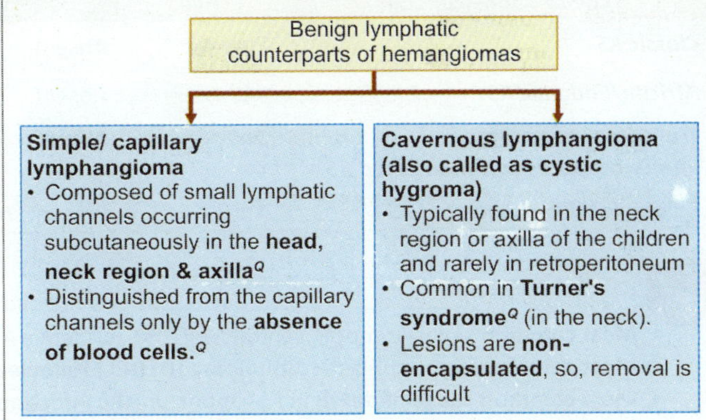

Glomus Tumor (Glomangioma)

- **Benign tumor**[Q] arising from the smooth muscle cells of the glomus body
- Most commonly present in the **distal portion of the digits (under fingernails).**[Q]
- **Histologically**: branching vascular channels & stroma containing nests /aggregates of **glomus cells** around vessels.
- **Excision is curative**[Q]

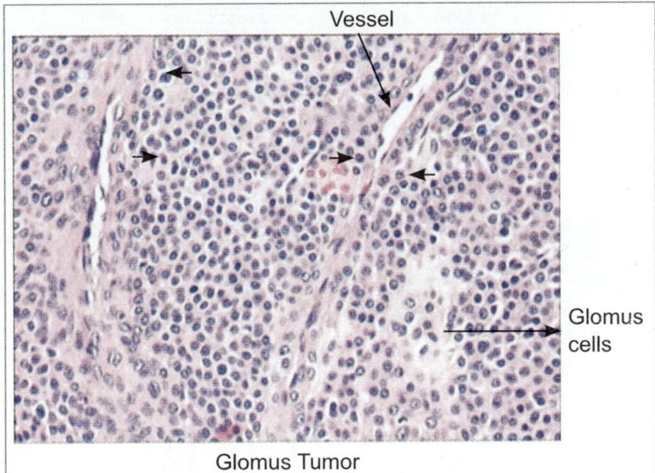

Glomus Tumor

Bacillary Angiomatosis

- **Vascular proliferation in immunocompromised hosts**[Q]
- Caused by opportunistic **Gram-negative bacilli of the Bartonella** family.
- Lesions can involve the **skin, bone, brain, and other organs**
- **Microscopy**: capillary proliferation with **epithelioid endothelial cells**[Q] exhibiting nuclear atypia and mitoses
- Stromal neutrophils, nuclear dust, and the causal bacteria can be identified

Intermediate/Borderline Tumors

Kaposi Sarcoma (KS)

- It is caused by KS Herpes virus or **Human herpes virus 8 (HHV8)**[Q]

- Characterized by proliferation of **spindle cells**[Q] which are of **vascular origin**[Q] and has the following 4 forms:

Type of Kaposi Sarcoma	Age	Association with HIV	Organs Affected
Classic KS	Elderly	Absent	Skin
African/Endemic KS	<40 yrs	Absent	**Lymph nodes** ± Viscera
Transplant associated/ Immunosuppression-associated KS	Any	Absent	Lymph nodes, mucosa & visceral organs
Epidemic/AIDS associated KS	Any	Present; **AIDS-defining illness**	**Lymph nodes & viscera** involved

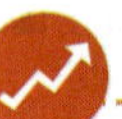

High Yield Facts

- **Most common** kaposi tumor in central Africa- KS (Endemic African KS in combination with AIDS-associated KS)
- **Most common immunoblastic lymphoma (DLBCL)** followed by AIDS associated (*epidemic*) *KS*[Q]
- **Most common cause of death** in KS- **opportunistic infections**[Q] rather than KS

Epithelioid Hemangioendothelioma

- Vascular tumor of adults occurring around medium and large-sized veins
- **20 % of these** can metastasize; cured by excision

Malignant Tumors

Angiosarcoma
- Malignant endothelial cell neoplasm **most commonly**[Q] seen in **skin,**[Q] **soft tissue,**[Q] **breast**[Q] and **liver**[Q]
- Hepatic angiosarcoma is associated with **arsenic, thorotrast** (a radioactive contrast) & **polyvinyl chloride** (PVC)[Q]
- Other important risk factor is **radiation**[Q]
- Endothelial cell origin is demonstrated by staining for CD31, CD34 or VWF. (Highly specific) FL$_1$/ERG
- Locally invasive; readily metastasize

Hemangiopericytoma
- Tumor derived from **pericytes**[Q]- **perivascular cells** that wrap around blood capillaries
- These tumors most commonly arise from **pelvic retroperitoneum**[Q] or the **limbs**[Q] (particularly thighs).
- Capillaries are arranged in **'fish-hook pattern;'**[Q] seen best with **silver stains**[Q]

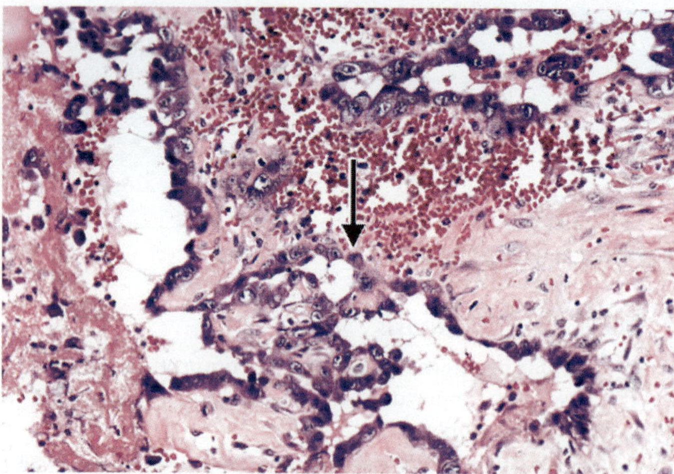

Angiosarcoma: Irregularly shaped vascular lumina lined by highly atypical endothelial cells S/o angiosarcoma

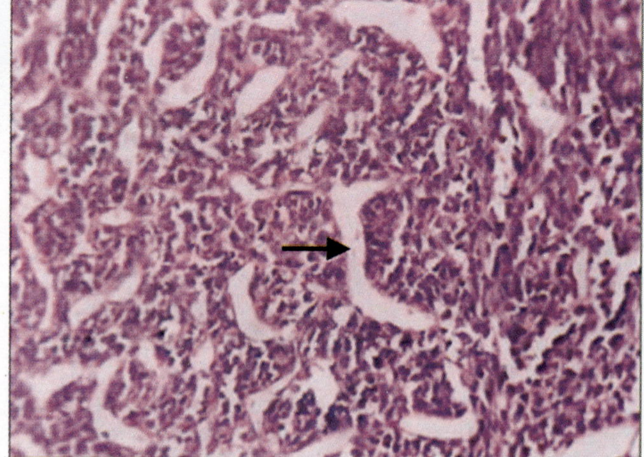

Hemangiopericytoma showing staghorn (fishhook pattern)

High Yield Facts

- **Lymphangiosarcoma** arises from dilated lymphatic vessels;[Q] most common site: post mastectomy arm[Q]
- **Rouget cells** –other name of **pericytes**[Q]

- **Pericytic (perivascular) tumors**-Glomus tumor, Hemangiopericytoma, Myopericytoma & PEComa(Perivascular epitheliod cell tumor)

CARDIOVASCULAR SYSTEM

HEART

Valves

- The four cardiac valves—tricuspid, pulmonary, mitral, and aortic—maintain unidirectional blood flow.
- **Cardiac valves:** Lined by endothelium and have similar, tri-layered architecture:
  - A dense collagenous core (fibrosa) at the outflow surface
  - A central core of loose connective tissue (spongiosa)
  - A layer rich in elastin on the inflow surface
- Pathologic changes of valves are largely of three types:
  - Damage to collagen that weakens the leaflets, exemplified by mitral valve prolapse
  - Nodular calcification beginning in interstitial cells, as in calcific aortic stenosis
  - Fibrotic thickening, the key feature in rheumatic heart disease

> **$R9^{th}$ Latest Update**
>
> - Cardiac stem cells are present **within the myocardium[Q]**, they are the **greatest in neonates**, and constitute up to **5% to 10% of normal atrial cellularity[Q]** and **1 in 100,000 cells [Q] in a normal ventricle[Q].**
>
> **Effects of Aging on Heart**
> - Epicardial fat increases
> - **Basophilic degeneration** within cardiac myocytes
> - **Intracellular lipofuscin deposits**

- **Sigmoid septum** [Q] bulging of the basal ventricular septum into the left ventricular outflow tract
- **Lambl's excrescences** [Q] small filiform processes on **closure lines[Q]** of aortic mitral valves: due to **organization of small thrombi.[Q]**
- Aorta becomes progressively **stiffer**-due to accumulation of **atherosclerotic plaque**
- Myocytes decrease in number, and deposition of **extracellular amyloid (most commonly due to poorly catabolized transthyretin[Q])**

Cardiac Hypertrophy

Cardiac myocytes which cannot undergo hyperplasia in response to stress, so the only adaptation seen in a cardiac muscle can be hypertrophy[Q] which can be of the following types:

Types	Concentric hypertrophy	Eccentric hypertrophy
Pathophysiology	Pressure overload	Volume overload
Definition	Deposition of the sarcomeres in parallel[Q] to the long axis of the cells	Dilatation with increased ventricular diameter [Q]
Cause	• Aortic stenosis [Q] • Hypertension [Q]	• Valvular regurgitation [Q] (mitral/aortic) • Thyrotoxicosis[Q] • Severe anemia[Q]

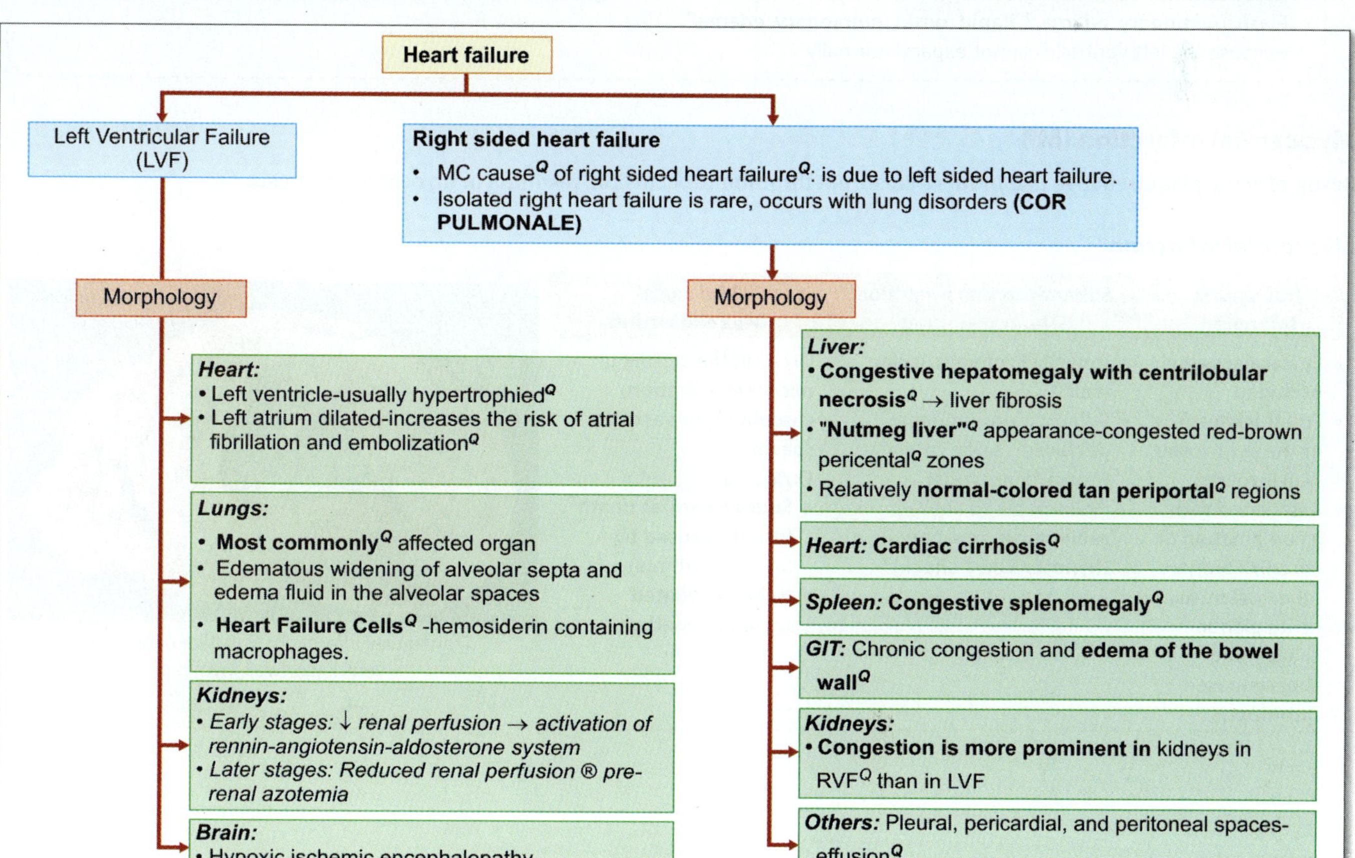

Morphologic Findings in Heart failure

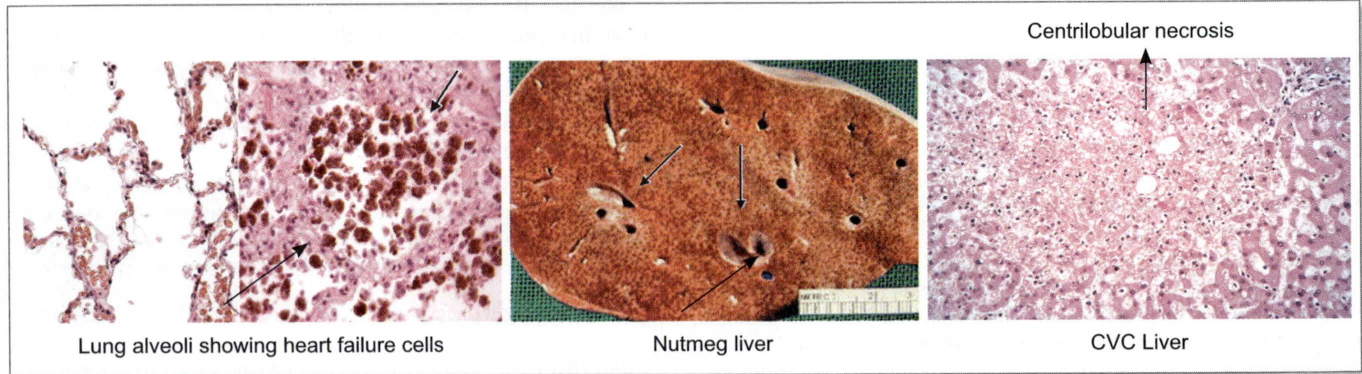

Lung alveoli showing heart failure cells

Nutmeg liver

Centrilobular necrosis

CVC Liver

ISCHEMIC HEART DISEASE

- Imbalance between **perfusion & demand** of heart for oxygenated blood.
- IHD can present as one or more of the following clinical syndromes:
  - **Angina pectoris**-where ischemia is **not severe** to cause infarction, but the **symptoms show infarction risk**[Q]
  - **Myocardial infarction (MI)** where ischemia causes frank cardiac necrosis
  - **Chronic IHD with heart failure**
  - **Sudden cardiac death (SCD)**

High Yield Facts

- **No hypertrophy or dilation of left ventricle**-In cases of failure caused by **mitral valve stenosis or unusual restrictive cardiomyopathies** [Q]
- **Most common**[Q] underlying etiology of LVF-**Hypertension**[Q]
- **Flash pulmonary edema,**[Q] **Rapid onset pulmonary edema**[Q] because the left ventricle cannot expand normally

- **Most common cause of ischemic heart disease**[Q]- Atherosclerotic narrowing resulting in coronary arterial obstruction
- **The level of cardiac markers remain unchanged in stable angina**[Q]

Myocardial Infarction (MI)

Result of acute plaque change that induces an abrupt thrombotic occlusion, resulting in myocardial necrosis.

Myocardial Infarction

Transmural Infarction	Subendocardial Infarction (Nontransmural)	Multifocal Microinfarction
• **Epicardial vessel occluded** • **Full thickness**[Q] of the ventricular wall involved • Associated with a combination of chronic coronary atherosclerosis, acute plaque change and superimposed thrombosis	• **Inner 1/3rd of ventricular wall**[Q] • Subendocardium-**least perfused**[Q]region of myocardium: **most** [Q]**vulnerable** to any reduction in coronary flow **(hypotension / shock)**[Q]	Occur in the setting of **microembolization, vasculitis**[Q], or vascular spasm[Q] **Outcome:** • **Sudden cardiac death**[Q] (usually caused by a fatal arrhythmia) • **Ischemic dilated cardiomyopathy**[Q]

Transmural infarction: Full thickness of the ventricular wall involved

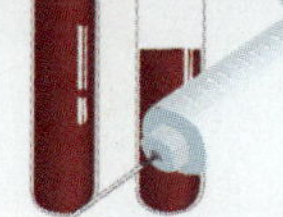

Myocardial Response[Q]

Feature	Time
• Onset of *ATP depletion*	Seconds[Q]
• **Loss of contractility**[Q]	**<2 min**[Q]
• ATP reduced to **50%** of normal[Q]	**10 min**[Q]
• ATP reduced **to 10%** of normal[Q]	**40 min**[Q]
• **Microvascular injury**[Q]	**>1 hr**[Q]

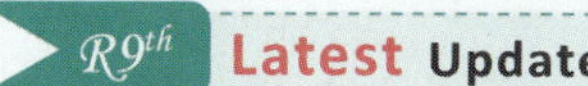

TAKOTSUBO cardiomyopathy [Q]: (also called "**broken heart syndrome**" because of the association with emotional distress) - **ischemic dilated cardiomyopathy**[Q]

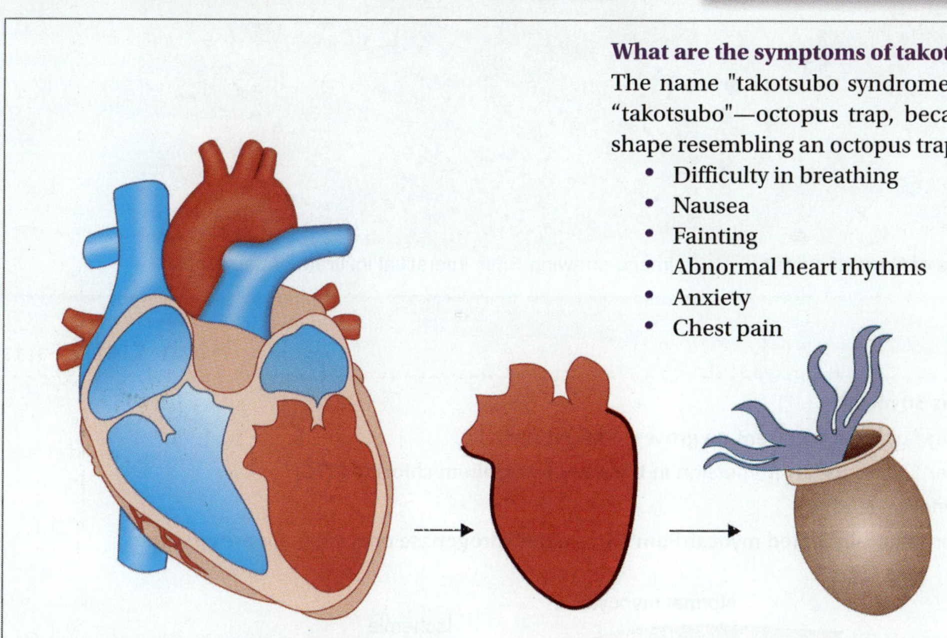

What are the symptoms of takotsubo cardiomyopathy?

The name "takotsubo syndrome" comes from the Japanese word "takotsubo"—octopus trap, because the left ventricle takes on a shape resembling an octopus trap.

- Difficulty in breathing
- Nausea
- Fainting
- Abnormal heart rhythms
- Anxiety
- Chest pain

Evolution of Morphological Changes in MI[Q]

Time	Gross	Light Microscopy	Electron microscopy
Reversible injury *0-30 min.*	None	None	• **Relaxation of myofibrils**[Q] • Glycogen loss • **Mitochondrial swelling**[Q]
Irreversible injury			
30 min-4 hr	None	**Waviness of fibers at border**[Q] (earliest microscopic change)	• **Sarcolemmal disruption**[Q] • **Mitochondrial amorphous densities**[Q]
4-12 hr	Dark mottling **appears**[Q]	**Beginning of coagulative necrosis**[Q]	
12-24 hr	Dark mottling	• **Neutrophilic infiltration** [Q] • **Myocyte hypereosinophilia**[Q] • Marginal **contraction band necrosis**	
1-3 days	**Yellow tan infarct center**[Q]	Brisk interstitial infiltrate of neutrophils	
3-7 days	**Hyperemic borders**[Q], central yellow tan softening	**Macrophages**[Q] at infarct border	
7-10 days	**Maximum**[Q] **yellow tan**	Early **formation of fibrovascular granulation tissue**[Q] at margins	
10-14 days	Red gray infarct borders	**Well established granulation tissue**[Q] Collagen deposition[Q]	
2-8 weeks	**Gray-white scar**[Q]	**Collagen deposition**[Q]	
>2 months	Scarring complete	**Dense collagenous scar**[Q]	

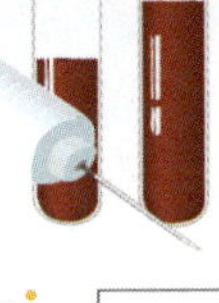

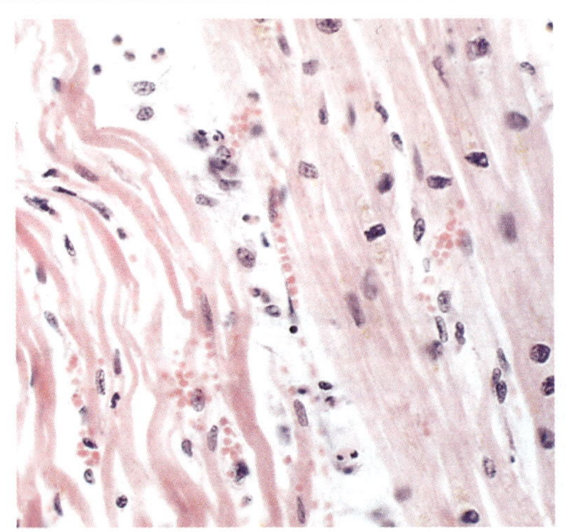

Image showing Waviness of fibers at border

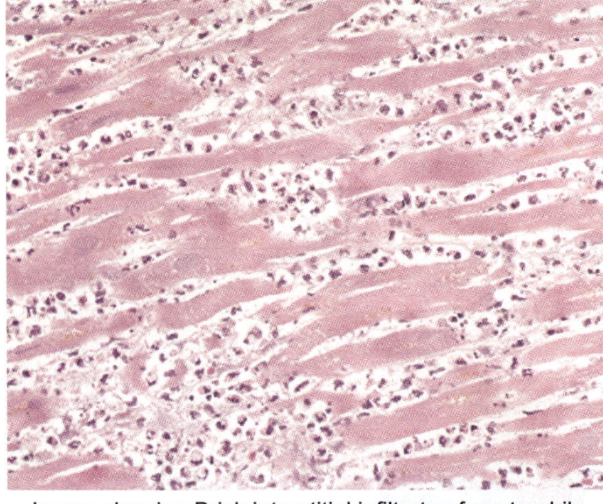

Image showing Brisk interstitial infiltrate of neutrophils

High Yield Facts

- **Time for reversible injury in heart is 30 mins[Q]**
- Myocardial infarct **less than 12 hours[Q]** old- **not apparent on gross examination[Q]**.
- **N**ecrotic area can be **visualized after 2–3 hours[Q]** by immersion in **triphenyltetrazolium chloride (TTC)[Q]**
- **Infarcted area** is revealed as **unstained pale zone[Q]**
- TTC imparts brick red magenta color to **non-infarcted myocardium[Q]** where **dehydrogenase enzymes[Q]** are preserved.

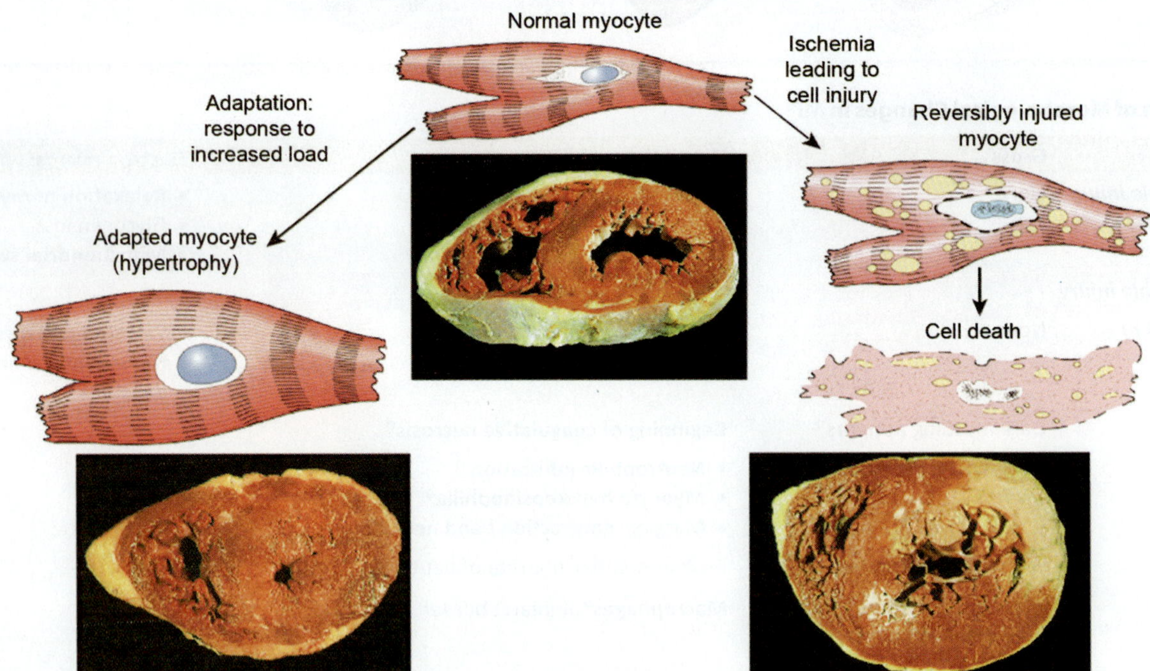

Triphenyltetrazolium chloride, an enzyme substrate that colors viable myocardium magenta.
Failure to stain is due to enzyme loss after cell death

- **Most common cause of SCD[Q]-malignant ventricular arrhythmias[Q]**-myocardial ischemia-induced irritability.

Complication of MI (Mnemonics – ACT RAPID)

- **Arrhythmia:**
  - **Most common** within one hour[Q]-**Ventricular fibrillation**[Q]
  - **Most common** after one hour[Q]-**Supraventricular tachycardia**[Q]
- **Contractile dysfunction**
  - Leads to Cardiogenic shock
- **Mural Thrombus**
- **Myocardial Rupture**
  - **Most common** - Rupture of **ventricular free wall**[Q]
  - **Most common** site for **free wall rupture- anterolateral wall at the midventricular level**[Q]
  - **Most frequent** 3 to 7 days after MI[Q]
  - **Least common-rupture of papillary muscles**[Q]
- **Ventricular Aneurysm**
  - **False aneurysm**[Q] - **localized hematoma**[Q] communicating with the ventricular cavity
  - **Wall of a false aneurysm** consists only of **epicardium and adherent parietal pericardium**[Q]
- **Pericarditis**
  - **Post MI pericarditis-Dressler syndrome or post MI syndrome**[Q]
    - **Autoimmune reaction**[Q]
    - **Fibrinous or fibrinohemorrhagic pericarditis**[Q]
    - Develops **second or third day**[Q] following a transmural infarct
- **Infarct expansion**
  - **Seen with** anteroseptal infarcts
  - Papillary muscle **Dysfunction**: Leads to Post infarct mitral regurgitation.
  - *Progressive late heart failure (chronic IHD)*

R9[th] Latest Update

Infarct Modification by Reperfusion.
- **Reperfusion Injury:** [Q]**Damage** that occurs **after restoration of flow to "vulnerable" myocardium**[Q] that is ischemic but not irreversibly damaged
- **Stunned Myocardium:**[Q] State of prolonged **cardiac failure**[Q] induced by short-term ischemia that usually recovers after several days
- **Hibernation:**[Q] Myocardium that is subjected to **chronic, sublethal ischemia** may also enter into a **state of lowered metabolism**[Q]
- **Reperfused infarcts are usually hemorrhagic**[Q]
- Irreversibly injured myocytes exhibit[Q]: **Contraction bands (intensely eosinophilic intracellular stripes), composed of closely packed sarcomeres**[Q] due to exaggerated contraction of sarcomeres when perfusion is re-established because of high concentration of **calcium ions**[Q] from the plasma.

Chronic Ischemic Heart Disease

- Also called **ischemic cardiomyopathy**
- **Progressive congestive heart failure**[Q] as a consequence of **accumulated ischemic myocardial damage**[Q]
- Appears post infarction due to the **functional decompensation of hypertrophied noninfarcted myocardium**[Q]
- Chronic IHD patients account for **50% of cardiac transplant recipients.**[Q]
- Microscopic findings include **myocardial hypertrophy**[Q], **diffuse subendocardial vacuolization**[Q] **& fibrosis.**[Q]

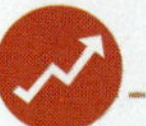

High Yield Facts

- **Most commonly** affected valve in RHD is **mitral valve**[Q]
- **Least commonly** affected in RHD is **pulmonary valve.**[Q]
- In acute rheumatic heart disease, the **most common valvular lesion is mitral regurgitation**[Q]
- In chronic rheumatic heart disease, **most common valvular lesion** is mitral stenosis.[Q]
- **Mac-callum patches-** map-like areas of **thickened part of the endocardium in the posterior wall of left atrium**[Q] - caused by **regurgitant jets of blood flow**[Q], due to incompetence of the mitral valve.

RHEUMATIC FEVER AND RHEUMATIC HEART DISEASE (RHD)

- An acute **immunologically** mediated **multisystem inflammatory disease**[Q] that occurs **few weeks** after an attack of **group Aβ- hemolytic streptococcal pharyngitis.**[Q]
- **Most common age group** affected is children between of **5-15 years**[Q].
- It is **not an infective** disease[Q].
- **Type II hypersensitivity reaction**
- Antibodies against '**M' protein** of some streptococcal strains **cross-react with the glycoprotein antigens in the heart**, joints and other tissues (molecular mimicry).

Salient Features of the Major Criteria

Carditis

Pancarditis: **Involves** pericardium, myocardium and endocardium

- **Endocardium:**
  - **Fibrinoid necrosis**[Q] within the cusps or tendinous cords.
  - **Verrucae-** small (1 to 2 mm) vegetations **along the lines of closure**[Q]
- **Myocardium-** has **Aschoff's bodies**[Q] in the **perivascular location**
- **Pericarditis** is associated with **fibrinous/serofibrinous**[Q] exudates-'**bread and butter' pericarditis.**[Q]

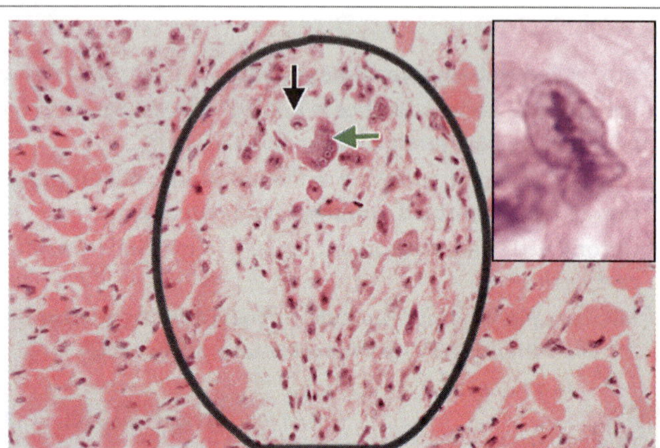

Aschoff Bodies: Here u can see collection of foci of swollen eosinophilic collagen surrounded by Lymphocytes, giant cells[Q] (marked with green arrow) and Antischkow cells (cells with caterpillar like chromatin shown in the inset)

Migratory Polyarthritis

- **Most commonly seen manifestation; More commonly seen in the adults[Q]** as compared to children
- Involvement of the large joints of the body; Arthritis involves **one joint after the other[Q]** (migratory)
- Subsides **spontaneously without any residual deformability[Q]** in the joints (**non-erosive arthritis**).

Subcutaneous Nodules

Painless subcutaneous lesions on **extensor surface of elbows, shin and occiput[Q]**.

Erythema Marginatum

Red macular rash more easily appreciated in fair skinned individuals **sparing the face[Q]**

Syndenham's Chorea

Involuntary, purposeless movements[Q] associated with **emotional lability of patient**

Chronic RHD

- Mitral valve is always involved
- **Cardinal anatomic changes in mitral valve**- leaflet thickening, **commissural fusion and shortening**, thickening & fusion of the tendinous cords.
- **Fibrosis produces Mitral stenosis [Q]**also known as 'fish-mouth' or 'button-hole' stenosis.[Q]

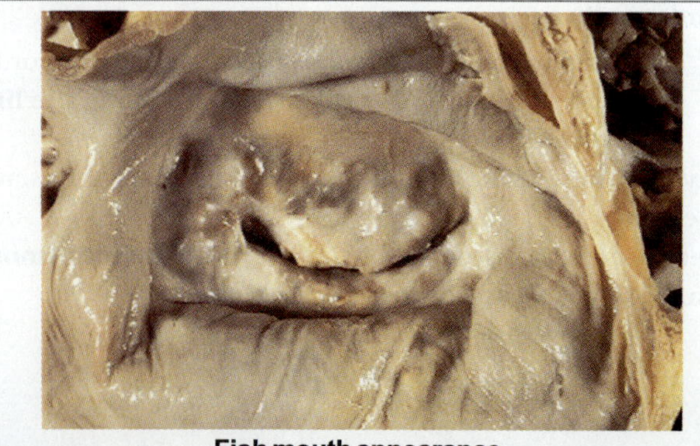

Fish mouth appearance

Aschoff Bodies:
- **Focal distinctive inflammatory lesions** seen **during acute rheumatic fever.[Q]**. They are **pathognomonic of RHD**
- Consist of **foci of swollen eosinophilic collagen[Q]** surrounded by:
  - Lymphocytes (primary T cells), Occasional plasma cells, Aschoff giant cells[Q] (macrophages of rheumatic fever)[Q], Antischkow cells (pathognomonic for RF)[Q]
    Antischkow cells - **modified macrophages with abundant cytoplasm** and central round to ovoid nuclei with **central wavy ribbon** like chromatin hence also called **caterpillar cells,[Q] seen in any of the 3 layers** of the heart[Q]

INFECTIVE ENDOCARDITIS (IE)

- Endocarditis-Inflammation of inner layer of heart

Acute Endocarditis	Subacute Endocarditis
• Infection of **Previously normal[Q]** valve.	• Infection of **Previously damaged valve[Q]**
• **Highly virulent[Q]** organisms	• **Low virulence[Q]** organisms
• Most common caused by **Staph. aureus[Q]**	• Most common **Hemolytic (viridans), Streptococcus[Q]**
• Produce necrotic and destructive lesions	• Produce less destruction of valves
• Death of the patient within **days to weeks**	• **Protracted cause of weeks and months-Recover after** antibiotic therapy

Morphology

- The friable, bulky destructive vegetations contain- **fibrin, bacteria and inflammatory cells** [Q]
- Found on the valve cusps, can also extend on to chordae.
- **Ring abscess[Q]**-When the vegetations erode into myocardium, they can form an abscess
- **Most commonly infected valve[Q]** - aortic valve and the mitral valve
- **Intravenous drug abusers[Q]** - **right side[Q]** of heart is affected

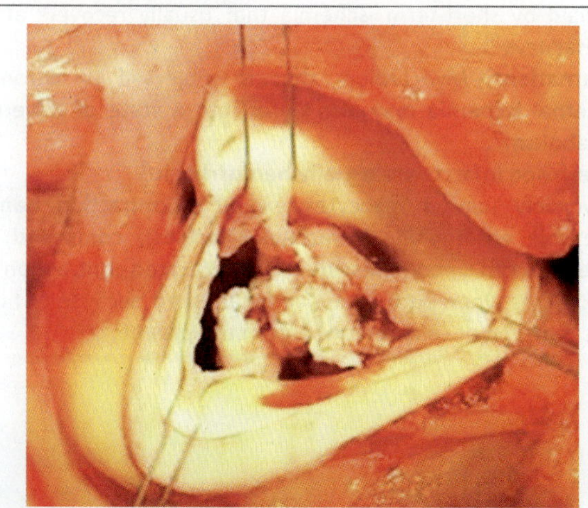

Image shows friable bulky vegetations

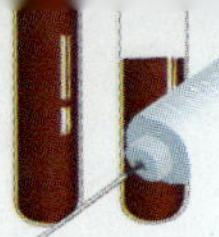

Clinical Features

- Fever is the **most consistent sign** of IE.
- The other features include weight loss, flu-like syndrome, microthromboemboli (manifest as **splinter or subungual** hemorrhages), erythematous or hemorrhagic non-tender lesions on palms or soles (**Janeway lesions**), subcutaneous nodules in the pulp of digits (**Osler nodes**), and retinal hemorrhages in the eyes (**Roth spots**).
- The disease is diagnosed by **Dukes criteria.**[Q]
- **Blood culture is the investigation of choice**[Q].

High Yield Facts

Most common site for vegetation in:
- **Libman Sack's endocarditis** are the **A-V valves**[Q], mitral and tricuspid.
- **NBTE** is **mitral**[Q] and less often aortic and Tricuspid.
- **RF** in **mitral**[Q] followed by combined mitral and aortic

Most frequent causes of the functional valvular lesions
- Aortic stenosis: **Calcification** of anatomically normal and **congenitally bicuspid aortic valves**
- Aortic regurgitation: Dilation of the ascending aorta due to **hypertension**[Q] and **aging**[Q]
- Mitral stenosis: **Rheumatic heart disease.**[Q]
- Mitral regurgitation: **Myxomatous degeneration** (mitral valve prolapse).[Q]

NONINFECTED VEGETATIONS

Nonbacterial Thrombotic Endocarditis (NBTE)/ Marantic Endocarditis

- Vegetations on heart valves are sterile and **do not contain microorganisms.**[Q]
- Small, present **along the line of closure, single or multiple.**[Q]
- **Not invasive, do not elicit any inflammatory reaction**[Q]
- **Loosely attached**, so can cause **systemic emboli**[Q] that produce significant infarcts in brain, heart, or elsewhere.

Predisposing Conditions
- Debilitated patients, such as those with cancer (Ca pancreas, mucinous adenoCa, APML) or sepsis—hence the previous term **marantic endocarditis**[Q]
- **Systemic hypercoagulable state**[Q]
- **Endocardial trauma**[Q], as from an indwelling catheter

Libman-sacks Endocarditis (seen in SLE)

- **Small** (1-4 mm), single or multiple, **sterile**[Q]**,** vegetations with a **warty (verrucous) appearance**[Q]
- Located on the **either or both sides of valve leaflets especially under surfaces of the atrioventricular valves**
- **Mitral and tricuspid valves** are involved
- Associated with an **intense valvulitis**[Q], characterized by **fibrinoid necrosis**[Q] of the valve substance
- Vegetations consist of **finely granular, fibrinous eosinophilic** material containing cellular debris & nuclear remnants

Diffrentiating Features of Various Types of Endocarditis

Rheumatic Fever (RF)	Non Bacterial Thrombotic (Marantic Endocarditis)	Libman Sack's Endocarditis	Infective Endocarditis
1. **Small, warty**[Q] 2. Firm 3. Friable	1. **Small, warty**[Q] 2. Friable	1. Medium sized (small) 2. Flat, Verrucous 3. Irregular	1. **Large**[Q] 2. **Bulky**[Q] 3. Irregular
Along line of closure[Q]	**Along line of closure**[Q]	1. On surface of cusps 2. (both surfaces may be involved but the **undersurface is more likely affected,**[Q] less commonly mural endocardium is involved) 3. **In pockets of valves**[Q]	1. Vegetations on the **valve cusps**[Q] 2. Less often on mural endocardium
Sterile (no organism)	Sterile	Sterile	**Non-sterile (bacteria)**[Q]
Embolization is uncommon	**Embolization is common**[Q]	Embolization is uncommon	**Embolization is very common (max chances)**[Q]
In **rheumatic heart disease**[Q]	**In cancers (like M3-AML, Ca pancreas), DVT, Trosseau's syndrome**[Q]	In SLE	In infective endocarditis

CARDIOMYOPATHIES

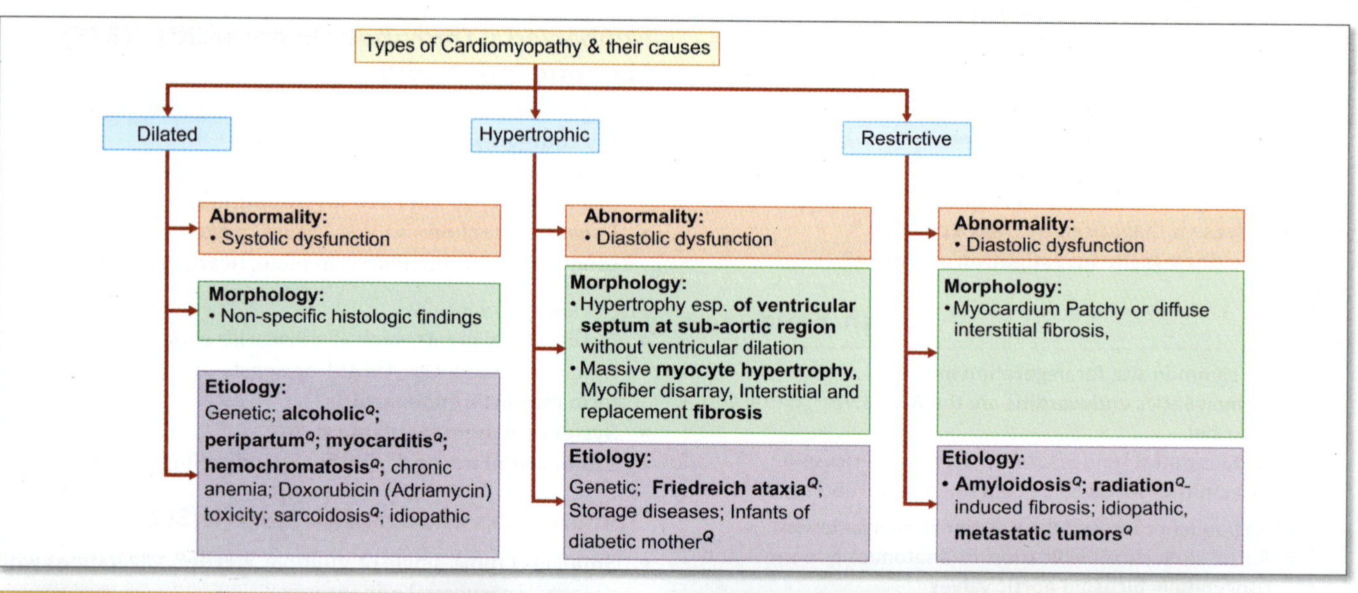

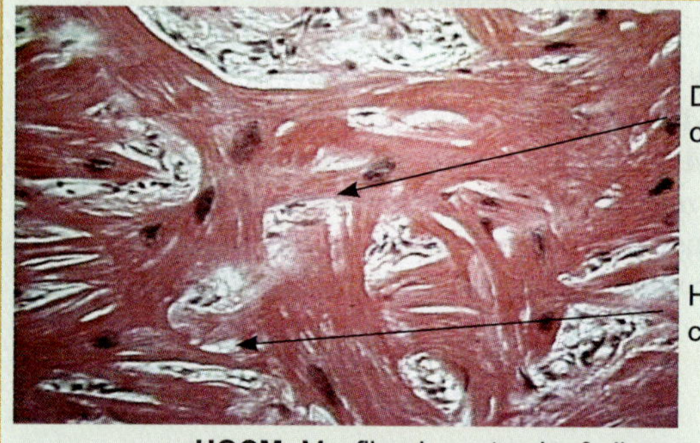

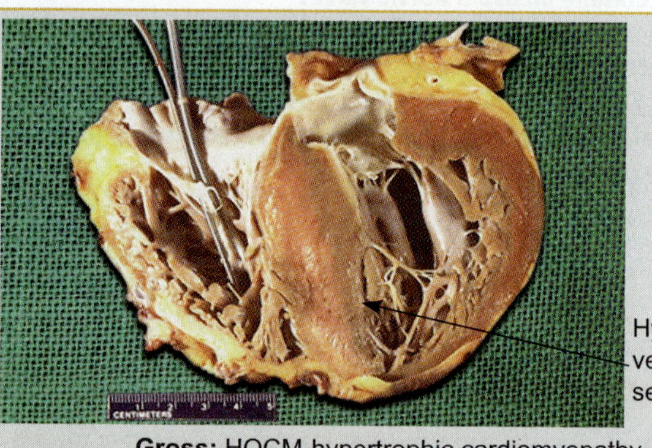

PERICARDITIS

- Normally, visceral pericardium is separated from the parietal pericardium by a **small quantity (15–50 mL) of fluid**^Q
- **Inflammation of pericardium is called pericarditis**^Q

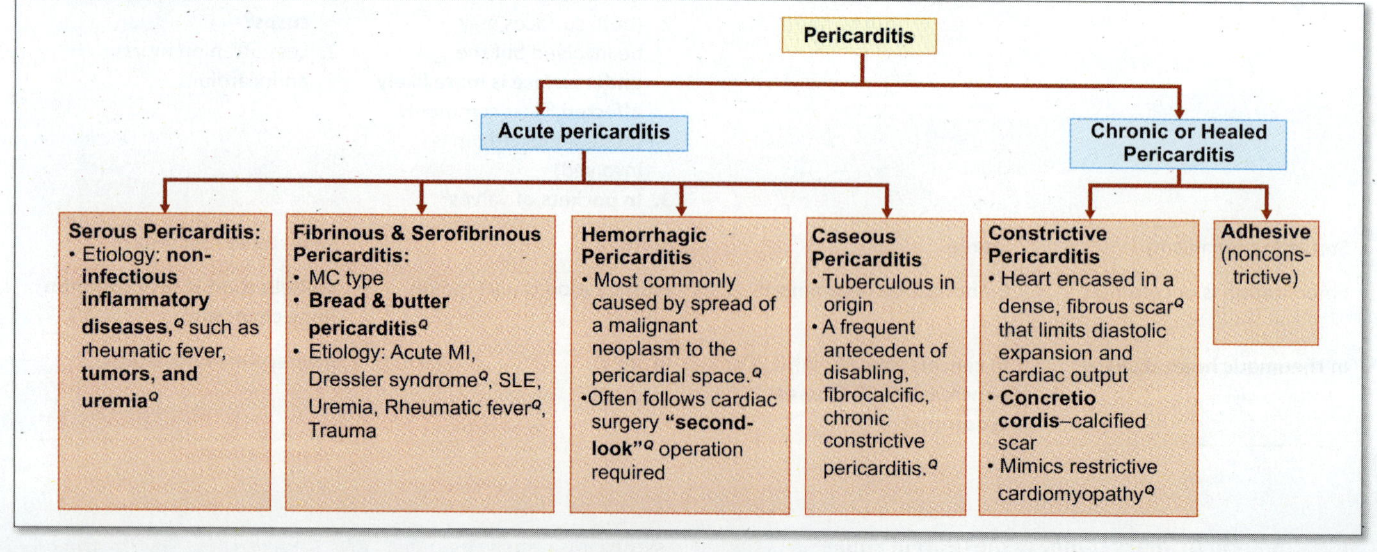

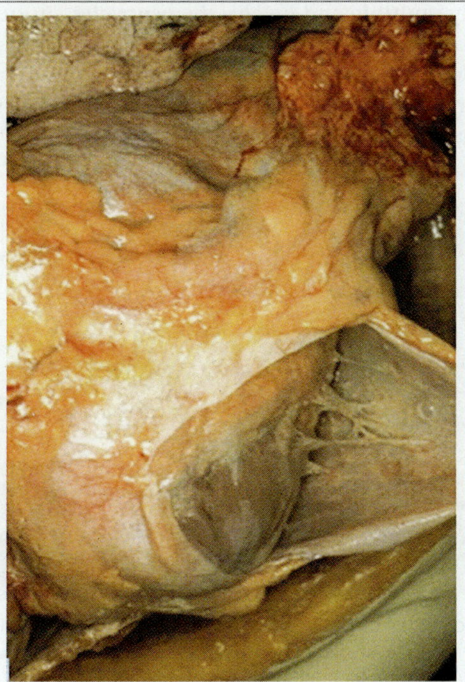

Fibrinous pericarditis

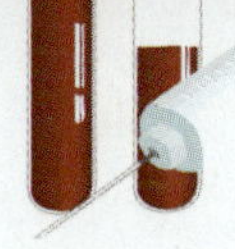

- Dilated cardiomyopathy is **most common**[Q] (90% of cases). Most cases are due to mutations in titin (largest known human protein)
- Restrictive cardiomyopathy is the **least frequent**[Q]
- **Naxos syndrome:**[Q] characterized by **arrhythmogenic right ventricular cardiomyopathy**[Q] **& hyperkeratosis**[Q] of plantar palmar skin, associated with mutation in gene encoding the desmosome-associated protein **plakoglobin**[Q]
- **HOCM** is the **leading cause of unexplained left ventricular hypertrophy**
- **HOCM** is Most common cause of **sudden death** in **young athletes**[Q]
- **Most common genetic mutation in HOCM**[Q] - gene encoding β-myosin heavy chain (β-MHC)[Q]
- **Loeffler's endomyocarditis:** Peripheral eosinophilia & **eosinophilic infiltrates in multiple organs, including heart**[Q]
- **Endocardial fibroelastosis:** Most common in the **first 2 years**[Q] of life
- **Endocardial fibroelastosis** morphologic end-point of different insults including viral infections (e.g., **intrauterine exposure to mumps**[Q]) or mutations in the gene for **tafazzin**[Q], which affects **mitochondrial inner membrane integrity**[Q]

MYOCARDITIS

- Myocarditis, i.e., cardiac inflammation, is most commonly caused by viral infections.
- *Coxsackieviruses A*[Q] *and B*[Q] *and other enteroviruses*[Q] account for most of the cases.
- **Most common helminth causing myocarditis-Trichinella**[Q]
- **Most common bacterial** infection associated with myocarditis- **Diphtheria**[Q]

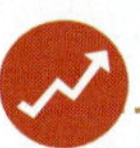

High Yield Facts

- **Most common** cause of pericarditis is **viral causes** [Q]
- **Mulibrey nanism-autosomal recessive**[Q] syndrome is characterized **by growth failure, muscle hypotonia, hepatomegaly, ocular changes, enlarged cerebral ventricles, mental retardation, ventricular hypertrophy & chronic constrictive pericarditis**[Q]
- **Most frequent type of pericarditis is fibrinous pericarditis**

Giant-cell Myocarditis

- Characterized by inflammatory infiltrate containing **multinucleate giant cells** with lymphocytes, eosinophils, plasma cells, and macrophages.
- Focal to frequently extensive **necrosis** is present.
- This variant carries a **poor prognosis.**[Q]

CARDIAC TUMORS

Myxoma

- **Most common primary tumor** of the heart in adults.[Q]
- **Benign** neoplasms

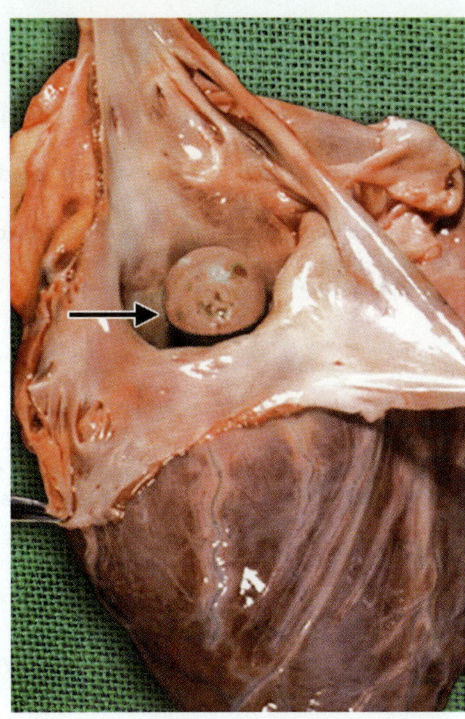

Myxoma

- Arise from **primitive multipotent mesenchymal cells** 90% are located in the atria, with a **left-to-right ratio of approximately 4:1 (atrial myxomas).**
- Major clinical manifestations are due to valvular "ball-valve" obstruction, embolization, or a syndrome of constitutional symptoms, such as fever and malaise the latter **most commonly due to cytokine interleukin-6.**

Morphology

- Always **single**
- **Fossa ovalis** in the **atrial septum** is the favored site of origin.
- Histologically, myxomas are composed of stellate or globular myxoma (**"lepidic"**) cells, embedded within an abundant acid **mucopolysaccharide ground substance** and covered on the surface by endothelium

Papillary Fibroelastoma

- Incidental, **sea-anemone-like lesions**, most often identified at autopsy[Q]
- >80% located on **valves**[Q] (**ventricular surfaces of semilunar valves & atrial surfaces of AV valves**)[Q]
- Resemble the much smaller, usually trivial, lambl excrescences

Rhabdomyoma

- **Most frequent primary tumor of the pediatric heart**[Q]
- Most common discovered in **first years** of life because of **obstruction of a valvular orifice**
- **Actually hamartomas**[Q] rather than true neoplasms as they **regress spontaneously.**[Q]
- 50% cases associated with **tuberous sclerosis**[Q]

- Usually **multiple** and involve the **ventricles**, protruding into the lumen
- **Histologically**: large, rounded, or polygonal cells containing numerous **glycogen-laden vacuoles** separated by strands of cytoplasm (**spider cells**)[Q]

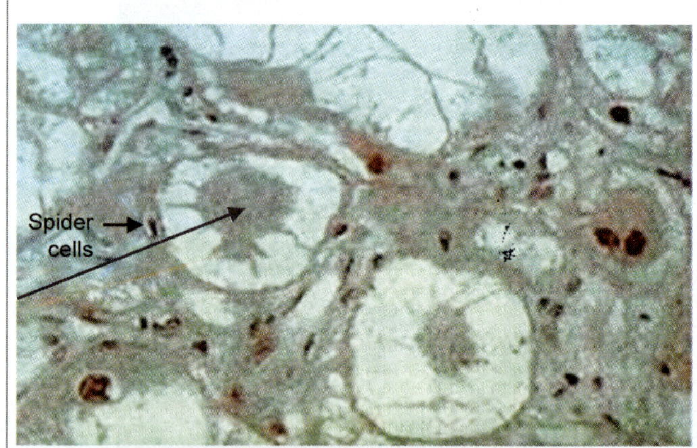

Large, polygonal cells ("spider cells") with glycogen vacuoles separated by strands of cytoplasm extending between cell membrane and nucleus

High Yield Facts

- The most common cardiac tumor is the **secondaries or metastasis.**[Q]
- The most common primary cardiac tumor in the adults is **the myxoma.**[Q]
- The most common cardiac tumor in the children is the **rhabdomyoma.**[Q]
- **Carney syndrome:** multiple cardiac & extracardiac myxomas, spotty pigmentation & endocrine overactivity
- **Carcinoid heart disease**[Q] typically causes abnormalities of the **right side of the heart.**[Q]
- **Familial syndromes associated with myxomas**
  - Activating mutations in the GNAS1 gene (in association with McCune-Albright syndrome)
  - Null mutations in PRKAR1A (Carney complex)[Q]

High Yield Facts

MC cause of *aortic aneusrysm*	Atherosclerosis[Q]	MC site of *Tuberculous aneurysms*	Thoracic aorta. (T for T)[Q]
MC *site of aneurysm caused by atherosclerosis*	Abdominal aorta (below renal artery and above bifurcation)[Q]	MC cause of *descending aortic aneusrysm*	Atherosclerosis[Q]
		MC site of *Syphilitic aneurysm*	Ascending aorta[Q]
MC cause of Thoracic Aortic Aneurysm	Hypertension[Q]	MC cause of *mycotic abdominal aneusrysm*	Salmonella gastroenteritis[Q]
MC cause of *ascending aortic aneusrysm*	Cystic medial degeneration[Q]/Systemic hypertension[Q]	MC site of *Traumatic aneurysms*	Descending thoracic aorta just below the site of insertion of ligamentum arteriosum.[Q]
MC cause of *aortic arch aneurysm*	Atherosclerosis[Q]	*Nutritional basis* for aneurysm formation	Scurvy[Q] Due to altered collagen cross-linking[Q] True aneurysm[Q]
MC site of *takayasu arteritis aneurysm*	Aortic arch[Q]		

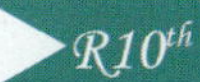 *R10th* **Latest** Update

c-ANCA and p-ANCA Disease Associations

Disease	c-ANCA (PR3) (%)	p-ANCA (MPO) (%)
GPA (WG)	66	24
MPA	26	58
EGPA (CSS)	<5	40

c-ANCA, cytoplasmic antineutrophil cytoplasmic antibody, EGPA (CSS), eosinophilic granulomatosis with polyangiitis (Churg-Strauss syndrome); GPA (WG), granulomatosis with polyangiitis (Wegener's granulomatosis); MPA, microscopic polyangiitis; MPO, myeloperoxidase; PR3, peroxidase-3.

 # NEXT Pattern Questions

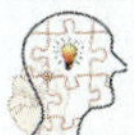 **Q's**

1. **A 32-year-old patient underwent renal Biopsy for nephrotic syndrome. Along with glomerular pathology, arterioles show the lesions as depicted in the histopathological picture. Identify the lesion.**

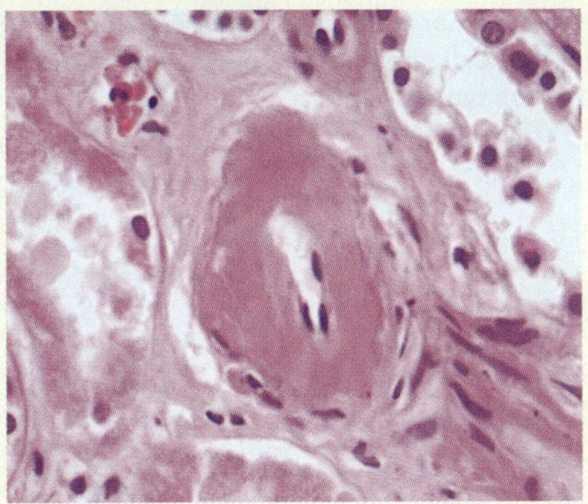

   a. Hyperplastic arteriolosclerosis
   b. Mönckeberg medial Sclerosis
   c. Hyaline arteriolosclerosis
   d. Atherosclerosis

Ans. (c) **Hyaline arteriolosclerosis**
   • Renal arterioles in diabetes show homogeneous pink deposits suggestive of **Hyaline arteriolosclerosis**

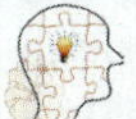 **Q's**

2. **A 40-year-old male patient presented with hypertension due to renal artery involvement, histological examination of the vessel is shown in the diagram. False statement regarding histological features is:**

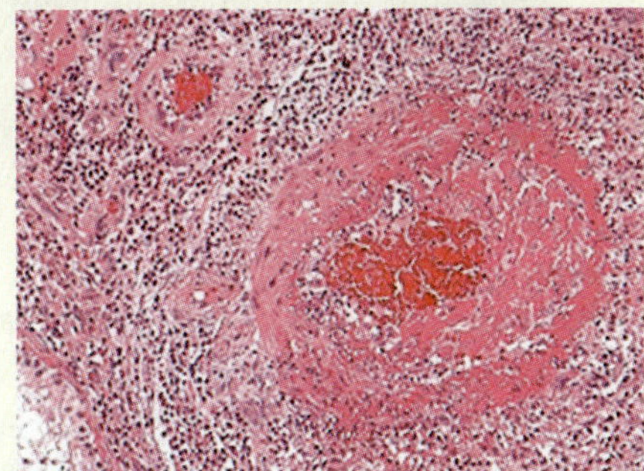

   a. Segmental transmural necrotizing inflammation of small- to medium-sized arteries
   b. In acute phase Fibrinoid necrosis can be seen
   c. Late stage show fibrosis, thrombosis
   d. All vessel or single vessel will be in same stage of inflammation

Ans. (d) **All vessel or single vessel will be in same stage of inflammation**
   • Here all stages of inflammation is seen, suggestive of PAN single stage of activity is seen in microscopic polyangitis.

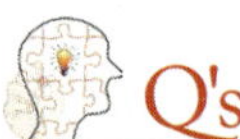

Q's

3. At what duration of myocardial infarction light microscopy demonstrate myocyte necrosis, hypereosinophilia, contraction band necrosis and intense neutrophil infiltrate

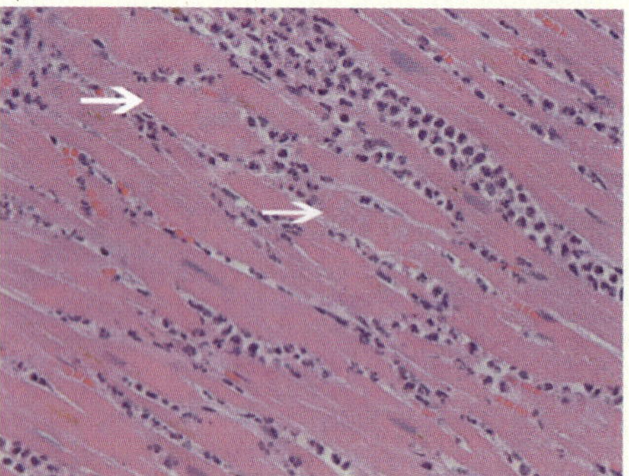

a. 4-6 hours	b. 12-24 hours
c. 1-3 days	d. 3-7 days

Ans. (c) 1-3 days

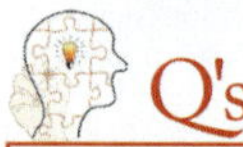

Q's

4. A 30-year-old male presented with severe dyspnea and fatigue. X-ray showed left atrial enlargement. Physician suspects the patient of having mitral stenosis and gets a histopath examination done, the image of which is shown, it shows?

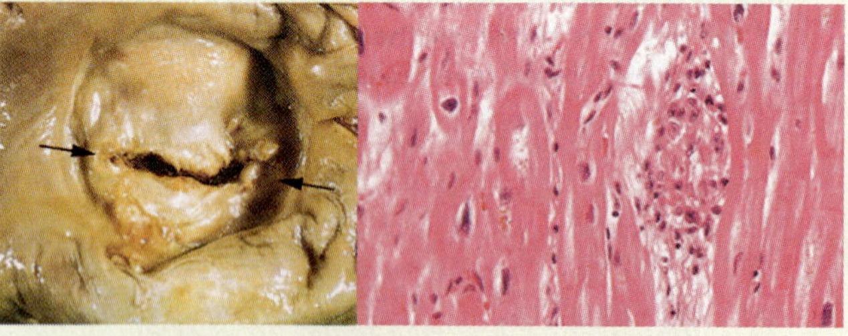

a. Sarcoidosis	b. Tuberculosis
c. Aschoff bodies	d. Fungal granuloma

Ans. (c) Aschoff bodies

- As you see the history of severe dyspnea and fatigue, X-ray showed left atrial enlargement, patient of having mitral stenosis. The gross image of valve shows fish mouth appearance and histopathology of the same shows Aschoff bodies.

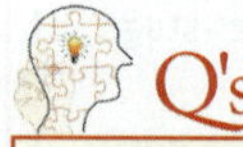

Q's

5. Vegetations of the following endocarditis has the maximum chances of embolization:
   a. Rheumatic heart disease
   b. Infective endocarditis
   c. Libman–Sacks endocarditis
   d. Subacute bacterial endocarditis

Ans. (b) Infective endocarditis

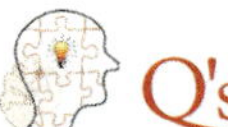

Q's

6. The swelling of size 1.5 cm is seen over chest of 20-year-old, soft to firm reddish swelling, progressing in size. Histopathological examination showed the following. What could be your possible diagnosis?

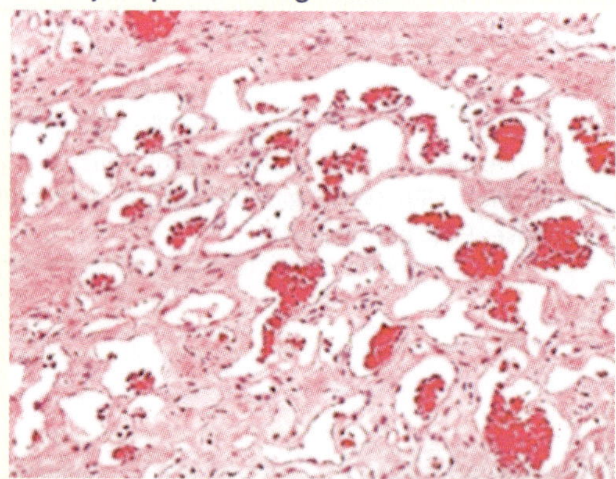

a. Hemangioma	b. Fibroadenoma
c. Lipoma	d. Dermatofibroma

Ans. (a) Hemangioma

- Soft to firm reddish swelling, progressing in size suggestive of hemangioma.

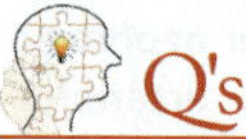

Q's

7. A 55-year-old female patient having large adnexal mass with raised inhibin level. Histopathology shows cord and sheets of tumor cell, often showing nuclear groove as shown in the diagram, based on the above clinical features identify the type of tumor.

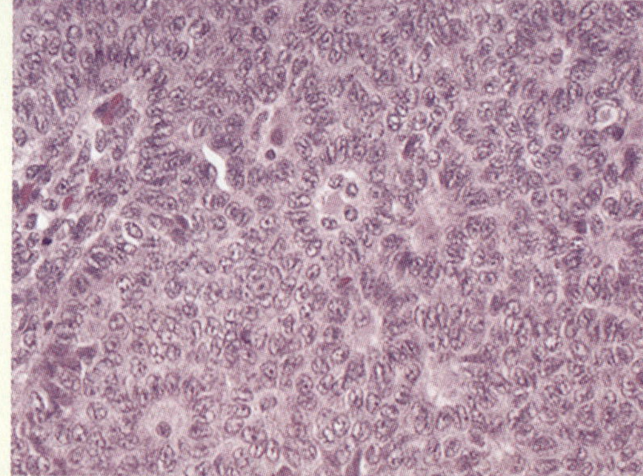

a. Choriocarcinoma
b. Granulosa cell tumor
c. Yolk sac tumor
d. Leydig cell tumor

Ans. (b) Granulosa cell tumor

- Large adnexal mass with raised inhibin level is suggestive of granulosa cell tumor. Histopathology shows cord and sheets of tumor cell, often showing nuclear groove suggestive of Call-Exner body seen in Granulosa cell tumor.

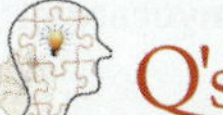

8. Post surgery image of a tumor in scrotum is shown below along with its histology. What could be your possible diagnosis?

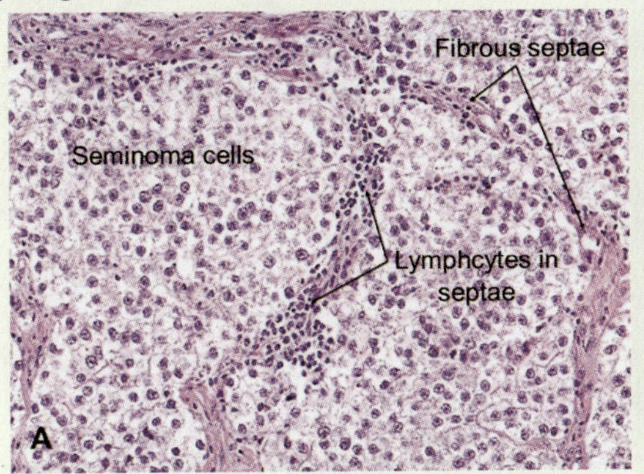

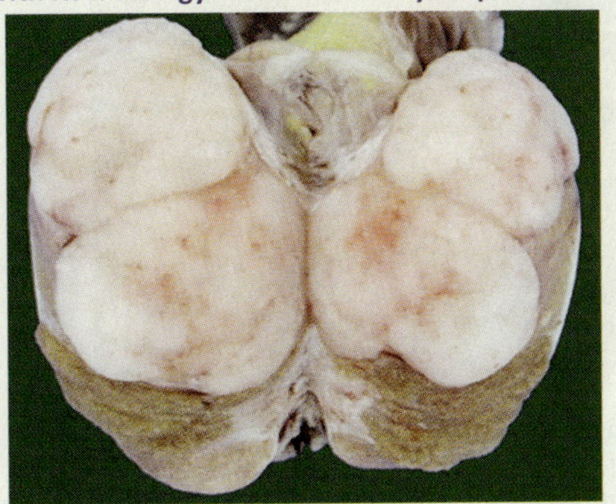

a. Teratoma   b. Seminoma   c. Yolk sac tumor   d. Lymphoma

Ans. (b) Seminoma

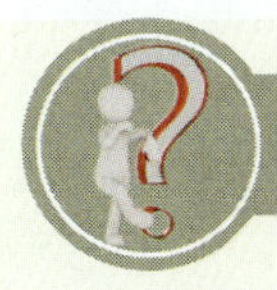

Image-Based Questions

1. A 45-year-old male presented with pulseless disease. On examination, following histopathological finding will be seen

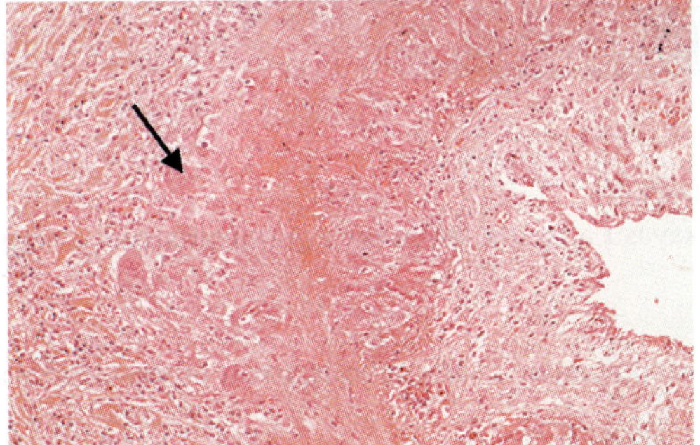

a. Granulomatous vasculitis   b. Fibrinoid necrosis
c. Leucocytoclastic vasculitis   d. Thromboangitis obliterans

2. A patient is a known case of polyarteritis nodosa. On examination of biopsy, accumulation of amorphous, basic, proteinaceous material in the vessel wall was seen. This finding is suggestive of:

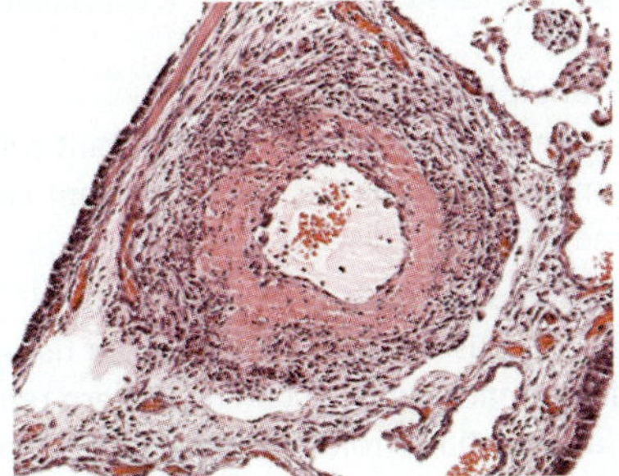

a. Fibrinoid necrosis   b. Leucocytoclastic vasculitis
c. Hyaline arteriosclerosis   d. Caseous necrosis

3. **A 34-year-old male patient presented with following clinical feature. Diagnosis**

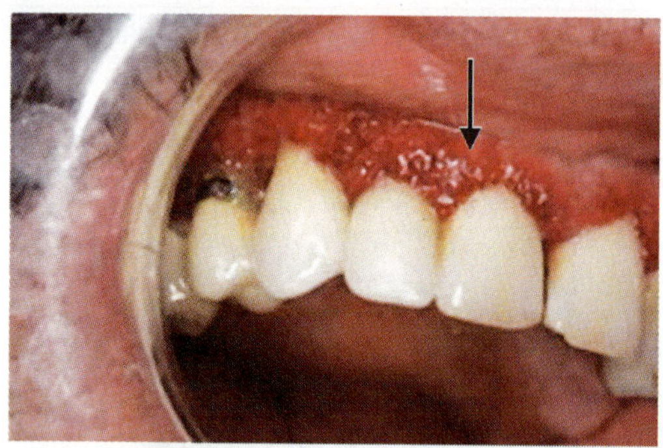

a. Kawasaki disease   b. PAN
c. MicroPAN   d. Wegener's granulomatosis

4. **A 15-year-old boy presented with pancarditis, on myocardial biopsy, following finding was seen. Diagnosis?**

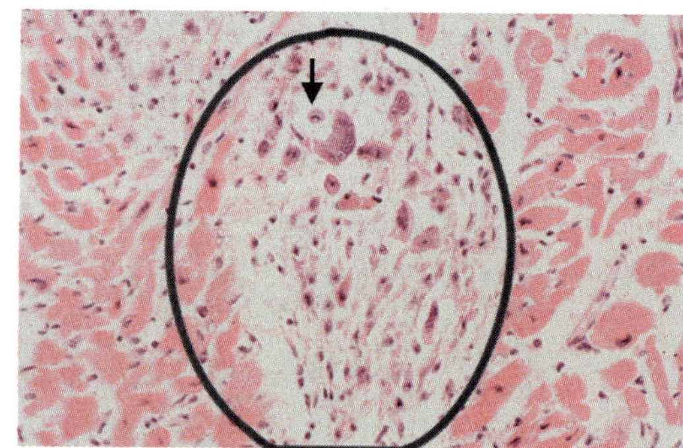

a. Aschoff nodule   b. TB
c. FB giant cells   d. None

5. **A 25-year-old male presented with growth in left atrium. Diagnosis?**

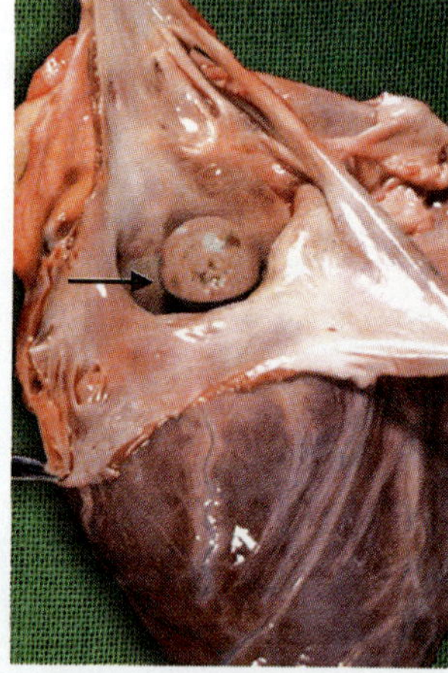

a. Rhabdomyoma   b. Myxoma
c. Metastasis   d. Papillary elastosis

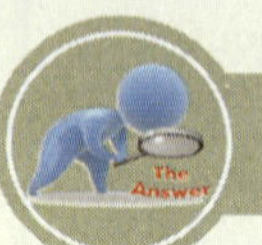

Answers of Image-Based Questions

1. **Ans. (a) Granulomatous vasculitis**
   - Here we can see epithelioid cells and giant cells s/o granulomatous vasculitis
   - Granulomatous vasculitis is seen in : Giant cell (temporal) arteritis, Takayasu arteritis, Wegener's granulomatosis, Churg-Strauss syndrome, Buerger's disease

2. **Ans. (a) Fibrinoid necrosis**
   - Fibrinoid necrosis is a form of necrosis, or tissue death, in which there is accumulation of amorphous, basic, proteinaceous material in the tissue matrix with a staining pattern reminiscent of fibrin.
   - How to differentiate from hyaline arteriosclerosis?- please remember in fibrinoid necrosis, pink material has fibrin like quality as opposed to glassy homogenous hyaline in hyaline arteriosclerosis. (refer to image 2)

3. **Ans. (d) Wegener's granulomatosis**
   - This is strawberry gums, seen in wegener's granulomatosis

4. **Ans. (a) Aschoff nodule**
   - Here one can see collection of foci of swollen eosinophilic collagen surrounded by : Lymphocytes (primary T cells), Occasional plasma cells, Aschoff giant cells[Q] (macrophages of rheumatic fever)[Q] and Antischkow cells (cells with caterpillar like chromatin marked with an arrow)

5. **Ans. (b) Myxoma**
   - The left atrium has been opened to reveal the most common primary cardiac neoplasm-an atrial myxoma. These benign masses are most often attached to the atrial wall. They can produce a "ball valve" effect by intermittently occluding the atrioventricular valve orifice.

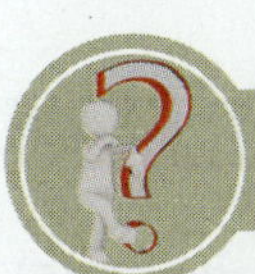

Multiple Choice Questions

BLOOD VESSELS

SCLEROSIS INCLUDING ATHEROSCLEROSIS

1. Cleft like space in atheromatous plaque mainly contains? *(Recent Question 2016)*
a. Smooth muscle cell
b. Fibrous tissue
c. Cholesterol
d. Macrophages

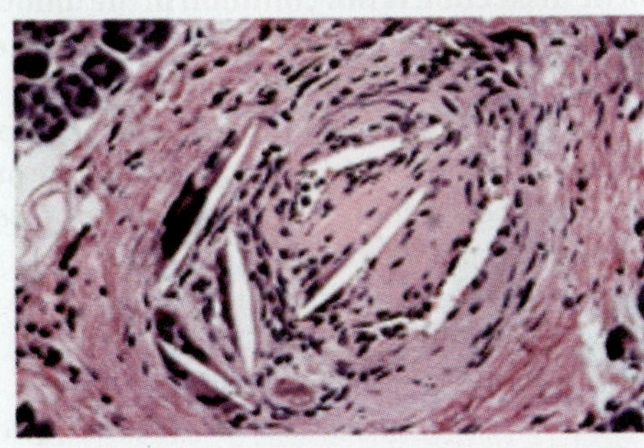

2. Atherosclerosis causes fibroblast plaque formation by injury to? *(Recent Question 2015)*
a. Endothelium
b. Fibroblast
c. Macrophage
d. Smooth muscle cells

3. The following arteries are usually spared from extensive atherosclerosis *(Recent Question 2015)*
a. Popliteal artery
b. Internal carotid artery
c. Arteries of circle of willis
d. Mesenteric arteries

4. The necrotic core of an atherosclerotic plaque contains
a. T cells
b. Collagen
c. Lipid
d. None of the above

5. True about atherosclerosis *(Recent Question 2014-15)*
a. Chronic inflammatory disorder of vessel wail
b. Not lead to complications of vessel wall
c. Thoracic aorta more than abdominal aorta
d. Atherosclerostic plaques do not demonstrate extracellular matrix deposition

6. The coronary artery most commonly involved in atherosclerosis *(Recent Question 2015)*
a. Left anterior descending artery
b. Left main coronary artery
c. Right coronary artery
d. Circumflex coronary artery

7. Not true about monkeberg medial sclerosis *(Recent Question 2015)*
a. Calcification of the walls of muscular arteries
b. Typically involving the internal elastic membrane
c. Persons older than age 50 are most commonly affected
d. Calcifications cause significant narrowing of vessel lumen

8. Foam cells in atherosclerosis contain lipid in the form of *(Recent Question 2014-15)*
a. Oxidized LDL
b. Reduced LDL
c. Oxidized VLDL
d. Reduced VLDL

9. Following are the modifiable risk factor of atherosclerosis except *(Recent Question 2014-15)*
a. Physical inactivity
b. Family history
c. Diabetes
d. Hypertension

10. True about the basic structure of artherosclerosis plaque is- *(Recent Question 2014-15)*
a. Concave part formed by fibrous cap
b. Convex part formed by tunica media of the vessel
c. Convex part formed by fibrous cap
d. Necrotic core contains collagen, elastin and proteoglycans

11. Atherosclerosis initiation by fibroblast plaque is mediated by injury to *(Recent Question 2014-15)*
a. Smooth muscle
b. Media
c. Adventitia
d. Endothelium

12. Atheromatous changes of blood vessels affects early in: *(Recent Question 2015)*
a. Kidney
b. Heart
c. Liver
d. Spleen

13. Medial calcification is seen in: *(Recent Question 2015)*
a. Atherosclerosis
b. Arteriolosclerosis
c. Monckebergs sclerosis
d. Dissecting aneurysm

14. Changes seen in-atherosclerotic plaque at the time of rupture, are all except: *(Recent Question 2014)*
a. Thin fibrotic cap
b. Multiple foam cap
c. Smooth muscle cell hypertrophy
d. Cell debris

15. Infective agent causing atherosclerosis *(Recent Question 2014)*
a. M. Pneumoniae
b. C. Pneumoniae
c. H. Influenza
d. C. Diphtheriae

16. In atherosclerosis, increased LDL in monocyte macrophage due to: *(DPG 10, PGI June 99)*
a. LDL receptors on macrophage
b. LDL receptors on endothelium
c. Lipids in LDL get oxidized
d. All of the above

HYPERTENSION

17. Characteristic histological finding in benign hypertension *(Recent Question 2015)*
a. Proliferative end arteritis
b. Necrotizing arteriolitis
c. Hyaline arteriosclerosis
d. Cystic medial necrosis

18. Which of the following is seen in kidney in malignant hypertension? *(Recent Question 2014-15)*
a. Hyaline necrosis
b. Fibrinoid necrosis
c. Medial wall hyperplasia
d. Microaneurysm

19. Onion peeling of renal vessels is seen in: *(Recent Question 2014)*
a. Benign hypertension
b. Malignant hypertension
c. Diabetic nephropathy
d. SLE

20. In a specimen of kidney, fibrinoid necrosis is seen and onion peel appearance is also present. Most probable pathology is: *(AIIMS May 2013)*
- a. Hyaline degeneration
- b. Hyperplastic arteriosclerosis
- c. Glomerulosclerosis
- d. Fibrillary glomerulonephritis

21. Typical histology in benign hypertension? *(JIPMER 2013)*
- a. Intimal proliferation and hyalinization of media of medium arteries
- b. Fibrinoid necrosis of small arteries
- c. Loss of endothelial cells of arterioles
- d. Formation of new vessels

22. Onion skin thickening of arteriolar wall is seen in:
- a. Atherosclerosis *(Recent Question 2013, DNB 10)*
- b. Median calcific sclerosis
- c. Hyaline arteriosclerosis
- d. Hyperplastic arteriosclerosis

ANEURYSMS

23. Syphilitic aneurysm is seen most commonly in? *(Recent Question 2016-17)*
- a. Ascending aorta
- b. Arch of aorta
- c. Descending aorta
- d. Abdominal aorta

24. Which of the following causes pseudoaneurysm?
- a. Trauma *(Recent Question 2015)*
- b. Atherosclerosis
- c. Congenital disease
- d. Infection

25. In Marfan syndrome, rupture of aortic aneurysm usually occurs at *(Recent Question 2015)*
- a. Ascending aorta
- b. Descending aorta
- c. Arch of aorta
- d. Abdominal aorta

26. For asymptomatic abdominal aortic aneurysm surgery is indicated if the size is greater than *(Recent Question 2015)*
- a. 4 cm
- b. 4.5 cm
- c. 5 cm
- d. 5.5 cm

27. Risk of aneurysm rupture is > 25% per year when the size is greater than *(Recent Question 2015)*
- a. 4 cm
- b. 6 cm
- c. 7 cm
- d. 8 cm

28. Most common cause of aneurysm *(Recent Question 2015)*
- a. Syphillis
- b. Atherosclerosis
- c. Cystic medial necrosis
- d. Hypertension

29. Which of the following is not a cause of aneurysm?
- a. Atherosclerosis *(Recent Question 2014)*
- b. Cystic medial necrosis
- c. Syphillis
- d. Mockenbergs sclerosis

30. Visceral aneurysm is most commonly seen in: *(Recent Question 2013)*
- a. Splenic
- b. Renal
- c. Hepatic
- d. Coronary

DISSECTIONS

31. IOC for acute aortic dissection
- a. MRI *(Recent Question 2015)*
- b. MD- CT scan
- c. Transesophageal echocardiography
- d. X-ray

32. Most common predisposing factor for aortic dissection *(Recent Question 2015)*
- a. Atherosclerosis
- b. Syphilis
- c. Hypertension
- d. Smoking

33. Aortic dissection is not common in the following disease *(Recent Question 2015)*
- a. Marfan syndrome
- b. Hypertension
- c. Cystic medial necrosis
- d. Secondary syphilis

34. Classification of aortic dissection depends upon-
- a. Cause of dissection *(Recent Question 2014)*
- b. Level of aorta affected
- c. Percentage of aorta affected
- d. None

35. Cystic medical necrosis is seen in- *(Recent Question 2013)*
- a. Marfans
- b. Friedrichs ataxia Pattern
- c. Downs
- d. Kawasaki

36. Most common cause of dissecting hematoma is because of- *(Recent Question 2016-17)*
- a. Hypertension
- b. Marfan's
- c. Iatrogenic
- d. Kawasaki

VASCULITIS

37. Small vessel vasculitis is/are? *(PGI May 2017)*
- a. Anti GBM ab
- b. Takayasu arteritis
- c. Kawasaki disease
- d. Carcinoma induced vasculitis
- e. IgA vasculitis

38. True about Takayasu is all except? *(PGI Nov 2016)*
- a. Causes transmural granuloma
- b. Granulomatous vasculitis
- c. Medium to small vessel
- d. Called aortoarteritis

39. All are true about Kawasaki disease except?
- a. Thrombocytopenia *(Recent Question 2016)*
- b. Dequamation rashes on trunk
- c. Fever
- d. Conjunctival congestion

40. Berger disease does not involve *(Recent Question 2016)*
- a. Artery
- b. Veins
- c. Nerve
- d. Lymphatics

41. Which one is found in HSP? *(Recent Question 2016)*
- a. IgA
- b. IgM
- c. Ig G
- d. IgE

42. Which of the following is non-granulomatous arteritis? *(Recent Question 2016)*
- a. Takayasu
- b. Wegeners
- c. Churgstrauss
- d. Classical PAN

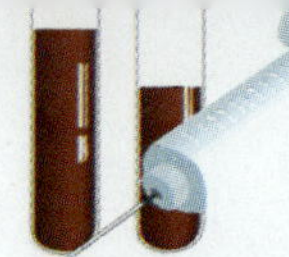

43. **HSP is characterized by all except?** *(APPGMEE 2015)*
   a. Glomerulonephritis
   b. Hematochezia
   c. Thrombocytopenia
   d. Palpable purpura

44. **c-ANCA is positive in** *(Recent Question 2015)*
   a. Microscopic Polyangitis
   b. Wegener's Granulomatosis
   c. Churg Strauss Syndrome
   d. Behcet's syndrome

45. **Arterial biopsy of elderly male shows fragmentation of elastic lamina, lymphocyte infiltration and giant cells**
   (Recent Question 2014-15)
   a. Temporal arteritis
   b. Takayasu disease
   c. Polyarteritisnodosa
   d. Kawasaki disease

46. **Temporal arteritis all are associated except**
   a. Elderly patient *(Recent Question 2014-15)*
   b. Low ESR
   c. Giant cells
   d. Polymyalgia rheumatica

47. **Fibrinoid necrosis is seen in** *(Recent Question 2014-15)*
   a. Polyarteritis nodosa
   b. SLE
   c. HIV
   d. Sarcoidosis

48. **Silk Road disease is** *(Recent Question 2015)*
   a. Behçet's syndrome
   b. Giant cell arteritis
   c. Henoch schonlein purpura
   d. Wegener's granulomatosis

49. **Which is not a characteristic of wegeners granulomatosis:**
   a. Granuloma in vessel wall *(Recent Question 2015)*
   b. Focal necrotising glomerulonephritis
   c. Positive for cANCA
   d. Involves large vessels

50. **Frequency of renal involvement in HSP**
   (Recent Question 2015)
   a. 20-40%
   b. >80%
   c. 40-60%
   d. 10%

51. **ANCA positive vasculitis –** *(Recent Question 2014)*
   a. Henoch schonlein purpura
   b. Behcet's syndrome
   c. Wegener's granulomatosis
   d. None

52. **Fibrinoid necrosis with neutrophilic infiltration is seen in:**
   a. PAN *(Recent Question 2014)*
   b. Giant cell arteritis
   c. Takayasu arteritis
   d. Wegener's granulomatosis

53. **Necrotizing arterioritis with fibrinoid necrosis is:**
   a. Immediate hypersensitivity *(Recent Question 2014)*
   b. Cell mediated immunity
   c. Antigen-antibody complex mediated
   d. Cytotoxic cell mediated

54. **Which is associated with vasculitis of medium size vessels** *(Recent Question 2014)*
   a. Temporal arteritis
   b. Wegners granulomatosis
   c. Classic PAN
   d. Tuberous sclerosis

55. **All is true about Giant cell arteritis except**
   (Recent Question 2014)
   a. Involves large to small sized areteries
   b. Granulomatous inflammation
   c. Most commonly involved artery is abdominal aorta
   d. Segmental nature of the involvement

56. **In Wegener's granulomatosis cytoplasmic anti neutro-philic antibodies are directed against**
   (Recent Question 2014)
   a. Proteinase 1
   b. Proteinase 2 June 08
   c. Proteinase 3
   d. Proteinase 4

57. **Microscopic polyangiitis is characterized by the following features EXCEPT** *(APPGMEE 14)*
   a. Involves small and medium sized arteries and veins
   b. 75% cases are associated with ANCA positivity
   c. Palpable purpura, ulcers and vesiculo bullous lesion
   d. Unlikely to cause pulmonary renal syndrome

58. **In PAN, cysts are seen in all except:**
   (Recent Question 13, AI 00,95)
   a. Lung
   b. Pancreas
   c. Liver
   d. Heart

59. **In Wegeners glomerulonephritis characteristic feature seen is:** *(AIIMS Nov 10, Nov 09)*
   a. Granuloma in the vessel wall
   b. Focal necrotizing glomerulonephritis
   c. Nodular glomerulosclerosis
   d. Interstitial granuloma

60. **Which of the following is not a common cause of vasculitis in adults:** *(DNB June 10)*
   a. Giant cell arteritis
   b. Kawasaki disease
   c. Henoch schonlein purpura
   d. Polyarteritis nodosa

VASCULAR TUMORS

61. **The swelling of size 1.5 cm is seen over chest of 20 year old, soft to firm reddish swelling, progressing in size. Histopathological examination showed the following. What could be your possible diagnosis?**
   (Recent exam 2018)

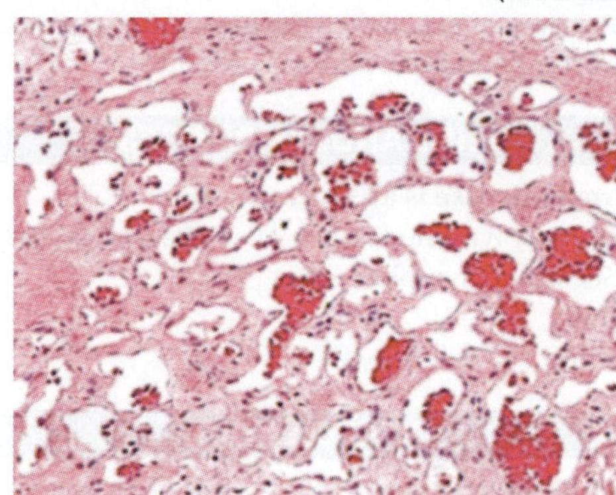

   a. Hemangioma
   b. Fibroadenoma
   c. Lipoma
   d. Dermatofibroma

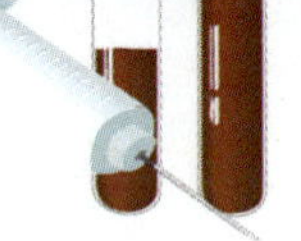

62. Kaposi sarcoma true is? *(PGI Nov 2015)*
a. Causative agent HHV 8
b. Can be Seen in depressed cell mediated immunity
c. Treatment is chemotherapy and surgery
d. Vascular tumor

63. Portwine stain is *(Recent Question 2015)*
a. Capillary hemangioma
b. Cavernous hemangioma
c. Lymphangioma
d. Vascular ectasias

64. Multifocal tumor of vascular origin in a patient with AIDS: *(Recent Question 2015)*
a. Astrocytoma
b. Gastric Carcinoma
c. Kaposi sarcoma
d. Primary CNS lymphoma

65. Find the true statement *(Recent Question 2015)*
a. Classic Kaposi sarcoma is associated with HIV
b. HAART therapy has decreased AIDS associated KS
c. Transplant associated AIDS-visceral involvement
d. Lymphadenopathic KS–extensive skin lesions

66. Fish hook pattern of capillaries is seen in *(Recent Question 2015)*
a. Capillary hemangioma
b. Cavernous hemangioma
c. Angiosarcoma
d. Hemangiopericytoma

67. Pathological feature of pyogenic granuloma: *(Recent Question 2015)*
a. Epitheloid cells
b. Capillary hemangioma
c. Granulation tissue
d. Giant cells

68. Most common site of Angiosarcoma is: *(Recent Question 2014)*
a. Liver
b. Lung
c. Kidney
d. Lip

69. CD marker of Angiosarcoma is? *(Recent Question 2013)*
a. CD 10
b. CD 19
c. CD25
d. CD 31

70. Spontaneous regression can occur with:
a. Cavernous hemangioma *(Recent Question 2013)*
b. Strawberry angioma
c. Nevus flemes
d. None of the above

71. True about Giant aneurysm: *(Recent Question 2013)*
a. Rarely rupture
b. Most common in middle cerebral artery
c. Pressure effect is often the presenting symptom
d. Thromboembolic phase is present

VEINS AND LYMPHATICS

72. Milroy's disease is an example of:
a. Primary lymphedema *(Recent Question 2015)*
b. Secondary lymphedema
c. Both
d. None

MISCELLENOUS

73. The following in not an aging change in heart
a. Increased LA cavity size *(Recent Question 2015)*
b. Increased LV cavity size
c. Sigmoid-shaped ventricular septum
d. Lambl excrescences

74. Raynaud's phenomenon what change is seen in vessels initial stage: *(Recent Question 2014)*
a. No change
b. Thrombosis
c. Fibrinoid necrosis
d. Hyaline sclerosis

75. Raynaud's phenomenon is seen in: *(PGI May 10)*
a. SIB
b. Systemic sclerosis
c. DM
d. Hypertension

CARDIOVASCULAR SYSTEM

HEART FAILURE

76. Heart failure cells are seen in *(Recent Question 2015)*
a. Kidney
b. Heart
c. Lungs
d. Brain

77. Commonest cause of right ventricular failure is:
a. Cor pulmonale *(AIIMS 14)*
b. Pulmonary involvement
c. Endomyocardial fibrosi
d. Left ventricular failure

78. Heart failure cells are: *(Recent Question 2013)*
a. Lipofuscin granules in cardiac cells
b. Pigmented alveolar macrophages
c. Pigmented pancreatic acinar cells
d. Pigment cells seen in liver

ISCHEMIC HEART DISEASE

79. Cardiac biopsy of a patient who died following myocardial infarction is shown below. What is the finding is a feature of reperfusion injury?
(Recent Pattern Question 2020)

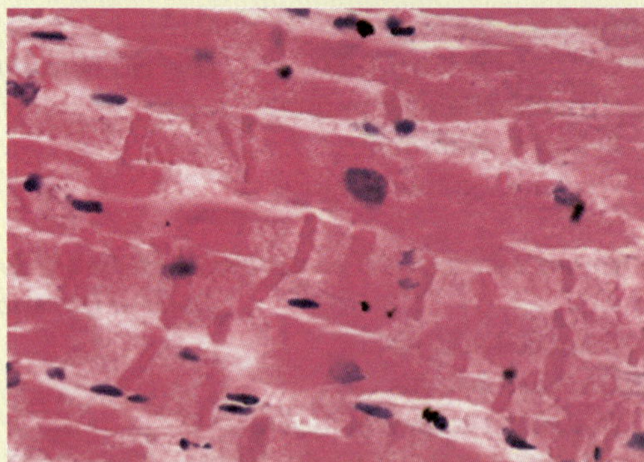

a. Waviness of fibers
b. Neutrophils in cardiac muscle
c. Eosinophilic contraction bands
d. Swelling of cells

80. Autopsy specimen of the heart of a patient who died due to myocardial infraction was stained with triphenyltetrazolium chloride dye. Colour of normal part of the heart will be:- *(AIIMS Nov 16)*
a. Blue
b. White
c. Red
d. Dark brown

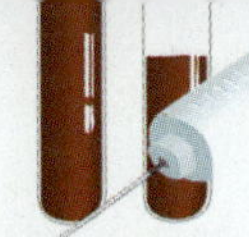

81. **Given below is the histology of heart from a patient who died of Myo cardial infarction. What is the time elapsed after MI?** *(AIIMS May 16)*

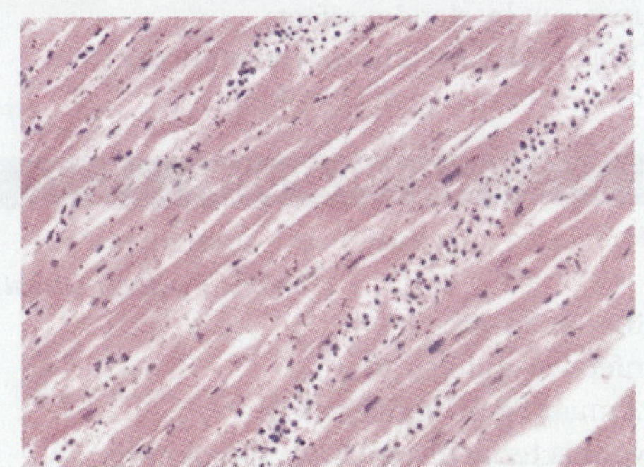

   a. 1-2 days   b. 7 days
   c. 6 hr   d. 2-3 weeks

82. **A 55 years old male presents with severe chest pain radiating to the left arm. ECG shows ST segment elevation in the V4, V5 and V6 leads. CK-MB and troponin levels are found to be increased. The most likely cause for the increase in enzyme in serum is** *(Recent Question 2016-17, JIPMER May 2015)*
   a. Clumping of nuclear chromatin
   b. Lysosomal Autophagy
   c. Mitochondrial swelling   d. Cell membrane defects

83. **Irreversible change in ischemia of heart occurs in?** *(Recent Question 2016-17)*
   a. 10 min   b. 30 min
   c. 60 min   d. 90 min

84. **Recurrent ischaemic events following thrombosis have been pathophysiologically linked to** *(Recent Question 2016)*
   a. Antibodies to thrombolytic agents
   b. Fibrinopeptide A
   c. Lipoprotein A   d. Triglycerides

85. **Post mortem finding in a case of death due to myocardial infarction is?** *(Recent Question 2015)*
   a. Fat necrosis   b. Caseous necrosis
   c. Liquefactive necrosis   d. Coagulative necrosis

86. **Autopsy diagnosis of myocardial infarction can be done by immersion of tissue slices in a solution of** *(Recent Question 2015)*
   a. Triphenyl tetrazolium chloride
   b. 100% alcohol
   c. Orcein stain
   d. Crystal violet

87. **Due to ischemia, irreversible cell injury to cardiac myocytes occur in** *(Recent Question 2015)*
   a. <2 minutes   b. 10-20 minutes
   c. 20-40 minutes   d. >1 hour

88. **Earliest light microscopic change in myocardial infarction** *(Recent Question 2015)*
   a. Waviness of fibres   b. Neutrophilic infiltration
   c. Coagulation necrosis   d. Contraction band necrosis

89. **The cells seen after 14 hours in the infarcted area in MI are:** *(Recent Question 2015)*
   a. Neutrophils   b. Lymphocytes
   c. Macrophages   d. Monocytes

90. **The type of necrosis in myocardial infarction is** *(APPGMEE 14)*
   a. Caseous   b. Coagulative
   c. Liquefactive   d. Fibrinoid

91. **Which of the following is a non-modifiable risk factor for CHD:** *(Recent Question 2013)*
   a. Diabetes   b. Smoking
   c. Hypertension   d. Old age

92. **Most common site of artery of atherosclerosis:** *(Recent Question 2013)*
   a. LAD   b. RCA
   c. LCX   d. Diagonal branch of LAD

93. **Fatal arrythmias are seen if myocardial infarction is:** *(Recent Question 2013)*
   a. Posterior   b. Inferior
   c. Anterolateral   d. Subendodardial

94. **A 45 years old male had severe chest pain and was admitted to the hospital with a diagnosis of acute myocardial infarction. Four days later he died and autopsy showed transmural coagulative necrosis. Which of the following microscopic features will be seen on further examination?** *(AIIMS May 11, AI 09)*
   a. Fibroblast and collegen
   b. Granulation tissue
   c. Neutrophilic infiltration surrounding coagulatives
   d. Granulomatous inflammation

95. **Approximate time, at the end of which the quantity, of ATPwithin ischemic cardiac myocytes is reduced to 10% of original is:** *(Karn 11)*
   a. <2 minutes   b. 10 minutes
   c. 20 minutes   d. 40 minutes

96. **Autopsy finding after 12 hrs in a case of death due to M.1.** *(MAHE 05, DPG 10)*
   a. Caseous necrosis
   b. Coagulative necrosis
   c. Fat necrosis
   d. Liquefactive necrosis

RHEUMATIC FEVER AND RHEUMATIC HEART DISEASE

97. **30 years old male presented with severe dyspnoea and fatigue. X-ray showed left atrial enlargement. Physician suspects the patient of having mitral stenosis and gets a histopath exam ination done, the image of which is shown, it shows?** *(AIIMS Nov 2017)*

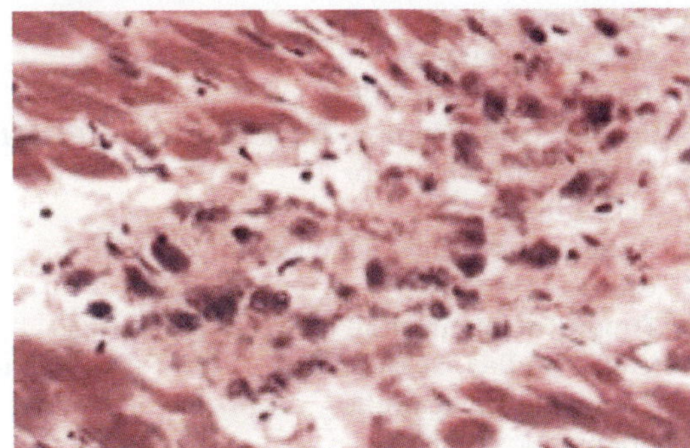

   a. Sarcoidosis   b. Tuberculosis
   c. Aschoff bodies   d. Fungal granuloma

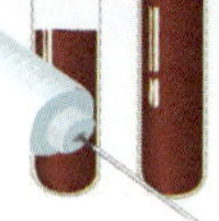

98. Pathological feature(s) of rheumatic heart disease is/ are? *(PGI Nov 2017)*
a. Widened mitral annulus
b. McCallum plaques
c. Rupture of papillary muscle
d. Aschoff nodules

99. Gross findings of heart form a 18 yrs /F presented with history of sore throat 3m back & joint pains has been shown below . On auscultatory finding a murmer was noted. What is your diagnosis. *(AIIMS May 16)*

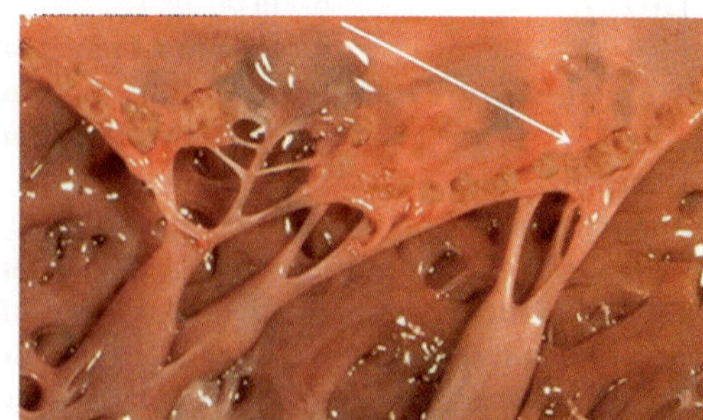

a. Libman sach endocarditis
b. Infective endocarditis
c. Rheumatic carditis
d. Marantic carditis

100. In Rheumatic carditis, Mc callums patch is seen in sub-endothelium of? *(Recent Question 2015)*
a. Right atrium
b. Right Ventricle
c. Left atrium
d. Left ventricle

101. Cells forming aschoff nodules are all the following except *(Recent Question 2015)*
a. T cells
b. B cells
c. Plasma cells
d. Macrophages

102. Causative organism of rheumatic fever *(Recent Question 2014-15)*
a. Group A Streptococci
b. Staphylococci
c. Group B Streptococci
d. Group D Streptococci

103. Anitschkow cells are found in? *(Recent Question 2014)*
a. Rheumatoid nodule
b. Rheumatic myocarditis
c. Bacterial Endocarditis
d. Libman sachs endocarditis

104. McCallum's patch is diagnostic of *(Recent Question 2013)*
a. Infective endocarditis
b. Rheumatic endocarditis
c. Myocardial infarction
d. Tetralogy of Fallot (ToF)

105. Feature of acute rheumatic fever includes: *(PGI May12)*
a. Carey coombs murmur
b. Pancarditis
c. Always cause residual it disease
d. Chorea
e. Streptococcal infection

106. Aschoff's bodies are seen in: *(Jipmer 11)*
a. Rheumatic myocarditis
b. Rheumatic arthritis
c. Bacterial endocarditis
d. Marantic endocarditis *Endocarditis*

107. What is the mechanism of acute rheumatic fever *(AIIMS May 10)*
a. Cross reactivity with endogenous antigen
b. Innocent by slender effect
c. Due to toxin secretion by streptococci
d. Release of pyrogenic cytokines

ENDOCARDITIS

108. Bulky friable vegetations are seen in: *(Recent Pattern Question 2020)*
a. Rheumatic carditis
b. Infective endocarditis
c. Libman-Sacks endocarditis
d. Nonbacterial thrombotic endocarditis

109. Libman-Sacks endocarditis most commonly causes *(Recent Question 2015)*
a. Mitral regurgitation
b. Mitral stenosis
c. Tricuspid regurgitation
d. Aortic regurgitation

110. Small warty vegetations seen on the under surfaces of AV valves, valvular endocardium, chords or mural endocardium of atria or ventricles is characteristic of
a. Libman sack endocarditis *(Recent Question 2015)*
b. Nonbacterial thrombotic endocarditis
c. Infective endocarditis
d. Rheumatic fever

111. Vegetations of the following endocarditis has the maximum chances of embolization
a. Rheumatic heart disease *(Recent Question 2015)*
b. Infective endocarditis
c. Libman-sacks endocarditis
d. Subacute bacterial endocarditis

112. Non-bacterial thrombotic endocarditis is seen in
a. Rheumatic fever *(Recent Question 2015)*
b. Systemic lupus erythematosus
c. Rheumatoid arthritis
d. Mucinous adenocarcinoma of pancreas

113. Non sterile vegetation is seen in
a. Libmann sack's endocarditis *(Recent Question 2015)*
b. Marantic endocarditis
c. Infective endocarditis
d. Rheumatic heart disease

114. Libmann sack endocarditis is seen in
a. Rheumatic fever *(Recent Question 2015)*
b. SLE
c. AML M3
d. Mucinous adenocarcinoma of pancreas

115. Which type of endocarditis has vegetation on both sides of the valves: *(Recent Question 2015)*
a. Infective endocarditis
b. Libman Sack'endocarditis
c. RF
d. None

116. Sterile vegetations are seen in all except- *(DNB Nov. 12 Pattern)*
a. SLE
b. Infective endocarditis
c. Rheumatic fever
d. Marantic endocarditis

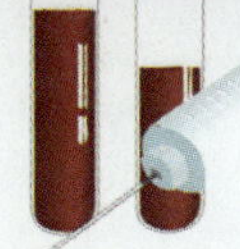

117. Which of the following is associated with destruction of valves? *(Recent Question 2016-17)*
a. Acute infective endocarditis
b. Libman sach's endocarditis
c. Rheumatic Heart disease
d. All

118. Flat vegetations in pockets of valves are due to
a. Rheumatic heart disease *(DNB Dec 11)*
b. Libman sacks Endocarditis
c. NBTE
d. Infective endocarditis

119. In which of the following vegetation are friable and easily detachable from the cardiac valves: *(AI 10)*
a. Rheumatic fever   b. Rheumatoid heart
c. SIB   d. Infective endocarditi

CARDIOMYOPATHY

120. Match the followings: *(AIIMS Nov 2019)*

Column A	Column B
a. Box car nuclei	1. HOCM
b. Myocyte disarray	2. Hypertension
c. Vacuolation in myocytes	3. DCM
	4. Subendothelial ischemia
d. Myocyte hypertrophy	5. Hypersensitive myocarditis

121. A patient had a quarrel with his brother with heightened emotion and falls suddenly and died. Most likely Cause of death in this case is ? *(AIIMS May 18)*
a. Arrhythmogenic right ventricle cardiomyopathy
b. Takotsubo cardiomyopathy
c. Dilated cardiomyopathy
d. Chronic ischemic cardiomyopathy.

122. Dilated cardiomyopathy, gene altered is? *(WBPGMEE 2016, MHPGMEE 2016)*
a. Dystrophin   b. Titin
c. Sarcomere   d. Mitochondrial genes

123. Pathological features of hypertrophic cardiomyopathy?
a. Death occurs in young athletes *(PGI Nov 2015)*
b. Mostly are genetic
c. LV septa is involved
d. RA is involved
e. Treatment is ablation of septa

124. Histological finding of hypertrophic cardiomyopathy includes: *(PGI May 2015)*
a. Myocyte disaaray
b. Interstitial fibrosis
c. Amyloid deposition in muscle
d. Myocyte hypertrophy
e. Myocardial fibers are arranged in parallel pattern

125. True about features of Hypertrophic cardiomyopathy: *(PGI Nov 2011)*
a. Hypertrophy of ventricles without dilatation
b. Myocytolysis
c. Irregular arrangement of fibers
d. Asymmetrical septal hypertrophy
e. Myocarditis

126. Dilated cardiomyopathy is/are seen in infection with:
a. Ischemic heart disease *(PGI May 2011)*
b. Amyloidosis
c. Viral myocarditis
d. Alcoholic liver disease
e. Thyroid disease

127. Which one of the following is not a cause for restrictive cardiomyopathy: *(DNB Dec 11, AIIMS May 04)*
a. Alcohol
b. Hemochromatosis
c. Amyloidosis
d. Sarcoidosis

CARDIAC TUMORS

128. Two most common tumors of heart in adult are: *(PGI May 2019)*
a. Myxoma
b. Fibroma
c. Angiosarcoma
d. Metastatic tumors
e. Rhabdomyoma

129. Most common primary tumor of heart is? *(Recent Question 2016)*
a. Myxoma   b. Liposarcoma
c. Rhabdomyoma   d. Lipoma

130. Carcinoid of heart involves? *(Recent Question 2015)*
a. Valvular endocardium of right atrium
b. Valvular endocardium of left atrium
c. Mural endocardium
d. Myocardium

131. False statement regarding cardiac myxoma *(Recent Question 2015)*
a. Most common primary tumor of heart
b. Most common in left atrium
c. More common in females
d. 90% familial

132. Most common primary tumor of heart in children
a. Myxoma *(Recent Question 2015)*
b. Rhabdomyoma
c. Lipoma
d. Fibroma

133. Spider cells are seen in *(Recent Question 2015)*
a. Papillary fibroelastoma
b. Tako-tsubo cardiomyopathy
c. Rhabdomyoma
d. Myxoma

134. Carcinoid heart disease affects which part:
a. Valvular endocardium *(Recent Question 2014-15)*
b. Pericardium
c. Myocardium
d. Epicardium

135. Lepidic cells are characteristic of?
a. Bronchio loaveolar carcinoma *(AP PGMEE 14)*
b. Mesothehioma
c. small cell cancer of lung
d. Myxoma of heart

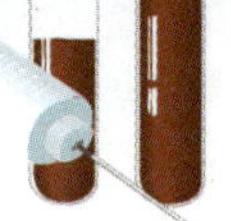

136. Characteristic pathological finding in carcinoid of heart: *(AI 10)*
a. Fibrous endocordial thickening of right ventricle and tricuspid valve
b. Collagen deposition in wall of right ventricle
c. Interstitial fibrous thickening of right ventricles
d. Mononuclear inflammatory infiltrate in the wall

137. Which carcinoma metastasizes to heart?
a. CA breast   *(PGI May 2010)*
b. CA stomach
c. CA lung
d. CA urinary bladder
e. Osteosarcoma

MYOCARDITIS AND PERICARDITIS

138. Hemopericardium is seen in-   *(Recent Question 2014)*
a. Chest injury
b. MI
c. Ruptured Aortic aneurysm
d. All

139. The causes of pericarditis are: *(Recent Question 2013)*
a. Infection
b. Trauma
c. Neoplasia
d. Acute mycardial infarction
e. Any of the above

140. Which worm causes myocarditis: *(Recent Question 2013)*
a. Trichomonas   b. Trichinella
c. Enterobius   d. Strongyloides

MISCELLANEOUS

141. Tigered effect in myocardium is due to:
a. Malignant change   *(Recent Question 2015)*
b. Fatty change in heart
c. Seen in rheumatic fever
d. Associated with myocarditis

142. Commonest complication of prosthetic valve is:
a. Embolism   *(Recent Question 2015)*
b. Subacute bacterial endocarditis
c. Rejection
d. Infarction CNS

143. A young female patient came for routine examination. On examination a mid systolic click was found. There is no history of RHD. The histopathological examination is most likely to show-   *(AIIMS May 12)*
a. Myxomatous degeneration and prolapse of the valve
b. Fibrinous deposition on the tipofpapillarymuscle
c. Rupture of chordae tendinae
d. Aschoff nodule on the mitral valve

144. What does "cardiac polyp" mean?   *(AIIMS May 11)*
a. Acute infarct   b. Cardiac aneurysm
c. Benign tumor   d. Fibrinous clot

145. True about subendocardial hemorrhage is all except-
a. May be seen after head injury   *(AIIMS Nov 10)*
b. Involves RV wall
c. Continous pattern of sheetlike
d. Flame shaped hemorrhages

146. Factor responsible for Cardiac Hypertrophy is?
a. ANF   b. TNF alpha   *(DNB Dec 10)*
c. c-myc   d. TGF beta

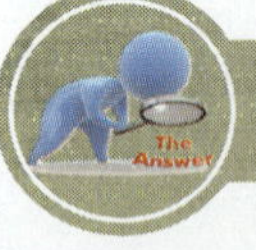

Answers with Explanations

1. Ans. (c) Cholesterol

(Ref: Robbins 9th/pg 496; 8th/pg 500)
Cholesterol clefts: space caused by the dissolving out of cholesterol crystals in sections of tissue embedded in paraffin.

2. Ans. (a) Endothelium

(Ref: Robbins 9th/pg 498-499; 8th/pg 505; Harrison 18th/pg 1503)
Pathogenesis of atherosclerosis best explained by the '**Response to Injury hypothesis to endothelium**

3. Ans. (d) Mesenteric arteries

(Ref: Robbins 9th/pg 498-499; 8th/pg 502)
Spared vessels are:
1. Upper extremities vessels
2. Mesenteric and renal arteries except at their ostia

4. Ans. (c) Lipid *(Ref: Robbins 9th/pg 496; 8th/pg 500)*

5. Ans. (a) Chronic inflammatory disorder of vessel wail

(Ref: Robbins 9th/pg 494; 8th/pg 500)

6. Ans. (a) Left anterior descending artery

(Ref: Robbins 9th/pg 498-499; 8th/pg 502)

7. Ans. (d) Calcifications cause significant narrowing of vessel lumen

(Ref: Robbins 9th/pg 491-492; 8th/pg 496-497)
Mönckeberg medial sclerosis
- **Calcification of the walls (media)**[Q] of muscular arteries, typically involving the internal elastic membrane[Q]
- **Do not encroach**[Q] on the vessel lumen

8. Ans. (a) Oxidized LDL

(Ref: Robbins 9th/pg 496; 8th/pg 500)
With chronic hyperlipidemia, lipoproteins accumulate within the intima, there they aggregate and become **oxidized** by **free radicals** produced by **inflammatory cells.**
These cannot be completely degraded, hence their ingestion by **macrophages/smooth muscle cells** leads to formation of **foam cells**

9.   **Ans. (a) Physical inactivity**

(Ref: Robbins 9th/pg 496; 8th/pg 500)

Physical inactivity

10. **Ans. (c) Convex part formed by fibrous cap**

(Ref: Robbins 9th/pg 496; 8th/pg 500)

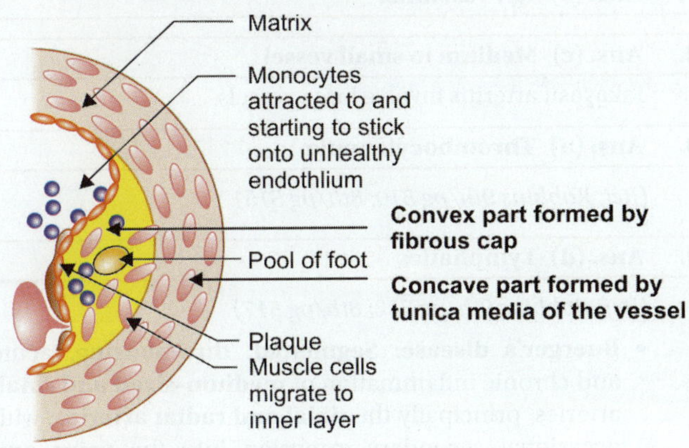

11. **Ans. (d) Endothelium**

(Ref: Robbins 9th/pg 498-499; 8th/pg 505; Harrison 18th/pg 1503)

12. **Ans. (b) Heart** *(Ref: Robbins 9th/pg 498-499; 8th/pg 502)*

13. **Ans. (c) Monckebergs sclerosis**

(Ref: Robbins 9th/pg 491-492)

14. **Ans. (c) Smooth muscle cell hypertrophy**

(Ref: Robbins 9th/pg 498-499; 8th/pg 505; Harrison 18th/pg 1503)

15. **Ans. (b) C. Pneumoniae** *(Ref: R 9th/pg 496; 8th/pg 1182)*

Infection. Although circumstantial evidence has been presented linking atherosclerosis **to herpesvirus, cytomegalovirus, and Chlamydophila pneumoniae,** there is no established causal role for infection.

16. **Ans. (c) Lipids in LDL get oxidized**

(Ref: Robbins 9th/pg 496; 8th/pg 500)

With chronic hyperlipidemia, lipoproteins accumulate within the intima, there they aggregate and become **oxidized** by **free radicals** produced by **inflammatory cells.**

17. **Ans. (c) Hyaline arteriosclerosis**

(Ref: Robbins 9th/pg 490, 938-939; 8th/pg 495)

a. Also called obliterative endarteritis seen in syphilis/ TB/radiation, poisoning, etc
b. Malignant MT
c. Benign HT
d. MC in marfan syndrome

18. **Ans. (b) Fibrinoid necrosis**

(Ref: Robbins 9th/pg 490, 938-939; 8th/pg 495)

19. **Ans. (b) Malignant hypertension**

(Ref: Robbins 9th/pg 490; 8th/pg 495)

20. **Ans. (b) Hyperplastic arteriosclerosis**

(Ref: Robbins 9th/pg 490)

21. **Ans. (a) Intimal proliferation and hyalinization of media of medium arteries**

(Ref: Robbins 9th/pg 490; 8th/pg 495)

There is increased myofibroblastic tissue in the intima along with hyaline deposits in benign hypertension. Intimal proliferation is usually the universal response of a vessel to injury.

22. **Ans. (d) Hyperplastic arteriosclerosis**

(Ref: Robbins 9th/pg 490)

23. **Ans. (a) Ascending aorta**

(Ref: Robbins 9th/pg 503)

Syphilis usually affects proximal ascending aorta (esp aortic ring) > aortic arch.

24. **Ans. (a) Trauma**

(Ref: Robbins 9th/pg 501-502; 8th/pg 506-507)

25. **Ans. (a) Ascending aorta** *(Ref: Robbins 9th/pg 501-502)*

MC cause of ascending aortic aneusrysm	Marfan's Syndrome Cystic medial degeneration[Q] / Systemic hypertension[Q]

26. **Ans. (d) 5.5 cm**

(Ref: Guidelines for the treatment of abdominal aortic aneurysms. J Vasc Surg. 2003;37(5):1106)

Aneurysm repair is the primary treatment for aneurysms that are symptomatic or at a high risk for rupture

Most people with an aneurysm less than 4.0 cm (1.6 inches) in diameter are advised not to have immediate surgery, but rather to follow the aneurysm over time; this is known as watchful waiting

On the other hand, most patients with an **asymptomatic aneurysm greater than 5.5 cm (2.2 inches) in diameter or that expands more than 0.5 cm within a six-month period** are advised to have repair.

27. **Ans. (c) 7 cm**

(Ref: Guidelines for the treatment of abdominal aortic aneurysms. J Vasc Surg. 2003;37(5):1106)

The annual risk of rupture based upon aneurysm size is estimated as follows:

- Less than 4.0 cm in diameter = –0%
- Between 4.0 to 5 cm in diameter = 1%
- Between 5.0 to 6 cm in diameter = 11%
- > 6.0 cm in diameter = 25%

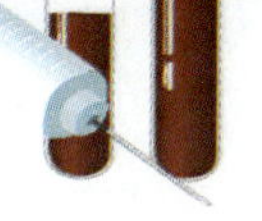

28.   **Ans. (b) Atherosclerosis** *(Ref: Robbins 9th/pg 501-502)*

29.   **Ans. (d) Mockenbergs sclerosis**

(Ref: Robbins 9th/pg 501-502; 8th/pg 506-507)

30.   **Ans. (a) Splenic**

(Ref: Semin Intervent Radiol. 2009 Sep; 26(3): 196–206)

- Visceral artery aneurysms (VAAs) and visceral artery pseudoaneurysms (VAPAs) frequently present as life-threatening emergencies
- **Splenic artery aneurysms- most common VAA**
- **Hepatic artery aneurysms (HAAs)- second most common VAA**
- Clinically, the patients with VAPAs, typically present with an antecedent history of arterial trauma or surgical manipulation

31.   **Ans. (c) Transesophageal echocardiography**

(Ref: Radiographics.rsna.org MARCH-APRIL 2010, Circulation: Cardiovascular Imaging (November 2009 vol. 2 no. 6 499-506, Harrison 17th ed table 242A))

The dissection is termed *acute* when it is diagnosed **within 14** days after the first symptoms appear

	Unstable/Critical Conditions	Stable Clinical Condition
Diagnostic modality	TEE with color Doppler	MD-CT with CTA (CT angiography) or MRI with MRA

32.   **Ans. (c) Hypertension** *(Ref: Robbins 9th/pg 504; 8th/pg 509)*

MC cause of dissection is hypertension[Q]

33.   **Ans. (d) Secondary syphilis**

(Ref: Robbins 9th/pg 504; 8th/pg 509)

MC cause of dissection is hypertension, seen in men between 40-60 yrs of age.
2nd MC cause of dissection is cystic medial necrosis(CMN)
Marfan's syndrome causes CMN hence dissection
Syphilis- Aneurysm of the aorta was the most common complication of syphilitic aortitis.
Syphilis will only potentially cause aortic dissection in its tertiary stage

34.   **Ans. (b) Level of aorta affected**

(Ref: Robbins 9th/pg 504)

35.   **Ans. (a) Marfans** *(Ref: Harrison 18th pg 206)*

Cystic medial necrosis (CMN)
- Disorder of **large arteries, in particular the aorta,[Q]**
- Characterized by an accumulation of **basophilic ground substance in the media[Q]** with cyst-like lesions.
- Diseases causing CMN
  - **Marfan's syndrome[Q], Chronic aortic dissection[Q], Congenital heart disease especially bicuspid aortic valve[Q], Scurvy[Q], Aortic aneurysm[Q], Atheroslerotic disease[Q], Hypertension[Q], Ehler danlos syndrome (type IV)[Q]**

36.   **Ans. (a) Hypertension**

(Ref: Robbins 9th/pg 504; 8th/pg 509)

MC cause of dissection is hypertension, seen in men between 40-60 yrs of age.
2nd MC cause of dissection is cystic medial necrosis. (option B).

37.   **Ans. (e) IgA vasculitis**

38.   **Ans. (c) Medium to small vessel**

Takayasu arteritis involve large vessels

39.   **Ans. (a) Thrombocytopenia**

(Ref: Robbins 9th/pg 510; 8th/pg 515)

40.   **Ans. (d) Lymphatics**

(Ref: Robbins 9th/pg 512; 8th/pg 517)

- **Buerger's disease: Segmental, thrombosing**, acute and chronic inflammation of **medium-sized and small** arteries, principally the **tibial and radial arteries**, with occasional secondary extension into the **veins and nerves** of the extremities

41.   **Ans. (a) IgA** *(Ref: Robbins 9th/pg 926; 8th/pg 934)*

- Most common antibody seen in these immune complexes is **IgA[Q]** (IgA levels are elevated)
- The **microscopic hallmark** of HSP is the deposition of **IgA in the walls[Q]** of involved blood vessels.

42.   **Ans. (d) Classical PAN**

(Ref: Robbins 9th/pg 506; 8th/pg 511)

43.   **Ans. (c) Thrombocytopenia**

(Ref: Robbins 9th/pg 926; 8th/pg 934)

- **HSP:** Purpura not due to a low platelet count but due to **vasculitis[Q]**
- Platelet count is normal or elevated[Q]

44.   **Ans. (b) Wegener's Granulomatosis**

(Ref: Robbins 9th/pg 507, Harrison 18thed p-2786-87)

- **C-ANCA (proteinsase 3[Q]** is the target antigen)
- Typically seen in Wegner's Granulomatosis[Q]

45.   **Ans. (a) Temporal arteritis**

(Ref: Robbins 9th/pg 507-8,510)

- **Biopsy and histological confirmation** of temporal artery is the **investigation of choice.**
- It shows **Granulomatous inflammation with giant cells & fragmentation of internal elastic lamina.[Q]**

46.   **Ans. (b) Low ESR** *(Ref: R 9th/pg 507-8,510; 8th/pg 512-13)*

47.   **Ans. (d) Sarcoidosis**

(Ref: Robbins 9th/pg 507-8,510; 8th/pg 512-13)

Fibrinoid necrosis is seen in Pan
- Aschoff Nodule, SLE, HIV and Malignant Hypertension

48. Ans. (a) Behçet's disease

(Ref: Robbins 9th/pg 511, www.behcets.com/american behcet disease association)

Behçet's disease is considered more prevalent in the areas surrounding the old silk trading routes in the Middle East and in Central Asia. Thus, it is sometimes known as **Silk Road Disease**

Linkage between the disease and **HLA-B51** is seen.

49. Ans. (d) Involves large vessels *(Ref: R 9th/pg 511-512)*

50. Ans. (c) 40-60%

(Ref: Hepinstall pathology of kidney volume 1- pg 463, JASN May 1, 2002 vol. 13 no. 5 1271-1278)

- **Incidence of Renal Involment in HSP (different in various studies, depends on** data of patients and the definition of renal involvement)
- **Adults : 45 to 85%**
- **Children-20-56%**

51. Ans. (c) Wegener's granulomatosis

(Ref: Robbins 9th/pg 507, Harrison 18thed p-2786-87)

Option a and b are **immune-mediated small-vessel systemic vasculitis. C-ANCA positive vasculitis**

52. Ans. (a) PAN *(Ref: Robbins 9th/pg 509; 8th/pg 511)*

PAN is characterized by **segmental transmural necrotizing inflammation**[Q] frequently accompanied by **fibrinoid necrosis.**[Q]

OPTION B, C, D are granulomotous vasculitis.

53. Ans. (c) Antigen-antibody complex mediated

(Ref: Robbins 9th/pg 509; 8th/pg 511)

PAN-Necrotising vasculitis with fibrinoid necrosis which is a type of **immune complex mediated vasculitis**[Q]

54. Ans. (c) Classic PAN (Ref: Robbins 9th/pg 506-7,510)

55. Ans. (c) Most commonly involved artery is abdominal aorta *(Ref: Robbins 9th/pg 507-8,510; 8th/pg 512-13)*

56. Ans. (c) Proteinase 3

(Ref: Robbins 9th/pg 507, Harrison 18thed p-2786-87)

- **C-ANCA (proteinsase 3**[Q] is the target antigen)
- Typically seen in Wegner's Granulomatosis[Q]

57. Ans. (d) Unlikely to cause pulmonary renal syndrome

(Ref: Robbins 9th/pg 510-11; 8th/pg 515)

Microscopic polyangiitis (MP)

- **Option a true- MP is small vessel vasculitis**
- Typically **spare medium-sized and larger arteries**
- **Option b is true- P-ANCA is present is majority of the** patients.
- **Option c is true- major clinical features include he-moptysis, hematuria and proteinuria, bowel pain or** bleeding, muscle pain or weakness, and palpable cutaneous purpura.

Skin findings are as follows:

- **Palpable purpura** (41%), Leukocytoclastic angiitis, livedo reticularis (12%), skin ulcerations, necrosis and gangrene, necrotizing nodules and digital ischemia (7%)
- **Urticaria** - Vasculitis-associated urticaria that lasts longer than 24 hours **Option d is false- Necrotizing glomerulonephritis** (90% of patients) and **pulmonary capillaritis** are **common**.

58. Ans. (a) Lung *(Ref: Robbins 9th/pg 509-510; 8th/pg 514-5)*

PAN Typically involving renal and visceral vessels but **sparing the pulmonary circulation.**

59. Ans. (b) Focal necrotizing glomerulonephritis

(Ref: Robbins 9th/pg 511-512; 8th/pg 516)

- **Wegner's granulomatosis** now called **Granulomatosis with Polyangiitis**
- Focal necrotizing, often crescentic, glomerulonephritis along with Necrotizing or granulomatous vasculitis affecting small to medium-sized vessels.

Option a- granulomas in vessel wall alone is not characteristic of wegners. It should be granulomatous or necrotizing vasculitis

60. Ans. (b, c) b. Kawasaki disease; c. Henoch schonlein purpura *(Ref: Robbins 9th/pg 508,510-12; 8th/pg 511-13)*

- Option a - Giant cell arteritis-vasculitis in a patient over the age of 50 years
- Option b - **Kawasaki disease**-vasculitis in **infancy and childhood**
- Option c - **Henoch schonlein purpura**-vasculitis in children
- Option d- Polyarteritis nodosa-vasculitis in 4th or 5th decade

61. Ans. (a) Hemangioma *(Ref: Robbins 9th ed p 516)*

Hemangiomas are very common tumors characterized by increased numbers of normal or abnormal vessels filled with blood. These lesions constitute 7% of all benign tumors of infancy and childhood; most are present from birth and initially increase in size, but many eventually regress spontaneously. While hemangiomas typically are localized lesions confined to the head and neck, they can occasionally be more extensive (angiomatosis) and can occur internally.

62. Ans. (a, b, c, d); a. Causative agent HHV 8, b. Can be Seen in depressed cell mediated immunity, c. Treatment is chemotherapy and surgery, d. Vascular tumor

(Ref: Robbins 9th/pg 518.; 8th/pg 523)

KAPOSI SARCOMA

- It is caused by KS Herpes virus or **Human herpes virus 8 (HHV8)-*option a is true***
- Characterized by proliferation of **spindle cells**[Q] which are of **vascular origin**[Q] (Option d is correct)

Transplant and HIV associated Kaposi usually occur in immunosupressed individuals. (Option b is correct)

Treatment – (Option c is correct)

- HAART is the best way to treat HIV associated Kaposi's sarcoma
- **Topical retinoid treatment**
- Cryosurgery (cryotherapy)
- Surgery; Radiation therapy
- Intralesional chemotherapy

**63.	Ans. (d)	Vascular ectasias** *(Ref: Robbins 9th/pg 515-516)*

Port-wine stain or **nevus flammeus**

- It is the **most common form** of **Vascular ectasias;** it persist throughout life[Q]
- Caused by a somatic activating c.548G→A mutation in the **GNAQ[Q]** gene
- Part of Sturge–Weber syndrome[Q] or Klippel–Trénaunay–Weber syndrome

**64.	Ans. (c)	Kaposi sarcoma** *(Ref: Robbins 9th/pg 518)*

**65.	Ans. (b)	HAART therapy has decreased AIDS associated KS**

(Ref: Robbins 9th/pg 518.; 8th/pg 523)

**66.	Ans. (d)	Hemangiopericytoma**

(Ref: Sternberg's Diagnostic Surgical Pathology, 5th Edition, table 5 11)

Hemangiopericytoma

- Tumor derived from **pericytes[Q]**- **perivascular cells** that wrap around blood capillaries
- These tumors most commonly arise from **pelvic retroperitoneum[Q] or the limbs[Q]** (particularly thighs).
- Capillaries are arranged in **'fish-hook pattern;'[Q] seen best with silver stains[Q]**

**67.	Ans. (b)	Capillary hemangioma**

(Ref: Robbins/pg 515-516)

PYOGENIC GRANULOMAS-lobular capillary hemangioma

Capillary hemangiomas[Q] that grows rapidly

Presents as red pedunculated lesions on the **skin, gingival, or oral mucosa[Q]**

Lesions **bleed easily[Q]**

**68.	Ans. (a)	Liver**

(Ref: Robbins 9th/pg 519; 8th/pg 523)

Angiosarcoma

- Malignant endothelial cell neoplasm most commonly seen in **skin, soft tissue, breast and liver[Q]**
- **Hepatic angiosarcoma** is associated with carcinogens including arsenic, thorotrast (a radioactive contrast) and polyvinyl chloride (PVC; a plastic)

**69.	Ans. (d)	CD 31** *(Ref: Robbins 9th/pg 591,519.; 8th/pg 523)*

- Endothelial cell origin of angiosarcoma is demonstrated by staining for **CD31, CD34 or VWF[Q].**
- CD10 – CALLA (common acute lymphoblastic leukemia antigen)

- CD19- pan B marker
- CD25- alpha chain of the IL-2 receptor

**70.	Ans. (b)	Strawberry angioma**

(Ref: Robbins 9th/pg 515-516)

Lesion	Features
Capillary hemangiomas	• **Strawberry hemanigioma** or **juvenile hemangioma** is a type • **Completely regress**
Port-wine stain or *nevus flammeus*	• Caused by a somatic activating c.548G→A mutation in the **GNAQ[Q]** gene • **Persist throughout life[Q]**
Cavernous hemangiomas	• **Do not[Q]** spontaneously regress.

**71.	Ans. (c, d); c. Pressure effect is often the presenting symptom; d. Thromboembolic phase is present**

(Ref: Neurosurgery [SHC Suppl 3]:SHC1289–SHC1299, 2008, Harrison 18th ed: 2262)

GIANT ANEURYSMS

- Definition
  - Diameter of greater than 25 mm
- Most common clinical presentation
  - Mass effect- most common
  - Subarachnoid hemorrhage, intracerebral hemorrhage, or both -
- Most common site
  - Internal carotid artery segments vertebrobasilar region- OPTION b is false
- Other features
  - Seizures
  - High risk for rupture- OPTION A is false
  - **Intraluminal thrombus-occlusion of perforating vessels**
  - **Distal embolic events are common**- OPTION d is true.

**72.	Ans. (a)	Primary lymphedema**

(Ref: Harrison 17th ed table 243-3)

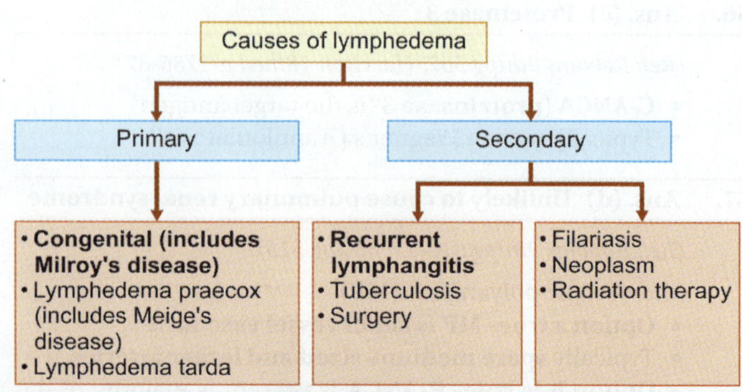

**73.	Ans. (b)	Increased LV cavity size**

(Ref: Robbins 9th/pg 526)

74.   **Ans. (a)** **No change**

(Ref: Harrison 17th ed Table 243-1)

Most common cause of Raynaud's Phenomenon -Primary or idiopathic.

In initial stages of Raynaud's phenomenon no changes is seen late stages may show atherosclerosis or thrombosis

75.   **Ans. (b)** **Systemic sclerosis**

(Ref: Harrison 17th ed Table 243-1, Robbins 9th/pg 513)

76.   **Ans. (c)** **Lungs**

(Ref: Robbins 9th/pg 529; 8th/pg 535)
Morphology in Lungs in LVF
Lungs: Most commonly affected organ
Heart failure cells[Q]-hemosiderin containing macrophages. Edematous widening of alveolar septa and -Edema fluid in the alveolar spaces.

77.   **Ans. (a)** **Cor pulmonale** *(Ref: R 9th/pg 530; 8th/pg 536)*

Isolated right-sided heart failure[Q] is very rare,, occurs with lung disorders. This is referred to as cor pulmonale[Q] The **common feature** of these disorders is **pulmonary hypertension**[Q]

78.   **Ans. (b)** **Pigmented alveolar macrophages**

(Ref: Robbins 9th/pg 529; 8th/pg 535)

79.   **Ans. (c)** **Eosinophilic contraction bands**

(Ref: R 9th pg 544)

80.   **Ans. (b)** **White**

(Ref: Robbins 9th/pg 544; 8th/pg 550)

- **N**ecrotic area can be **visualized after 2-3 hours**[Q] by immersion in **triphenyltetrazolium chloride (TTC)**[Q]
- **Infarcted area** is revealed as **unstained pale zone**[Q]
- TTC imparts brick red colour to **non-infarcted myocardium**[Q] where **dehydrogenase enzymes**[Q] are preserved.

81.   **Ans. (a)** **1–2 days**

(Ref: Robbins 9th/pg 544)

Image is neutrophil infiltrate which is seen 2–24 hr after infarction

82.   **Ans. (d)** **Cell membrane defects**

Cell membrane damage leads to leakage of enzymes from the cell; which can be detected in serum.

83.   **Ans. (b)** **30 min**

(Ref: Robbins 9th/pg 544)

- **Time for reversible injury in heart is 30 mins**[Q]

84.   **Ans. (c)** **Lipoprotein A**

(Ref: Circulation June 29, 2004 vol. 109)

Novel Biomarkers in the Prediction of Future Cardiovascular Events
Lipoprotein(a)

Homocysteine
High-sensitivity C-reactive protein (hsCRP)

85.   **Ans. (d)** **Coagulative necrosis** *(Ref: Robbins 9th/pg 544)*

The type of necrosis in myocardial infarction is – **Coagulative**

86.   **Ans. (a)** **Triphenyl tetrazolium chloride**

(Ref: Robbins 9th/pg 544)

(Refer Answer 121)

87.   **Ans. (c)** **20-40 minutes** *(Ref: R 9th/pg 544; 8th/pg 550)*

88.   **Ans. (a)** **Waviness of fibres**

(Ref: Robbins 9th/pg 544; 8th/pg 550)

Waviness of fibers at border[Q] **(earliest microscopic change)**

89.   **Ans. (a)** **Neutrophils**

(Ref: Robbins 9th/pg 544; 8th/pg 550)

90.   **Ans. (b)** **Coagulative (Ref: Robbins 9th/pg 539-40)**

91.   **Ans. (d)** **Old age** *(Ref: Robbins 9th/pg 492; 8th/pg 497)*

92.   **Ans. (a)** **LAD** *(Ref: Robbins 9th/pg 542; 8th/pg 549)*

Most common site of artery of atherosclerosis: LAD

93.   **Ans. (b)** **Inferior** *(Ref: Robbins 9th/pg 549; 8th/pg 555)*

"Location of portions of the atrioventricular conduction system (bundle of His) in the inferoseptal myocardium, infarcts of this region may also be associated with heart block."

94.   **Ans. (b)** **Granulation tissue**

(Ref: Robbins 9th/pg 544; 8th/pg 550)

95.   **Ans. (d)** **40 minutes** *(Ref: Robbins 9th/pg 541; 8th/pg 550)*

96.   **Ans. (b)** **Coagulative necrosis**

(Ref: Robbins 9th/pg 544)

97.   **Ans. (c)** **Aschoff bodies**

98.   **Ans. (b, d) b. McCallum plaques; d. Aschoff nodules**

(Ref: R 559)

- **Aortic valve thickening**
The cardinal anatomic changes of the mitral valve in chronic RHD are leaflet thickening, commissural fusion and shortening, and thickening and fusion of the tendinous cords along with increase in calcific aortic stenosis.

99.   **Ans. (c)** **Rheumatic carditis**

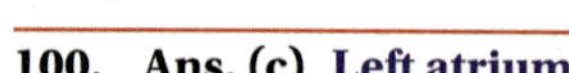

100. Ans. (c) Left atrium

(Ref: Robbins 9th/pg 557-559; 8th/pg 565-66)

Mac-callum patches-map-like areas of **thickened and wrinkled part of the endocardium in the left atrium**[Q]
- Caused by **regurgitant jets of blood flow**[Q], due to incompetence of the mitralvalve
- Seen in **Rheumatic endocarditis**

101. Ans. (b) B cells

(Ref: Robbins 9th/pg 557-559; 8th/pg 565-66)

102. Ans. (a) Group A Streptococci *(Ref: R 9th/pg 557-559)*

Rheumatic heart disease is a An acute **immunologicaly** mediated **multisystem inflammatory disease**[Q] that occurs **few weeks** after an attack of **group A β-hemolytic streptococcal pharyngitis**

103. Ans. (b) Rheumatic myocarditis *(Ref: R 9th/pg 557-559)*

104. Ans. (b) Rheumatic endocarditis *(Ref: R 9th/pg 557-559)*

105. (a, b, d, e); a. Carey coombs murmur; b. Pancarditis; d. Chorea; e. Streptococcal infection

(Ref: Robbins 9th/pg 557-559)

Option a-true: Carey coombs murmur- occurs in patients with mitral valvulitis due to acute rheumatic fever
Option b-true Pancarditis
Option c-false: Migratory polyarthritis
- Subsides **spontaneously without any residual deform-ability**[Q] in the joints (non-erosive arthritis).
Option d-true: Syndenham's chorea
Late manifestation of the disease

106. Ans. (a) Rheumatic myocarditis *(Ref: R 9th/pg 557-559)*

107. Ans. (a) Cross reactivity with endogenous antigen

(Ref: Harrison 18th ed:2552; Robbins 9th/pg 557-559; 8th/pg 565-66)

108. Ans. (b) Infective endocarditis *(Ref: R 9th pg 560)*

109. Ans. (a) Mitral regurgitation

(Ref: Robbins 9th/pg 560; 8th/pg 567)

110. Ans. (a) Libman sack endocarditis *(Ref: R 9th/pg 560)*

111. Ans. (b) Infective endocarditis *(Ref: Robbins 9th/pg 560)*

112. Ans. (d) Mucinous adenocarcinoma of pancreas

(Ref: Robbins 9th/pg 560; 8th/pg 567)

113. Ans. (c) Infective endocarditis *(Ref: Robbins 9th/pg 560)*

114. Ans. (b) SLE *(Ref: Robbins 9th/pg 560; 8th/pg 567)*

115. Ans. (b) Libman-Sacks endocarditis *(Ref: R 9th/pg 560)*

116. Ans. (b) Infective endocarditis *(Ref: Robbins 9th/pg 560)*

117. Ans. (d) All *(Ref: Robbins 9th/pg 560,562; 8th/pg 567,569)*

A. **Maximum valve damage:** Acute infective endocarditis
B. Libman sach's endocarditis - Associated with an **intense valvulitis**[Q], characterized by **fibrinoid necrosis**[Q] **of the valve substance**
C. Rheumatic Heart disease - The valves show leaflet thickening, commissural fusion and shortening, thickening & fusion of the tendinous cords seen in chronic RHD.

118. Ans. (b) Libman sacks Endocarditis *(Ref: R 9th/pg 560)*

119. Ans. (d) Infective endocarditis *(Ref: Robbins 9th/pg 560)*

120. Ans. (a) 2, (b) 1, (c) 4, (d) 3 *(Ref: R 9th pg/568-569)*

Myocyte hypertrophy seen in hypertension is best evaluated in correlation with heart size. The classic histologic description is rectangular, hyperchromatic nuclei, often called "box-car" nuclei. In HOCM, histological features include cardiomegaly with left ventricular hypertrophy, hypertrophic myocytes, and myocyte disarray and/or myofiber bundle disorder. Myocyte degeneration with vacuolation is a feature of Arrhythmogenic cardiomyopathy and subendocardial ischemia. The diagnosis of dilated cardiomyopathy is not made histologically. The microscopic findings are very nonspecific and consist of myocyte hypertrophy and myocardial fibrosis.

121. Ans. (b) Takotsubo cardiomyopathy

122. Ans. (b) Titin

(Ref: Robbins 9th/pg 565-566; 8th/pg 573-574)

- DCM is familial in at least 30% to 50% of cases
- Autosomal dominant inheritance is the predominant pattern;
- Most common- mutations in TTN, a gene that encodes titin (20% of all cases of DCM)

123. Ans. (a, b, c, e) a. Death occurs in young athletes; b. mostly are genetic; c. LV septa is involved; e. treatment is ablation of septa

(Ref: Robbins 9th/pg 568-569; 8th/pg 575-576)

124. Ans. (a, b, d); a. Myocyte disaaray; b. Interstitial fibrosis; d. Myocyte hypertrophy

(Ref: Robbins 9th/pg 568-569)

The **histologic features** of HOCM myocardium are
1. Massive myocyte hypertrophy, transverse myocyte diameters **greater than 40 μm**[Q] (normal, approximately 15 μm);
2. **Myofiber disarray**[Q]
3. Interstitial and replacement **fibrosis**[Q]

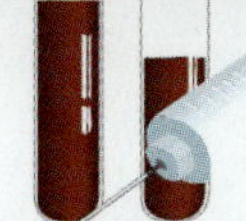

125. Ans. (a, c, d); a. Hypertrophy of ventricles without dilatation; c. Irregular arrangement of fibers; d. Asymmetrical septal hypertrophy

(Ref: Robbins 9th/pg 568-569)

126. Ans. (c, d, e); c. Viral myocarditis; d. Alcoholic liver disease; e. Thyroid disease *(Ref: Robbins 9th/pg 565-566)*

Causes of Phenotype
- Genetic; **alcoholic[Q]; peripartum[Q]; myocarditis[Q]; hemochromatosis[Q]**; chronic anemia; doxorubicin (Adriamycin) toxicity; sarcoidosis[Q]; idiopathic

127. Ans. (a) Alcohol *(Ref: R 9th/pg 565-566; 8th/pg 573-574)*

128. Ans. (a) Myxoma; (d) Metastatic tumors

(Ref: R 9th pg 575)

129. Ans. (a) Myxoma *(Ref: Robbins 9th/pg 575; 8th/pg 583)*

130. Ans. (a) Valvular endocardium of right atrium

(Ref: Robbins 9th/pg 562; Heart 2004;90:1224-1228 doi:10.1136/hrt.2004.040329)

- **Carcinoid heart disease[Q]** typically causes abnormalities of the **right side of the heart.[Q]**
- Preferential **right heart involvement[Q]** is most likely related to **inactivation of the vasoactive substances by the lungs[Q]**
- The two key investigations for the diagnosis of carcinoid heart disease are **24 hour urinary excretion of 5-hydroxyindole acetic acid (5-HIAA) and transthoracic echocardiography.**

131. Ans. (d) 90% familial

(Ref: Robbins 9th/pg 575; 8th/pg 583)

Option a –true- Myxomas are the most common primary tumor of the adult heart

Option b –true- About 90% of myxomas arise in the atria, with a left-to-right ratio of approximately 4 : 1.

Option c –true- Approximately 75% of sporadic myxomas occur in females

Option d-false- Most cardiac myxomas are sporadic and arise as isolated masses in the left atrium.

Familial syndromes associated with myxomas have activating mutations in the GNAS1 gene or null mutations in PRKAR1A, encoding a regulatory subunit of a cyclic-AMP-dependent protein kinase (Carney complex).

132. Ans. (b) Rhabdomyoma *(Ref: Robbins 9th/pg 575)*

133. Ans. (c) Rhabdomyoma *(Ref: R 9th/pg 575; 8th/pg 583)*

134. Ans. (a) Valvular endocardium

(Ref: Robbins 9th/pg 562; Heart 2004;90:1224-1228 doi:10.1136/hrt.2004.040329)

135. Ans. (d) Myxoma of heart

(Ref: Robbins 9th/pg 575; 8th/pg 583)

136. Ans. (a) Fibrous endocordial thickening of right ventricle and tricuspid valve

(Ref: Robbins 9th/pg 562; Heart 2004;90:1224-1228 doi:10.1136/hrt.2004.040329)

Carcinoid heart disease:
- **Characteristic** pathological findings are **endocardial plaques of fibrous tissue** that may involve the **tricuspid valve[Q], pulmonary valve[Q]**, cardiac chambers, venae cavae, pulmonary artery, and coronary sinus.

137. Ans. (a, c) a. CA breast; c. CA lung

(Ref: Cancers and heart by Reynolds 2nd pg 316)

Tumors that are likely to involve heart and pericardium
- **Ca lung**
- **Ca esophagus**
- **Lymphoma**
- **Ca breast**
- **Melanoma**
- **Leukemia**

138. Ans. (d) All

(Ref: Robbins 9th/pg 573-574; 8th/pg 581-82)

Hemopericardium: Causes
- Cardiac rupture after transmural myocardial infarction (especially day 5)
- Aortic aneurysm rupture, chest trauma, anticoagulation, leukaemia and TB Pericarditis

139. Ans. (e) Any of the above

(Ref: Robbins 9th/pg 573-574)

140. Ans. (b) Trichinella

(Ref: Robbins 9th/pg 570-71; 8th/pg 578)

MC helminth causing myocarditis- trichinella[Q]

141. Ans. (b) Fatty change in heart

Fatty change of heart: band of yellow (fatty) myocardium along with red (normal myocardium)

142. Ans. (a) Embolism *(Ref: Robbins 9th/pg 563; 8th/pg 570)*

Thromboembolism is the commonest complication of prosthetic valves.

143. Ans. (a) Myxomatous degeneration and prolapsed of valve

(Ref: Robbins 9th/pg 556; 8th/pg 563)

Mitral valve prolapse (MVP)
- One or both mitral valve leaflets are "floppy" and prolapse, or balloon back, into the left atrium during systole
- Associated with Marfan syndrome, caused by fibrillin-1 (FBN-1) mutations
- Key histologic change in the tissue is marked thickening of the spongiosa layer with deposition of mucoid (myxomatous) material, called myxomatous degeneration
- Most individuals diagnosed with MVP are asymptomatic
- Discovered incidentally by auscultation of mid-systolic clicks, sometimes followed by a mid to late systolic murmur.

144. Ans. (d) Fibrinous clot

(Ref: Textbook of Practical Histology 2nd pg 28-29)

Post mortem fibrinous clot of heart is called cardiac polyp

145. Ans. (b) Involves RV wall

(Ref: Forensic Pathology Reviews Volume 2, 2005, pp 293-306)

Subendocardial haemorrhage

Causes	• Cardiac injuries and resuscitation • Secondary to noncardiac injuries comprising **head injuries**, infectious diseases, intoxications, hemorrhagic diathesis, abdominal trauma, asthma, and **hypovolemic shock**[Q].- *option a -true*
Pathophysiology	• Mediated by the autonomic nervous system via hypersecretion of catecholamines[Q]
MC sites	• Located in **the upper part of the interventricular septum,** the opposing papillary muscles, and adjacent trabeculae carneae of the **free wall of the left ventricle**[Q]
Pattern	• **Flame shaped, confluent. Sheet like**[Q]- *option c and d -true*

146. Ans. (c) c-myc *(Ref: Robbins 9th/pg 527; 8th/pg 532)*

Cardiac Hypertrophy: Pathophysiology
Molecular changes include the expression of immediate-early genes (e.g., FOS, JUN, MYC, and EGR1)

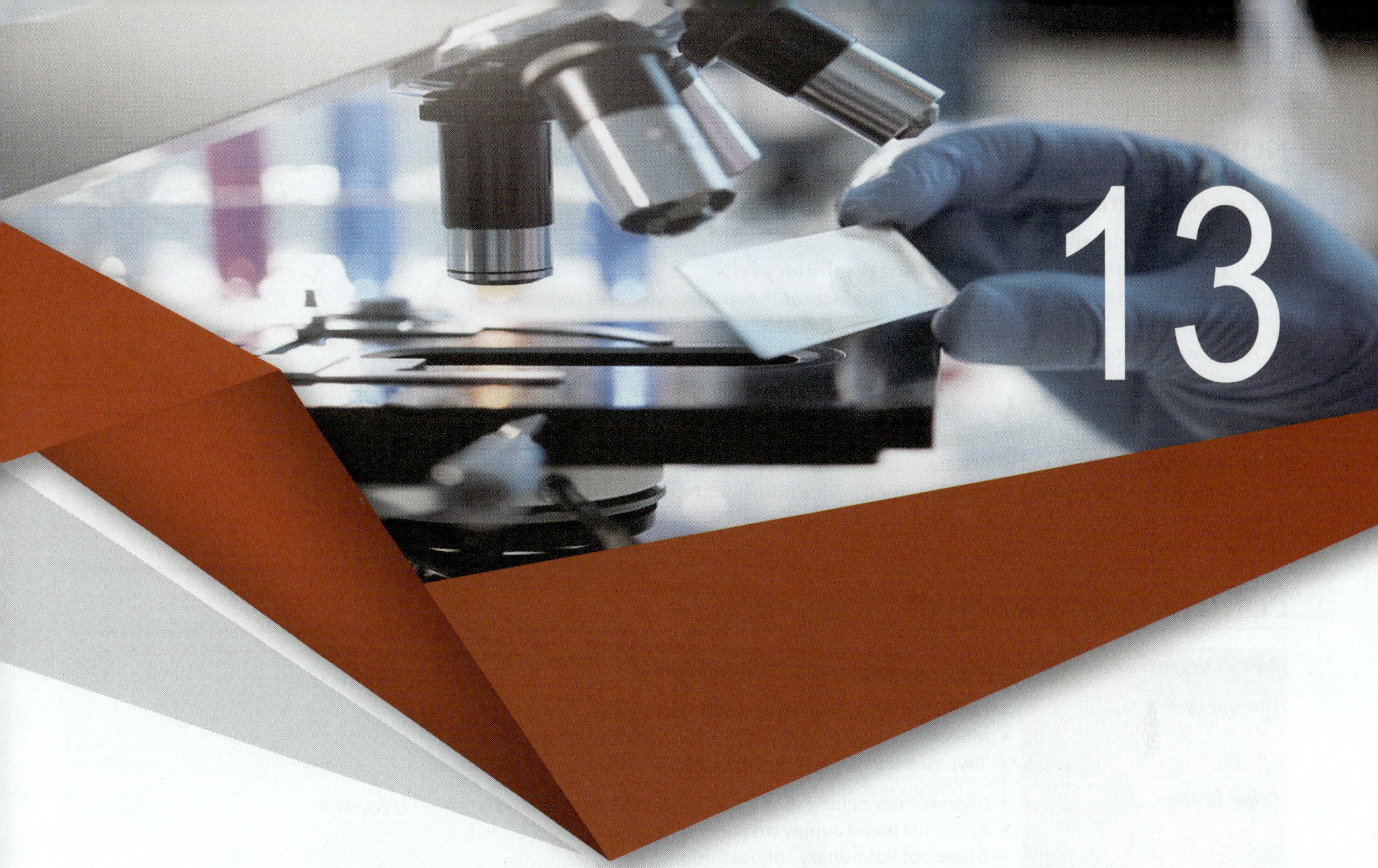

13

Respiratory System and its Disorders

Key Points

- » **Respiratory system develops** from: **ventral wall of foregut**[Q]
- » Sequence of division: Trachea → 2 bronchi → **B**ronchioles → **T**erminal Bronchiole → **R**espiratory Bronchiole → Alveolar duct → Alveolar **S**ac[Q] **(B-T-R-S – "Bu T teRS")**
- » **Bronchi** have **cartilage** and abundant **subepithelial glands** that produce mucus
- » **Bronchioles: Do not** have **cartilage**[Q], goblet cells and **submucosal glands**[Q]
- » **Acinus:** Part of the lung **distal to terminal bronchiole**[Q] (composed of respiratory bronchioles, alveolar ducts, and alveolar sacs)
- » **Pulmonary lobule**[Q]**:** Cluster of **3 to 5 terminal bronchioles**
- » Entire respiratory tree (larynx, trachea & bronchioles), is lined by **pseudostratified**[Q]**, tall, columnar and ciliated**[Q] **epithelial cells**
- » Exception to above rule are **vocal cords:** lined by **stratified squamous epithelium.**[Q]
- » Bronchial mucosa also contains neuroendocrine cells that have neurosecretory-type granules releasing: **serotonin**[Q]**, calcitonin**[Q] **and gastrin-releasing peptide (bombesin)**[Q]

Key Recent Updates

- » Basaloid carcinoma is new subtype added to SCC lung
- » NUT carcinoma of lung is very aggressive neoplasm of lung.

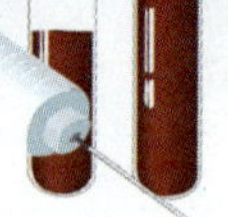

NORMAL ANATOMY

Microscopic Structure of the Alveolar Wall

- Alveolar epithelium:
  - **Type I pneumocytes** (95%)[Q] flattened **respiratory cells**
  - **Type II pneumocytes**: Synthesize **surfactant,**[Q] **repair type I cells**
- **Alveolar macrophages:** Loosely attached or lying free within the alveolar spaces
- **Pores of Kohn**[Q]: Permit the passage of **bacteria** and **exudate** between adjacent alveoli.
- Basement membrane and interstitial tissue
- Network of anastomosing capillaries lined with **endothelial cells**

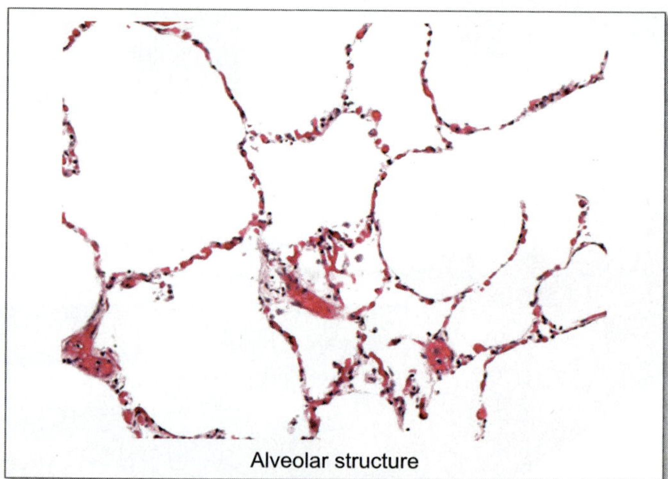

Alveolar structure

CONGENITAL MALFORMATIONS OF LUNGS

Pulmonary hypoplasia	Defective development of **one or both lungs**
Foregut cysts	• **Abnormal detachments of primitive foregut** • Most often located in the **hilum**[Q] or middle **mediastinum**. • 3 types: **Bronchogenic (most common),**[Q] Esophageal or Enteric
Sequestration	• Discrete area of **lung tissue that lacks any connection**[Q] to the airway system • Abnormal **blood supply arising from aorta**[Q] • 2 types of Pulmonary sequestration:

Extralobar sequestration	Intralobar sequestration
• **External** to lungs	• **More common**[Q]
• With pleural cover	• Occur **within** the lung **without pleural cover**
• Causing mass effect.	• Localized **infection** or **bronchiectasis**[Q]
• **Venous return** to **right** side of heart through **IVC**	• Associated with diaphragmatic hernia, colonic duplication, vertebral abnormalities, and pulmonary hypoplasia
	• Venous drainage through pulmonary veins

Congenital cystic adenomatoid malformation (CCAM)	**Hamartomatous**[Q] or **dysplastic** lung tissue, usually confined to one lobe.

ATELECTASIS

Incomplete expansion[Q] of the lungs (neonatal atelectasis) or **collapse of previously inflated lung**, producing areas of relatively **airless pulmonary parenchyma.**[Q]

Three types:

Type	Pathophysiology
Resorption atelectasis	Due to complete **obstruction**[Q] of an airway.
Compression atelectasis	Results when **fluid** (transudate, exudate or blood), **tumor, or air**[Q] (pneumothorax) accumulate within the pleural cavity.
Contraction atelectasis	Occurs when focal or generalized pulmonary or pleural **fibrosis**[Q] prevents full lung expansion

PULMONARY EDEMA

- Results from **increased hydrostatic pressure**[Q] (left-sided **congestive heart failure**)[Q]
- Histologically:
  - Alveolar **capillaries are engorged**
  - Intra-alveolar **transudate**[Q] appears as finely **granular pale pink**[Q] material.
  - **Alveolar micro-hemorrhages & hemosiderin-laden macrophages**[Q] ("heart failure" cells)[Q] may be seen

ACUTE LUNG INJURY (ALI) & ACUTE RESPIRATORY DISTRESS SYNDROME (ARDS)

Acute lung injury (ALI) (also called **non-cardiogenic pulmonary edema**) is characterized by the **sudden onset** of *significant hypoxemia and bilateral pulmonary infiltrates* on CXR, **without cardiac failure.**[Q]

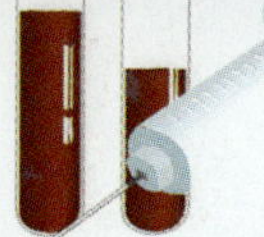

Diagnostic Criteria for ALI and ARDS

Oxygenation	Features	Absence of Left Atrial Hypertension
ALI: $PaO_2/FIO_2 < 300$ mm Hg[Q] ARDS: $PaO_2/FIO_2 < 200$ mm Hg[Q]	• Bilateral alveolar or interstitial infiltrates on CXR • Lung Biopsy: Diffuse alveolar damage with hyaline membrane disease	PCWP <18 mm Hg or no clinical evidence of increased left atrial pressure

Etiology of ARDS & ALI

Infections	Physical/Injury	Chemical injury	Hematologic conditions
• **Sepsis**[Q] • **Gastric aspiration**[Q] • Diffuse pulmonary infections • **Viral**[Q], *Mycoplasma*, *Pneumocystis,*[Q] • **Miliary tuberculosis**[Q]	• Mechanical trauma, including **head injury**[Q] • Pulmonary contusions, • Fractures with fat embolism • **Near-drowning**[Q], **Burns**[Q] • Ionizing radiation • **Hypothermia**[Q]	• **Oral:** Heroin / Barbiturate overdose, Acetylsalicylic acid • **Inhaled:** O_2 toxicity, **Smoke,**[Q] Irritant gases & chemicals • Pancreatitis • Uremia	• **Multiple transfusions (TRALI)**[Q] • **DIC**[Q] • Cardiopulmonary bypass • Hypersensitivity reactions

Pathogenesis

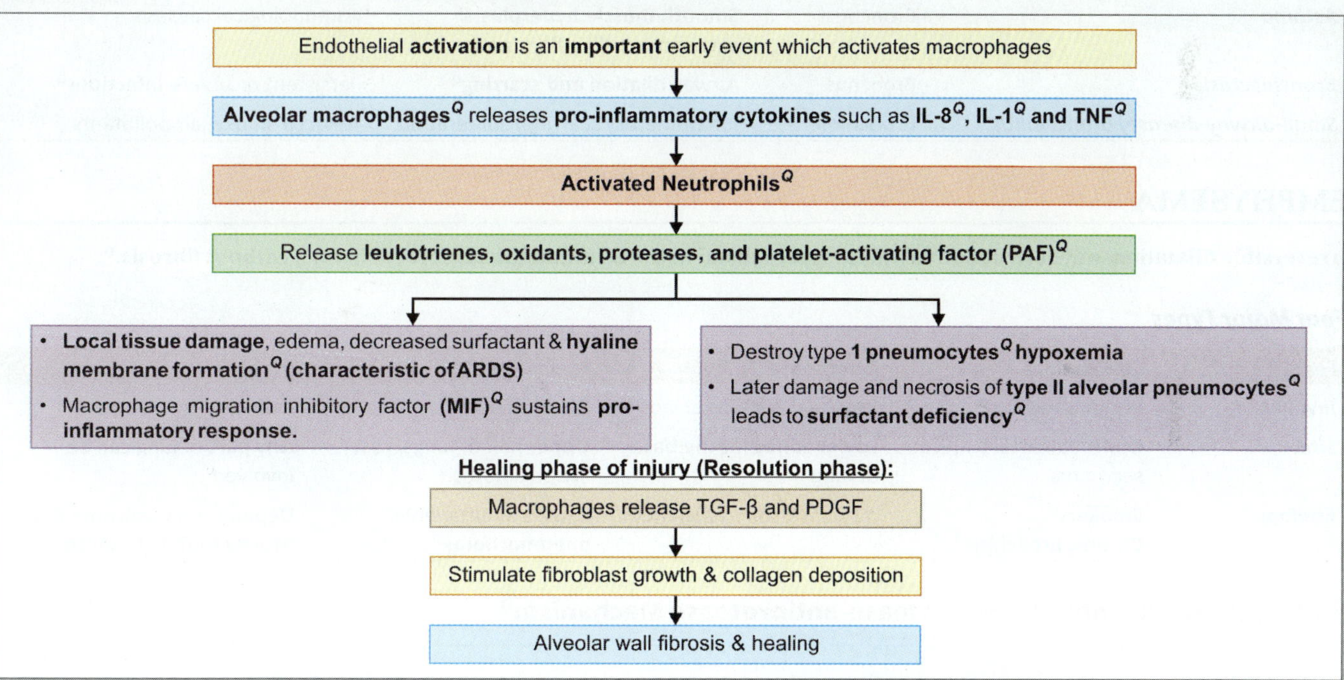

Lung Morphology in ARDS & ALI

- *Early stage:*
  - Interstitial and intraalveolar **edema**[Q] & **inflammation**[Q]
  - **Diffuse alveolar damage or necrosis**[Q]
  - **Fibrin deposition** → Alveoli become lined by **waxy hyaline membranes** (fibrin-rich edema fluid with **necrotic epithelial cells**).[Q]
- *Late organizing stage:*
  - **Type II pneumocytes proliferate**
  - **Granulation tissue**[Q] forms in the alveolar walls and spaces.

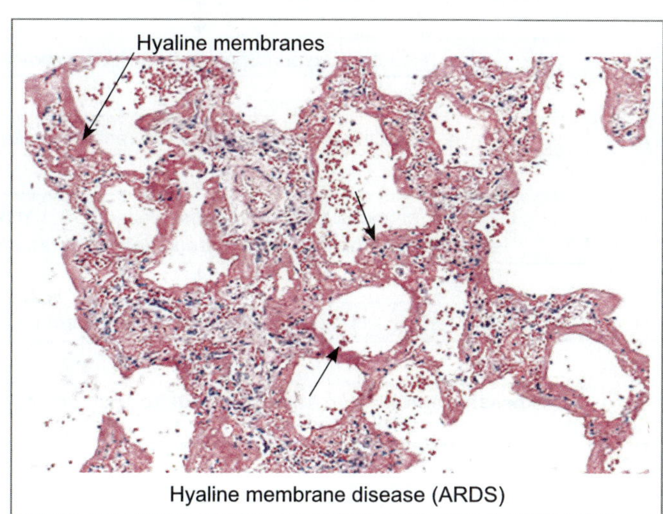

Hyaline membrane disease (ARDS)

- **ARDS** is also called **"shock lung"**[Q]
- **Earliest event** of ARDS is: diffuse **damage of alveolar capillary wall**[Q]
- Most important **cellular mediator** of ARDS is **Neutrophil**[Q]
- Most important **cytokine** involved in ARDS is **IL8**[Q]
- Histological **diagnostic hallmark** of ARDS is **Diffuse alveolar damage + Hyaline Membrane**[Q]

OBSTRUCTIVE LUNG DISEASE

Definition: Increase in **resistance**[Q] **to airflow** due to **partial or complete obstruction**[Q] at any level of airway.

Spectrum of Chronic Obstructive Pulmonary Disease

Clinical Term	Primary Site	Major Pathologic Changes	Etiology
Emphysema (pink puffers)[Q]	**Acinus**[Q]	Airspace **dilatation**[Q] & wall **destruction**[Q]	**Tobacco smoke**[Q]
Chronic bronchitis ("blue bloaters")[Q] *(B-B)*	**Bronchus**[Q]	**Mucous gland hyperplasia,**[Q] hypersecretion	**Tobacco smoke**[Q], air pollutants
Asthma	Bronchus	**Smooth muscle hyperplasia**[Q], **excess mucus**[Q], **inflammation**[Q]	Immunological causes
Bronchiectasis	Bronchus	Airway **dilation and scarring**[Q]	Persistent or severe **infections**[Q]
Small-airway disease, Bronchiolitis	**Bronchiole**[Q]	Inflammatory scarring/obliteration	Tobacco smoke, air pollutants

EMPHYSEMA

Irreversible dilatation and destruction[Q] of the airspaces **distal to the terminal bronchiole (acinus)**[Q]**, without fibrosis.**[Q]

Four Major Types

Features	Centriacinar	Panacinar	Paraseptal	Irregular
Involves	**Proximal** acinus[Q]	**Proximal** & **distal** acinus[Q]	**Distal** acinus[Q]	**Irregular**[Q] involvement
Site	**Upper lobes**[Q] esp apical segments	**Lower zones**[Q] at the base of lung	**Upper** half of lungs, cyst-like structures.	**Any part** of lung can be involved
Etiology	**Smokers**[Q] **Chronic bronchitis**[Q]	*α1-antitrypsin* **deficiency**[Q]	Causes Spontaneous **pneumothorax**[Q]	Depends on involvement, **Mostly found at autopsy**

Pathogenesis of Emphysema: Protease-antiprotease Mechanism[Q]

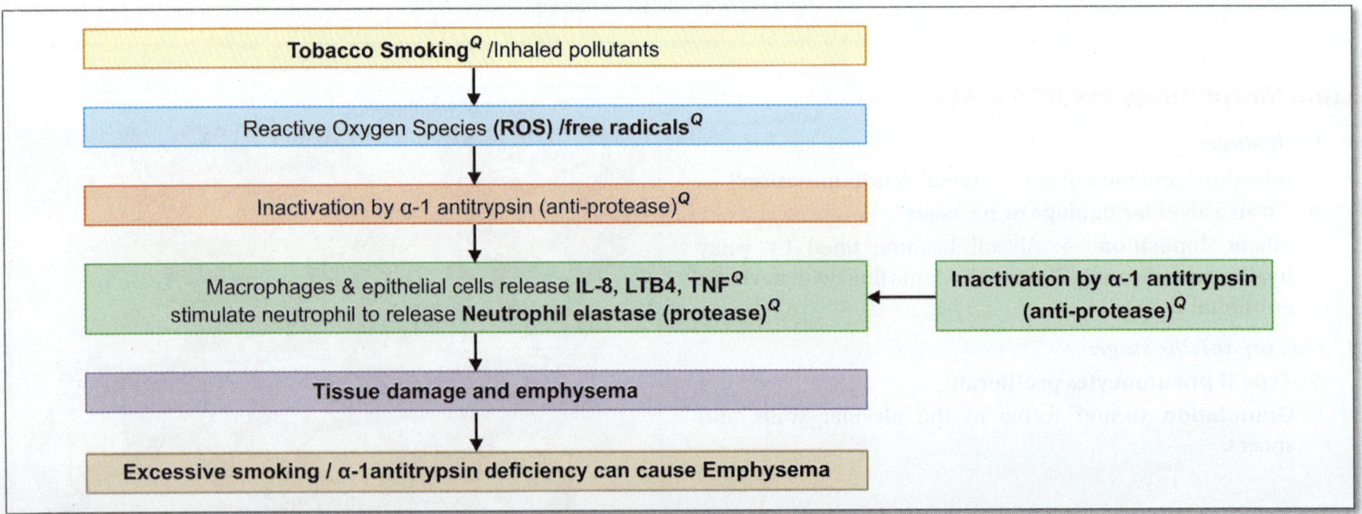

Morphology in Emphysema

- **Over inflated**[Q] voluminous lungs, often overlapping the heart
- **Large apical blebs** or **bullae**- more common in **irregular and distal**[Q] emphysema
- **Microscopically:** abnormally **large alveoli**[Q] are **separated by thin septa**[Q] with only **focal centriacinar fibrosis**[Q]
- **Enlarged pores of Kohn**[Q], with septa appearing **floated or protrude blindly** into alveolar spaces with a **club-shaped end.**

CHRONIC BRONCHITIS

- *Definition:*
  - **Persistent cough** with **sputum production**[Q] for at least **3 months**[Q] in at least **2 consecutive years,**[Q] in **the absence of any other identifiable cause.**[Q]
- *Pathogenesis:*
  - **Initiating factor** is **exposure to noxious or irritating inhaled substances**[Q] such as **tobacco smoke**[Q] (90% are smokers) and **dust from grain, cotton, and silica.**[Q]
- *Morphology:*
  - Increase in size of **mucous glands (hyperplasia) with mild hypertrophy**[Q]
  - **Reid index**[Q] or ratio of *thickness of mucous gland layer: thickness of wall between epithelium & cartilage* is **increased > 0.4**[Q]
  - **Goblet cell hyperplasia**[Q] and **chronic inflammation**[Q]
  - **Bronchiolar wall fibrosis (bronchiolitis obliterans).**[Q]

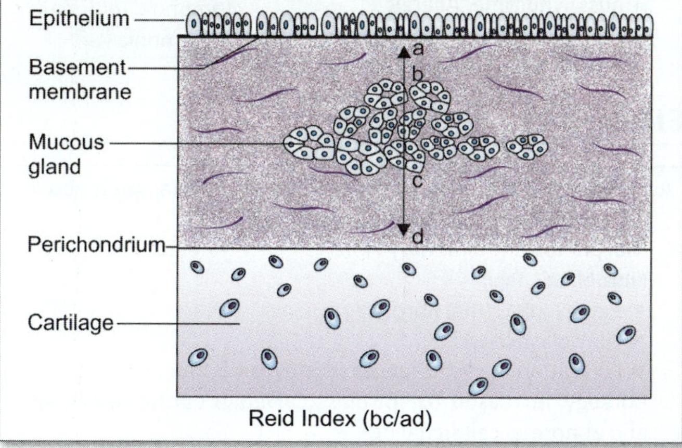

Reid Index (bc/ad)

ASTHMA

- *Definition:*
  - **Reversible bronchoconstriction** of conducting airways, along with **inflammation**[Q] & **increased mucus secretion**[Q] usually caused by an **immunological reaction**[Q], due to increased **airway sensitivity** to a variety of stimuli;
- *Genetic basis:*
  - **Chr 5q** polymorphisms in the **IL13 gene**[Q] (**strongest & most consistent association**)[Q]
  - Polymorphisms in the gene encoding **ADAM33**[Q]
  - **Class II HLA alleles → Increased IgE**
  - **IL-4 receptor gene** variants
  - Increased serum levels and lung expression of **YKL-40** (a chitinase-like glycoprotein) correlate with disease severity, airway remodeling and decreased pulmonary function [Q^{gs}]
- *Pathogenesis:*
  - Exaggerated **TH2 response**[Q] to normally harmless environmental antigens. Type 1 hypersensitivity
- *Morphology:*
  - **Gross: Occlusion of bronchi** and **bronchioles** by **thick, tenacious** mucus plugs
- *Sputum or bronchoalveolar lavage (" 3-Cs"):*
  - Curschmann spirals: extrusion of **mucus plugs** from subepithelial mucous gland ducts or bronchioles.[Q]
  - Charcot-Leyden crystals-composed of eosinophil protein called **galectin-10**[Q]
  - Creola bodies: ciliated columnar cells sloughed from the bronchial mucosa[Q]
- *Histologic findings:*
  - **Thickening of airway wall**
  - **Sub-basement membrane fibrosis**[Q] (due to deposition of **type I and III collagen**)
  - Increased **vascularity**[Q]
  - Increase in the **size of sub-mucosal glands**[Q] and **number of airway goblet cells**[Q]
  - **Hypertrophy** and/or **hyperplasia** of the **bronchial wall muscle**[Q]

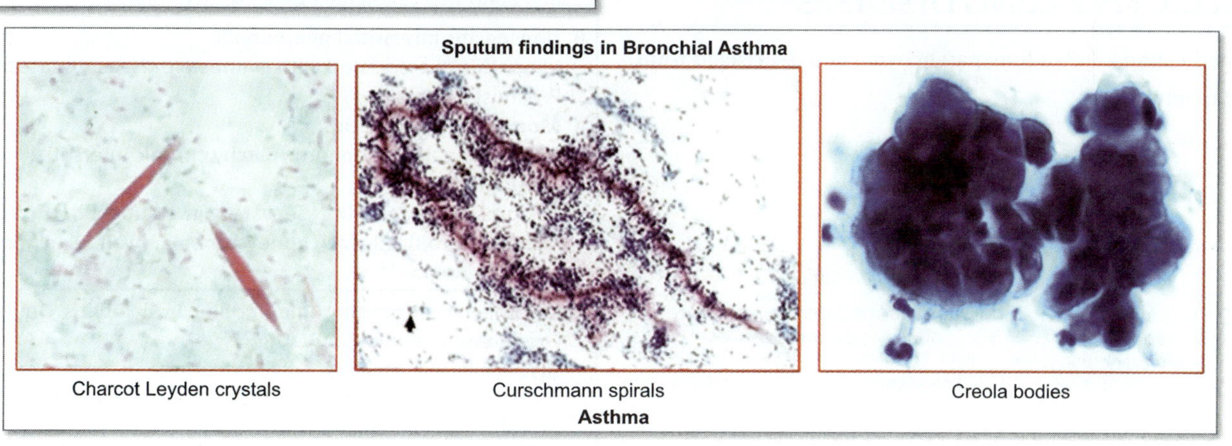

Sputum findings in Bronchial Asthma

Charcot Leyden crystals | Curschmann spirals | Creola bodies

Asthma

BRONCHIECTASIS

- *Definition:*
  - **Destruction of smooth muscle and elastic tissue** by chronic necrotizing infections leads to **permanent**[Q] **dilation of bronchi and bronchioles.**[Q]
- *Etiology:*
  - Idiopathic
  - Congenital/hereditary: e.g. **cystic fibrosis,**[Q] **intralobar sequestration,**[Q] primary ciliary dyskinesia & **Kartagener's syndrome**[Q]
  - Infections- Bacterial (Tuberculosis[Q], *Staph aureus*), viral (*Influenza*) and **fungal (*Aspergillus*)**
  - Bronchial **obstruction**-tumor, mucus plug, **Foreign body**[Q]
  - Others-**Rheumatoid Arthritis**[Q], SLE, IBD, **GVHD**[Q]
- *Gross Morphology:*
  - Involves **lower**[Q] lobes **bilaterally**[Q]
  - **Airways are dilated**, sometimes up to **four times normal size**[Q]
- *Microscopy:*
  - **Acute & chronic inflammatory exudates** within walls of bronchi & bronchioles
  - **Fibrosis**[Q] may occur

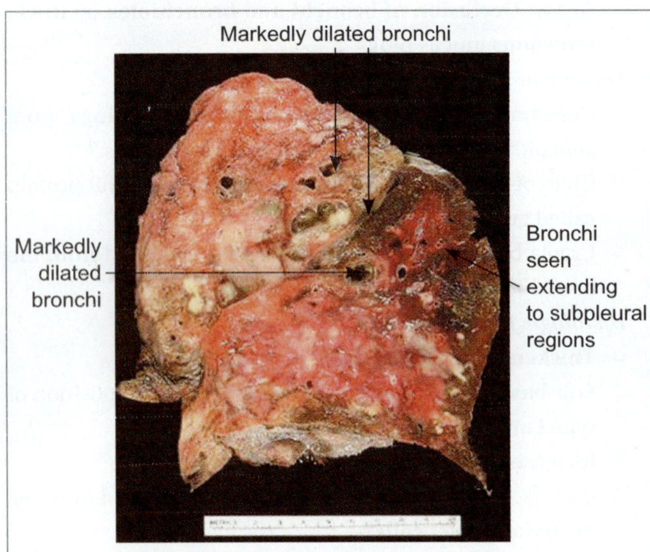

RESTRICTIVE LUNG DISEASES

Reduced expansion[Q] of lung parenchyma and **decreased total lung capacity.**[Q]

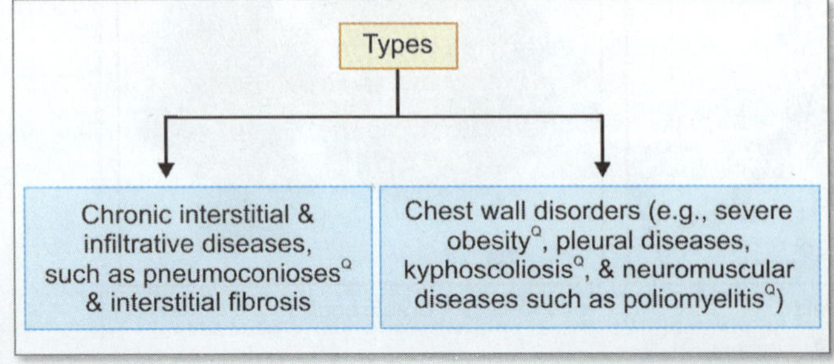

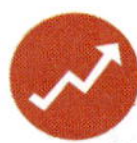

- **Kartagener's syndrome**-bronchiectasis, sinusitis, and situs **inversus**[Q]
- **Kartagener's syndrome** is seen in **50% patients** with primary ciliary dyskinesia
- **Reid index is increased in chronic bronchitis**

CHRONIC DIFFUSE INTERSTITIAL (RESTRICTIVE) DISEASES

Major Categories

Fibrosing	Granulomatous
• **Usual interstitial pneumonia (idiopathic pulmonary fibrosis)**[Q] • **Nonspecific interstitial pneumonia**[Q] • **Cryptogenic organizing pneumonia**[Q] • Associated with connective tissue diseases-**RA, SLE**[Q] • **Pneumoconiosis**[Q] • Drug reactions • Radiation pneumonitis	• **Sarcoidosis**[Q] • **Hypersensitivity pneumonitis**[Q] **Smoking related** • **Desquamative interstitial pneumonia**[Q] • Bronchiolitis-associated interstitial lung disease
Eosinophilic	**Others**
• Idiopathic **chronic eosinophilic pneumonia** • Other causes of pulmonary eosinophilia are: Churg-Strauss syndrome, Allergic Bronchopulmonary Aspergillosis	• **Pulmonary alveolar proteinosis**[Q] • Langerhans cell histiocytosis [R9j] Lymphoid interstitial pneumonia [R9j]

FIBROSING DISEASES

A. Idiopathic pulmonary fibrosis /Usual interstitial pneumonia:
Prototype of restrictive lung diseases
Morphology: (Pulmonary Fibrosis ← **P F** → Patchy Fibroblastic foci)[Q]
- **P**atchy interstitial fibrosis[Q]
- **F**ibroblastic foci[Q]
- Formation of **cystic spaces (honeycomb lung)**[Q]

Etiology: Increased TGF-β[Q] due to **alveolar epithelial damage** and abnormal cell signaling

B. Nonspecific interstitial pneumonia:
Idiopathic or associated with **connective tissue diseases**[Q]
Prognosis: **Good**[Q]
Morphology: 2 varieties
- **Cellular pattern:** Uniform/patchy chronic interstitial **inflammation**
- **Fibrosing pattern:** Diffuse/patchy interstitial **fibrotic** lesions

Absent: Fibroblastic foci, honeycombing, hyaline membranes and granulomas[Q]

C. Cryptogenic Organizing Pneumonia/Bronchiolitis Obliterans Organizing Pneumonia (BOOP)[Q]
Histology: Presence of polypoid plugs of loose organizing connective tissue **(Masson bodies)**[Q] within **alveolar ducts, alveoli, and bronchioles**

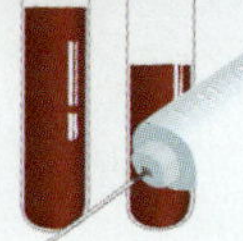

PNEUMOCONIOSIS

Definition: Diseases induced by organic as well as inorganic particulates and chemical fumes and vapors.

Characteristics	Anthracosis	Silicosis	Asbestosis
Exposure	**Coal mining**[Q] (particularly hard coal)	Foundry work, **sandblasting**, hard rock mining, **stone cutting**[Q]	**Mining, milling**, fabrication, and installation and removal of **insulation**[Q]
Type of Mineral dust	**Coal particles**	**Amorphous forms & crystalline forms (Quartz, cristobalite, and tridymite) –more fibrogenic**[Q]	**Serpentine**[Q] **(M.C)** and **Amphibole**[Q] **(more pathogenic)**
Site of involvement	**upper lobes**[Q] and **upper zones** of the lower lobes	**upper lobes**[Q] and **upper zones** of the lower lobes	**Lower lobes**[Q] and subpleurally.
Caplan syndrome[Q]	+	+	+
Lung lesions	**Coal macules**[Q] (1-2 mm) Larger **coal nodules**[Q] **Complicated coal workers' pneumoconiosis**[Q] Progressive **massive fibrosis**[Q] (1-10cm)	**Discrete nodules in hilar nodes & upper zones of lungs**[Q] **Hard, collagenous scars** Fibrotic lesions in nodes & pleura (pleural thickening) **Eggshell calcification**[Q] **Hallmark: Central collagen** with **peripheral zone** of **dust-laden macrophages**[Q] Progressive **massive fibrosis**[Q] (1-10cm) **Lung Ca**[Q] **(2 fold risk)**	**Asbestos bodies**[Q] **Ferruginous bodies**[Q] Localized fibrous plaques **Diffuse pleural fibrosis**[Q] Pleural effusions Parenchymal interstitial fibrosis (asbestosis) **Lung carcinoma**[Q] Mesotheliomas[Q] **Laryngeal, ovarian, colon ca**[Q]

OTHER LUNG DISEASES CAUSED BY AIR POLLUTANTS

Agent	Disease	Exposure
	Mineral dusts	
Beryllium	Acute berylliosis, Beryllium granulomatosis[Q], Lung carcinoma[Q]	Mining, fabrication
Iron oxide	**Siderosis**[Q]	Welding
Barium sulfate	**Baritosis**[Q]	Mining
Tin oxide	**Stannosis**[Q]	Mining
	Organic dusts that induce hypersensitivity pneumonitis	
Moldy hay	Farmer's lung[Q]	Farming
Bagasse	Bagassosis[Q]	Manufacturing wallboard, paper
Bird droppings	Bird-breeder's lung[Q]	Bird handling

GRANULOMATOUS DISEASES

Sarcoidosis

- *Definition:*
  - A **systemic disease** characterized by **non-caseating granulomas** in tissues and organs.
- *Epidemiology:*
  - **Females more commonly** affected than males
- *Genetic basis:*
  - Associated with **HLA-A1 and HLA-B8**[Q]
- *Etiology and Pathogenesis:*
  - **Disordered immune regulation** in **genetically predisposed** individuals exposed to certain environmental agents.
  - **Cell-mediated response**[Q] to an unidentified antigen by **CD4+ helper T cells.**
  - Intra-alveolar and interstitial **CD4/CD8** T-cell ratios = **5 : 1 to 15 : 1**[Q]
  - Increased **T cell–derived TH$_1$** cytokines: **IL-2 and IFN-γ** →T-cell expansion and **macrophage activation**
  - Increased levels of **IL-8, TNF, macrophage inflammatory protein 1**α that favor recruitment of **T cells** & **monocytes** and contribute to the formation of **granulomas**.
  - **TNF** concentration in the **bronchoalveolar lavage (BAL)** fluid is a **marker of disease activity**[Q]
- *Clinical features:*
  - Most commonly presents with **bilateral hilar lymphade-nopathy** or **lung** involvement[Q] (90% cases) followed by **Skin** > Extrathoracic lymph nodes > Eye > Liver > Spleen > Neurologic >**Heart** > **Kidney (least common)**[Q]

- **Histology:**
  - All involved tissues show **well-formed non-caseating granulomas**[Q] composed of **epithelioid cells**[Q], with **Langhans or foreign body–type giant cells**[Q]
  - Central necrosis is **unusual.**[Q]
  - **Schaumann bodies**[Q]: laminated concretions composed of **calcium and proteins**[Q]
  - **Asteroid bodies**[Q]: **Stellate inclusions** enclosed within **giant cells**[Q]

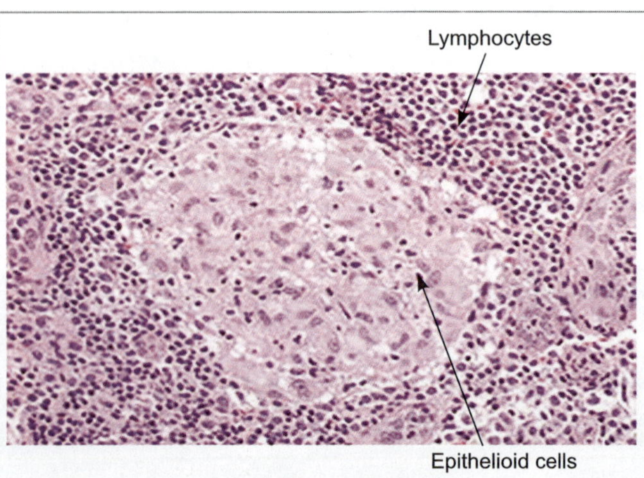

Non-caseating granuloma

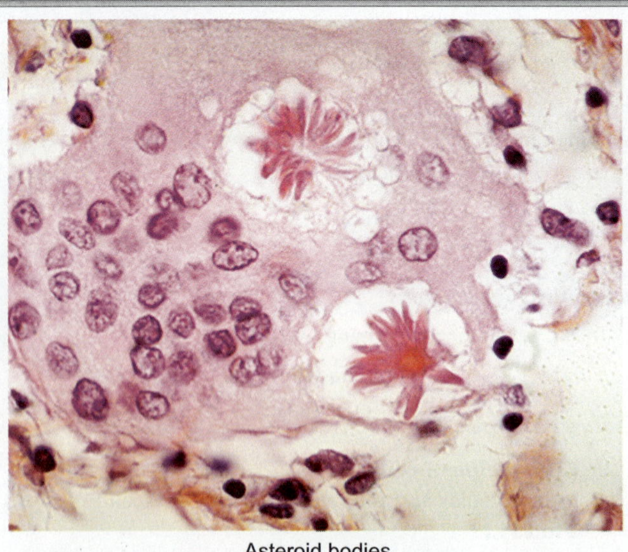

Asteroid bodies

- **Diagnosis:**
  - EXCLUDE infections and malignancy
  - **Elevated ACE level**[Q] (elevated in other granulomatous diseases but not in malignancy).
  - **Positive gallium scan:** Increased activity in
    - Parotids and lacrimal glands (**panda sign**)[Q]
    - Right paratracheal and left hilar area (**lambda sign**)[Q].
  - **Bronchoalveolar lavage (BAL)** shows **increase in lymphocytes**
  - **CD4/CD8 ratio**[Q] of lymphocytes in BAL > **3.5:1**[Q] is **strongly supportive** of Sarcoidosis

- Kviem-Siltzbach procedure (**specific diagnostic test, no longer used**): Non-caseating granulomas seen **4–6 weeks** after **Intradermal injection** of splenic tissue extract of a known sarcoidosis patient, is **highly specific** for the diagnosis of Sarcoidosis.
- **Hypercalcemia and/or hypercalciuria** (10% cases) due to increased production of **1,25-dihydroxyvitamin D$_3$** by the granuloma.

High Yield Facts

- **Caplan Syndrome (Rheumatoid pneumoconiosis)**[Q] is a combination of **rheumatoid arthritis (RA)**[Q] and **pneumoconiosis** that manifests as **intrapulmonary nodules**[Q]
- **Silicosis** is **M.C** pneumoconiosis in the world[Q]
- **Crystalline silica** (e.g., quartz) is **most dangerous** silica particle[Q]
- In patients with **Silicosis**, there is increased susceptibility to **tuberculosis**[Q]
- **Silicosis** is **progressive** even after exposure stops[Q]
- **Asbestos bodies:** golden brown, **fusiform or beaded rods** with a translucent center and consists of **asbestos fibers coated** with an **iron-containing proteinaceous material**[Q]
- **Ferruginous bodies:** **Inorganic particulates** coated with **iron-protein complexes**[Q]
- **Lung Ca** and **mesotheliomas (pleural and peritoneal)** develop in workers exposed to asbestos.
- **Amphibole**[Q] variety of asbestos though less prevalent, are **more pathogenic** than chrysotiles, to cause **mesothelioma**
- **Risk of Lung Ca** is increased about **five-fold**[Q], while that of **mesothelioma is 1000-fold**[Q] greater in **Asbestos** exposure

HYPERSENSITIVITY PNEUMONITIS

- **Also called:**
  - Also called **Extrinsic allergic alveolitis**[Q]
- **Definition:**
  - **Immunologically mediated**, predominantly **interstitial** lung disorder due to prolonged exposure to inhaled organic antigens.
- **Pathogenesis:**
  - Involves **type IV**[Q] > **type III**[Q] hypersensitivity reaction (*Harrison's 18th ed, Chapter 255*)
- **Morphology:**
  - **Interstitial pneumonitis:**[Q] lymphocytes, plasma cells & macrophages (**eosinophils rare**)
  - **Non-caseating granulomas**[Q] in 2/3rd of patients
  - **Interstitial fibrosis, fibroblastic foci, honeycombing & obliterative bronchiolitis** (in **late** stages)
  - Intra-alveolar infiltrates in more than half of patients

PULMONARY INFECTIONS

Pneumonia

- **Definition:** Infection of the **lung parenchyma;**[Q]
- Can be Typical (airway involvement) or Atypical (interstitial involvement)

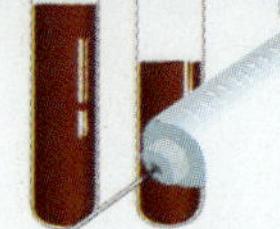

Typical Pneumonia

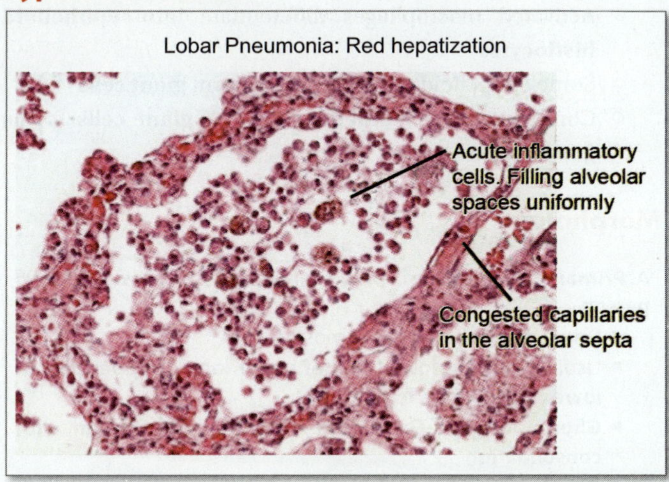

- *2 patterns*
  - **Broncho**pneumonia (**Patchy consolidation** of the lung)[Q]
  - **Lobar** pneumonia (fibrino-suppurative consolidation of **a part of lobe** or **entire lobe**)[Q]

- *Etiology*
  - **Bacterial:**[Q] *Streptococcus pneumonia,*[Q] *H. influenzae, Moraxella catarrhalis, S. aureus, K. pneumoniae, Pseudomonas spp.*
- *Morphology*
  - In **lobar pneumonia**, 4 stages have been described; see below
  - **In Bronchopneumonia:**
  - Scattered a**reas of acute suppurative inflammation,**[Q] usually multilobar, **frequently bilateral**[Q] & **basal**[Q] because of the tendency of secretions to gravitate to lower lobes;
  - **Histologically: neutrophil-rich exudate**[Q] that fills the bronchi, bronchioles and adjacent alveolar spaces.
- *Complications*
  - **Abscess formation**[Q] (common with **type 3** *Pneumococci* or *Klebsiella* infections)
  - **Empyema:** Due to spread of infection to **pleural cavity**[Q]
  - **Bacteremic dissemination**[Q] to the heart valves, pericardium, brain, kidneys, spleen, or joints, causing **metastatic abscesses**, endocarditis, meningitis, or suppurative arthritis.

Stages of Lobar Pneumonia[Q]

Stage	Characteristics
Congestion (1-2 days)[Q]	• **Grossly:** Lung is heavy, boggy & red. • **Microscopically: Vascular engorgement,**[Q] intra-alveolar fluid with **neutrophils**[Q] & bacteria.
Red hepatization (2-4 days)[Q]	• **Grossly: Red**, firm & **airless**, with a **liver-like consistency**[Q], hence the term **hepatization**. • **Microscopically**: Confluent **exudation** with neutrophils, **RBCs, fibrin**[Q] filling alveoli;
Gray hepatization (5-8 days)[Q]	• **Grossly: Grayish brown**, dry surface. • **Microscopically: Disintegration of RBCs** & persistence of a **fibrinosuppurative exudate**
Resolution (8-9 days)	• Exudates within alveoli broken down by enzymatic digestion to produce **granular debris**[Q] • Debris may be reabsorbed/ingested by macrophages/expectorated/**organized by fibroblasts**[Q]

High Yield Facts

- MC cause of **Community-acquired pneumonia** is *Streptococcus pneumoniae*[Q] followed by *H. influenza*
- Most common cause of **Community-acquired atypical pneumonia** is *Mycoplasma pneumonia*[Q]> *Chlamydia*
- Most common cause of **Hospital-acquired pneumonia** are **Gram-negative rods**[Q], Enterobacteriaceae (*Klebsiella spp., Serratia marcescens, Escherichia coli*) and *Pseudomonas spp.*
- Most common cause of **Aspiration pneumonia** are **Anaerobic**[Q] oral flora (*Bacteroides*[Q], *Prevotella,*

Fusobacterium, Peptostreptococcus), admixed with aerobic bacteria (*Streptococcus pneumoniae, Staphylococcus aureus, Haemophilus influenzae,* and *Pseudomonas aeruginosa*)
- Defects in **innate immunity**[Q] & **humoral immunodeficiency**[Q] → Increased infections with **pyogenic** bacteria.
- **Cell-mediated** immune[Q] defects → Infections with **Mycobacteria**[Q], *Herpes* viruses, *Pneumocystis jiroveci.*[Q]

Atypical Pneumonia

- *Definition:*
  - Acute febrile respiratory disease characterized by **patchy inflammatory changes** in the lungs, largely confined to the **alveolar septa**[Q] and **pulmonary interstitium**[Q].
- *Differences of atypical from typical pneumonia:*
  - **Moderate** amount of **sputum**[Q]
  - **No physical findings** of consolidation[Q]
  - Only **moderate elevation of WBCs**[Q]
  - **Lack of alveolar exudate**[Q]

- *Etiology:*
  - **Atypical organisms:** *Mycoplasma pneumoniae* (MC)[Q], *Chlamydia pneumonia, C burnetii* (Q-fever)
  - **Viruses:** *Influenza* **virus types A and B**, *Respiratory syncytial viruses (RSV), Parainfluenza (children), Human metapneumovirus, Adenovirus, Rhinoviruses, Rubeola, Varicella* viruses
- *Risk Factors:*
  - Extremes of age[Q], malnutrition[Q], alcoholism[Q] & underlying debilitating illnesses
- *Morphology:*
  - **Interstitial**[Q] **inflammatory reaction**, virtually **localized within the walls**[Q] of alveoli.

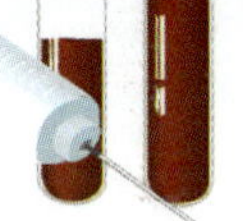

- ○ **Alveolar septa** are **widened and edematous**[Q] and usually have a **mononuclear inflammatory infiltrate**[Q] of lymphocytes, macrophages, and occasionally plasma cells.
- ○ Superimposed bacterial infection → **ulcerative bronchitis, bronchiolitis & bacterial pneumonia**.
- ○ *Herpes simplex, Varicella & Adenovirus*, may be associated with **necrosis of bronchial and alveolar epithelium**[Q] and **acute inflammation.**[Q]

Tuberculosis

Causative agent: M*ycobacterium tuberculosis*

- Weakly **Gram positive**[Q] bacilli
- **Acid fast (resists decoloration with acid & acid-alcohol)**[Q] on **Ziehl Neelsen (ZN)**[Q] **staining**, due to a cell wall composed of glycolipids & **mycolic acid**[Q]
- **Group specificity** is due to **polysaccharide**[Q]
- **Type specificity** is due to **protein antigen**[Q].

Main source of transmission: Person to person transmission of **air-borne**[Q] organisms

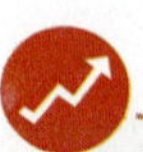

High Yield Facts

- • **Mycobacterium tuberculosis** enters into macrophages with the help of **mannose binding lectin**[Q] and **CR3.**[Q]
- • **Macrophages**[Q] are the **primary cells infected** by M. tuberculosis.
- • **IFN-γ**[Q] **is the critical mediator** that enables macrophages to contain the M. tuberculosis infection.
- • **NK T cells**[Q] & γδ **T-cells**[Q] also produce IFN-γ.
- • People with genetic **deficiencies in IL-12 & IFN-γ pathway**, including STAT1 a signal transducer for IFN-γ, are **vulnerable to severe Mycobacterial infections**.
- • **Polymorphisms in genes for HLA, IFN-γ, IFN-γ receptor & TLR2** are associated with **increased susceptibility** to TB
- • Factors contributing in pathogenesis of TB: **Cord factor, Lipoarabinomannan**[Q], **Complement system**, M. tuberculosis **heat shock proteins**.
- • **Risk of acquiring TB infection** is determined mainly by **exogenous factors**[Q] while **risk of developing TB disease** depends largely on **endogenous factors**[Q].

Pathogenesis

- ■ *Entry & replication in macrophages:*
  - ○ By **inhibition** of **phagolysosome** formation[Q]
- ■ *TH1 response:*
  - ○ **Alveolar macrophages** that **present TB antigen** to T cells, also secrete **IL-12** which activates T cells to differentiate to **TH1 cells.**
- ■ *Macrophage activation & bacteria killing:*
  - ○ IFN γ[Q] produced by **TH1 cells** – Stimulates: **Maturation of phago-lysosome**
  - ○ Stimulates production of **NO à reactive nitrogen intermediates**
  - ○ Mobilizes antimicrobial peptides (**defensins**) against *M. tuberculosis*
  - ○ Stimulates **autophagy** to destroy *M. tuberculosis*.

- ■ *Granulomatous inflammation & tissue damage:*
  - ○ Activated macrophages differentiate into '**epithelioid histiocytes'**
  - ○ Some epithelioid cells may fuse to form **giant cells**[Q]
  - ○ Combination of **epithelioid cells & giant cells forms granulomas**[Q]

Morphology

A. Primary Tuberculosis: in **previously unexposed (unsensitized)**[Q] **person.**

- ■ **Primary organ** involved is mostly **lungs**[Q]
- ■ Usually involves **lower part of upper lobe** or **upper part of lower lobe**[Q] (close to pleura)[Q]
- ■ **Ghon's focus**[Q] : Grey white area of **inflammation with consolidation**
- ■ **Ghon's complex:**[Q] Ghon's focus + inflamed regional lymph nodes
- ■ **Histology:** Granulomatous inflammatory reaction with both **caseating & non-caseating** tubercles
- ■ **Simon's Focus**[Q] : Occult hematogenous dissemination to apex of lung

Fate of primary TB:

- ■ **95% cases:** controlled by immunity Calcified healed lesions & hilar lymph nodes **(Ranke complex)**
- ■ **5% cases:** Primary tuberculosis is progressive **(Progressive Primary TB)**
  - → resembles acute bacterial pneumonia
  - → **Lymphohematogenous dissemination** may cause **tuberculous meningitis** &/or **miliary TB**

B. Secondary Tuberculosis: in a **previously sensitized host**[Q]

Also called 'adult type' or **'reactivation tuberculosis'** or 'chronic pulmonary TB'

- ■ Involves **apical & posterior segments of upper lobe** due to high O_2 concentration (**Puhl's lesion**[Q])
- ■ **Infraclavicular lesion** is called **Assman's Focus**[Q]
- ■ **Regional lymph node involvement is late**[Q]
- ■ **Cavitation occurs readily**[Q] with erosion of the cavities into an airway
- ■ **Histology:** Active lesions show **coalescent tubercles** with central caseation **(Caseous Necrosis)**[Q]
- ■ **AFB** can be seen **in early phase** of granuloma formation but usually not seen in late fibro-calcific stage

C. Extrapulmonary TB:

- ■ **MC site is lymph node**[Q], MC cervical & supraclavicular (**"Scrofula"**)[Q]
- ■ **Pleural TB: Exudative**[Q] Pleural effusion, tuberculous empyema, or obliterative fibrous pleuritic;
- ■ **Renal TB: sterile pyuria**[Q]
- ■ **Genital TB:** Preferentially involves **fallopian tube**[Q] in females & **epididymis**[Q] in males
- ■ **Skeletal TB:** Most common site **spine**[Q] **(Pott's disease)**[Q] > hip > knee
- ■ **Paravertebral cold abscess** may form;
- ■ **TB meningitis** (paresis of cranial nerves especially ocular, is frequent finding)[Q]
- ■ **GI TB (MC site terminal ileum and caecum)**[Q]

- **Tuberculous pericarditis (MC cause of chronic constrictive pericarditis)**[Q]
- **Endobronchial, endotracheal & laryngeal tuberculosi**s may develop by spread through lymphatic channels or from expectorated infectious material.

RECENT EXAM[Q]

- **Miliary/Disseminated TB:** When bacteria disseminate through systemic **arterial system** & involve **lungs** ± multiple organs. Most prominent in the **liver**, bone marrow, spleen, adrenals and meninges.

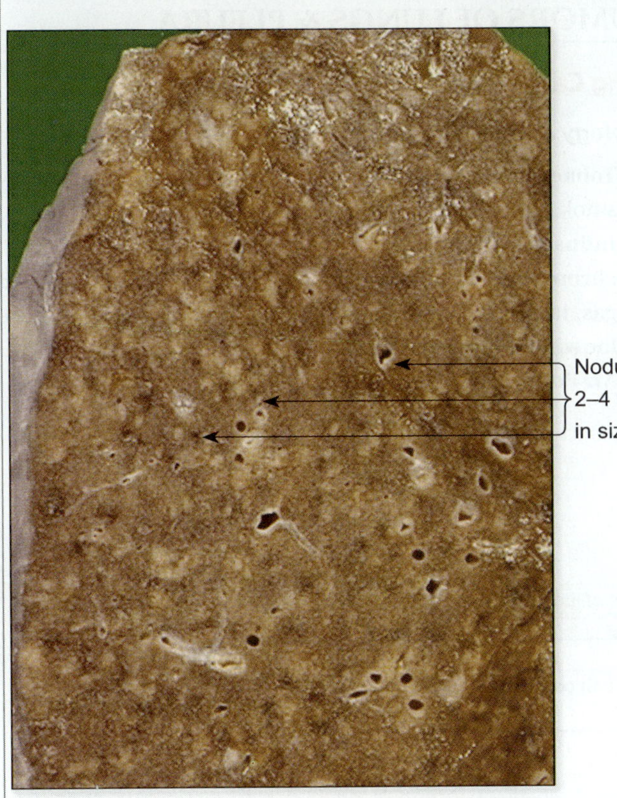

Here one can see multitude of small tan(-) yellow granulomas, about 2 to 4 mm in size, scattered throughout the lung parenchyma. The miliary pattern gets its name from the resemblence of the granulomas to millet seeds. Diagnosis miliary–TB.

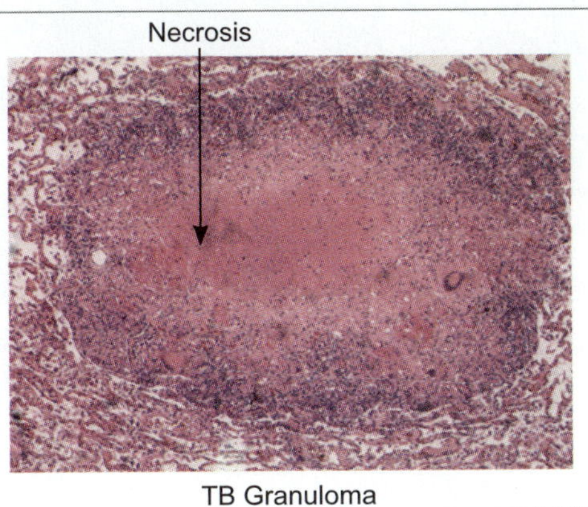

TB Granuloma

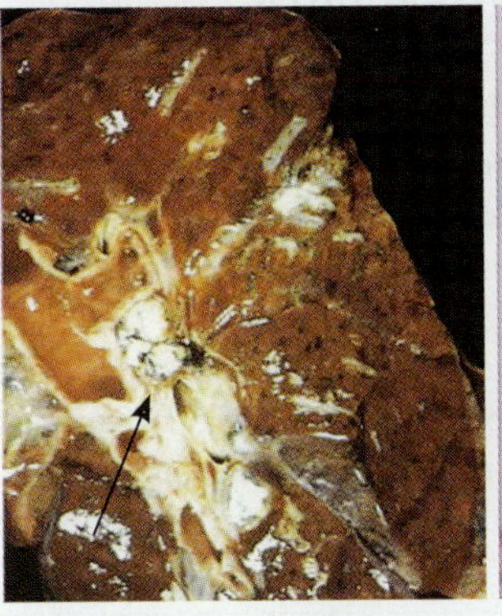

Ghon's focus

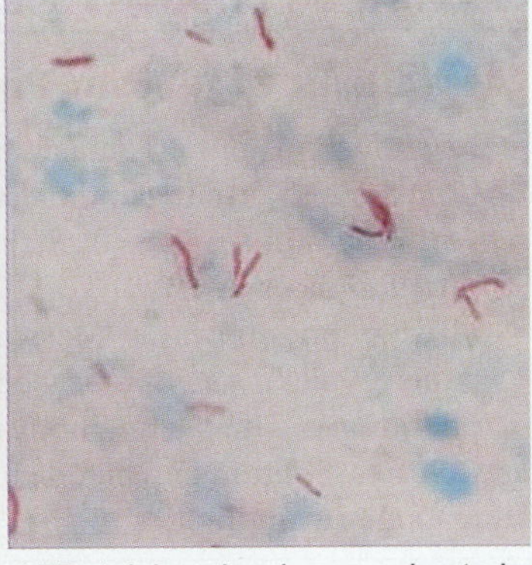

AFB staining showing mycobacteria

- In **congenital TB**, primary organ involved is **liver**[Q]. Cantwell revised criteria for congenital TB.

Cantwell criteria

- **Presence of proven Tuberculous disease with atleast 1 of the following:**
  1. Lesions in the newborn baby during the first week of life.
  2. Primary hepatic complex or caseating hepatic granuloma.
  3. Tuberculous infection of the placenta or maternal genital tract.
  4. Exclusion of possibility of postnatal transmission by investigation of contacts, including hospital staff.

Diagnosis

- **Mantoux (Tuberculin test)**[Q] & **IFN-γ release assay (IGRA)**[Q] indicate **infection with TB** & **not TB disease**[Q]
- **Sputum Microscopy** by **ZN staining**[Q]
- **Petroff's method**[Q] is best suited for decontamination of sputum
- **Auramine Rhodamine**[Q] stain **more sensitive** than ZN staining
- **Culture** media for TB are: **LJ media, Middlebrook** media
- **Bactec/MGIT** method may be used for early diagnosis
- **Rapid** diagnostic tests for TB include: **PCR, Line probe assay**[Q], **GeneXpert**[Q]
- **FNAC/Biopsy** of involved organ shows **caseating/non-caseating granuloma with/without AFB**[Q]

High Yield Facts

- **"Primary"** TB occurs in **non-immune** host & **"secondary"** TB occurs in a **host immune** to *M. tuberculosis*.
- **Immunocompromised** people **do not form granulomas** & their macrophages **contain many AFB**[Q]
- **Hemoptysis** (in 20–30% cases) may result from rupture of a dilated vessel in a cavity **(Rasmussen's aneurysm)**[Q] or from **Aspergilloma** formation in an old cavity
- Adenosine deaminase **(ADA) level** in pleural fluid **> 40 IU/L**[Q] indicates Tuberculosis.
- **Causes of Necrotizing epithelioid cell granulomas:**

• Tuberculosis	• Tuberculoid leprosy	• Wegener's Granulomatosis[Q]
• Cat's scratch disease	• Syphilis	

OTHER TYPES OF PNEUMONIA

Cryptogenic Organizing Pneumonia (COP)

- Noninfectious pneumonia characterized by inflammation of bronchioles and surrounding structure
- Formerly known as: Bronchiolitis obliterans organizing pneumonia or BOOP
- Micrograph shows a Masson body (pale circular and paucicellular), as may be seen in cryptogenic organizing pneumonia. The Masson body plugs the airway
- Cultures: Sputum and blood cultures are negative and has no response to antibiotics

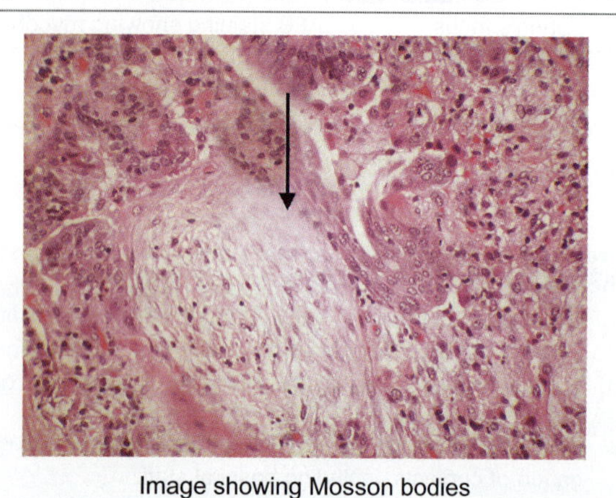
Image showing Mosson bodies

LUNG ABSCESS

- *Definition:*
  - **Local suppurative**[Q] process **within the lung**, characterized by **necrosis** of lung tissue.
- *Etiology:*
  - *Bacteroides*[Q], *Fusobacterium*[Q], *& Peptococcus*[Q] (3 **most common** bacteria), Aerobic and anaerobic *Streptococci, S. aureus* & gram -ve organisms.
- *Risk factors:*
  - **Aspiration of infective material**[Q] **(Most common cause)**

TUMORS OF LUNGS & PLEURA

Lung Carcinoma

Etiology and Pathogenesis

1. **Tobacco Smoking: 60 times**[Q] greater among habitual heavy smokers (2 packs/day for 20 years)
2. **Industrial Hazards**: Exposure to **asbestos**[Q], **arsenic**[Q], **chromium**[Q], **uranium, nickel, vinyl chloride and mustard gas**, increase the risk of developing lung cancer. High-dose **ionizing radiation** is carcinogenic.
3. **Air Pollution:** Radon

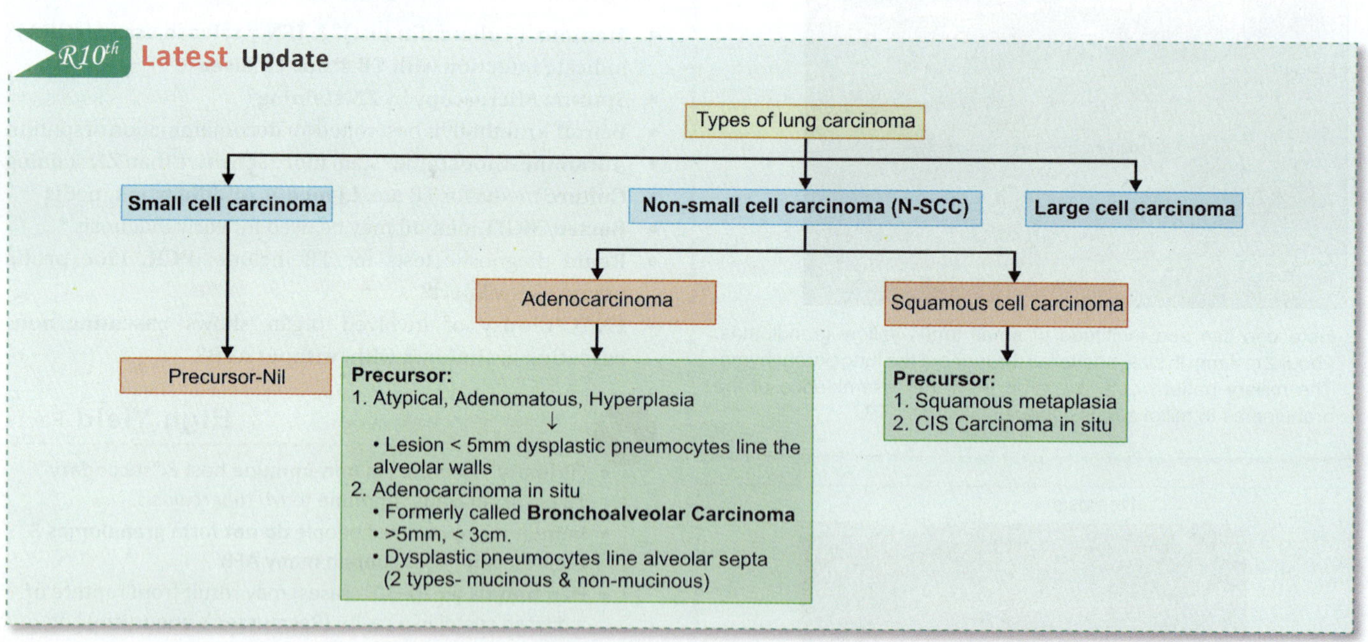

Types of Lung Ca

- **Adenocarcinoma:**
  - **Peripherally** located[Q]
  - **Well-differentiated tumors** with obvious glandular element
  - Express thyroid transcription factor-1 **(TTF-1)[Q]** and Napsin **A**
  - Electron Microscopy shows **short, plump microvilli[Q]**
  - 2 subtypes:
    - **Microinvasive:** ≤3 cm in size and ≤5 mm invasion[Q]
    - **Mucinous:** Tend to **spread aerogenously[Q]** forming **satellite tumors[Q]**

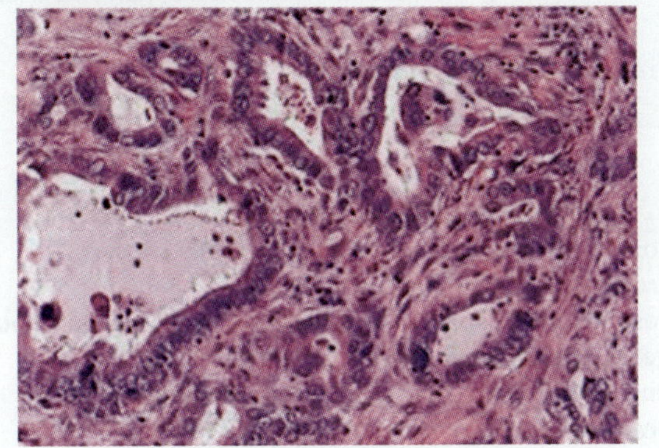

Adenocarcinoma

- **Squamous cell carcinoma:**
  - **Strongly associated with smoking[Q]**
  - **Central in location[Q]**
  - Precursor lesions- **Squamous metaplasia** or **dysplasia** of bronchial epithelium
  - Mass like lesion which may infiltrate surrounding areas
  - **Hemorrhage** or **necrosis** which may also form **cavity lesions[Q]**
  - **Keratinization ("squamous pearls")[Q]** on **light microscopy** and/or **Intercellular bridges[Q]** on **electron microscopy** is diagnostic

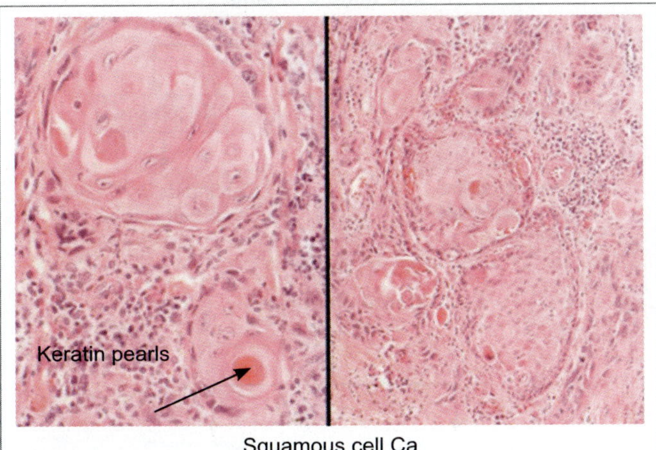

Squamous cell Ca

- **Small cell carcinoma:**
  - **Most malignant Lung Ca[Q]**, most **aggressive,[Q]** wide **metastasis[Q]** and **fatal[Q]**

- **Strongest** relationship to **cigarette smoking[Q]**
- **Central > peripheral** in location[Q]
- No preinvasive phase.
- **Light Microscopy:**
  - Small cells with **salt and pepper pattern[Q]**, **nuclear molding[Q]** is prominent

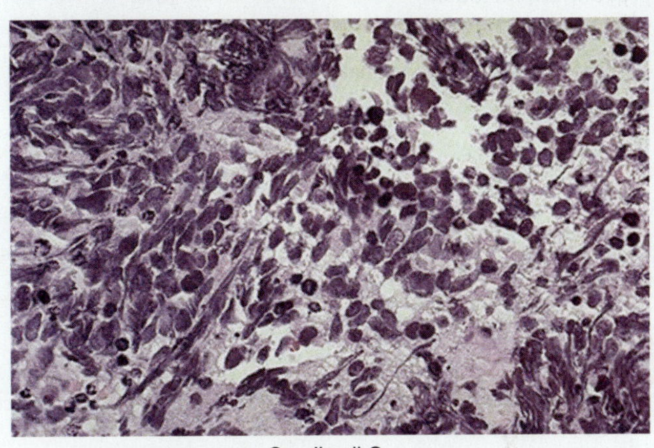

Small cell Ca

- **Basophilic staining** of vascular walls due to encrustation by DNA from necrotic tumor cells **(Azzopardi effect)[Q]**

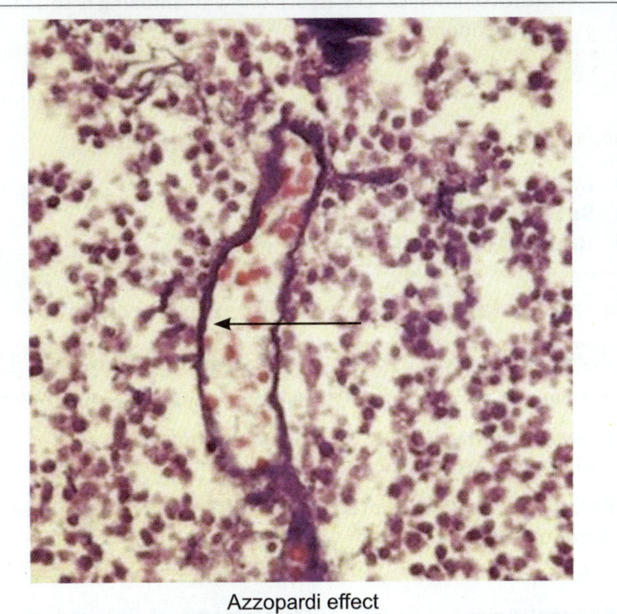

Azzopardi effect

  - **Electron microscopy: Dense-core neurosecretory granules[Q]** releasing neuroendocrine markers such as **chromogranin[Q]**, **synaptophysin[Q]** and **CD57[Q]**, para-thormone-related protein[Q]
  - **Most common lung Ca** associated with **ectopic hormone production[Q]**
  - Immunohistochemistry: **BCL2[Q]** in 90% of tumors
- **Large cell carcinoma:**
  - Diagnosis of exclusion
  - **Large nuclei,[Q]** prominent nucleoli,[Q] and a moderate amount of cytoplasm

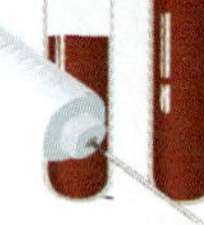

Differences between Small Cell and Non-small Cell Lung Carcinoma

Features	Small cell lung carcinoma	Non-Small cell lung carcinoma
Tumor Suppressor gene abnormalities		
3p deletions	>90%	>80%
RB mutations	−90%	−20%
p(6KDKN2A) mutation	−10%	>50%
TP53 mutation	>90%	>50%
Dominant oncogene abnormalities		
KRAS mutations	Rare	−30% (adenocarcinoma)
EQR mutations	Absent	−20% (adenocarcinoma, non-smokers, woman)
ALK rearrangements	Absent	4%–6% adenocarcinoma, non-smokers, often have signet ring morphology
Responses to chemotherapy and radiotherapy	Often complete response but recur invariably	Incomplete

High Yield Facts

- **Lung Carcinoma is most frequently diagnosed**[Q] major cancer in the world
- **Lung Carcinoma is most common cause of cancer mortality**[Q] worldwide
- Most common Lung Ca **world-wide is Adenocarcinoma**[Q]
- Most common lung Ca in **India** is **Squamous cell Ca**[Q]
- Most common cancer associated with **smoking** is squamous cell carcinoma
- Most specifically associated with smoking: small cell carcinoma
- Most common cancer in **non-smokers**[Q] and **women**[Q], **young age**[Q] is Adenocarcinoma
- Lung Ca with **best prognosis- Adenocarcinoma**[Q]
- Lung Ca with **worst prognosis- Small Cell Ca**[Q]
- **Lung Carcinoids may occur in patients with MEN type I**
- Most common paraneoplastic manifestations of Bronchoalveolar carcinoma is systemic sclerosis

Metastasis from Lung Ca to Other Organs

- Lymphatic and hematogenous pathways[Q]
- **Sq cell Ca shows late metastasis**[Q]
- **Brain > Adrenals**, Liver, and bone

Paraneoplastic Syndromes in Lung Carcinoma

Hormone Secreted	Clinical Manifestations
Antidiuretic hormone (ADH)[Q]	**Hyponatremia** due to **SIADH**[Q]
Adrenocorticotropic hormone (ACTH)[Q]	**Cushing syndrome**[Q]
Parathormone, PTH -related peptide, PGE	**Hypercalcemia**[Q] [Most commonly seen with SCC lung]
Calcitonin	**Hypocalcemia**
Gonadotropins	**Gynecomastia** [Most commonly seen with large cell carcinoma lung]
Serotonin and bradykinin	**Carcinoid syndrome**[Q]

Other Systemic Manifestations of Lung Carcinoma

- **Lambert-Eaton myasthenic syndrome**[Q]
- **Peripheral neuropathy**[Q]
- **Acanthosis nigricans**[Q]
- Leukemoid reactions
- **Trousseau syndrome** (deep vein thrombosis and thromboembolism)[Q]

- **Hypertrophic pulmonary osteoarthropathy**, associated with **clubbing of the fingers**.[Q]
- Apical lung cancers (**Pancoast tumors**): Severe pain along ulnar nerve
- **Horner syndrome**[Q] (enophthalmos, ptosis, miosis, and anhidrosis) on the same side as the lesion

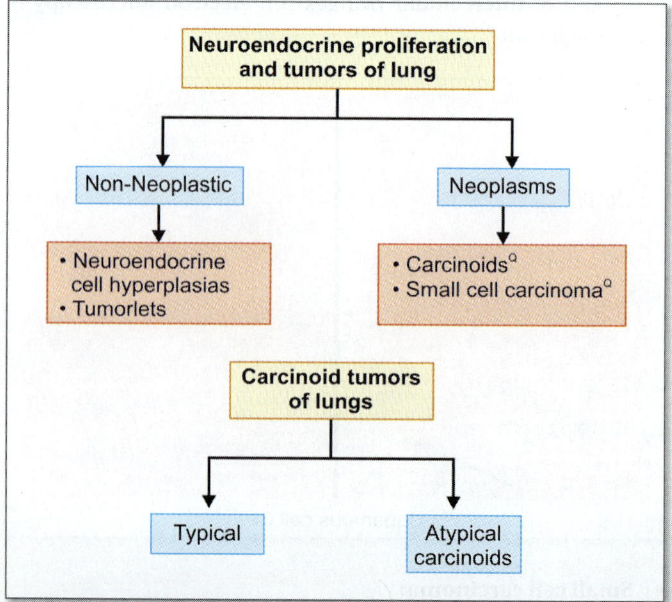

Theory

Carcinoid Tumors of Lungs

- **Epidemiology:**
  - **1% -5% of all lung tumors**[Q]
  - **Age of Onset: < 40 years**[Q] of age, **Male is equally involved to females**[Q]
  - **20% - 40%** of patients are **non-smokers**[Q]
- **Classification:**
  - **Classical carcinoid:** <2 mitosis/10 hpf (high power fields) and **lack necrosis**[Q]
  - **Atypical carcinoid:** 2-10 mitosis/hpf with increased **pleomorphism, necrosis, prominent nucleoli**[Q], may cause **Carcinoid syndrome**[Q]
- **Clinical Features:**
  - Obstructive line **bronchiectasis, emphysema** & **atelectasis**[Q]
  - **Elaboration of vasoactive amines:** Carcinoid syndrome characterized by **diarrhea, flushing & cyanosis**.[Q]
- **Gross Morphology:**
  - Carcinoids may arise **centrally** or may be **peripheral**
  - **Spherical polypoid masses**[Q] (3-4 cm) that project into the **lumen of bronchus**
  - Some tumors **penetrate bronchial wall** (invasive)[Q] to fan out in the peribronchial tissue, producing 'collar-button lesion'.[Q]
- **Light Microscopy:**
  - **Nest/rosette-like** arrangements of cells separated by a delicate fibrovascular stroma[Q]
- **IHC:**
  - Stains positive for **Serotonin**[Q], **Neuron-specific enolase**[Q], **Bombesin**[Q], **Calcitonin**[Q]
- **Electron microscopy:**
  - **Dense-core granules**,[Q] characteristic of all neuroendocrine tumors
- **Reported 5-year survival rates:**
  - Typical carcinoids **(Best Prognosis)**[Q],
  - Small cell carcinoma **(Worst prognosis)**[Q]

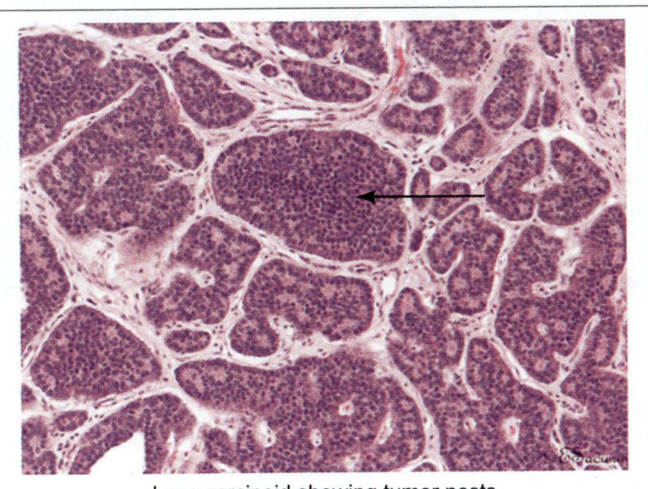

Lung carcinoid showing tumor nests

Metastatic Tumors

Lung is the most common site of metastatic neoplasms[Q]

Pleural Tumors

Solitary Fibrous Tumor

- **Definition:**
  - Soft-tissue tumor of the **pleura**[Q] and, less commonly, in the lung
- **Epidemiology:**
  - No relationship to asbestos exposure.[Q]
- **Genetics:**
  - Cryptic inversion of **chr 12 involving NAB2-STAT6 fusion gene**[Q]
- **Gross Morphology:**
  - May be attached to the **pleural surface** by a pedicle, **dense fibrous tissue** with occasional cysts filled with viscid fluid
- **Microscopy:**
  - Tumor shows **whorls of reticulin**[Q] and **collagen fibers**[Q] with interspersed **spindle cells**[Q] resembling fibroblasts
  - Tumor cells are CD34+ve[Q] and keratin -ve[Q] by immunostaining

Malignant Mesothelioma

- **Epidemiology:**
  - **Rare tumor** but risk of mesothelioma in heavily asbestos exposed individuals **(25-45 yrs)**.
  - **No increased risk of mesothelioma in asbestos workers who smoke**[Q]
  - **SV40 (simian virus 40)** is often associated[Q]
- **Gross Morphology:**
  - **Diffuse lesion** arising either from visceral or parietal pleura
  - May cause extensive **pleural effusion & direct invasion of thoracic structures**
- **Light Microscopy:**
  - **Epithelioid (60%) Most common variety**[Q], Sarcomatoid (20%), Mixed (20%)
- **IHC:**
  - Strong positivity for keratin proteins, **calretinin,**[Q] **WT-1,**[Q] **cytokeratin 5/6**[Q] & **D2-40**[Q]
- **Electron microscopy:**
  - **Long microvilli** & **abundant tonofilaments** but **absent microvillous rootlets** and **lamellar bodies**[Q]
- MC gene mutated is BAP_1

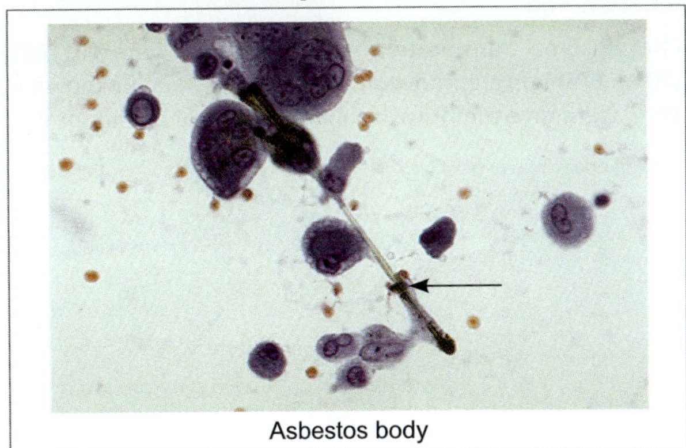

Asbestos body

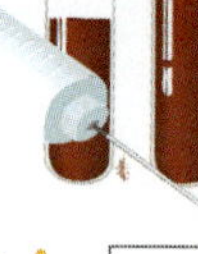

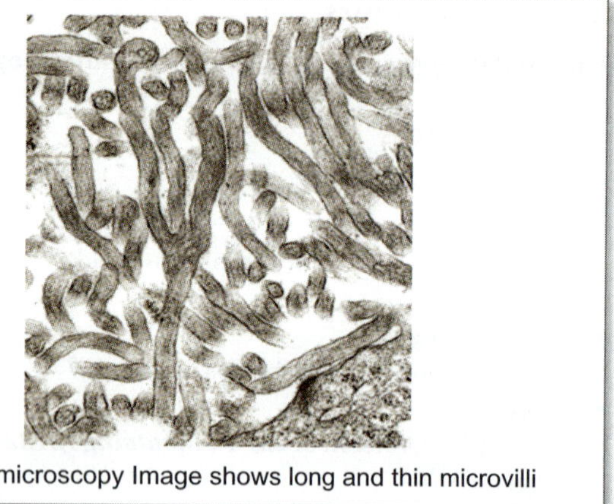

Electron microscopy Image shows long and thin microvilli

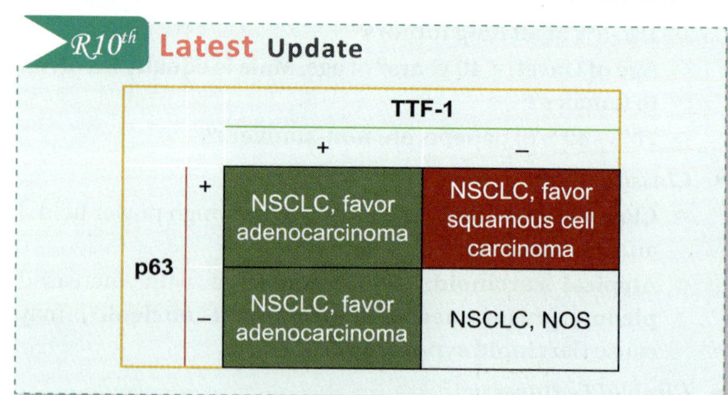

		TTF-1	
		+	−
p63	+	NSCLC, favor adenocarcinoma	NSCLC, favor squamous cell carcinoma
	−	NSCLC, favor adenocarcinoma	NSCLC, NOS

R10th Latest Update

Squamous cell carcinoma - 2015 UPDATES

> **Number of subtypes have been reduced to three, which makes the diagnosis easier and avoids rare subtypes with confusing names**

- Keratinizing
- Non-keratinizing
- Basaloid squamous cell carcinoma **(new category added)**

Note The Terminologies:
- Basaloid squamous cell carcinoma -if this component is >50% of the tumor, regardless of the presence of any keratinization.
- In tumors with <50% basaloid component, this can be acknowledged in the diagnosis "with basaloid features".

Neuroendocrine Tumors-2015 Updates

- They are grouped into high grade tumors (small cell and large cell neuroendocrine carcinoma), intermediate and low grade tumors (atypical and typical carcinoids), and the preinvasive diffuse idiopathic pulmonary neuroendocrine cell hyperplasia (DIPNECH), and for each of these, there are characteristic molecular alterations

Small cell carcinoma
Large cell neuroendocrine carcinoma
Carcinoid tumor
Diffuse idiopathic pulmonary neuroendocrine cell hyperplasia

The following entities are listed according to the new WHO classification:
- NUT CARCINOMA
- Lymphoepithelioma-like carcinoma

Nut Carcinoma

- Chromosomal translocation between the **NUT gene (NUTM1) on chromosome 15q14** and other genes: BRD4 on chromosome 19p13.1 (70%), BRD3 on chromosome 9q34.2 (6%), or an unknown partner gene (24%)
- Very aggressive tumor with a median survival of 7 months

NEXT Pattern Questions

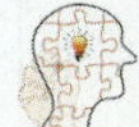 **Q's**

1. A 45-year-old male presented with severe respiratory distress. O/E he had pedal edema, bilateral crepitation on auscultation. He was admitted to emergency department and expired 2 days of admission. Lung biopsy done suggested the following. What is your diagnosis?

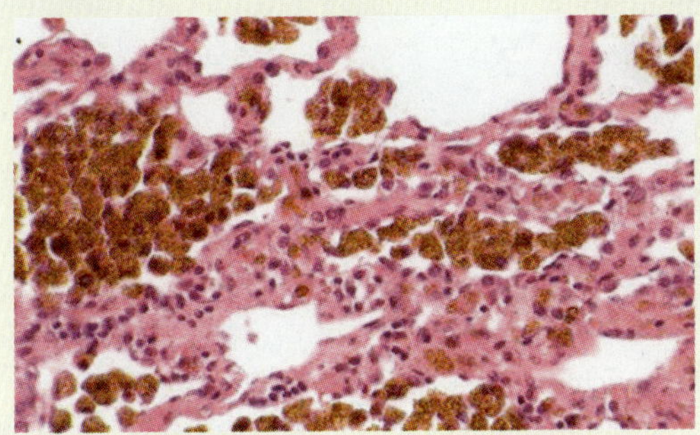

   a. CMV pneumonitis   b. Small cell Ca lung
   c. Tuberculosis   d. Heart failure cells

Ans. (d) Heart failure cells

- With the history of heart failure symptoms, notice the brown colored macrophages with hemosiderin called heart failure cells.

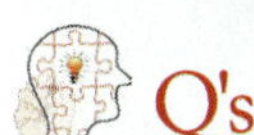 **Q's**

2. A Factory worker was working in a factory from past 20 years, and now presenting with pleural thickening and fibrosis. Histopathology of lesion is shown in below image. Most likely diagnosis is:

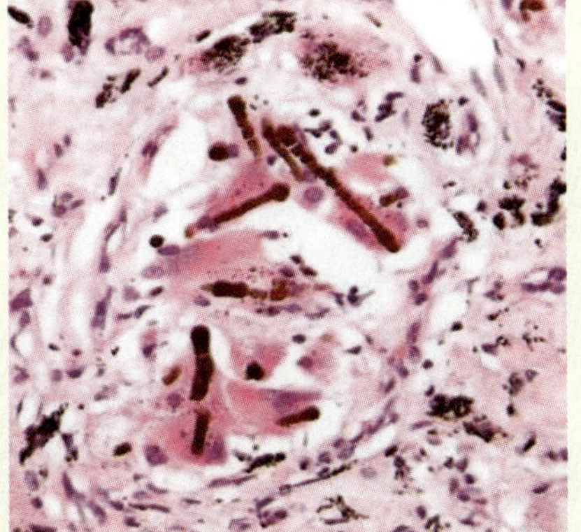

   a. Asbestosis
   b. Byssinosis
   c. Coal Worker Pneumoconiosis
   d. Silicosis

Ans. (a) Asbestosis

- Note the brown colored the alveoli suggestive of Asbestosis.

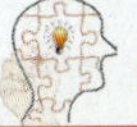 **Q's**

3. A middle aged immunocompromised male came with fever and breathlessness. HRCT showed a middle lobe lesion with infiltration. Lung biopsy from the lesion is shown in image. Most likely Diagnosis is:

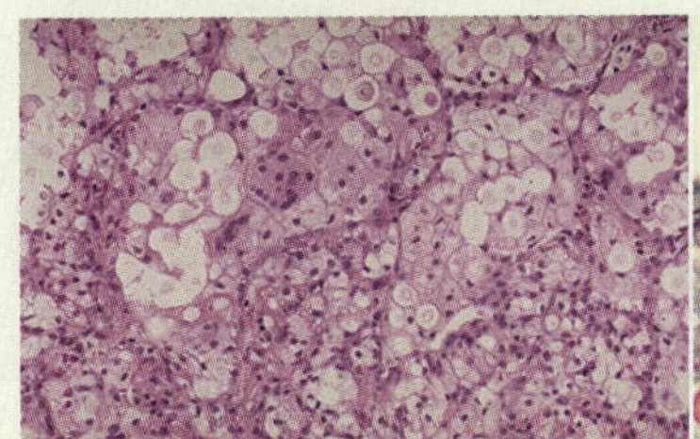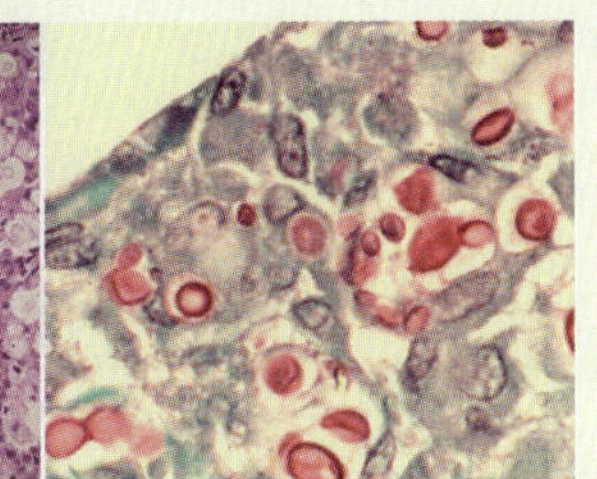

   a. Tuberculosis Pneumonia
   b. Cryptococcus pneumonia
   c. Small cell carcinoma lung
   d. CMV pneumonia

Ans. (b) Cryptococcus pneumonia

- Cryptococcus pneumonia is common in HIV immunocompromised patients. Notice the clear capsulated cryptococcus and the PAS + stained capsule of the same.

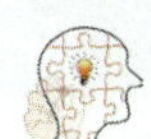 **Q's**

4. A 58-year-old female presents with difficulty of breathing. CT scan show peripherally located mass lesion. Histopathological diagram of lung biopsy is shown below, based on it what is your diagnosis?

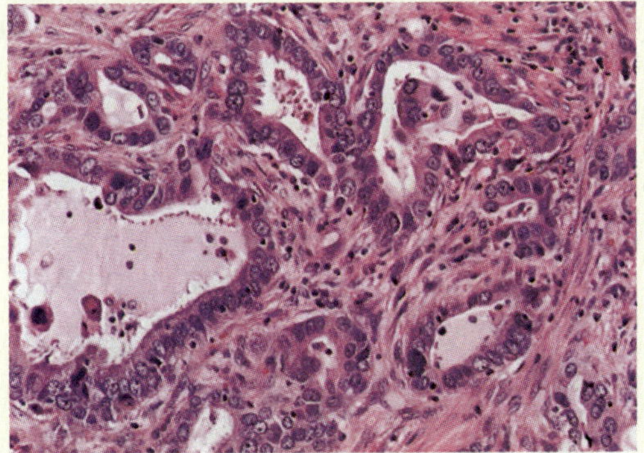

   a. Adenocarcinoma
   b. Squamous cell carcinoma
   c. Carcinoid tumor
   d. Small cell carcinoma

Ans. (a) Adenocarcinoma

- The mass in the bronchus which is peripherally located, shows malignant invasive glands suggestive of adenocarcinoma

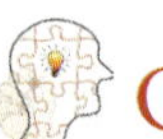

Q's

5. Which of the following disease is classically associated with the following?

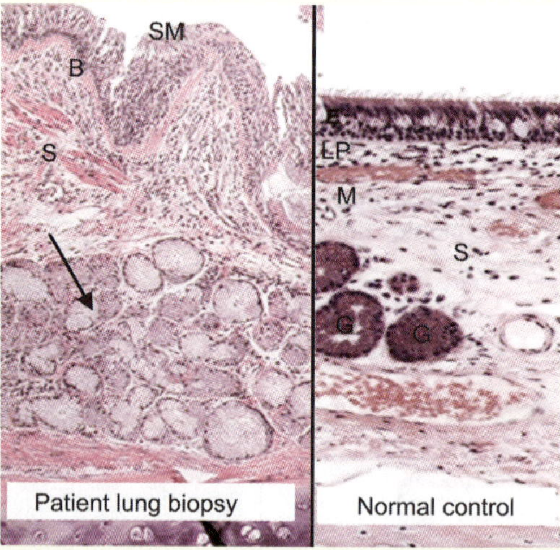

a. Bronchiectasis   b. Interstitial lung disease   c. Chronic Bronchitis   d. Emphysema

Ans. (c) Chronic Bronchitis

- In chronic bronchitis, there is increase in Reid index which means the ratio of submucosal mucin gland layer by bronchial wall layer is more than 0.4.

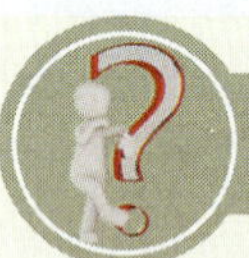

Image-Based Questions

1. A 45-year-old male presented with severe respiratory distress. O/E he had pedal edema, bilateral crepitation on auscultation. He was admitted to emergency department and expired 2 days of admission. Lung biopsy done suggested the following. What is your diagnosis?

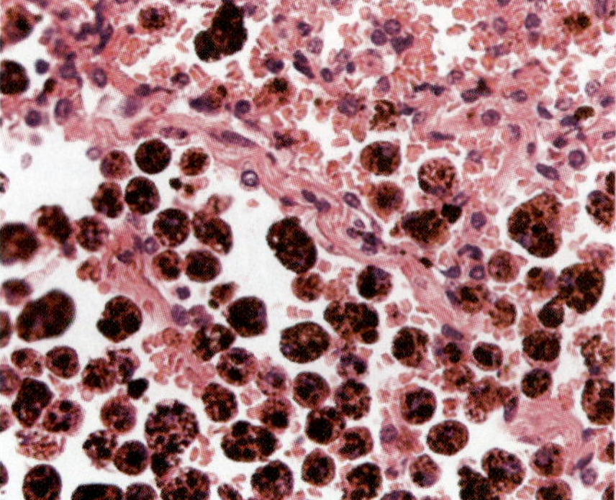

  a. CMV pneumonitis
  b. Small cell Ca lung
  c. Tuberculosis
  d. Heart failure cells

2. A 50-year-old male chronic smoker who smokes 20 cigarettes/ day for last 15 years died of severe respiratory distress. His lung autopsy shows the following. Identify the lesion?

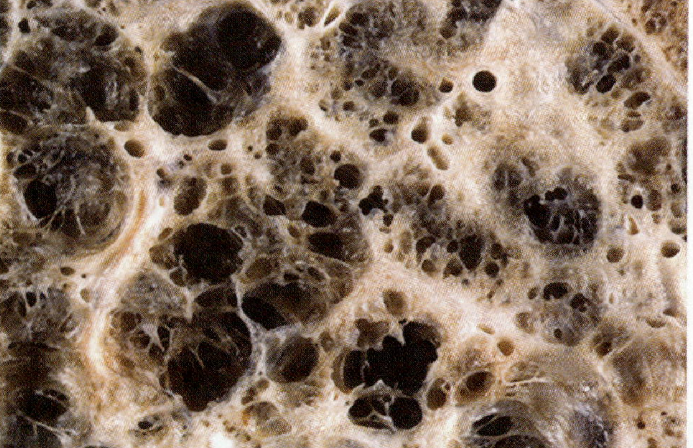

  a. Centriacinar emphysema
  b. Panacinar Emphysema
  c. Chronic bronchitis
  d. Bronchiectasis

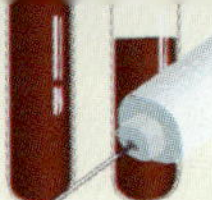

3. Autopsy gross specimen from lungs suggested the following, What is your interpretation?

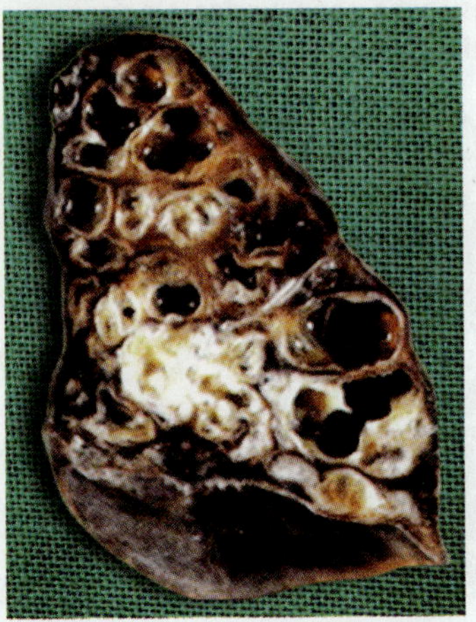

a. Chronic bronchitis
b. Bronchiectasis
c. Lung Ca
d. Pleural mesothelioma

5. Identify the given test being shown and its importance?

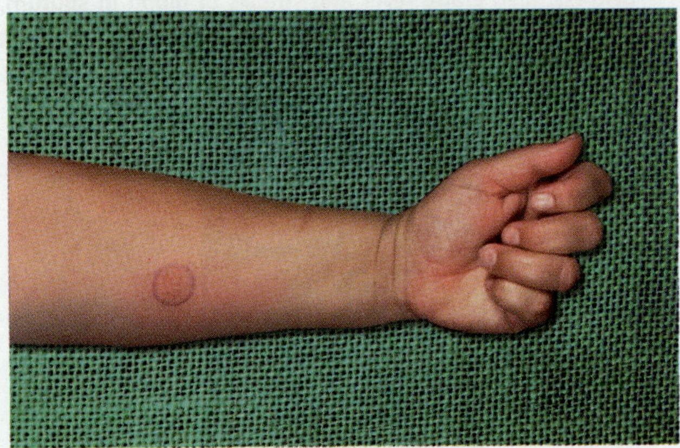

a. Schick Test, Confirmed TB diagnosis
b. Mantoux test, latent Tb diagnosis
c. Mantoux test, TB disease
d. Mantoux test, Prior TB exposure

4. A full term neonate rapidly develops progressive respiratory distress shortly after birth. lung biopsy done post-mortem reveals the following, what is your diagnosis?

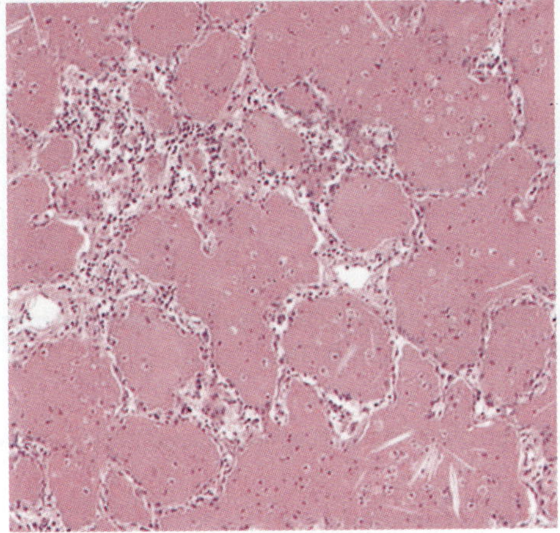

a. Pulmonary hemorrhage
b. Pulmonary alveolar proteinosis
c. Pneumonia
d. Pulmonary edema

6. A 40-year-old female was admitted to hospital with fever, loss of appetite and weight, cough and weakness of 3 months duration. A chest X-ray showed consolidation at the upper part of lung. She died a few days after admission. Autopsy findings of gross lung and its biopsy findings have been shown. What is your diagnosis?

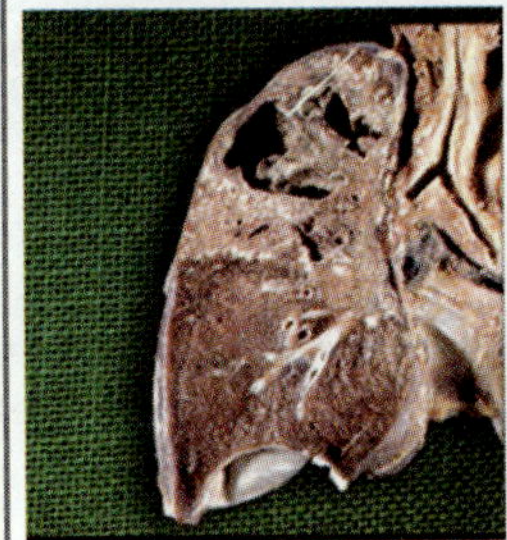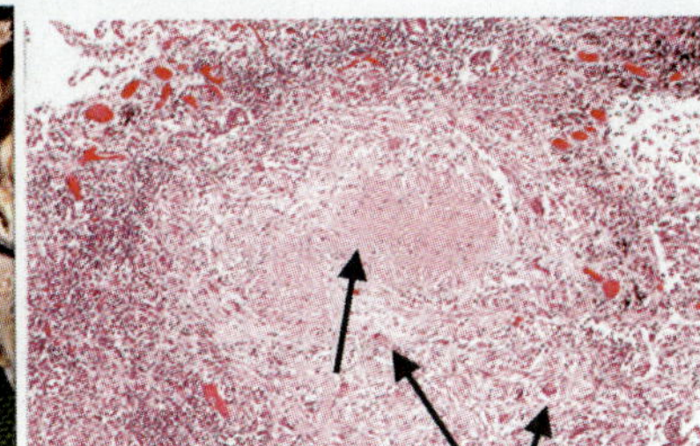

a. Sarcoidosis
b. Ca lung
c. Tuberculosis Lung
d. Bronchiectasis

7. A 56-year-old male who presented with severe respiratory distress, high grade fever and streaks of blood in sputum, died 7 days after hospitalization in AIIMS ICU. The lung autopsy has been shown, Identify the pathology?

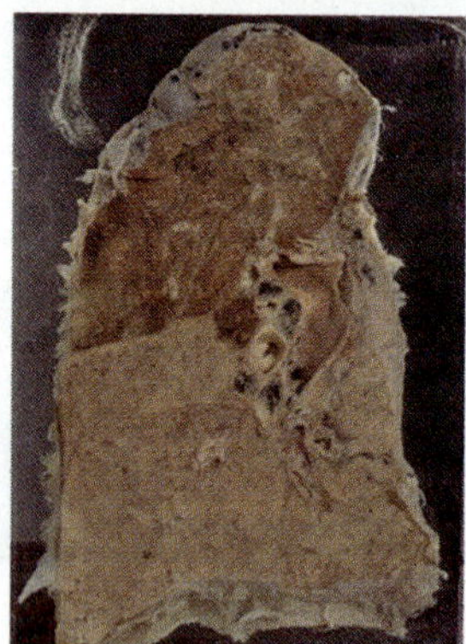

a. Lobar pneumonia   b. Bronchopneumonia
c. Tuberculosis   d. Bronchogenic Carcinoma

8. A 56-year-old male presented with lesion at the lung apex. He was working in asbestos factory for last 20 years. The lung biopsy was seen under electron microscope which revealed the following. What is your diagnosis?

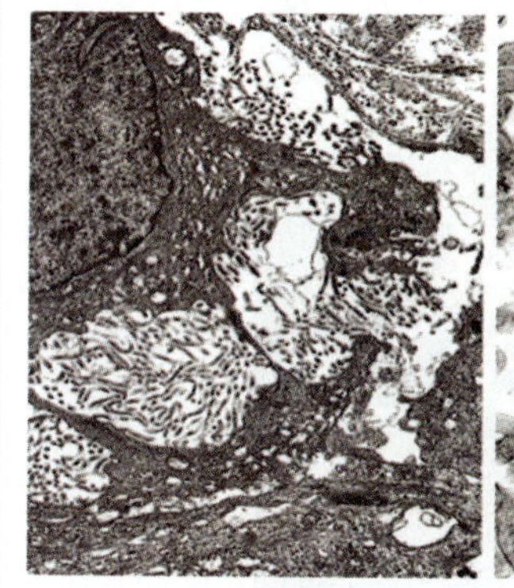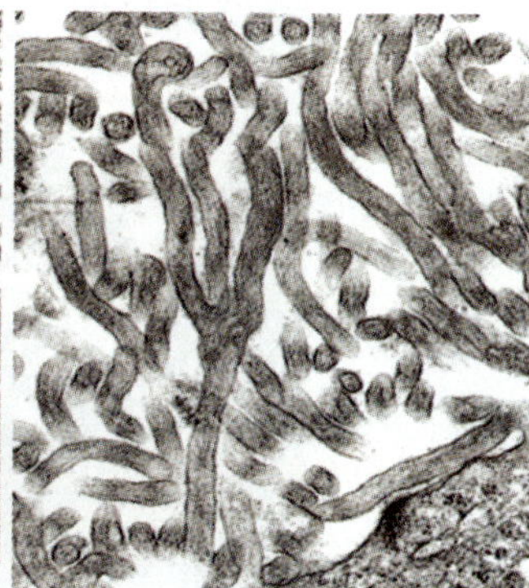

a. Adenocarcinoma Lung   b. Mesothelioma
c. Lung metastasis   d. Benign pleural fibroma

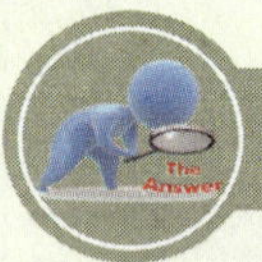

Answers of Image-Based Questions

1. **Ans. (d) Heart failure cells**
   - The lung biopsy shows intra-alveolar **transudate granular pale pink** material along with **alveolar micro-hemorrhages & hemosiderin-laden macrophages ("heart failure" cells)** seen in left-sided congestive heart failure.

2. **Ans. (a) Centriacinar emphysema**
   - Central areas in the lung specimen shows marked emphysematous damage surrounded by relatively spared alveolar spaces.

3. **Ans. (b) Bronchiectasis**
   - Cut surface of lung shows markedly distended peripheral bronchi upto four times the normal size.

4. **Ans. (b) Pulmonary alveolar proteinosis**
   - The alveoli are filled with a dense, amorphous, protein-lipid granular precipitate, while the alveolar walls are normal.

5. **Ans (d) Mantoux test, Prior TB exposure**
   - **Mantoux (Tuberculin test)** indicate **infection with TB and Type IV hypersensitivity to antigens but not TB disease.**

6. **Ans. (c) Tuberculosis lung**
   - Gross lung shows upper lobe cavitations and its biopsy findings shows caseating granuloma suggestive of Tuberculosis.

7. **Ans. (a) Lobar pneumonia**
   - The gross specimen of lung shows consolidation of a large portion of an entire lower lobe .

8. **Ans. (b) Mesothelioma**
   - **Electron microscopy shows long microvilli & abundant tonofilaments** but **absent microvillous rootlets** and **lamellar bodies.**

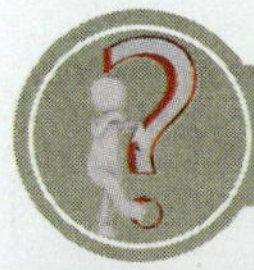

Multiple Choice Questions

RESPIRATORY SYSTEM AND ITS CONGENITAL MALFORMATIONS

1. Ciliocytophthoria is seen in: *(AIIMS Nov 2019)*
a. Kartagener
b. Situs inversus
c. Acute respiratory infection
d. Cystic fibrosis

2. True about pulmonary sequestration: *(PGI May 2019)*
a. Female preponderance
b. Supplied by bronchial supply
c. May have independent venous drainage
d. Intralobular variety more common
e. May be associated with other congenital anomalies

3. Kartageners syndrome cause of infertility is?
a. Oligospermia　　　　　*(AIIMS May 18)*
b. Asthenospermia
c. Undescended testis
d. Epididymis obstruction

4. Bronchial mucosa secretes all except?
a. Bombesin　　　　*(Recent Question 2015)*
b. Calcitonin
c. Serotonin
d. Bradykinin

5. Most common type of foregut cysts are?
　　　　　　　　　　(Recent Question 2014)
a. Bronchogenic　　　　b. Esophageal
c. Enteric　　　　　　　d. Mixed type

6. Blood supply of bronchogenic sequestration is?
　　　　　　　　　　(Recent Question 2014)
a. Aorta　　　　　　　　b. Pulmonary artery
c. Pulmonary Vein　　　　d. Bronchogenic artery

7. Hamartomatous lung tissue is? *(Recent Question 2015)*
a. Hypoplasia of lung
b. Congenital cyst
c. Lobar sequestration
d. Congenital cystic adenomatoid malformation

8. Respiratory system develops from?
　　　　　　　　　　(Recent Question 2013)
a. Ventral wall of foregut　　b. Dorsal wall of foregut
c. Ventral wall of midgut　　d. Dorsal wall of midgut

9. Bronchogenic cyst is lined by? *(Recent Question 2013)*
a. Stratified Squamous epithelium
b. Squamous epithelium
c. Non ciliated pseudostratified columnar epithelium
d. Ciliated pseudostratified columnar epithelium

10. Which cells produce surfactant in conducting part of the lung?　　　*(MAHA 2015)*
a. Goblet cells　　　　b. Brush cells
c. Basal cells　　　　d. Clara cells

11. Pores of Kohn are present in? *(Recent Question 2013)*
a. Bronchioles
b. Alveoli
c. Bronchus
d. Terminal bronchiloes

ARDS AND PNEMONIA

12. A middle aged immunocompromised male came with fever and breathlessness. HRCT showed a middle lobe lesion with infiltration in the lung as shown in image. Most likely Diagnosis is? *(AIIMS May 18)*

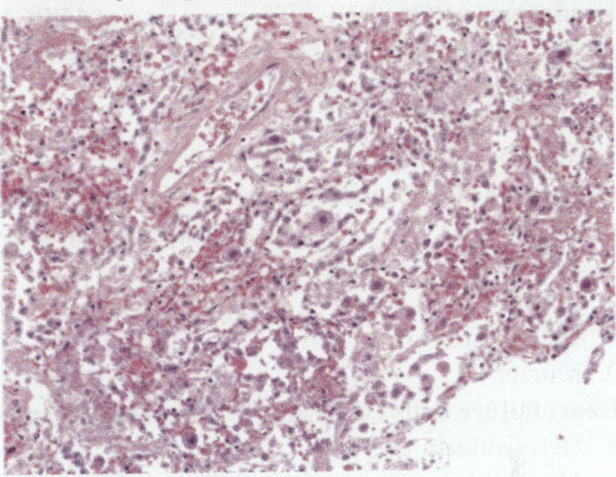

a. Tuberculous Pneumonia
b. Cryptogenic organizing pneumonia
c. Small cell carcinoma lung
d. CMV pneumonia

13. The following are true regarding hyaline membrane disease except: *(APPGMEE 2015)*
a. Basic abnormality is deficiency of surfactant
b. Prenatal diagnosis by low amniotic fluid L/S ratio
c. Intratracheal surfactant helps
d. Occurs in babies born post-dates

14. What is false about ARDS? *(Recent Question 2016)*
a. Mucus plug in alveoli
b. Interstitial edema
c. Hyaline membrane present
d. Interstitial infiltrates by cells

15. Etiology of ARDS are all except? *(Recent question 2015)*
a. Multiple transfusion
b. Sepsis
c. Aspiration of gastric contents
d. Fat embolism

16. Characteristic feature of best sputum sample is /are?
a. Presence of leukocytes　　*(PGI Nov 2015)*
b. Respiratory epithelium
c. Neutrophils
d. Mucus with inflammatory cells
e. Presence of alveolar macrophages

17. Heart failure cells are actually? *(Recent Question 2015)*
a. Alveolar macrophages　　b. Type I pneumocytes
c. Type 2 pneumocytes
d. Pulmonary edema fluid cells

18. Heart Failure cells are: *(Recent Question 2014, 2013)*
a. Lipofuscin granules in cardiac cells
b. Pigmented alveolar macrophages
c. Pigmented pancreatic acinar cells
d. Pigment cells seen in liver

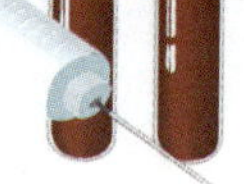

19. Terminal stage of pneumonia is: *(Recent Question 2014)*
a. Congestion
b. Red hepatization
c. Gray hepatization
d. Resolution

20. ARDS is due to defect in? *(AIIMS May 2014)*
a. Type 1 pneumocytes
b. Type 2 pneumocytes
c. Endothelial cells
d. Clara cells

21. All are recognized causes of Adult Respiratory Distress Syndrome (ARDS) EXCEPT: *(APPGMEE 14)*
a. Smoke inhalation
b. Malignant hypertension
c. Hypothermia
d. Viral pneumonias

22. In Hyaline Membrane Disease the pathology in the lung consists of: *(Recent Question 2013)*
a. Albumin and complement
b. Fibrin
c. Precipitated surfactant
d. Mucus

23. Heart failure cells contain: *(Recent Question 2013)*
a. Hemosiderin
b. Lipofuscin
c. Myoglobin
d. Albumin
e. Pneumonia

24. Patient with h/o long standing depressive illness come to emergency with acute breathlessness. The X-ray shows diffuse infiltrates with predominance in right middle lobe and right lower lobe. The patient did not survive and the following picture in the lungs was seen on autopsy? *(AIIMS Nov 2017)*

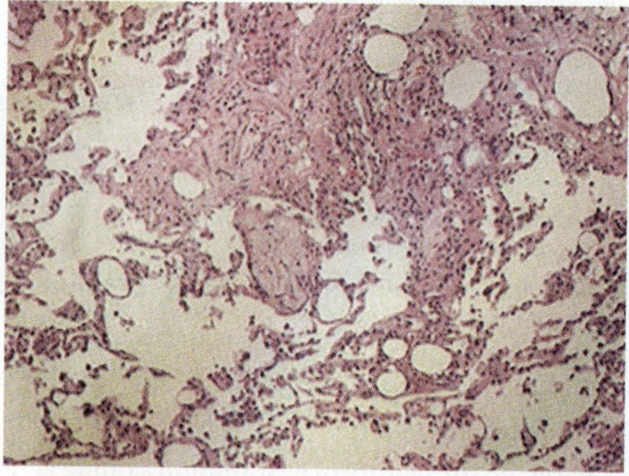

a. Severe necrosis with fungal hyphae, severe fungal pneumonia
b. Coagulation necrosis, Tuberculosis
c. Vegetable matter; Aspiration pneumonia
d. Severe necrosis; severe necrotizing pneumonia

25. In the stage of Grey hepatization:
a. WBCs fill the alveoli *(Recent Question 2013)*
b. RBCs fill the alveoli
c. Organisms fillthealveoli
d. Accumulation of fibrin in alveoli

26. The most common fate of lobar pneumonia is: *(Recent Question 2013)*
a. Consolidation
b. Resolution
c. Abscess formation
d. Empyema

27. Characteristic histopathological finding in SHOCK Lung: *(AI 12, AIIMS Nov 07, May 08)*
a. Diffuse alveolar necrosis
b. Interstitial pulmonary edema
c. Diffuseinterstitialinflammatin
d. Intra-cellular debris

28. Histological picture of a lesion excised from the right cervical region is shown below. What is your diagnosis? *(Recent Pattern Question 2020)*

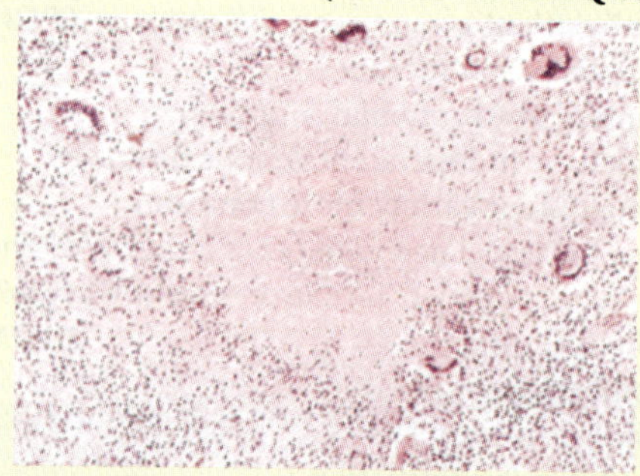

a. Necrotizing granulomatous inflammation
b. Neurofibroma
c. Schwannoma
d. Hodgkin lymphoma

29. A patient underwent lung transplantation. The resected lung from the patient showed following features. What could be your possible diagnosis? *(Recent exam 2018)*

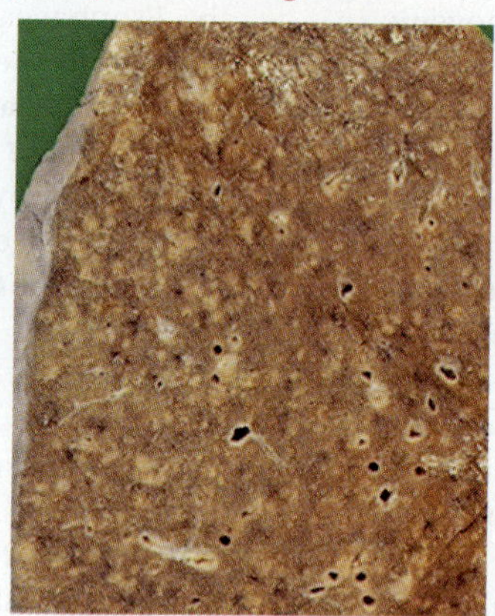

a. Bronchiectasis
b. Lung abscess
c. Lung carcinoma
d. Miliary tuberculosis

30. True about miliary tuberculosis: *(PGI May 2016)*
a. Occur primarily due to hematogenous spread
b. Miliary lesion is generally of size 1-2 mm
c. Diffuse bilateral crepitation is always present
d. Onset is generally acute
e. Sputum smear microscopy is negative in 80% of cases

31. MC site of TB reactivation in lung is? *(Recent Question 2016)*
a. Apex
b. Base
c. Subpleural
d. Near bronchus

32. TB infects which cell *(Recent Question 2016)*
a. Macrophage
b. Lymphocyte
c. Neutrophils
d. Eosinophils

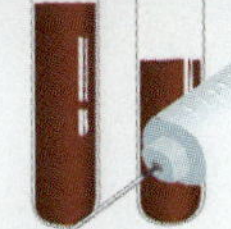

33. Miliary TB is: *(Recent Question 2014)*
a. Primary
b. Post-primary
c. Extra-pulmonary
d. None

34. All of the following are lesions seen in primary tuberculosis except: *(Recent Question 2015)*
a. Simon's focus
b. Ghon's focus
c. Ranke complex
d. Puhl's lesion

35. Primary site of involvement in congenital TB:
a. Lungs *(Recent Question 2015)*
b. Liver
c. Lymph nodes
d. Stomach

36. Most common site of gastrointestinal TB:
(Recent Question 2014)
a. Stomach
b. Duodenum
c. Terminal ileum
d. Colon

37. Miliary TB occurs due to spread via:
a. Arteries *(Recent Question 2014)*
b. Veins
c. Lymphatics
d. Direct invasion

38. Ghons complex refers to: *(Recent Question 2013)*
a. Healed parenchymal lesions
b. Necrotic lymph nodes
c. Parenchymal lesion along with inflamed lymph nodes
d. Complication in enlarged hilar lymph nodes

39. In TB, cytokine which plays a major role in conversion of macrophage to epithelioid cell is? *(JIPMER 2013)*
a. IFN-γ
b. TNF
c. IL-12
d. Macrophage chemoattractant protein

40. Infraclavicular lesion of tuberculosis is known as:
(AIIMS 11)
a. Ghon's focus
b. Puhl's focus
c. Assmans focus
d. Simmon's focus

41. All of the following statements about Interferon gamma release assays are true (IGRA) except? *(DNB June 2012)*
a. More specific than tuberculin skin testing
b. ESAT-6 and CFP-10 are the antigens used
c. Quantitative and qualitative measurement of Interferon gamma released by mycobacterium tuberculosis in the body
d. Lesser cross-reactivity to BCG than tuberculin testing

42. The most important function of epithelioid cells in tuberculosis is: *(DPG 10)*
a. Phagocytosis
b. Secretory
c. Antigenic
d. Healing

43. A 30-year-old male presented with history of dyspnea, cough and sputum production. The patient died of respiratory failure. Gross image of lung is shown below. What is the likely etiology?
(Recent Pattern Question 2020)

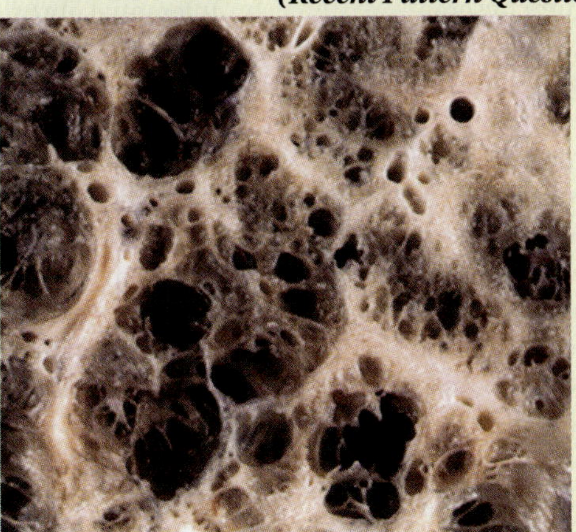

a. Cystic fibrosis
b. Mutation in dynein arms
c. Alpha 1 antitrypsin deficiency
d. Antibodies against type IV collagen

44. A 75-year-old male, known smoker presented to pulmonology department with history of cough. Biopsy was taken which showed the following. What is the change shown? *(Recent Pattern Question 2020)*

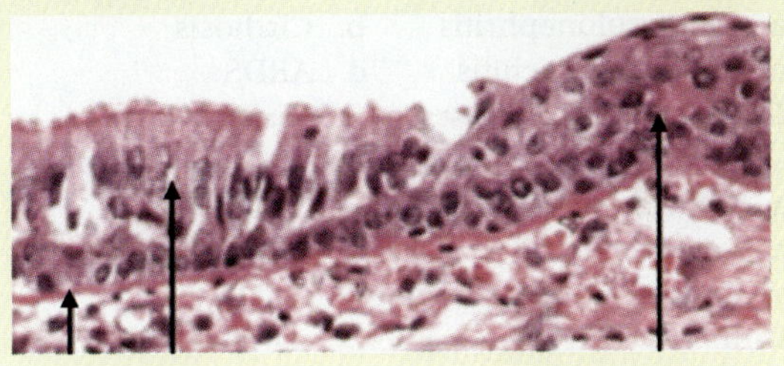

a. Dysplasia
b. Metaplasia
c. Hyperplasia
d. Atrophy

45. The main diagnostic criteria of ABPA are all except?
(APPGMEE 2015)
a. Pulmonary infiltrates
b. Bronchial asthma
c. Distal bronchiectasis
d. Eosinophilia

46. Which of the following structures in the lung is likely to be affected the most in a patient who smoked a pack and half of cigarettes per day for 30 years and developed centrilobular emphysema? *(AP 2013)*
a. Alveolar sac
b. Terminal bronchiole
c. Alveolar duct
d. Respiratory bronchiole

47. Chronic bronchitis can be a premalignant condition, which involves: *(Recent Question 2015)*
a. Columnar to squamous
b. Squamous to columnar
c. Squamous to cuboidal
d. Cuboidal to squamous

48. Emphysema pathologically involves beyond the:
(Recent Question 2015)
a. Bronchi
b. Terminal bronchiole
c. Respiratory bronchiole
d. Alveolar Sac

49. Commonest type of emphysema is:

(Recent Question 2014)

a. Centriacinar b. Obstructed
c. Irregular d. Panacinar

50. All are obstructive lung disease except:

(Recent Question 2014)

a. Emphysema b. Interstitial fibrosis
c. Asthma d. Bronchitis

51. Curshmann's crystals are seen in:

(Recent Question 2014)

a. Bronchial asthma b. Bronchiectasis
c. Chronic bronchitis d. Wegener's granulomatosis

52. Which of the following finding, composed of shed epithelium with thick mucus are seen in bronchial asthma? *(JIPMER 2014)*

a. Creola body b. Councilman body
c. Curshmann spirals d. Charcot leyden crystals

53. Hyperplasia of smooth muscle of airway is seen in?

(Recent Question 2013)

a. Emphysema b. Asthma
c. Alveolar proteinosis d. Brochiectasis

54. Creola bodies are seen in: *(Recent Question 2013)*

a. Bronchial asthma b. Chronic bronchitis
c. Emphysema d. Bronchiectasis

55. Bronchiectasis means --------of bronchi:

(Recent Question 2013)

a. Inflammation b. Dilatation
c. Cavitation d. All

56. Reid index is useful in: *(AI 12)*

a. Glomerulonephritis b. Cirrhosis
c. Chronic bronchitis d. ARDS

57. Centriacinar emphysema primarily involves:

(PGI Nov 2011)

a. Upper lobe b. Middle lobe
c. Lower lobe d. All lobes
e. Lower part of upper lobe

58. Difference between bronchial asthma and COPD is:
a. Reversible bronchoconstriction *(Jipmer 11)*
b. Hyperventilation on chest X ray
c. Acute exacerbation by URTI
d. Decreased FEV1/FVC

59. Which of the following is NOT a complication of bronchiectasis: *(AIIMS Sep 10)*
a. Lung abscess b. Lung cancer
c. Amyloidosis d. Empyema

60. Reid's Index is? *(DNB Dec 10)*
a. Increased in Chronic Bronchitis
b. Decreased in Chronic Bronchitis
c. Increased in Bronchial Asthma
d. Decreased in Bronchial Asthma

61. Which one of the following is NOT a feature of Kartagener's syndrome: *(UPSC 09), (WBPG 2016)*
a. Bronchiectasis
b. Ciliary dyskinesia
c. Dysphagia
d. Situs inversus

62. A Factory worker was working in a factory from past 20 years , and now presenting with pleural thickening and fibrosis. Histopathology of lesion is shown in below image. Most likely diagnosis is? *(AIIMS May 18)*

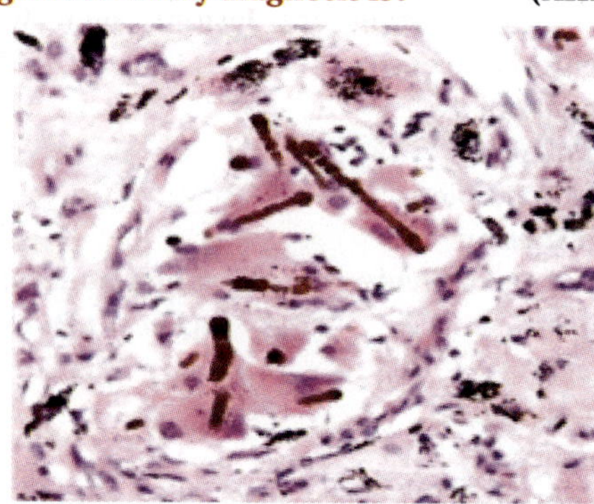

a. Asbestosis
b. Cotton Fiber
c. Coal Worker Pneumoconiosis
d. Silicosis

63. Silicosis biopsy features and radiological correlation?
a. Lower lobe involved *(AIIMS May 2017)*
b. Dense collagen and calcifications in the lymph nodes seen
c. Progressive massive fibrosis can be seen as late complication
d. Immune granuloma can be seen
e. Macules may be seen

64. The lung pathology occurring in persons working in cotton- wool industries is *(Recent Question 2016-17)*
a. Asthma like features
b. Hypersensitivity pnemonitis
c. Lung Ca
d. Chronic bronchitis

65. Bagassosis occurs in people working in which industry?

(Recent Question 2016-17)

a. Silica b. Wallboard paper
c. Cotton d. Asbestosis

66. Most common cause for lung abscess?

(Recent Question 2016-17)

a. Staph aureus b. Staph pyrogen
c. Bacteroids d. Klebsiella

67. APBA is associated with? *(Recent Question 2016-17)*
a. Central bronchiectasis
b. Bronchitis
c. Midlung bronchiectasis
d. Peripheral bronchiectasis

68. All are true about hypersensitivity pneumonitis except:

(Recent Question 2016-17)

a. Type IV Hypersensitivity reaction
b. More common in smoker
c. Bronchoalveolar lavage shows CD4+ and CD8+ T lymphocytes
d. May presents with cough, dyspnea & breathlessness

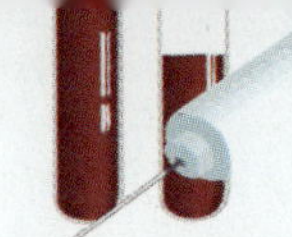

69. **Cavitatory lesion in right lower lung with dyspnoea with following histopathological appearance**

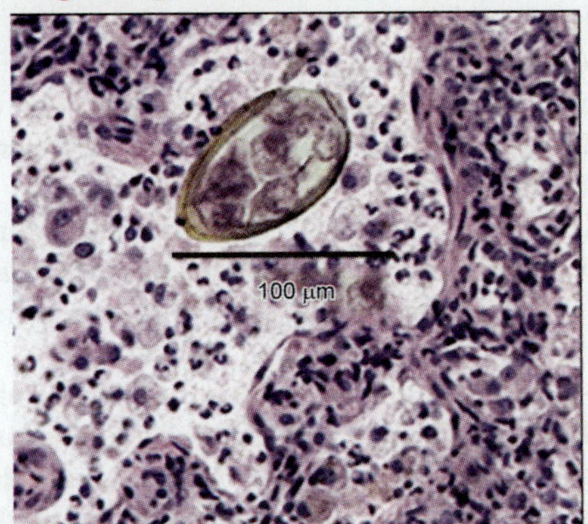

Most likely diagnosis: *(AIIMS Nov 2015)*
a. Echinococcus with 2 layers
b. Strongyloides with 2 layers
c. Paragonimus with 2 layers
d. Cysticercosis with 3 layers

70. **Causative agent of Farmer's lung is:**
a. Themophilus actinomyces *(Recent Question 2015)*
b. Aspergillus
c. Penicilliumglabrum
d. Rhizopus

71. **Causative particle in asbestosis is?**
(Recent Question 2015)
a. Amphibole
b. Crysolite
c. Tridymite
d. Gristobalite

72. **All are true about silicosis except?** *(PGI Nov 2015)*
a. Bifringent crystals seen
b. Pleural plaque seen
c. Lower lobe is ussualy involved
d. Most common pnemoconiosis

73. **Asbestosis causes?** *(Recent Question 2014)*
a. Lymphoma
b. Leukaemia
c. Renal cell carcinoma
d. Mesothelioma

74. **Anthracosis is due to inhalation of:**
(Recent Question 2013)
a. Coal dust
b. Asbestos dust
c. Silica dust
d. Berylium dust

75. **Ferruginous bodies are seen in?** *(DNB Aug 12)*
a. Sarcoidosis
b. Silicosis
c. Asbestosis
d. Coal worker's pneumoconiosis

76. **A female presents with history of progressive breathlessness. Histology shows heterogenous patchy fibrosis with several fibroblastic foci. The most likely diagnosis is:** *(AI 11)*
a. Cryptogenic organizing pneumonia
b. Non specific interstitial pneumonia
c. Usual interstitial pneumonia
d. Desquamative interstitial pneumonia

77. **Schaumann bodies are seen in:** *(AIIMS 11)*
a. Sarcoidosis
b. Chronic bronchitis
c. Asthma
d. Syphilis

78. **Asteroid bodies are seen in?** *(DNB Dec 11, June 10)*
a. Sarcoidosis
b. Syphilis
c. Chromoblastomycosis
d. Sporotrichosis

79. **The following does not occur with asbestosis:**
(DPG 11, DNB Dec 08)
a. Methemoglobinemia
b. Pneumoconiosis
c. Pleural mesothelioma
d. Pleural calcification

80. **Laminated concretions of calcium and proteins are:**
(Maharashtra 10)
a. Schaumanns bodies
b. Ferrugenious bodies
c. Asteroid bodies
d. Gamma Gandy bodies

81. **The dangerous particle size causing pneumoconiosis varies from:**
a. 100-150 µm
b. 50-100 µm
c. 10-50 µm
d. 1-5 µm

TUMORS OF LUNGS & PLEURA

82. **WHO 2015 new inclusion in lung squamous cell carcinoma is/are?** *(AIIMS May 2017)*
a. Basaloid type
b. Lymphoephtheliod type
c. Papillary type
d. Clear cell variety
e. Small cell variety

83. **Tumor marker for lung adenocarcinoma?**
a. ck7
b. ck20 *(AIIMS May 2017)*
c. TTF1
d. CK 11
e. Berep-4

84. **A 34 yr women presented with coughing, dyspnea, flushing, diarrhea, hypotension, hematemesis for 3 months, Bronchoscopy shows large intraductal mass. Histopathology of the mass is given below. Mitosis was 5/hpf and is chromogranin positive. What is your diagnosis?** *(AIIMS May 2016)*

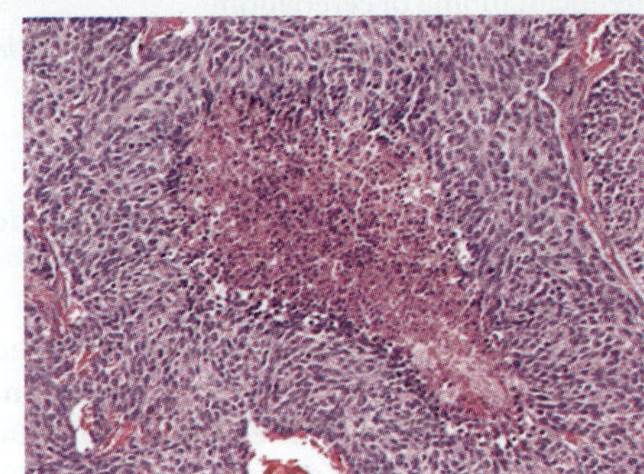

a. Small cell CA
b. Large cell CA
c. Typical carcinoid tumor stage IV
d. Atypical carcinoid Stage IV

85. **Most common lung malignancy in woman and with smokers less than 10 packet cigarette per year?**
(Recent Question 2016-17)
a. Small cell Ca
b. Sq cell Ca
c. Adenoca
d. Carcinoids

86. **Mutations associated with nonsmall cell Lung ca is?**
(Recent Question 2016-17)
a. p 53
b. EGFR
c. Rb
d Myc

87. **Lung Ca metastasize early is?** *(Recent Question 2016-17)*
a. Adeno ca
b. Sq cell Ca
c. Small cell Ca
d. Large cell ca

88. **Carcinoid of lung (bronchial adenoma) arise from**
(JIPMER 2015)
a. Ciliated cell
b. Kulchitsky cell
c. Type 2 pnemocytes
d. Clara cell

89. Lymphoma like picture in lung cancer is seen in which subtype? *(Recent Question 2015)*
   a. Squamous cell carcinoma
   b. Adenocarcinoma
   c. Small cell carcinoma
   d. Large cell carcinoma

90. Which of the following is the marker for mesothelioma: *(Recent Question 2015)*
   a. ck7
   b. ck22
   c. ck 5/6
   d. TTF-1

91. Which of these is used as a marker in mesothelioma? *(Recent Question 2015)*
   a. Calretinin
   b. TTF-1
   c. CK-8/9
   d. Glypican

92. Most common posterior mediastinal tumor is? *(Recent Question 2015)*
   a. Thymoma
   b. Neuroma
   c. Chordoma
   d. Pleuroma

93. Which malignancy is most commonly associated with asbestos? *(Recent Question 2015)*
   a. Malignant mesothelioma
   b. Benign Pleural fibroma
   c. Squamous Cell Ca Lung
   d. Carcinoids

94. Ectopic ACTH production is seen in:
   a. Small cell carcinoma is lung *(Recent Question 2014)*
   b. Anaplastic carcinoma of lung
   c. Squamous cell carcinoma of lung
   d. Adenocarcinoma of cerebellum

95. Primary pleural tumor is: *(Recent Question 2014)*
   a. Mesothelioma
   b. Myxoma
   c. Lipoma
   d. Fibroma

96. Most common mediastinal tumor is: *(Recent Question 2014)*
   a. Neurogenic tumor
   b. Pericardial cyst
   c. Hernia
   d. Teratoma

97. A 60 yr old person presents with a mass located at central bronchus causing distal bronchiectasis and recurrent pneumonia. Which of the following findings is expected from biopsy of the mass? *(AIIMS Nov 14)*
   a. Abundant osteoid matrix formation
   b. Contains all three germ layers
   c. Spindle cells with abundant stromal matrix
   d. Small round cells and hyperchromatic nuclei with nuclear moulding

98. A hyperplastic mass containing neuroendocrine cells in an area of chronic inflammation and scarred tissue of lung is called? *(JIPMER 2014)*
   a. Carcinoid
   b. Tumorlet
   c. Hamartoma
   d. Teratoma

99. Small cell cancer commonly metastasizes to: *(Recent Question 2014)*
   a. Brain
   b. Liver
   c. Adrenal
   d. Kidney

100. Most common type of carcinoma lung is:
   a. Small cell carcinoma *(Recent Question 2013)*
   b. Adenocarcinoma
   c. Squamous cell carcinoma
   d. Large cell carcinoma

101. Marker of small cell cancer of lung is: *(Recent Question 2013)*
   a. Chromogranin
   b. Cytokeratin
   c. Desmin
   d. Vimentin

102. Which paraneoplastic syndrome is not seen with Small Cell Ca Lung: *(Recent Question 2013)*
   a. PTH
   b. ACTH
   c. ADH
   d. Carcinoid syndrome

103. Carcinoid tumor develops from: *(Recent Question 2013)*
   a. Enterochromaffin cells
   b. Neuroectoderm
   c. J cells
   d. Goblet cells

104. A 60-year-old male had a chronic history of exposure of asbestosis. He now presents with a mass in the apex of right lung. Which of the following would be seen on electron microscopy of a biopsy from the lesion? *(AIIMS Nov 2013)*
   a. Melanosomes
   b. Neurosecretory granules
   c. Numerous long slender microvilli
   d. Desmosomes with secretory endoplasmic reticulum

105. True about lung carcinoma: *(PGI Dec 13)*
   a. Squamous cell Ca is most common carcinoma
   b. Squamous cell Ca cause myopathy
   c. Small cell Ca has best prognosis
   d. BronchoalveolarCa involves proximal airways
   e. Hypercalcemia is common with Small cell Carcinoma

106. Immunohistochemical marker used for detection of AdenoCa lung? *(JIPMER 2013)*
   a. TTF
   b. GFAP
   c. Progesterone Receptors
   d. AFP

107. Paraneoplastic syndromes are most commonly associated with? *(JIPMER 2013)*
   a. Bronchial adenoCa
   b. BroncoalveolarCa
   c. Small cell Ca
   d. Bronchial Carcinoid

108. Incorrect statement about Small cell Ca of lung: *(PGI May 12)*
   a. Not associated with smoking
   b. Surgical resection alone is the treatment of choice
   c. Associated with paraneoplastic syndrome
   d. Most patients have distantmetastasesondiagnosis
   e. Contain neurosecretory granules

109. Which of the following causes malignant mesothelioma? *(DNB Aug 12)*
   a. Smoking
   b. Asbestosis
   c. Silicosis
   d. Pneumoconiosis

110. Histological findings inbronchoalveolar carcinoma includes: *(PGI Nov 2011)*
   a. Clara cells
   b. Adenosquamous
   c. Mucin secreting cells
   d. Type II pneumocytes
   e. Neuroendocrine cells

111. Following is true about bronchial carcinoids:
   a. Highly radiosensitive *(JIPMER 11)*
   b. Metastasis common
   c. Carcinoid syndrome does not manifest
   d. Commonly arise from terminal bronchioles

112. PTH like substance is produced by which type of lung malignancy: *(JIPMER 11)*
   a. Squamous cell carcinoma
   b. Oat cell carcinoma
   c. Adeno carcinoma
   d. Large cell carcinoma

113. True about lung carcinoma: *(AI 10)*
   a. More than 75% of lung cancers are squamous cell type
   b. Oat cell carcinoma frequently show cavitation
   c. Lung calcification is characteristically seen in oat cell carcinoma
   d. Oat cell carcinoma is commonly associated with bilateral hilar lymphadenopathy

114. On biopsy, characteristic finding of malignant mesothelioma is: *(AIIMS May 10)*
   a. Myelin
   b. Desmin
   c. Weibel-palade bodies
   d. Branching microvilli
   e. Fibrosis

115. Which of the following is not true about Bronchoalveolar carcinoma: *(Maharashtra 10)*
   a. Adenocarcinoma
   b. Stromal invasion with desmoplasia
   c. Preservation of alveolar structure
   d. Grows along pre-existing anatomical structures

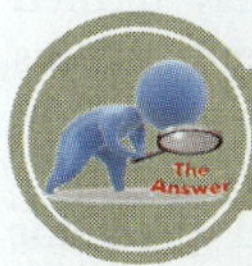

Answers with Explanations

1. Ans. (c) Acute Respiratory infection

Ciliocytophthoria (CCP) defines a degenerative process of the ciliated cells consequent to viral infections after acute respiratory infections, and it is characterized by typical morphological changes.

2. Ans. (c) May have independent venous drainage; (d) Intralobular variety more common; (e) May be associated with other congenital anomalies
(Ref: Robbins 9th/pg 670)

Sequestration
- Discrete area of lung tissue that lacks any connection to the airway system
- Abnormal blood supply arising from the aorta
- Venous return to the right side of the heart through IVC (extralobar) or pulmonary veins (intralobar)

3. Ans. (b) Asthenospermia

Asthenozoospermia (or asthenospermia) is the medical term for reduced sperm motility due to defect in ciliary movement

4. Ans. (d) Bradykinin *(Ref: Robbins 9th/pg 669-670)*

Bronchial mucosa contains **neuroendocrine cells** that have neurosecretory-type granules releasing: **serotonin**[Q], **calcitonin**[Q]**, and gastrin-releasing peptide (bombesin)**[Q]

5. Ans. (a) Bronchogenic *(Ref: Robbins 9th/pg 670; 8th/pg 679)*

6. Ans. (a) Aorta *(Ref: Robbins 9th/pg 670; 8th/pg 679)*

7. Ans. (d) Congenital cystic adenomatoid malformation

(Ref: Robbins 9th/pg 670; 8th/pg 679)

Congenital cystic adenomatoid malformation (CCAM): **Hamartomatous**[Q] or **dysplastic** lung tissue, usually confined to one lobe.

8. Ans (a) Ventral wall of foregut *(Ref: R 9th/pg 669-670)*

- **Respiratory system develops** from: **ventral wall of foregut (formed** when embryo is 4 weeks old) while Cartilagenous, muscular & connective tissue of trachea and lungs are derived from splanchnic mesoderm.

9. Ans. (d) Ciliated pseudostratified columnar epithelium

(Ref: Robbins 9th/pg 670; 8th/pg 679)

- A **bronchogenic cyst is rarely connected to the tracheobronchial tree**.
- Microscopically, the cyst is lined by ciliated pseudostratified columnar epithelium with squamous metaplasia occurring in areas of inflammation. The wall contains bronchial glands, cartilage, and smooth muscle.

10. Ans. (d) Clara cells *(Ref: Robbins 9th/pg 670; 8th/pg 679)*

Club cells, also known as **bronchiolar exocrine cells**, originally known as **Clara cells**, are **dome-shaped cells** with **short microvilli,** found in the **small airways (bronchioles)** of the lungs, produce substances similar to surfactant.

11. Ans. (b) Alveoli *(Ref: Robbins 9th/pg 669-670; 8th/pg 678)*

Pores of Kohn[Q]- permit the passage of **bacteria** and **exudate** between adjacent alveoli.

12. Ans. (d) CMV pneumonia

Large cell with basophilic intranuclear inclusion is the clue

13. Ans. (d) Occurs in babies born post-dates

(Ref: Robbins 9th/pg 672)

14. Ans. (a) Mucus plug in alveoli *(Ref: R 9th/pg 672-673)*

15. Ans. (d) Fat embolism *(Ref: Robbins 9th/pg 672-673)*

Etiology of ARDS & ALI

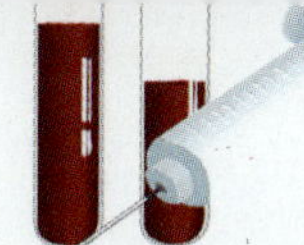

16. **Ans. (a, d) a. Presence of leukocytes; d. Mucus with inflammatory cells**

(Ref: Mayo Clin Proc. 1975 Jun; 50(6):339-44)

Good quality sputum samples have:
- Should not be contaminated by oropharyngeal flora
- ≥10 leukocytes with mucus, but <25 squamous epithelial cells per low-power field (LPF, ×100),

17. **Ans. (a) Alveolar macrophages** *(Ref: R 9th/pg 669-670)*

18. **Ans. (b) Pigmented alveolar macrophages**

(Ref: Robbins 9th/pg 669-670; 8th/pg 678)

19. **Ans. (d) Resolution** *(Ref: Robbins 9th/pg 704-705)*

20. **Ans. (a) Type 1 pneumocytes**

(Ref: Robbins 9th/pg 672-673)

In ARDS
- Initially, there is destruction of **type 1 pneumocytes^Q →hypoxemia**
- Later damage and necrosis of **type II alveolar pneumocytes^Q →** leads to **surfactant deficiency^Q**

21. **Ans. (b) Malignant hypertension** *(Ref: R 9th/pg 672-673)*

22. **Ans. (b) Fibrin** *(Ref: Robbins 9th/pg 672-673)*

Hyaline membrane consists of fibrin-rich edema fluid with **necrotic epithelial cells.**

23. **Ans. (a) Hemosiderin** *(Ref: Robbins 9th/pg 669-670)*

24. **Ans. (c) Vegetable matter; Aspiration pneumonia**

25. **Ans. (d) Accumulation of fibrin in alveoli**

(Ref: Robbins 9th/pg 704-705; 8th/pg 712-713)

26. **Ans. (b) Resolution** *(Ref: Robbins 9th/pg 704-705)*
- In **most cases of pneumonia, resolution** occurs;
- <10% of patients have pneumonia severe enough to merit hospitalization & in most such instances death results from a complication, as stated below;

27. **Ans. (a) Diffuse alveolar necrosis**

(Ref: R 9th/pg 672-673)

ARDS is also called **"shock lung"**

28. **Ans. (a) Necrotizing granulomatous inflammation**

(Ref: Rob^{bi}ns 9th/pg 376)

29. **Ans. (d) Miliary tuberculosis**

(Ref: Robbins 9th ed p376)

Miliary pulmonary disease occurs when organisms draining through lymphatics enter the venous blood and circulate back to the lung. Individual lesions are either microscopic or small, visible (2-mm) foci of yellow-white con-solidation scattered through the lung parenchyma (the adjective "miliary" is derived from the resemblance of these foci to millet seeds). Miliary lesions may expand and coalesce, resulting in consolidation of large regions or even whole lobes of the lung. With progressive pulmonary tuberculosis, the pleural cavity.

30. **Ans. (a, b, e) a. Occur primarily due to hematogenous spread, b. Miliary lesion is generally of size 1-2 mm, e. Sputum smear microscopy is negative in 80% of cases**

(Ref: Robbins 9th/pg 375-376; 8th/pg 370-371)

31. **Ans. (a) Apex**

Postprimary (Adult-Type) Disease
- Also referred to as *reactivation* or *secondary TB*, postprimary TB is probably most accurately termed *adult-type TB*, since it may result from endogenous reactivation of distant latent infection or recent infection (primary infection or reinfection).
- It is usually localized to the apical and posterior segments of the upper lobes, where the substantially higher mean oxygen tension (compared with that in the lower zones) favors mycobacterial growth

32. **Ans. (a) Macrophage**

(Ref: Robbins 9th/pg 375; 8th/pg 370)
- **Mycobacterium tuberculosis**enters into macrophages with the help of **mannose binding lectin^Q**and **CR3.^{Q}**
- **Macrophages^Q** are the **primary cells infected** by M. tuberculosis

33. **Ans. (b) Post-primary** *(Ref: Robbins 9th/pg 375-376)*

Fate of primary TB:
- **95% cases:** Cell mediated immunity controls infection → Calcified healed lesions & hilar lymph nodes formed **(Ranke complex).**
- **5% cases:** Primary tuberculosis is progressive **(Progressive Primary TB)** → resembles acute bacterial pneumonia → **Lympho-hematogenous dissemination** may cause **tuberculous meningitis** &/or **miliary tuberculosis.**

34. **Ans. (d) Puhl's lesion** *(Ref: Robbins 9th/pg 375-376)*

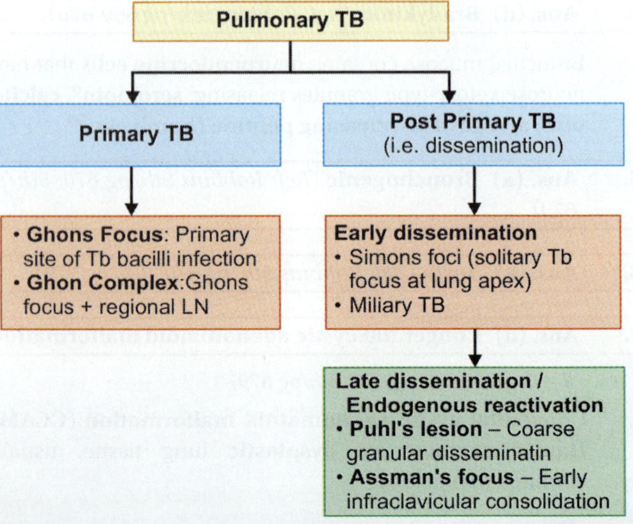

35. **Ans. (b) Liver** *(Ref: Nelson 19 ed Chap 212)*

In congenital TB, primary organ involved is liver.

- Congenital tuberculosis is rare because the most common result of female genital tract tuberculosis is infertility.
- Congenital transmission usually **occurs from a lesion in the placenta** through the umbilical vein.
- **Primary infection in the mother** just before or during pregnancy is more likely to cause congenital infection than is reactivation of a previous infection.
- The tubercle bacilli **first reach the fetal liver**, where a primary focus with periportal lymph node involvement may occur.

Organisms pass through the liver into the main fetal circulation and infect many organs.

36. **Ans. (c) Terminal ileum** *(Ref: Robbins 9th/pg 375-376)*

Extrapulmonary TB:

- **MC site is lymph node**^{Q}, MC cervical & supraclavicular **("Scrofula")**^{Q}
- **Pleural involvement: Exudative**^{Q} **Pleural effusion,** tuberculous empyema, or obliterative fibrous pleuritic

Genitourinary *TB*: **sterile pyuria**^{Q}; *Preferentially involves* fallopian tube^Q *in females &*epididymis^Q *in males*

- **Skeletal** TB: Most common site **spine**^{Q} **(Pott's disease)** ^{Q}> hip > knee
- **TB meningitis** (paresis of cranial nerves especially ocular, is frequent finding)^Q
- **In Gastro-intestinal (GI) TB: MC site terminal ileum and caecum**^{Q}

37. **Ans. (a) Arteries** *(Ref: Robbins 9th/pg 375-376)*

- Miliary TB is due to **hematogenous spread** of tubercle bacilli.
- Although in **children** it is often the consequence of **primary infection**, in **adults** it may be due to either **recent infection or reactivation of old disseminated foci.**
- Lesions are usually yellowish **1–2 mm granulomas** that resemble millet seeds (thus the term *military*)
- **Miliary pulmonary disease** occurs when organisms draining through lymphatics enter the venous blood and circulate back to the lung
- **Systemic miliary tuberculosis** occurs when bacteria disseminate through the **systemic arterial system.**
- Miliary tuberculosis is most prominent in the **liver, bone marrow, spleen, adrenals, meninges, kidneys, fallopian tubes, and epididymi**s, but could involve any organ

38. **Ans. (c) Parenchymal lesion along with inflamed lymph nodes** *(Ref: Robbins 9th/pg 375-376; 8th/pg 370-371)*

- **Ghon's focus**^{Q}: Grey white area of **inflammation with consolidation**
- **Ghon's complex:**^{Q}**Ghon's focus + inflamed regional lymph nodes**

39. **Ans. (a) IFN-g** *(Ref: Robbins 9th/pg 371-372; 8th/pg 368)*

40. **Ans. (c) Assmans focus** *(Ref: Robbins 9th/pg 375-376)*

- Classically involves **apical and posterior segments of upper lobe** due to high O_2 concentration **(Puhl'slesion**^{Q}**)** **Infraclavicular lesion** is called **Assman's Focus;** Refer to Ans 44 above;

41. **Ans. (c) Quantitative and qualitative measurement of Interferon gamma released by mycobacterium tuberculosis in the body** *(Ref: Harrison 18th/chapter 165)*

- **IGRAs are more specific** than the TST as a result of **less cross-reactivity due to BCG vaccination** and sensitization by **non-tuberculous mycobacteria**
- Measure **T cell release of IFN**- in response to stimulation with the highly **TB-specific antigens ESAT-6 and CFP-10**
- This test is **performed in vitro**& not in vivo, hence the answer is option C

42. **Ans. (b) Secretory**

(Ref: Immunology, 8th edition, by David Male; pg 427)

- **Epithelioid cells** are transformed macrophages that have **lost their phagocytic function** but **retained their secretory activity.**
- Epithelioid cells contain **numerous endoplasmic reticulum & golgi bodies.**
- They **secrete IL10, TNF alpha, TGF beta;**

43. **Ans. (c) Alpha 1 antitrypsin deficiency** *(Ref: R 9th pg 675)*

Features are suggestive of Emphysema

44. **Ans. (b) Metaplasia** *(Ref: Robbins 9th/pg 675)*

45. **Ans. (c) Distal bronchiectasis** *(Ref: Harrison 18th/pg 2120)*

46. **Ans. (d) Respiratory bronchiole**

(Ref: Robbins 9th/pg 675)

Cigarette smoking is most likely to cause damage to smaller segments of airway like acinus

47. **Ans. (a) Columnar to squamous**

(Ref: Robbins 9th/pg 679)

Chronic bronchitis is an example of squamous metaplasia in which normal columnar epithelium of respiratory tract is replaced by squamous epithelium;

48. **Ans. (b) Terminal bronchiole**

(Ref: Robbins 9th/pg 675-676)

Emphysema is defined as **irreversible dilatation and de-struction**^{Q} of the airspaces **distal to the terminal bronchiole (acinus)**^{Q}**, without fibrosis.**^{Q}

49. **Ans. (a) Centriacinar** *(Ref: Robbins 9th/pg 675-676)*

Centriacinar emphysema is the most common form, constituting more than 95% of clinically significant cases.

50. **Ans. (b) Interstitial fibrosis**

(Ref: Robbins 9th/pg 674-675)

Obstructive lung diseases include: Emphysema, Chronic Bronchitis, Asthma, Bronchiectasis,

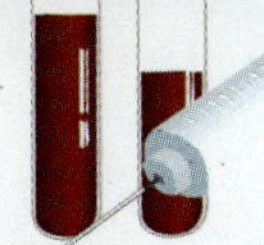

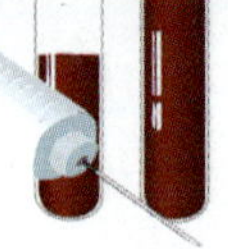

51. **Ans. (a)** **Bronchial asthma** *(Ref: Robbins 9th/pg 679-680)*
- Curschmann spirals: extrusion of **mucusplugs** from subepithelial mucous gland ducts or bronchioles.[Q]

52. **Ans. (c)** **Curshmann spirals**

(Ref: Robbins 9th/pg 679-680)

53. **Ans. (b)** **Asthma** *(Ref: Robbins 9th/pg 679-680)*

Characteristic histologic findings ("airway remodeling") of asthma include: Hypertrophy and/or hyperplasia of the bronchial wall muscle[Q]

54. **Ans. (a)** **Bronchial asthma** *(Ref: Robbins 9th/pg 679-680)*

55. **Ans. (b)** **Dilatation** *(Ref: Robbins 9th/pg 683-684)*

Bronchiectasis refers to **destruction of smooth muscle and elastic tissue** *by chronic necrotizing infections leading to* permanent[Q] *dilation of bronchi and bronchioles.*[Q]

56. **Ans. (c)** **Chronic bronchitis** *(Ref: Robbins 9th/pg 679)*

57. **Ans. (a)** **Upper lobe** *(Ref: Robbins 9th/pg 675-676)*

58. **Ans. (a)** **Reversible bronchoconstriction**

(Ref: Robbins 9th/pg 674-675; 8th/pg 683-684)

59. **Ans. (b)** **Lung cancer** *(Ref: Robbins 9th/pg 683-684)*

60. **Ans. (a)** **Increased in Chronic Bronchitis**

(Ref: Robbins 9th/pg 679; 8th/pg 687-688)

61. **Ans. (c)** **Dysphagia** *(Ref: Robbins 9th/pg 683-684)*
- **Kartagener syndrome** refers to **bronchiectasis, sinusitis, and situsinversus;**[Q]
- It is seen in **50% patients** with primary ciliary dyskinesia

62. **Ans. (a)** **Asbestosis**

Look at knobbed ends and brown colour , this is suggestive of asbestos bodies. As they also contain iron, so they take blue colour on perls stain

63. **Ans. (b, c, d) b. Dense collagen and calcifications in the lymph nodes seen; c. Progressive massive fibrosis can be seen as late complication; d. Immune granuloma can be seen**

64. **Ans. (a)** **Asthma like features** *(Ref: Robbins 9th 689)*
- In 10–25% cases, disease may be progressive, with chest tightness recurring or persisting throughout the workweek.
- After >10 years of exposure, workers with recurrent symptoms are more likely to have an **obstructive pattern** on pulmonary function testing.

65. **(b)** **Wallboard paper** *(Ref: Robbins 9th/pg 688*

66. **Ans. (a)** **Staph aureus** *(Ref: Robbins 9th pg)*

67. **Ans. (a)** **Central bronchiectasis**

(Ref: Robbins 9/683)

Predominant involvement of the central airways is reported in association with allergic bronchopulmonary aspergillosis (ABPA), in which an immune-mediated reaction to *Aspergillus* damages the bronchial wall.

68. **Ans. (b)** **More common in smoker**

(Ref: Robbins 9th/694-95; Davidson 22nd/719-20; Harrison 19th/ 1681-83)

69. **Ans. (c)** **Paragonimus with 2 layers**

(Ref Harrison's 19thed/1429; CDC website)

The figure shows: ***Eggs of Paragonimus sp. taken from a lung biopsy stained with hematoxylin and eosin***

70. **Ans. (a)** **Themophilus actinomycetes**

(Ref: Robbins 9th/pg 689; 8th/pg 687)

In *farmer's lung*, inhalation of proteins, such as thermophilic actinomyces bacteria and fungal spores that are present in moldy bedding and feed, are most commonly responsible for the development of Hypersensitivity pneumonitis.

71. **Ans. (a)** **Amphibole** *(Ref: Robbins 9th/pg 689)*

Serpentine[Q] **(M.C)** and **Amphibole**[Q] **(more pathogenic)** as particles are asbestor particle associated with asbestosis.

72. **Ans. (c)** **Lower lobe is ussualy involved**

(Ref: Robbins 9th/pg 689; 8th/pg 687)

Silicosis involves upper lobe more commonly than lower lobe. Examination of the nodules by polarized microscopy reveals the birefringent silicate particles (silica is weakly birefringent).

73. **Ans. (d)** **Mesothelioma** *(Ref: Robbins 9th/pg 691-692)*

74. **Ans. (a)** **Coal dust** *(Ref: Robbins 9th/pg 689; 8th/pg 697)*

75. **Ans. (c)** **Asbestosis** *(Ref: Robbins 9th/pg 691-692)*

76. **Ans. (c)** **Usual interstitial pneumonia** *(Ref: R 9th/pg 685)*

77. **Ans. (a)** **Sarcoidosis** *(Ref: Robbins 9th/pg 693-694)*

Histology in Sarcoidosis:
- Well-formed non-caseating granulomas[Q] composed of an aggregate of tightly clustered epithelioid cells[Q], with Langhans or foreign body–type giant cells; Central necrosis is unusual.[Q]
- Schaumann bodies: laminated concretions composed of calcium and proteins[Q]
- Asteroid bodies: Stellate inclusions enclosed within giant cells[Q]

78.   **Ans. (a) Sarcoidosis** *(Ref: Robbins 9th/pg 693-694)*

79.   **Ans. (a) Methemoglobinemia**

(Ref: Robbins 9th/pg 691-692)

80.   **Ans. (a) Schaumanns bodies**

(Ref: Robbins 9th/pg 693-694)

81.   **Ans. (d) 1-5 μm** *(Ref: Robbins 9th/pg 689; 8th/pg 697)*

For pneumoconiosis, the most dangerous particles are from **1 to 5 μm** in diameter, because particles of this size may reach the **terminal small airways and air sacs and settle in their linings.**

82.   **Ans. (a) Basaloid type**

Squamous Cell Carcinoma - 2015 UPDATES

Number of subtypes have been reduced to three, which makes the diagnosis
- Keratinizing
- Non-keratinizing
- Basaloid squamous cell carcinoma (new category added)

83.   **Ans. (a, c, e) a. ck7; b. TTF1; e. Berep-4**

Adenocarcinoma lung is positive for TTF-1, BerEP-4, CK 7+/ CK 20-. They have EGFR, K-RAS & ALK gene mutation.

84.   **Ans. (d) Atypical carcinoid Stage IV**

(Ref: Robbins 9th / pg 231-234; 8th / pg 221-229)

- In the given question features like **coughing, dyspnea, flushing, diarrhea, hypotension, haematemesis** for 3 months is suggestive of **a neu roendocrine tumor** most likely to be **carcinoid.**
- **Morphology of a typical carcinoid tumor:** Nests or trabeculae of medium sized polygonal cells with lightly eosinophilic cytoplasm, low nuclear grade, round to oval finely granular nuclei; may have rosettes or small acinar structures with variable mucin.
- **Also remember:**
    - **Typical- <2 mitosis/10 hpf** (high power fields) and lack Necrosis; **Atypical carcinoids- 2-10 mitosis/hpf** with increased pleomorphism, necrosis, prominent nucleoli[Q], may cause Carcinoid syndrome[Q]

85.   **Ans. (c) Adenoca** *(Ref: Robbins 9th/pg 701; 8th/pg 710)*

86.   **Ans. (b) EGFR**

Mutations in small cell Ca lung include *TP53* (75% -90%), *RB* (~100%), chr 3p deletions and *MYC* family.

87.   **Ans. (c) Small cell Ca (Ref:** *Robbins 9th/716)*

88.   **Ans. (b) Kulchitsky cell** *(Ref: Robbins 9th/pg 719)*

- Enterochromaffin (EC) cells, or "Kulchitsky cells", are a type of enteroendocrine and neuroendocrine cell occurring in the epithelia lining the lumen of the digestive tract and the respiratory tract that release serotonin.
- Tumors from these cells results in carcinoid.

89.   **Ans. (d) Large cell carcinoma** *(Ref: Robbins 9th/pg 715)*

Large cell carcinoma is an undifferentiated malignant epithelial tumor that lacks the cytologic features of other forms of lung cancer. The cells typically have large nuclei, prominent nucleoli, and a moderate amount of cytoplasm. This gives a lymphoma like picture.

90.   **Ans. (c) ck 5/6** *(Ref: Robbins 9th/pg 723-724)*

Morphology of Malignant mesothelioma:

IHC Shows: Strong positivity for keratin protein, **calretinin**[Q], **Wilmstum or 1 (WT-1)**[Q], **cytokeratin 5/6**[Q], and D2-40[Q].

91.   **Ans. (a) Calretinin** *(Ref: Robbins 9th/pg 723-724)*

92.   **Ans. (b) Neuroma** *(Ref: Robbins 9th/pg 721; 8th/pg 731)*

93.   **Ans. (a) Malignant mesothelioma**

(Ref: R 9th/pg 723-724)

Rare tumor but risk of developing mesothelioma in heavily asbestos exposed individuals is as high as **7% to 10%.**

94.   **Ans. (a) Small cell carcinoma is lung**

(Ref: R 9th/pg 715-717)

Small cell lung ca is the most common lung Ca associated with **ectopic hormone production like ADH, ACTH, PTH.**

95.   **Ans. (a) Mesothelioma** *(Ref: Robbins 9th/pg 723-724)*

Pleural tumors:
- Solitary fibrous tumor
- Malignant mesothelioma

96.   **Ans. (a) Neurogenic tumor** *(Ref: Robbins 9th/pg 721)*

Neurogenic tumor is the most common mediastinal tumor.

97.   **Ans. (d) Small round cells and hyperchromatic nuclei with nuclear moulding** *(Ref: Robbins 9th/pg 715-717)*

This typical presentation of 60 yr/M presenting with a **mass located at central bronchus** causing distal **bronchiectasis and recurrent pneumonia** is suggestive of small cell Carcinoma.

In Small cell Ca lung, location in lungs are most commonly central and usually presents with mass within the bronchus.

Light Microscopy feature of Small cell Ca is:

- Small cells with **salt and pepper pattern, hyperchromatic nuclei,**[Q] **nuclear molding**[Q] is prominent
- **Basophilic staining** of vascular walls due to encrustation by DNA from necrotic tumor cells **(Azzopardi effect)**[Q]

About other options:

A. Abundant **osteoid matrix** formation points towards **metastatic Osteosarcoma;**

B. Contains **all three germ layers:** is consistent with a **Teratoma;**

C. **Spindle cells with abundant stromal matrix** is suggestive of **Sarcoma;**

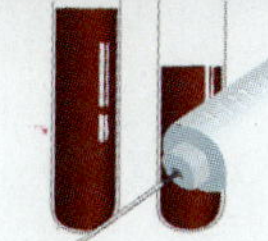

98. Ans. (b) Tumorlet

(Ref: Robbins 9th/pg 719-720; 8th/pg 729)

Benign tumorlets of lungs are **small,** insignificant, **hyperplastic nests**[Q] of neuroendocrine cells seen in areas of **scarring or chronic inflammation**[Q]

99. Ans. (c) Adrenal

(Ref: Robbins 9th/pg 717; 8th/pg 725)

Metastasis from Lung Ca to other organs:
- Lymphatic andhematogenous pathways[Q]
- Sq cell Ca shows late metastasis[Q]
- **Adrenals** (>50%), Liver(30%- 50%),Brain (20%) and bone (20%)

100. Ans. (b) Adenocarcinoma *(Ref: Robbins 9th/pg 715)*

101. Ans. (a) Chromogranin *(Ref: Robbins 9th/pg 717)*

Electron microscopy of Small cell Carcinoma lung: dense-core neurosecretory granules[Q] releasing neuroendocrine markers such as **chromogranin**[Q], **synaptophysin**[Q], **and CD57**[Q], **parathormone-related protein**[Q]

102. Ans. (a) PTH *(Ref: Robbins 9th/pg 715-717)*

Most common variety causing **hypercalcemia** is **Squamous cell Ca, while all other hormones are usually secreted by small cell Ca**

103. Ans. (a) Enterochromaffin cells *(Ref: R 9th/pg 719-720)*

Carcinoid tumor develops from **Enterochromaffin cells which contains** neuroendocrine hormones.

104. Ans. (c) Numerous long slender microvilli

(Ref: Robbins 9th/pg 723-724; 8th/pg 733-734)

Prolonged asbestos exposure increases the risk of **mesothelioma**, which presents as a localized gray-white pleural mass.

Features	Adenocarcinoma	Malignant Mesothelioma
Immunohis-tochemistry	Carcinoembryonic antigen (CEA), CD15, **Ber-EP4, MUC4,** thyroid transcription factor 1 **(TTF-1),** Napsin A	Calretinin, WT1, keratin 5/6, claudin-4, thrombomodulin, D2-40/ podoplanin, h-caldesmon, caveolin-1,vimentin
Electron microscopy	Short & plump microvilli	longer and more slender microvill

About other options,
A. **Melanosomes:** Seen in **Malignant Melanoma**
B. **Neurosecretory granules**: Seen in **Small Cell Carcinoma of lung**
D. Desmosomes with secretory endoplasmic reticulum: can suggest Adenocarcinoma

105. Ans. (a) Squamous cell Ca is most common carcinoma

(Ref: Harrison 18th/chapter 89Robbins 9th/pg 715-717)

A.	True	Most common Lung Ca in India is Squamous cell ca, while Adenocarcinoma world wide
B.	**False**	**Lambert-Eaton myasthenic syndrome is a paraneoplastic syndrome associated with Small cell Lung Ca**
C.	False	Small cell Ca has the poorest prognosis
D.	**False**	BronchoalveolarCa mostly involves distal airways while Small cell & Squamous cell Carcinoma involve proximal airways
E.	False	Hypercalcemia is common with Squamous cell Carcinoma

106. Ans. (a) TTF

(Ref: Robbins 9th/pg 715-717; 8th/pg 724-725)

Adenocarcinoma expressthyroid transcription factor-1 **(TTF-1);** Refer to Ans 136 above;

107. Ans. (c) Small cell Ca *(Ref: Robbins 9th/pg 715-717)*

108. Ans. (a,b) a. Not associated with smoking; b. Surgical resection alone is the treatment of choice

(Ref: Robbins 9th/pg 715-717; 8th/pg 724-725)

Small Cell Carcinoma (SCC) is the most common lung Ca associated with smoking
Since, SCC is highly malignant, Surgery with chemotherapy is the treatment of choice

109. Ans. (b) Asbestosis *(Ref: Robbins 9th/pg 723-724)*

Malignant mesothelioma is associated with **Asbestosis. Smoking does NOT increase the risk of malignat mesothelioma.**

110. Ans. (a,c,d) a. Clara cells; c. Mucin secreting cells; d. Type II pneumocytes *(Ref: Robbins 9th/pg 715-717)*

Bronchoalveolar Ca
- Previously a subtype of Adenocarcinoma is now classified as **premalignant lesion of Lung Ca**
- Has **no invasion** and produces **pneumonia like consolidation,** hence called **"Lepedic"**[Q]
- Consists of mucin secreting **bronchiolar cell**[Q], **Clara cells**[Q], **Type II pneumocytes**[Q]

111. Ans. (c) Carcinoid syndrome does not manifest

(Ref: Robbins 9th/pg 719-720; 8th/pg 729)

112. Ans. (a) Squamous cell carcinoma

(Ref: R 9th/pg 715-717)

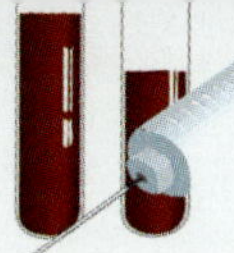

113. Ans. (d) Oat cell carcinoma is commonly associated with bilateral hilar lymphadenopathy

(Ref: R 9th/pg 715-717)

Oat cell Ca is the other name for small cell ca

a.	False, as **most common lung Ca is Adenoca**
b.	False as **cavitations are most common in squamous cell Ca**
c.	False as **Squamous cell ca is most often associated with calcification**
d.	True as **metastasis in small cell ca is common to hilar nodes & distant sites like adrenal & CNS**

114. Ans. (d) Branching microvilli *(Ref: R 9th/pg 715-717)*

Short Branching microvilli is the finding in electron microscopy

115. Ans. (b) Stromal invasion with desmoplasia

(Ref: Robbins 9th/pg 715-717; 8th/pg 724-725)

Note

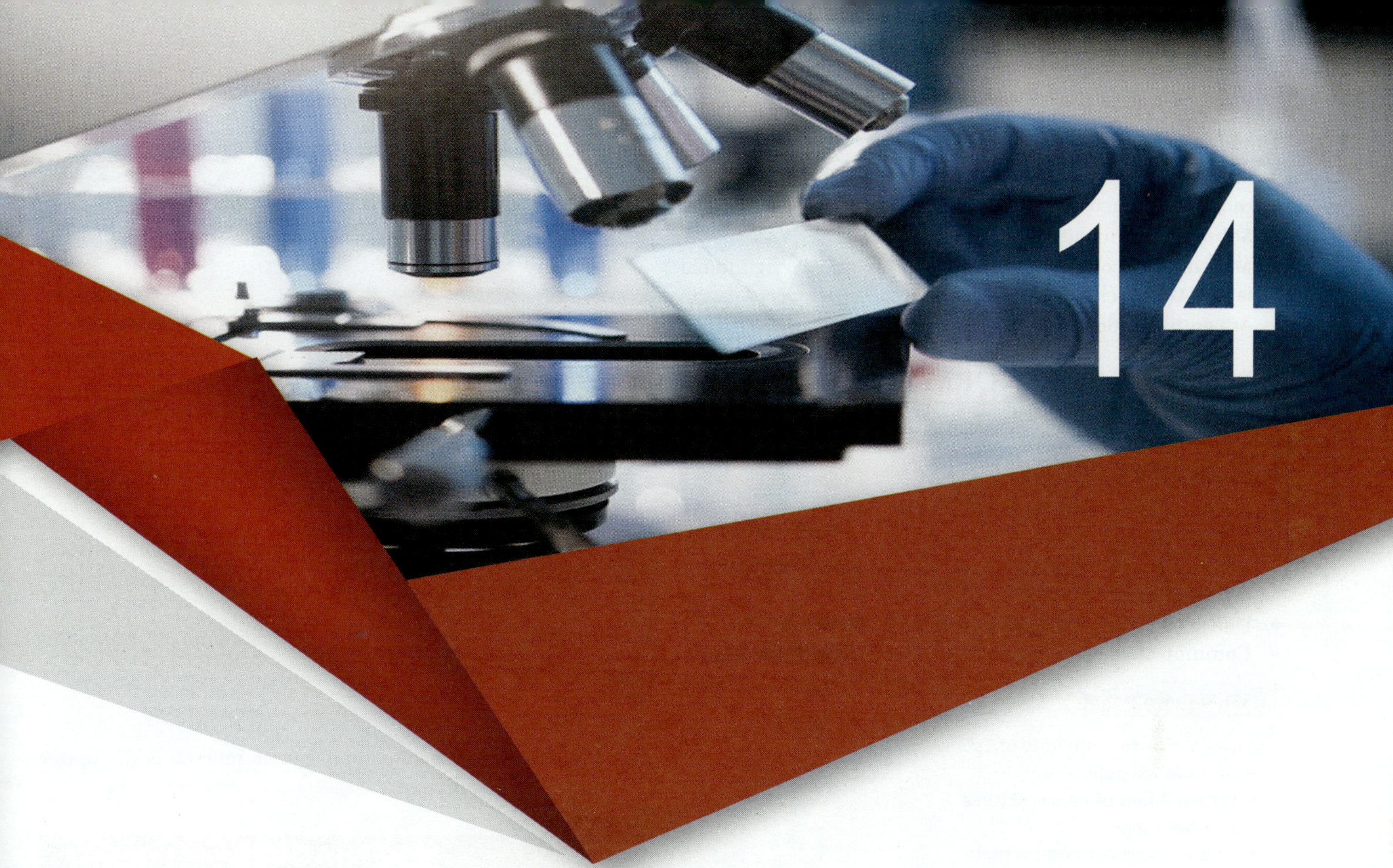

14

Gastrointestinal Tract and its Disorders

- Esophagus does not have serosa
- Most common fungal organism causing Esophageal infections is Candida
- Barret esophagus is characterized by intestinal metaplasia within the esophageal squamous mucosa
- Most common esophageal cancer in India is Squamous cell Carcinoma
- Most important risk factors for Adenocarcinoma is Barrett's esophagus
- Curling ulcers-Ulcers occurring in the proximal duodenum and associated with severe burns or trauma
- Hallmark of Crohn disease-non-caseating granulomas
- Most common site of carcinoid tumor: Tracheobronchial tree followed by ileum, followed by rectum
- Classic FAP at least 100 polyps are necessary for a diagnosis
- Squamous cell carcinoma most common tumor of anal canal

- Dysbiosis is seen in pseudomembranous colitis
- Combination of strong crypt CG3 staining and loss of DAS 1 stain is seen in 45% UC. Hence, these are new markers of UC.

The GI tract contains four layers:-

- **Mucosa** consisting of lining epithelium, **lamina propria** and muscularis mucosae
- **Submucosa**-mucous secreting glands, **Meissner's plexus**
- **Muscularis propia** (inner circular layer, outer longitudinal layer)-**Auerbach's plexus** in between these two layers.
- **Adventitia or Serosa**

CONGENITAL ABNORMALITIES[Q]

Diverticulum

Meckel's Diverticulum

Most **common true diverticulum** which occurs in the **ileum**. (antimesenteric side)

True diverticulum is defined by the presence **of all three layers** of the bowel wall.[Q]

- Due to failed involution of the **vitelline duct**[Q]
- **Common site** of gastric ectopia, can cause **occult bleeding.**[Q]

Mnemonic

Meckel's diverticulum Rule of 2s"
- Occur in **2%** population
- **Within 2 feet of** ileocecal valve
- **2 inches** long
- 2 times more common in males
- Symptomatic by **age 2**

Acquired Diverticulum

Most common in sigmoid colon

Hirschsprung Disease (Congenital Aganglionic Megacolon[Q])

- Normal migration of **neural crest cells from cecum to rectum is arrested prematurely**
- Distal intestinal segment lacks **both the Meissner's submucosal and the Auerbach myenteric plexus.**[Q]
- **Proximal to aganglionic segment, colon undergoes progressive dilation**[Q]
- Defect always **begins at the rectum**,[Q] but extends proximally for variable lengths.
- **Aganglionic region** may have a grossly **normal or contracted appearance.**[Q]
- In contrast, **the normally** innervated proximal colon may undergo **progressive dilation (megacolon)**[Q]
- Heterozygous **loss of function mutations** in **RET gene causes most of** familial cases & 15% of sporadic cases[Q]

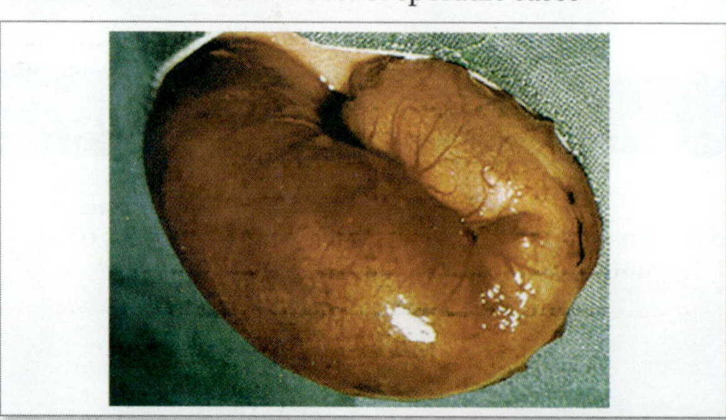

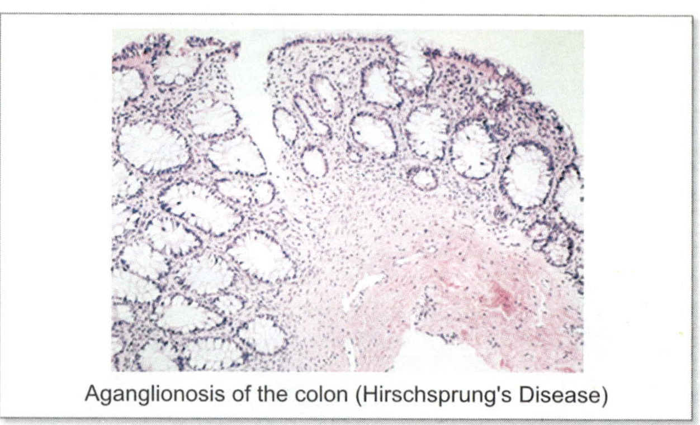

Aganglionosis of the colon (Hirschsprung's Disease)

Omphalocele

- Abdominal viscera herniating into a ventral membranous sac.

Gastroschisis

- Herniation of **all layers**[Q] of the abdominal wall, from peritoneum to skin.

Ectopia

- **M**ost **frequent site** of ectopic gastric mucosa is the **upper third of the esophagus**

ESOPHAGUS

ACHALASIA CARDIA

- Occurs due to selective **loss of function of inhibitory neurons** like those secreting vasoactive intestinal peptide and nitric oxide which causes relaxation of LES whereas cholinergic innervations is intact

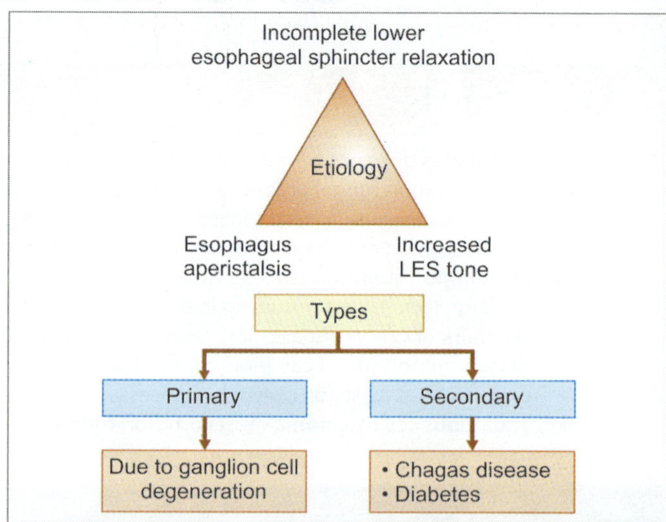

Screening Test

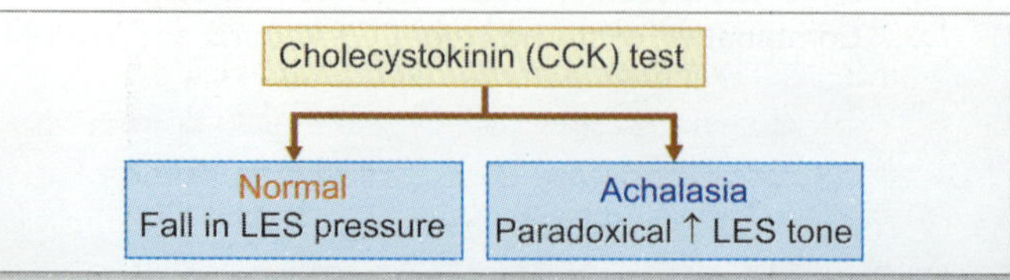

High Yield Facts

- Achlasia differs from Hirschsprung's disease since dilated esophagus contains less ganglion cells whereas dilated colon contains normal ganglion cells proximal to constricted aganglionic segment in Hirschsprungs.
- Inlet patch:[Q] Ectopic gastric mucosa is the upper third of the esophagus

Diagnosis

- Barium swallow shows **bird beak appearance** of the esophagus
- Method of choice-Manometry[Q]

LACERATIONS

Mallory-Weiss Tears	Boerhaave Syndrome
• Longitudinal **mucosal** tears • These tears usually **cross the gastroesophageal junction** • Associated with **severe retching or vomiting**[Q] secondary to acute alcohol intoxication. • Generally require **surgical intervention**[Q]	• **Transmural** tearing[Q] • Most common location: **left posterolateral part 3–5 cm above the gastroesophageal junction.** • **Require surgical intervention**

ESOPHAGITIS

- Inflammation of the esophageal mucosa is known as esophagitis
- **Most common cause**[Q]-Reflux of gastric contents into the lower esophagus due to **transient lower esophageal sphincter relaxation**[Q]
- **Gold standard** for the diagnosis of reflux esophagitis **is 24 hours pH study**[Q].

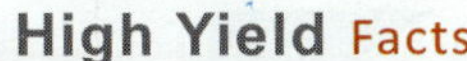

High Yield Facts

Esophageal infection
- **Herpes viruses** typically cause **punched-out ulcers**[Q]
- **CMV** causes **shallower ulcerations**[Q] with nuclear & cytoplasmic inclusions **within capillary endothelium and stromal cells**[Q]
- **M.C fungal** organism causing Esophageal infections is **Candida**[Q] followed by mucormycosis and Aspergillus.

BARRETT'S ESOPHAGUS

- Characterized by **intestinal metaplasia** within the esophageal squamous mucosa.[Q]
- Occurs due to **chronic gastroesophageal reflux disease (GERD).**[Q]
- Risk of **dysplasia correlates with length of esophagus affected. Long segment has the higher risk**[Q]
- Confers an **increased risk of esophageal adenocarcinoma**.[Q]
- Classified as long segment (if >3 cm is involved) or short segment (if <3 cm is involved).

- Diagnosis: Endoscopy and biopsy.
- Microscopically, **lower** esophageal squamous epithelium is replaced by columnar epithelium
- **Definite diagnosis is made only when columnar mucosa contains the intestinal goblet cells which show distinct mucous vacuoles that stain pale blue by hematoxylin and eosin.**[Q]

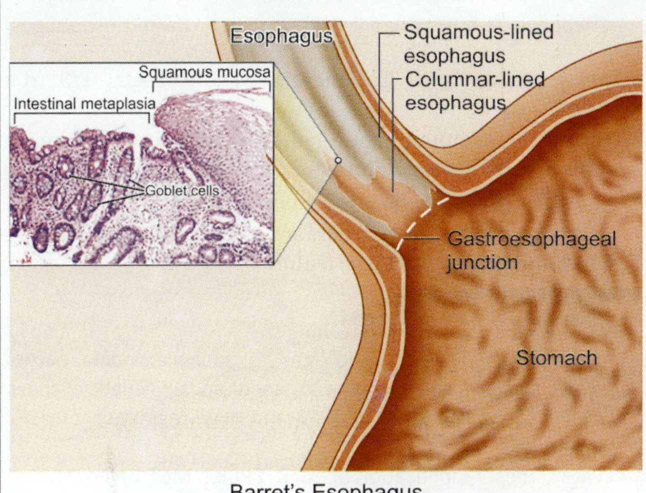

Barret's Esophagus

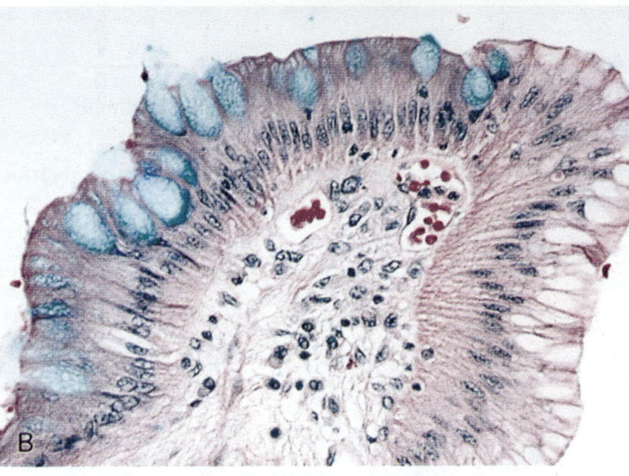

Alcian Blue Positivity in Barrets Esophagus

R9th Latest Update

Dysplasia is detected in 0.2%–2% of persons with Barrett's esophagus each year
- **Barrett's ulcer is the ulcer in the columnar lined portion of Barrett's esophagus.**[Q]

ESOPHAGEAL TUMORS

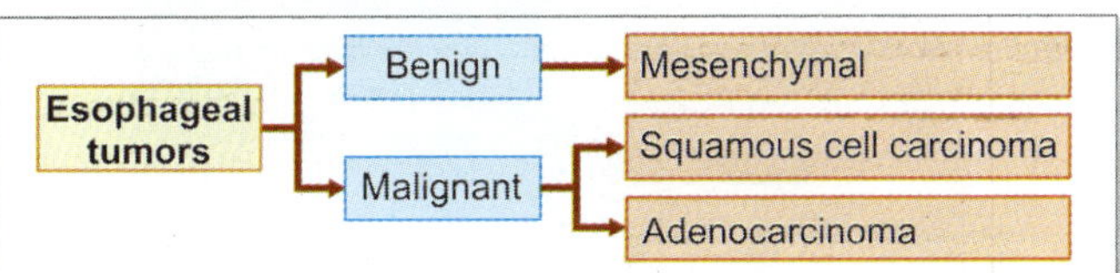

Adenocarcinoma

Risk factors for Adenocarcinoma	Risk is reduced by
• **Barrett's esophagus (Most important)**, Tobacco exposure, Radiation, Obesity, Gastroesophageal reflux disease (GERD), **Scleroderma**[Q], **Alcohol**[Q], Medications : Long term use (> 5 yr) of Theophylline & Beta-agonists	• Fresh fruits and vegetables, **Helicobacter pylori**[Q] (reduces incidence of Barrett esophagus)

- Most frequently in **Caucasians**, M > F, Distal 1/3 rd of esophagus[Q]
- By the time symptoms appear, the tumor has usually spread to **submucosal lymphatic vessels**;
- Overall 5-year survival is less than 25%.
- Microscopically, most cancers are mucin producing glandular tumors with intestinal type features

> **R9th — Latest Update**
>
> Progression of Barrett's esophagus to adenocarcinoma occurs through the stepwise acquisition of genetic and epigenetic changes
> - **Early stages:** Mutation of TP53 and downregulation of p16/INK4a
> - **Late stages:** Amplification of EGFR, ERBB2, MET, cyclin D1, and cyclin E genes.

Squamous Cell Carcinoma

- **Most common site: middle third**[Q] of the esophagus
- More common in **African Americans**[Q]
- Foci of **dysplastic epithelium as well as in situ carcinoma are present adjacent**[Q] to the mucosa

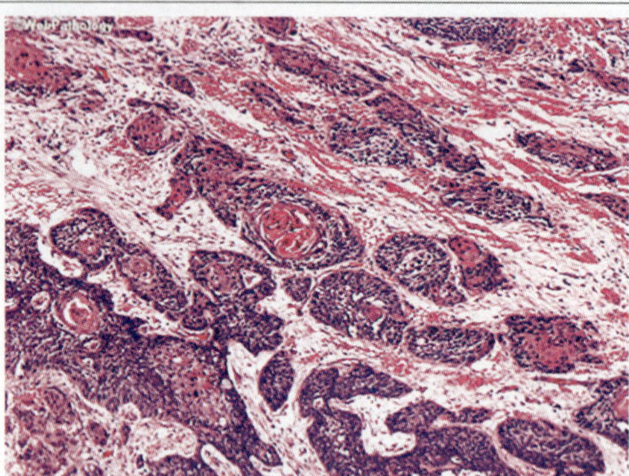

Squamous cell carcinoma

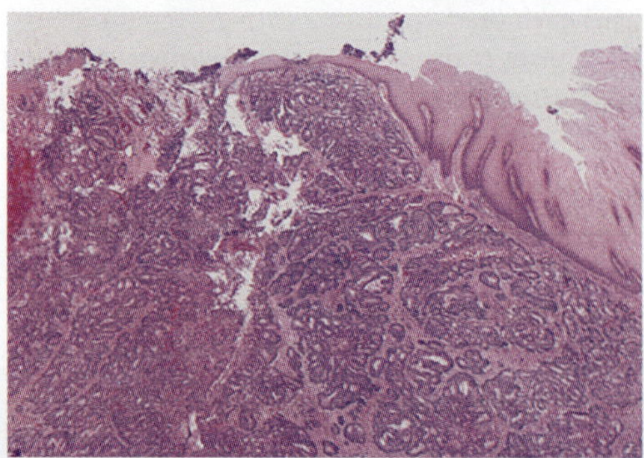

Adeno carcinoma

> **R9th — Latest Update**
>
> Mutations with SCC esophagus[Q]
> - Amplification of the transcription factor gene SOX2[Q]
> - Overexpression of the cell cycle regulator cyclin D1; and loss-of-function mutations in the tumor suppressors TP53, E-cadherin, and NOTCH1.[Q]

Risk Factors for Squamous Cell Carcinoma

- Tobacco and alcohol consumption[Q]
- Poverty
- Caustic esophageal injury
- Chronic achalasia[Q]
- Tylosis et plamaris
- Plummer Vinson syndrome
- Hot beverages or food
- Radiation-tumor occurs 5 to 10 or more years[Q] after exposure
- Long-standing esophagitis
- Human papillomavirus (HPV) infection (in high-risk areas but not in low-risk regions)[Q]
- Polycyclic hydrocarbons, nitrosamines
- Nutritional deficiency of vitamin A, vitamin C, riboflavin, zinc, molybdenum
- Long-standing celiac disease[Q]
- Ectodermal dysplasia[Q] and epidermolysis bullosa

High Yield Facts

- **Most Common benign tumor of esophagus leiomyomas**[Q]
- Most Common esophageal cancer worldwide is squamous cell carcinoma[Q] (Robbins 9th ed pg 758) **R9th**
- **Most Common esophageal cancer in India is Squamous cell Carcinoma**[Q]
- Most prevalent esophageal cancer worldwide (**old + new cases**) is **squamous cell carcinoma**[Q]

Most Common esophageal cancer worldwide (**new cases**) is **Adenocarcinoma**[Q]

- Most important risk factors for Adenocarcinoma is **Barrett's esophagus**[Q]
- **Most Common site of esophageal carcinoma- middle 1/3rd of the esophagus**
- **Most Common site of esophageal carcinoma in India is middle one-third of the esophagus**
- Most Common type of esophageal cancer in **upper 1/3rd of esophagus**: Squamous cell cancer[Q]
- Most Common type of esophageal cancer in **middle 1/3rd of esophagus**: Squamous cell cancer[Q]
- Most Common type of esophageal cancer in **lower 1/3rd of esophagus**: Adenocarcinoma[Q]
- **Milk, termed mursik, which contains the carcinogen acetaldehyde:** Esophageal squamous cell carcinoma
- **Plummer Vinson syndrome (also known as Patterson Kelly syndrome):** Triad of iron-deficiency anemia, esophageal webs and glossitis
- **Tylosis et plamaris: Hyperkeratosis and pitting of palms and soles**

STOMACH

Anatomic regions of Stomach and types of cells in them

Cardia	Fundus	Body	Antrum
• Mucin-secreting[Q] Foveolar cells[Q]	• Chief cells[Q] • Parietal cells[Q]	• Chief cells[Q] • Parietal cells[Q]	• Mucin-secreting foveolar cells[Q] • Endocrine cells, such as G cells[Q]

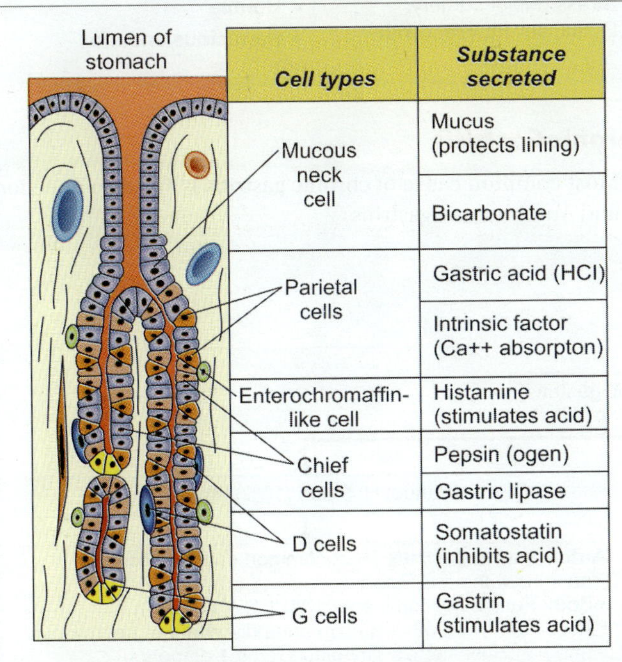

Cell types	Substance secreted
Mucous neck cell	Mucus (protects lining)
	Bicarbonate
Parietal cells	Gastric acid (HCl)
	Intrinsic factor (Ca++ absorpton)
Enterochromaffin-like cell	Histamine (stimulates acid)
Chief cells	Pepsin (ogen)
	Gastric lipase
D cells	Somatostatin (inhibits acid)
G cells	Gastrin (stimulates acid)

- **Gastropathy-When inflammatory cells are rare or absent.[Q]**
  - 2 types:

Ménétrier disease	Zollinger-ellison syndrome
• Characterised by the hypertrophy of gastric mucosa and not by **exophytic growth.[Q]** • Associated with excessive secretion of transforming growth factor **α (TGF-α)** a ligand for the tyrosine kinase epidermal growth factor receptor, resulting in selective expansion of surface foveolar mucous cells and hypersecretion of mucus • Risk of gastric **adenocarcinoma is increased** in adults with Ménétrier disease[Q]	• Caused by **gastrin-secreting tumors.[Q]** • These gastrinomas are most commonly found in the **small intestine or pancreas[Q]** • **Most remarkable feature is a doubling of oxyntic mucosal thickness due to a five-fold increase in the number of parietal cells.[Q]**

Gastropathy

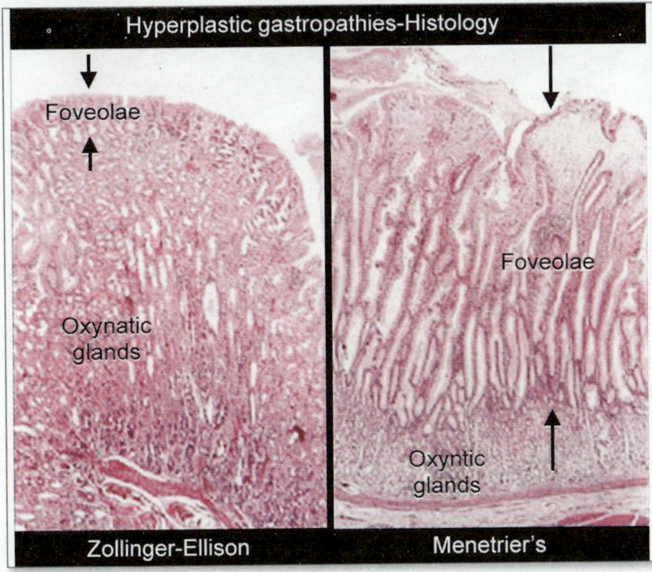

GASTRITIS

Gastritis is the **inflammation of the gastric mucosa.**

It can be divided into:

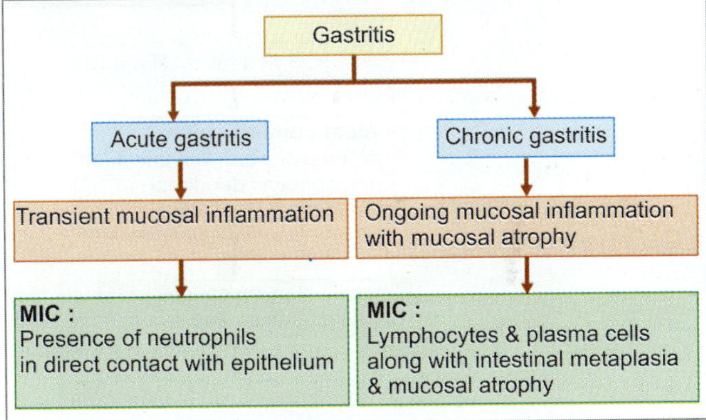

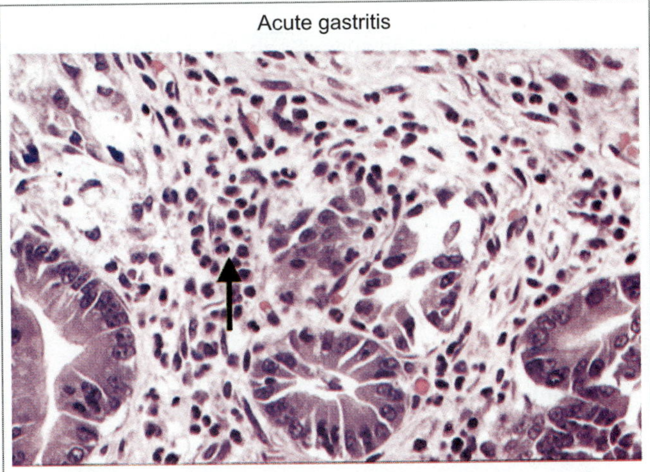

Neutrophilic infiltration of gastric mucosa S/o acute gastritis.

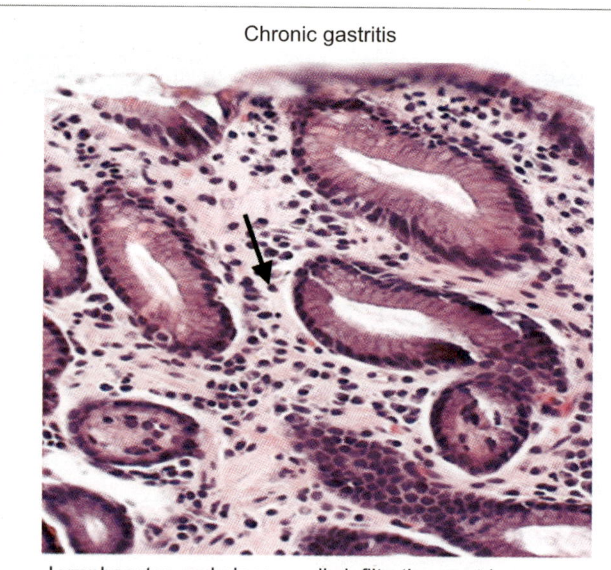

Chronic gastritis

Lymphocytes and plasma cells infiltrating gastric mucosa
S/o chronic gastric

Risk factors of

Acute gastritis	Chronic gastritis
• Heavy smoking • Excessive Alcohol • Excessive NSAID-aspirin Ibuprofen, Naproxen • **Uremia** • **Ischemia and shock** • Stress (Major surgery, Burns, severe infections)	• Drugs-NSAIDS • **H. pylori** • Alcohol and smoking • Radiation • **Gastrectomy with gastroenterostomy** • **Uremia** • **Pernicious anemia**

Chronic Gastritis

- Most common cause of chronic gastritis is *H.pylori* infection and Autoimmune gastritis

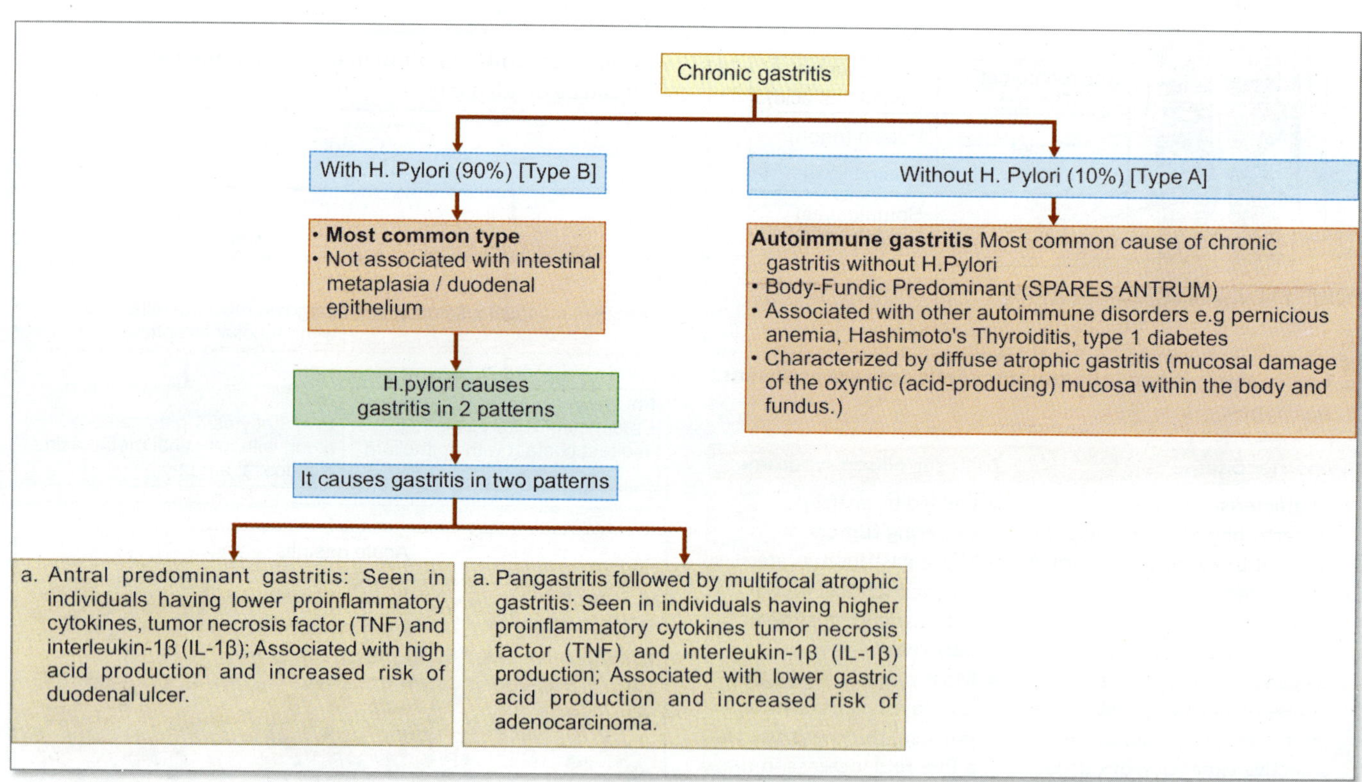

Chronic Gastritis Associated with H. pylori (in 90% Patients)

- Intraepithelial neutrophils and subepithelial plasma are characteristic of H. pylori gastritis

- Special stains **non-silver stains**[Q] (like Giemsa, Diff-Quick, Acridine orange) and **silver stain**[Q] (like warthin-Starry, Steiner Stain).

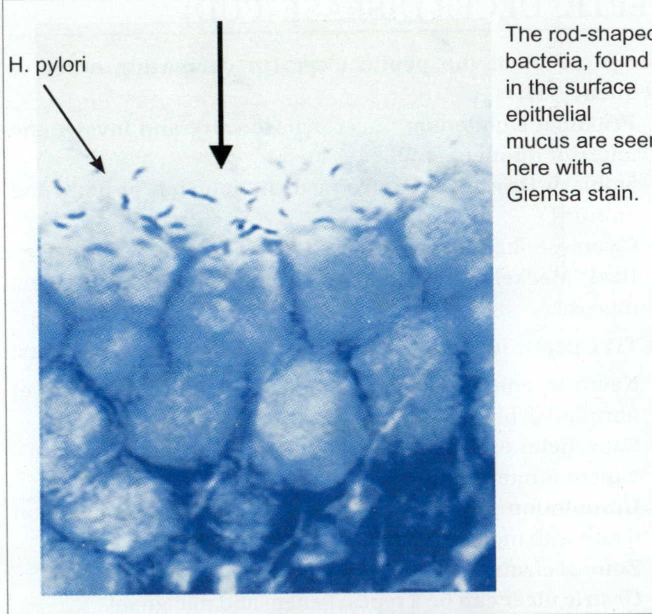

The rod-shaped bacteria, found in the surface epithelial mucus are seen here with a Giemsa stain.

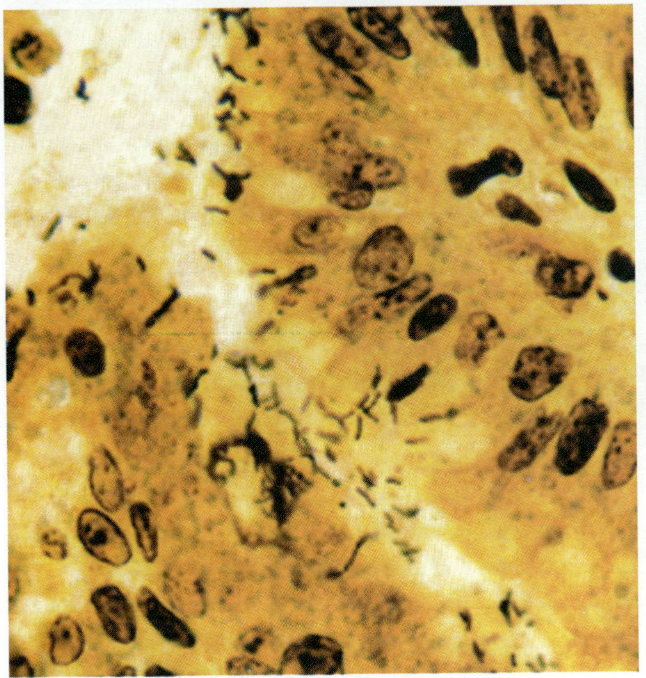

Helicobacter pylori on Warthin-Starry silver stain

H. pylori Causes

- Gastritis
- Peptic ulcer disease
- Gastric cancer - **Iron deficiency may also be a risk factor for H. pylori–associated gastric cancer.**[Q]
- Gastric lymphoma especially MALT lymphoma

Virulence Factors of H. pylori

- H. pylori is a Gram-negative flagellated bacteria

- **Flagella:** Allows the bacteria to be motile in viscous mucus
- **Urease:** Produces ammonia from endogenous urea-elevates local gastric pH and enhances bacterial survival
- **Adhesins:** Like **BabA** (responsible for enhanced binding in people with blood group O)
- **Toxins:** cytotoxin-associated gene A (CagA) and VacA

Diagnosis

- **Screening test:** Serum ELISA for antibodies against *H. pylori*
- **Urea breath test** (radiolabeled urea is broken down to radiolabeled CO_2 by urease enzyme which is detected, thus suggesting presence of *H.pylori* infection)
- **Gold standard: antral biopsy showing the bacilli**[Q], highlighted by Warthin-Starry silver stain.
- **Most specific investigation: Culture of bacteria (done on Skirrow's medium)**[Q]

Autoimmune Gastritis

- **Most common** form of chronic gastritis in patients **without H. pylori infection.**[Q]
- **Most common cause of diffuse atrophic gastritis**[Q]
- *No link to* HLA alleles.
- *Median age at diagnosis is 60.*
- Autoimmune gastritis is characterized by: Antibodies to **parietal cells** (most **prominently the H+, K+- ATPase, or proton pump,**[Q]) and **intrinsic factor**[Q] -present in 80% patients, detected in serum and gastric secretions
- **CD4+ T cells** directed against parietal cell components, including the H+, K+-ATPase- **principal agents** of injury
- **Defective gastric acid secretion (achlorhydria)**[Q] **hypergas-trinemia**
- **Hyperplasia of gastrin producing G cells** in the antral mucosa may result in **gastric carcinoid tumor**[Q]

STRESS-RELATED MUCOSAL DISEASE

Stress-related mucosal disease occurs in patients with severe trauma, extensive burns, intracranial disease, major surgery, other forms of severe physiologic stress.

- Gastric lesions usually develop during the **first 3 days** of their illness
  - **Stress ulcers:** Most common in individuals with shock, sepsis, or severe trauma.
  - **Curling ulcers:** Ulcers occurring in the proximal duodenum and associated with severe burns or trauma
  - **Cushing ulcers:** Gastric, duodenal, and esophageal ulcers arising in persons with intracranial disease. These have high incidence of perforation
    - **Most commonly**[Q] occurs due to local ischemia
    - **Most common**[Q] complication- **Bleeding** followed by perforation
    - **Recover completely** with treatment

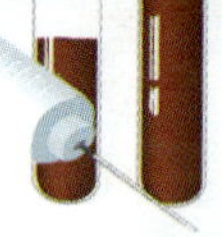
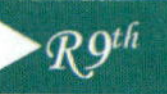

$R9^{th}$ Latest Update

Non-stress-related causes of gastric bleeding:

- **Dieulafoy lesion**: submucosal artery that **does not branch properly** within the wall of the stomach and thus has diameter of up to 3 mm, or 10 times the size of mucosal capillaries.
  - Found along the lesser curvature, near the gastroesophageal junction
  - Bleeding is often associated with NSAID use and may be recurrent
- **GAVE (watermelon stomach):** Longitudinal stripes of edematous erythematous mucosa alternate with less severely injured and paler mucosa. The erythematous stripes are created by **ectatic mucosal vessels**. Most common cause-idiopathic, others being cirrhosis and systemic sclerosis.[Q]

COMPLICATIONS OF CHRONIC GASTRITIS

1. Peptic Ulcer Disease
2. Gastritis Cystica

PEPTIC ULCER DISEASE (PUD)

The location of the peptic ulcer (in decreasing order of frequency) is:

- **Proximal Duodenum** : near **pyloric valve and involve the anterior duodenal wall.**[Q]
- Stomach (**lesser curvature** near the junction of body and antrum)
- Gastroesophageal junction in **GERD or Barrett's esophagus**
- **Ileal Meckel's diverticulum** containing ectopic gastric mucosa.

ACTIVE peptic ulcers are made up of following histogical layers:

- **Necrotic zone**[Q]-Base of peptic ulcers has thin layer of fibrinoid debris[Q]
- **Superficial exudative zone**[Q] -Zone of neutrophil predominant infiltrate[Q]
- **Granulation tissue zone**[Q] -Base having active granulation tissue with mononuclear leukocytes[Q]
- **Zone of cicatriaztion**[Q]-Zone of fibrous or collagenous scar[Q]
- **Gastric ulcer can be 2 types:** benign and malignant

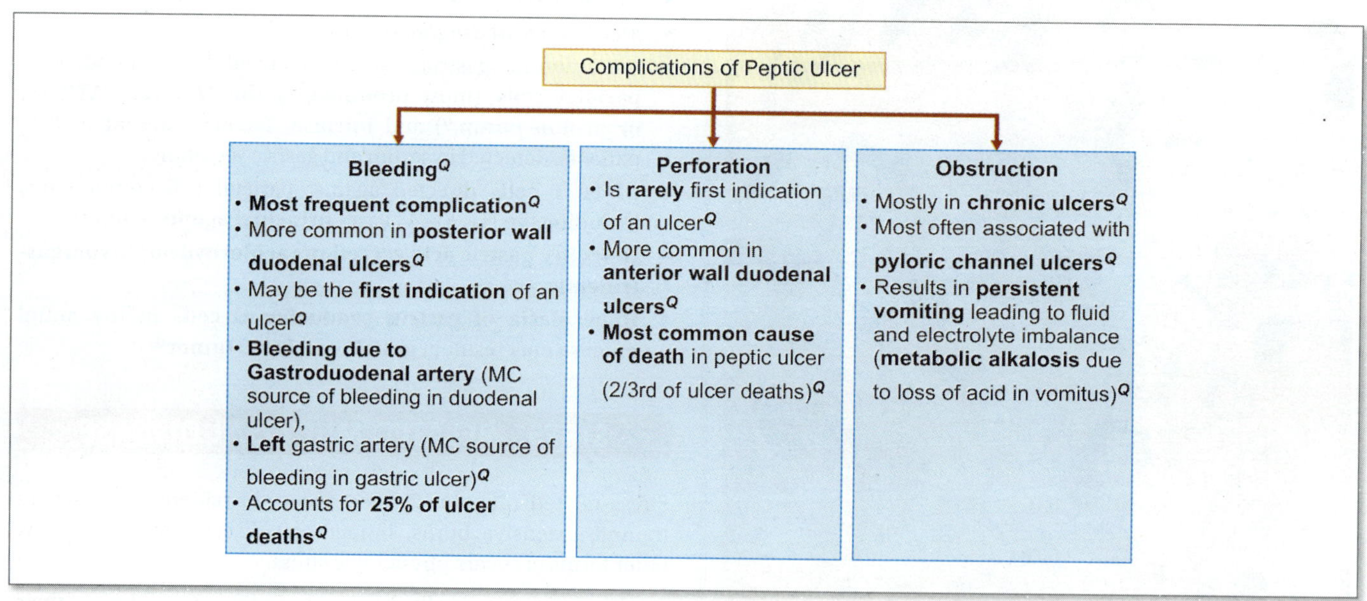

High Yield Facts

- **PUD does not impart an increased risk of gastric cancer**[Q], but patients who have had partial gastrectomies for PUD have a slightly higher risk of developing cancer **in the residual gastric stump, possibly due to hypochlorhydria, bile reflux, and chronic gastritis.**[Q]

- **Most common cause of PUD older than 60 years of age** is increased **NSAID use**[Q] (especially low-dose aspirin combined with other NSAIDs.)

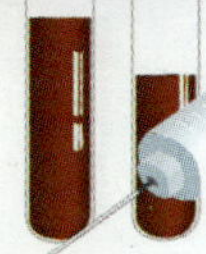

Benign Gastric Ulcer	Malignant Gastric Ulcer
• Generally at lesser curvature[Q] • Smooth radiating folds[Q] with Hampton line & collar[Q] • Overhanging margins[Q] showing regeneration • Mucosal rugae projects outwards from the margins of ulcer[Q] • Huge base[Q] • Preserved peristalsis[Q] • Heals within 8-10 weeks[Q]	• At greater curvature[Q] • Interrupted nodular, clubbed folds with Lasman Kirklin complex[Q] (malignant ulcer with no mass) • Eccentric with heaped up and everted margins[Q] • Mucosal rugae stop far of the ulcer[Q] • Necrotic base[Q] • No peristalsis[Q] • No healing[Q]

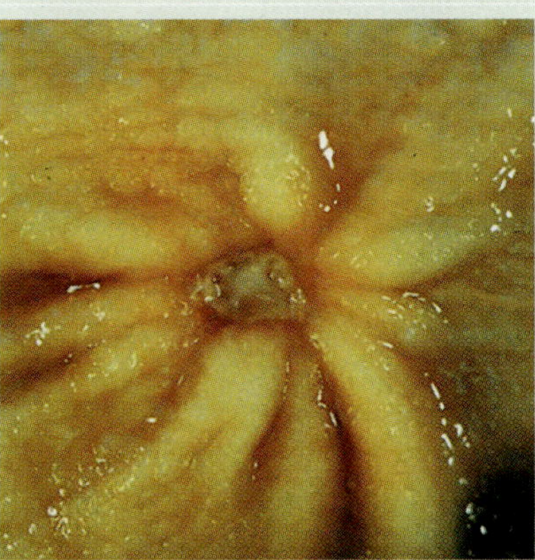

Benign gastric ulcer

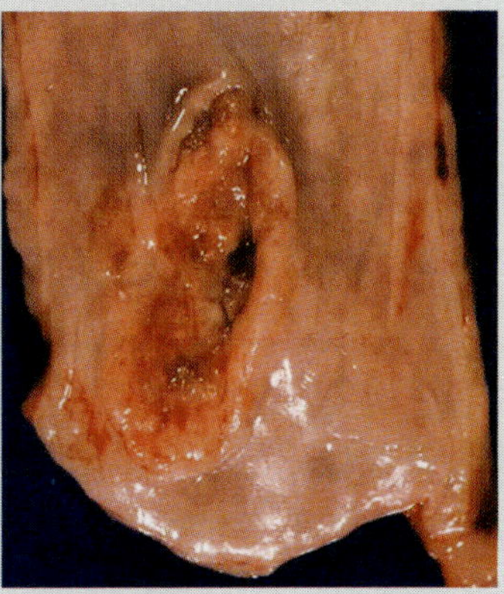

Malignant gastric ulcer

Gastritis Cystica

- Exuberant reactive epithelial proliferation associated with entrapment of epithelial-lined cysts
- May be found within the **submucosa (gastritis cystica polyposa)**[Q] or deeper layers of the gastric wall **(gastritis cystica profunda)**[Q]

GASTRIC POLYPS

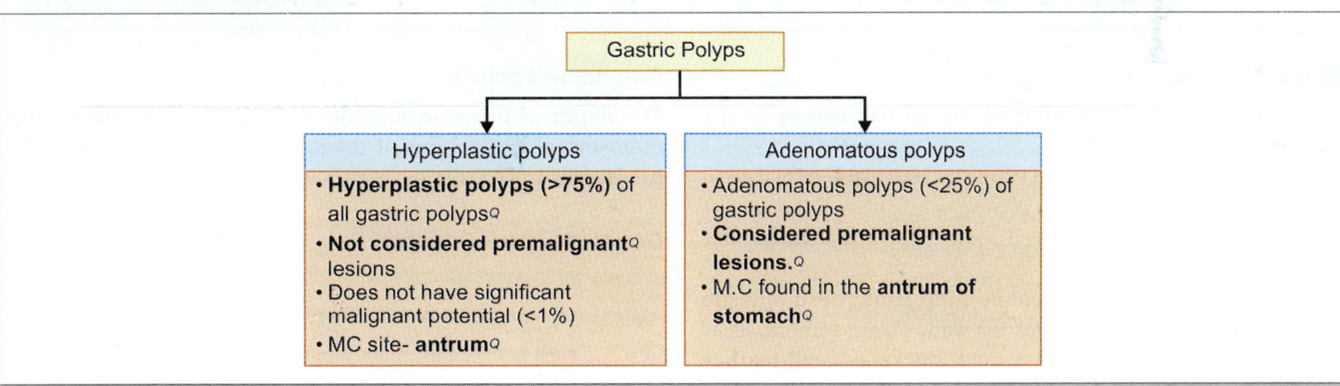

High Yield Facts

- **Hyperplastic gastric polyps** are called inflammatory polyps[Q] & usually associated with H. pylori[Q]
- **Fundic gastric polyp** usually is associated with familial adenomatous polyposis (FAP)[Q]
- **Fundic gastric polyp** has increased due to proton pump inhibitor therapy[Q]. It is glandular hyperplasia due to gastrin oversecretion in response to reduced acidity[Q].
- Gastric dysplasia and adenomas[Q] are recognizable precursor lesions associated with gastric adenocarcinoma.
- Most common site of Gastric Adenocarcinoma secondary to H. pylori infection is **Antrum**[Q]
- Most common site of Gastric Adenocarcinoma secondary to Pernicious anemia is **Fundus and Body**[Q]
- **Linitis plastica-** leather bottle appearance-seen in diffuse gastric cancer[Q], it is also seen in metastasis from cancers of breast and lung[Q].

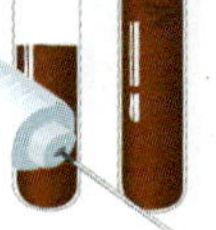

GASTRIC MALIGNANCIES

Gastric Adenocarcinoma[Q]: Most Common Gastric Malignancy

Classification of Gastric Adenocarcinoma

Gastric malignancies
Adenocarcinoma (MC)	Lymphoma	GIST

Based on Depth of invasion	Based on Lauren's histological classification

• Early gastric cancer (superficial spreading type[Q]):
  ■ Involvement of **mucosa and the submucosa**[Q] irrespective of the involvement of perigastric lymph nodes
  ■ **Associated with best prognosis.**[Q]
• Late gastric cancer:
  ■ Involvement of the **muscle layer** of the stomach
  ■ **Poor prognosis**
	• **Intestinal type**: composed of the **neoplastic intestinal glands**[Q]
	• **Diffuse type**: *linitis plastica*
	  ■ Non-cohesive cells which do not form glands
	  ■ "Signet ring"[Q] appearance (because mucin in the cell pushes the nucleus to the periphery)
	  ■ **Worst prognosis**[Q]
	  ■ **E-cadherin mutation frequently associated**[Q]

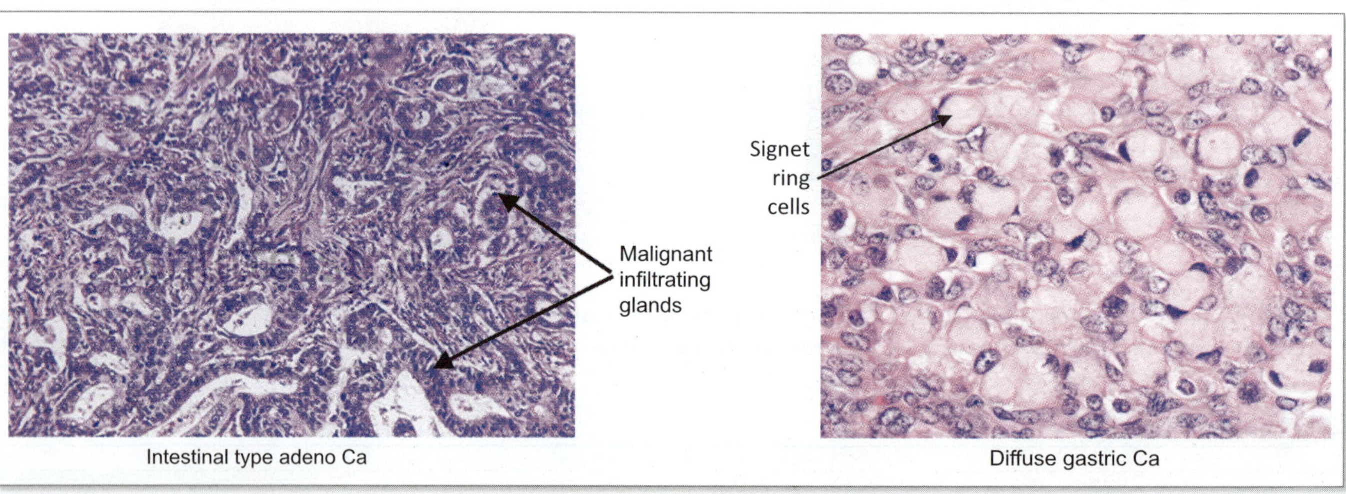

Intestinal type adeno Ca

Diffuse gastric Ca

Clinical Features

■ The most common location of the gastric cancer is the **antrum of the stomach.**[Q]

■ Cancer of the **gastric cardia is on the rise especially due to Barrett's esophagus**[Q]

■ **Lesser curvature**[Q] is involved more often than the greater curvature.

■ **Diffuse gastric cancer**-no definite lump, strong **desmoplastic reaction** that stiffens the gastric wall. These tumors show diffuse rugal flattening and a rigid, thickened wall-**leather bottle appearance termed linitis plastica**[Q].

Investigation of Choice

Endoscopy with Biopsy of Lesion[Q]

Metastasis

■ Occurs to the liver (**first organ to be affected**) followed by lungs, bone, ovary (where it is known as **Krukenberg's tumor**), periumbilical lymph nodes (Sister Mary Joseph nodule), peritoneal cul-de-sac (**Blumer's** shelf palpable on rectal or vaginal examination) and **left supraclavicular lymph node (Virchow's lymph node).**[Q]

Prognostic Factors

The **depth of invasion and the extent of nodal and distant metastases** at the time of diagnosis are the **most powerful prognostic indicators** in gastric cancer[Q]

Genes in Gastric Cancer

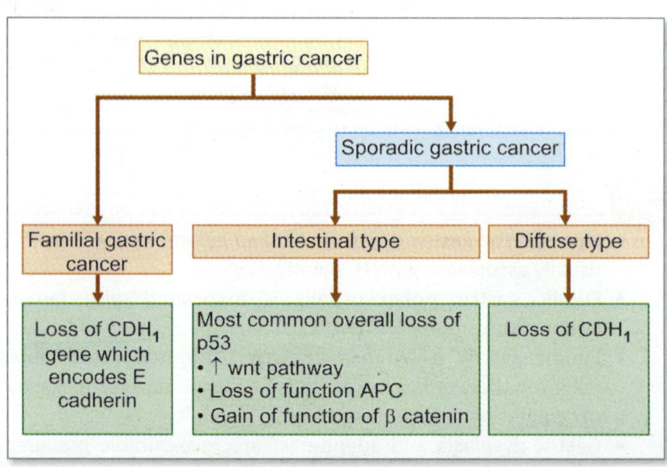

GI Lymphomas

- Gastrointestinal tract is the most common extranodal site involved by lymphoma
- Most common lymphomas are **NHL**
- Most frequent sites in order of its occurrence are the **stomach followed by small intestine and ileocecal region**[Q]
- 90% of the primary gastrointestinal lymphomas are of B- cell lineage with very few T-cell lymphomas and Hodgkin's lymphoma

Gastric Lymphoma

- Stomach is a **common site** for extranodal lymphomas
- Accounts for 5% of all gastric malignancies
- **MC: Indolent extranodal marginal zone B-cell lymphomas (**mucosa-associated lymphoid tissue (MALT)
- M**ost common** inducer: **H. pylori**[Q]
- M**ost common presenting symptoms are dyspepsia and epigastric pain**[Q]
- **Diagnostic lesions** on biopsy-**lymphoepithelial lesions**[Q]
- **Translocations** are associated with gastric MALToma, t(**11;18**)(**q21;q21**)[Q] & t(1;14)(p22;q32) and t(14;18)(q32;q21).

Gastrointestinal Stromal Tumor (GIST)

- **Most common mesenchymal tumor** of the abdomen with mean age of 60 yrs
- **Most common site (> 50%) is stomach; > small intestine (30%) colon and rectum**
- **Most common mutation is KIT (80%) > PDGFRA (8%) > SDH mutations (SDH deficient)**
- Arise from **interstitial cells of Cajal,** or pacemaker cells, of the gastrointestinal muscularis propria
- Increased incidence of GIST is seen in **NF-1**
- M**ost useful diagnostic marker** is **c-kit (CD117)** detectable in 95% of the patients.
- Microscopically the tumor may show either epithelioid cells, spindle cells or mixed (both the epithelioid cells and spindle cells).
- **Size and mitotic rate** are predictive of behavior[Q]
- Those with mutations in **KIT or PDGFRA** often respond to the tyrosine kinase inhibitor **imatinib.**

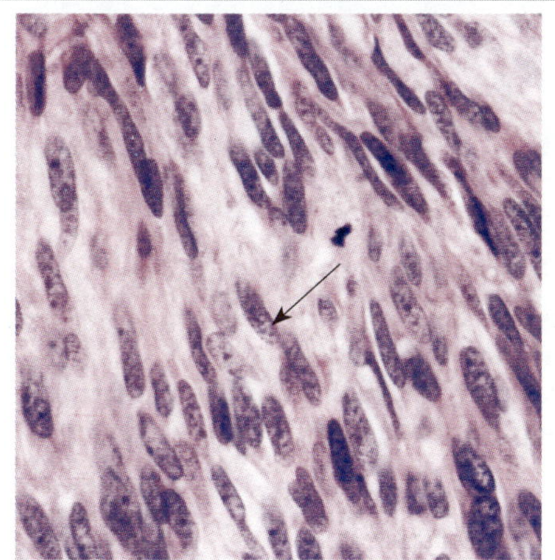
GIST–Microscopy shows spindle cells

SDHB deficient (pediatric type) GIST	Usual GIST, (SDHB POSITIVE)
• Predominantly pediatric and young adult • F:M ratio as high as 9:1 • All are gastric, most in antrum • Frequently multiple, simultaneous or metachronous[Q] • Lymph node metastases common[Q] • Poor response to imatinib • No CKIT or PDGFRA mutations[Q] • Protracted course (e.g. 15 years), even if metastatic	• Predominantly older adults • M = F • May occur throughout gastrointestinal tract • Usually solitary[Q] • Lymph node metastases rare • Responsive to imatinib • CKIT or PDGFRA mutations (90%)[Q] • Poor prognosis if metastatic

R9th **Latest** Update

SDH-deficient GISTs are located exclusively in the stomach, showing predilection for children and young adults with female preponderance.
- The tumor generally pursues an indolent course and exhibits primary resistance to imatinib therapy in most cases.

Carney-Stratakis Syndrome
- Germline mutations in **succinate dehydrogenase genes SDHB, SDHC or SDHD**[Q]
- **No germline or somatic KIT or PDGFRA mutation**[Q]
- **Familial paraganglioma and GIST**[Q]
- **Associated with Carney's triad:** Carney's triad is gastric GIST + paraganglioma + pulmonary chondroma.

SMALL INTESTINE AND COLON

ANGIODYSPLASIA

- Occurs in 6th decade, in cecum/right colon
- Important cause of **major episodes of lower intestinal bleeding**[Q]
- Malformed **submucosal and mucosal blood vessels,**[Q]

MALABSORPTION SYNDROMES

- Presents **most commonly as chronic diarrhea**[Q]
- **Hallmark: Steatorrhea,** characterized by **excessive fecal fat and bulky, frothy, greasy, yellow or clay-colored stools.**[Q]

Celiac Disease (Celiac Sprue or Gluten Sensitive Enteropathy)

- Fundamental disorder is **sensitivity to gluten**[Q]
- Gluten is protein component (gliadin) of **wheat**[Q] related grains (**Oat, barley & rye**)[Q].
- **Hallmark: T-cell mediated chronic inflammatory reaction**[Q] with an autoimmune component
- Almost all individuals share **HLA-DQ2** or **HLA-DQ8**[Q] haplotype.
- The **epithelial cells secrete** excess **IL-5** that **activates CD8+ T cells** & increases the **risk of lymphoma**[Q]

Mnemonic

Gluten
- **B** – Barley
- **R** – Rye
- **O** – Oat
- **W** – Wheat

High Yield Facts

Serology of Celiac disease
- **Latent celiac disease**-in which positive serology is not accompanied by villous atrophy
- **M**ost **sensitive tests** are the **measurement of IgA antibodies against tissue transglutaminase (tTG) or IgA or IgG antibodies to deamidated gliadin peptide (DGP)**[Q]
- **Specific test** but not sensitive-**IgA anti-endomysial antibodies**[Q]

High Yield Facts

- Most common **chronic malabsorptive disorders: Pancreatic insufficiency, Celiac disease, Crohn disease**[Q]
- Intestinal GVHD is an important cause of malabsorption and diarrhea after allogenic hematopoietic stem cell transplantation.[Q]
- In **celiac disease, proximal intestine**[Q] is involved whereas in **tropical sprue, whole of the intestine**[Q] is involved

Clinical Features

- Classic presentation includes **diarrhea, flatulence, weight loss and fatigue**[Q]
- **Associations: Dermatitis herpetiformis**[Q], Auto immune diseases, Downs & Turner syndrome, IgA, nephropathy
- **Dramatic improvement** in features of malabsorption **after withdrawal of gluten**[Q] containing substances from diet
- On long term, increased risk of **malignancy**[Q] - **enteropathy-associated T-cell lymphoma**[Q] > *Small intestinal adenocarcinoma*

Diagnosis

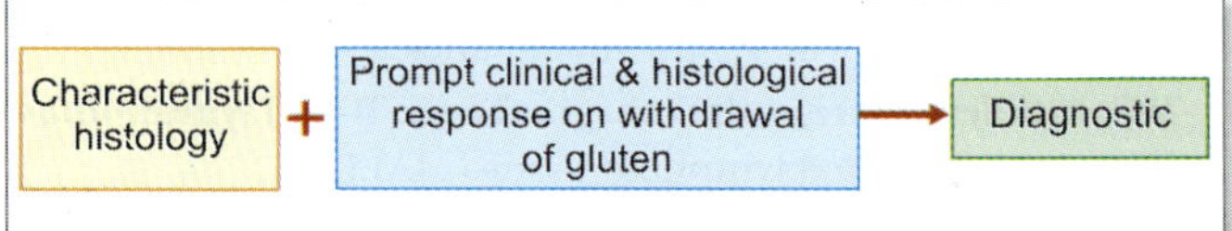

- **Morphology Biopsy:** from **second portion of the duodenum or proximal jejunum are diagnostic are diagnostic**
- Overall mucosal thickness remains same in celiac sprue
- **Diffuse enteritis**, with **marked atrophy or total loss of villi**[Q]
- **Hyperplastic, elongated, tortuous crypts** with **increased mitotic activity**[Q]
- Increased numbers of **intraepithelial CD8+ T lymphocytes**[Q]

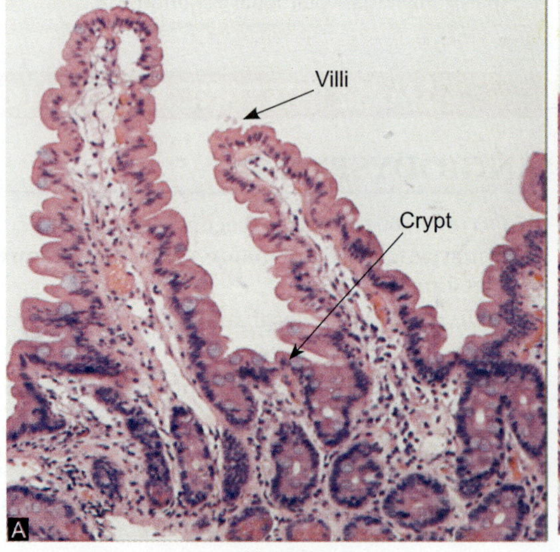

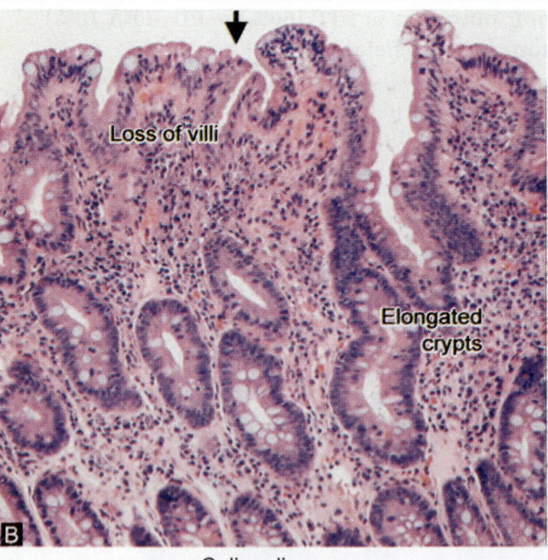

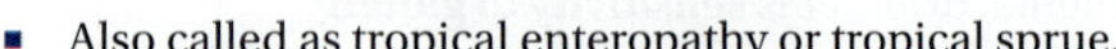

Environmental Enteropathy

- Also called as tropical enteropathy or tropical sprue.
- No accepted criteria for diagnosis of environmental enteropathy.
- **No single infectious agent** has been linked.
- Biopsy of the intestine shows the **diffuse enteritis with atrophy of the villi.**[Q]

Whipple's Disease

- **Multisystem illness** caused by Gram +ve actinomycete **"Trophyrema whippeli"**[Q]
- May involve any organ of the body but principally affects the **intestine, CNS and joints**[Q].

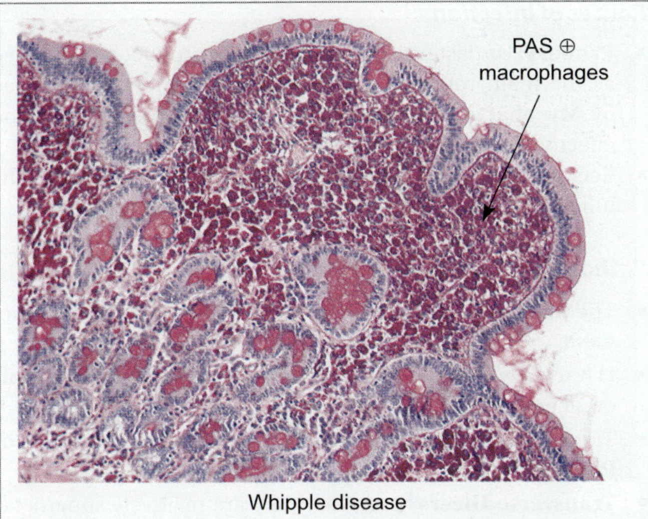

Whipple disease

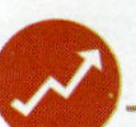

High Yield Facts

- **Hallmark** of Whipple's disease had been presence **of PAS positive macrophages** containing the characteristic bacilli. But, similar picture (PAS +ve macrophages with bacilli) can also be seen with **M. avium complex** (cause of diarrhea in AIDS)
- Acid-fast stain are helpful, since **mycobacteria stain positively while T. whippelii do not**[Q].
- Patients with sickle cell disease are particularly susceptible to Salmonella osteomyelitis.[Q]
- The development of dementia is a relatively late symptom and is extremely poor prognostic sign[Q] of whipple's disease.

Clinical Features

- Malabsorption[Q]
- Multisystem involvement along with fever, lymphadenopathy and arthralgias[Q]
- CNS involvement (10%) dementia, seizures, coma, myoclonus[Q]

Diagnosis

- **Morphologic hallmark:** Duodenal biopsy showing PAS positive diastase resistant macrophages showing characteristic granules (**lysosome stuffed with partially digested microorganisms**[Q]).
- Election microscopy shows **rod shaped microorganisms**[Q].
- Diagnosis is **confirmed by** identification of **T. whipplei** by polymerase chain reaction **(PCR).**[Q]

Treatment

- **Prolonged use** of **double-strength trimethoprim/sulfamethoxazole** for approximately **one year**[Q].
- PAS positive macrophages can persist following successful treatment, and the **presence of bacilli outside of macrophages** is indicative of **persistent infection** or an early sign of **recurrence**[Q].

MICROSCOPIC COLITIS

Two Types

- **Collagenous colitis:** Presence of **a dense subepithelial collagen layer**, increased numbers of intraepithelial lymphocytes, and a mixed inflammatory infiltrate within the lamina propria
- **Lymphocytic colitis**:
  - Increase in intraepithelial lymphocytes > **T lymphocyte/5 colonocyte**[Q]
  - **Strong association with celiac disease and autoimmune diseases**[Q].

> **R9th Latest Update**
>
> - **Autoimmune enteropathy**[Q] is an X-linked disorder characterized by severe persistent diarrhea and autoimmune disease that is caused by mutation in **FOXP3 gene,**[Q] resulting in defective function of regulatory T cells.

INFECTIOUS DISEASES

The important causes of infections in the intestine are as follows:

Enteric Fever (Typhoid)

- It is caused by infection with **Salmonella enterica** & its two subtypes, typhi (most common in endemic countries) and paratyphi (most common travellers)
- Clinically-**step-ladder pyrexia,** rose spots (erythematous macular lesions on chest and abdomen), abdominal pain, vomiting
- **Characteristic: Hypertrophy of Peyer patches in the terminal ileum and their ulceration, presence of longitudinal ulcers (oval ulcers with long axis along the long axis of the ileum)**[Q].
- Microscopic-macrophages having bacteria and red blood cells (**erythrophagocytosis**)
- **Gallbladder colonization** with **S. typhi** or **S. paratyphi** is associated with gallstones and the **chronic carrier state**.
- Liver, Bone marrow and lymph node shows small, randomly scattered foci of parenchymal necrosis in which hepatocytes are replaced by macrophage aggregates, called **typhoid nodules**[Q];
- Complications include hemorrhage and perforation.
- Extraintestinal complications - encephalopathy, meningitis, seizures, endocarditis, myocarditis, pneumonia & cholecystitis
- **Blood culture is the diagnosis of choice**[Q]
- **Widal test** is used for measuring the antibody titer

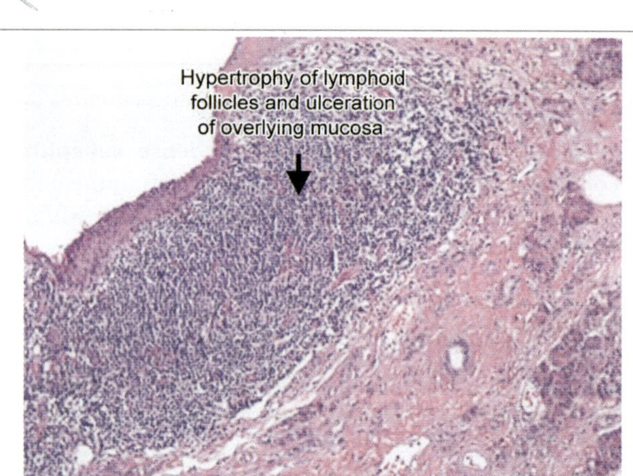

Enteric fever

Mnemonic

Tie Typhoid → (Tie) → Longitudinal ulcers

TB – Transverse ulcers

Amoebiasis – flask shaped ulcers

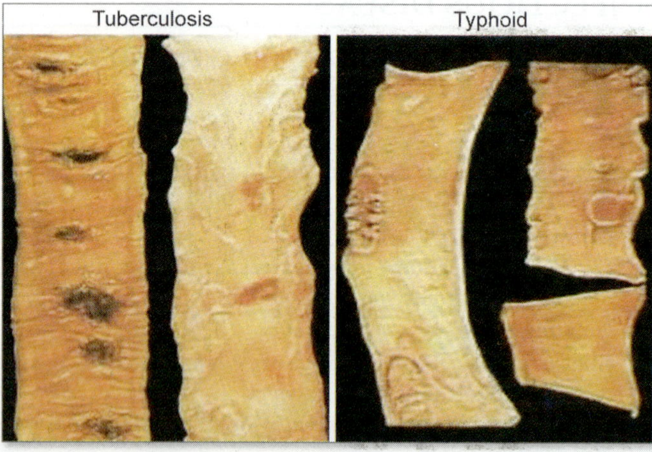

Intestinal Tuberculosis (ITB)

It can present itself in two of the following forms:

- Primary infection
- Secondary following reactivation, usually from a primary pulmonary focus

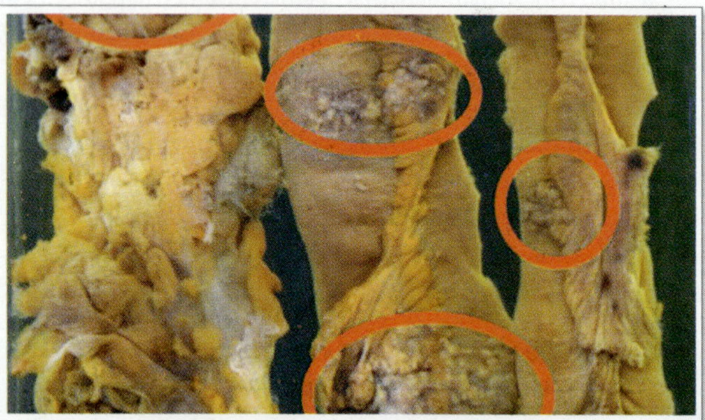

Distribution of tuberculous lesions

Ileum > cecum > ascending colon > jejunum > appendix > sigmoid > rectum > duodenum > stomach > esophagus

Routes of Infection

- **Primary:** Unpasteurized milk and milk product are regarded as the main route of transmission of zoonotic. TB caused by **Mycobacterium bovis** in countries where there are no effective eradication programs.
- **Secondary:** Ingestion, sputum from an active focus in the lung, Hematogenous, Direct spread from adjacent organs

Pathology

- The **ileocecal region** is the **most common site**[Q] of involvement
- ITB usually has one of three forms: ulcerative, hypertrophic or ulcerohypertrophic or fibrous
- Tuberculous granulomas initially form in the **mucosa or Peyer's patches**[Q]
- **Transverse Ulcers**[Q] are seen, they are relatively superficial, with a different appearance from those in Crohn's disease
- ITB progresses slowly and presents late with complications, acute or subacute obstruction due to mass (tuberculoma), stricture formation in the ileocecal region or perforation leading to peritonitis
- The mesenteric lymph nodes are enlarged; matted and caseous. **Tabes mesenterica.**[Q]
- Diagnosis – widening of the ileocecal angel (known as "**pulled up cecum**"[Q] on barium radiography,
  - Histological evidence of caseating epithelloid cell granulomas along with langhan giant cells
  - Confirmation of acid fast bacilli on **Ziehl-Neelsen and culture/PCR positivity**[Q]

Amebiasis

- It is caused by infection with an anaerobic protozoa **E. histolytica**[Q]
- **Flask-shaped ulcers**[Q] (ulcer with a broad base but narrow neck).
- **Cecum and ascending colon**[Q]
- The ulcers usually involve the mucosa and the submucosa (not the muscle layer)
- Microscopy shows presence of **trophozoites**[Q] in the ulcer
- **Liver** shows hepatic abscess (called as "**anchovy sauce pus**").[Q]

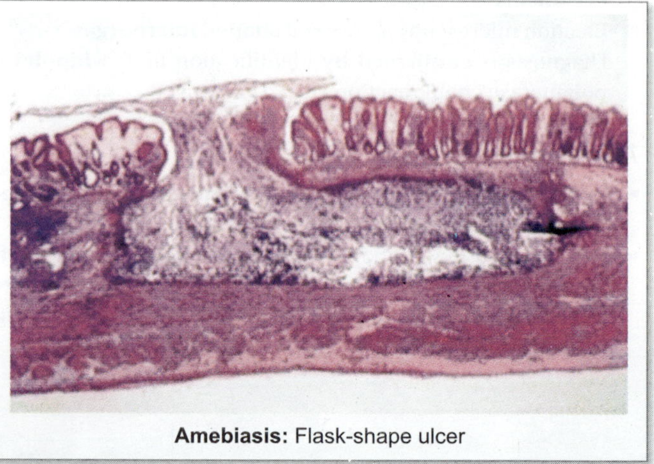

Amebiasis: Flask-shape ulcer

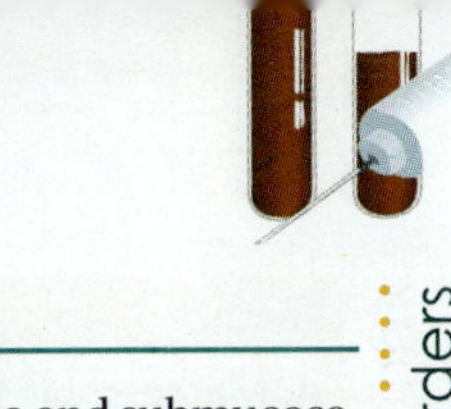

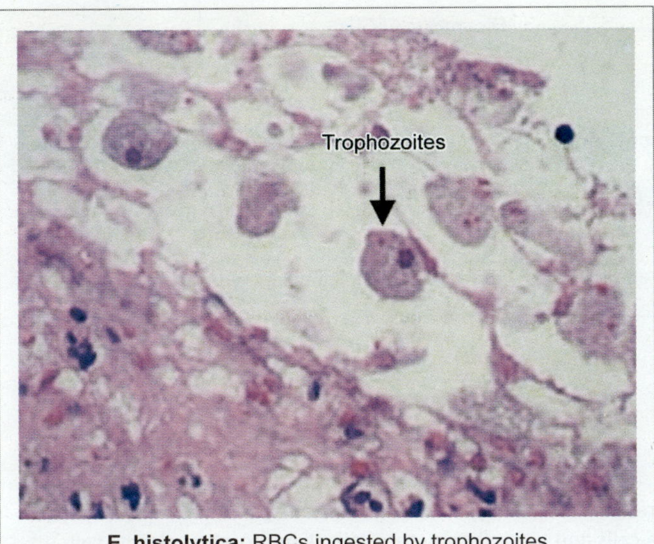

E. histolytica: RBCs ingested by trophozoites

INFLAMMATORY BOWEL DISEASE (IBD)

Inflammatory bowel disease (IBD) is a chronic condition resulting from **inappropriate mucosal immune** activation.

It is primarily of two types: Crohn's disease and ulcerative colitis.

Crohn's Disease

- **Sharply delineated and transmural involvement of bowel by inflammatory process**
  - ○ **Any portion of intestine can be involved (most common site: ileum)**
  - ○ Associated with HLA-DR1/DQw5 and an abnormal T-cell response TH1 cells.

Hallmark of crohn's disease- non-caseating granulomas.

High Yield Facts

- Earliest change in **Crohn's disease** is Apathoid ulceration[Q].
- Earliest change in **Ulcerative colitis** is Blurring of mucosal stripe and granular appearance[Q].

Metastatic Crohn's disease
- A misnomer since there is no cancer
- Described when cutaneous granulomas form nodules

ULCERATIVE COLITIS

- Ulcerative colitis extends only into the mucosa and submucosa.
- **Mural thickening is not present, the serosal surface is normal, and strictures do not occur**
- Associated with **HLA-DR2, polymorphism in IL-10 gene** and an **abnormal T-cell response particularly of Th2 cells.**[Q]
- **Always involves the rectum** and extends proximally in a **continuous fashion** to involve part or all of the colon. Disease of the entire colon is termed **pancolitis.**[Q]
- In severe cases of pancolitis, mild mucosal inflammation of the distal ileum is termed as backwash Ileitis[Q]

Mnemonic

Extraintestinal manifestations of UC-SEAS
- **S**kin manifestations: erythema nodosum, pyoderma gangrenosum
- **E**ye inflammation: iritis, episcleritis
- **A**rthritis
- **S**clerosing cholangitis

- Approximately **2.5% to 7.5%** of individuals with ulcerative colitis also have **primary sclerosis cholangitis**[Q]

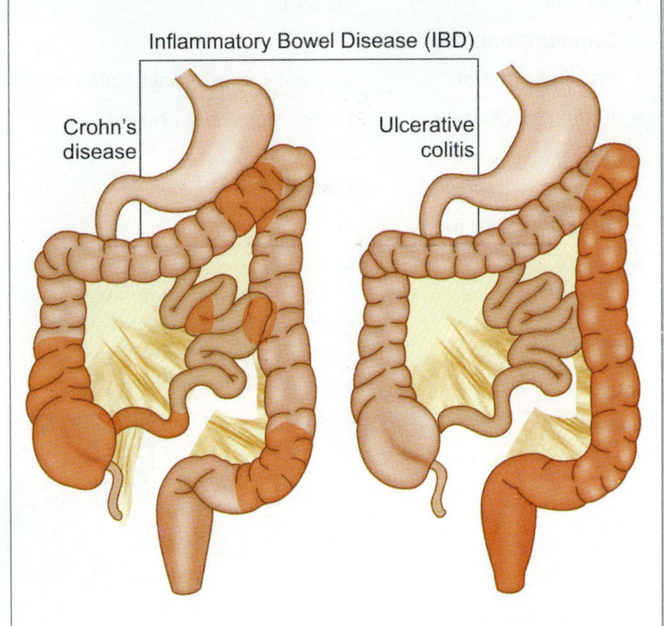

Feature	Crohn's Disease	Ulcerative Colitis
A. Macroscopic features		
• Distribution	Segmental with **skip areas**[Q]	**Continuous** without skip areas[Q]
• Location	Commonly **terminal ileum (most common) and/or ascending colon**	Commonly **rectum sigmoid colon and extending upwards**
• Extent	Usually involves the **entire thickness of the affected segment of bowel wall**	Usually superficial, **confined to mucosal layers**
• Ulcers	**Serpiginous ulcers**, that develop into deep **fissures**[Q]	Superficial mucosal ulcers without fissures
• **Pseudopolyps**	Rarely seen	**Commonly present**[Q]
• Fibrosis	**Common**	Rare
• Shortening	Due to fibrosis	Due to contraction of muscularis
B. Microscopic features		
• Depth of inflammation	Typically **transmural**[Q]	**Mucosal**[Q] **and Submucosal**
• Type of inflammation	**Non-caseating granulomas**[Q] and infiltrate of mononuclear cells (lymphocytes, plasma cells and macrophage)	Crypt abscess and non-specific acute and chronic inflammatory cells (lymphocytes, plasma cells neutrophils, eosinophils, mast cells)
• Mucosa	Patchy ulceration	Hemorrhagic mucosa with ulceration
• Submucosa	**Widened** due to edema and lymphoid aggregates	Normal or reduced in width
• Muscularis	Infiltrated by inflammatory cells	Usually spared, except in cases of **Toxic Megacolon**[Q]
• Fibrosis	Present	Usually absent
C. Complications		
• Fistula formation	Internal and external fistulae in 10% case	Extremely **rare**[Q]
• Malignant changes	Less common but present	May occur in disease of more than 10 years duration (**more common**[Q])
• **Fibrous strictures**	**Common**[Q]	Never[Q]
• **Toxic megacolon**	–	**Risk present**[Q]
• Features	• Hose pipe appearance[Q] • Cobble-stone appearance[Q] • Halo sign on CT[Q] • String sign of cantor[Q] • Raspberry/rosethorn appearance[Q]	• Garden hose appearance[Q] • **Pseudopolyps**[Q] • **Pipestem colon (Ahaustral)**[Q]

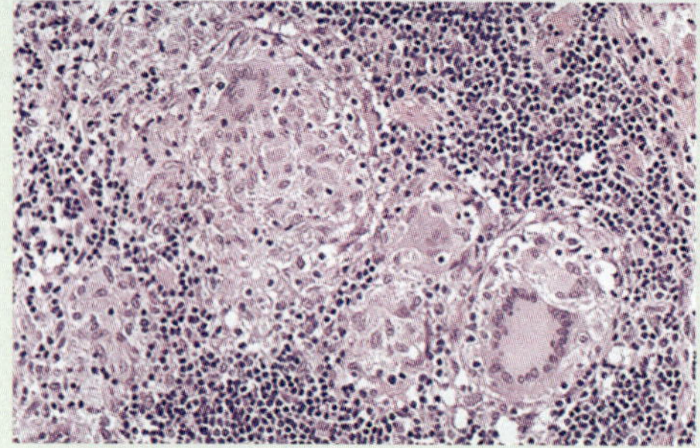

Histological findings are suggestive of non-caseating granuloma. It is a hallmark of Crohn's disease

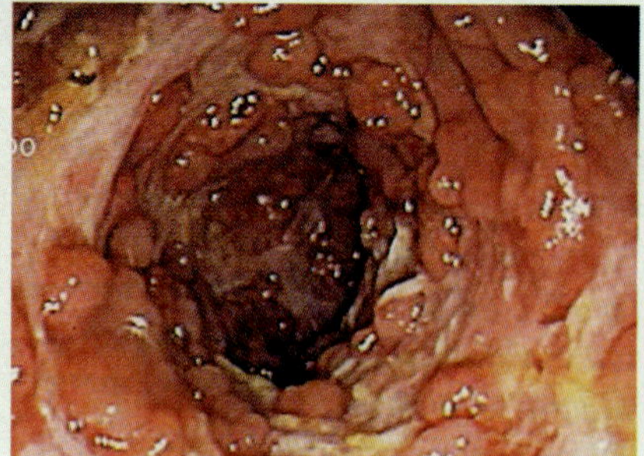

Cobblestone appearance Crohn's disease

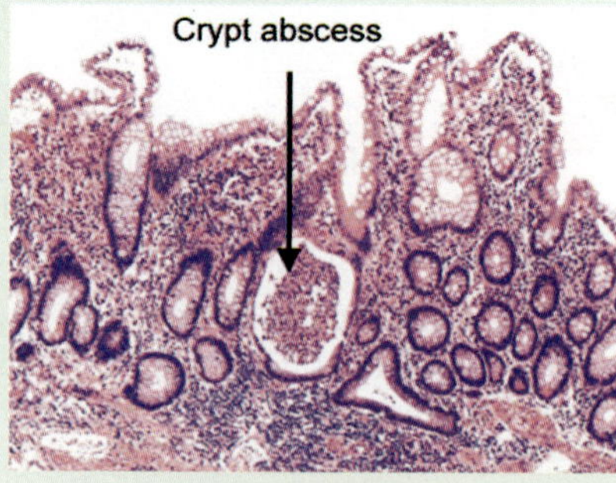

Crypt abscess
(ulcerative colitis) > Crohns disease

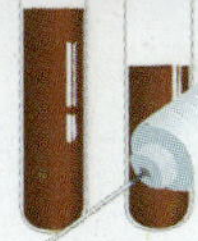

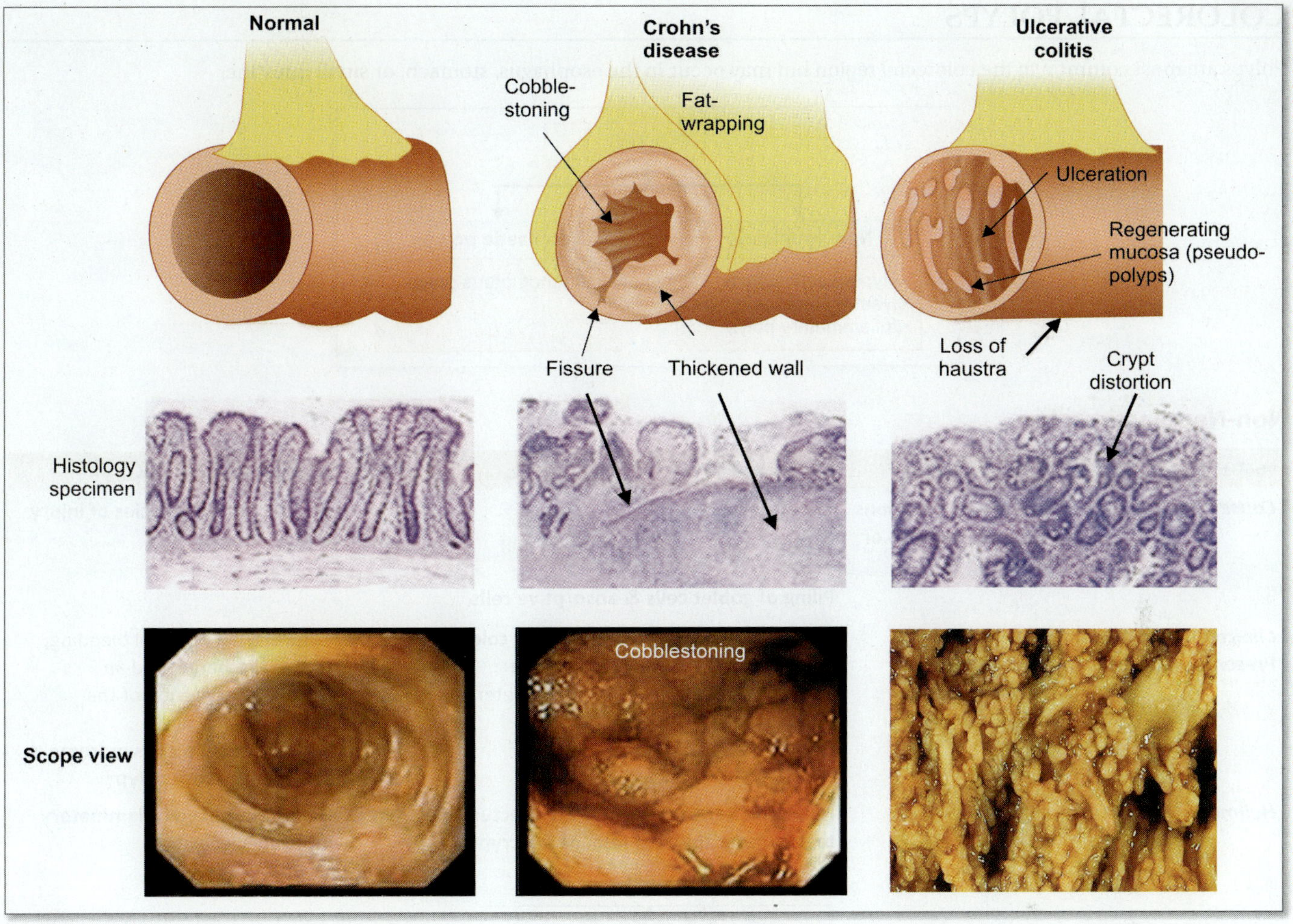

High Yield Facts

- Extraintestinal manifestations of Crohn's disease include uveitis, migratory polyarthritis, sacroiliitis, ankylosing spondylitis, erythema nodosum, and clubbing of the fingertips, any of which may develop before intestinal disease is recognized.[Q]
- Approximately 2.5–7.5% of individuals with ulcerative colitis also have primary sclerosis cholangitis.
- Polymorphism of the IL-23 receptor is **protective** in both the types of inflammatory bowel disease.
- Autosomal recessive mutations of the **IL-10 and IL-10 receptor genes** are linked to severe, early onset IBD
- Smoking is a strong exogenous risk factor for development of CD whereas smoking partly relieves symptoms in UC.[Q]
- Anti-flagellin antibodies are common in Crohn's disease and uncommon in ulcerative colitis patients.[Q]
- Gene assoicated with chrons disease NOD2 > ATG16L1 and IRGM R9th

R9th Latest Update

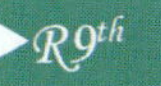

Colitis-Associated Neoplasia

Depends on following parameters:

- ***Duration of the disease:*** Risk increases 8 to 10 years after disease onset.
- Extent of disease: Pancolitis > Left side
- Nature of inflammation - ↑ neutrophils more risk
- ***Duration of the disease:*** Risk increases 8 to 10 years after disease onset.

High Yield Facts

Antibody	GI Disorder
Antiendomysial antibody[Q]	*Celiac sprue*
Antisaccharomyces cerevisiae antibody[Q]	*Crohn's disease*
p-Antineutrophil cytoplasmic antibody[Q]	*Ulcerative colitis*

COLORECTAL POLYPS

Polyps are most common in the colorectal region but may occur in the esophagus, stomach, or small intestine.

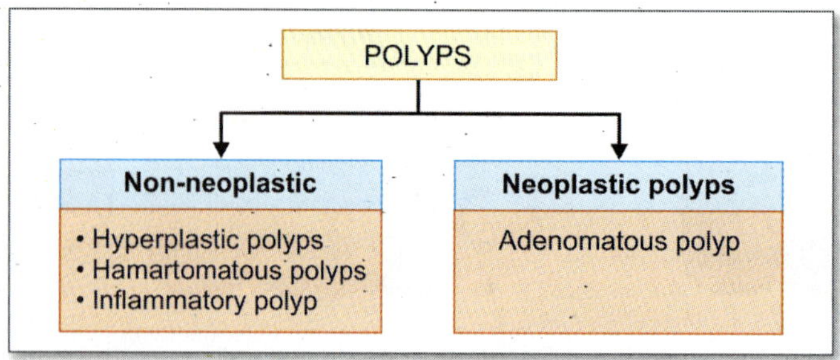

Non-Neoplastic Polyp

Features	Hamartomatous Polyps	Hyperplastic Polyps	Inflammatory Polyps
Cause	Caused by **germline mutations in tumor suppressor genes or proto-oncogenes.**[Q]	↓ **Epithelial turnover** — Delayed surface epithelial shedding **Piling of goblet cells & absorptive cells**	Result of **chronic cycles of injury and healing.**[Q]
Clinical Presentation	Types: • Juvenile polyp • Peutz Jegher's syndrome (Discussed below)	• Most commonly found in the **left colon** • Sixth and seventh decades of life • Typically less than 5 mm in diameter	Clinical triad of rectal bleeding, mucus discharge, and an inflammatory lesion of the anterior rectal wall. **Solitary rectal ulcer syndrome is an inflammatory polyp**[Q]
Hallmark	discussed below separately	**Hallmark: Serrated surface architecture. Restricted to the upper third, or less, of the crypt.**[Q]	**Hallmark: Mixed inflammatory infiltrates, erosion.**
Malignant potential	Associated with increased cancer risk, **either within the polyps or at other intestinal or extra-intestinal sites**[Q]	**Non-neoplastic**[Q]	**Non-neoplastic**[Q]

Hyperplastic polyp. (60-70years) Due to ↓ epithelial turnover

Piling goblet cells

Serrated surface in upper third of crypt

Lumen is not round

10X- surface mucosal ulceration

Types of Hamartomatous Polyps

Features	Juvenile Polyps	Peutz Jegher's Syndrome
Age	Children younger than 5 years of age	Median age of 11 years
Site	Rectum	Jejunum
Symptoms	**Rectal bleeding**[Q] Most juvenile polyps are less than 3 cm in diameter	They come to attention for following • Intussception, Mucocutaneous pigmentation, Secondary cancers
Morphology	• Sporadic single, called **retention polyps.** • Juvenile polyposis syndrome (JPS): autosomal dominant syndrome, 3 to as many as 100 polyps	• Multiple GI hamartomatous, **polyps and mucocutaneous hyperpigmentation (especially lips, buccal mucosa,**[Q] • **Hallmark histology: The arborization and presence of smooth muscle intermixed with lamina propria.**
Mutation	**SMAD4**[Q]	Heterozygous loss-of-function of **STK11**[Q]

Malignant potential	• **Dysplasia is extremely rare in sporadic juvenile polyps**[Q]
	 • Juvenile polyposis syndrome is associated with dysplasia and 30 to 50% develop colonic adenocarcinoma by age 45.
		• Markedly increased risk of several malignancies
		 • Surveillance is recommended
		   ■ **At birth, for sex cord tumors of the testes;**
		   ■ **Late childhood for gastric and small intestinal cancers;**[Q]
		   ■ **Second and third decades of life for colon, pancreatic, breast, lung, ovarian, and uterine cancers.**[Q]

Other Syndromes with Hamartamotous Polyps[Q]

- **Cowden Syndrome and Bannayan-Ruvalcaba-Riley Syndrome**: Autosomal dominant hamartomatous polyp syndromes associated with loss-of-function mutations in *PTEN* hence also known as **PTEN hamartoma syndrome**.
- **Cronkhite-Canada Syndrome: Nonhereditary** and develops in individuals over 50 years of age

Neoplastic Polyps

- Any tumor mass lesion in the GI tract like this includes adenocarcinomas, neuroendocrine (carcinoid) tumors, stromal tumors, lymphomas, and even metastatic cancers from distant sites) can produce a mucosal protrusion or polyp.

- The most common neoplastic polyps are colonic adenomas. Adenomas are intraepithelial neoplasms like small pedunculated, polyps to large sessile lesions
- Colorectal adenomas are characterized by the presence of epithelial dysplasia
- Colonic adenomas are classified as tubular, tubulovillous, or villous based on their architecture
- Tubular adenomas- **most common**[Q] adenoma
- Villous adenomas contain foci of invasion more frequently
- **The size of the adenoma is the most important characteristic which correlates with the risk of malignancy.**[Q]

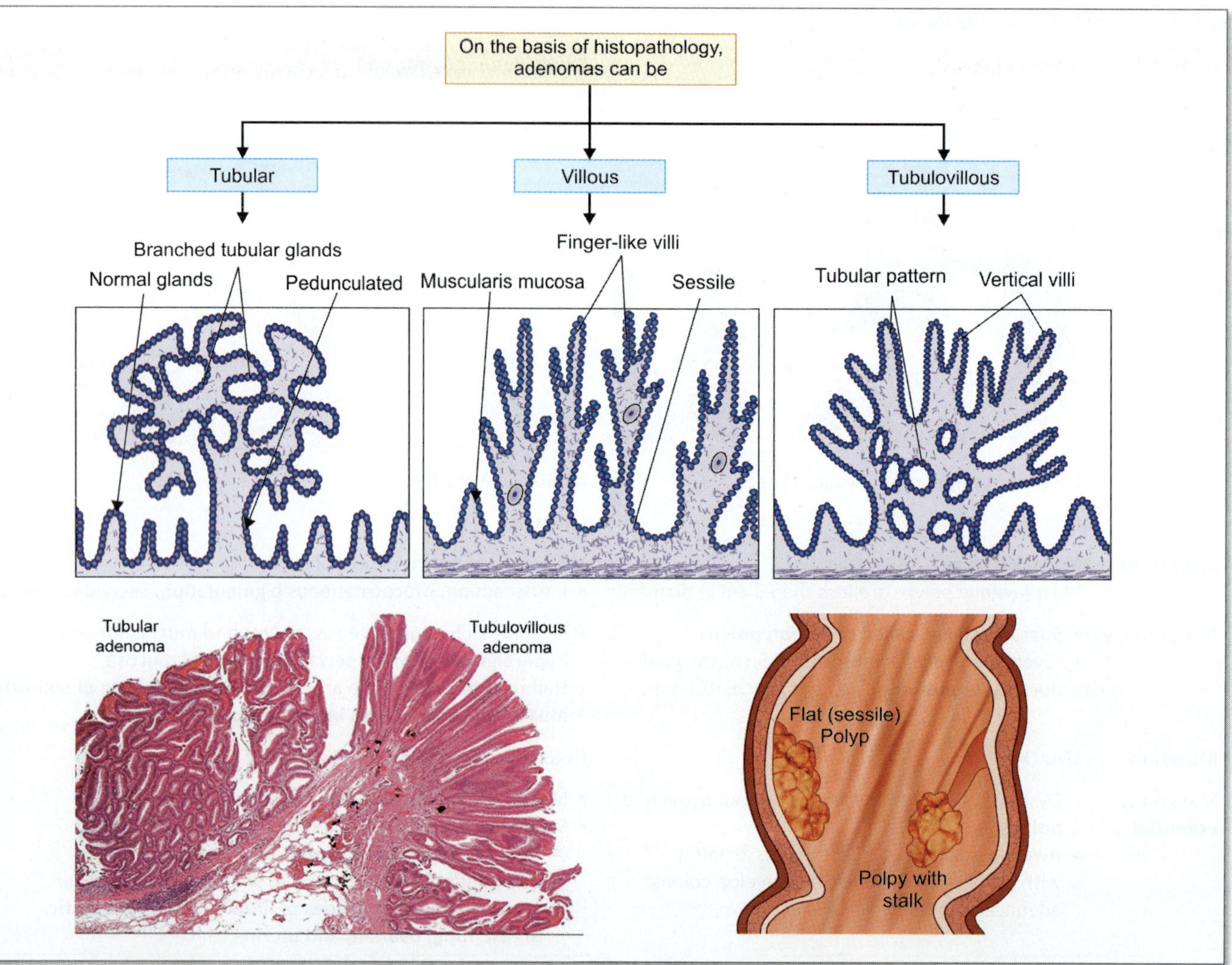

Sessile Serrated Adenomas

- **Lack cytologic dysplasia^Q** and share morphologic features with hyperplastic polyps, more at right colon.
- Differs from **hyperplastic polyps** by serrated architecture throughout the **full length^Q** of the glands
- **Intramucosal carcinoma:** When dysplastic epithelial cells breach the basement membrane to invade the lamina propria or muscularis mucosae.
- **Intramucosal carcinomas** have little or no metastatic potential as functional lymphatic channels are absent in the colonic mucosa.

FAMILIAL ADENOMATOUS POLYPOSIS (FAP)

- *Inheritance:*
  - AD
- *Cause:*
  - Adenomatous polyposis coli (APC; 5q21) mutation
- *Predominant Site(s):*
  - None

- *Syndromes associated:*
  - **Gardner syndrome**
  - **Turcot syndrome**
- *Extraintestinal manifestations*
  - **Congenital hypertrophy of retinal pigment epithelium^Q**
- **MYH-associated polyposis**
  - Autosomal recessive
  - Some polyposis patients without APC loss have mutations of the base-excision repair gene MYH (also referred to as MUTYH). In these cases, polys are similar to attenuated FAP, with polyp development at later ages, the presence of fewer than 100 adenomas, and the delayed appearance of colon cancer, often at ages of 50 or older.
- **Lynch syndrome OR Hereditary Non-Polyposis Colorectal Cancer**
  - **Inheritance:** AD
  - **Cause:** Mutations in **DNA repair genes. MSH2, MLH1** leading to **microsatellite instability**
  - Predominant site: Right colon

High Yield Facts

- Most common extra intestinal manifestation of fivenile polyposis is pulmonary A-V malformation
- **Classic FAP: At least 100 polyps are necessary for a diagnosis**[Q]
- **Attenuated FAP: Lower number of adenomatous polyps (around 30)**
- **Gardner syndrome**: osteomas of mandible, skull, and long bones, epidermal cysts, desmoid tumors, thyroid tumors, and dental abnormalities, including **unerupted and supernumerary teeth**
- **Turcot syndrome**: Intestinal adenomas and tumors of the central nervous system (**Most common-Medulloblastoma or Glioblastoma**)
- **Squamous cell carcinoma- most common** tumor of anal canal, most common HPV

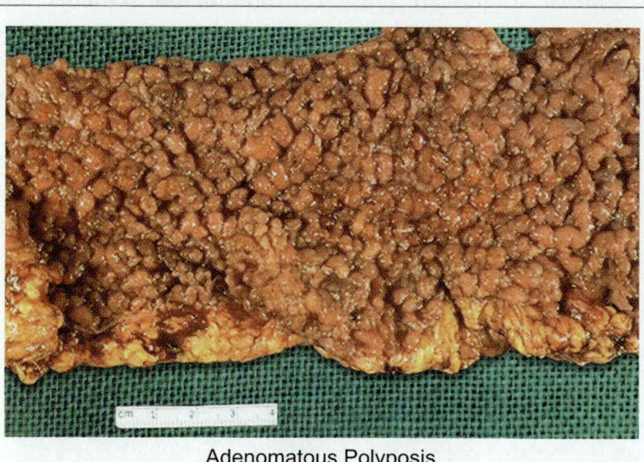

Adenomatous Polyposis

COLORECTAL MALIGNANCY

Adenocarcinoma

- **Most common malignancy of the GI tract**[Q]
- Colorectal cancer incidence peaks at 60 to 70 years of age.
- The **risk factors** for the colon cancer are:
- **Etiology (MNEMONIC: CRAPS)**
  - **C**hronic ulcerative colitis
  - **R**atio of animal fat: fibre diet
  - **A**denomatous polyps
  - Familial **P**olyposis
  - **S**trong family history of colon cancer.

High Yield Facts

- **Intramucosal carcinoma**- when dysplastic epithelial cells breach the basement membrane to invade the **lamina propria or muscularis mucosae.**[Q]
- Have **no metastatic potential**[Q] as **functional lymphatic channels are absent** in the colonic mucosa
- NSAIDS ↓ risk of colon cancer c̄ pharmacologic chemoprevention

Genetic Mutations in Colon Carcinoma

- **APC/β-catenin pathway (mc;80%)** followed by late event mutations like activating mutations in KRAS then SMAD2 and SMAD4 and later in 70% to 80% of colon cancers. Telomerase re-activation can futher progress the tumor
- **Microsatellite instability pathway:** Occurs due to DNA mismatch repair deficiency. Mutations accumulate in microsatellite repeats, referred to as microsatellite instability (MSI). Tumors with this pathway - MSI high, or MSI-H, tumors. Common genes where this occurs are : type II TGF-β receptor. pro-apoptotic protein BAX[Q]
- **Microsatellite instability** without mutations in DNA mismatch repair enzymes[Q] with CpG island hypermethylation phenotype (CIMP). Often show BRAF gene mutation
- **Increased CpG island methylation (CIMP)** in the absence of microsatellite instability. Often they have K-RAS mutation
- **No CpG island methylation (CIMP)** show p53 mutation

Prognosis

Depth of invasion and the presence or absence of lymph node metastases[Q]

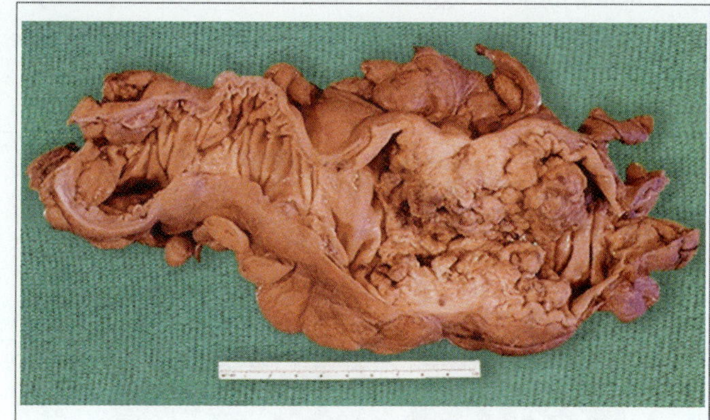

Colon Carcinoma (Gross)

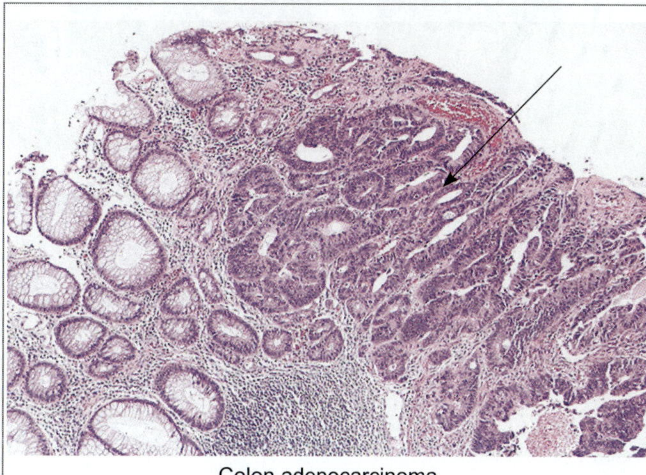

Colon adenocarcinoma

TUMORS OF THE APPENDIX

- Most common tumor of the appendix is the **well differentiated neuroendocrine (carcinoid) tumor**.[Q]
- Forms a solid bulbous swelling at the **distal tip**[Q] of the appendix.
- Nodal metastases are very infrequent[Q], and distant spread is exceptionally rare.

UPDATE ON CARCINOID TUMOR

Carcinoid Tumor

- Arises from the **endocrine cells called as argentaffin tissue** (also called as Kulchitzsky cells of crypts of Lieberkuhn) now properly referred to as **well-differentiated neuroendocrine tumors**[Q]
- The carcinoid tumors can be of the following types:
  - **Foregut carcinoid tumors**: Arise from the esophagus, stomach and the duodenum proximal to the ligament of Trietz, these are usually **benign.**
  - **Midgut carcinoid tumors**: Arise from the jejunum and ileum; these are **aggressive and metastasize frequently.**[Q]
  - **Hindgut carcinoid tumors**: Arise from the **appendix, colon and rectum; usually benign.**[Q]

- Grossly, carcinoids are **intramural or submucosal** masses that create small polypoid lesions, which on cut section gives yellow tan color.
- On electron microscopy, the tumor cells show **dense core granules** in the cytoplasm
- Immunohistochemistry-these granules stain positively with **chromogranin A, neuron-specific enolase and synaptophysin**

Carcinoid Syndrome (5% Cases of Carcinoid Tumor)

- Manifest when vasoactive substances from the tumor enters systemic circulation escaping hepatic degradation.
- It is strongly associated with **metastatic disease.**
- **Clinical features** are **Intestinal hypermotility** (Vomiting, diarrhea), **Vasomotor symptoms** like flushing and cyanosis of the skin, **Systemic fibrosis** (Affect cardiac valves, endocardium, retroperitoneal and pelvic fibrosis)
- Cardiac lesions are present in **50% of the patients** with the carcinoid syndrome. Most common is **tricuspid regurgitation (not tricuspid stenosis) followed by pulmonary stenosis. (TIPS- Tricuspid insufficiency and pulmonary stenosis)**[Q]

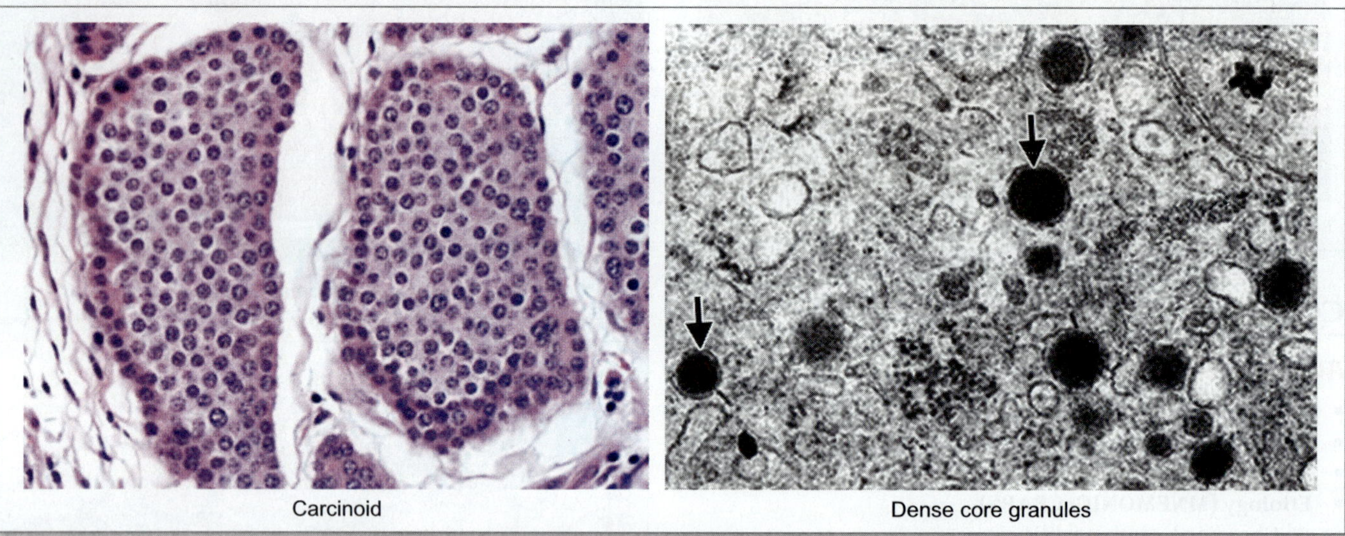

Carcinoid

Dense core granules

Diagnosis

- **Serum chromogranin A** levels ($\uparrow$ in 56–100% of carcinoid tumors) and the level correlates with tumor bulk
- The levels of 5-HT and its metabolite 5-hydroxyindoleacetic acid (5-HIAA) is elevated in the urine. Measurement of **5HIAA is most frequently used.**

- Most common site of carcinoid tumor: Tracheobronchial tree followed by ileum followed by rectum[Q]
- Most common site of carcinoid tumor in foregut[Q]-Bronchus, lung, trachea[Q] (27.9%) > Stomach (4.6 %) > Duodenum (2.0%)
- Most common site of carcinoid tumor in midgut[Q] - Appendix (4.8%) > Ileum[Q] (14.9%) > Colon (8.6%)
- Most common site of carcinoid tumor in hindgut[Q] – rectum[Q] (13.6%)
- At Presentation, most common symptom of carcinoid syndrome is diarrhea and flushing and during the course of disease most common symptom is flushing[Q]
- The cardiac changes are largely **right sided** due to inactivation of both serotonin and bradykinin in the blood during passage through the lungs by the **monoamine oxidase present in the pulmonary vascular endothelium.**[Q]

R10ᵗʰ Latest Update

Pseudomembranous Colitis Antibiotic-associated colitis or antibiotic-associated diarrhea

- Most commonly caused by **Clostridium difficile**[Q]
- **Hallmark: Adherent layer of inflammatory cells and necrotic debris at sites of colonic mucosal injury (pseudomembrane)**[Q]
- Occurs due to disruption of the normal colonic microbiota due to antibiotics, which allows **C. difficile** overgrowth to produce large amounts of **two toxins, toxin A and toxin B**[Q].
- Toxins released by **C. difficile** cause the **ribosylation of small GTPases**
- **Diagnosis: detection of C. difficile toxin (Not Culture)**[Q] and is supported by the characteristic histopathology

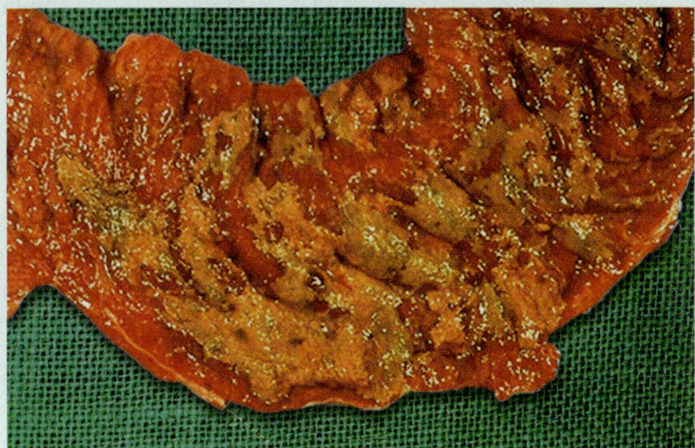

Peudomembranous enterocolitis

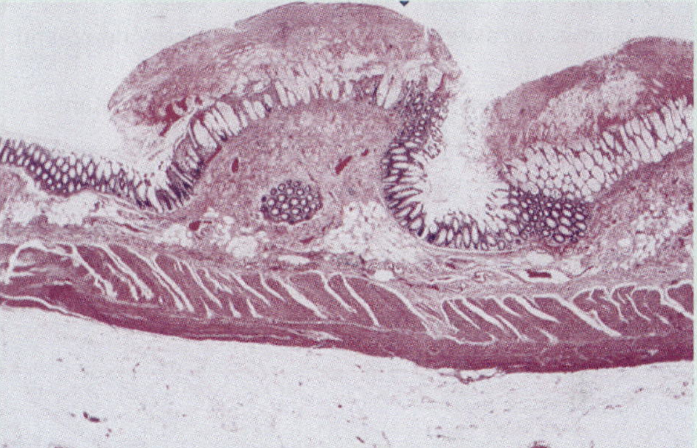

Mucopurulent exudate erupting from crypts to form mushroom like cloud on surface

R10ᵗʰ Latest Update

Microbiome and Dysbiosis

- The microbiome is the diverse microbial population of bacteria, fungi, and viruses found in or on the human body (e.g., in the intestinal tract, skin, upper airway, and vagina)
  Dysbiosis refers to changes in composition of the microbiome that are associated with disease. These changes may result from therapies or various pathophysiologic conditions.
- Use of some antibiotics is an important risk factor for intestinal infections caused by toxin-producing Clostridium difficile. These antibiotics kill or inhibit normal commensal bacteria, allowing overgrowth of C. difficile.
- Restoration of the microbiome by duodenal infusion of stool containing commensal flora from healthy donors successfully treats C. difficile infection in many individuals who have relapsed after antibiotic therapy

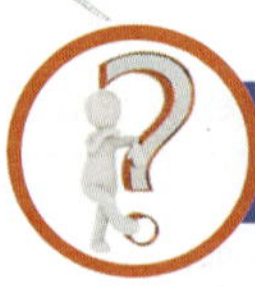
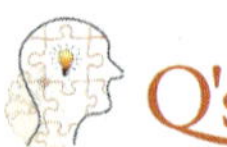

NEXT Pattern Questions

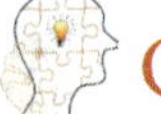

Q's

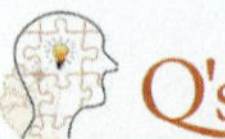

1. A 45/m presented with abdominal pain. Endoscopy shows a mass in stomach following which a biopsy was taken as shown below. Which of the following statement is not true about the case?

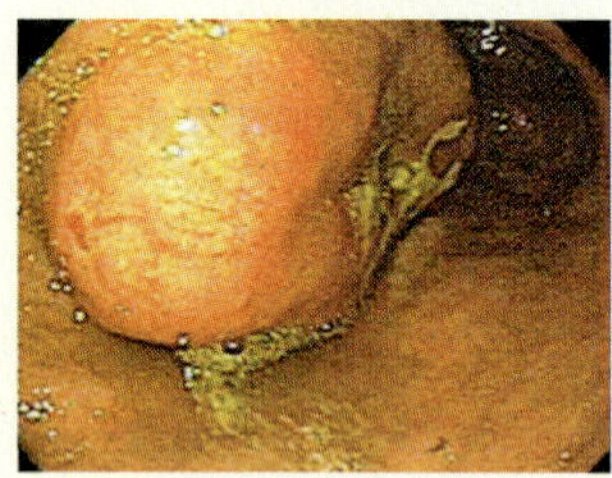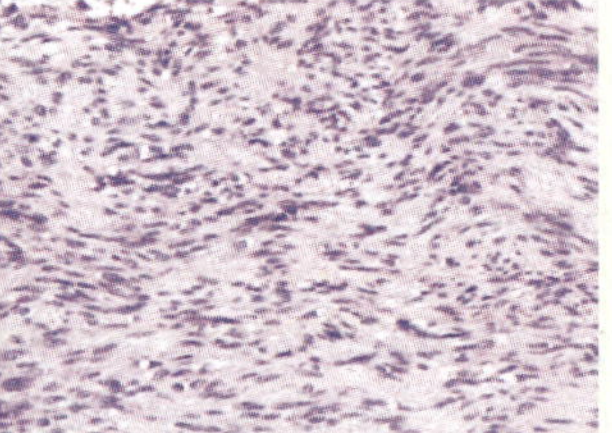

a. GISTs without mutated KIT or PDGFRA have mutations in succinate dehydrogenase complex
b. Mutation of KIT or PDGFRA is an early event in sporadic GISTs
c. Prognosis correlates with tumor size, mitotic index, and location
d. Patients having mutations in KIT are Imatinib resistant

Ans. (d) Patients having mutations in KIT are Imatinib resistant

- The given image shows the histopath of spindle cells and with the biopsy taken from stomach, its GIST. Now, the cases of GIST have mutation in KIT, PDGFR-a. Otherwise, they have SDH loss mutation. Kit mutation is important as these cases are sensitive to Imatinib.

Q's

3. A 30-year-old presented with malabsorption with diarrhea, weight loss, abdominal pain, Occasionally polyarthritis, CNS complaints. Duodenal biopsy shows the following. Which is the correct statement?

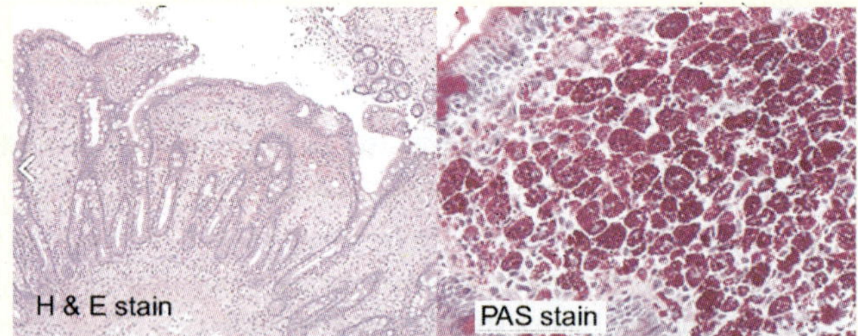

a. Infiltration of histiocytes with RBCs in the lamina propria
b. Granuloma in the lamina, can be intestinal TB
c. Macrophages with PAS (+) ve material inside the lamina propria representing Whipples disease
d. Eosinophils in the lamina propria

Ans. (c) Macrophages with PAS (+) ve material inside the lamina propria representing Whipples disease

- Malabsorption with diarrhea, weight loss, abdominal pain and occasionally polyarthritis, CNS complaints are seen in Whipples disease. Remember, these cases show PAS (+) ve material inside macrophages in the lamina propria layer.

Q's

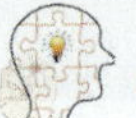

2. A 50-year-old male presented with recurrent bloody diarrhea. Colonoscopy was done followed by histopathology as shown below. What is your diagnosis?

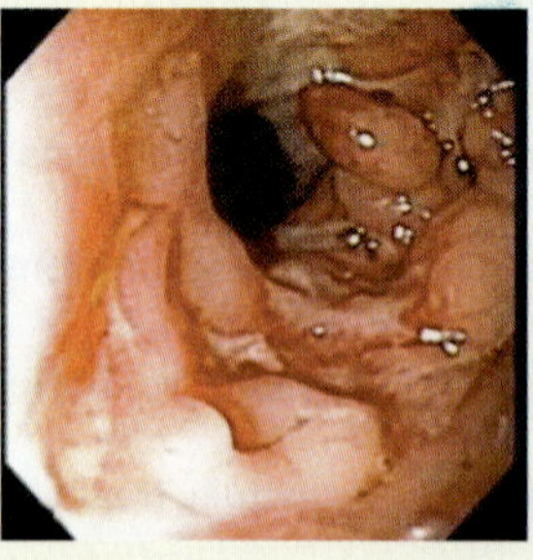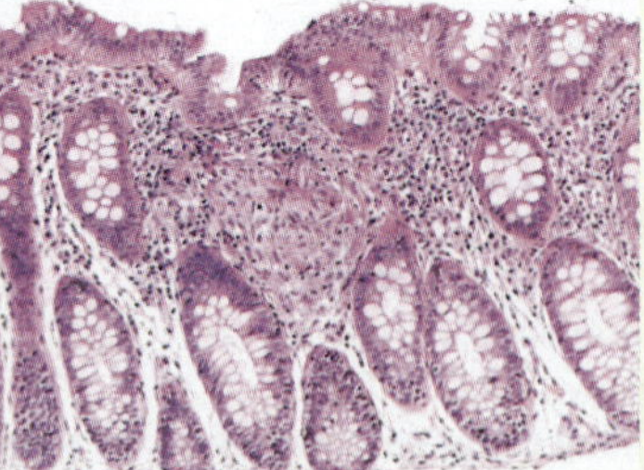

a. Pseudomembranous colitis
b. Non-Hodgkin lymphoma colon
c. Ulcerative colitis
d. Crohns disease

Ans. (d) Crohns disease

- Non caseating granuloma as seen in the histopathology is virtually the hallmark of Crohns disease.

Q's

4. All of the following statements are true regarding colonic polyposis shown below except ?

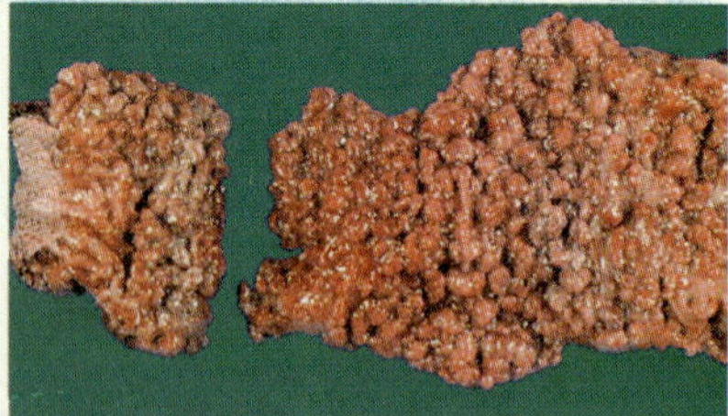

a. FAP without mutation in APC gene have another target of MYH gene
b. Untreated case develop malignancy
c. Prophylactic colectomy prevent the risk of development of cancer in other organ as well
d. Gardner syndrome encompasses the subset of FAP patients with brain tumor medulloblastma

Ans. (d) Gardner syndrome encompasses the subset of FAP patients with brain tumor medulloblastma

- The colonic polyposis syndrome in FAP is Turcot syndrome which has FAP with brain tumor and not Gardner syndrome.

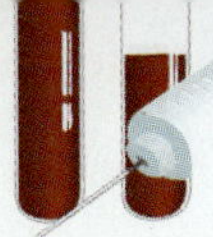

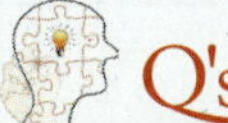 **Q's**

5. Intestinal biopsy from a patient A 25-year-old male presenting with symptoms of fatigueness, chronic diarrhea, bloating, or chronic fatigue. What is not true about the given condition?

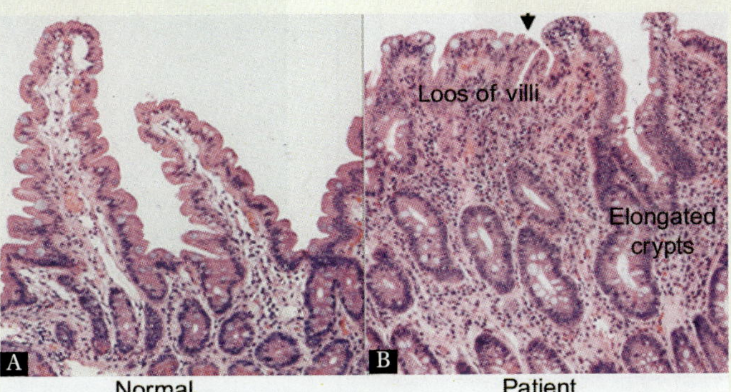

a. Characteristic itchy, blistering skin lesion, is seen in 10% cases
b. Most sensitive tests are the measurement of IgA antibodies against tissue transglutaminase
c. Most common celiac disease-associated cancer is adenocarcinoma colon
d. Hla-DQ 2 and HLA DQ-8/ B8 is useful for its high negative predictive value

Ans. (c) Most common celiac disease-associated cancer is adenocarcinoma colon

- The symptoms of fatigueness, chronic diarrhea, bloating, or chronic fatigue are suggestive of malabsorption. Histopath shows loss of villi and so is Celiac disease. Remember, Celiac disease causes T cell lymphoma and not adenoma as the most common tumor.

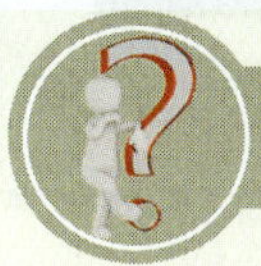

Image-Based Questions

1. A 45-year-old male complained of dysphagia. On investigation, he was HIV positive. He underwent endoscopy and biopsy. Endoscopy findings and histological findings are suggestive of?

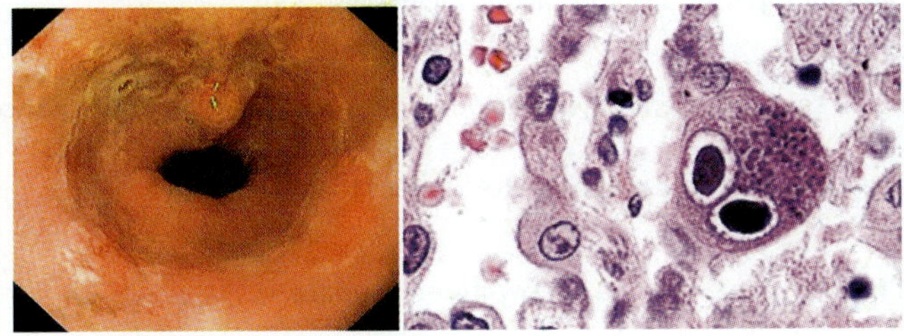

a. Herpes
b. CMV
c. Candida
d. Pseudomonas

2. A 50-year-old male with Gastroesophageal reflux disease– Diagnosis?

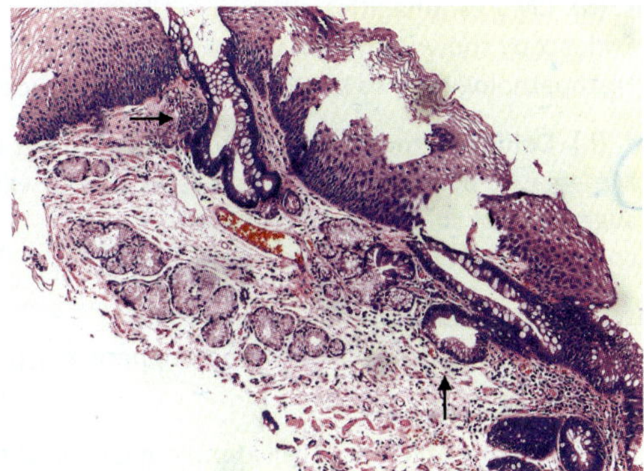

a. Squamous metaplasia
b. Columnar metaplasia
c. Dysplasia
d. Malignancy

3. Old male with H/O long intake of antibiotics. Diagnosis:

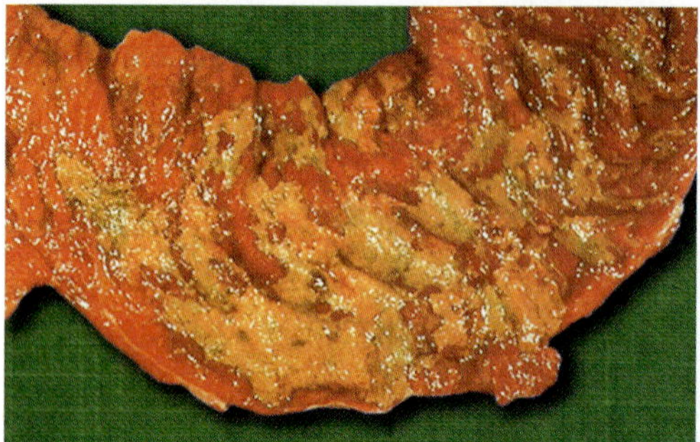

a. Pseudomembranous Colitis
b. Chrons
c. Ulcerative colitis   d. Amoebic colitis

4. Histological findings are suggestive of non-caseating granuloma. It's a hallmark of:

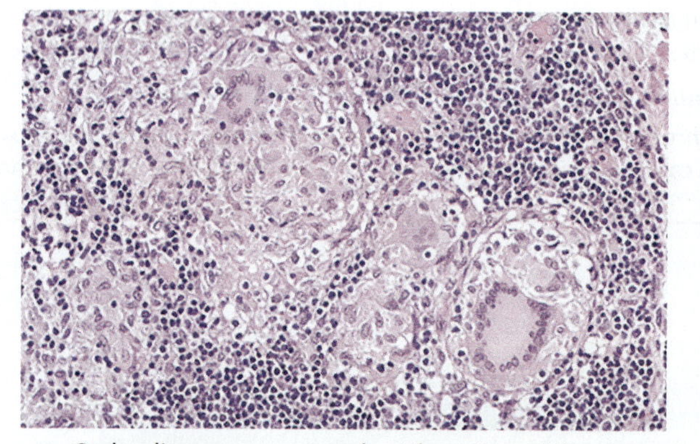

a. Crohn disease   b. Ulcerative colitis
c. Salmonella   d. Amoebiasis

5. Gross findings are suggestive of:

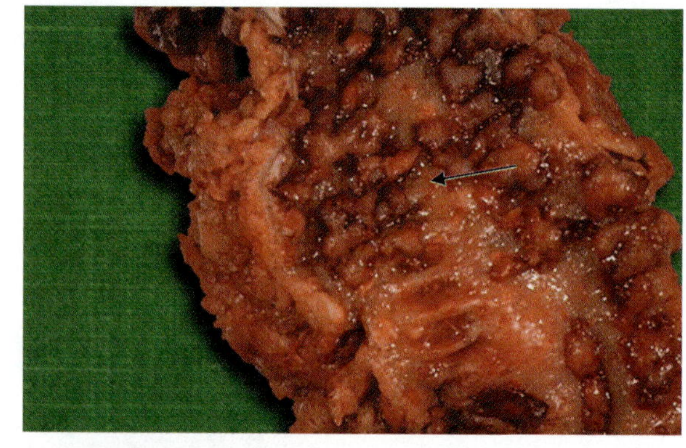

a. Pseudopolyps   b. Pseudopipe
c. Cobblestone   d. Ulcers

6. A 20-year-old male with osteomas of the skull.

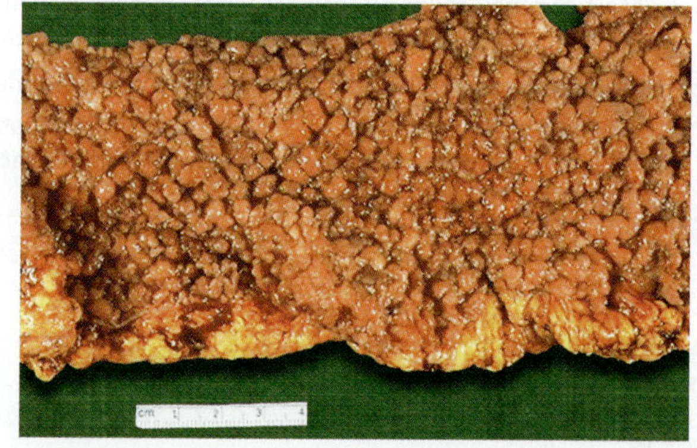

a. Adenomatous Polyposis   b. Crohn's disease
c. Ulcerative colitis   d. None

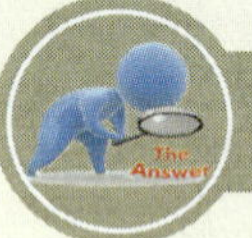

Answers of Image-Based Questions

1. Ans. (b) CMV esophagitis
- Endoscopy showed shallow ulcera at lower end of esophagus
- Histopathology shows large eosinophilic intranuclear inclusion and multiple small cytoplasmic inclusions

2. Ans. (b) Columnar metaplasia Histological findings of barrett esophagus
- Metaplastic columnar epithelium (specialized) with goblet cells is seen adjacent to squamous epithelium of esophagus hence suggestive of columnar metaplasia
- Long-segment: Barrett's mucosa extends 3 cm or more. Short-segment: Barrett's mucosa extends less than 3 cm

3. Ans. (a) Pseudomembranous enterocolitis
- The mucosal surface of the colon seen here is hyperemic and is partially covered by a yellow-green exudate.

4. Ans. (a) Crohn's disease
- Non caseating epithelioid cell granuloma. Look at the presence of giant cells and lot of lymphocytes

5. Ans. (a) Pseudopolyps suggestive of ulcerative colitis
- Pseudopolyps can be seen clearly as raised red islands of inflamed mucosa.

6. Ans. (a) Adenomatous Polyposis
- Gross picture shows multiple polyposis with numerous small polyps covering the colonic mucosa.
- A 20-year-old male should be suspected as having faulty APC gene as he is having multiple polyps and also having osteomas of skull. Other extra colonic manifestations should be looked for.

Multiple Choice Questions

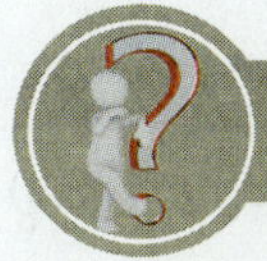

1. A 40-year-old immunocompromized patient presented with complaints of dysphagia. UGI scopy showed multiple ulcers in the distal esophagus. Biopsy from the esophagus showed the following. What is the diagnosis?

(Recent exam 2018)

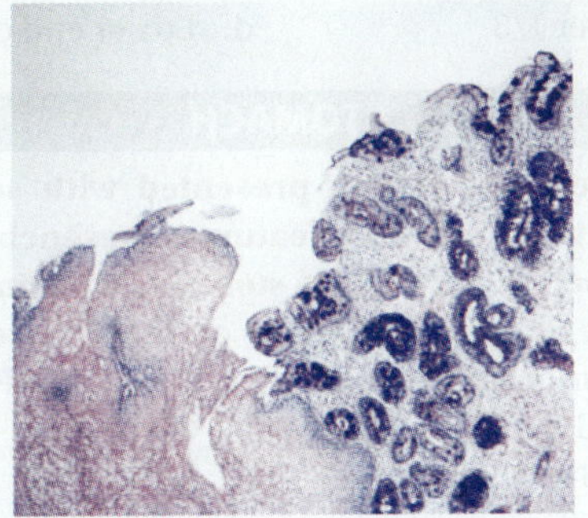

a. Candida
b. Cytomegalovirus
c. Herpes
d. Eosinophilic esophagitis

2. On endoscopy and barium swallow the following findings are seen, which of the following will be seen on histopathology?

(AIIMS Nov 2017)

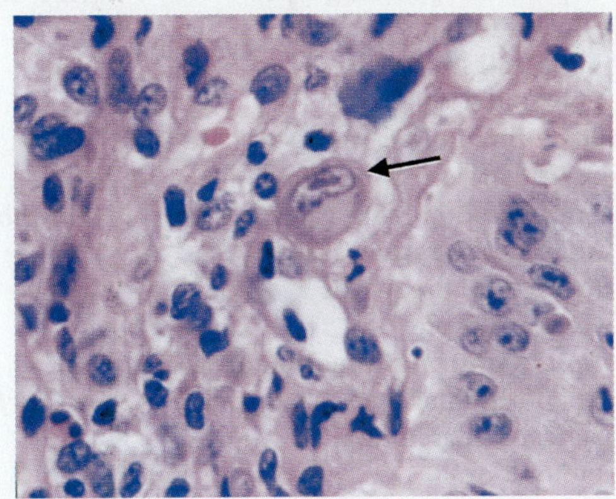

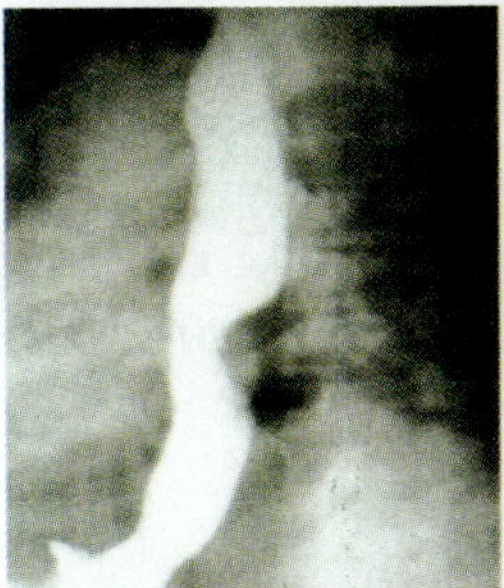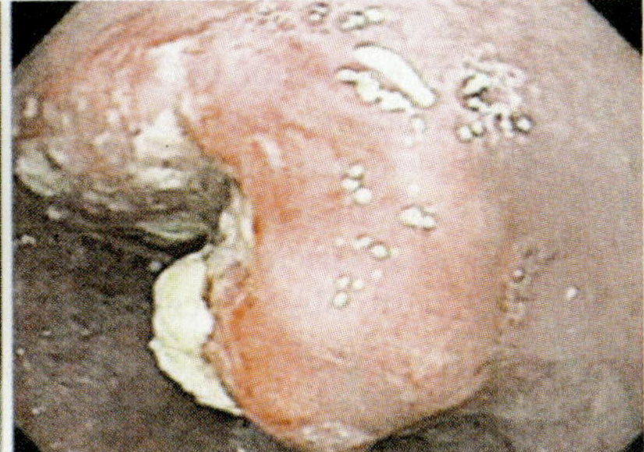

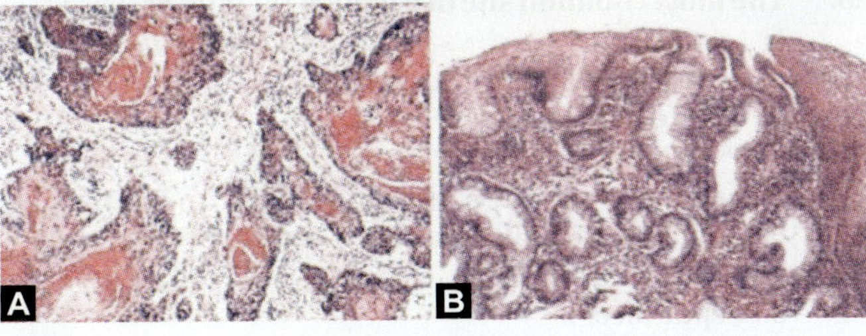

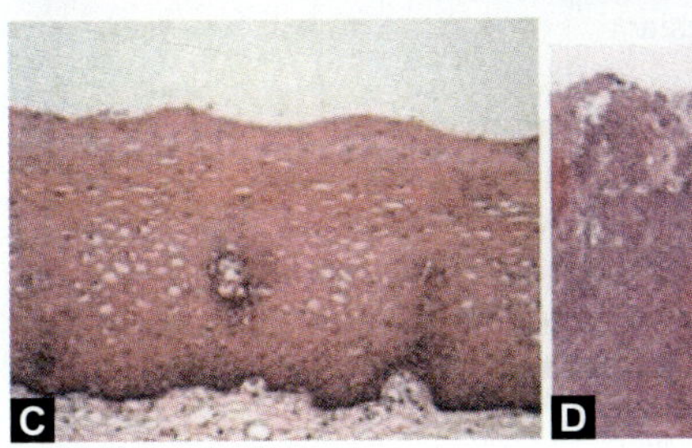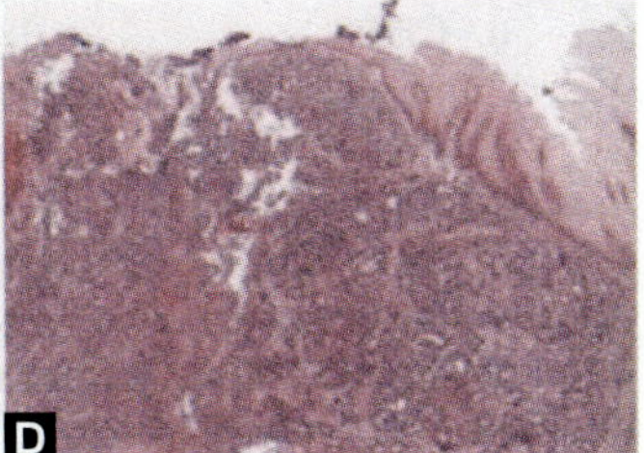

3. A 40-year-old patient presented with heart burn and increased salivation. UGE scopy was done and biopsy was taken and is as shown below. Which of the is the diagnosis?

(AIIMS May 2017)

a. Barret esophagus
b. Adenocarcinoma
c. Esophagitis
d. Squamous cell carcinoma

4. Prognostic factors for carcinoma esophagus is/are:

(PGI May 16)

a. Depth of invasion   b. Lymph node status
c. Tumour grading   d. Stage of the disease

5. Layer absent in esophagus   *(Recent Question 2016)*
a. Mucosa   b. Serosa
c. Muscularis   d. lamina propria

6. A 30-year-old software engineer came to OPD with chief complains of heartburn. On endoscopic biopsy, the lesion shows the following (figure below). Idenfity the lesion, stain has been done for what and what additional features should be looked for?

(AIIMS Nov 2015)

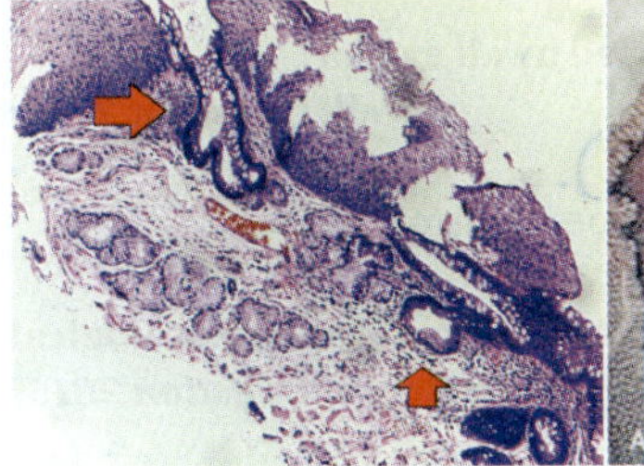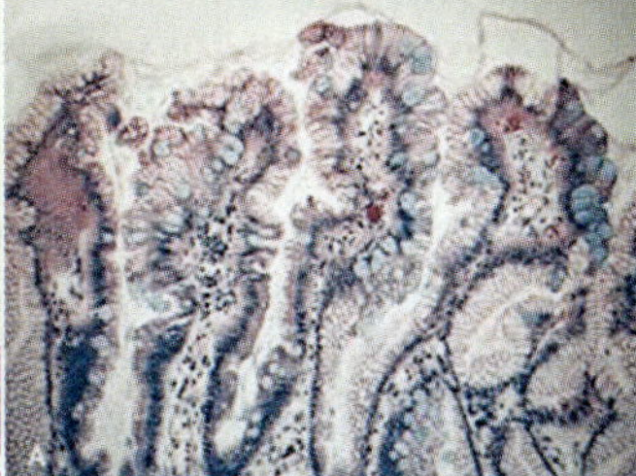

a. Adenocarcinoma; PAS; malignancy
b. Barretts oesophagus; mucin stain; dysplasia
c. Squamous cell carcinoma; cytokeratin, squamous pearls
d. Infection; fungal stain; inclusion body

7. Most frequent site of ectopic gastric mucosa is:
a. Upper third of esophagus   *(Recent Question 2015)*
b. Middle third of esophagus
c. Lower third of esophagus
d. Duodenum

8. Achalasia cardia: *(Recent Question 2015)*
a. Absence of nerves   b. Absence of muscles
c. Hypertrophy of nerves   d. None

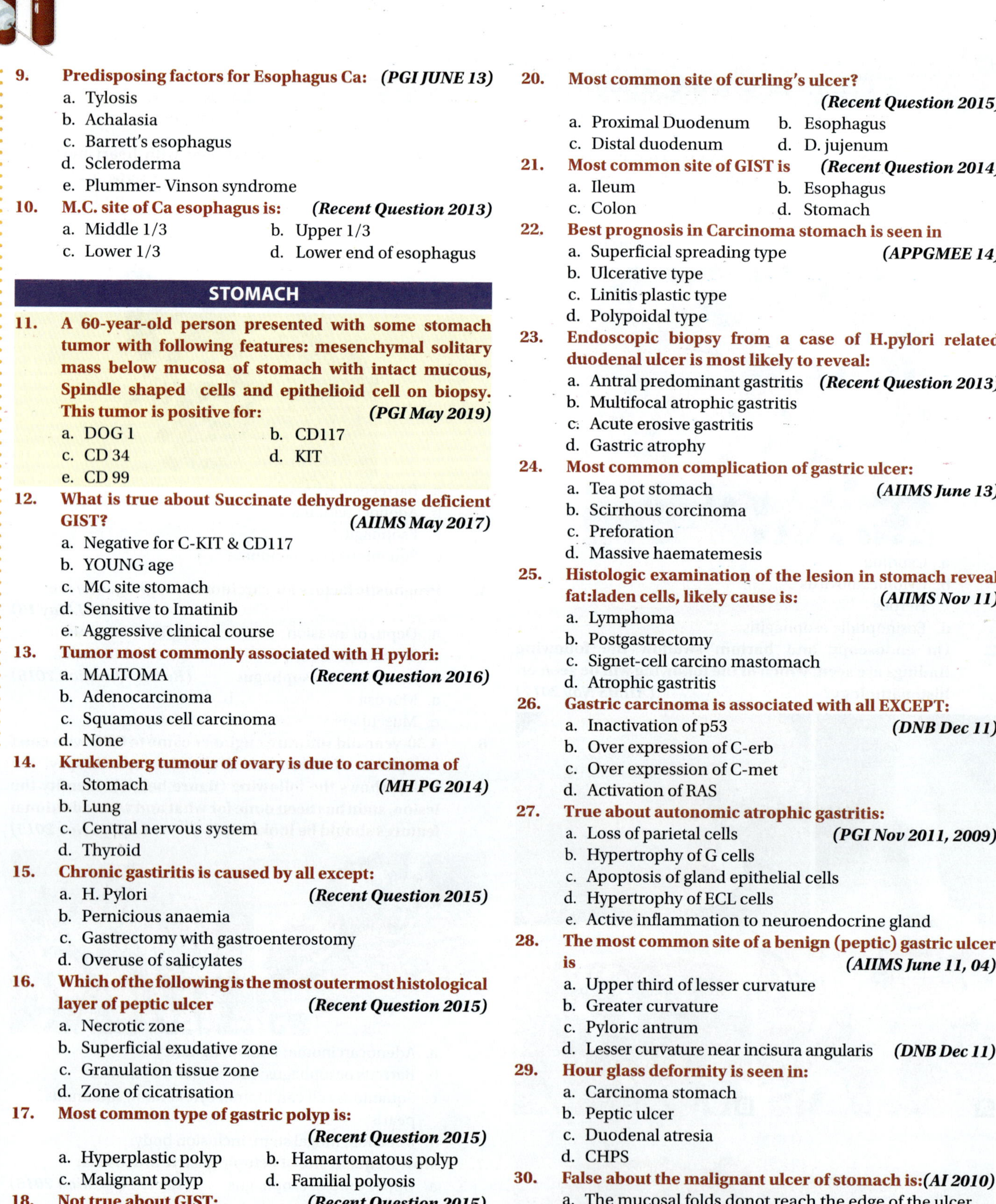

9. Predisposing factors for Esophagus Ca: *(PGI JUNE 13)*
 a. Tylosis
 b. Achalasia
 c. Barrett's esophagus
 d. Scleroderma
 e. Plummer- Vinson syndrome

10. M.C. site of Ca esophagus is: *(Recent Question 2013)*
 a. Middle 1/3   b. Upper 1/3
 c. Lower 1/3   d. Lower end of esophagus

STOMACH

11. A 60-year-old person presented with some stomach tumor with following features: mesenchymal solitary mass below mucosa of stomach with intact mucous, Spindle shaped cells and epithelioid cell on biopsy. This tumor is positive for: *(PGI May 2019)*
 a. DOG 1   b. CD117
 c. CD 34   d. KIT
 e. CD 99

12. What is true about Succinate dehydrogenase deficient GIST? *(AIIMS May 2017)*
 a. Negative for C-KIT & CD117
 b. YOUNG age
 c. MC site stomach
 d. Sensitive to Imatinib
 e. Aggressive clinical course

13. Tumor most commonly associated with H pylori:
 a. MALTOMA   *(Recent Question 2016)*
 b. Adenocarcinoma
 c. Squamous cell carcinoma
 d. None

14. Krukenberg tumour of ovary is due to carcinoma of
 a. Stomach   *(MH PG 2014)*
 b. Lung
 c. Central nervous system
 d. Thyroid

15. Chronic gastiritis is caused by all except:
 a. H. Pylori   *(Recent Question 2015)*
 b. Pernicious anaemia
 c. Gastrectomy with gastroenterostomy
 d. Overuse of salicylates

16. Which of the following is the most outermost histological layer of peptic ulcer *(Recent Question 2015)*
 a. Necrotic zone
 b. Superficial exudative zone
 c. Granulation tissue zone
 d. Zone of cicatrisation

17. Most common type of gastric polyp is:
 (Recent Question 2015)
 a. Hyperplastic polyp   b. Hamartomatous polyp
 c. Malignant polyp   d. Familial polyosis

18. Not true about GIST: *(Recent Question 2015)*
 a. Stomach is the most common site
 b. High propensity of malignant change
 c. Associated with c-KIT mutation
 d. Histology shows epithelioid and spindle shaped cells

19. MC site for stomach Ca: *(Recent Question 2015)*
 a. Lesser curvature   b. Antrum
 c. Greater curvature   d. Pylorus

20. Most common site of curling's ulcer?
 (Recent Question 2015)
 a. Proximal Duodenum   b. Esophagus
 c. Distal duodenum   d. D. jujenum

21. Most common site of GIST is *(Recent Question 2014)*
 a. Ileum   b. Esophagus
 c. Colon   d. Stomach

22. Best prognosis in Carcinoma stomach is seen in
 a. Superficial spreading type   *(APPGMEE 14)*
 b. Ulcerative type
 c. Linitis plastic type
 d. Polypoidal type

23. Endoscopic biopsy from a case of H.pylori related duodenal ulcer is most likely to reveal:
 a. Antral predominant gastritis   *(Recent Question 2013)*
 b. Multifocal atrophic gastritis
 c. Acute erosive gastritis
 d. Gastric atrophy

24. Most common complication of gastric ulcer:
 a. Tea pot stomach   *(AIIMS June 13)*
 b. Scirrhous corcinoma
 c. Preforation
 d. Massive haematemesis

25. Histologic examination of the lesion in stomach reveal fat:laden cells, likely cause is: *(AIIMS Nov 11)*
 a. Lymphoma
 b. Postgastrectomy
 c. Signet-cell carcino mastomach
 d. Atrophic gastritis

26. Gastric carcinoma is associated with all EXCEPT:
 a. Inactivation of p53   *(DNB Dec 11)*
 b. Over expression of C-erb
 c. Over expression of C-met
 d. Activation of RAS

27. True about autonomic atrophic gastritis:
 a. Loss of parietal cells   *(PGI Nov 2011, 2009)*
 b. Hypertrophy of G cells
 c. Apoptosis of gland epithelial cells
 d. Hypertrophy of ECL cells
 e. Active inflammation to neuroendocrine gland

28. The most common site of a benign (peptic) gastric ulcer is *(AIIMS June 11, 04)*
 a. Upper third of lesser curvature
 b. Greater curvature
 c. Pyloric antrum
 d. Lesser curvature near incisura angularis   *(DNB Dec 11)*

29. Hour glass deformity is seen in:
 a. Carcinoma stomach
 b. Peptic ulcer
 c. Duodenal atresia
 d. CHPS

30. False about the malignant ulcer of stomach is: *(AI 2010)*
 a. The mucosal folds donot reach the edge of the ulcer
 b. Mucosal folds are thickened and fused
 c. Ulcer crator is eccentric
 d. Margins of the ulcer are overhanging

31. Which of the following markers is specific for gastro-intestinal stromal tumor (GIST): *(AI 10, 09)*
 a. CD 117   b. CD 34
 c. CD123   d. S-100

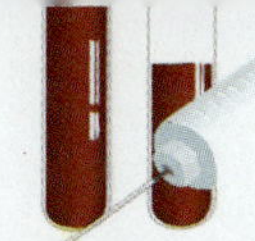

32. When carcinoma of stomach develops secondarily to pernicious anemia, it is usually situated in the:

a. Prepyloric region   b. Pylorus   *(DNB 2010)*

c. Body   d. Fundus

33. True about H. pylori infection:

a. Gram +ve aerobe   *(WB PGMEE 2016, PGI Nov 2009)*

b. Invade gastric mucosa and cause ulcer

c. Rapid urease test on endoscopy is diagnostic

d. Serology confirms eradication

e. Causes MALT lymphoma of stomach

SMALL INTESTINE

34. A 23-year-old lady presented with diarrhea, vomiting and poor appetite. Biopsy showed crypt hyperplasia, villous atrophy and CD8+ cells in the lamina propria. Skin manifestations have been shown. What could be the diagnosis?   *(Recent Pattern Question 2020)*

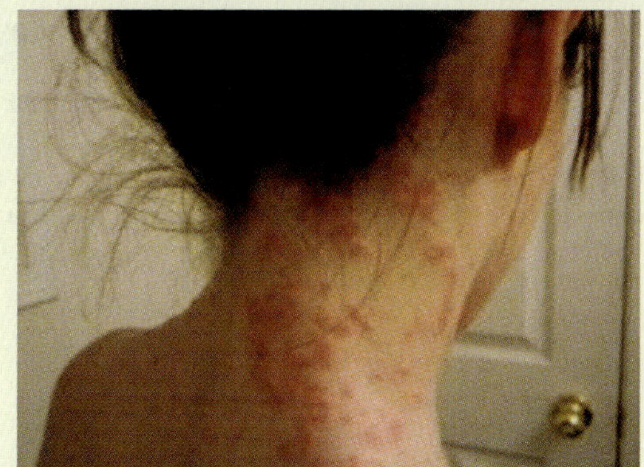

a. Whipple's disease

b. Chronic pancreatitis

c. Environmental enteropathy

d. Celiac disease

35. Which of the following is associated with PAS positive macrophages?   *(Recent exam 2018)*

a. Whipple disease   b. Abetalipoproteinemia

c. Crohns disease   d. Ulcerative colitis

36. A patient presented with complains of chronic constipation and diarrhoea. There was excessive associated weight loss. Intestinal biopsy was obtained and it showed the following findings. What is your diagnosis?   *(AIIMS Nov 16)*

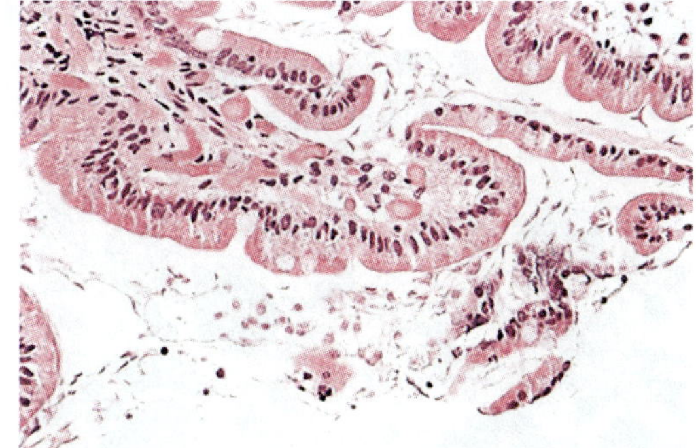

a. Giardia   b. Entamoeba

c. Whipple's disease   d. CMV

37. Which sugar is used to diagnose intestinal malabsoption?   *(Recent Question 2016-17)*

a. Xylose   b. Glucose

c. Amylase   d. Lactose

38. Duodenal villous atrophy is seen in   *(Recent Question 2016-17)*

a. Crohn's disease

b. Ulcerative colitis

c. Celiac disease

d. Cystic fibrosis

39. All are true about Peutz Jegher's syndrome except: *(WBPGMEE 2016, Recent Question 2015)*

a. Autosomal dominant

b. Hamartomatous polyps do not develop into adenocarcinoma

c. Gain of function mutation in LKB1/STK11

d. Chance of fatal intussusceptions

40. True about gluten sensitive enteropathy: *(PGI May 2015)*

a. Diet should exclude barley, wheat and rye

b. Intestinal biopsy is diagnostic

c. Anti IgA endomycial antibody is specific

d. Mucosal hyperplasia

41. Pathologist examines biopsy from a patient presenting with bleeding per rectum with a past history of intussuption for the past 6 months. Histopathology obtained has been shown below. Identify the Pathology?   *(AIIMS NOV 2015)*

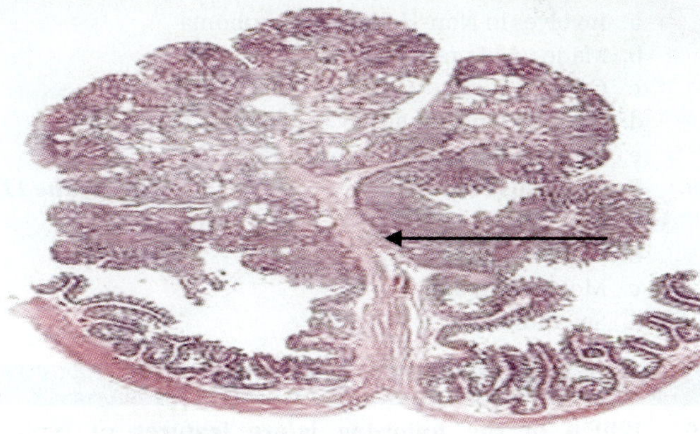

a. Tubule villous adenoma

b Adeno carcinoma

c. Hamartoma

d. Juvenile polyposis syndrome

42. Celiac sprue is associated with   *(Recent Question 2014-15)*

a. HLA DQ1

b. HLA DQ2

c. HLA DQ3

d. HLA DQ4

43. Characteristic histopathology finding in Whipples disease is :   *(Recent Question 2014-15)*

a. PAS positive macrophages and rod shaped bacilli in lamina propria

b. Shortened thickened villi with increased crypt depth

c. Blunting and flattening of mucosal surface and absent villi

d. Mononuclear infiltration at base of crypts

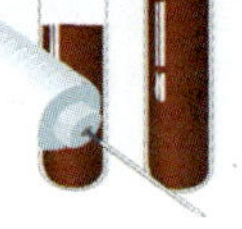

44. A 2-year-old male presented with abdominal distension, chronic diarrhea, severe anemia and failure to thrive? Which of the following is the investigation of choice?
a. Anti milk protein antibody *(Recent Question 2015)*
b. Anti endomysial antibody
c. Antinuclear antibody   d. Intestinal biopsy

45. True about Peutz-jeghers syndrome: *(PGI May 2013)*
a. Pigmentary changes in skin and mucous membrane around mouth
b. Adenomatous polyp in intestine
c. Most common of pattern inheritance is autosomal recessive
d. 20-30% premalignant
e. May presents as anemia in children

46. Whipple's disease is characterized by?
a. Foamy macrophages   *(Recent Question 13)*
b. AFB posititve
c. Papillary projections
d. Villous atrophy

47. True about abdominal lymphoma: *(PGI Nov 2011)*
a. GIT lymphoma most commonly has polypoid appearance
b. Primary small intestinal lymphoma are most common
c. Lymphoma is most common primary malignant neoplasm of colon
d. Stomach is most common site for extranodal lympoma
e. MALT lymphoma isassociated with H .pylori infection

48. True about intestinal lymphoma: *(PGI Nov 2010)*
a. Involves in Non-Hodgkin's lymphoma
b. Made up of predominantly T cells
c. C-kit positive
d. Most common at ileocecal junction
e. Lymphadenectomy is always done

49. Paneth cells contain: *(DNB June 11)*
a. Zinc
b. Copper
c. Molybdenum
d. Selenium

LARGE INTESTINE

50. Which of the following is/are features of typical Ulcerative colitis: *(PGI May 2019)*
a. Crypt distortion
b. Chronic inflammatory cells in the lamina propria
c. Crypt abscess
d. Granuloma
e. Crypt branching

51. Which of the following is a feature of Crohn's disease?
a. Pseudopolyps can be seen   *(Recent exam 2018)*
b. Non-caseating granulomas are present
c. Backwash ileitis may be associated with Crohn's disease
d. Both b and c

52. Which of the following is the earliest change in intestine which occurs in Crohn's disease?   *(Recent exam 2018)*
a. Cobblestone appearance
b. Aphthous ulcer
c. Perforation
d. Stricture

53. A 50-year-old male presented with recurrent bloody diarrhea. Colonoscopy showed geographical ulcers. Histopathology is shown below. What is your diagnosis?

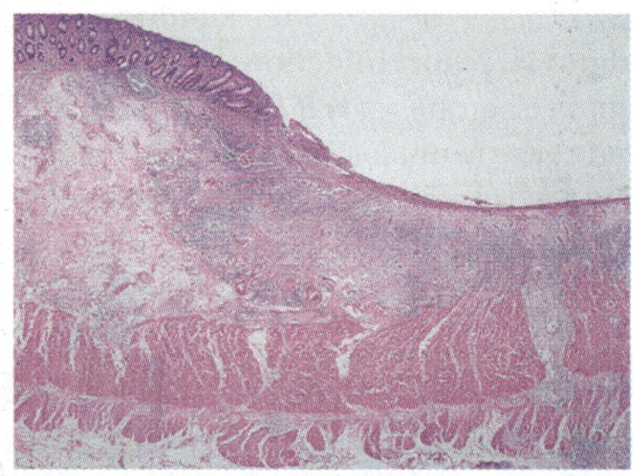

a. Pseudomebranous colitis   *(AIIMS May 2017)*
b. Non-hodgkin lymphoma colon
c. Adenocarcinoma colon
d. Crohn disease

54. About Crohn's disease true is?   *(AIIMS May 2017)*
a. Loss of haustration   b. Linear fissure
c. Cobblestone colon   d. String sign of kantor
e. Pipe stem colon

55. Identify the parasite in the intestinal biopsy of a HIV positive patient.   *(Recent Pattern Question 2020)*

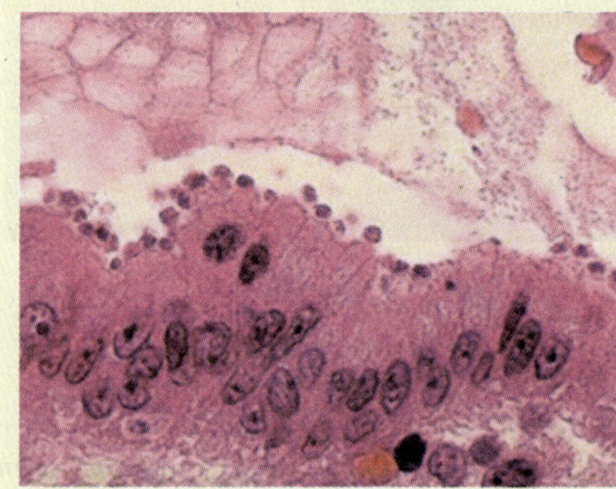

a. Giardia
b. CMV
c. Amoebic colitis
d. Cryptosporidium

56. A 26-year-old male presented with abdominal pain and bloody diarrhea of one week duration. The following colonoscopic biopsy is diagnostic of infection with   *(AIIMS May 16)*

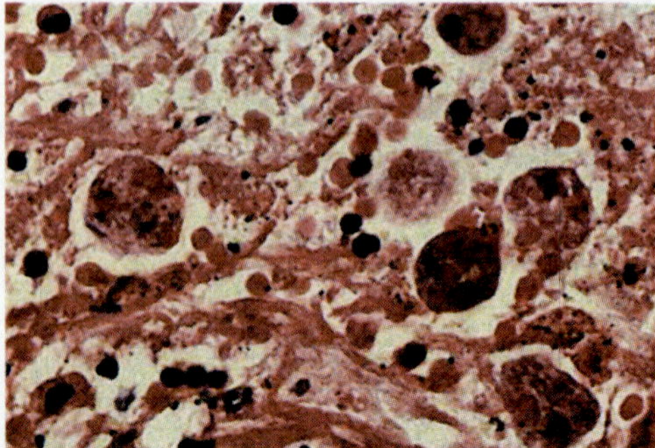

a. Giardiasis   b. Amoebiasis
c. Enterobius   d. Severe bacterial infection

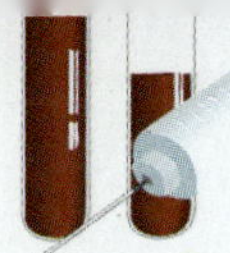

57. Extraintestinal manifestations of Crohn disease include ALL EXCEPT *(JIPMER 2016)*
a. Uveitis
b. Migratory polyarthritis
c. Sacroiliitis
d. Pericholangitis

58. Which gene involved in colonic adenoma to colonic carcinoma? *(Recent Question 2016-17)*
a. TP 53 (Protoncogene mutation)
b. Rb
c. K RAS (Protoncogene mutation)
d. EGFR

59. Which of the following is NOT associated with an increased risk of Gastrointestinal malignancy? *(Recent Question 2015)*
a. Cowden's syndrome
b. Lynch syndrome
c. Gardner's syndrome
d. HNPCC

60. In carcinoma of unknown primary, if the tissue marker CDX-2 is positive, it indicates: *(Recent Question 2015)*
a. Bladder cancer
b. Gastrointestinal cancer
c. Lung cancer
d. Thyroid cancer

61. All the following conditions are characterized by neoplastic polyps except: *(MHPGMEE 2016, Recent Question 2015)*
a. Peutzjehers syndrome
b. Gardner syndrome
c. Turcot syndrome
d. Lynch syndrome

62. An 11-year-old girl presents with abdominal pain, no diarrhea, freckles lips, nostrils, buccal mucosa, palmar surfaces of the hands. Likely diagnosis:
a. Gardner syndrome *(Recent Question 2015)*
b. Cowden syndrome
c. Peut zjeghers syndrome
d. Cronkhite Canada sydrome

63. Not true about Cowden syndrome:
a. Mutation of PTEN gene *(Recent Question 2015)*
b. Multiple hamartomas
c. Increased risk of Gl maliganancy
d. Risk of follicular thyroid cancer

64. Most common site of carcinoid tumor in hindgut: *(Recent Question 2015)*
a. Caecum
b. Rectum
c. Transverse colon
d. Descending colon

65. Pseudopolyps are features of: *(Recent Question 2015)*
a. Crohn's disease
b. Ulcerative colitis
c. Celiac sprue
d. Whipple's disease

66. True about ulcerative colitis, all except: *(Recent Question 14)*
a. Rectum involved
b. Pseudopolyps
c. Pancolitis
d. Noncaseating granuloma

67. Inheritance of Gardner syndrome is: *(Recent Question 2014)*
a. Autosomal recessive
b. Autosomal dominant
c. X linked
d. None of the above

68. Aganglionic seqment is encountered in which part of colon in case of Hirschsprung disease: *(AIIMS Nov 14)*
a. Distal to dilated segment
b. In Whole colon
c. Proximal to dilatedsegment
d. In the dilated segment

69. Acquired diverticulum most common site is: *(Recent Question 2015)*
a. Sigmoid colon
b. Ileum
c. Ascending colon
d. Transverse colon

70. Regarding FAP all true except- *(JIPMER 2017)*
a. Autosomal recessive
b. Duodenal polyp
c. More than 100 polyps
d. Extraintestinal manifestations

71. A 5 year-old boy presented with bleeding per rectum. PR showed rectal polyp, biopsy showed the following. What is your diagnosis? *(Recent Pattern Question 2020)*

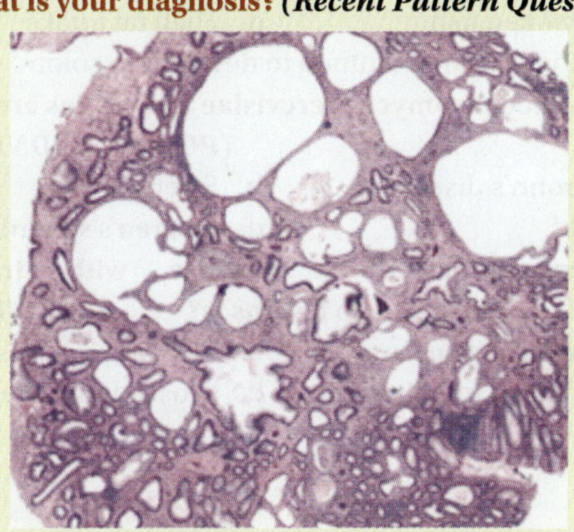

a. Villous adenoma
b. Peutz-Jeghers polyp
c. Juvenile polyp
d. Serrated adenoma

72. Which polyp has got the maximum risk of turning into malignancy: *(Recent Question 2014)*
a. Pseudopolyp
b. Hyperplastic polyp
c. Tubular villous adenomas (multiple)
d. Adenomatous polyps

73. Gene involved in HNPCC is: *(Recent Question 2014)*
a. APC
b. PTEN
c. HLH1
d. SKTH

74. FALSE statement regarding Hirschprung disease is *(AP-PGMEE 14)*
a. Aganglionosis always involves distal rectum
b. Non passage of meconium in first 24 hours is a cardinal feature
c. Diagnosis is established by Suction rectal biopsy
d. No passage ofstools after per rectal examination

75. The minimum number of polyps necessary for a diagnosis of Familial Adenomatous Polyposis (FAP) is:
a. 05
b. 10 *(APPGMEE 14)*
c. 50
d. 100

76. Premalignant conditions of the GIT are: *(PGI 13)*
a. Ileocaecal TB
b. Familial polyposis
c. Villous adenomas
d. Ulcerative colitis

77. True about Carcinoembryonic antigen (CEA): *(PGI May 2013)*
a. Used for monitoring of recurrence of coloncancr
b. Specific for colon cancer
c. Increased in smokers
d. Increased in colon cancer

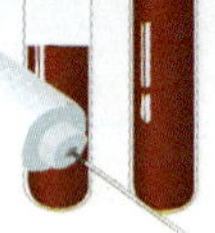

78. In Hirschsprung's disease, staining used for diagnosis is? *(Recent Question 2013)*
a. Fontana stain
b. Trichome stain
c. AChE
d. Auramine Rhodamine stain

79. Osteomas, adenomatous polyps of intestine and periampullary carcinomas are seen in: *(Recent Question 2013)*
a. Cowden syndrome
b. Peutz Jeghers syndrome
c. FAP
d. Gardener syndrome

80. Dietery factors associated with colon carcinoma:
a. High fiber
b. Low fiber *(PGI Dec 12)*
c. Smoked fish
d. High fat intake
e. Japanese are common to develop Ca colon

81. Anti-Saccharomyces cercvisiae antibodies are seen in? *(PGI Dec 12, DNB June 11)*
a. Crohn's disease
b. Scleroderma
c. SLE
d. Sjogren's syndrome

82. Inflammatory bowel disease with transmural involvement and skip lesions is? *(DNB June 11)*
a. Crohn's disease
b. Ulcerative colitis
c. Shigella infection
d. Clostridium infection

83. Not true about familial polyposis colon cancer syndrome?
a. Autosomal recessive *(Jipmer 11)*
b. Associated with fibromas and osteomas
c. Associated with brain tumors
d. 100% incidence of colon ca

84. True about intestinal lymphoma: *(PGI Nov 10)*
a. Involved in non-Hodgkins lymphoma
b. Made up of predominantly T cells
c. C-kit positive
d. Most common site is ileocaecaljunction
e. Lymphadenopathy always seen

MISCELLANEOUS

85. Least predilection for distal ileum:
a. Carcinoid syndrome *(Recent Question 2014)*
b. Meckel diverticulum
c. Chrons disease
d. Zollinger Ellison syndrome

86. Mesenteric tumours are: *(Recent Question 2013, Karnat 05)*
a. Usually solid
b. Usually cystic
c. Highly malignant
d. Highly vascular

Answers with Explanations

1. **Ans. (b)** **Cytomegalovirus** *(Ref: Robbins 9th ed p 755)*

CMV causes shallower ulcerations and characteristic nuclear and cytoplasmic inclusions within capillary endothelium and stromal cells. Infected cells are strikingly enlarged, often to a diameter of 40 μm, and show cellular and nuclear pleomorphism. Prominent intranuclear basophilic inclusions spanning half the nuclear diameter are usually set off from the nuclear membrane by a clear halo

2. **Ans. (a)** **A**

- The gross morphology in the lower part of esophagus shows tumor masses that may be polypoid, or exophytic, and protrude into and obstruct the lumen suggestive of carcinoma A.

3. **Ans. (a)** **Barret esophagus** *(Ref: R 9/ p 757)*

- Barrett's esophagus is the metaplastic change in the esophageal lining in which the normal squamous epithelium is changed to columnar epithelium due to prolonged gastroesophageal reflux (GERD)
- Columnar metaplasia, glandular metaplasia, goblet cell metaplsia.
- Definite diagnosis is made only when columnar mucosa contains **the intestinal goblet cells, which will be positive for PAS, Alcian blue (mucin stain)**

4. **Ans. (a, b, c, d)** **a. Depth of invasion; b. Lymph node status c. Tumour grading d. Stage of the disease**

5. **Ans. (b)** **Serosa** *(Ref: Robbins 9th/pg ; 8th/pg 768)*

6. **Ans. (b)** **Barretts oesophagus; mucin stain; dysplasia**

(Ref: Robbin's 9th/ 757)

- There are two figures given in this question.
- The first figure shows **lower oesophagus, in which normal squamous epithelium has been replaced by columnar epithelium**.
- This type of replacement of one mature tissue by another is called as **Metaplasia.**
- Now since in this case, **squamous epithelium is getting replaced by columnar epithelium; this is referred to as Columnar metaplasia** referred to as **Barrett's esophagus**.
- This can be diagnosed by H& E stain (1st picture) which shows **when columnar mucosa contains the intestinal goblet cells which show distinct mucous vacuoles that stain pale blue by hematoxylin and eosin.**
- **For specific staining of mucus, mucin stain can be used (2nd picture)**

7. **Ans. (a)** **Upper third of esophagus**

(Ref: R 9th/pg ; 8th/pg 768)

Ectopic gastric mucosa is seen most commonly in the **upper third of the esophagus**
This is known as inlet patch.

8. **Ans. (a)** **Absence of nerves**

(Ref: Robbins 9th/pg ; 8th/pg 768)

Achalasia cardia is caused by selective **loss of function of inhibitory neurons** like those secreting vasoactive intestinal peptide and nitric oxide which causes relaxation of LES whereas cholinergic innervations is intact

9. **Ans. (a, b, c, d, e); a. Tylosis; b. Achalasia; c. Barrett's esophagus; d. Scleroderma; e. Plummer-Vinson syndrome** *(Ref: Robbins 9th/pg 758-59; 8th/pg 773)*

10. **Ans. (c)** **Lower 1/3**

(Ref: Robbins 9th/pg 759, Bailey & love 24th ed: 1009)

11. **Ans. (a) DOG 1; (b) CD117; (c) CD 34; (d) KIT**

(Ref: R 9th pg 785)

The findings are suggestive of GIST, IHC for GIST are DOG 1, CD117, CD 34, KIT

12. **Ans. (a, b, c) a. Negative for C-KIT & CD117; b. YOUNG age; c. MC site stomach**

Most gastrointestinal stromal tumors (GISTs) are characterized by KIT or platelet-derived growth factor alpha (PDGFRA) activating mutations. However, there are still 10%-15% of GISTs lacking *KIT* and *PDGFRA* mutations, called wild-type GISTs (WT GISTs). Among these so-called WT GISTs, a small subset is associated with succinate dehydrogenase (SDH) deficiency, known as SDH-deficient GISTs. In addition, GISTs that occur in Carney triad and Carney-Stratakis syndrome represent specific examples of SDH-deficient GISTs. SDH-deficient GISTs locate exclusively in the stomach, showing predilection for children and young adults with female preponderance. The tumor generally pursues an indolent course and exhibits primary resistance to imatinib therapy in most cases.

13. **Ans. (a)** **MALTOMA** *(Ref: Robbins 9th/pg 773; 8th/pg 786)*

- H. pylori gastritis induces mucosa-associated lymphoid tissue (MALT) that can give rise to B cell lymphomas (MALTomas).
- Histologically, gastric MALToma takes the form of a dense lymphocytic infiltrate in the lamina propria. Characteristically, the neoplastic lymphocytes infiltrate the gastric glands focally to create diagnostic **lymphoepithelial lesions**

14. **Ans. (a)** **Stomach** *(Ref: Robbins 9th/pg 771; 8th/pg 785)*

Metastasis from stomach cancer Occurs to the liver **(first organ to be affected)** followed by lungs, bone, **ovary (where it is known as Krukenberg's rumor)**, periumbilical lymph nodes (Sister Mary Joseph nodule), peritoneal cul-de-sac (**Blumer's** shelf palpable on rectal or vaginal examination) and **left supraclavicular lymph node (Virchow's lymph node**

15. **Ans. (d)** **Overuse of salicylates (Ref: R** *9th/pg ; 8th/pg 775)*

16. **Ans. (d)** **Zone of cicatrisation** *(Ref: Robbins 9th/pg 766)*

17. **Ans. (a)** **Hyperplastic polyp**

(Ref: Robbins 9th/pg 769; 8th/pg 783)

18. **Ans. (b)** **High propensity of malignant change**

(Ref: Robbins 9th/pg 775; 8th/pg 789)

19. **Ans. (b)** **Antrum** *(Ref: Robbins 9th/pg 771; 8th/pg 785)*

- The most common location of the gastric cancer is the **antrum of the stomach.**[Q]
- Cancer of the **gastric cardia is on the rise especially due to Barrett esophagus**[Q]
- **Lesser curvature**[Q] is involved more often than the greater curvature.
- **Hence the most common site is lesser curvature of anteropyloric region**[Q]

20. **Ans. (a)** **Proximal duodenum** *(Ref: Robbins 9th/pg 762)*

Curling ulcers-Ulcers occurring in the proximal duodenum and associated with severe burns or trauma

21. **Ans. (d)** **Stomach** *(Ref: Robbins 9th/pg 775; 8th/pg 789)*

22. **Ans. (a)** **Superficial spreading type** *(Ref: R 9th/pg 771)*

The **depth of invasion and the extent of nodal and distant metastases** at the time of diagnosis remain the **most powerful prognostic indicators** in gastric cancer.

23. **Ans. (a)** **Antral predominant gastritis**

(Ref: Harrison 18th ed: 2458, 17th ed:1870)

- The **most common cause** of chronic gastritis- **H. pylori**[Q]
- Within the stomach, H. pylori are **most often found in the antrum – antral predominant gastritis**[Q] *or type B gastriris*[Q]

24. **Ans. (d)** **Massive haematemesis**

(Ref: Robbins 9th/pg 767)

25. **Ans. (d)** **Atrophic gastritis**

(Ref: Odze RD, Goldblum JR (2009). Surgical Pathology of the GI Tract, Liver, Biliary Tract, and Pancreas. Philadelphia, PA: Saunders, http://www.histopathology-india.net/gaxan.htm, Gastrointestinal Pathology: an atlas and text. Philadelphia, PA: Lippincott Williams & Wilkins)

Collection of lipid laden macrophages within the lamina propria is defined as **gastric xanthoma**

Associated with pathological lesions such as **chronic gastritis** & intestinal metaplasia, **atrophic gastritis,** and gastric ulcer. **Rarely these are also seen in dudenogastric reflux after gastric surgery hence d> b**

Usually located at the antral and the lesser curvature

Positive with Sudan black, oil red O (on frozen section), and CD68

Differential diagnosis

Signet ring carcinoma-**mucin laden tumor cells** infiltrate gastric wall. PAS/alcian blue positive

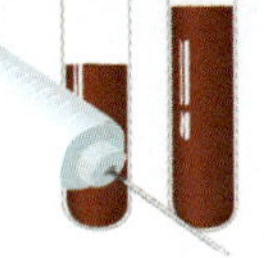

26.   **Ans. (d)**   **Activation of RAS** *(Ref: Robbins 9th/pg 771)*

- MC mutations seen in gastric carcinoma- **p53**
- Least common mutation seen in gastric carcinoma- K-Ras
- MC mutations seen in diffuse type gastric carcinoma- CDH1 gene mutations
- MC mutations seen in intestinal type gastric carcinoma- **Wnt pathway, APC, β-catenin, e-erb 2 amplification**
- Mutations seen in both intestinal and diffuse type gastric cancers- **p53, Cmet and cyclin E genes amplification**

27.   **Ans. (a, b, d);   a. Loss of parietal cells; b. Hypertrophy of G cells; d. Hypertrophy of ECL cells** *(Ref: R 9th/pg 764)*

28.   **Ans. (d)   Lesser curvature near incisura angularis**

(Ref: Robbins 9th/pg 766; 8th/pg 776)

29.   **Ans. (b)   Peptic ulcer**

(Ref: Robbins 9th/pg 766; 8th/pg 776)

30.   **Ans. (d)   Margins of the ulcer are overhanging**

(Ref: Chandrasoma Taylor 3ed: 582,587) Read Pretext

31.   **Ans. (a)   CD 117** *(Ref: Robbins 9th/pg 775; 8th/pg 789)*

Most **useful diagnostic marker** is **c-kit (CD117)** detectable in 95% of the patients.

32.   **Ans. (d)   Fundus** *(Ref: Robbins 9th/pg 771; 8th/pg 785)*

- **Most common site of Gastric Adenocarcinoma secondary to H. pylori infection is Antrum**[Q]
- **Most common site of Gastric Adenocarcinoma secondary to Pernicious anemia is Fundus and Body**[Q]

33.   **Ans. (e)   Causes MALT lymphoma of stomach**

(Ref: Robbins 9th/pg 764; 8th/pg 777)

- Option a false-H.pylori is a gram-negative flagellated bacteria
- Option b false-The organism is concentrated within the **superficial mucus**[Q] overlying epithelial cells
- Option c–true, rapid urease test has high sensitivity and specificity, can be **false negative**[Q] with recent use of PPIs.**Gold standard test is : antral biopsy showing the bacilli**[Q]
- Option d: Serology- Cannot be used for early follow-up Urea breath test- useful for follow-up after treatment
- Option e-true- **M**ost **common** inducer of gastric MALToma –**H Pylori**

34.   **Ans. (d)   Celiac disease** *(Ref: R 9th pg 782)*

35.   **Ans. (a)   Whipple disease** *(Ref: Robbins 9th ed p 792)*

36.   **Ans. (a)   Giardia** *(Ref: www.ncbi.nihgov/pubmed/104699)*

This image shows Giardia lamblia infection of the small intestine. The small pear-shaped trophozoites live in the duodenum and become infective cysts that are excreted. They produce a watery diarrhea. A useful test for diagnosis of infectious diarrheas is stool examination for ova and parasites.

37.   **Ans. (a)   Xylose**

(Ref: https://en.wikipedia.org/wiki/D-xylose_absorption_test)

D-xylose is a monosaccharide, that does not require enzymes for digestion prior to absorption. Its absorption requires an intact mucosa only. In contrast, polysaccharides require enzymes, such as amylase, to break them down so that they can eventually be absorbed as monosaccharides. This test was previously in use but has been made redundant by antibody tests.

In normal individuals, a 25 g oral dose of D-xylose will be absorbed and excreted in the urine at approximately 4.5 g in 5 hours. A decreased urinary excretion of D-xylose is seen in conditions involving the GI mucosa, such as small intestinal bacterial overgrowth and Whipple's disease if the D-xylose urinary excretion is not normal after a course of antibiotics, then small intestinal bacterial overgrowth is ruled out and non-infectious cause of malabsorption (i.e., celiac disease) is suggested.

38.   **Ans. (c)   Celiac disease** *(Ref: R9/ 1782)*

D Xylose absorption test is a medical test to diagnose condition that cause malabsorption of proximal small intestine.

39.   **Ans. (c)   Gain of function mutation in LKB1/STK11**

(Ref: Robbins 9th/pg 806; 8th/pg 817)

40.   **Ans. (a, c)   a. Diet should exclude barley, wheat & rye;   c. Anti IgA endomycial antibody is specific**

(Ref: Robbins 9th/pg 782; 8th/pg 795)

41.   **Ans. (c)   Hamartoma**

(Ref: Robbins 9th/pg 806; SEE ans 57 Above)

Clinically history of intussuption and pathologically we see **arborization and presence of smooth muscle intermixed with lamina propria- marked with an arrow, both are suggestive of peutz jegher polyp which is a hamartomatous polyp.**

42.   **Ans. (b)   HLA DQ2** *(Ref: Robbins 9th/pg 782; 8th/pg 795)*

43.   **Ans. (a)   PAS positive macrophages and rod shaped bacilli in lamina propria**

(Ref: Robbins 9th/pg 783; 8th/pg 796)

44.   **Ans. (b)   Anti endomysial antibody**

(Ref: http://emedicine.medscape.com/article/932104-clinical, Robbins 9th/pg782;8th/p795)

45.   **Ans. (a, e);   a. Pigmentary changes in skin and mucous membrane around mouth; e. May presents as anemia in children** *(Ref: Robbins 9th/pg 806; 8th/pg 817)*

PJ Syndrome come to attention for following
- Intussception
- Mucocutaneous pigmentation
- Secondary cancers
- Hematochezia can present in 14% cases – can present as anemia

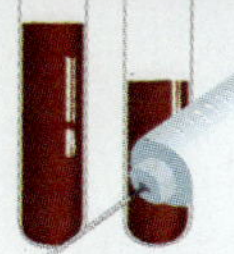

46. Ans. (a) Foamy macrophages *(Ref: Robbins 9th/pg 783)*

47. Ans. (d, e); d. Stomach is most common site for extranodal lympoma; e. MALT lymphoma is associated with H. pylori infection

(Ref: http://www.ncbi.nlm.nih.gov/pmc/articles/PMC3042647/)

48. Ans. (a) Involves in Non-Hodgkin's lymphoma

(Ref: http://www.ncbi.nlm.nih.gov/pmc/articles/C30426L47/; See Ans 66)

49. Ans. (a) Zinc

(Ref: Ross histology; 4th ed, Pathology of stomach and duodenum: 320)

50. Ans. (a) Crypt distortion; (b) Chronic inflammatory cells in the lamina propria; (c) Crypt abscess; (e) Crypt branching

(Ref: R 9th pg 799)

Noncaseating granuloma is the hallmark of Crohn's disease.

51. Ans. (c) Non-caseating granulomas are present

(Ref: Robbins 9th ed p 799)

52. Ans. (b) Aphthous ulcer (Ref: Robbins 9th ed p 799)

The earliest lesion in crohn disease, the aphthous ulcer, may progress, and multiple lesions often coalesce into elongated, serpentine ulcers oriented along the axis of the bowel.

53. Ans. (d) Crohn disease (Ref: R 9/ 798)

The picture shows – transmural inflammation(blue part) and a overlying ulcer. The best option here is Crohns disease.

54. Ans. (c, d) c. Cobblestone colon; d. String sign of kantor

Aphthoid ulcers develop into linear ulcers and fissures to produce an ulceronodular or "cobblestone" appearance.

55. Ans. (d) Cryptosporidium *(Ref: R 9th pg 800)*

56. Ans. (b) Amoebiasis *(Ref: https://msu.edu)*

57. Ans. (d) Severe bacterial infection

(Ref: Gut liver 2010, 4 (3): 338-344)

Uveitis and polyarthritis are common extra intestinal manifestation of crohn's disease.

Sacroiliitis is more common in crohn's disease (21%) as compared to U.C (12.2%) especially in patients with upper CaI or personal involvement.

Pre cholangitis is common extra intestinal manifestation of U.C.

58. Ans. (c) K RAS (Protoncogene mutation)

Normal colon	APC at 5q21	Germline (inherited) or somatic (acquired) mutations of cancer suppressor genes **("first hit")**
Mucosa at risk	APC b-catenin	Methylation abnormalities Inactivation ofnormal alleles **("second hit")**
Adenomas	K-RAS at 12p12	Protooncogene mutations
Adenomas	TP53 at 17p13 LOH at 18q21 (SMAD 2 and 4)	Homozygous loss of additional cancer suppressor genes
Carcinoma	Telomerase,	Additional mutations Gross chromosomal alterations

Remember both p53 & KRAS mutations occur, However p53 to tumor suppressor gene (not oncogene)

59. Ans. (a) Cowden's syndrome *(Ref: Robbins 9th/pg 1316)*

All are neoplastic polyp except cowden syndrome
In Cowden syndrome –there is no increased risk of GI malignancy but other organ malignancies can develop
Cowden Syndrome and Bannayan-Ruvalcaba-Riley Syndrome- autosomal dominant hamartomatous polyp syndromes associated with loss-of-function mutations in *PTEN* hence also known as **PTEN hamartoma syndrome**.

60. Ans. (b) Gastrointestinal cancer

(Ref: Am J Surg Pathol 2003;27:303)

- CDX2: Also called caudal-related homeobox gene 2, caudal type homeobox transcription factor 2
- Fairly specific marker of GI origin for adenocarcinomas

61. Ans. (a) Peutz jehers syndrome *(Ref: Robbins 9th/pg 806)*

Syndromes with hamartamotous polyps-
Cowden Syndrome and Bannayan-Ruvalcaba-Riley Syndrome- autosomal dominant hamartomatous polyp syndromes associated with loss-of-function mutations in *PTEN hence* also known as **PTEN hamartoma syndrome**.
Cronkhite-Canada Syndrome- contrasts sharply with other hamartomatous polyposis syndromes as it is nonhereditary and develops in individuals over 50 years of age

62. Ans. (c) Peutz jeghers syndrome

(Ref: Robbins 9th/pg 806)

63. Ans. (c) Increased risk of Gl maliganancy

(Ref: Robbins 9th/pg 1316)

64. Ans. (b) Rectum *(Ref: Harrison 18th ed: 350-3)*

65. Ans. (b) Ulcerative colitis

(Ref: Robbins 9th/pg 798; 8th/pg 810, harshmohan 4th ed:543)

66. **Ans. (d)** **Noncaseating granuloma**

(Ref: Robbins 9th/pg 798-800; 8th/pg 810-811)

Noncaseating granuloma is seen in chrons

67. **Ans. (b)** **Autosomal dominant** *(Ref: Robbins 9th/pg 809)*

68. **Ans. (a)** **Distal to dilated segment**

(Ref: Robbins 9th/pg 751)

69. **Ans. (a)** **Sigmoid colon** *(Ref: Robbins 9th/pg 751)*

- True diverticulum is defined by the presence **of all three layers** of the bowel wall.[Q]
- **Most common true diverticulum** is the Meckel diverticulum, which occurs in the **ileum**.
- **Acquired diverticula:** Most common site: **sigmoid colon**[Q]

70. **Ans. (a)** **Autosomal recessive**

71. **Ans. (c)** **Juvenile polyp** *(Ref: R 9th pg 808)*

72. **Ans. (d)** **Adenomatous polyps**

(Ref: Robbins 9th/pg 808,809)

Option a is pseudopolyp in inflammatory condition-are not premalignant condition

Option b- hyperplastic polyp is **Non-neoplastic polyp**

Here the doubt arises between 2 options:option c and d

Option d-adenomatous polyposis (FAP) is an autosomal dominant disorder in which patients develop numerous colorectal adenomas as teenagers

Colorectal adenocarcinoma develops in 100% of untreated FAP patients, often before age 30 and nearly always by age 50

Option c- adenomas- The most common neoplastic polyps are colonic adenomas, which are precursors to the majority of colorectal adenocarcinomas.

73. **Ans. (a)** **APC** *(Ref: Robbins 9th/pg 809; 8th/pg 820-824)*

74. **Ans. (d) No passage of stools after per rectal examination**

(Ref: http://www.aafp.org/afp/2006/1015/p1319.html)

- Most cases of Hirschsprung disease are diagnosed in the newborn period. Hirschsprung disease should be considered in any newborn that fails to pass meconium within 24-48 hours of birth-option b true
- Distal intestinal segment that lacks both the Meissner submucosal and the Auerbach myenteric plexus. - option a is true
- Proximal to aganglionic segment, colon undergoes progressive dilation
- Rectal examination may demonstrate a tight anal sphincter and explosive discharge of stool and gas - option d is false
- A rectal suction biopsy can detect hypertrophic nerve trunks and the absence of ganglion cells in the colonic submucosa, confirming the diagnosis.- option c is true

- Down syndrome (trisomy 21) is the most common chromosomal abnormality associated with the disease, accounting for approximately 10 percent of patients

75. **Ans. (d)** **100** *(Ref: Robbins 9th/pg 809; 8th/pg 820-824)*

- **Classic FAP -At least 100 polyps are necessary for a diagnosis**[Q]
- **Attenuated FAP-lower number of adenomatous polyps (around 30)**

76. **Ans. (b, c); b. Familial polyposis; c. Villous adenomas**

(Ref: Robbins 9th/pg 808,809)

77. **Ans. (a, c, d); a. Used for monitoring of recurrence of coloncaner; c. Increased in smokers; d. Increased in colon cancer**

(Ref: De Mais, Daniel. ASCP Quick Compendium of Clinical Pathology, 2nd Ed. ASCP Press 2009)

CEA-Carcinoembryonic antigen (CEA) is a **glycoprotein**[Q] CEA measurement is mainly used as a **tumor marke**r to monitor colorectal carcinoma treatment, to identify **recurrences** after surgical resection, for **staging** or to localize cancer spread through measurement of biological fluids.

78. **Ans. (c)** **AChE**

(Ref: http://ajcp.ascpjournals.org/content/126/1/9.full.pdf)

In addition to absent intrinsic ganglion cells in hirschsprung disease, most striking and diagnostically useful finding is the presence of hypertrophic nerve fibers in the myenteric and submucosal plexuses.

The diagnostic approach in hirschsprung is:

- Identify ganglion cells.- H & E stain
- Acetylcholinesterase histochemistry (AChE staining), -
  - **Hirschsprung disease**-abnormally thick and numerous nerve fibers in the muscularis mucosa and lamina propria
  - **Normal rectal mucosa**-relatively sparse, thin AChE-positive nerve fibers that are limited largely to the deep muscularis mucosa

79. **Ans. (d)** **Gardener syndrome** *(Ref: Robbins 9th/pg 1316)*

- **Gardner syndrome**: osteomas of mandible, skull, and long bones, epidermal cysts, desmoid tumors, thyroid tumors, and dental abnormalities, including **unerupted and supernumerary teeth**
- **Turcot syndrome**- intestinal adenomas and tumors of the central nervous system (**MC- Medulloblastoma or Glioblastoma**)
- **Both gardener and turcot syndrome have mutated APC gene and are associated with FAP**

80. **Ans. (b, d); b. Low fiber; d. High fat intake**

(Ref: Robbins 9th/pg 811; 8th/pg 822)

81. **Ans. (a)** **Crohn's disease** *(Ref: Robbins 9th/pg 798)*

82. **Ans. (a)** **Crohn's disease** *(Ref: Robbins 9th/pg 798)*

83.   **Ans. (a) Autosomal recessive (Ref: Robbins 9th/pg 809)**

84.   **Ans. (a) Involved in non-Hodgkins lymphoma**

(Ref: http://www.ncbi.nlm.nih.gov/pmc/articles/PMC3042647)

85.   **Ans. (d) Zollinger Ellison syndrome**

(Ref: Robbins 9th/pg 798; 8th/pg 810)

Option a, b, c occur ileum. Option d –ZES (gastrinoma) does not occur in distal ileum

86.   **Ans. (b) Usually cystic**

(Ref: World J Surg Oncol. May 19 2009;7:47)

Mesenteric tumors have been described as cystic in 40-60% of cases- **option b is true**

Solid primary tumors of the mesentery are rare- **option a is false**

Option c is false- Malignant primary mesenteric tumors are extremely uncommon

Option d is false -Two thirds of malignant mesenteric tumors are mesenchymatous (most characterized as leiomyosarcoma or liposarcoma), while the remainder are primarily lymphomas.

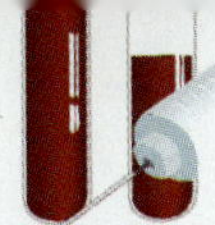

Answers with Explanations

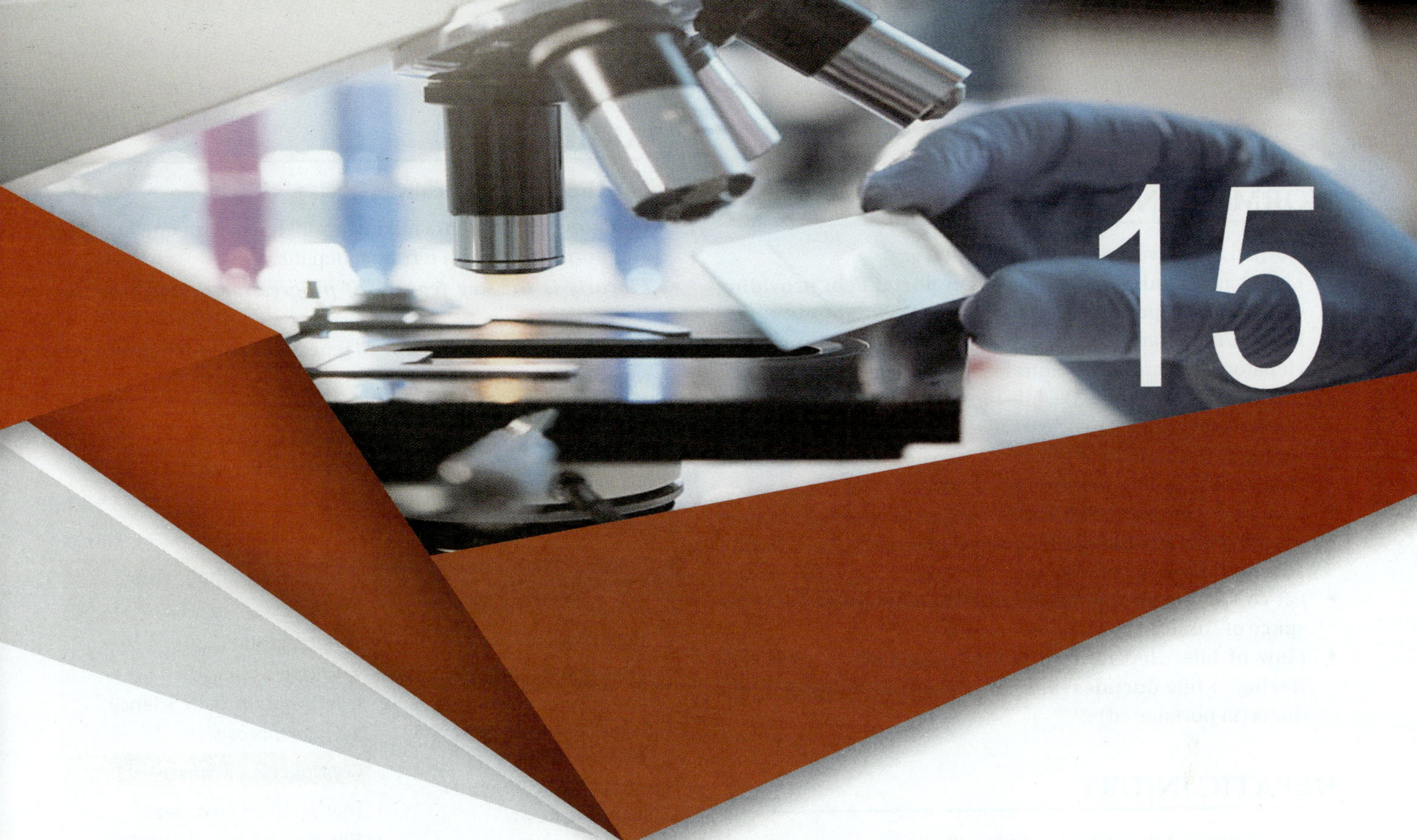

15

Liver, Gallbladder, Pancreas and its Disorders

- Normal adult liver weighs **1400 to 1600 gm & has** a **dual blood supply** from **portal vein** & **hepatic artery**
- **Kupffer cells** are **modified macrophages of the liver**
- **Acetaminophen poisoning** is the most common cause of hepatic toxicity in **Western countries**
- **Capillarization of Sinusoids is the Hallmark of Cirrhosis**
- **Proliferation & activation** of hepatic stellate cells is caused by **PDGF-β and TNF**
- Most common **mode of Hepatitis B transmission** in **India** is **Horizontal**
- **20%** of individuals **with chronic HCV** infection progress to cirrhosis
- HEV infection has the **highest mortality rate** among **pregnant** women
- Diagnostic hallmark of **Chronic Hepatitis B** is "ground-glass" hepatocytes
- Anti–liver kidney microsome-1 **(anti-LKM-1) is seen in type II autoimmune hepatitis**
- **Alcoholic liver disease begins in acinus zone 3** & extends outwards toward the portal tracts
- Most common acquired metabolic disorder is non-alcoholic fatty liver disease
- Peliosis hepatitis is associated with anabolic steroids, Danazol, OCPs and tamoxifen
- **Hepatoblastoma is the most common liver tumor of early childhood**
- **Fibrolamellar Carcinoma** is variant of HCC, associated with a generally favorable prognosis
- **Metastasis to Liver are the most common malignant tumors in liver**
- *Pancreas divisum* is the **most common^Q** congenital anomaly of the pancreas

- NASH is a component of metabolic syndrome.
- Pediatric NAFLD shows diffuse steatosis, portal fibrosis and portal and parenchymal mononuclear cells.

LIVER

NORMAL ANATOMY OF LIVER

- Normal adult liver weighs **1400 to 1600 g.**
- Liver has a **dual blood supply**, with **portal vein providing 60%-70%** & **hepatic artery** supplying **30%-40%.**
- Hepatic micro-architecture is based on the **lobular model.**
- Hepatocytes around central hepatic vein are called **"centrilobular" (zone 3)** while those near the portal tract are **"periportal"(zone 1)**
- Between the trabecular plates of hepatocytes are **vascular sinusoids,** lined by fenestrated endothelial cells.
- **Space** between **sinusoids and hepatocytes is Space of Disse.**
- **Kupffer cells** are **modified macrophages of the liver** that are attached to the sinusoids
- Fat-containing myofibroblastic **stellate cells** are found in the **space of Disse.**
- **Flow of bile:** Hepatocytes → **bile canaliculi** → **canals of Hering** → **bile ductules** (periportal region) → **terminal bile ducts** (in portal triad)

HEPATIC INJURY

Occurs in two forms: Necrosis and Apoptosis

Necrosis	Apoptosis
• Due to **ischemic** or **hypoxic** injury & **oxidative stress**[Q] • Can be Confluent, Zonal or Bridging Necrosis	• Apoptotic hepatocytes in **yellow fever** are called **'Councilman bodies'**[Q] • **Apoptotic bodies** in **acute & chronic hepatitis** are termed **acidophil bodies**[Q] (due to deep eosinophilic staining)

LIVER FAILURE

Acute Liver Failure

Acute liver illness associated with **encephalopathy and coagulopathy** that occurs **within 26 weeks** of the initial liver injury in the absence of pre-existing liver disease.

Morphology: Depends on the duration and nature of injury: shows **Massive hepatic necrosis** with **parenchymal loss** with **regenerating hepatocytes.**

High Yield Facts

- **M.C cause** of acute liver failure is massive hepatic necrosis induced by **drugs or toxins.**
- **Acetaminophen poisoning** is the most common cause in **Western countries** followed by **autoimmune hepatitis**
- In Asia, **acute hepatitis B & E** are the M.C cause of acute liver failure

CIRRHOSIS

Defined histopathologically by:

- *Bridging fibrous scars* linking portal tracts with one another and portal tracts with terminal hepatic veins.[Q]
- *Fibrosis is the key feature of progressive damage to the liver.*[Q]
- *Parenchymal nodules*: due to repeated cycles of **hepatocyte regeneration and scarring**
  - ○ <3 mm –micronodules[Q]
  - ○ >3 mm – macronodules[Q]
- *Disruption of the architecture* of the entire liver.

Causes

Acquired Causes	Inherited Metabolic Liver Disease

• **Alcoholism**
 • **Chronic viral hepatitis** (Hepatitis B & C)
 • **Non-Alcoholic Steato-Hepatitis** (NASH)
 • Autoimmune hepatitis
 • Biliary cirrhosis
   ■ Primary biliary cirrhosis
   ■ Primary sclerosing cholangitis
   ■ Autoimmune cholangiopathy
 • Cardiac cirrhosis
	• Hemochromatosis
	 • Wilson's disease
	 • α1-Antitrypsin deficiency
	 • Cystic fibrosis

	Cryptogenic Cirrhosis
	Many patients who were thought to have cryptogenic cirrhosis are ultimately found to have nonalcoholic steatohepatitis

Pathogenesis

The central pathogenic processes in cirrhosis are:

- *Death of hepatocytes*
- *Extracellular matrix (ECM) deposition* [q]
- *Vascular reorganization*[Q]

R9th Latest Update

In cirrhosis, Kupffer cell activation leads to:

Functions performed	Cytokines involved
Proliferation & activation of hepatic stellate cells	**PDGF-β and TNF**
Contraction of **myofibroblasts**	**Endothelin-1** (ET-1)
Fibrosis	**TGF-β, Metalloproteinase** 2 (MMP-2); Tissue inhibitors of MMP 1 & 2 (TIMP-1 & -2)
Chemotaxis to areas of injury	**PDGF** & monocyte chemot-actic protein-1 (**MCP-1**).

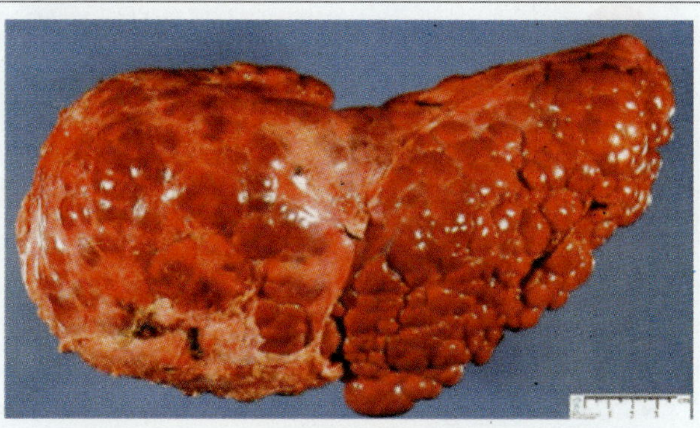

Gross liver showing nodular surface S/o Cirrhosis

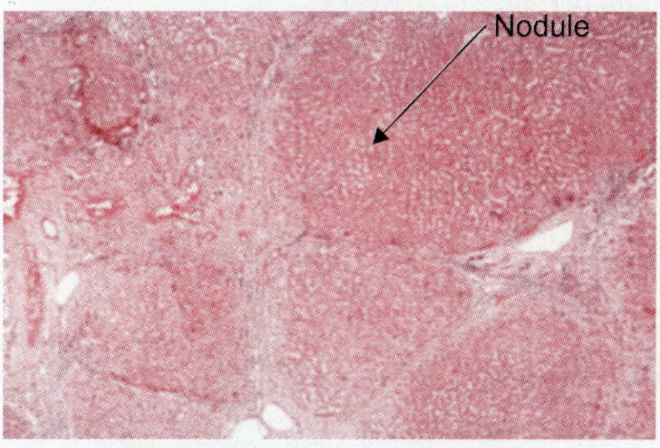

Mic of cirrhotic liver showing nodules

- **Capillarization of Sinusoids is the Hallmark of Cirrhosis[Q]**
  - **Normally** collagen **types I & III** are concentrated in portal tracts and around central veins while **type IV collagen** are present in the **space of Disse.**
  - **In cirrhosis**, types I and III collagen are deposited in the **space of Disse**
  - Leads to **loss of fenestrations** of **sinusoids (Capillarization of sinusoids)**, impairing the function of sinusoids as channels that permit the exchange of solutes between hepatocytes and plasma.

Scar Formation

- Principal cell type involved in scar deposition is the **hepatic stellate cell (ITO cells)[Q]**
- **ITO cells** are **Vitamin-A storage** cells[Q]
- In acute & chronic injury, the **stellate cells** get activated to **highly fibrogenic** cells called **myofibroblasts[Q]**

HEPATITIS

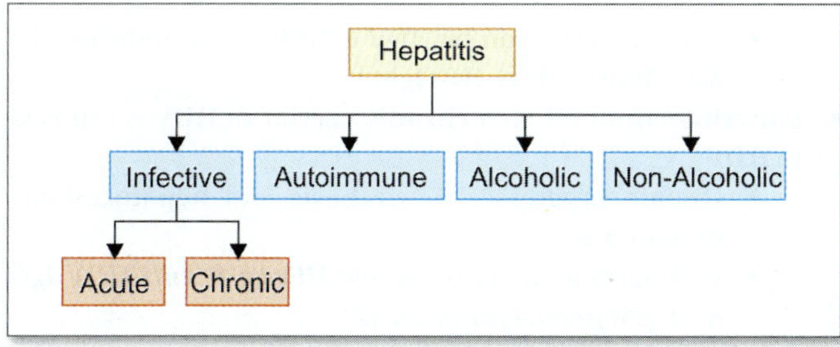

Acute Infective Hepatitis

- **Etiology: Hepatotrophic viruses**: Hep A, B, C, D and E[Q].
  - **Other Systemic Viruses which can cause hepatitis: EBV, CMV, Herpes virus and Adenovirus Yellow fever (yellow fever virus)**

Hepatitis A

- *Causative organism:* Hepatitis A virus (HAV)-Non-enveloped 27-nm, heat-, acid- & ether-resistant **RNA virus** in the *Hepatovirus* genus of the **Picornavirus** family[Q]

- *Mode of transmission:* Feco-oral[Q] (**most common**), Sexual ±[Q], Percutaneous route
- *Incubation period:* **2 to 6 weeks**[Q]
- *Clinical course*
  - **Fulminant hepatitis:** 0.1%
  - **Progression to chronicity**: None[Q]
  - **Carrier state:** None[Q]
  - **Prognosis**: Excellent
- *Serology*
  - **Early fecal shedding** of HAV **2-3 weeks before & 1 week after**[Q] the onset of jaundice.
  - **Diagnosis**: IgM anti-HAV[Q]
  - **Previous infection:** IgG anti-HAV[Q]

Hepatitis B

- *Causative organism:*
  Hepatitis B virus (HBV): Hepadna virus family
  - 42 nm double-shelled virion with spherical 3.2-kb **DNA**, circular, ss/ds **(incomplete ds)**[Q]
  - Hepatitis B has eight subtypes and eight genotypes (A–H)
  - Genotypes **B (*adw*) and C (*adr*) predominate in Asia**[Q]
- *HBV Genes & Antigens*

Gene	Antigen produced
C gene	**HBcAg**, hepatitis B core antigen
C & Pre C genes	**HBeAg** (hepatitis B e antigen)
S gene	**HBsAg,** (hepatitis B surface antigen): large, middle, and small HBsAg
P gene	**DNA polymerase (pol)** and **reverse transcriptase**
X gene	HBx Ag: virus **replication** and **transcriptional transactivator**

- *Mode of transmission*
  - In **High prevalence** regions (≥8%): **Perinatal (most important)**[Q]
  - In **Intermediate prevalence** areas **(2-7%; India)**[Q]: **Horizontal**- Blood products, percutaneous- minor breaks in the skin/mucous membranes, perinatal (vertical)
  - In **Low prevalence** areas **(<2%)**: Sexual and intravenous drug abuse.

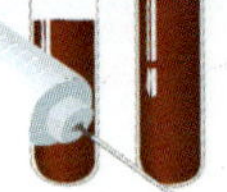

- *Incubation period:* 2 to 26 weeks
- *Clinical course in Hep B can be presented as:*

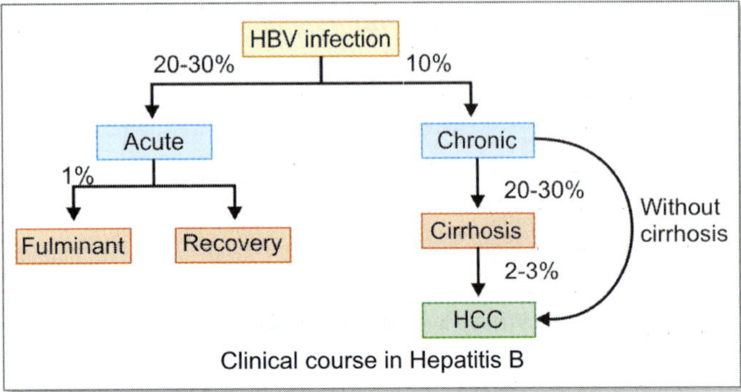

Clinical course in Hepatitis B

Serologic Patterns of Hepatitis B Infection

HBsAg	Anti-HBs	Anti-HBc	HBeAg	Anti-HBe	Interpretation
+	–	IgM	+	–	**Acute** hepatitis B, **high infectivity**[Q]
+	–	IgG	+	–	**Chronic** hepatitis B, high infectivity
+	–	IgG	–	+	**"Precore–mutant"** (HBeAg –ve)
+	+	+	+/–	+/–	**(Surface mutant)**[Q] Seroconversion from HBsAg to anti– HBs
–	–	IgM	+/–	+/–	1. Acute hepatitis B 2. Anti–HBc "window"[Q]
–	–	IgG	–	+/–	Hep B in remote past
–	+	IgG	–	+/–	Recovery from hepatitis B
–	+	–	–	–	**After Hep B vaccination**

- The most common **mode of Hepatitis B transmission in India** is: **Horizontal**[Q]
- **Age** at the time of onset of infection is the **best predictor of chronicity**
- **Younger** the age at the time of HBV infection, **higher is the probability of chronicity**
- **Prognosis** of Hepatitis B worsens with age
- **Pre-core Mutants** are strains of HBV that **do not produce HBeAg** despite HBV DNA.
- **Vaccine-induced escape mutant:** replicate in the presence of vaccine-induced immunity.

Incidence of Fulminant Hepatitis in:
- Hep A-0.1%
- Hep-B ~1%
- Hep C-0.1%
- Hep D-5.20%
- Hep E-1-2% (20% in pregnancy)

Hepatitis C

- *Causative organism:* 40–60 nm enveloped virus, 9.4-kb RNA, linear, ss**RNA** virus of **Hepacivirus** family
- *Mode of transmission:* IV drug abuse, sexual, needle-stick injury, blood products (horizontal), perinatal ±
- *Incubation period:* 15–160 days
- *Clinical course:*
  - **Fulminant hepatitis:** 0.1%[Q]
  - **Progression to chronicity:** common **upto 85%**[Q]
  - **Cirrhosis: 20%** of individuals **with chronic HCV** infection.[Q]
- *Prognosis:* Moderate

Hepatitis D

- *Causative agent:* **Hepatitis D virus (HDV) or "the delta agent," is a unique RNA virus that is dependent for its life cycle on HBV**
- *Mode of transmission:*
  - Percutaneous >Sexual> Perinatal
  - *More common in* **IV drug abusers** & *multiple blood transfusions.*[Q]
- *2 types of infection:*
  - **Co-infection:** Due to exposure to serum containing **both HDV & HBV** at the **same time**.
    - Higher rate of acute hepatic failure in intravenous drug users.
    - Acute co-infection by HDV & HBV is best indicated by **Anti-HDV & Anti-HBcIgM**[Q]
- **Superinfection:** When a **chronic carrier of HBV** is exposed to **HDV**
    - Disease progresses to **cirrhosis** and **hepatocellular carcinoma**
    - With chronic delta hepatitis, *HBsAg & anti-HDV IgG and IgM persist for months*[Q]
- *Incubation period:* 30–180 days
- *Clinical course:*
  - **Progression to chronicity: Common**[Q]
- *Prognosis:* Acute → good, but Chronic → poor
- *Prevention:* **Vaccination for HBV also prevents HDV infection**[Q]

- **Persistent infection** and **chronic hepatitis** are the **hallmarks** of HCV infection
- Due to changing structure of **HCV RNA polymerase, multiple genotypes** of viruses are found in the same patient after some duration of Hep C infection —"**Quasi-species**"
- **E2 protein** of the envelope **most variable region** of the entire viral genome → escape from neutralizing antibodies
- **Genomic instability** & **antigenic variability** are responsible for **persistent infection** & **ineffective HCV vaccine**.
- Hepatitis C (especially **HCV genotype 3**) infection is the association with **metabolic syndrome**
- HCV can give rise to **insulin resistance** & **non-alcoholic fatty liver disease** (NAFLD)

Hepatitis E

- **Causative organism:** 32–34 nm non-enveloped icosahederal 7.6 kb ss linear **RNA** of **Hepevirus family**
- **Mode of transmission:** Faeco-oral^Q
- **Incubation period:** 14–60 days
- **Clinical course:**
  - **Progression to chronicity:** None^Q (**Seen** in **AIDS** & immunosuppressed **transplant** patients)^Q
- **Prognosis:** Good (except in pregnant women)^Q

- **HEV infection** accounts for more than **30%– 60% cases of sporadic acute hepatitis** in **India, exceeding the frequency of HAV.**^{Q}
- Characteristic feature of HEV infection is the **high mortality rate** among **pregnant** women, approaching **20%.**^{Q}
- **Carrier state:** Individual who **harbors** and can **transmit** an organism, but has **no symptoms**.

Morphology of Acute Viral Hepatitis

- **Gross:** Normal or slightly mottled and in **severe cases liver may shrink** greatly.^{Q}
- **Microscopically**
  - **"Ballooning degeneration":**^{Q} Diffuse swelling due to hepatocyte injury
  - **"Dropout" of hepatocytes**: cytoplasm looks empty & is surrounded by scavenger macrophages
  - **Lymphoplasmacytic** (mononuclear) infiltrate (also seen in chronic hepatitis)
  - **Minimal** or absent **portal-inflammation**
  - **"Spotty necrosis"/lobular hepatitis:**^{Q} Scattered parenchymal injury throughout hepatic lobule
  - **Councilman body:**^{Q} Intensely eosinophilic apoptotic hepatocytes with pyknotic nucleus
  - **Confluent necrosis in severe acute hepatitis**^{Q}
  - **Central to portal bridging necrosis:**^{Q} with increasing severity
  - **Parenchymal collapse:**^{Q} In **most severe** cases

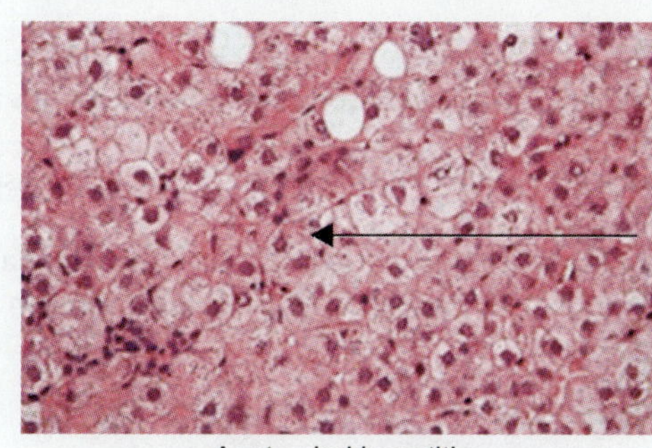

Acute viral hepatitis

Chronic Hepatitis

- **Definition:** Symptomatic, **biochemical**, or **serologic** evidence of **continuing or relapsing** hepatic disease for **more than 6 months**^{Q}

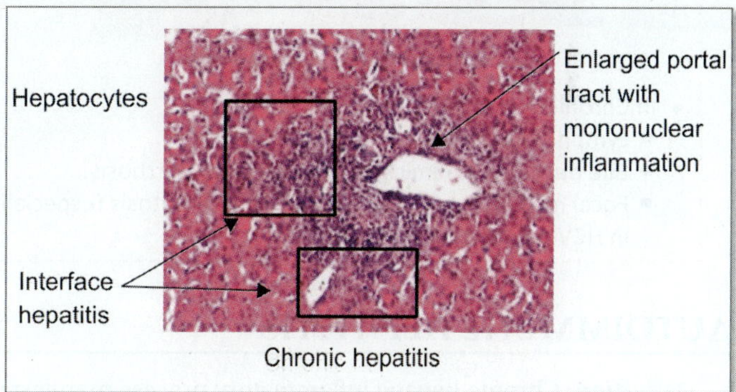

Chronic hepatitis

- **Morphology**
  - **Defining histologic feature** is **mononuclear portal infiltration**^{Q}
  - **Interface hepatitis**: Inflammatory infiltrate **at the interface** between hepatocellular **parenchyma & portal tract** stroma, along with lobular hepatitis
  - **Hallmark** of **progressive chronic liver damage** is deposition of **fibrous tissue (scarring)**^{Q}
  - May progress to **bridging fibrosis**
  - **Cirrhosis (scarring with nodule formation)** in most severe cases
- **Histologic grading & staging:** Histologic activity index (HAI) & METAVIR score: Based on Biopsy assessment-
  - Grading is based on inflammation & Necrosis
  - Staging is based on fibrosis
  - **Type of Necrosis:**
    - Periportal necrosis, including piecemeal necrosis and/or bridging necrosis
    - Intralobular necrosis: Confluent/ Focal
- **Type of Inflammatory Activity** (grade)
  - Portal Inflammation: Mild, moderate or Severe
  - **Type of Fibrosis:** Portal, Bridging, Cirrhosis

- Inflammatory cells in both **acute and chronic** viral hepatitis are **mainly T cells**
- **In Acute Hepatitis A**: mononuclear infiltrate is rich in **Plasma cells**
- Diagnostic hallmark of **Chronic Hepatitis B** is "ground-glass" **hepatocytes** (cells with **endoplasmic reticulum swollen by HBsAg**) (arrow head)

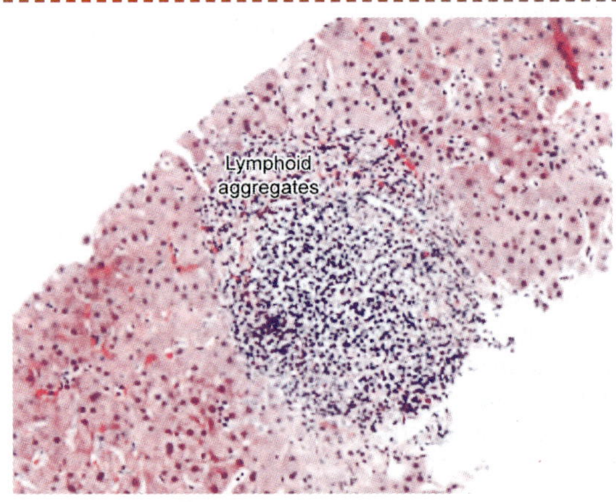

Lymphoid Aggregates in Portal Tracts

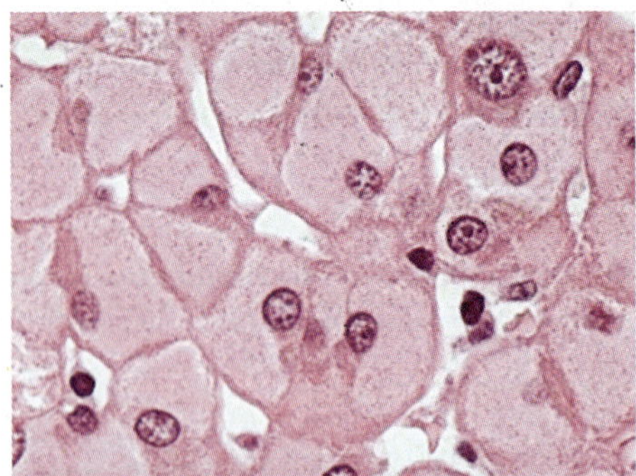

Ground Glass Hepatocytes

- In Chronic hepatitis C:
  - Lymphoid aggregates
  - Bile duct injury mimicking primary biliary cirrhosis.
  - Focal mild to moderate macrovesicular steatosis (especially in HCV genotype 3 infections)

- **Etiology** rather than the histologic pattern is the **most important determinant** of the probability of developing **progressive chronic hepatitis.**
- **Piecemeal necrosis or interface hepatitis- disruption of the limiting plate** of periportal hepatocytes by inflammatory cells[Q]
- **Piecemeal necrosis is an** important diagnostic criterion in Chronic active hepatitis
- **Bridging necrosis:** confluent necrosis that **bridges vascular structures**—between **portal tract** or between **portal tract and central vein**[Q]

AUTOIMMUNE HEPATITIS

- *Definition:* Chronic hepatic inflammatory process manifested by **elevated serum AST**, liver-associated serum **autoantibodies** and **hypergammaglobulinemia**[Q]
- *Classification: (based on serology)*

Features	Type I	Type II	Type III
Characteristic auto-antibodies	• Antinuclear **(ANA)**, • Anti–smooth muscle actin **(SMA)** • Anti–soluble liver antigen/liver-pancreas antigen **(anti-SLA/LP)** antibodies[Q] • Anti-mitochondrial **(AMA)** antibodies[Q]	• Anti–liver kidney microsome-1 **(anti-LKM-1) (directed against CYP2D6)**[Q] • Anti–liver cytosol-1 (ACL-1) antibodies	• **Absent ANA & anti-LKM1** but **anti-SLA/LP present**
Age at presentation	**Middle-aged to older individuals**[Q]	Predominantly childhood and young adulthood	More severe than type I, but is now considered a part of type I
Treatment failure	Infrequent	Frequent; relapse common	

- *Morphology (On Microscopy)*
  - **Parenchymal destruction followed rapidly by scarring:** Extensive interface hepatitis, **(perivenular or bridging necrosis)**
  - **Plasma cell predominance**[Q] in the mononuclear inflammatory infiltrates
  - Hepatocyte **"rosettes"**[Q] in areas of marked activity.

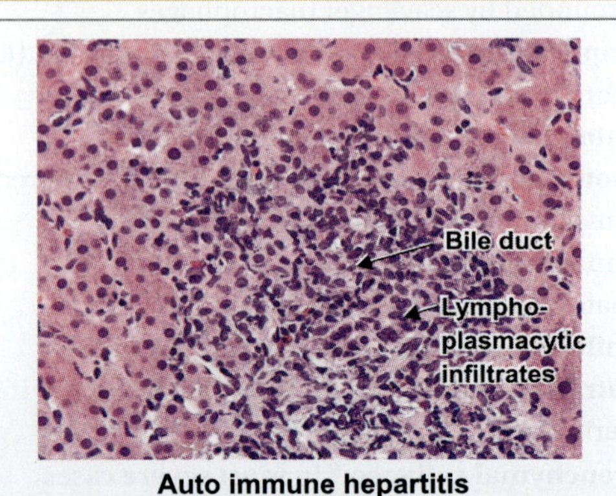

Auto immune hepartitis

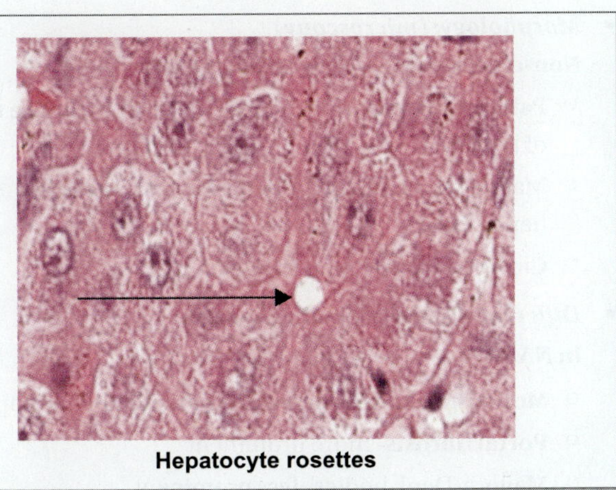

Hepatocyte rosettes

- **Prognosis**
  - Better in adults than in children
  - **Immunosuppressive** therapy leads to **remissions in 80%** of patients.[Q]

DRUG AND TOXIN INDUCED LIVER DISEASE

A diagnosis of drug or toxin-induced liver injury may be made on the basis of:

- **Temporal association** of liver damage with drug toxin exposure
- **Recovery** (usually) **upon removal** of the inciting agent
- **Exclusion** of other potential causes

Patterns of Injury in Drug- and Toxin-Induced Hepatic Injury: (Refer Answers of this Chapter)

High Yield Facts

- Alcohol produces more toxic liver injury than any other agent
- Most common hepatotoxin causing **acute liver failure** is **acetaminophen** (centrilobular hepatic necrosis)
- Most common hepatotoxin causing **chronic liver disease** is **alcohol**

ALCOHOLIC LIVER DISEASE

- **Epidemiology:**
  - Excessive ethanol consumption is the **leading cause of liver disease in the West**
  - Alcohol is the eighth highest risk factor for death
- **Dose dependent severity:**
  - In men, **>60–80 g/d** of alcohol for 10 years produces fatty liver[Q]
  - **160 g/d** for **10–20 years** causes **hepatitis or cirrhosis**
  - Only **15%** of alcoholics develop **alcoholic liver disease**.[Q]
  - Risk of developing **HCC is 1% to 6%** of cases annually[Q]
- **Risk Factors:**

- **Females are more susceptible**[Q] to hepatic injury than men
- **African Americans** are more prone. **ALDH*2**, a variant of aldehyde-dehydrogenase (ALDH), found in 50% of Asians are more prone
- **Iron overload,**[Q] infections with **HCV and HBV**[Q] synergize with alcohol.
- Concurrent **Hepatitis C** infection is associated with **younger age** for severity, more **advanced histology, decreased survival.**[Q]

- **Pathogenesis: Alcohol causes-**
  - Changes in **lipid metabolism &** decreased export of lipoproteins
  - Cell injury by **reactive oxygen species** and cytokines.
- **Clinical & Laboratory features:**
  - AST:ALT Ratio = 2:1 or 3:1[Q]
  - Increased GGT (non-specific), Bilirubin, Alkaline phosphatase
- **Morphology:** Liver disease **begins in acinus zone 3**[Q] & extends outwards toward the portal tracts.
  - **Fatty liver** (Hepatocellular steatosis):
    - Macroscopically, liver is large (4-6 kg), soft, **yellow and greasy.**
    - **Fatty change is completely reversible** if there is abstention from further intake of alcohol[Q]
    - **Microscopically, Microvesicular** fatty change that coalesces to **Macrovescicular change.**
  - **Alcoholic Steatohepatitis:**
    - Hepatocyte swelling and necrosis
    - **Mallory-Denk bodies** (previously called **Mallory Hyaline bodies**):[Q] Clumped, amorphous, eosinophilic material in ballooned hepatocytes.
    - **Neutrophilic reaction** around hepatocytes.

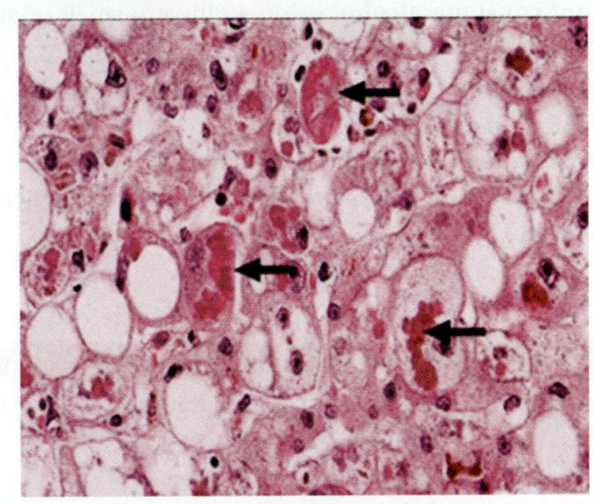

Mallory-Denk body (eosinophilic inclusions)

- **Morphology: Alcoholic steatofibrosis:**
  - Fibrosis begins with sclerosis of central veins
  - Perisinusoidal scar accumulates in the space of Disse spreading outward, encircling in a **chicken wire fence pattern**[Q]

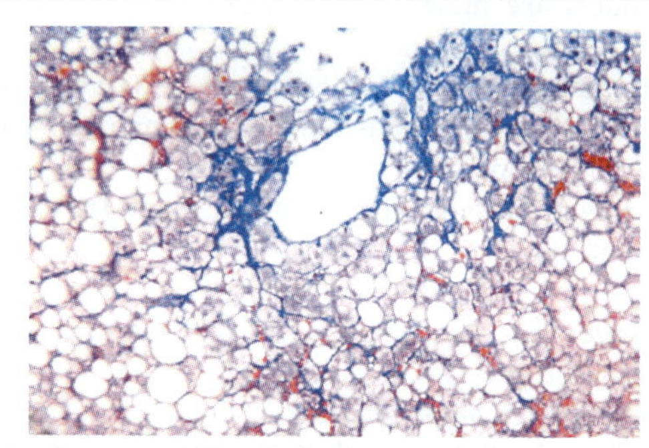

Fatty change and fibrosis (stained blue) in a characteristic perisinusoidal chicken wire fence pattern (Masson trichrome stain)

○ **Perisinusoidal scarring** leads to a classic **micronodular**[Q] or **Laennec cirrhosis**.

High Yield Facts

- **Mallory-Denk bodies** are composed of Intermediate filaments-**keratins 8 and 18 with ubiquitin.**
- **Causes of Mallory-Denk bodies: "WAIT in PHC"**
  - W : **W**ilson disease
  - A : **A**lcoholic liver disease
  - I : **I**ndian Childhood Cirrhosis
  - T : Alpha1 anti-**T**rypsin deficiency
  - P : **P**rimary Biliary Cirrhosis
  - HC : **H**epatocellular **C**arcinoma

METABOLIC LIVER DISEASE

Non-Alcoholic Fatty Liver Disease (NAFLD)

- **Definition: Hepatic steatosis** (fatty liver) in individuals **who do not consume alcohol** or do so in very small quantities (less than 20 g of ethanol/week).[Q]

- **Pathogenesis:**
  Two hit model for NAFLD.
  1. **Insulin resistance**[Q] gives rise to **hepatic steatosis**.
  2. Hepatocellular **oxidative injury**[Q] resulting in liver cell necrosis and inflammatory reactions

- **Morphology: (microscopy)**
  Non-alcoholic steatohepatitis (NASH)
  ○ Pathologic **steatosis** is defined as involving **more than 5%** of hepatocytes[Q]
  ○ Macrovesicular and microvesicular steatosis seen in hepatocytes
  ○ Cirrhosis may be seen in later stages

- **Difference from Alcoholic hepatitis:**
  In NASH:
  ○ **Mononuclear cells more** prominent than neutrophils
  ○ **Portal fibrosis**- more prominent
  ○ Mallory-Denk bodies- less prominent
  ○ Hepatocyte ballooning - less prominent

High Yield Facts

- Most common cause of **chronic liver disease** in West: **NAFLD**[Q]
- Most common cause of **metabolic liver disease**[Q] is **NAFLD**[Q]
- Most common acquired metabolic disorder is **non-alcoholic fatty liver disease**[Q]
- Histologic hallmarks of **NAFLD**[Q] are most consistently associated with the **metabolic syndrome**
- **Cardiovascular disease** is a frequent cause of **death** in patients with NASH[Q]
- Level of **hedgehog pathway activity**[Q] correlates with stage of **fibrosis** in NAFLD
- NASH has increased risk of **hepatocellular carcinoma.**[Q]
- **>90%** of previously described "**cryptogenic cirrhosis**"[Q] (i.e., cirrhosis of unknown cause) is now thought to represent such "**burned out**" NAFLD[Q]

Inherited Metabolic Diseases

- Hemochromatosis
- Wilson's disease
- α_1-antitrypsin deficiency

	Hemochromatosis	Wilson's disease	α_1-antitrypsin deficiency
Genetic Defect	HFE[Q](C282Y) gene mutation, Chr 6p21.3[Q]	ATP7B gene[Q] mutation on Chr 13[Q]	• Deficiency of α_1-antitrypsin which is a "protease inhibitor" (Pi) • Gene on **Chr 14**[Q]
Mode of Inheritance	Autosomal Recessive	Autosomal Recessive	Autosomal Recessive
Pathophysiology	Excessive iron absorption	• Decrease in copper transport into bile • Impaired incorporation of Cu into ceruloplasmin • Impaired ceruloplasmin secretion into the blood	Increased protease enzymes (neutrophil elastase, cathepsin G, and proteinase 3) released from neutrophils

Contd...

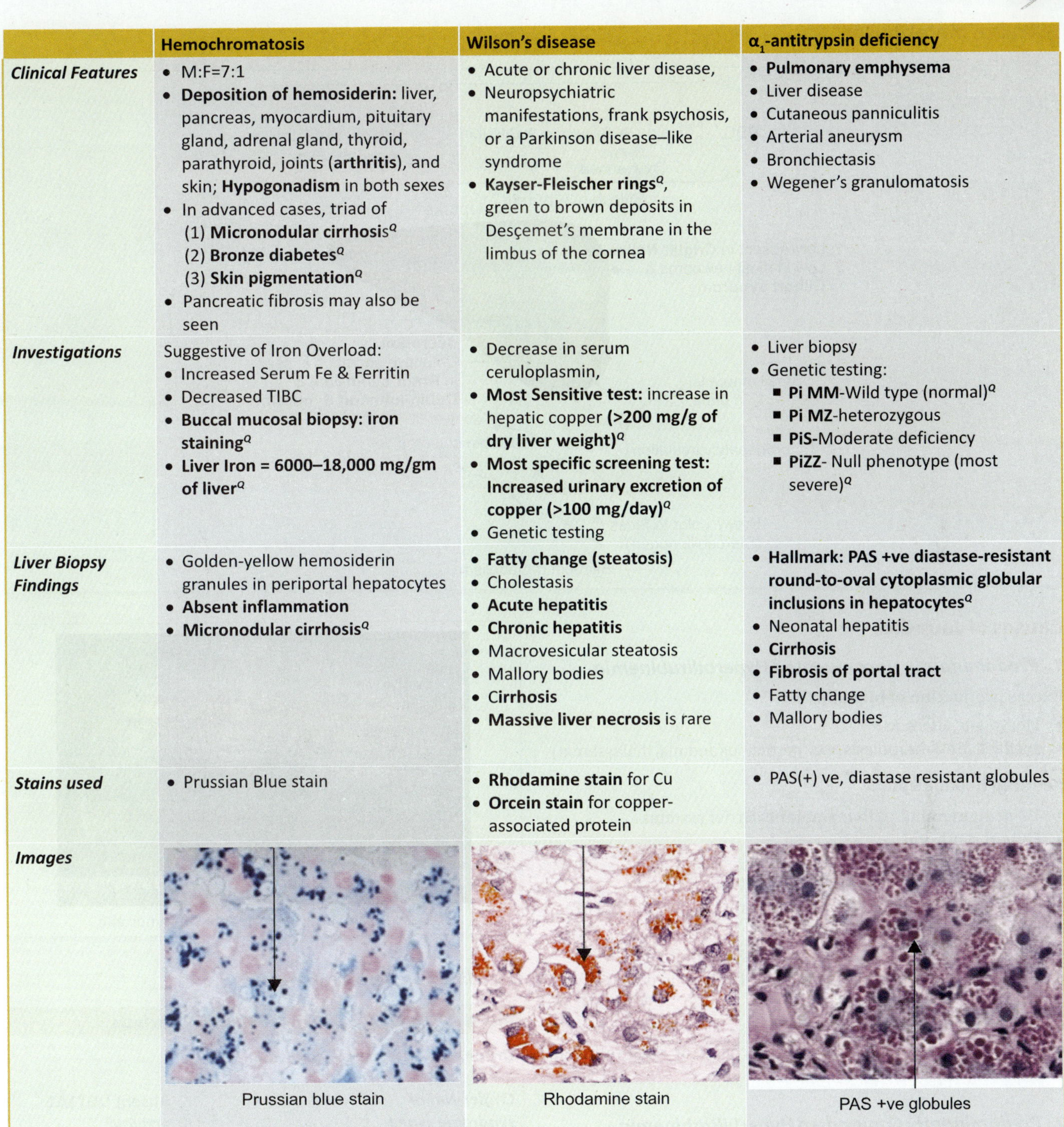

	Hemochromatosis	Wilson's disease	α₁-antitrypsin deficiency

Clinical Features	• M:F=7:1
	• **Deposition of hemosiderin:** liver, pancreas, myocardium, pituitary gland, adrenal gland, thyroid, parathyroid, joints (**arthritis**), and skin; **Hypogonadism** in both sexes
	• In advanced cases, triad of
	  (1) **Micronodular cirrhosis**[Q]
	  (2) **Bronze diabetes**[Q]
	  (3) **Skin pigmentation**[Q]
	• Pancreatic fibrosis may also be seen
		• Acute or chronic liver disease,
		• Neuropsychiatric manifestations, frank psychosis, or a Parkinson disease–like syndrome
		• **Kayser-Fleischer rings**[Q], green to brown deposits in Desçemet's membrane in the limbus of the cornea
			• **Pulmonary emphysema**
			• Liver disease
			• Cutaneous panniculitis
			• Arterial aneurysm
			• Bronchiectasis
			• Wegener's granulomatosis

Investigations	Suggestive of Iron Overload:
	• Increased Serum Fe & Ferritin
	• Decreased TIBC
	• **Buccal mucosal biopsy: iron staining**[Q]
	• **Liver Iron = 6000–18,000 mg/gm of liver**[Q]
		• Decrease in serum ceruloplasmin,
		• **Most Sensitive test:** increase in hepatic copper (>200 mg/g of dry liver weight)[Q]
		• **Most specific screening test: Increased urinary excretion of copper (>100 mg/day)**[Q]
		• Genetic testing
			• Liver biopsy
			• Genetic testing:
			  ▪ **Pi MM**-Wild type (normal)[Q]
			  ▪ **Pi MZ**-heterozygous
			  ▪ **PiS**-Moderate deficiency
			  ▪ **PiZZ**- Null phenotype (most severe)[Q]

Liver Biopsy Findings	• Golden-yellow hemosiderin granules in periportal hepatocytes • **Absent inflammation** • **Micronodular cirrhosis**[Q]	• **Fatty change (steatosis)** • Cholestasis • **Acute hepatitis** • **Chronic hepatitis** • Macrovesicular steatosis • Mallory bodies • **Cirrhosis** • **Massive liver necrosis** is rare	• **Hallmark: PAS +ve diastase-resistant round-to-oval cytoplasmic globular inclusions in hepatocytes**[Q] • Neonatal hepatitis • **Cirrhosis** • **Fibrosis of portal tract** • Fatty change • Mallory bodies
Stains used	• Prussian Blue stain	• **Rhodamine stain** for Cu • **Orcein stain** for copper-associated protein	• PAS(+) ve, diastase resistant globules
Images	Prussian blue stain	Rhodamine stain	PAS +ve globules

CHOLESTATIC DISEASES

Jaundice

Yellow discoloration of the sclera, skin, and mucous membranes indicating Hyperbilirubinemia.

Jaundice occurs when there is any one or more of following:

- Bilirubin overproduction
- Hepatitis
- Obstruction to the flow of bile

Bilirubin Metabolism

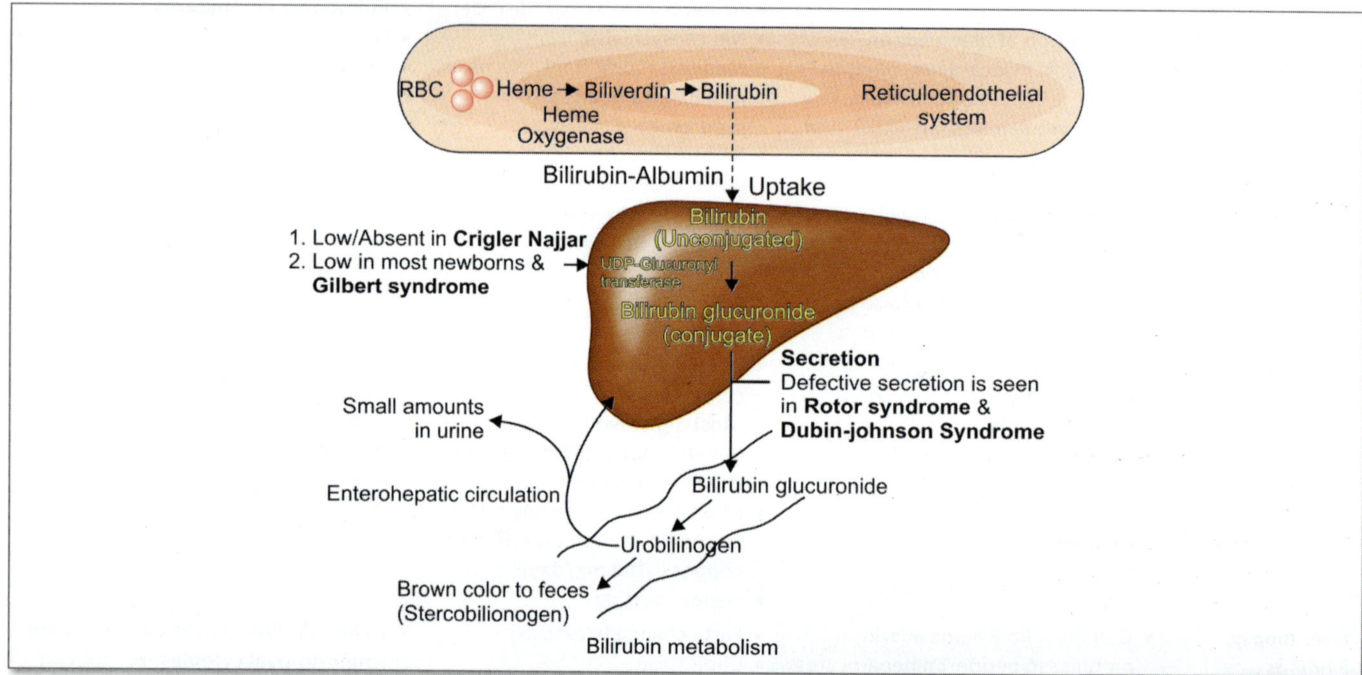

Causes of Jaundice

1. Predominantly Unconjugated Hyperbilirubinemia

Excess production of bilirubin

- Hemolytic anemias
- Ineffective erythropoiesis (e.g., pernicious anemia, thalassemia)

Reduced hepatic uptake

- Drug interference with membrane carrier systems
- Gilbert syndrome

Impaired bilirubin conjugation

- Physiologic jaundice of the newborn (decreased UGT1A1 activity, decreased excretion)
- Breast milk jaundice (β-glucuronidases in milk)
- Crigler-Najjar syndrome types I and II: Genetic deficiency of UGT1A1 activity
- Gilbert syndrome
- Diffuse hepatocellular disease (e.g., viral or drug-induced hepatitis, cirrhosis)

2. Predominantly Conjugated Hyperbilirubinemia

a. Defective secretion
- Rotor syndrome
- Dirbin johnson syndrome

b. Cholestasis
- Intrahepatic prile duct obstruction
- Extrahepatic Bile duct obstruction.

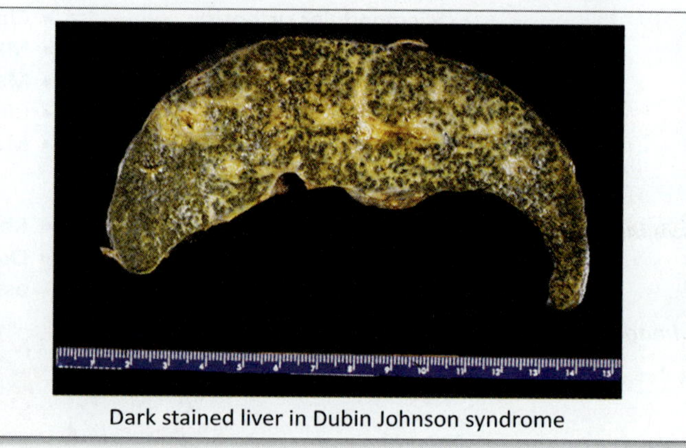

Dark stained liver in Dubin Johnson syndrome

Hereditary Hyperbilirubinemias

Disorder	Inheritance	Defects
Unconjugated Hyperbilirubinemia		
Crigler-Najjar syndrome type I	AR[Q]	Absent UGT1A1 activity[Q]
Crigler-Najjar syndrome type II	AD[Q] with variable penetrance	Decreased UGT1A1 activity[Q]
Gilbert syndrome	Promoter mutation: AR Missense mutations: AD	Decreased UGT1A1 activity[Q]

Contd...

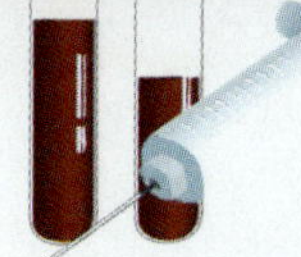

Conjugated Hyperbilirubinemia		
Dubin-Johnson syndrome	AR; mutation in canalicular multidrug resistance protein 2 **(MRP2)**[Q]	Impaired bilirubin glucuronide excretion
Rotor syndrome	AR	Decreased hepatic uptake, storage & biliary excretion
Progressive Familial Intrahepatic Cholestasis (PFIC)	AR	**PFIC1- ATP8B1** **PFIC2- ABCB11** **PFIC3- ABCB4**

Neonatal Cholestasis

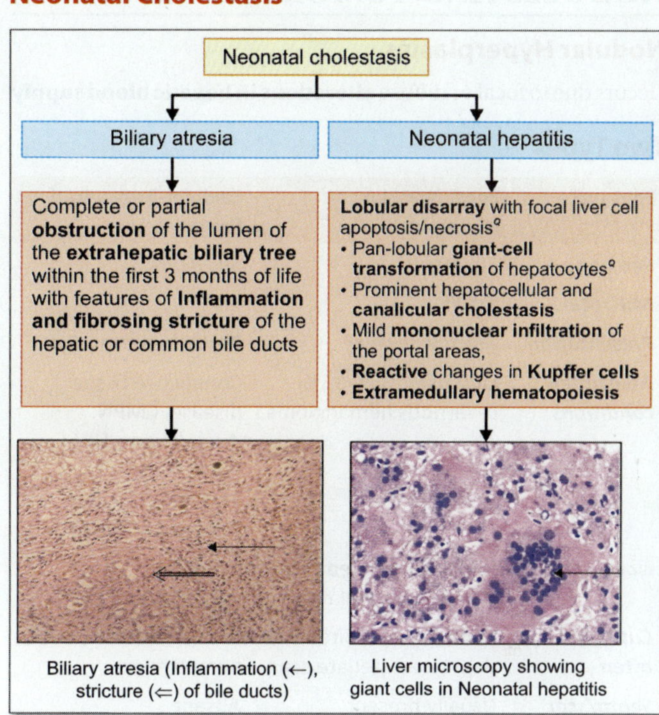

Biliary atresia (Inflammation (←), stricture (⇐) of bile ducts)

Liver microscopy showing giant cells in Neonatal hepatitis

AUTOIMMUNE CHOLANGIOPATHIES

Two Types

- Primary biliary cirrhosis
- Primary sclerosing cholangitis

Intrahepatic Biliary Disease Tract

Features	Primary Biliary Cirrhosis	Secondary Biliary Cirrhosis	Primary Sclerosing Cholangitis
Involvement	**Intrahepatic**[Q] biliary tree	**Extrahepatic**[Q] biliary tree	**Both extrahepatic**[Q] **& intrahepatic**[Q] biliary tree
Etiology	• **Sjögren syndrome**[Q] • Scleroderma • Thyroid disease	• Biliary Atresia • Gallstones • Stricture • Carcinoma of pancreatic head	• **Inflammatory bowel disease**[Q] • Retroperitoneal fibrosis
Sex predilection	F:M = 6 : 1	None	**F:M = 1 : 2**[Q]
Clinical features	**Pruritus, jaundice**, malaise, dark urine, light stools, hepatosplenomegaly		
Lab findings	**Conjugated hyperbilirubinemia, increased Alkaline Phosphatase**, bile acids, cholesterol		
Autoantibodies	**95% AMA-positive**[Q]	None; as it is not an autoimmune disease	**65% Atypical p-ANCA positive**[Q]
Important pathologic findings	**Florid duct lesions** (lympho-plasmacytic inflammation & loss of **small ducts only**	**Prominent bile stasis**[Q] in bile ducts, bile **ductular proliferation** with surrounding neutrophils, portal tract edema	**Inflammatory destruction**; fibrotic obliteration of bile ducts (**"onion-skin" fibrosis**)[Q]

NODULES AND TUMORS

Nodular Hyperplasias

Occurs due to focal or diffuse **alterations in hepatic blood supply**

Two Types

Features	Focal Nodular Hyperplasia	Nodular Regenerative Hyperplasia
Peak age	30–40 yrs	50–70 yrs
M:F ratio	**1:10[Q]**	1:1
Presentation	**Asymptomatic[Q]**	**Portal hypertension**
Associated conditions	**OCP use[Q]** (66%-95%), cavernous hemangioma	Connective tissue disease, CMPN, drugs/toxins, HIV, Post-transplant, vascular disorders, Rheumatoid arthritis
Nodules	**Well-demarcated but poorly encapsulated[Q]**	Numerous **micronodular**
Cut surface often	Central gray-white, **depressed stellate scar**	Tan-white, rarely hemorrhagic
Septa/scar	Usually present	Absent

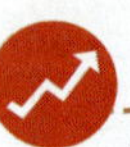

High Yield Facts

- Peliosis hepatitis is associated with **anabolic steroids, Danazol, OCPs and tamoxifen**
- Von Meyenburg Complexes are "bile duct hamartomas," mimic metastases to the liver
- **Primary Sclerosing Cholangitis is an autoimmune disease that predominantly occurs in males**
- **Primary Sclerosing Cholangitis** is associated with inflammatory bowel disease in 70% cases.
- Prevalence of PSC in persons with ulcerative colitis is about 4%
- **AMA**-Anti-mitochondrial Ab directed against **E2 component of the pyrurate dehydrogenase[Q]** complex (PDC-E2)
- **Atypical p-ANCA (perinuclear staining pattern)[Q]** seen in **Primary Sclerosing Cholangitis**, is directed **against a nuclear envelope protein[Q]**, instead of myeloperoxidase**)**.

Benign Tumors

- **M**ost **common benign liver tumor** is **Cavernous hemangioma.[Q]**

Hepatocellular Adenomas

- Benign neoplasms developing from hepatocytes.
- **Associated with: Oral contraceptives[Q] (estrogen rich) and anabolic steroids**.
- **Morphology of Hepatic adenoma: Cords of hepatocytes, with an arterial vascular supply without portal tracts.[Q]**

Latest Update

Classification of adenomas

- **HNF1-α inactivated adenomas**
  - No risk of malignant transformation
  - Often associated with OCP use
  - In individuals with MODY-3
- **β-Catenin activated adenoma:** Mutation in the β-catenin gene
  - Diagnostic hallmark: Nuclear translocation for β-catenin
  - Leading to marked atypia
  - Very high risk for malignant transformation
- **Inflammatory adenomas:**
  - Associated with non-alcoholic fatty liver disease
  - Characterized by activating mutations in gp130, a co-receptor for IL-6 leading to JAK-STAT signaling and overexpression of acute phase reactants (C-reactive protein & serum amyloid-A)
  - 10% have β-catenin activating mutations
  - Risk for malignant transformation is intermediate

Malignant Tumors

Hepatoblastoma

- **Most common liver tumor of early childhood.[Q]**
- Rarely occurs beyond the age of 3 years.
- Characterized by: Activation of the **WNT signaling pathway[Q]** (APC gene)
- Associated with **Beckwith-Wiedemann syndrome[Q]**

Hepatocellular Carcinoma (HCC)

- *Epidemiology:*
  - Peak incidence age: 20-40 yrs; M:F = 4-8:1
- Factors associated with increased risk of HCC
  - *Common*
    - **Cirrhosis (M.C)[Q]**
    - **Hepatitis B >>C** chronic infection
    - Chronic Alcoholism
    - **NASH/NAFLD**
    - Aflatoxin B_1 or other mycotoxins
  - *Less common causes*
    - Primary biliary cirrhosis **Hemochromatosis,** α1 Anti-trypsin deficiency
    - Glycogen storage diseases
    - Citrullinemia, Porphyria cutanea tarda, **Hereditary tyrosinemia,**
    - **Wilson's disease**

Latest Update

Genetic Factors:

- **Activation of β-catenin** (40% cases) & **inactivation of p53** (60% cases) are the 2 most common early mutational events
- Activation of **IL-6/JAK STAT pathway** suppress hepatocyte differentiation & promote their proliferation by regulating function of transcription factor HNF4-α

- **Gross Morphology:**
  - Unifocal (usually large) mass or Multifocal, Diffusely infiltrative
- **Light Microscopy**
  - Pattern of growth can be **trabecular, solid, or tubular with Mallory hyaline bodies**
- **Ultrastructural findings:**
  - Malignant hepatocyte with **numerous mitochondria,**[Q] **microbodies** & abundant **glycogen.**[Q] Cells also contain intracytoplasmic bile products
- **Immunohistochemistry**
  - **HepPar-1**[Q] is a **monoclonal antibody** that reacts to a cytoplasmic marker of normal & neoplastic hepatocytes

- **Glypican-3**[Q] - stains most **hepatocellular carcinomas** (especially those associated with cirrhosis) and **high-grade dysplastic nodules**, but not normal liver (**most specific**)
- **Serum markers**
  - **p-CEA (canalicular staining): 100% specificity;**[Q] often **negative in Poorly Differentiated**-HCC
  - **AFP:** 90-95% specificity, Arginase-1, TTF-1, **PIVKA-2**[Q], **DCP (Des CarboxyProthrombin)**[Q]
- **Metastasis from HCC:**
  - **Intrahepatic metastases,** by either vascular invasion or direct extension
  - **Hematogenous metastases** (extrahepatic): occurs to **lung** & portal vein and **right side of heart** via IVC

R10th Latest Update

Precursor Lesions of Hepatocellular Carcinoma (HCC)

Characteristics	Hepatocellular Adenoma	Small cell change	Large cell change	Low-grade Dysplastic Nodule	High-Grade Dysplastic Nodule
Focality in liver	Single or multiple	Diffuse	Diffuse	Single or multiple	Single or multiple
Premalignant	Yes	Yes	In Some HBV	Uncertain	Yes
Association with cirrhosis	Rare	Common	Common	Usual	Usual

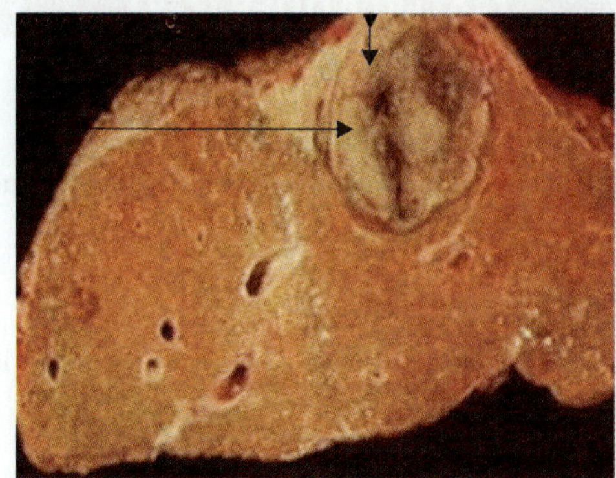

Gross showing gray white growth in liver S/o HCC

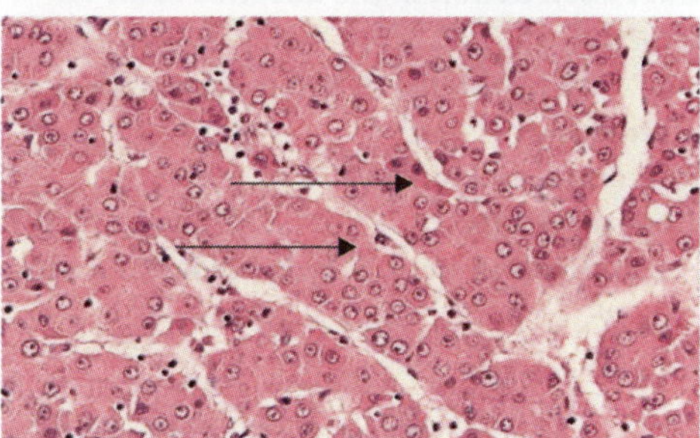

Trabecular pattern in HCC

Fibrolamellar Variant of HCC

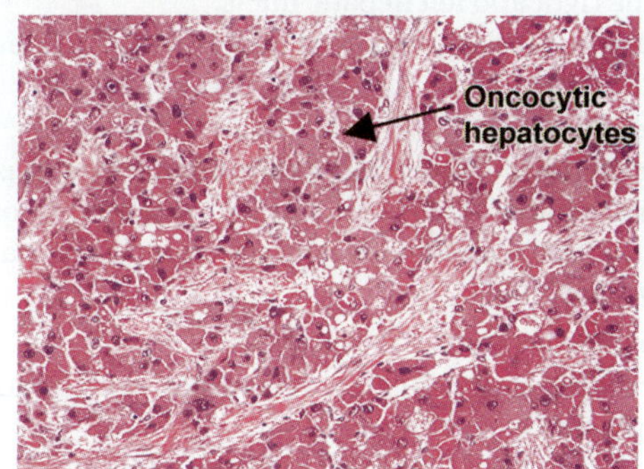

Nests and cords of malignant-appearing, oncocytic hepatocytes separated by dense bundles of collagen

Hepatocellular Carcinoma vs Fibrolamellar Variant of Hepatocellular Carcinoma

	Hepatocellular Carcinoma	Fibrolamellar variant of HCC
Age	70 years	20-30 years
Male : Female	3-4:1	1 : 1
Tumour marker	Alphafetoprotein (AFP) very high	AFP Normal, but **Neurotensin** elevated
Prognosis	Poor	Good

Cholangiocarcinoma (CCA)

- **Origin:** Biliary tree, arising from bile ducts within and outside liver.
- **Risk Factors**
  - Chronic inflammation, cholestasis, hepatolithiasis & fibropolycystic liver disease and primary sclerosing cholangitis
  - Liver flukes (Opisthorchis and Clonorchis species)
  - Hepatitis B and C

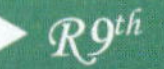

$R9^{th}$ Latest Update

Precursor Lesions of Cholangiocarcinoma

Characteristics	Biliary intraepithelial neoplasia, high grade (BilIN-3)	Mucinous cystic Neoplasm	Intraductal papillary Biliary Neoplasia
Focality in liver	Diffuse or multifocal	Single	Focal or diffuse
Commonly associated diseases	PSC, Hepatolithiasis, Liver flukes	None	None
Association with cirrhosis	Sometimes	No	No

- **Site**
  - **Extrahepatic forms:**[Q]
    - 50-60 % **perihilar (Klatskin tumor)**[Q]: At the junction of the right and left hepatic ducts.
    - 20% to 30% are distal and posterior to the duodenum.
  - Intrahepatic-10%.
- **Clinical Features:**
  - **Intrahepatic:** Cholestasis, symptomatic liver mass
  - **Extrahepatic** (hilar & distal): symptoms of biliary obstruction, cholangitis, right upper quadrant pain.
- **Morphology**
  - **Gross:** Small to massive lesions
  - **Microscopically: Adenocarcinoma**[Q] with marked **desmoplasia**[Q]
- **Prognosis:** Poor

High Yield Facts

- **Metastasis to Liver are the most common malignant tumors in liver (more common than primary).**[Q]
- Common primary sites from where **Metastasis occurs to Liver are colon, breast, lung, and pancreas.**[Q]
- **Biliary intraepithelial neoplasias** (BilIN-1, -2, or -3: low to high grade,) are premalignant for **cholangiocarcinoma**
- **BilIN-3**, the highest grade lesion, incurs the **highest risk** of malignant transformation
- **Cholangiocarcinoma is the second** most common **primary malignant tumor** of the liver after HCC[Q]

$R9^{th}$ Latest Update

Other Primary Hepatic Malignant Tumors

Tumors	Characteristics
Combined hepatocellular & cholangiocarcinoma	Originates from a multipotent stem cell.
Mucinous cystic neoplasms & Intraductal papillary biliary neoplasia	May occur as in situ lesions or as invasive cholangiocarcinoma.
Angiosarcoma of liver	Associated with **vinyl chloride, arsenic, or Thorotrast exposure**, poor prognosis
Epithelioid hemangioendo-thelioma	Endothelial malignancy, better prognosis
Hepatic lymphomas	Most are **diffuse large B-cell lymphomas**> MALT lymphomas. Seen in middle aged men Associated with Hep B, Hep C, HIV, and PBC.
Hepatosplenic delta-gamma T cell lymphoma	Most common in young adult males, has a predilection for **hepatic & splenic sinusoids** as well as the marrow.

GALLBLADDER (GB)

Acute Cholecystitis

- **Definition:** Acute inflammation of GB
- **Etiology:** 90% cases caused by obstruction **(stone); 10% Acalculous**

Acalculous Cholecystitis

- **Definition:** Inflammation of GB resulting from ischemia (cystic artery is an end artery)
- **Pathophysiology: Inflammation and edema** of the GB wall, GB **stasis,** accumulation of biliary sludge & mucus, causing **cystic duct obstruction** in the **absence of stone**.
- **Risk factors**
  - **Sepsis**[Q] with hypotension and multisystem organ failure;
  - **Immunosuppression**[Q]
  - Major trauma and **burns**
  - **Diabetes mellitus**[Q]
  - Infections: **Salmonella, Staphylococci, E.coli**[Q]

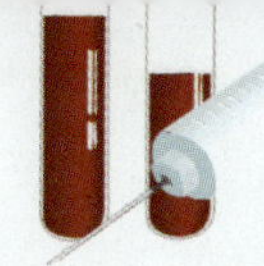

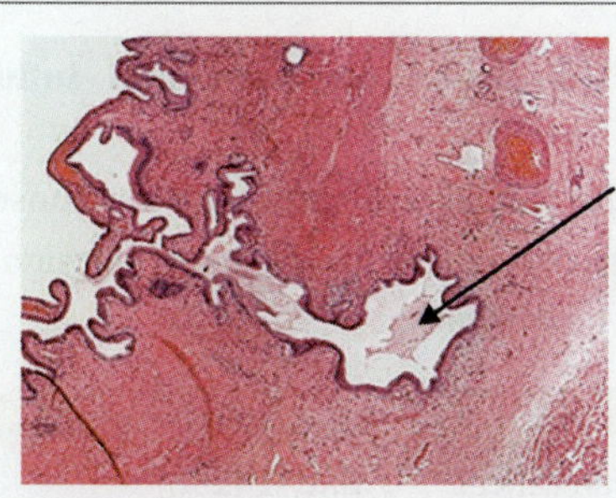

Rokitansky-Aschoff sinus Chronic cholecystitis

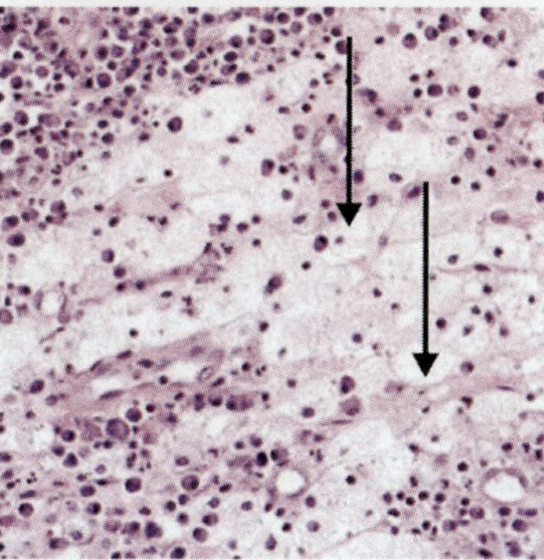

Image shows infiltrate of foam cells S/o xanthogranulomatous cholecystitis

Chronic Cholecystitis

- *Definition:* Chronic inflammation of GB which may be a **sequel** to repeated bouts of acute cholecystitis, or in absence of antecedent attacks.
- *Etiology:* Associated with ***cholelithiasis in more than 90% of cases***[Q]
- *Morphology:*
  - **Rokitansky-Aschoff sinuses**[Q]**:** Outpouchings of the mucosal epithelium through the wall
  - **Porcelain gallbladder:**[Q] **Dystrophic calcification** within GB wall, Increased **GB cancer**.[Q]
  - **Xanthogranulomatous cholecystitis**:·
    - Massively thickened, shrunken, nodular wall, chronically inflamed with foci of necrosis & hemorrhage
    - **Triggered by rupture** of **Rokitansky-Aschoff sinuses** into wall of GB, followed by accumulation of **lipid laden foamy macrophages (xanthoma cells)** 
- **Hydrops of GB:** Atrophic, chronically obstructed gallbladder containing clear secretions

Adenomyomatosis GB

Benign proliferation of gallbladder surface epithelium with gland-like formation, extramural sinuses, transverse strictures, and/or fundal nodule ("adenoma" or "adenomyoma") formation.

High Yield Facts

- In the West, 90% of gallstones are cholesterol stones, rest are pigment stones composed of bilirubin calcium salts
- **Carcinoma gallbladder is the most common malignancy of the extrahepatic biliary tract**.[Q]

Carcinoma Gallbladder

- *Epidemiology*
  - Occurs most frequently in the **seventh decade** of life
  - It is slightly **more common in women** (M:F = 1:2)
- *Risk factors:* Gallstones (cholelithiasis)[Q]
- *Genetics:* ERBB2 (Her-2/neu) mutation
- *Gross Morphology*
  - Most common sites of involvement are the fundus and the neck;
  - Only 20% involve the lateral walls.
  - **Infiltrating (more common)**[Q] or **exophytic**.
- *Microscopy:* **Adenocarcinoma**[Q] > Squamous cell Ca> Carcinosarcoma
- *Prognosis:* **Papillary tumors** have a **better prognosis**[Q].

PANCREAS

CONGENITAL ANOMALIES

- *Pancreas Divisum*
  - **Most common**[Q] congenital anomaly of the pancreas
  - **Failure of fusion** of the fetal duct systems of the dorsal and ventral pancreatic primordia
  - Predisposes to **chronic pancreatitis**[Q]
- *Annular Pancreas:* **Band-like ring** of normal pancreatic tissue that encircles the 2nd part of duodenum
- *Ectopic Pancreas:* In sites like **stomach & duodenum**[Q], followed by the jejunum, Meckel diverticula & ileum
- *Agenesis of Pancreas:* Due to mutation in **PDX1 gene**, encoding a homeobox transcription factor that is critical for pancreatic development

High Yield Facts

- **Pancreas is a retroperitoneal organ** extending from the C-loop of the duodenum to the hilum of the spleen.
- Pancreas develops from dorsal & ventral pancreatic primordial buds.
- Pancreas consists of an:
  - Exocrine part (80% to 85%) that secrete enzymes, stored in granules as proenzymes (zymogens)[Q]
  - Endocrine part: that secretes important hormones
- Somatostatin is also secreted by extra-islet neuroendocrine cells

ACUTE PANCREATITIS

- *Definition:* **Reversible** pancreatic parenchymal injury associated with inflammation.
- *Etiology:*
  - **Excessive alcohol intake (most common)**[Q]
  - Pancreatic duct obstruction (e.g. **gallstones**)
  - Traumatic injuries
  - **Drugs:** Azathioprine, L-Asparaginase, Furosemide, estrogens, Dideoxyinosine
  - Infections e.g. **mumps**[Q]

- ○ Metabolic disorders leading to **hypercalcemia**^{Q}
- ○ Ischemia
- ○ Hereditary factors
- *Genetic factors:*

Gene (chr)	Protein product	Function / Characteristics
CFTR (7q31)	Cystic fibrosis transmembrane conductance regulator	**Loss-of-function mutations** limit HCO_3 secretion → inspissation of secreted fluids & **duct obstruction**
PRSS1 (17q34)	Serine protease 1 (trypsinogen 1)	Cationic trypsin, **Gain-of – function mutations prevent self-inactivation of trypsin**
SPINK1 (5q32)	Serine protease inhibitor, kazal type 1	Inhibitor of trypsin, **Mutations cause** loss-of-function, **increasing trypsin activity**

- *Morphology:*
  - ○ **Inappropriate activation** of digestive **enzymes within** the substance of the **pancreas** leads to:
    - • Microvascular leak and edema, Fat necrosis, Acute inflammation, Destruction of pancreatic parenchyma, Destruction of blood vessels and interstitial hemorrhage

PANCREATIC CYSTIC NEOPLASMS

- **Serous cystic neoplasms: (also known as serous cystadenomas): VML gene:** always Benign
- **Mucinous Cystic Neoplasms: 1/3rd** associated with **invasive adenocarcinoma**^{Q}
- **Intraductal papillary mucinous neoplasms (IPMNs): Can progress to an invasive cancer.**^{Q}
- **Solid-pseudopapillary neoplasms: Wnt signaling pathway (β-catenin)**^{Q} **oncogene**

PANCREATIC CARCINOMA

- *Precursor lesions:* "Pancreatic intraepithelial neoplasias" (PanINs)
- *Molecular Alterations:*

Gene	Chr	%	
KRAS	12p	90	**Most commonly involved Oncogene**^{Q}
p16/CDKN2A	9p	95	**Most commonly involved Tumor suppressor gene**^{Q}
TP53	17p	50-70	**Involved in Response to DNA damage**
SMAD4	18q	55	**TGF β pathway**
BRCA2	13q	10	**Germ-line mutation**^{Q}

- *Etiology:*
  - ○ **Cigarette smoking (strongest environmental influence)**^{Q}**, Fat rich diet**
  - ○ **Chronic pancreatitis** & diabetes mellitus (new-onset diabetes mellitus in an older patient may be the first sign)
- *Inherited Predisposing conditions:*

Disorder	Gene (Chromosome)
Hereditary breast and ovarian cancer	BRCA2 (13q)
Familial atypical multiple-mole melanoma syndrome	p16/CDKN2A (9p)
Hereditary pancreatitis	PRSS1 (7q) and SPINK1
Peutz-Jeghers syndrome (maximum risk of Pancreatic Ca)	LKB1 (19p)
Hereditary Non polyposis Colorectal Cancer (HNPCC)$^{R9^{th}}$	MLH1, MSH2 (2p) $^{R9^{th}}$

- *Site:* **Pancreatic Head (most common)**^{Q} > Body > Tail
- *Clinical features:*
  - ○ 50% **Pancreatic Head** Carcinoma develop **jaundice**
- *Important Characteristics*
  - ○ **Mostly adenocarcinoma**^{Q}**, Highly invasive**

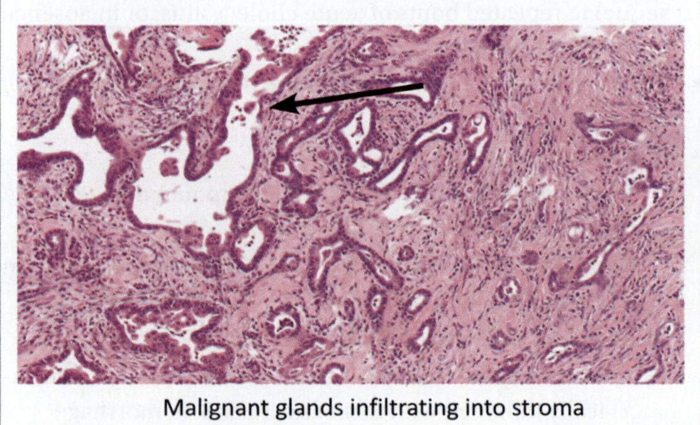
Malignant glands infiltrating into stroma

- ○ Elicits "**desmoplastic** response" (dense fibrosis).
- ○ **Migratory thrombophlebitis (Trousseau sign)**^{q}**, 10%**- due to release of **Platelet activating factor** and procoagulants from carcinoma or its necrotic products.

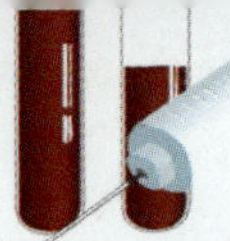

R10ᵗʰ Latest Update

Molecular serum markers of liver fibrosis

Marker	Function
Liver function	
ALT	Metabolic enzymes in the liver
AST	Metabolic enzymes in the liver
ECM formation	
PHINP	Propeptide of collagen type III
PINP	Propeptide of collagen type I
Type IV collagen	Basement membrane formation
P4NP 7S	N-terminal pro-peptides of type IV collagen 7S domain
PVCP	Propeptide of collagen type V
HA	Component of ECM
YKL-40	Glycoprotein involved in ECM turnover
MFAP	Glycoprotein involved in ECM turnover
Fibrinolytic process	**Neo-epitope**
MMP-1/MMP-13	Degrade fibrotic matrix
MMP-2	Degrades basal membranes and fibrotic matrix
MMP-9	Degrades basal membranes
TIMP-1	Inhibits MMP-1 activity

Marker	Function
ECM degradation	
CO3-610	Collagen type III fragment generated by MMP-9
CO6-MMP	Collagen type VI fragment generated by MMP-2,9
CO1-764	Collagen type I fragment generated by MMP-2,9,13
C4M	Collagen type IV fragment generated by MMP-9
Cytokines	
TGF-β	Growth factor stimulates production of ECM by HSC
CTGF	Potent pro-fibrogenic factor
PDGF	Growth factor stimulates proliferation of HSC
TNF-α	Inflammatory cytokine involved in fibrogenesis
IL-4, 6, 8, 18	Inflammatory cytokine involved in fibrogenesis

R10ᵗʰ Latest Update

Laboratory Evaluation of Liver Disease

Test Category	Blood Measurement*
Hepatocyte integrity	Cytosolic hepatocellular enzymes 1. *Serum aspartate aminotransferase* (AST) 2. *Serum alanine aminotransferase* (ALT) 3. Serum lactate dehydrogenase (LDH)
Biliary excretory function	Substances normally secreted in bile† • *Serum bilirubin* • *Urine bilirubin* • *Serum bile acids* • Plasma membrane enzymes (from damage to bile canaliculus) *Serum alkaline phosphatose* *Serum, γ-glutamyl transpeptidase* (GGT)
Hepatocyte function	Proteins secreted into the blood • *Serum albumin* • *Prothrombin time* (PT) • *Partial thromboplastin time* (PTT) Hepatocyte metabolism • Serurn ammonia • Aminopyrine breath test (hepatic demethvlation)

R10ᵗʰ Latest Update

World Health Organization Criteria for the Metabolic Syndrome

One of	Diabetes mellitus *or* Impaired glucose tolerance *or* Impaired fasting glucose *or* Insulin resistance
and two of:	• **Blood pressure:** ≥ 140/90 mm Hg • **Dyslipidemia:** Triglycerides (TG): ≥1.695 mmol/L and high-density lipoprotein cholesterol (HDL-C) ≤ 0.9 mmol/L (male), ≤1 mmol/L (female) • **Central obesity:** waist-hip ratio> 0.90 (male); > 0.85 (female), or body mass index > 30 kg/m² • **Microalbuminuria:** urinay albumin excretion rate of ≥ 20 µg/min of albumin-to-creatinine ≥30 mg/gm

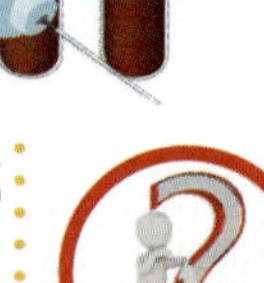

NEXT Pattern Questions

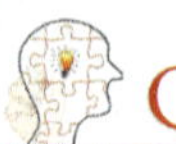 Q's

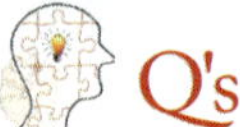 Q's

1. A 44-year-old patient presented with jaundice and had needle prick injury 2 years back and liver biopsy shown below. Based on the histological features what classify type of hepatitis?

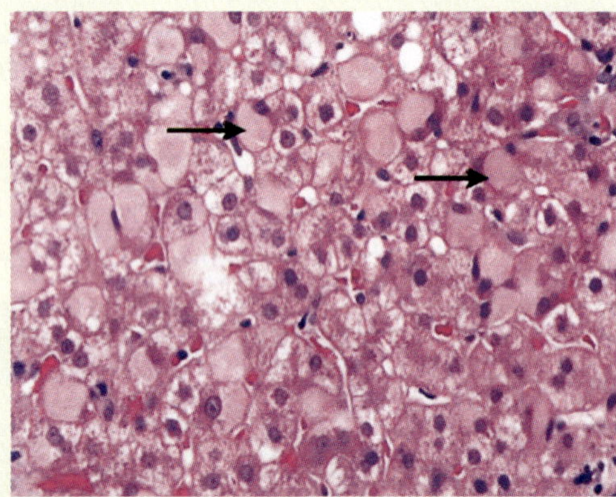

a. Hepatitis B virus induced hepatitis
b. Hepatitis C virus induced hepatitis
c. Hepatitis A virus induced hepatitis
d. Hepatitis E virus induced hepatitis

Ans. (a) Hepatitis B virus induced hepatitis

- With a history of Jaundice for last 2 years and the liver biopsy showing homogeneous pink color suggestive of ground glass appearance, this is most likely to be the case of Hepatitis B infection.

2. A 54-year-old patient presented with jaundice (raised direct bilirubin) and presence of pANCA antibody. Liver biopsy shows the following. Which of the following statement are true regarding the condition?

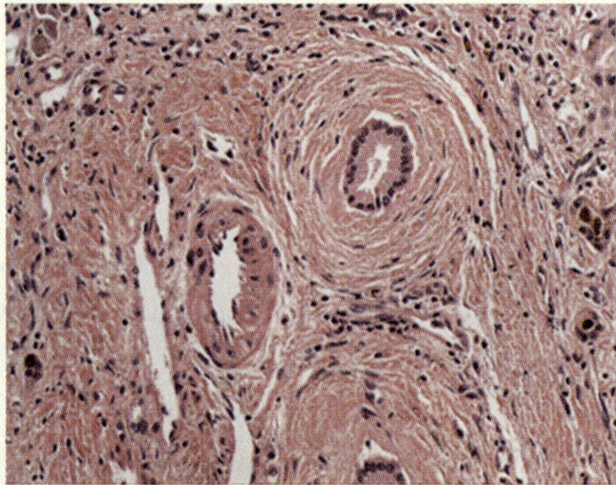

a. Most common antibody seen is pANCA
b. It is associated with ulcerative colitis
c. On histology it shows circumferential onion skin fibrosis around duct
d. All of the above

Ans. (d) All of the above

- Obstructive jaundice (raised direct bilirubin) and presence of pANCA antibody is suggestive of primary sclerosing cholangitis. 70% cases are often seen with ulcerative colitis. Biopsy of liver will show circumferential onion skinning appearance.

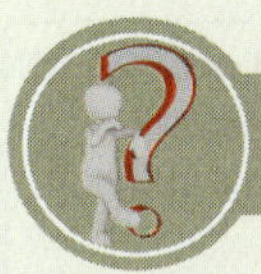

Image-Based Questions

1. Liver biopsy from a patient shows dark brownish-black deposits in hepatocytes, canaliculi, Kupffer cells, and ductules. Polarised microscopy of the same shows maltese cross picture of red birefringence in the larger deposits. What is your diagnosis?

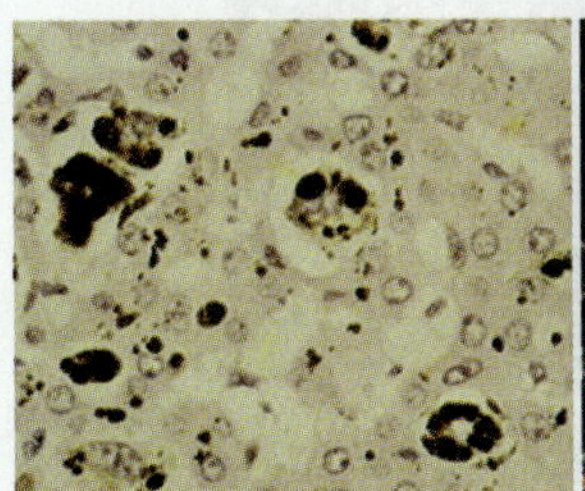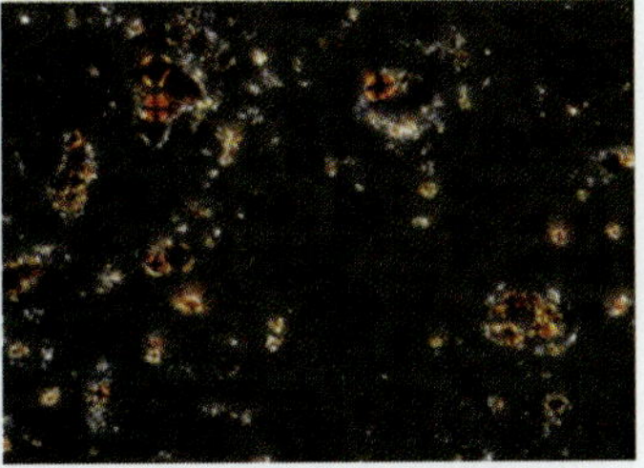

a. Melanosis
b. Cholestasis
c. Erythropoietic protoporphyria
d. Hepatitis B

2. A 61-year-old man had leg swelling with grade 2 pitting edema upto the knees, prominent jugular venous distention to the level of the mandible & increasing levels of serum AST and ALT. A diagnosis of congestive heart failure was made. The gross appearance of the liver has been shown in the figure. Identify the condition?

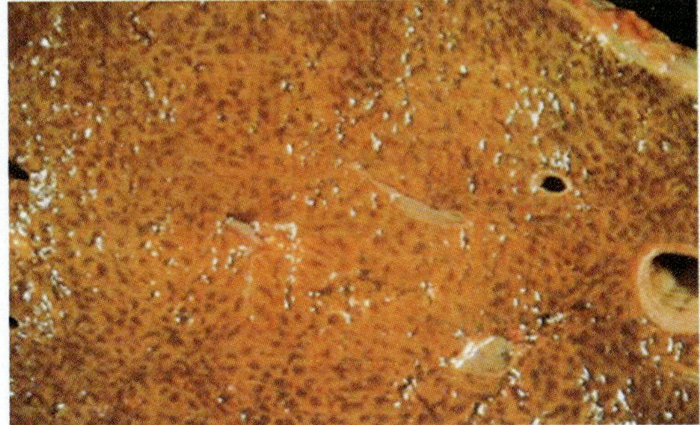

a. Portal vein thrombosis
b. Cirrhosis
c. Fatty liver
d. Chronic venous congestion

3. Identify the areas Labeled 1, 2 and 3?

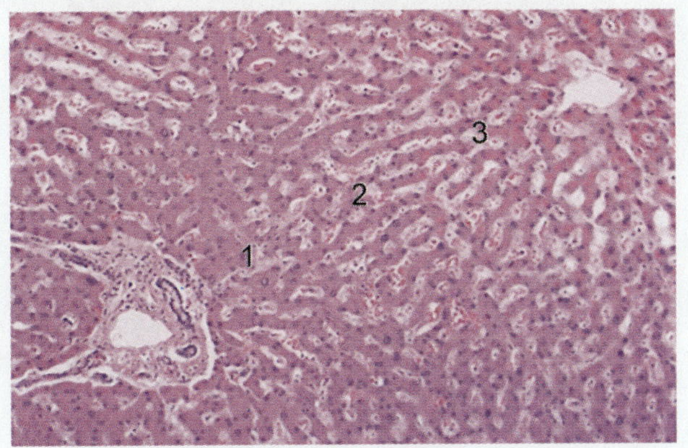

a. Periportal, Midzonal, Centrilobular
b. Periportal, Centrilobular, Midzonal
c. Midzonal, Centrilobular, Midzonal
d. Periportal, Centrilobular, Midzonal

4. 45/M chronic alcoholic presented with pain abdomen, USG suggested fatty liver. Liver biospsy done has been shown below. What is your interpretation and likely diagnosis?

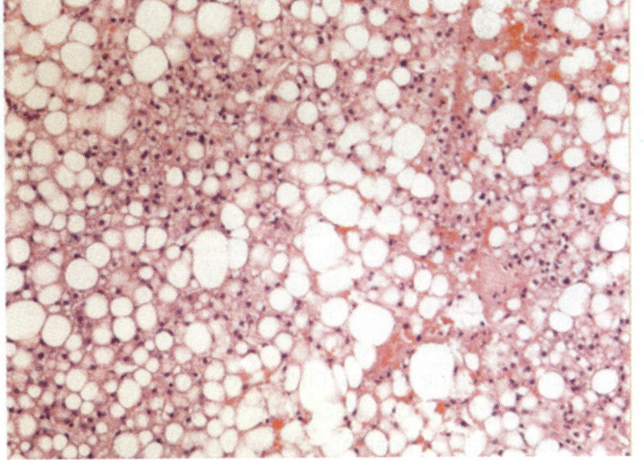

a. Lymphocytic infiltrate, Hep C
b. Neutrophillic Infiltrate, Hep B
c. Macrovesicular steatosis, Alcoholic liver disease
d. Squamous pearls, Metastasis

5. A 6-week-old infant presented with conjugated Hyper-bilirubinemia. HIDA scan done was not suggestive of Extrahepatic biliary atresia. Liver biopsy showed the following finding. Identify the underlying Etiology?

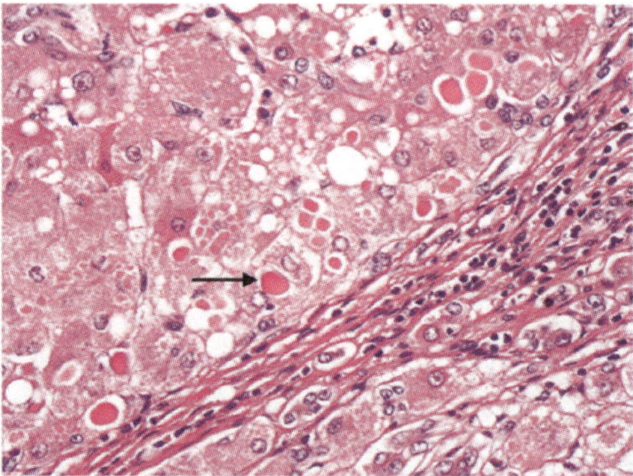

a. Wilson's disease
b. Cystic fibrosis
c. α1 antitrypsin deficiency
d. Idiopathic neonatal hepatitis

6. 45/M, a chronic alcoholic presented to Med OPD of AIIMS with Jaundice. S. Bilirubin was 4.5 mg% with direct Bilirubin being 3mg%. Liver biopsy was done which suggested the following. What is your interpretation and likely diagnosis?

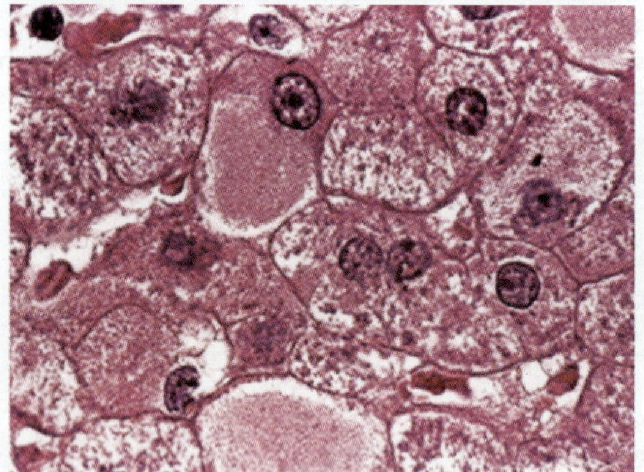

a. Malory Hyaline bodies, HCC
b. Malory Hyaline bodies, Chronic Hepatitis B
c. Ground glass appearance, HCC
d. Ground Glass appearance, Chronic Hepatitis B

7. 25/M presented with jaundice, clay coloured stool and pruritus. Bilirubin was 7 gm%, Direct Bilirubin 5gm%, ALP 500 IU/L. Biopsy from biliary tract revealed the following. What is your diagnosis?

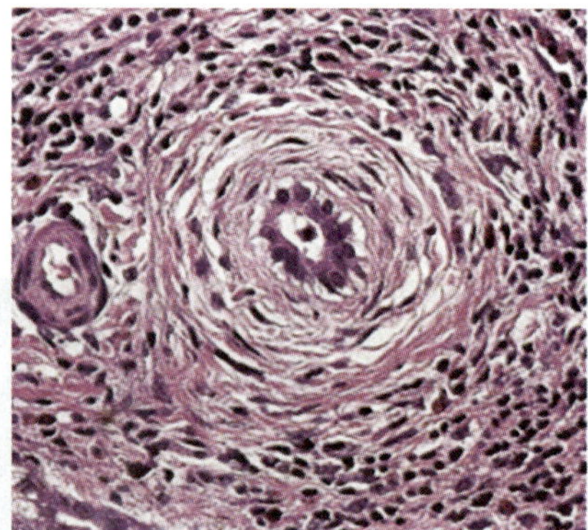

a. PSC   b. SBC
c. PBC   d. Bile duct stones

8. The condition associated with their formation is:

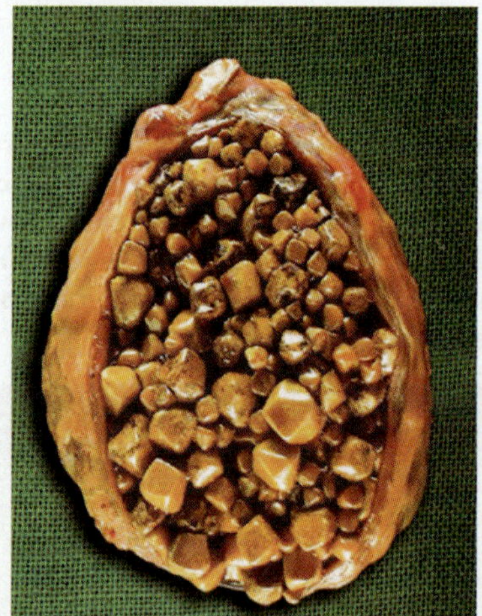

a. Hypomotility of gall bladder
b. Accelerated cholesterol crystal nucleation
c. Hypersecretion of mucus
d. All of the above

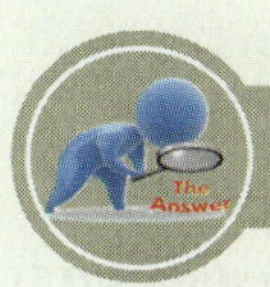

Answers of Image-Based Questions

1. **Ans. (c) Erythropoietic protoporphyria**
   - Liver biopsy showing dark brownish-black deposits in hepatocytes, canaliculi, Kupffer cells, and ductules with polarised microscopy of the same showing maltese cross picture of red birefringence in the larger deposits, a characteristic of Erythropoietic protoporphyria.

2. **Ans. (d) Chronic venous congestion**
   - The cut surface of the liver has a variegated mottled red appearance, representing congestion and hemorrhage in the centrilobular regions of the parenchyma. Also note that on microscopic examination, the centrilobular region is suffused with red blood cells and atrophied hepatocytes are not easily seen. Portal tracts and the periportal parenchyma are intact.

3. **Ans. (a) Periportal, Midzonal, Centrilobular**
   - Liver is divided histologically into lobules. The center of the lobule is the central vein. At the periphery of the lobule are portal triads. Functionally, the liver can be divided into three zones, based upon oxygen supply. Zone 1 encircles the portal tracts where the oxygenated blood from hepatic arteries enters. Zone 3 is located around central veins, where oxygenation is poor. Zone 2 is located in between.

4. **Ans. (c) Macrovesicular steatosis, Alcoholic liver disease**
   - Liver with mixed small and large fat droplets (white round structures, steatosis) a feature seen in alcoholic liver disease.

5. **Ans. (c) α1 antitrypsin deficiency**
   - The history given is that of neonatal hepatitis. Liver biopsy here shows Periodic acid–Schiff (PAS) stain after diastase digestion of the liver, characteristic magenta cytoplasmic granules seen in hepatitis due to α1 antitrypsin deficiency.

6. **Ans. (d) Ground Glass appearance, Chronic Hepatitis B**
   - The microscopic section of liver hepatocytes here show large pale, finely granular pink cytoplasmic inclusions on hematoxylin and eosin staining.

7. **Ans. (a) PSC**
   - Clinical feature of jaundice, clay coloured stool and pruritus is suggestive of obstructive jaundice. Biopsy showing fibrotic obliteration of bile ducts ("onionskin" fibrosis) seen in primary biliary cirrhosis.

8. **Ans. (d) All of the above**
   - The figure shows gall bladder filled with gall stones. Causes of its formation can include
     a. Hypomotility of gall bladder
     b. Accelerated cholesterol crystal nucleation
     c. Hypersecretion of mucus.

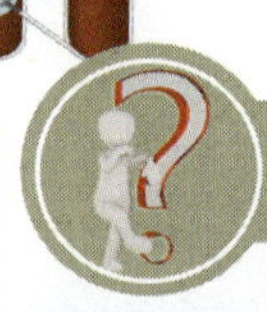

Multiple Choice Questions

STRUCTURE OF LIVER

1. In Obstructive jaundice, which of the following enzyme is elevated? *(Recent Question 2016-17)*
a. GGT
b. AST
c. ALT
d. LDH

2. The given figure shows which of the following? *(AIIMS Nov 2015)*

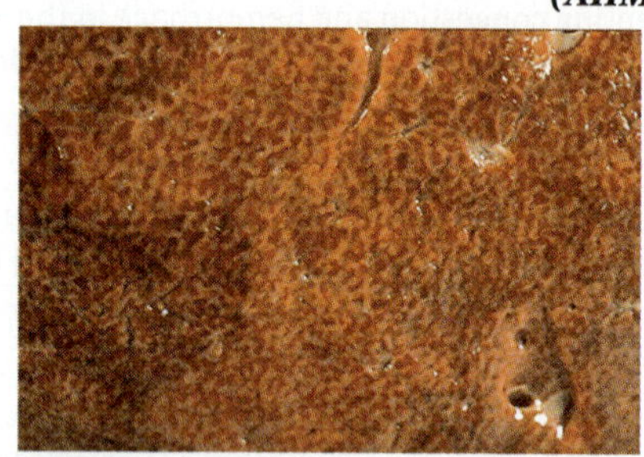

a. Amyloidosis: grey areas are viable; white areas are necrotic
b. Nutmeg liver: red areas are viable pericentralareas; white areas are periportal necrotic areas
c. Nutmeg liver: Red areas are pericental necrotic areas, white areas are viable fibrotic periportal area
d. Amyloidosis - necrotic white periportal viable grey pericentral areas

3. Absent urobilinogen in urine with icterus indicates? *(AIIMS Nov 2015)*
a. Perihepatic obstruction
b. Hemolysis
c. Hepatitis
d. Liver failure

4. Massive hepatocellular necrosis is seen with *(Recent Question 2015)*
a. Tetracycline
b. Macrolides
c. Methyldopa
d. Acetaminophen

5. Liver damage in shock *(Recent Question 2015)*
a. Centrilobular necrosis
b. Diffuse necrosis
c. Periportal necrosis
d. Spotty necrosis

6. Nutmeg liver is seen in *(Recent Question 2015)*
a. Chronic venous congestion of liver
b. Portal vein obstruction
c. Hepatic artery obstruction
d. Non-alcoholic hepatic steatosis

7. False statement about alagille syndrome *(Recent Question 2015)*
a. Complete absence of bile ducts
b. Normal liver
c. Mutations in Jagged 1 gene
d. No Risk of hepatocellular carcinoma

8. Most common hepatotoxin causing acute liver injury *(Recent Question 2015)*
a. Acetaminophen
b. Alcohol
c. Paracetamol
d. Halothane

9. Fibrin ring granuloma in liver is caused by *(Recent Question 2015)*
a. Sulphonamides
b. Amlodarone
c. Isoniazid
d. Allopurinol

10. Peliosis hepatis is caused by *(Recent Question 2015)*
a. Contraceptives
b. Anabolic steroids
c. Erythromycin
d. Ezetemibe

11. Steatohepatitis with mallory-Denk bodies is caused by *(Recent Question 2015)*
a. Alcohol
b. Enalapril
c. Vitamin A
d. Methotrexate

12. Periportal fibrosis is caused by? *(Recent Question 2015)*
a. Alcohol
b. Methotrexate
c. Rifampicin
d. OCPs

13. The following is not a feature of non-cirrhotic portal fibrosis *(Recent Question 2015)*
a. Intimal fibroelastosis
b. Lymphocytic infiltration
c. Portal fibrosis
d. Bridging fibrosis

14. Perivenular fibrosis is caused by *(Recent Question 2015)*
a. Methotrexate
b. Alcohol
c. OCPs
d. Amiodarone

15. In cirrhosis, the proliferation and activation of the following cell results in fibrosis *(Recent Question 2015) (WB PG 2016)*
a. Hepatocytes
b. Stellate cells
c. Kuptter cells
d. Bile duct epithelium

16. Centrilobular necrosis of liver may be seen with- *(Recent Question 2014)*
a. Phosphorus
b. Arsenic
c. CCl_4
d. Ethanol

17. Mallory bodies contain - *(Recent Question 2013)*
a. Vimentin
b. Cytokeratin
c. Keratin
d. Collagen

18. Which substance is/are not deposited in hepatocyte? *(PGI May 10, June 01)*
a. Lipofuscin
b. Pseudomelanin
c. Bile pigment
d. Iron
e. Melanin

19. On stopping Alcohol, all the following changes are reversible EXCEPT - *(DNB Dec 10)*
a. Hepatitis
b. Cirrhosis
c. Microvesicular fatty change
d. Macrovesicular fatty change

20. Which one of the following is not a feature of liver histology in non-cirrhotic portal fibrosis (NCPF)'? *(AI 05, DPG 10)*
a. Fibrosis in and around the portal tracts
b. Thrombosis of the medium and small portal vein branches
c. Non-specific inflammatory cell infiltrates in the portal tracts
d. Bridging fibrosis

21. Bile infarct is related to: *(PGI Nov 10)*
a. Hepatitis B
b. Dubin Johnson syndrome
c. Extrahepatic cholestasis
d. Intrahepatic cholestasis
e. Occlusion of hepatic artery

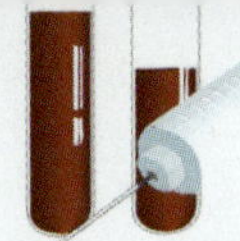

HEPATITIS SEROLOGY & CLINICAL FEATURES

22. A patient presented with fibrosis of liver. ALT 40IU/uL. Serology report suggested: *(AIIMS Nov 2016)*

HbeAg –ve   Anti HBc Ab +ve
Anti HCV Ab +ve

Next line of investigation will be?
a. Liver biopsy
b. HBsAg
c. HBV DNA
d. HCV RNA

23. Which hepatitis marker can be used to diagnose Acute Hepatitis B? *(Recent Question 2016-17)*
a. HBc Ag
b. Anti HBc Igm
c. HBs Ag
d. HBe Ag

24. Which of the following viral markers signifies the ongoing viral replication in the case of Hepatitis-B infection? *(Recent Question 2016-17)*
a. Anti-HBs
b. Anti-HBc
c. HBe Ag
d. HBs Ag

25. Serology profile of a patient suggested the following, what is your diagnosis? *(AIIMS Nov 2015)*

- Hbs Ag: non reactive
- IgG anti Hbc: reactive
- HbeAg: Non reactive
- Hep B viral DNA: undetectable

a. Window period
b. Chronic hepatitis inactive stage
c. Recovery from remote infection
d. Recovery from acute infection

26. Reverse transcriptase is a RNA dependent DNA polymerase. Which of these use it ? *(AIIMS May 2015)*
a. Hepatitis A virus
b. Hepatitis B virus
c. Hepatitis E virus
d. Hepatitis C virus

27. Which hepatitis causes more morbidity in pregnant female? *(Recent Question 2016)*
a. Hep A
b. Hep B
c. Hep C
d. Hep E

28. Fecooral transmission is seen in? *(Recent Question 2016)*
a. Hep A
b. Hep B
c. Hep C
d. Hep E

29. HBV DNA polymerase is encoded by which of the following gene? *(Recent Question 2015)*
a. P
b. X
c. C
d. S

30. Calciviridae is? *(Recent Question 2015)*
a. Hepatitis A
b. Hepatitis E
c. Hepatitis C
d. Hepatitis D

31. In Chronic Hepatitis B (HBV) infection presence of HBeAg (Hepatitis B e antigen) suggests which of the following? *(MAHA 16)*
a. Ongoing viral replication
b. Resolving infection
c. Development of cirrhosis
d. Development of Hepatoma

32. Most common route hepatitis E transmission is? *(Recent Question 2015)*
a. Sexual
b. Faeco-oral
c. Horizontal
d. Vertical

33. Gene responsible for mutation of HBV is? *(Recent Question 2015)*
a. X gene
b. S gene
c. P gene
d. C gene

34. A nurse got a needle prick injury. Which of the following suggests active phase of hepatitis? *(AIIMS Nov 14)*
a. IgM Ab of HBc
b. IgG Ab of HBc
c. IgG of HBs
d. Anti HbeAb

35. Most common subtype of Hepatitis B in North India is? *(Recent Question 2014)*
a. adr
b. adw
c. ayw
d. ayr

36. Acute hepatitis 'B' can be diagnosed by: *(PGI May 12)*
a. HBsAg
b. IgM anti-HBcAb
c. HBeAg
d. IgG anti-HBcAb
e. Core antigen

37. Hepatitis virus that causes chronic liver disease is? *(DNB Aug. 12 Pattern) (WBPG 2016)*
a. Hepatitis A
b. Hepatitis B
c. Hepatitis C
d. Hepatitis D

38. Not a complication of acute viral Hepatitis? *(DNB Aug 12 Pattern)*
a. Aplastic anemia
b. Acute pancreatitis
c. Autoimmune hepatitis
d. Hepatocellular carcinoma

39. A 25-year-old person presents with mild icterus. His HBsAg +ve, HBeAg –ve with SGOT and SGPT raised 5-6 times the original value. HBV DNA levels were>1,00,000/ml. What is your diagnosis? *(AI 2010)*
a. Wild type HBV
b. Surface mutant HBV
c. Precore mutant HBV
d. Active HBV carrier

HEPATITIS HISTOLOGY

40. Which of the following is/are features of acute hepatitis?
a. Interface hepatitis *(PGI May 18)*
b. Mononuclear cell infiltration
c. Apoptosis of hepatocyte
d. Portal tracts Inflammation
e. Bridging fibrous

41. Hepatitis infection persists in 3% asymptomatic individuals. Why is there an increased risk of developing liver cancer in these patients? *(AIIMS Nov 2017)*
a. Inability to induce inflammation to remove organism
b. Increased liver transaminases
c. High rate of hepatocyte proliferation
d. Integration of viral DNA to host DNA

42. Hallmark of chronic hepatitis *(Recent Question 2015)*
a. Interface hepatitis
b. Ballooning degeneration of hepatocytes
c. Cholestasis
d. Periportal fibrosis and bridging fibrosis

43. Ground glass hepatocyte is seen in which hepatitis? *(Recent Question 2015)*
a. Hepatitis A
b. Hepatitis B
c. Hepatitis D
d. Hepatitis E

44. Councilman bodies are seen in- *(Recent Question 2014, DNB Dec 09)*
a. Alcoholic cirrhosis
b. Wilson's disease
c. Acute viral hepatitis
d. Autoimmune hepatitis

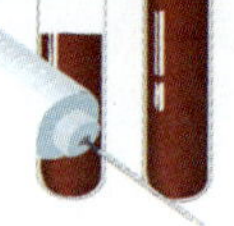

45. Microvesicular fatty change in hepatocytes is seen due to infection with: *(Recent Question 2014)*
a. Hepatitis A
b. Hepatitis B
c. Hepatitis C
d. Hepatitis D

46. Histopathology of chronic hepatitis shows -
a. Ballooning of hepatocytes *(Recent Question 2013)*
b. Councilman bodies
c. Bridging fibrosis
d. All of the above

47. Chronic persistent hepatitis and chronic active hepatitis are differentiated by - *(DNB June 11)*
a. Anti-Smith Ab
b. C-Reactive Protein
c. Arthritis
d. Liver biopsy

48. Which of the following is single most important indicator of likelihood of progression of hepatitis to liver cirrhosis - *(MH 10)*
a. Etiology
b. Associated serological findings
c. Presence of bridging necrosis
d. Presence of mallory hyaline bodies

49. Chronic Active Hepatitis is most reliably distinguished from chronic Persistent hepatitis by the presence of -
a. Extrahepatic manifestations *(UPSC 05, 10)*
b. Significant titre of anti-smooth muscle antibody
c. Characteristic liver histology
d. Hepatitis B surface antigen

ALCOHOLIC LIVER DISEASE

50. The specific marker for alcoholic hepatitis? *(AIIMS Nov 18)*
a. GGT
b. Alanine transaminase
c. Alkaline phosphatase
d. LDH

51. Alcohol is a risk factor for which of the following cancers? *(PGI May 18)*
a. Liver
b. Esophagus
c. Gastric
d. Cervical
e. Breast

52. True about morphological feature(s) of alcoholic steatosis? *(PGI Nov 2017)*
a. Fat droplet in hepatocyte
b. Mallory body may be seen
c. May cause hepatic necrosis
d. Perisinusoidal fibrosis may be seen
e. Macro-nodule formation

53. Malory Hyaline body is seen in? *(Recent Question 2016-17)*
a. Acute Hep A
b. Chronic Hep A
c. Acute Hep B
d. Chronic Hep B

54. Ground glass hepatocytes are seen in ? *(Recent Question 2016-17)*
a. Hep A
b. Hep B
c. Hep C
d. Hep D

55. Malory Denk bodies are not seen in?
a. Non alcoholic liver disease *(Recent Question 2016-17)*
b. Wilsons
c. Indian childhood cirrhosis
d. Chronic hep B

56. Focal or confluent periportal necrosis along with ballooning degeneration of hepatocytes with or without Mallory bodies and megamitochondriais suggestive of? *(Recent Question 2015/WBPG 2014)*
a. Acute Hepatitis B
b. Chronic Hepatitis B
c. Alcoholic liver injury
d. Primary HCC

57. Which of the following is not a feature of Alcoholic liver disease? *(WBPG 2015)*
a. Macrovesicular fat within hepatocytes
b. Lipogranuloma
c. Lymphocytic infiltration of portal tracts
d. Portal & sinusoidal collagen deposits

58. The sign of reversible injury in a case of alcoholic liver disease - *(Recent question 2014)*
a. Loss of cell membrane
b. Nuclear karyolysis
c. Cytoplasmic vacuole
d. Pyknosis

59. An obese female presented with features of hepatitis. She is a known diabetic. Which of the following would be the liver biopsy feature? *(AIIMS May 2014)*
a. NASH
b. Hepatocyte necrosis
c. Cirrhosis
d. Lipoid necrosis

60. A child presented with viral fever followed by unconsciousness. CT scan was suggestive of cerebral edema. Which of the following would be a finding on liver biopsy? *(AIIMS May 2014)*
a. Peacemeal necrosis
b. Microvesicular steatosis
c. Bridging fibrosis
d. Ballooning degeneration

61. Pathological manifestation of chronic alcoholism include all of the following except -
a. Piecemeal necrosis *(Recent Question 2013)*
b. Ballooning degeneration
c. Microvesicular fatty changes
d. Central hyaline sclerosis

62. If a patient has bilirubin 20 mg/dl, AST=313 IU/L, ALT=103 IU/L & GGT=44 IU/L. Most probable diagnosis is: *(PGI May 2013)*
a. Viral hepatitis
b. Alcoholic hepatitis
c. Billiary atresia
d. Drugs
e. Autoimmune hepatitis

FATTY LIVER

63. Microvesicular fatty liver is caused by- *(Recent Question 2014)*
a. DM
b. Valproate
c. Starvation
d. IBD

64. Which does not cause microvesicular steatosis -
a. Alcoholic fatty liver *(Recent Question 2013)*
b. Tetracycline toxicity
c. Acute fatty liver of pregnancy
d. Reyes syndrome

AUTOIMMUNE HEPATITIS

65. About autoimmune hepatitis, which of the following is true? *(PGI Nov 2017)*
a. More common in female
b. Anti–liver kidney microsome-1 (anti-LKM-1) antibody is found in type I subtype only
c. Oral corticosteroids are given in severe cases
d. Associated with other autoimmune disease
e. Rarely lead to cirrhosis

66. **Characteristic antibodies of autoimmune hepatitis include all of the following except:** *(APPGMEE 2015)*
    a. ANAs
    b. Anti-CCP antibodies
    c. Smooth muscle antibodies
    d. Anti LKM antibodies

67. **Antibody present in autoimmune hepatitis type 2**
    a. Anti-LKM1 antibody *(Recent Question 2015)*
    b. Anti-nuclear antibody
    c. Anti-endomysial antibody
    d. Anti-mitochondrial antibody

68. **40/male presented with fever and jaundice. The clinical picture improved on immunosuppressive therapy, what is the most likely diagnosis?** *(AIIMS May 2014)*
    a. Autoimmune hepatitis
    b. Primary biliary cirrhosis
    c. Infectious hepatitis
    d. Secondary biliary cirrhosis

69. **Most common antibody in autoimmune hepatitis is?** *(DNB Aug 12)*
    a. U1 RNP
    b. Anti-Sm
    c. ANA
    d. Anti-LKM

70. **In adults, most common autoimmune disease of liver is?** *(DNB Aug 12)*
    a. Autoimmune hepatitis
    b. Sclerosing cholangitis
    c. α-1 antitrypsin deficiency
    d. Primary biliary cirrhosis

71. **Autoimmune hepatitis has the following Antibodies except?**
    a. ANA
    b. ANCA
    c. Anti LKM-1
    d. Anti- SLA

HYPERBILIRUBINEMIA

72. **Causes of unconjugated hyperbilirubinemia is/are?**
    a. Hemolysis due to ABO incompatibility *(PGI May 18)*
    b. Criggler-Najar syndrome
    c. Gilbert syndrome
    d. Sepsis
    e. Roter's syndrome

73. **True about surgical jaundice:** *(PGI May 2016)*
    a. Increase of serum bilirubin
    b. Increase acid phosphatase
    c. Increase alkaline phosphatase
    d. Urine bilirubin is absent
    e. Stool sterocobilinogen absent

74. **Regarding Gilbert's syndrome, which one of the following statements is not correct?** *(Recent Question 2016-17)*
    a. Jaundice becomes severe with time.
    b. Hyperbilirubinemia increases after fasting.
    c. Inheritance of disease is autosomal dominant.
    d. Liver histology is normal.

75. **A 55-year-old gentleman presented with history of right upper quadrant discomfort, jaundice, pruritis, fever, fatigue and weight loss. His serum bilirubin and** alkaline phosphatase levels are raised and he also gives history of treatment for inflammatory bowel disease. He is most likely to be suffering from: *(Recent Question 2016-17)*
    a. Benign bile duct stricture with cholangitis
    b. Biliary worms
    c. Bile duct malignancy
    d. Primary sclerosing cholangitis

76. **True about primary biliary cirrhosis:**
    a. More common in female *(PGI May 2015)*
    b. Periportal fibrosis
    c. May be ssociated with Rheumatoid arthritis & crohn's disease
    d. Jaundice may be present
    e. Autoimmune disease are seen

77. **Florid duct lesions are diagnostic of**
    a. Klatskin tumor *(Recent Question 2015)*
    b. Primary sclerosing cholangitis
    c. Primary biliary cirrhosis
    d. Secondary biliary cirrhosis

78. **False statement regarding alagille syndrome**
    a. Mutation in jagged-1-gene *(Recent Question 2015)*
    b. Portal and bile ducts are completely absent
    c. Micronodural cirrhosis of liver
    d. All of the above

79. **Onion skin fibrosis is seen in** *(Recent Question 2015)*
    a. Primary biliary cirrhosis
    b. Secondary biliary cirrhosis
    c. Primary sclerosing cholangitis
    d. Progressive familial intrahepatic cholestasis

80. **Which of the following does not cause cholestasis in new-born?** *(Recent Question 2016)*
    a. ABO incompatibility
    b. Sepsis
    c. Tyrosenemia
    d. Biliary atresia

81. **All of the following are autosomal recessive except:** *(Recent Question 2015)*
    a. Gilbert's syndrome
    b. CrigglerNajjar type I
    c. CrigglerNajjar type II
    d. Dubin Johnson syndrome

82. **Antimitochondrial antibodies are positive in** *(Recent Question 2015)*
    a. Primary sclerosing cholangitis
    b. Secondary biliary cirrhosis
    c. Primary biliary cirrhosis
    d. Primary hemochromatosis

83. **Which one of the following inherited conditions causes direct hyperbilirubinemia:** *(APPGMEE 2015)*
    a. Gilbert syndrome
    b. Type I Criglernajjar syndrome
    c. Rotor syndrome
    d. Type II Criglernajjar syndrome

84. **About Gilbert syndrome, true are all except-**
    a. Causes cirrhosis *(Recent Question 2014)*
    b. Autosomal dominant
    c. Normal liver function test
    d. Normal histology

85. **Unconjugated hyperbilirubinemia is seen in -**
    a. Rotor syndrome *(Recent Question 2014)*
    b. Dubin-Johnson syndrome
    c. Gilbert syndrome
    d. Bile duct obstruction

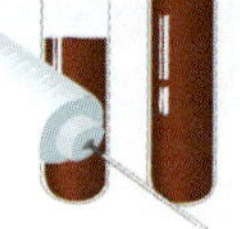

86. Feature of unconjugated bilirubin is/are:
(PGI Nov 2011)
a. Water soluble
b. Fat soluble
c. Direct reaction with Van den Bergh reaction
d. Affinity for brain tissue
e. Increased in hemolytic anemia

87. Pigment stone is composed of? *(Recent Question 2015)*
a. Ca bilirubinate
b. Ca phosphate
c. Ca carbonate
d. Ca gluconate

88. Sclerosing cholangitis is associated with-
(Recent Question 2014)
a. Ulcerative colitis
b. Celiac sprue
c. Wilson's disease
d. Whipple's disease

89. Conjugated hyperbilirubinemia is seen in?
a. Dubin Johnson Syndrome *(Recent Question 2014)*
b. Gilbert syndrome
c. Criggler Najjar syndrome
d. Hemolysis

90. Grossly pigmented liver is seen in?
a. Criggler-Najjar Type I *(Recent Question 2014)*
b. Gilberts Syndrome
c. Dubin johnson Syndrome
d. Rotor's Syndrome

91. The following features differentiate Rotor syndrome from Dubin Johnson's syndrome EXCEPT
(APPGMEE 14)
a. Liver in patients with Rotor syndrome has no increased pigmentation and appears normal
b. In Rotor syndrome, Gall bladder is usually visualized on cholecystography
c. Total urinary coproporphyin is substantially increased in Rotor syndrome
d. Fraction of coproporphyin I in urine is elevated usually more than 80% of the total in Rotor syndrome

92. Which of the following statement(s) is/are true about primary sclerosing cholangitis? *(PGI Nov 2017)*
a. May be complicated by bacterial infection
b. Rarely progress to biliary cirrhosis
c. Involve only intrahepatic bile duct not extrahepatic bile ducts
d. Associated with Inflammatory bowel disease
e. Narrowing of bile duct

93. Primary biliary cirrhosis is positive for·
a. ANCA *(Recent Question 2013)*
b. Anti-mitochondrial antibody
c. Anti nuclear antibody
d. Anti-microsomal antibody

94. True about cholelithiasis is? *(PGI May 2013)*
a. Cholesterol stones are most common
b. 90% of gallstone are radio-opaque
c. Mirrizi syndrome is due to impaction of stone in hartmann's pouch
d. Hemolytic anaemia cause black colored stone
e. Carcinoma is not a risk associated with gallstone

95. All are true about ascending cholangitis except?
(PGI May 2013)
a. Most commonly caused by gram positive organisms
b. In severe cases collapse can occur
c. Urgent removal of stone by ERCP can be done
d. Cholecystectomy can be done
e. Commonly caused by obstruction of bile duct by stone

96. True about obstructive jaundice: *(PGI May 2011)*
a. Unconjugated bilirubin
b. Positive indirect Van den Bergh
c. Pruritus
d. Pale stools
e. Icterus

97. In post-hepatic jaundice, the concentration of conjugated bilirubin in the blood is higher than that of unconjugated bilirubin because: *(AIIMS Nov 10)*
a. There is an increased rate of destruction of red blood cells.
b. The unconjugated bilirubin is trapped by the bile stone produced in the bile duct.
c. The conjugation process of bilirubin in liver remains operative without any interference.
d. The UDP-glulcuronoyltransferase activity is increased manifold in obstructive jaundice.

METABOLIC LIVER DISEASE

98. Biochemical finding used for diagnosis of Wilson disease include(s): *(PGI May 2019)*
a. Increased serum ceruloplasmin
b. Increased urinary copper excretion
c. Increased serum copper
d. Increased liver copper content
e. Decreased serum copper

99. A 1-month-old child with conjugated bilirubinemia and intrahepatic cholestasis. On Liver biopsy and staining with PAS red coloured granules were seen inside the hepatocytes. Probable diagnosis is ? *(AIIMS May 2015)*
a. Alpha1 Antitrypsin deficiency
b. Congenital hepatic fibrosis
c. Wilson disease
d. hereditary hemochromatosis

100. PAS-positive, diastase-resistant globules in hepatocytes are seen in? *(Recent Question 2015)*
a. Hemochromatosis
b. Wilsons disease
c. Alpha 1 antitrypsin deficiency
d. Acute necrotic hepatitis

101. Hemochromatosis is a defect in metabolism of:
(Recent Question 2015)
a. Iron
b. Copper
c. Magnesium C
d. Calcium

102. Gene for Wilson's disease is located on chromosome-
(Recent Question 2014)
a. 7
b. 10
c. 13
d. 17

103. Wilson's disease is characterized by-
(Recent Question 2014), (WBPG 2016)
a. Increased serum ceruloplasmin
b. Decreased copper excretion in urine
c. ↑Ceruloplasmin
d. Low ↑Ceruloplasmin high urine copper

104. Diabetic patient with liver cirrhosis and hyperpigmentation, diagnosis is-
a. Wilson's disease *(Recent Question 2014)*
b. Hemochromatosis
c. Primary sclerosing cholangitis
d. Hepatitis B

105. **Type of inheritance in Wilson's disease-**
(Recent Question 2014)
   a. Autosomal dominant b. Autosomal recessive
   c. X-linked dominant d. X-linked recessive

106. **PAS positive intrahepatic globules are seen in:**
   a. Wilson disease *(Recent Question 2014)*
   b. Hemochromatosis
   c. Primary Sclerosing Cholangitis
   d. Alpha-1-antitrypsin deficiency

107. **ATP7B gene is present on chromosome:**
(Recent Question 2014)
   a. 5 b. 13
   c. 18 d. 21

108. **In Alpha-1 anti trypsin deficiency, hepatocytes are:**
   a. PAS + ve diastase resistant *(Recent Question 2014)*
   b. Diastase positive PAS resistant
   c. PAS –ve d. Oilred O positive

109. **Hemochromatosis leads to deposition of?**
(Recent Question 2014)
   a. Iron b. Copper
   c. Zinc d. Lead

110. **In Wilson's disease, hepatic copper content usually exceeds _______ μg per gram dry weight** *(MAHA 16)*
   a. 150 b. 250
   c. 350 d. 450

111. **Most common gene responsible for hereditary hemochromatosis is?** *(Recent Question 2013)*
   a. HJV gene b. HAMP gene
   c. TfR2 gene d. HFE gene

112. **Which of the following leads to chronic liver disease?**
   a. Hepatitis A *(DNB Aug 12 Pattern)*
   b. EBV
   c. Infectious mononucleosis
   d. α-l-antitrypsin deficiency

LIVER TUMORS

113. **Which of the infections is/are predisposes to cholangiocarcinoma?** *(PGI May 18)*
   a. Paragonimus westermani
   b. Fasiciola hepatica
   c. Schistosoma hematobium
   d. Opisthorchis viverrini
   e. Clonorchis sinensis

114. **Which of the following is true about Nodular Regenerative Hyperplasia?** *(JIPMER 18)*
   a. Nodule size 0.1 to 1 cm
   b. Fibrosis septa present
   c. Portal hypertension seen in 50% of patients
   d. AST and ALT are markedly elevated

115. **Vinyl chloride is associated with?** *(JIPMER 18)*
   a. Hemangiosarcoma b. Hepatoma
   c. Testicular carcinoma d. Thyroid malignancy

116. **True about liver haemangioma are all except?**
(PGI May 18)
   a. Most common benign tumor of liver
   b. Pregnancy is risk factor
   c. Thrombocytopenia may occur
   d. Diagnosis by MRI and CT scan
   e. Need surgical removal in every case because chances of rupture is high

117. **Which of the following has best prognosis?**
   a. Fibrolamellar Variant of HCC *(JIPMER 2016)*
   b. Hemangisarcoma
   c. Adenosarcoma
   d. Hepatocellular Ca

118. **True about fibrolamellar carcinoma of liver:**
(PGI May 2016)
   a. Better prognosis than typical hepatocellular carcinoma
   b. Associated with cirrhosis
   c. AFP-positive
   d. Occur in younger adults e. More common in females

119. **All are true about focal nodular hyperplasia except:**
   a. Multiple nodule may present *(PGI May 2016)*
   b. More common in male
   c. May be associated with contraceptive pills use
   d. Hypovascular on the arterial-phase and hypervascular on the delayed-phase CT images
   e. CT is less sensitive than MRI in depicting the characteristic central scar

120. **Regarding carcinoma gall bladder following features are true except:** *(Recent Question 2016-17)*
   a. One can have similar presentation with benign biliary disease
   b. Squamous cell carcinoma is 40% of all cases
   c. Most patients present with advanced disease
   d. Prognosis is poor

121. **Which of the following is not true about alcoholic cirrhosis?** *(Recent Question 2016-17)*
   a. On many occasions alcoholic hepatitis and alcoholic cirrhosis coexist.
   b. Concomitant HIV infection accelerates it.
   c. Starts with macronodular and later on changes to micronodular cirrhosis.
   d. 10 – 40 % remains clinically silent.

122. **Which of the following do not cause Hepatocellular Ca?**
   a. Hepatitis B *(Recent Question 2016)*
   b. Tyrosenemia
   c. Alcoholism
   d. Non alcoholic fatty liver disease

123. **Angiosarcoma of the liver can occur due to occupational exposure to:** *(Recent Question 2015)*
   a. Asbestos b. Benzene
   c. Vinyl chloride d. Toluene

124. **Hepatic adenoma is most common in**
(Recent Question 2015)
   a. Young males b. Young females
   c. Old males d. Old females

125. **Which liver tumor has the best prognosis**
   a. Hepatoceluler carcinoma *(Recent Question 2015)*
   b. Hemangiosarcoma
   c. Hemangioblastoma d. Fibrolamellar carcinoma

126. **Not true about HNF1-α Inactivated hepatocellular adenomas** *(Recent Question 2015)*
   a. Mostly in women
   b. High risk of malignant transformation
   c. Associated with MODY-3
   d. OCPs are implicated in pathogenesis

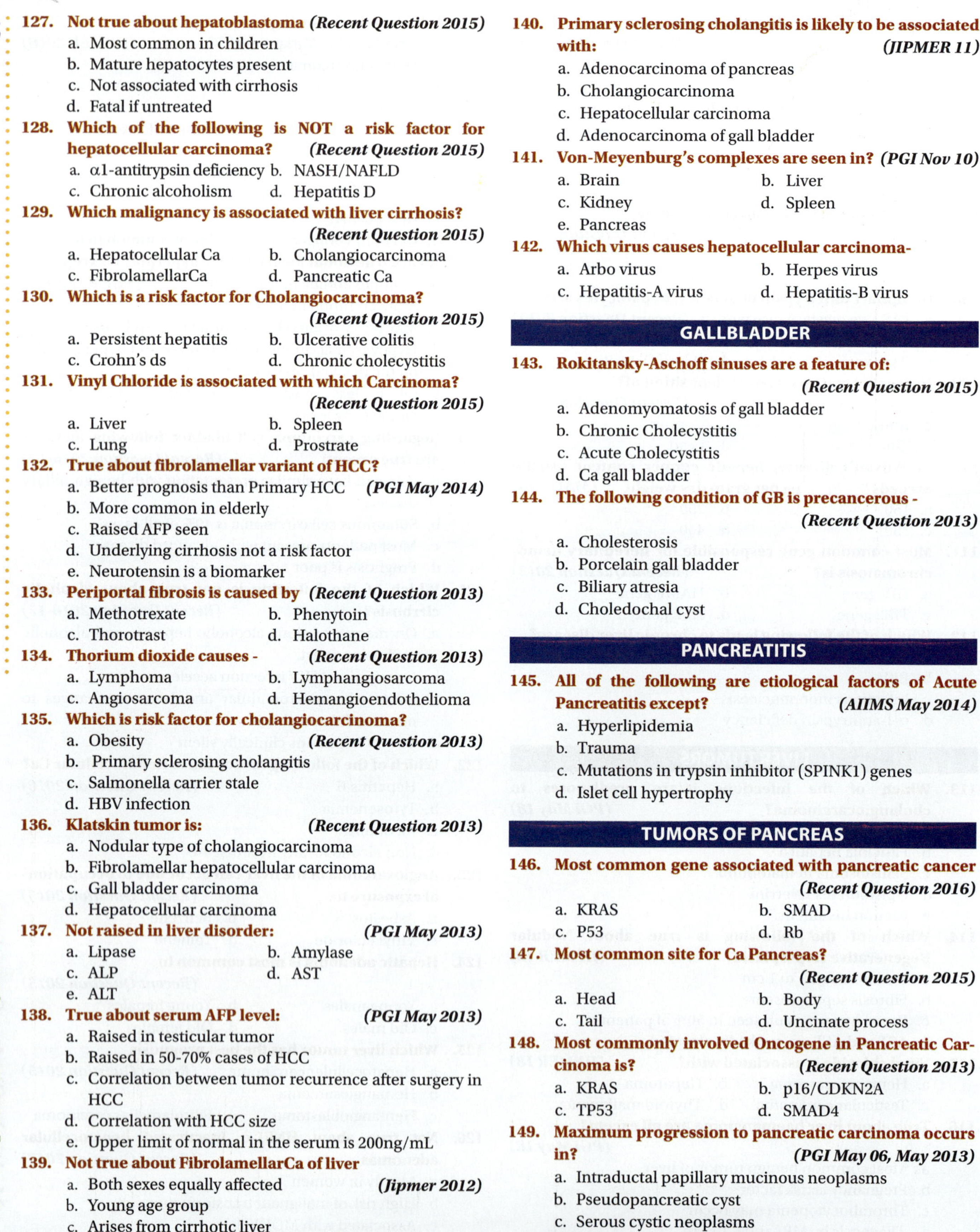

127. Not true about hepatoblastoma *(Recent Question 2015)*
a. Most common in children
b. Mature hepatocytes present
c. Not associated with cirrhosis
d. Fatal if untreated

128. Which of the following is NOT a risk factor for hepatocellular carcinoma? *(Recent Question 2015)*
a. α1-antitrypsin deficiency b. NASH/NAFLD
c. Chronic alcoholism   d. Hepatitis D

129. Which malignancy is associated with liver cirrhosis?
(Recent Question 2015)
a. Hepatocellular Ca   b. Cholangiocarcinoma
c. FibrolamellarCa   d. Pancreatic Ca

130. Which is a risk factor for Cholangiocarcinoma?
(Recent Question 2015)
a. Persistent hepatitis   b. Ulcerative colitis
c. Crohn's ds   d. Chronic cholecystitis

131. Vinyl Chloride is associated with which Carcinoma?
(Recent Question 2015)
a. Liver   b. Spleen
c. Lung   d. Prostrate

132. True about fibrolamellar variant of HCC?
a. Better prognosis than Primary HCC   *(PGI May 2014)*
b. More common in elderly
c. Raised AFP seen
d. Underlying cirrhosis not a risk factor
e. Neurotensin is a biomarker

133. Periportal fibrosis is caused by *(Recent Question 2013)*
a. Methotrexate   b. Phenytoin
c. Thorotrast   d. Halothane

134. Thorium dioxide causes - *(Recent Question 2013)*
a. Lymphoma   b. Lymphangiosarcoma
c. Angiosarcoma   d. Hemangioendothelioma

135. Which is risk factor for cholangiocarcinoma?
a. Obesity   *(Recent Question 2013)*
b. Primary sclerosing cholangitis
c. Salmonella carrier stale
d. HBV infection

136. Klatskin tumor is: *(Recent Question 2013)*
a. Nodular type of cholangiocarcinoma
b. Fibrolamellar hepatocellular carcinoma
c. Gall bladder carcinoma
d. Hepatocellular carcinoma

137. Not raised in liver disorder: *(PGI May 2013)*
a. Lipase   b. Amylase
c. ALP   d. AST
e. ALT

138. True about serum AFP level: *(PGI May 2013)*
a. Raised in testicular tumor
b. Raised in 50-70% cases of HCC
c. Correlation between tumor recurrence after surgery in HCC
d. Correlation with HCC size
e. Upper limit of normal in the serum is 200ng/mL

139. Not true about FibrolamellarCa of liver
a. Both sexes equally affected   *(Jipmer 2012)*
b. Young age group
c. Arises from cirrhotic liver
d. Good prognosis

140. Primary sclerosing cholangitis is likely to be associated with: *(JIPMER 11)*
a. Adenocarcinoma of pancreas
b. Cholangiocarcinoma
c. Hepatocellular carcinoma
d. Adenocarcinoma of gall bladder

141. Von-Meyenburg's complexes are seen in? *(PGI Nov 10)*
a. Brain   b. Liver
c. Kidney   d. Spleen
e. Pancreas

142. Which virus causes hepatocellular carcinoma-
a. Arbo virus   b. Herpes virus
c. Hepatitis-A virus   d. Hepatitis-B virus

GALLBLADDER

143. Rokitansky-Aschoff sinuses are a feature of:
(Recent Question 2015)
a. Adenomyomatosis of gall bladder
b. Chronic Cholecystitis
c. Acute Cholecystitis
d. Ca gall bladder

144. The following condition of GB is precancerous -
(Recent Question 2013)
a. Cholesterosis
b. Porcelain gall bladder
c. Biliary atresia
d. Choledochal cyst

PANCREATITIS

145. All of the following are etiological factors of Acute Pancreatitis except? *(AIIMS May 2014)*
a. Hyperlipidemia
b. Trauma
c. Mutations in trypsin inhibitor (SPINK1) genes
d. Islet cell hypertrophy

TUMORS OF PANCREAS

146. Most common gene associated with pancreatic cancer
(Recent Question 2016)
a. KRAS   b. SMAD
c. P53   d. Rb

147. Most common site for Ca Pancreas?
(Recent Question 2015)
a. Head   b. Body
c. Tail   d. Uncinate process

148. Most commonly involved Oncogene in Pancreatic Carcinoma is? *(Recent Question 2013)*
a. KRAS   b. p16/CDKN2A
c. TP53   d. SMAD4

149. Maximum progression to pancreatic carcinoma occurs in? *(PGI May 06, May 2013)*
a. Intraductal papillary mucinous neoplasms
b. Pseudopancreatic cyst
c. Serous cystic neoplasms
d. Mucinous cystic neoplasms

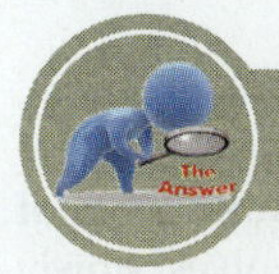

Answers with Explanations

1. Ans. (a) GGT

The activities of three enzymes—alkaline phosphatase, 5'-nucleotidase, and -glutamyl transpeptidase (GGT)—are usually elevated in cholestasis

2. Ans. (c) Nutmeg liver: Red areas are pericentral necrotic areas, white areas are viable fibrotic periportal area

(Ref: Robbins 9th/pg 863; 8th/pg 872)

The given picture shows **Chronic passive hepatic congestion,** The centrilobular regions are grossly red-brown and slightly depressed (because of cell death) and are prominently visible against the surrounding zones of uncongested tan liver (**nutmeg liver**).

3. Ans. (a) Perihepatic obstruction

(Ref: Robbin's 9th/830-840; Harrison's 18th/chapter 42)

Condition	Serum Bilirubin	Urine Urobilinogen	Urine Bilirubin	Fecal Urobilinogen
Normal	Direct 0.1-0.4 mg/dl Indirect 0.2-0.7 mg/dl	0.4 mg/24 h	Absent	40-280 mg/24h
Hemolytic anemia	↑Indirect	Increased	Absent	Increased
Hepatitis	↑Direct and indirect	Decreased if micro-obstruction is present	Present if micro-obstruction occurs	Decreased
Obstructive jaundice	↑Direct	Absent	Present	Trace to absent

4. Ans. (d) Acetaminophen *(Ref: Robbins 9th/pg 864)*

5. Ans. (a) Centrilobular necrosis *(Ref: R 9th/pg 864)*

Centrilobular zonal necrosis	Periportal injury
• Carbon tetrachloride (CCl$_4$) • Chloroform • Cardiac shock • Trichloroethylene	• Yellow phosphorus poisoning
	Midzonal necrosis
	• Yellow fever

6. Ans. (a) Chronic venous congestion of liver

(Ref: Robbins 9th/pg 863)

7. Ans. (d) No Risk of hepatocellular carcinoma

(Ref: Robbins 9th/pg 853; 8th/pg 854)

Alagille Syndrome (Syndromic Paucity of Bile Ducts; Arteriohepatic Dysplasia)

- An **autosomal dominant** disorder characterized by **absence of bile ducts in portal tracts**.
- Caused by mutations or deletion of gene encoding **Jagged1**, on chromosome 20p.
- Patients can survive into adulthood but **are at risk for hepatic failure & hepatocellular carcinoma**
- Major clinical features:
  - **Chronic cholestasis**
  - **Peripheral pulmonary artery stenosis**
  - **Butterfly-like vertebral arch defects**
  - An eye defect known as **posterior embryotoxon,**
  - A peculiar hypertelic, **triangular facies.**

8. Ans. (a) Acetaminophen *(Ref: Robbins 9th/pg 864)*

9. Ans. (d) Allopurinol *(Ref: Robbins 9th/pg 863)*

Fibrin Ring or "Doughnut" Granulomas

- Small, non-necrotizing granulomas with a very distinctive appearance that are usually found in the liver and bone marrow in patients with^Q fever.
- These granulomas characteristically contain a ring-like structure consisting of fibrinoid material; they may or may not have a centrally located fat vacuole(s).
- Other conditions: CMV, EBV, hepatitis A, infectious mononucleosis, visceral leishmaniasis, Lyme disease, toxoplasmosis, Hodgkin disease, non-Hodgkin lymphomas, and drug reactions like allopurinol.

10. Ans. (b) Anabolic steroids *(Ref: Robbins 9th/pg 863)*

Peliosis Hepatis

- **Peliosis hepatis** is a condition in which there is **primary hepatic sinusoidal dilation**; unknown pathogenesis
- **Sinusoidal dilation** occurs in any condition in which **efflux of hepatic blood is impeded**.
- Liver contains **blood-filled cystic spaces**, either unlined or lined with sinusoidal endothelial cells.
- Peliosis hepatis is associated with **cancer, tuberculosis, AIDS, or post-transplantation immunodeficiency**.
- Also associated with exposure to **anabolic steroids, oral contraceptives and danazol.**
- *Bartonella* species have been seen in the sinusoidal endothelial cells **in AIDS-associated peliosis**.
- Clinical signs are generally absent, but **fatal intra-abdominal hemorrhage** or **hepatic failure** may occur.

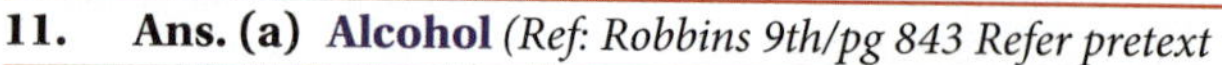

11. **Ans. (a)** **Alcohol** *(Ref: Robbins 9th/pg 843 Refer pretext)*

12. **Ans. (b)** **Methotrexate** *(Ref: Harrison 18th/ch 309)*

13. **Ans. (d)** **Bridging fibrosis** *(Ref: Robbins 9th/pg 863)*

Non-cirrhotic Portal Fibrosis (NCPF) and Idiopathic Portal Hypertension

Characterized by	Portal hypertension and a moderate **portal fibrosis without cirrhosis**.
Epidemiology	• NCPF is common in India • Idiopathic portal hypertension, described in Japan, has a female predominance
Clinical presentation	• **Upper gastrointestinal bleeding** • **Isolated splenomegaly**
Pathogenesis	• Idiopathic • Bacterial infection of gut causing septic embolization of portal vein. • Fibrosis of portal vein branches associated with increased expression of **vascular cell adhesion molecule-1 (VCAM-1)**.
Histology	• Increased **connective tissue deposition and fibrosis of portal tracts** with thrombotic obliteration of small branches of portal veins. • Infiltrates in portal tract • Also called **'hepatic sclerosis'** or **'obliterative portal venopathy'**

14. **Ans. (b)** **Alcohol** *(Ref: Robbins 9th/pg 837)*

- Alcoholic hepatitis is often accompanied by prominent activation of sinusoidal stellate cells and portal fibroblasts, giving rise to fibrosis.
- Fibrosis begins with sclerosis of central veins.
- **Perisinusoidal scar** then accumulates in the space of Disse of the centrilobular region, spreading outward, encircling individual or small clusters of hepatocytes in a **chicken wire fence pattern**

15. **Ans. (b)** **Stellate cells** *(Ref: Robbins 9th/pg 825; 8th/pg 837)*

16. **Ans. (c)** CCl_4 *(Ref: Robbins 9th/pg 864; 8th/pg 872)*

17. **Ans. (b)** **Cytokeratin** *(Ref: Robbins 9th/pg 843; 8th/pg 858)*

Mallory-Denk bodies (previously called **Mallory Hyaline bodies**[Q]): Clumped, amorphous, eosinophilic material in ballooned hepatocytes. Intermediate filaments-**keratins 8 and 18 with ubiquitin**.

18. **Ans. (b)** **Pseudomelanin** *(Ref: Sternburg /pg 1667-1670)*

Discussing options one by one,

A. **Lipofuscin:** Lipofuscinosis in centrilobular hepatocytes is induced by prolonged intake of Phenacetin, Aminopyrin, Chlorpromazine, Anticonvulsant therapy.

B. **Pseudomelanin is not deposited in liver but is seen in intestine in melanosis coli of intestine**

C. **Bile pigment in obstructive jaundice**

D. **Iron:** Dark brown or black **malarial pigment** in Kupffer cells & in **hemochromatosis**

E. **Melanin: deposits in hepatocytes in melanoma**

19. **Ans. (b)** **Cirrhosis** *(Ref: Robbins 9th/pg 842-844)*

- **Alcoholic Cirrhosis** is the **final & irreversible form of alcoholic liver disease** which usually evolves slowly and insidiously but may develop in 1 or 2 years in some cases of alcoholic liver disease.
- **Microvesicular & Macrovesicular fatty change is completely reversible** if there is abstention from further intake of alcohol.

20. **Ans. (d)** **Bridging fibrosis** *(Ref: Robbins 9th/pg 863)*

21. **Ans. (b, c, d); b. Dubin Johnson syndrome; c. Extrahepatic cholestasis; d. Intrahepatic cholestasis**

(Ref: Liver Pathology by Suriawinata & Thung, 2011/ pg 67)

Bile infarct is seen in **severe cholestatic disease**

Cholestasis is seen in **Dubin Johnson syndrome, Extrahepatic cholestasis & Intrahepatic cholestasis**

Bile infarcts:

- In **severe cholestasis**, extravasation of bile leads to hepatocyte necrosis & pale foamy macrophages, forming **bile infarct**s

- Although small bile infarcts may occur in any intense canalicular cholestasis, **large lesions**, especially around portal tracts, **suggest biliary obstruction**.

22. **Ans. (b)** **HBsAg**

(Ref: Robbins 9th/pg 831-832; 8th/pg 845-846; Harrison 19th/ Pg 2097)

The history in the question given is suggestive of Hepatitis C patient with concurrent Hepatitis B infection (HbcAb) but it is not enough to reliably tell us if it is acute infection or remote recovery as IgM or IgG is not mentioned in the question. So the next best logical step should be HbsAg followed by HBV DNA

23. **Ans. (b)** **Anti HBc IgM**

24. **Ans. (c)** **HBe Ag**

(Ref: Harrison 19th ed. Pg. 2007-2015; R9th 831-833)

25. **Ans. (c)** **Recovery from remote infection**

(Ref: Harrison 19th ed. Pg. 2007-2015; Robbins 9th 831-833)

26. **Ans. (b)** **Hepatitis B virus** *(Ref: Robbins 9th/pg 831-832)*

27. **Ans. (d)** **Hep E** *(Ref: Robbins 9th/pg 835; 8th/pg 849)*

A characteristic feature of HEV infection is the high mortality rate among pregnant women, approaching 20%

28. **Ans. (d)** **Hep E** *(Ref: Robbins 9th/pg 830; 8th/pg 840)*

Most common mode of Hep E transmission is Faeco-oral

Transmission	HAV	HBV	HCV	HDV	HEV
Fecal-oral	+++	–	–	–	+++
Percutaneous	Unusual	+++	+++	+++	–
Perinatal (Fetomaternal)	–	+++	±	+	–
Sexual	±	++	±	++	–

29. **Ans. (a)** **P** *(Ref: Robbins 9th/pg 831-832; 8th/pg 845-846)*

30. **Ans. (b)** **Hepatitis E**

- **HEV** was included in family **Caliciviridae** previously
- Although resembling caliciviruses, HEV is **now thought to be sufficiently distinct** from any known agent to merit a new classification of its own, as a unique genus, **Hepevirus,** within the family Hepeviridae.
- So the best answer here is HEV

31. **Ans. (a)** **Ongoing viral replication**

(Ref: R 9th/pg 831-832)

HBeAg
- The principal clinical usefulness of HBeAg is as an **indicator of relative infectivity**.
- **HBeAg, HBV-DNA & DNA polymerase appear in serum soon after HBsAg**, and **all signify active viral replication.**
- **Persistence of HBeAg** is an important indicator of **continued viral replication, infectivity, and probable progression to chronic hepatitis.**
- The appearance of **anti-HBe antibodies** implies that an **acute infection has peaked and is on the decline.**

32. **Ans. (b)** **Faeco-oral** *(Ref: Robbins 9th/pg 831-835)*

33. **Ans. (a)** **X gene** *(Ref: Robbins 9th/pg 831-832)*

Gene responsible for mutation of HBV is X gene
- **X gene** codes for **HBxAg**, that is capable of **transactivating transcription** of both viral & cellular genes
- HBxAg effects **calcium release from mitochondria →** **activates signal-transduction** pathways → stimulation of HBV reverse transcription & HBV **DNA replication**
- It also **enhances replication of HBV**, leading to severe **chronic hepatitis & hepatocellular carcinoma**.
- Can also enhance the transcription & replication of other viruses like **HIV**
- Cellular processes transactivated by X include human **interferon gene & class I MHC** genes
- These effects contribute to **enhanced susceptibility** of HBV-infected hepatocytes to cytolytic T cells.
- The expression of X can also **induce programmed cell death (apoptosis).**

34. **Ans. (a)** **IgM Ab of HBc**

(Ref: Robbins 9th/pg 831-832; 8th/pg 845-846; Harrison 18th/ Chapter 304)

35. **Ans. (c)** **ayw**

(Ref: Ismail et al. Molecular epidemiology & genetic characterization of hepatitis B virus in the Indian subcontinent. Int J Infect Dis. 2014 Mar; 20:1-10)

Hepatitis B has **eight subtypes and eight genotypes (A–H)**
This question can only be answered by a **recent publication on Hepatitis B**, mentioned above!
Most common genotype/subtype of Hepatitis B in:
- **North-Eastern India: D/ayw** followed by C / adr
- **Southern India: D/ayw**
- **Eastern India: C/adr**

36. **Ans. (a, b); a. HBsAg; b. IgM anti-HBc Ab**

(Ref: Robbins 9th/pg 831-832; 8th/pg 845-846)

37. **Ans. (c)** **Hepatitis C** *(Ref: Robbins 9th/pg 833-834)*

Progression to chronicity in **hepatitis C** is **upto 85% (maximum among the Hepatitis viruses)**

38. **Ans. (d)** **Hepatocellular carcinoma** *(Ref: R 9th/pg 837)*

- **Hepatocellular carcinoma is a complication of chronic hepatitis & not acute hepatitis.**
- Rare complications of acute viral hepatitis include pancreatitis, myocarditis, atypical pneumonia, aplastic anemia, transverse myelitis & peripheral neuropathy

39. **Ans. (c)** **Precore mutant HBV**

(Ref: Robbins 9th/pg 831-832)

Pre-core Mutant: Mutated strains of HBV emerge that **do not produce HBeAg despite the presence of serum HBV DNA.**

40. **Ans. (b, c, d) b. Mononuclear cell infiltration; c. Apoptosis of hepatocyte; d. Portal tracts Inflammation**

41. **Ans. (d)** **Integration of viral DNA to host DNA**

42. **Ans. (d)** **Periportal fibrosis and bridging fibrosis**

(Ref: Robbins 9th/pg 837; 8th/pg 850)

43. **Ans. (b)** **Hepatitis B** *(Ref: Robbins 9th/pg 837; 8th/pg 852)*

Diagnostic hallmark of **Chronic Hepatitis B** is "**ground-glass" hepatocytes** (cells with **endoplasmic reticulum swollen by HBsAg**)

44. **Ans. (c)** **Acute viral hepatitis** *(Ref: Robbins 9th/pg 837)*

- **Councilman bodies:** are intensely eosinophilic **a**poptotic hepatocytes with pyknotic nucleus, seen in acute viral hepatitis

45. **Ans. (d)** **Hepatitis D** *(Ref: Robbins 9th/pg 835; 8th/pg 849)*

Acute **HDV infection** has been associated with **microvesicular change** in hepatocytes; this **'spongiocytic change'** or **'morula cell degeneration'** was attributed to accumulation of **small lipid droplets** in damaged hepatocytes.

46. **Ans. (c)** **Bridging fibrosis** *(Ref: Robbins 9th/pg 837)*

- **Hallmark** of **progressive chronic liver damage** is deposition of **fibrous tissue (scarring)**[Q] bridgin fibrosis

47. **Ans. (d)** **Liver biopsy**

(Ref: Rosai and Ackerman's Surgical Pathology, Volume 1, chapter 13, Box 13.2)

Chronic hepatitis is classified on the basis of:
- Diagnosis of chronic hepatitis
- Etiology
- Grade of disease activity: evaluated by clinical symptoms, aminotransferase levels & liver biopsy
- Stage of disease progression

This classification system was used to distinguish between a **milder form (chronic persistent hepatitis** – CPH) with a

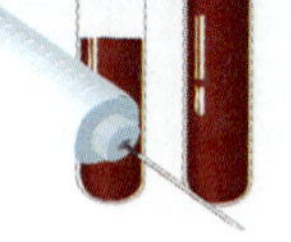

low degree of necro-inflammatory activity & **more severe variants (chronic aggressive or active hepatitis** – CAH) featuring higher degrees of necro-inflammatory lesions.

48. **Ans. (a)** **Etiology** *(Ref: Harrison 18th/Chapter 308)*

Single most important indicator of likelihood of progression of hepatitis to liver cirrhosis is etiology

49. **Ans. (c)** **Characteristic liver histology**

(Ref: Rosai and Ackerman's Surgical Pathology, Volume 1, chapter 13, Box 13.2)

50. **Ans. (a)** **GGT**

Serum levels of GGT differ from those of ALP during pregnancy, in which GGT remains normal even during cholestasis in pregnancy. GGT is often increased in alcoholics even without liver disease; in some obese people; and in the presence of high concentrations of therapeutic drugs, such as acetaminophen and phenytoin and carbamazepine (increased up to five times the reference limits), even in the absence of any apparent liver injury. Studies suggest that alcohol induces mitochondrial damage, resulting in the release of mitochondrial AST, which, besides being the predominant form of AST in hepatocytes, has a significantly longer half-life than do extramitochondrial AST and ALT. This frequently results in the disproportionate elevation of AST over ALT, yielding an AST/ALT quotient, also called the DeRitis ratio, of 3–4:1 in alcohol-induced liver disease

51. **Ans. (d)** **Cervical**

52. **Ans. (a, b, d) a. Fat droplet in hepatocyte; b. Mallory body may be seen; d. Perisinusoidal fibrosis may be seen**

(Ref: Robbins 9th ed p 845)

Perisinusoidal scarring leads to a classic micronodular or Laennec cirrhosis first described for end-stage alcoholic liver disease.

53. **Ans. (d)** **Chronic Hep B** *(Ref: Robbins 9th/pg 837)*

54. **Ans. (b)** **Hep B** *(Ref: Robbins 9th/pg 837; 8th/pg 850)*

55. **Ans. (d)** **Chronic hep B** *(Ref: Robbins 9th/pg 837)*

56. **Ans. (c)** **Alcoholic liver injury**

(Ref: Rosai and Ackerman's Surgical Pathology, Volume 1, chapter 13, Box 13.2)

- **Megamitochondria** appear as **eosinophilic, PAS–diastase-negative, round, oval, or cigar-shaped inclusions**
- Better visualized with **chromotrope–aniline blue (CAB) stain** & immunohistochemistry.
- They are **not specific for alcohol-induced liver disease**, but found more frequently in alcohol-related fibrosis

- **Oxyphilic granular hepatocytes or oncocytes** are a common, though not pathognomonic, cellular component in acute and chronic alcoholic liver disease.
- On Electron microscopy, Oncocytes are characterized by a **large number of mitochondria** (mitochondriosis).

57. **Ans. (c)** **Lymphocytic infiltration of portal tracts**

(Ref: Robbins 9th/pg 837; 8th/pg 850; Rosai and Ackerman's Surgical Pathology, Volume 1, chapter 13)

Lipogranuloma (or fat granuloma) represents a focal response to rupture of lipid-laden hepatocytes. It contains macrophages, occasional lymphocytes, eosinophils, and sometimes giant cells; It may be seen in

Alcoholic liver disease; Neutrophil rather than lymphocytic infiltration is seen in alcoholic liver disease

58. **Ans. (c)** **Cytoplasmic vacuole**

(Ref: Robbins 9th/pg 842-844)

- **Alcoholic liver disease is fully reversible in the steatosis stage.**
- In this stage fatty changes appear in the hepatocytes, represented by **cytoplasmic vacuoles** as the lipid is dissolved during processing
- Loss of cell membrane, nuclear karyolysis and pyknosis represents irreversible cell injury and so not reversible.

59. **Ans. (a)** **NASH** *(Ref: Robbins 9th/pg 845-846)*

Obesity and diabetes are two important risk factors for NASH

60. **Ans. (b)** **Microvesicular steatosis**

(Ref: Robbin's 8th/pg 857; Sternberg's 4th ed/ch 36)

The given clinical scenario and findings on CNS imaging are suggestive of Reyes Syndrome.

Reye syndrome (also called '**Jamshedpur fever'**)
- Occurs principally, but not exclusively, in **young children**
- Predisposing factors: **Salicylate** use, inherited **disorder of mitochondrial ß-oxidation**
- Presents clinically with an initial acute, mild viral illness, followed by **vomiting, lethargy & coma**
- Severe disease with **poor prognosis**, resulting in death in about one-third of patients.
- Histopathology of liver: **Panlobular microvesicular Steatosis**, with smaller droplets in centrilobular areas & larger fat vacuoles in periportal regions & **necrosis** of periportal hepatocytes
- **Glycogen depletion** is also a feature

61. **Ans. (a)** **Piecemeal necrosis** *(Ref: Robbins 9th/pg 837)*

Piecemeal necrosis is suggestive of chronic active hepatitis & not Alcoholic liver disease

62. **Ans. (b)** **Alcoholic hepatitis** *(Ref: Robbins 9th/pg 842-844)*

In the given scenario, the patient has Hyperbilirubinemia with AST: ALT ratio > 3:1 & GGT=44 IU/l. Most probable diagnosis is **Alcoholic liver disease.**

Features of Alcoholic liver disease:
- Clinical Features are usually non-specific.
- **AST:ALT Ratio =2:1 or 3:1**[Q] (In contrast to other etiologies where AST:ALT =1:1 or 1:2)
- Increased GGT (Normal 10-40 U/L), Bilirubin, Alkaline phosphatase

---

63. Ans. (b) Valproate

(Ref: Robbins 9th/pg 842-844; 8th/pg 857-858; Rosai and Ackerman's Surgical Pathology, Volume 1, chapter 13)

Steatosis refers to hepatocellular fat accumulation. **Macrovesicular steatosis is more commonly seen than Microvesicular steatosis.**

Features	Macrovesicular steatosis	Microvesicular steatosis
Histology	• Single large vacuole distends the hepatocyte & **displaces the nucleus to one side**	• **Fine-droplet fatty change** due to inhibition of mitochondrial fatty acid ß-oxidation & mitochondrial dysfunction
Etiology	• Alcoholic liver disease • Obesity; Diabetes. • Cachexia • PEM or Malnutrition (Periportal) • After total parenteral nutrition • Drugs: Steroid, Methotrexate • AIDS • Poisoning: phosphorus, CCl_4	• Alcoholic liver disease • Acute fatty liver of pregnancy • Severe liver injury • Jamaican vomiting sickness • Drugs: Tetracycline, Amiodarone, Valproate • Reye syndrome

---

64. Ans. (a) Alcoholic fatty liver

(Ref: Robbins 9th/pg 842-844)

Alcoholic fatty liver shows both microvesicular fatty change, initially, followed by macrovesicular fatty change; But rest of the options give rise to microvesicular steatosis only

---

65. Ans. (a, c, d, e) a. More common in female; c. Oral corticosteroids are given in severe cases; d. Associated with other autoimmune disease; e. Rarely lead to cirrhosis *(Ref: Robbins 9th ed p 855-857)*

Anti–liver kidney microsome-1 (anti-LKM-1) antibody is found in type II subtype.

---

66. Ans. (b) Anti-CCP antibodies *(Ref: R 9th/pg 839-840)*

Anti-CCP Ab seen in Rhemmatoid Arthritis

---

67. Ans. (a) Anti-LKM1 antibody

(Ref: Robbins 9th/pg 842; 8th/pg 857)

---

68. Ans. (a) Autoimmune hepatitis *(Ref: R 9th/pg 839-840)*

---

69. Ans. (c) ANA *(Ref: Robbins 9th/pg 839-840 8th/pg 855-856)*

---

70. Ans. (d) Primary biliary cirrhosis *(Ref: R 9th/pg 858-859)*

- **Most common autoimmune disease of liver in adults is Primary biliary cirrhosis**
- **Primary Sclerosing Cholangitis is an autoimmune disease that predominantly occurs in males**
- **Primary Sclerosing Cholangitis** is associated with inflammatory bowel disease in 70% cases.
- Prevalence of PSC in persons with ulcerative colitis is about 4%

---

71. Ans. (b) ANCA *(Ref: Robbins 9th/pg 839-840)*

---

72. Ans. (e) Roter's syndrome

---

73. Ans. (a) Increase of serum bilirubin, c. Increase alkaline phosphatase e. Stool sterocobilinogen absent

(Ref: PJM 20th/20;Harrison 19th/281; CMDT 2016/665)

---

74. Ans. (a) Jaundice becomes severe with time.

---

75. Ans. (d) Primary sclerosing cholangitis

The clinical feature of obstructive jaundice (jaundice, pruritis, raised bilirubin and alkaline phosphatase) along with Inflammtory bowel disease in an adult male is suggestive of Primary sclerosing cholangitis.

---

76. Ans. (a, b, d, e) a. More common in female; b. Periportal fibrosis; d. Jaundice may be present; e. Autoimmune disease are seen

(Ref: Robbins 9th/pg 858; 8th/pg 867)

---

77. Ans. (c) Primary biliary cirrhosis

(Ref: Robbins 9th/pg 858; 8th/pg 867)

In Primary biliary cirrhosis: Interlobular bile ducts are actively destroyed by lymphoplasmacytic inflammation with or without granulomas (**the *florid duct lesion***)

---

78. Ans. (c) Micronodural cirrhosis of liver

(Ref: Robbins 9th/pg 859; 8th/pg 869)

---

79. Ans. (c) Primary sclerosing cholangitis

(Ref: Robbins 9th/pg 859; 8th/pg 869)

---

80. Ans. (a) ABO incompatibility

(Ref: Robbins 9th/pg 852)

ABO incompatibility causes jaundice due to hemolysis and not cholestasis

---

81. Ans. (c) Criggler Najjar type II *(Ref: R 9th/pg 853-854)*

---

82. Ans. (c) Primary biliary cirrhosis

(Ref: Robbins 9th/pg 859)

---

83. Ans. (c) Rotor syndrome *(Ref: Robbins 9th/pg 853)*

84. **Ans. (a)** **Causes cirrhosis** *(Ref: Harrison 18th/Chapter 303)*

Gilbert Syndrome

Feature	Gilbert's Syndrome
Inheritance (all autosomal)	Promoter mutation: recessive Missense mutations: 7 of 8 dominant; 1 reportedly recessive
Total serum bilirubin	< 4 mg/dL in absence of fasting or hemolysis
Routine liver tests	Normal
Hepatic histology	Usually normal; increased lipofuscin pigment in some

85. **Ans. (c)** **Gilbert syndrome**

(Ref: Robbins 9th/pg 853-854)

86. **Ans. (b, d, e);** **b. Fat soluble; d. Affinity for brain tissue; e. Increased in hemolytic anemia**

(Ref: Robbins 9th/pg 852)

- Unconjugated bilirubin is **increased in hemolytic anemia**
- It is insoluble in water but **is fat soluble, so it can cross the blood brain barrier**
- It is **not filtered through the glomerulus, so does not appear in urine**.
- **Unconjugated bilirubin bound to albumin** is transported to the liver, where it is **taken up by hepatocytes** via a **carrier-mediated** membrane transport.

87. **Ans. (a)** **Ca bilirubinate**

(Ref: Robbins 9th/pg 877)

Two main types of gallstones:

- **Cholesterol stones** (**most common type in West**) containing crystalline cholesterol monohydrate.
- **Pigment stones** composed mainly of calcium bilirubinate; contain <20% cholesterol and are classified into "black" & "brown" types, the latter forming secondary to chronic biliary infection.

88. **Ans. (a)** **Ulcerative colitis** *(Ref: Robbins 9th/pg 859-860)*

- **PSC** is commonly seen in **association with** inflammatory bowel disease particularly **chronic ulcerative colitis**, which coexists in approximately **70%** of individuals with primary sclerosing cholangitis.
- Conversely, the **prevalence of PSC in persons with ulcerative colitis is about 4%.**

89. **Ans. (a)** **Dubin Johnson Syndrome**

(Ref: R 9th/pg 853-854)

90. **Ans. (c)** **Dubin Johnson Syndrome**

(Ref: R 9th/pg 853-854)

91. **Ans. (d)** **Fraction of coproporphyrin I in urine is elevated usually more than 80% of the total in Rotor syndrome**

(Ref: Harrison 18th/Chapter 303)

Differentiation between Dubin-Johnson syndrome & Rotor syndrome:

Characteristic	Dubin-Johnson syndrome	Rotor syndrome
Pigmentation of Liver	Pigmented cytoplasmic globules	Not seen; normal histology
Total urinary coproporphyrin excretion	Normal	Increased
Fraction of coproporphyrin I/III in urine	**> 80% of total**[Q]	**<70% of the total**[Q]
BSP clearance	**Normal**[Q], with reflux	**Delayed**[Q], No reflux

92. **Ans. (a, b, e)** **a. May be complicated by bacterial infection; b. Rarely progress to biliary cirrhosis; e. Narrowing of bile duct**

(Ref: Robbins 9th ed p 860)

PSC is characterized by inflammation and obliterative fibrosis of intrahepatic and extrahepatic bile ducts with dilation of preserved segments. Inflammatory bowel disease like ulcerative colitis is seen in 70% of individuals with PSC.

93. **Ans. (b)** **Anti-mitochondrial antibody**

(Ref: Robbins 9th/pg 859-860; 8th/pg 869)

94. **Ans. (a, c, d), a. Cholesterol stones are most common; c. Mirrizi syndrome is due to impaction of stone in hartmann's pouch; d. Hemolytic anaemia cause black colored stone**

(Ref: Robbins 9th/pg 876-877; 8th/pg 868; Harrison 18th/pg chapter 311)

a.	True	90% of gallstones are *cholesterol stones*
b.	False	10–15% of cholesterol stones and 50% of pigment stones are radiopaque
c.	True	In Mirizzi syndrome, a gallstone becomes impacted in cystic duct or neck of the gallbladder (**hartmann's pouch**) → compression & obstruction of CBD → jaundice.
d.	True	Pigment stones seen in Hemolytic anemia are black or brown in colour
e.	False	Gallstones are associated with an increased risk of gallbladder carcinoma

95. **Ans. (a) Most commonly caused by gram positive organisms** *(Ref: Harrison 18th/Chapter 42)*

Ascending cholangitis

- It is m**ost commonly caused by gram negative organisms like E. coli, Klebsiella spp**
- **Obstruction of bile duct by stone** is an important predisposing factor

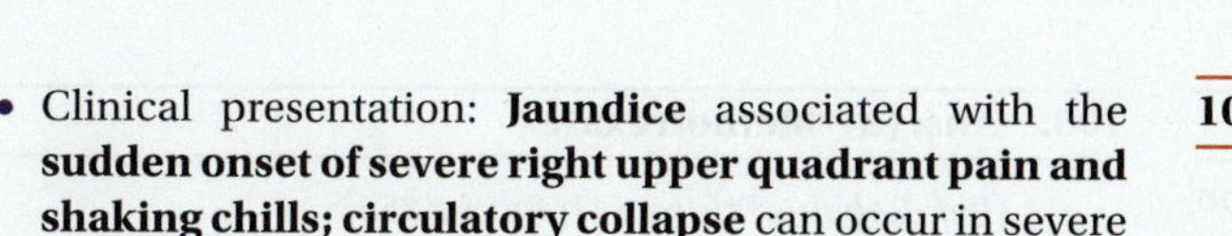

- Clinical presentation: **Jaundice** associated with the **sudden onset of severe right upper quadrant pain and shaking chills; circulatory collapse** can occur in severe cases
- **IV antibiotics, Urgent removal of stone by ERCP or Cholecystectomy** can be done

96. **Ans. (c, d, e); c. Pruritus; d. Pale stools; e. Icterus**

(Ref: Harrison 18th/Chapter 42)

Discussing options about obstructive jaundice one by one:

a.	False	Conjugated Hyperbilirubinemia is seen
b.	False	Positive direct Van den Bergh for conjugated bilirubin
c.	True	Pruritus occurs as bile salts irritates skin
d.	True	Absence of bilirubin excretion causes pale stools
e.	True	Icterus is a yellowish discoloration of tissue resulting from deposition of bilirubin; Scleral icterus indicates a serum bilirubin of at least 3 mg/dL

97. **Ans. (c) The conjugation process of bilirubin in liver remains operative without any interference**

(Ref: Harrison 18th/Chapter 42)

In post-hepatic jaundice, the concentration of conjugated bilirubin in the blood is higher than that of unconjugated bilirubin because:

- **The conjugation process of bilirubin in liver remains operative without any interference.**
- But there is **decreased excretion** of conjugated bilirubin into the bile ductules & **backward leakage** of the pigment into the circulation

98. **Ans. (b) Increased urinary copper excretion; (d) Increased liver copper content** *(Ref: R 9th pg 847)*

99. **Ans. (a) Alpha1 Antitrypsin deficiency**

(Ref: Robbins 9th/pg 847-851; 8th/pg 861-864; Refer to pretexts)

100. **Ans. (c) Alpha 1 antitrypsin deficiency**

(Ref: Robbins 9th/pg 847-851; 8th/pg 861-864)

101. **Ans. (a) Iron** *(Ref: Robbins 9th/pg 847-851; 8th/pg 861-864)*

102. **Ans. (c) 13** *(Ref: Robbins 9th/pg 847-851; 8th/pg 861-864)*

103. **Ans. (d) Low ↑ Ceruloplasmin high urine copper**

(Ref: Robbins 9th/pg 847-851; 8th/pg 861-864)

104. **Ans. (b) Hemochromatosis** *(Ref: Robbins 9th/pg 847-851)*

105. **Ans. (b) Autosomal recessive**

(Ref: Robbins 9th/pg 847-851)

106. **Ans. (d) Alpha-1-Antitrypsin deficiency**

(Ref: Robbins 9th/pg 847-851; 8th/pg 861-864)

107. **Ans. (b) 13** *(Ref: Robbins 9th/pg 847-851; 8th/pg 861-864)*

108. **Ans. (a) PAS + ve diastase resistant**

(Ref: R 9th/pg 847-851)

109. **Ans. (a) Iron** *(Ref: Robbins 9th/pg 847-851; 8th/pg 861-864)*

110. **Ans. (b) 250** *(Ref: Robbins 9th/pg 847-851; 8th/pg 861-864)*

111. **Ans. (d) HFE gene** *(Ref: Robbins 9th/pg 847-851)*

112. **Ans. (d) α-l-antitrypsin deficiency** *(Ref: R 9th/pg 847-851)* **Cirrhosis can occur due to alpha1 antitrypsin deficiency**

113. **Ans. (d, e) d. Opisthorchis viverrini; e. Clonorchis sinensis**

114. **Ans. (c) Portal hypertension seen in 50% of patients**

115. **Ans. (a) Hemangiosarcoma**

116. **Ans. (e) Need surgical removal in every case because chances of rupture is high**

117. **Ans. (a) Fibrolamellar Variant of HCC**

118. **Ans. (a) Better prognosis than typical hepatocellular carcinoma**

(Ref: Robbins (SEA) 9th/873; Harshmohan 7th/620; Harrison 19th/552)

119. **Ans. (b) More common in male**

(Ref: Robbins (SEA) 9th/867)

120. **Ans. (b) Squamous cell carcinoma is 40% of all cases**

(Ref: Robbins 9th pg 879-880)

Morphology of Gall bladder Ca is mostly Adenocarcinoma[Q] > Squamous cell Ca (5% cases)

121. **Ans. (c) Starts with macronodular and later on changes to micronodular cirrhosis.**

(Ref: Robbins 9th pg 842-844)

The three distinctive forms of alcoholic liver injury: (1) hepatocellular steatosis or fatty change, (2) alcoholic (or steato-) hepatitis, and (3) steatofibrosis (patterns of scarring typical for all fatty liver diseases including alcohol) up to and including cirrhosis in the late stages of disease.

Iron overload and infections with HIV, HCV and HBV synergize with alcohol, leading to increased severity of liver disease.

122. **Ans. (b)** **Tyrosenemia** *(Ref: Robbins 9th/pg 870)*

Among the given options, Tyrosenemia is the least common cause of HCC, so is the answer.

123. **Ans. (c)** **Vinyl chloride** *(Ref: Robbins 9th/pg 870)*

- **Angiosarcoma of liver** is associated with **vinyl chloride, arsenic or Thorotrast exposure** and has poor prognosis

124. **Ans. (b)** **Young females** *(Ref: Robbins 9th/pg 870)*

125. **Ans. (d)** **Fibrolamellar carcinoma**

(Ref: R 9th/pg 870)

Fibrolammellar Ca has a good prognosis while others behave as Malignant tumors.

126. **Ans. (b)** **High risk of malignant transformation**

(Ref: Robbins 9th/pg 870)

Features of **HNF1-α inactivated adenomas**
- Common in feamles
- Virtually **no risk of malignant** transformation,
- Often associated with **OCP** use
- In individuals with **MODY-3**

127. **Ans. (b)** **Mature hepatocytes present** *(Ref: R 9th/pg 870)*

Histology of Hepatoblastoma can be of 2 types:
- *Epithelial type*, composed of small polygonal fetal cells or smaller embryonal cells forming acini, tubules, or papillary structures
- *Mixed epithelial and mesenchymal type*, which contains foci of mesenchymal differentiation that may consist of primitive mesenchyme, osteoid, cartilage, or striated muscle.

Mature appearing hepatocytes are absent.

128. **Ans. (d)** **Hepatitis D** *(Ref: Robbins 9th/pg 838; 8th/pg 853)*

129. **Ans. (a)** **Hepatocellular Ca** *(Ref: Robbins 9th/pg 870)*

130. **Ans. (b)** **Ulcerative colitis** *(Ref: Robbins 9th/pg 874)*

Risk Factors for cholangiocarcinoma:
- Chronic inflammation eg Ulcerative colitis
- Cholestasis
- Primary sclerosing Cholangitis
- Liver flukes (particularly Opisthorchis and Clonorchis species)
- Hepatitis B and C
- Non-alcoholic fatty liver disease

131. **Ans. (a)** **Liver** *(Ref: Robbins 9th/pg 875; 8th/pg 856)*

- Oral contraceptives have been implicated in the development of hepatic adenoma and, rarely, hepatocellular carcinoma and hepatic vein occlusion (Budd-Chiari syndrome).

132. **Ans. (a, d, e)** **a. Better prognosis than Primary HCC; d. Underlying cirrhosis not a risk factor; e. Neurotensin is a biomarker** *(Ref: Robbins 9th/pg 873; 8th/pg 879)*

133. **Ans. (a)** **Methotrexate**

(Ref: Robbins 9th/pg 841; 8th/pg 856)

134. **Ans. (c)** **Angiosarcoma**

(Ref: Robbins 9th/pg 841; 8th/pg 856)

135. **Ans. (b)** **Primary sclerosing cholangitis**

(Ref: Robbins 9th/pg 874; 8th/pg 880)

136. **Ans. (a)** **Nodular type of cholangiocarcinoma**

(Ref: Robbins 9th/pg 874; 8th/pg 880)

(Klatskin tumor) is Nodular type of cholangiocarcinoma at the junction of the right and left hepatic ducts.

Intrahepatic-10%.

137. **Ans. (a, b)** **a. Lipase; b. Amylase**

(Ref: Robbins 9th/pg 884; 8th/pg 893)

Lipase and Amylase are raised in pancreatitis rather than liver disorder.

138. **Ans. (a, b, c, d); a. Raised in testicular tumor; b. Raised in 50-70% cases of HCC; c. Correlation between tumor recurrence after surgery in HCC; d. Correlation with HCC size** *(Ref: Harrison 18th/Chapter 92)*

AFP:
- Normal Range of AFP in adults: 0–8.5 ng/mL
- **It is a tumor marker for Liver Cancers**, non-seminomatous[Q] germ cell tumors of testis
- **Liver diseases with elevated AFP are:** Tumors like **Hepatocellular Carcinoma,[Q] Hepatoblastoma, Infantile hemangioendothelioma** & non-neoplastic lesions like **Amebic liver abscess[Q] & Hepatitis[Q]**
- Adverse prognostic factors in HCC include ascites, jaundice, vascular invasion, and elevated AFP; AFP correlates with HCC size
- **Postoperative AFP level** is a useful tool for **predicting recurrence after curative hepatectomy**.
- A positive level of AFP after operation might suggest a site of residual viable cancer.

139. **Ans. (c)** **Arises from cirrhotic liver** *(Ref: R 9th/pg 873)*

140. **Ans. (b)** **Cholangiocarcinoma** *(Ref: Robbins 9th/pg 874)*

141. **Ans. (b)** **Liver** *(Ref: Robbins 9th/pg 862; 8th/pg 869)*

Von Meyenburg Complexes
- Clusters of **dilated bile ducts** embedded in a fibrous, sometimes hyalinized, stroma located close to or within portal tracts.
- These lesions are often referred to as **"bile duct hamartomas"**
- They are without clinical significance except in the **differential diagnosis of metastases to the liver**

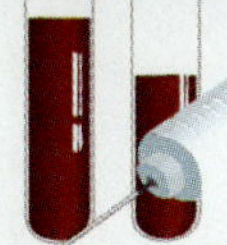

142. Ans. (d) Hepatitis-B virus

(Ref: Robbins 9th/pg 871-873)

Hepatitis-B & C virus are important risk factors of HCC

143. Ans. (a) Adenomyomatosis of gall bladder

(Ref: Robbins 9th/pg 879; 8th/pg 886)

Rokitansky-Aschoff sinuses[Q] are Outpouchings of the mucosal epithelium through the wall seen in adenomyomatosis of gall bladder

144. Ans. (b) Porcelain gallbladder

(Ref: Robbins 9th/pg 879)

Porcelain Gallbladder:
- **Calcium salt deposition within the wall of a chronically inflamed** gallbladder
- May be detected on the plain abdominal film.
- It is **associated with the development of carcinoma** of the gallbladder
- Cholecystectomy is advised in all patients with porcelain gallbladder

Limey Bile or Milk of Calcium Bile
- Calcium precipitation & diffuse, hazy opacification of bile due to calcium salts in the lumen of the gallbladder
- Produce or a layering effect on plain abdominal roentgenography.
- Usually clinically innocuous, but cholecystectomy is recommended, especially when it occurs in a hydropic gallbladder.

145. Ans. (d) Islet cell hypertrophy

(Ref: Robbins 9th/pg 884)

146. Ans. (a) KRAS *(Ref: Robbins 9th/pg 892-894)*

Gene	Chr	Percentage	
KRAS	12p	90	**Most commonly involved Oncogene[Q]**
p16/ CDKN2A	9p	95	**Most commonly involved Tumor suppressor gene[Q]**
TP53	17p	50–70	Involved in Response to DNA damage
SMAD4	18q	55	TGF β pathway
BRCA2	13q	10	**Germ-line mutation[Q]**

147. Ans. (a) Head *(Ref: Robbins 9th/pg 892-894; 8th/pg 900-903)*

Pancreatic Carcinoma is

Site of	Pancreatic Head (most common)[Q] > Diffuse > Body > Tail

148. Ans. (a) KRAS *(Ref: Robbins 9th/pg 892-894)*

149. Ans. (a) Intraductal papillary mucinous neoplasms

(Ref: Robbins 9th/pg 892-894; 8th/pg 900-903)

A.	Intraductal papillary mucinous neoplasms	IPMNs **progress to an invasive cancer**
B.	Solid-pseudopapillary neoplasms	Usually benign
C.	Serous cystic neoplasms	Always benign
D.	Mucinous cystic neoplasms	1/3rd associated with invasive adenocarcinoma

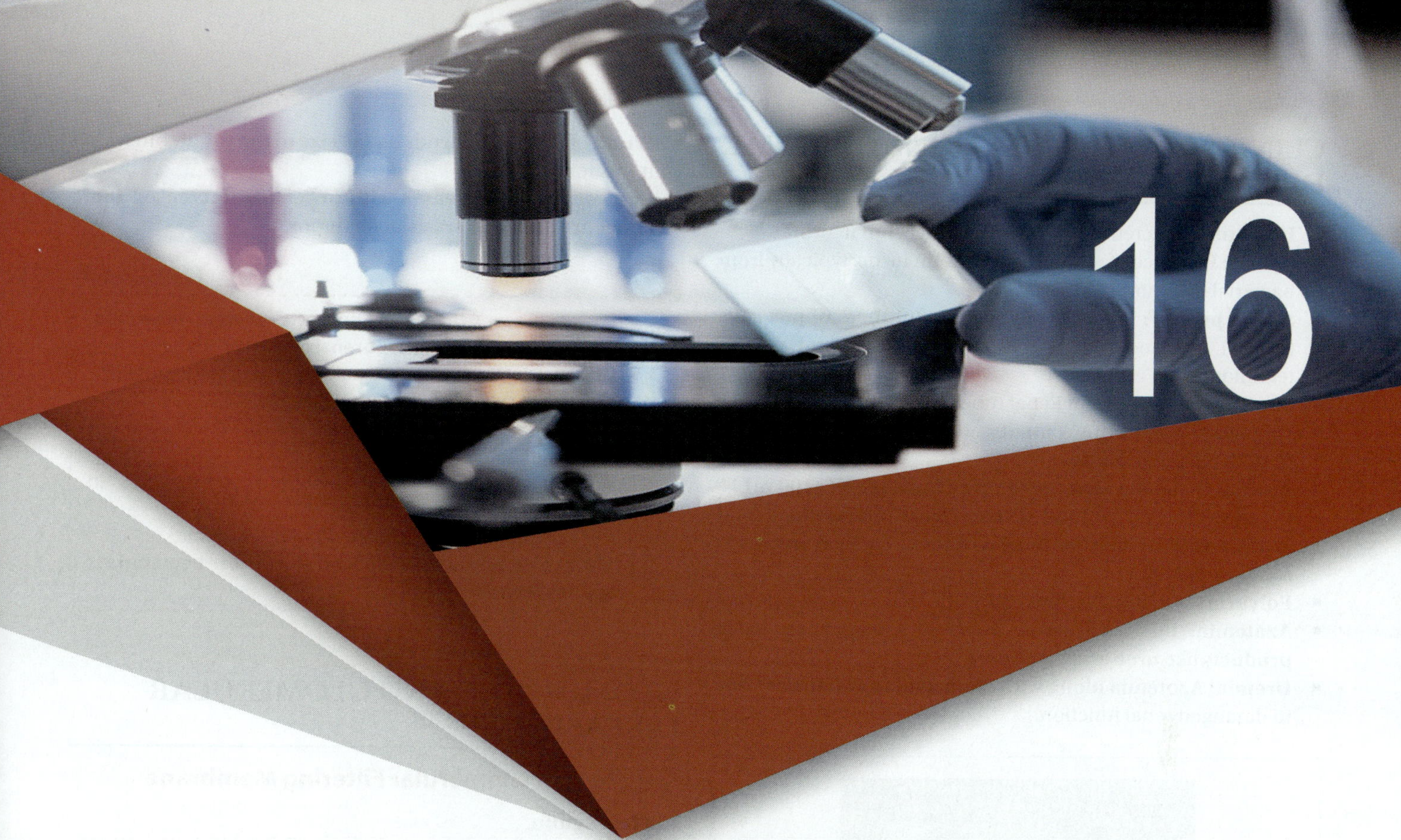

Renal System and its Disorders

16

Key Points

» **Hematuria** is excretion of **intact RBCs >3/hpf** in urine
» **Sterile pyuria:** presence of **elevated numbers of pus cells** (WBCs) in sterile urine (seen in Tuberculosis)
» Most common cause of **isolated glomerular hematuria** is IgA nephropathy
» **Mesangial cells are mesenchymal origin**, are **contractile, phagocytic**, and **capable of proliferation**
» **Crescents are seen in RPGN and suggest poor prognosis**
» **Microalbuminuria:** Excretion of **30–300 mg/day** of albumin in urine or **30–300 mg/g of creatinine in urine**
» **Focal Segmental Glomerulosclerosis (FSGS) is the most common cause of nephrotic syndrome in adults**
» **Minimal change disease is the most frequent cause of nephrotic syndrome in children**
» **Most specific histological lesion in diabetic nephropathy is Kimmelsteil -Wilson lesions**
» **Thyroidization of tubules is a feature of Chronic pyelonephritis**
» Major Causes of Papillary Necrosis is **analgesic nephropathy**
» **Clear cell Ca is the most common histological subtype of Renal cell Carcinoma (RCC)**
» Polycythemia and Hypertension **is the most common paraneoplastic feature of RCC**
» **Michaelis-Gutmann bodies are seen in Malacoplakia**

Key Recent Updates

» MPGN type II is now classified as C3 glomerulopathy
» Fibronectin glomerulopathy occurs due to mutation of FN_1 gene on chromosome 2q34.

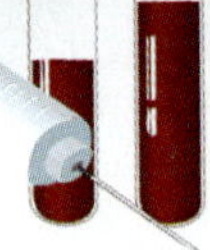

CLINICAL MANIFESTATIONS OF RENAL DISEASES

- **Hematuria:** Excretion of **intact RBCs > 3/ hpf** in urine[Q]
- **Pyuria:** Presence of **> 5 pus cells/hpf**[Q] in urine, typically from bacterial infection
- **Sterile pyuria**[Q]**:** Presence of **elevated numbers of pus cells** (WBCs) in urine which is **sterile** using standard culture techniques
- **Sterile pyuria** is seen in Renal tuberculosis
- **Oliguria**[Q]**:** 24-h urine output **<400 mL**[Q], usually due to underlying renal failure.
- **Anuria:** Complete **absence of urine formation (<100 mL).**[Q] It can be caused by **total urinary tract obstruction, total renal artery or vein occlusion, shock, cortical necrosis, ATN and RPGN.**[Q]
- **Polyuria:** 24-h urine output **>3 L**[Q]
- **Azotemia:** Increased serum levels of **nitrogenous waste products** like **urea and creatinine**[Q]
- **Uremia:** Azotemia along with clinical manifestations[Q] due to deranged renal function.

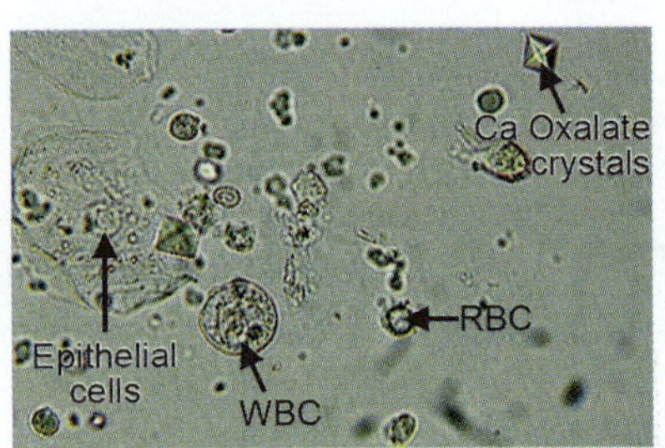

Normal urine microscopy

Urinary Casts (Refer Annexures for Images and Types)

- **Formed elements of urine**[Q] that have **kidney as their sole site of origin**[Q]
- **Tamm-Horsfall protein**, secreted from the **thick ascending loop of Henle**[Q] forms the **matrix of all casts**[Q]

- **Width** of the cast depends on the **size of the tubule**[Q] in which it was formed
- Cast formation **increases with lower pH, increased ionic concentration and stasis** in nephrons[Q]

High Yield Facts

- Eosinophils in the urine suggests **allergic interstitial nephritis or atheroembolic renal disease.**[Q]
- **Urinary Dipsticks** detect **only albumin as urinary protein**[Q]
- **Dipstick** gives **false-positive** results for:
  - Albumin: when pH >7.0, urine is very concentrated or contaminated with blood.[Q]
  - Hematuria: when myoglobinuria is present, as in rhabdomyolysis.[Q]
- RBCs of **glomerular origin** are often **dysmorphic**[Q]
- Most common cause of **isolated glomerular hematuria** is **IgA nephropathy**[Q]

GLOMERULUS AND GLOMERULAR DISEASES

Structure of Glomerular Filtering Membrane

- **Mesangium**
- **Visceral epithelial cells (podocytes)**[Q]**:**
  - **20-30-nm**–wide filtration slits → size selective barrier
  - Responsible for synthesis of GBM components
- **Glomerular basement membrane (GBM):**
  - Composed of collagen **type 4 (or COL4 α1 to α6)**[Q]
  - Each molecule consists of a **7S domain** at the **N terminus**, a triple-helical domain in the middle, and a globular **noncollagenous domain (NC1)** at the C terminus.
  - Other components are: **Laminin, polyanionicproteo-glycans (negatively charged), mostly heparan sulfate**, fibronectin, entactin and several other glycoproteins.
- **Fenestrated endothelial cells** (70-100 nm)[Q].

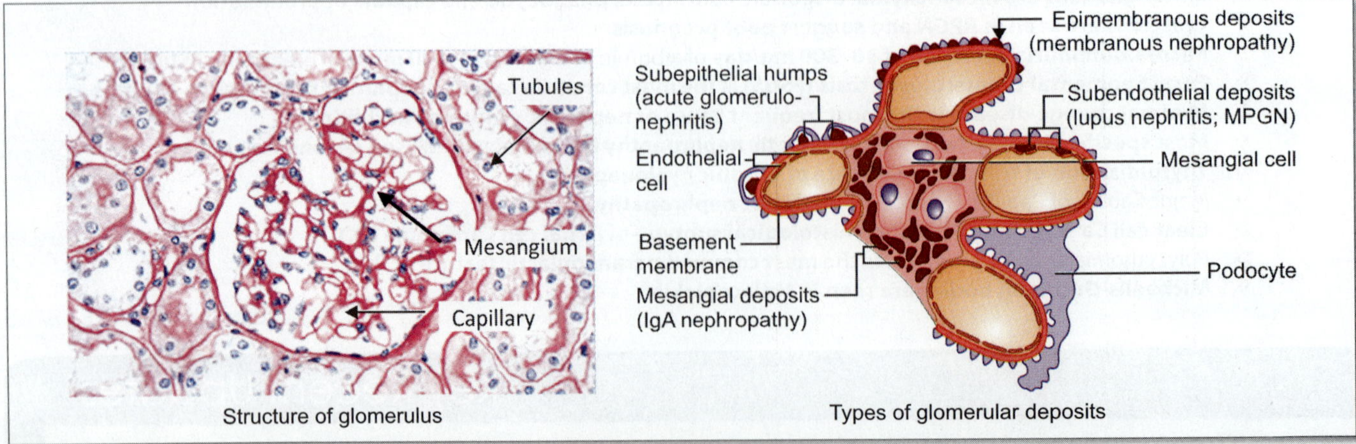

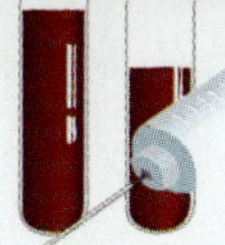

PATHOLOGIC RESPONSES OF THE GLOMERULUS TO INJURY

Site of glomerular deposits	Type of Glomerulonephritis
Subepithelial deposits	• PSGN • Membranous GN • RPGN • Heymann Nephritis
Subendothelial deposits	• Lupus nephritis • MPGN-I
Membranous deposits	• MPGN II
Mesangial deposits	• IgA nephropathy • HSP

Terminologies used in Kidney Biopsy	
Terminology	**Description**
Diffuse	Involving **>50%** of the glomeruli in the kidney[Q]
Global	Involving the glomerulus **completely**[Q]
Focal	Involving **<50%** of the glomeruli in the kidney
Segmental	Affecting **a part of each glomerulus**[Q]
Capillary loop Mesangial	Affecting predominantly **capillary or mesangial regions**[Q]

High Yield Facts

- Mesangial cells[Q]- **mesenchymal origin**, are contractile[Q], phagocytic[Q], and capable of proliferation[Q]
- Mesangial cells and mesangial matrix support the glomerular tuft
- Glomerular filtering membrane is a size- and charge-dependent barrier
- Neutral substance ≤ 4A can get freely filtered through GBM
- **GBM** is **negatively charged** due to **sialo-glycoprotein**
- All proteins (negatively charged) are normally repelled by GBM
- **Albumin** (smallest molecular wt, 70 kD) is the **1st protein to appear in urine in glomerulonephritis**
- **AN**ionic antigens form sub**EN**dothelial deposits
- **Cationic** antigens form **subepithelial** deposits
- **Neutral** antigens form **mesangial** deposits

PATHOGENESIS OF GLOMERULAR INJURY

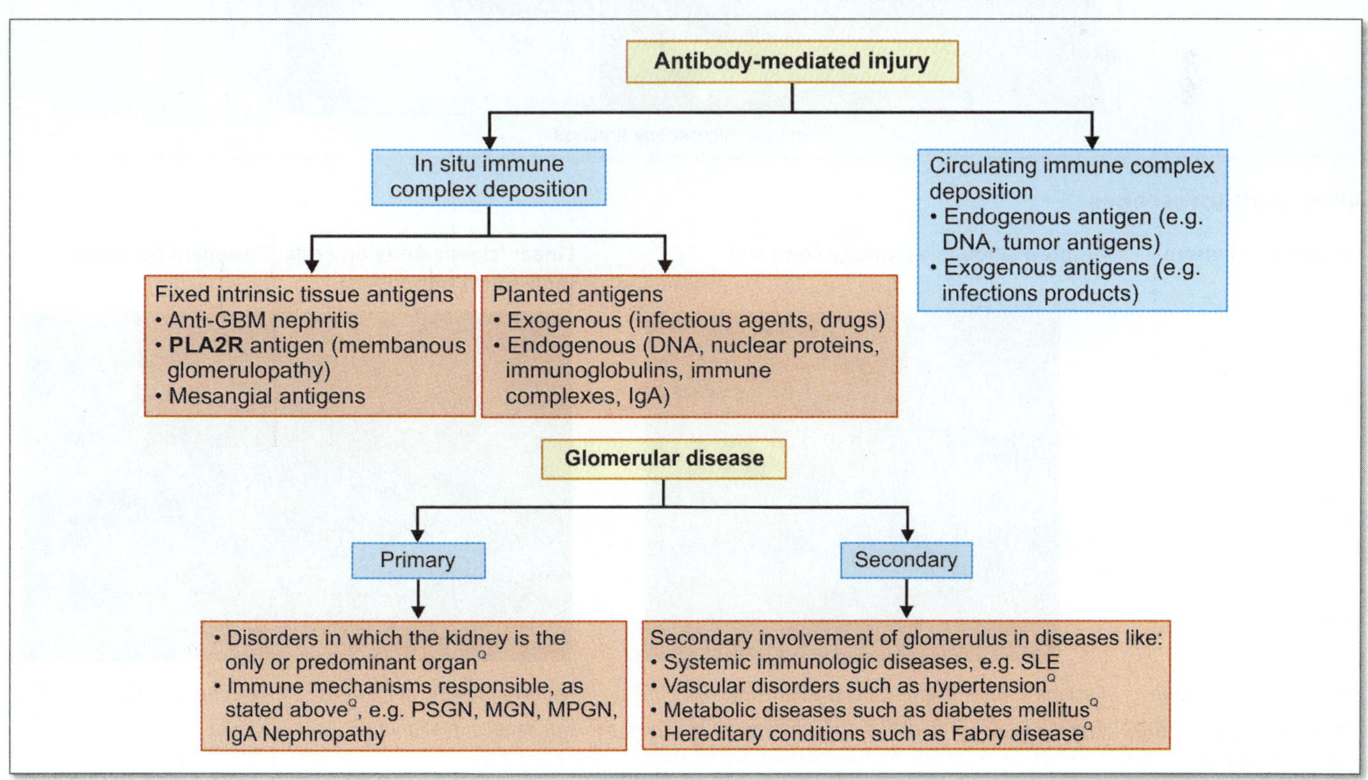

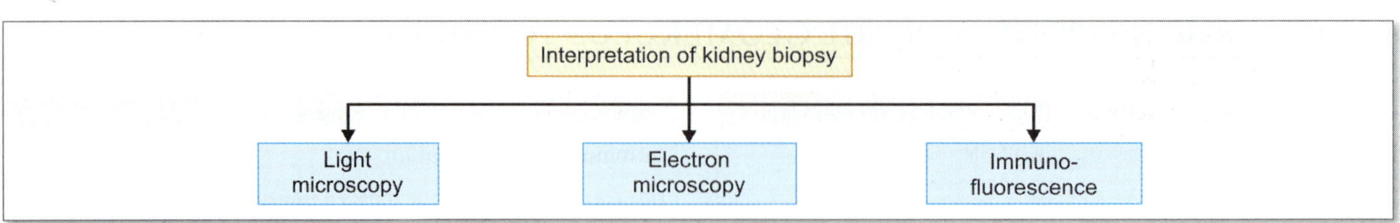

Electron Microscopy

Subepithelial	Intramembranous	Subendothelial	Mesangial	Combined Subendothelial, Subepithelial and Mesangial
Membranous GN	Dense-deposit disease	MPGN C3GN	IgA nephropathy	Lupus (WHO classes III and IV) C3GN
Lupus (WHO class V)	GN related to endocarditis, deep-seated abscesses	Lupus (WHO class III and IV)	Henoch-Schonlein purpura	MPGN type III
Postinfectious GN	Other infections	Cryoglobulinemic GN (microglobular structure)	Lupus (WHO class II) Clq nephropathy Rare other forms of mesangioproliferative GN	GN related to infections. Proliferative GN with monoclonal IgG deposit

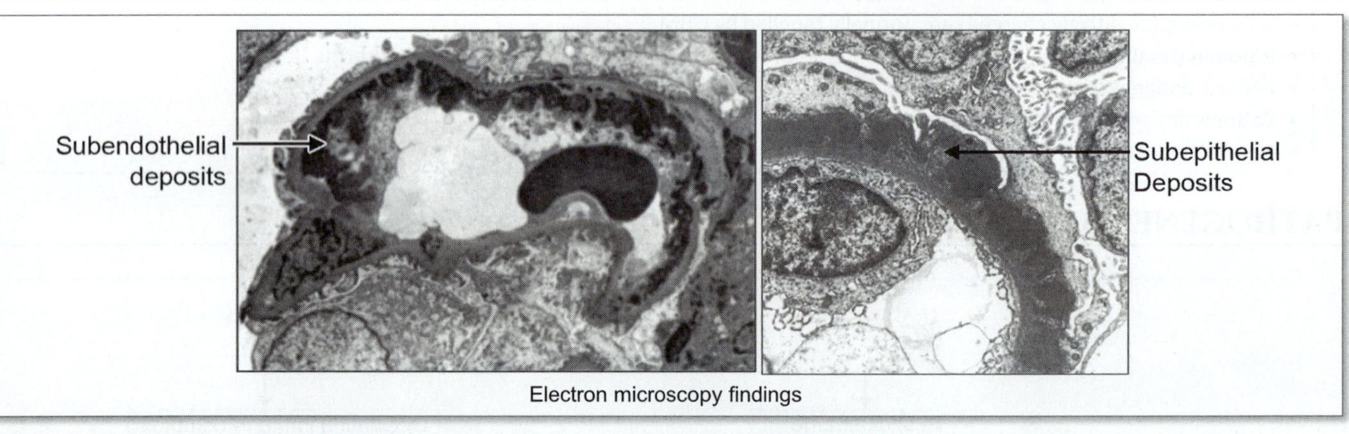

Electron microscopy findings

Immunofluorescence

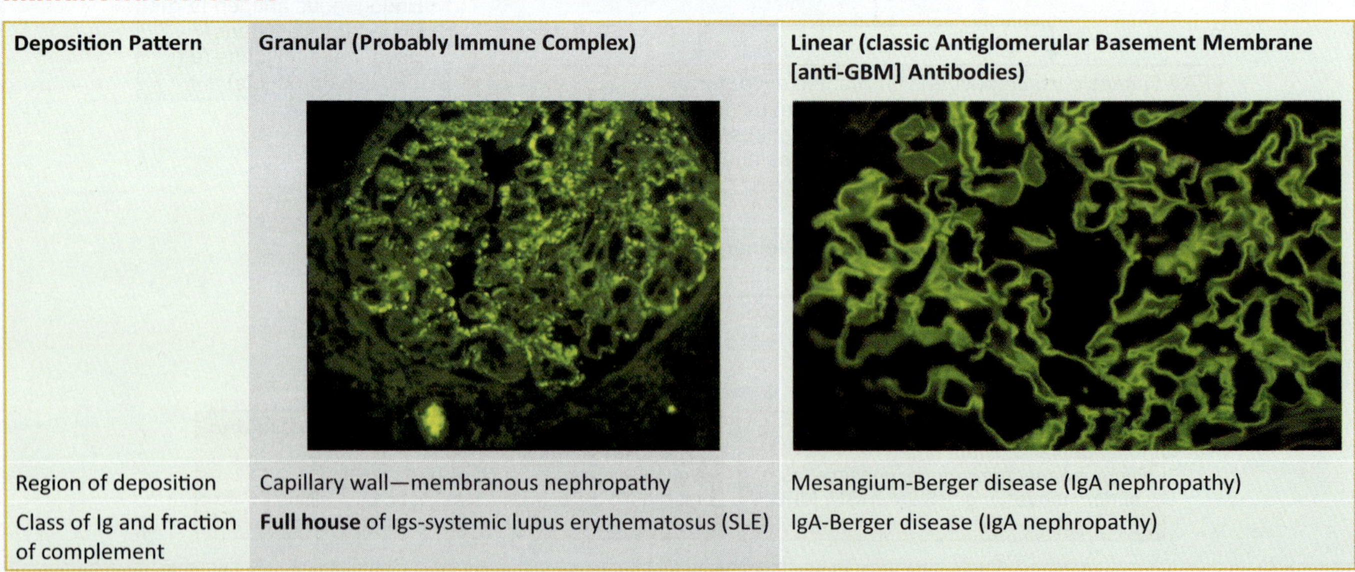

Deposition Pattern	Granular (Probably Immune Complex)	Linear (classic Antiglomerular Basement Membrane [anti-GBM] Antibodies)
Region of deposition	Capillary wall—membranous nephropathy	Mesangium-Berger disease (IgA nephropathy)
Class of Ig and fraction of complement	**Full house** of Igs-systemic lupus erythematosus (SLE)	IgA-Berger disease (IgA nephropathy)

NEPHRITIC SYNDROME

- **Definition: Sudden** onset of **gross hematuria, oliguria, nephritic range proteinuria**, mild **edema, hypertension, and renal insufficiency**[Q]
- Characterized by **inflammation** in the **glomeruli**[Q]

Difference between nephritic and nephrotic syndrome

Characteristic	Nephritic Syndrome	Nephrotic Syndrome
Hematuria and RBC casts	Present	Absent/few
Proteinuria	Nephritic range (<3.5g/day)[Q]	Nephrotic range (>3.5g/day)[Q] (>40 mg/m²/hr)
Hypertension	Present[Q]	Uncommon
Uremia	Present[Q]	Absent
Oliguria	Present[Q]	Absent

POSTSTREPTOCOCCAL GLOMERULONEPHRITIS (PSGN)

- **Time course**: **1 to 4 weeks** after a streptococcal infection (**sore throat or pyoderma**)[Q]
- **Age group**: most frequently, **children 6 -10 years**[Q]
- **Inciting agent**: **group A β-hemolytic streptococci**[Q] – nephritogenic strains (**12, 4, and 1**)[Q]
- **Complement levels C3 decrease Anti-Streptococcal-O (ASO) increase**s, normal levels of C4

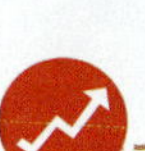

High Yield Facts

- In PSGN, Serum complement levels (C3): **transiently low**[Q]
- **Principal antigen in PSGN**: streptococcal pyogenic exotoxin B (Spe B)[Q]
- **Early treatment** of sore throat/pyoderma with antibiotics **does not**[Q] prevent PSGN
- Deposits seen in PSGN[Q]: **Subepithelial humps**, Subendothelial, mesangial

Morphology

Light Microscopy	Immunofluorescence Microscopy	Electron Microscopy
• Hypercellular glomeruli • Infiltration by WBCs, • Proliferation of endothelial and mesangia cells: **Endo- and exocapillary proliferation**[Q] • **Crescents**: Severe cases[Q]	Granular deposits of **IgG, and C3 in mesangium**[Q] and along GBM	Discrete, amorphous, electron-dense **SUBEPITHELIAL deposits ("Humps")**[Q]

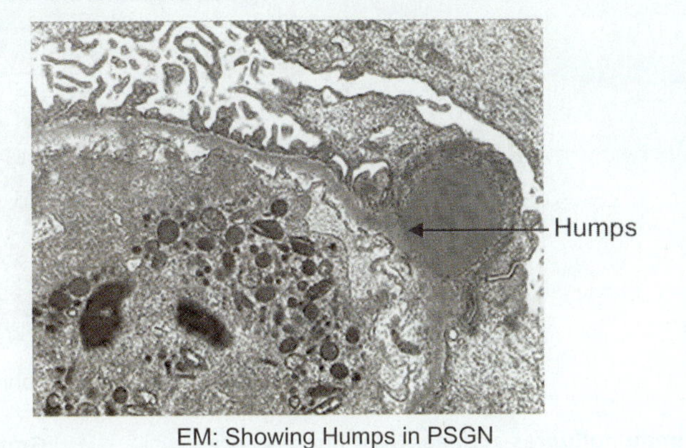

EM: Showing Humps in PSGN

Prognosis

In children:
- Self-recovery is seen in **95% (Good prognosis)**[Q]
- **1% become severely oliguric, and develop RPGN**[Q]
- **5%** undergo slow progression to **chronic glomerulonephritis**[Q]

RAPIDLY PROGRESSIVE GLOMERULONEPHRITIS (RPGN)

- Characterized by severe glomerular injury (**crescents**) leading to **rapid and progressive loss of renal function** associated with **severe oliguria** and signs of nephritic syndrome.[Q]
- If untreated, **death** from renal failure occurs **within weeks to months.**[Q]

Types of RPGN

Entity	Type I (20%)	Type II (25%)	Type III (55%)
Mechanism	Anti-GBM Antibody	Immune Complex	Pauci-immune, c-ANCA/p-ANCA mediated

Etiology	Renal limited
	Good pasture syndrome[Q]
	(Serum antibodies against **alpha 3 NC1 domain of collagen – IV**)
		• **Postinfectious**
		  ■ Poststreptococcal glomerulonephritis[Q]
		  ■ Bacterial endocarditis[Q]
		• **Noninfectious**
		  ■ SLE[Q], HSP[Q]
		  ■ Mixed cryoglobulinemia[Q]
		• **Primary Renal Disease**
		  ■ MPGN[Q]
		  ■ IgA nephropathy[Q]
			ANCA-associated
			• Idiopathic
			• **Granulomatosis with polyangiitis (Wegener granulomatosis)**[Q]
			• Microscopic polyangiitis[Q]
			• Hypersensitivity vasculitis[Q]

Grossly	Kidneys are enlarged and pale, often with **petechial hemorrhages** on the cortical surfaces. (FLEA-BITTEN KIDNEY)[Q]		
Light m/e	• **Glomeruli: Crescents** are Hallmark[Q] • Focal and segmental necrosis[Q], endothelial and mesangial proliferation[Q] • **Pauci-immune: Segmental glomerular necrosis** is characteristic[Q] 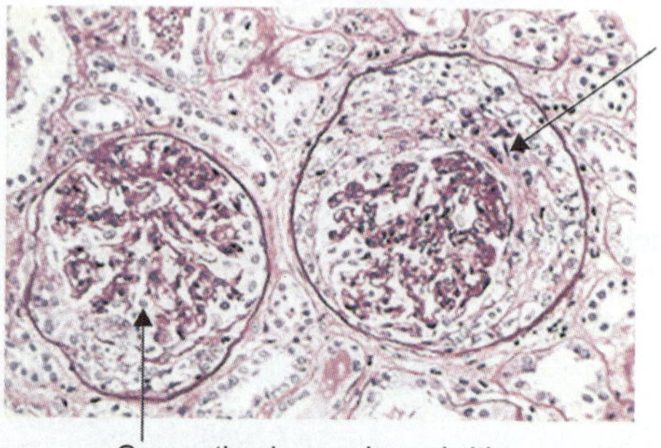		
Immunofluorescence m/e	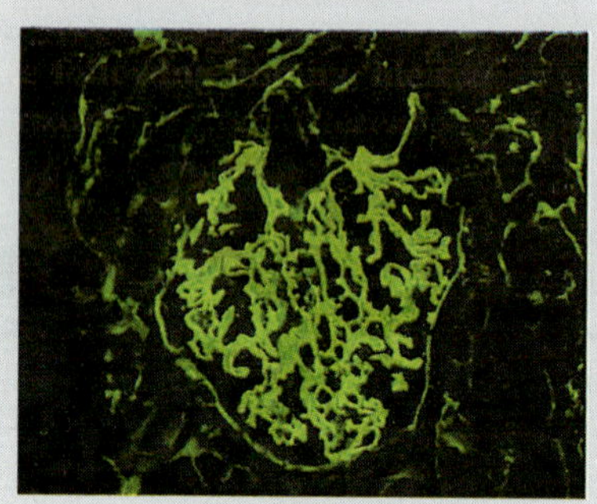 **Linear GBM fluorescence**[Q]	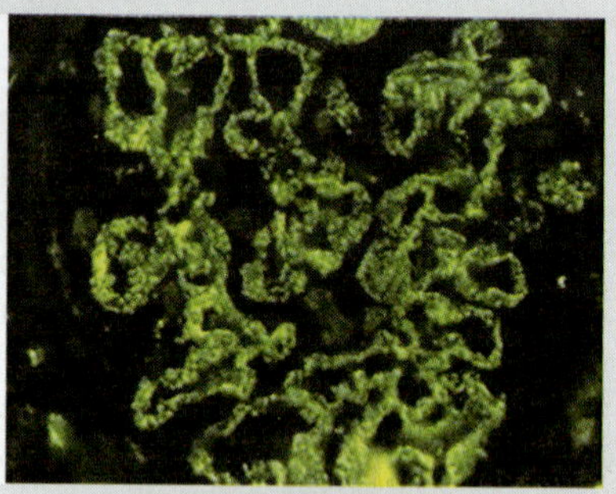 **Granular immune deposits**[Q]	**No** deposition of immune reactants[Q] **No Deposits seen** (Pauci-immune)
Electron m/e	**Ruptures in the GBM**[Q] may be present, Type II shows immune complex deposits		

Crescents- Formed by

- Proliferation of **parietal cells**[Q]
- Infiltration by **WBCs**[Q]
- **Fibrin strands.**[Q]

Crescents obliterate the urinary space and compress the glomerular tuft, hence **More the number of crescents → poorer the prognosis**[Q]

Cresentic glomerulonephritis

Type I RPGN (Linear)

Type II RPGN (Granular)

Clinical Course

- **Hematuria with RBC casts**[Q] in the urine, variable proteinuria, hypertension and edema.
- **Progressive over weeks** and ends in **severe oliguria/renal failure.**[Q]
- **Goodpasture syndrome**: Recurrent **hemoptysis** or even life-threatening pulmonary hemorrhage (**Necrotizting hemorrhagic interstitial pneumonitis**).[Q]

NEPHROTIC SYNDROME

The Manifestations of Nephrotic Syndrome Include

- **Massive proteinuria (>3.5 g/day)**[Q] (>40 mg/m^2/hr)
- **Hypoalbuminemia**[Q] (plasma albumin <3 g/dL)
- **Generalized edema** (due to **loss of oncotic pressure**[Q] > sodium and water retention)[Q]

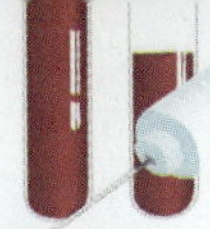

- **Hyperlipidemia:**[Q]-Increased synthesis of lipoproteins in the liver, abnormal transport of circulating lipid particles, and decreased lipid catabolism.
- **Lipiduria** (free fat or as oval fat bodies in urine)[Q]

Remember: Proteinuria can be

- **Selective proteinuria:** → Initially; consists mostly of **low-molecular-weight proteins (albumin, 70 kD; transferrin, 76 kD)**
- **Nonselective proteinuria:** → Later, in advanced disease, consists of higher molecular-weight globulins and albumin.

Causes of Nephrotic Syndrome

Primary Glomerular Disease	Systemic Diseases
• Membranous glomerulonephropathy (MGN)[Q] • Minimal-change disease (MCD)[Q] • Focal segmental glomerulosclerosis (FSGS)[Q] • Membranoproliferative glomerulonephritis (MPGN) • IgA nephropathy[Q]	• **Diabetes mellitus[Q], Amyloidosis[Q]** • Systemic lupus erythematosus (**SLE**)[Q] • Drugs (**NSAIDs, penicillamine, Lithium, Pamidronate, heroin injection**)[Q] • Infections (**hepatitis B and C, HIV, malaria, toxoplasmosis, syphilis**)[Q] • Malignant disease (**carcinoma, lymphoma**)[Q] • Hereditary nephritis, **Renal vein thrombosis**)

High Yield Facts

- **Microalbuminuria:** Excretion of **30–300 mg/day**[Q] of albumin in urine or **30–300 mg/g of creatinine in urine**[Q]
- **Macroalbuminuria:** Excretion of **300–3500 mg/day** of albumin in urine[Q]
- **Nephrotic range proteinuria:** Excretion of > **3.5 g/day**[Q] of albumin in urine
- **Selective proteinuria:** Selective excretion of **low-molecular-weight proteins** like **albumin and transferrin**[Q] by the kidney.

MEMBRANOUS NEPHROPATHY

- *Characterized by:* **Diffuse thickening** of glomerular capillary wall due to accumulation of deposits containing immune complex deposits along **sub-epithelial side** of basement membrane.[Q]
- *Etiology:*
  - **Primary: 75%:** Associated with **HLA-DQA1**[Q], Autoantigen: **phospholipase A2 receptor**[Q]
  - **Secondary: 25%**
    - Infections: Chronic hepatitis B, hepatitis C, Syphilis, Schistosomiasis, Malaria[Q]
    - Drugs: Penicillamine, Captopril, Gold, NSAIDs[Q]
    - Carcinoma lung, colon, and melanoma

- **Autoimmune diseases:** SLE (10–15%), Rheumatoid Arthritis, Primary biliary cirrhosis, Dermatitis herpetiformis
- **Systemic** diseases: Fanconi's syndrome, sickle cell anemia, diabetes, **Crohn's disease**, Sarcoidosis,

- *Morphology:*
  - **Light microscopy:** Uniform, diffuse **thickening of the glomerular capillary wall.**[Q]
  - **Immunofluorescence microscopy:** Granular/Lumpy bumpy[Q] electron dense immune complexes deposits
  - **Electron microscopy: Granular deposits, (Ig + complement)**
    - **Effacement of podocyte** foot processes[Q]
  - **On Silver methenamine stain-** prominent "**spikes**" and "**domes**"[Q] of silver-staining matrix

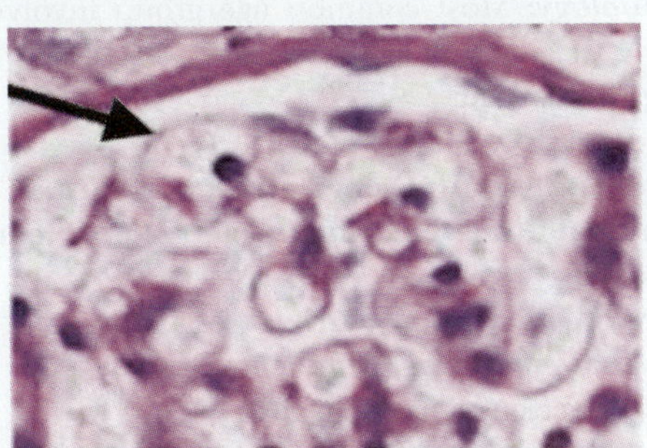

Normal capillary wall

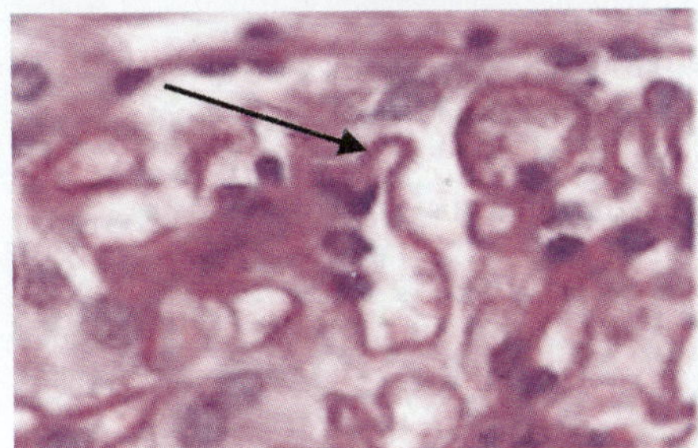

Thickened capillary wall

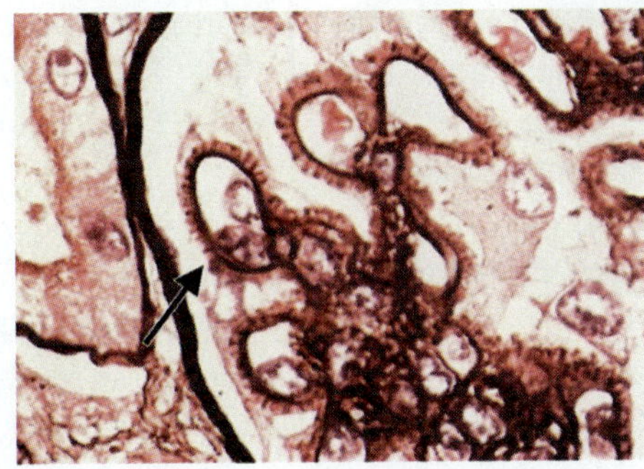

Spikes and domes on silver stain

- *Clinical course:*
  - **Persistent proteinuria** in **60%** of patients[Q]
  - **40%** develop severe CKD or ESRD[Q]
  - **40% recurs in patients who undergo transplantation**[Q]

- **Membranous nephropathy** is the **most frequent cause of** nephrotic syndrome in elderly[Q]
- **Focal segmental glomerulosclerosis (FSGS) is the most common cause of nephrotic syndrome in adults**[Q]
- **Minimal change disease is the most frequent cause of** nephrotic syndrome in children[Q]
- **Mutation in NPHS2 is the most common cause of Steroid Resistant Nephrotic syndrome**[Q]

MINIMAL CHANGE DISEASE

- *Characterized by:* **Absence of immune deposits** but has an immunologic basis.[Q]
- *Epidemiology:* Most common age group involved: **2 to 6** years[Q]
- *Etiology:* Idiopathic
- *Morphology:*
  - **Light microscopy: Glomeruli appear normal**[Q]
  - **Immunofluorescence microscopy: No Ig/ complement deposits**
  - **Electron microscopy: Diffuse effacement of foot processes of podocytes ("podocytopathy")**[Q]
    - No electron-dense deposits[Q]
  - **Proximal tubules** cells get **laden with lipid** and protein due to tubular reabsorption of lipoproteins: **Lipoid nephrosis**[Q]
- *Clinical course:*
  - **Excellent prognosis**: **>90% respond** rapidly to steroids[Q]
  - Renal function remains normal[Q]
  - No hypertension or hematuria.[Q]
  - Selective proteinuria is seen

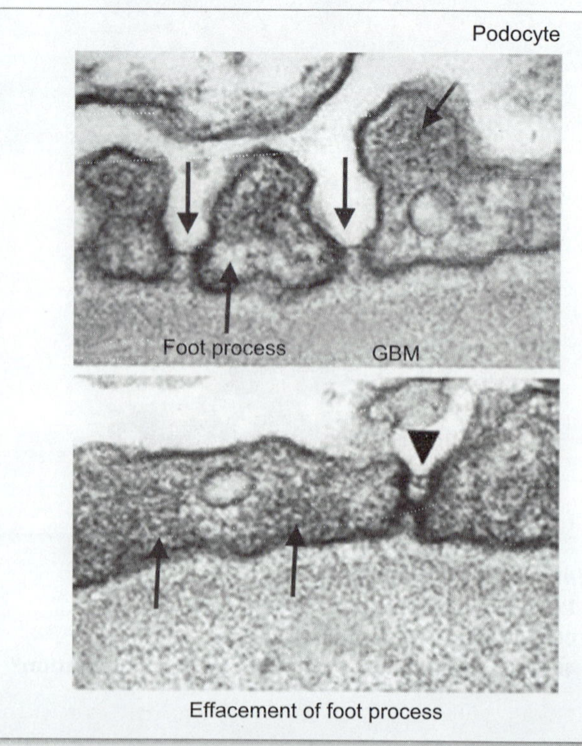

FOCAL SEGMENTAL GLOMERULOSCLEROSIS (FSGS)

- *Hallmark* **Disruption of visceral epithelial cells** with **effacement of foot processes (podocytopathy)**[Q]
- *Genetic basis:* **APOL1 gene** on **chr 22** is strongly associated
- *Etiology*
  - **Primary:** Idiopathic (10% in children and 35% in adults)[Q]
  - **Secondary: Due to underlying etiology**
    - **Reflux nephropathy**[Q]
    - Hypertensive nephropathy
    - **HIV infection (HIV-associated nephropathy)**[Q]
    - **Heroin addiction (heroin nephropathy)**[Q]
    - **Sickle-cell disease**[Q]
    - Massive obesity
    - Secondary event to focal glomerulonephritis (e.g. **IgA nephropathy**)[Q]
    - **Renal ablation/surgery**[Q]

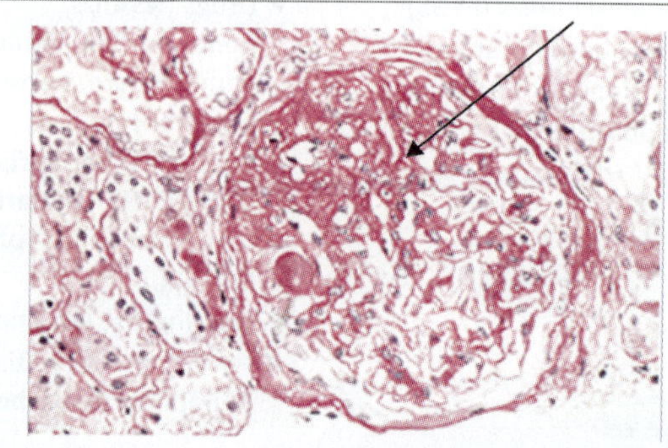

FSGS: Renal biopsy showing sclerosis of a part of glomerulus

- Congenital anomalies (unilateral **renal agenesis or renal dysplasia**)
- **Inherited forms** of nephrotic syndrome : mutation in **podocin,** α-actinin 4, and TRPC6 (transient receptor potential calcium channel-6)[Q]
- *Morphology*
  - **Light microscopy**
    - Collapse of capillary loops in sclerotic areas
    - Deposition of plasma proteins along capillary wall **(hyalinosis)**
  - **Immunofluorescence microscopy**
    - IgM + C3 deposition in sclerotic areas and/or in mesangium.
  - **Electron microscopy**
    - **Diffuse effacement** of foot processes of podocytes
    - **Focal detachment** of the epithelial cells
    - **Denudation** of the underlying GBM.
- *Clinical course*
  - 20% of patients follow rapid course, with massive proteinuria ending in renal failure within 2 years.
  - Histologic subtype (collapsing variant $\rightarrow$ unfavorable course; tip variant $\rightarrow$ good prognosis)
  - 25–50% recurs in patients who undergo transplantation

Nephrotic Syndrome in Children due to Genetic Disorders of the Podocytes

Gene	Name	Chr	Inheritance	Renal Disease
STEROID-RESISTANT NEPHROTIC SYNDROME				
NPHS1[Q]	**Nephrin[Q]**	**19q**	**Recessive[Q]**	**Finnish-type[Q] congenitalnephrotic syndrome**
NPHS2[Q]	**Podocin[Q]**	**1q**	**Recessive[Q]**	**FSGS[Q]**
FSGS1	α-actinin-4 (α*ACTN4*)	19q	**Dominant**	**FSGS[Q]**
FSGS2	Unknown	11q	**Dominant**	**FSGS**
WT1	**Wilms tumor-suppressor gene**	11p	Dominant	**Denys-Drash syndrome Frasier's syndrome[Q]**
LMX1BQ	LIM-homeodomain protein	9q	Dominant	Nail-patella syndrome[Q]
SMARCAL1	SW1/SNF2-related	2q	Recessive	Schimkeim- muno-osseous dysplasia with FSGS
STEROID-RESPONSIVE NEPHROTIC SYNDROME				
Unknown	Unknown	Unknown	Recessive	MCNS

HIV-associated Nephropathy (HIVAN)

- Associated with 5–10% of HIV-infected individuals

Morphology

Light microscopy	Electron microscopy
Collapsing variant of FSGS: ■ **Most characteristic lesion[Q]** ■ **Poor prognosis[Q]** Characterized by **collapse** of entire glomerular tuft along with **proliferation and hyper-trophy** of glomerular **visceral epithelial cells[Q]** (also seen in pamidronate toxicity).	● **Focal cystic dilation of tubule** segments filled with proteinaceous material, and inflammation and fibrosis ● **Tubuloreticular inclusions[Q]** within endothelial cells (also seen in SLE)

MEMBRANOPROLIFERATIVE GLOMERULONEPHRITIS (MPGN)

Etiology

Primary	Idiopathic	
Secondary	**Invariably type I:** More common in **adults[Q]**	
	Autoimmune diseases	**SLE[Q]**
	Infections	**Hep C** infection, usually with **cryoglobulinemia[Q]**, **Hep B, HIV, Schistosomiasis[Q]**
	Other causes	α1-Antitrypsin deficiency[Q], **CLL**

	MPGN I	MPGN II (Now called C3 glomerulopathy)
Complement activation	Both classical and alternate pathway	Only alternate pathway
Complement levels	All factors reduced	C1, C2 and C4 normal; C3 Nephritic factor seen;
Light Microscopy	Mesangial and GBM proliferation (tram track appearance)	Dense deposits (also called dense deposit disease)
Type of deposits	Subendothelial	Electron dense intram-embranous

ISOLATED GLOMERULAR DISEASES

IgA Nephropathy (Berger's Disease)

- Most common type of glomerulonephritis in adults, worldwide.
- Most common cause of gross hematuria

Characterized by: Recurrent hematuria and presence of IgA deposits in the **mesangium.[Q]**

Pathogenesis

- Aberrantly glycosylated **IgA-1** deposition in **mesangium[Q] or** Autoimmune response to IgA-1

Mesangial immune deposits **activate mesangial cells[Q]** to proliferate, produce increased amounts of **extracellular matrix**, and secrete numerous cytokines and growth factors.

Etiology

- **Primary:** Idiopathic
- **Secondary IgA nephropathy:** Due to underlying causes-
  - **Gluten enteropathy (celiac disease):** Intestinal mucosal defects[Q]
  - **Liver disease:** Defective hepatobiliary clearance of IgA[Q]

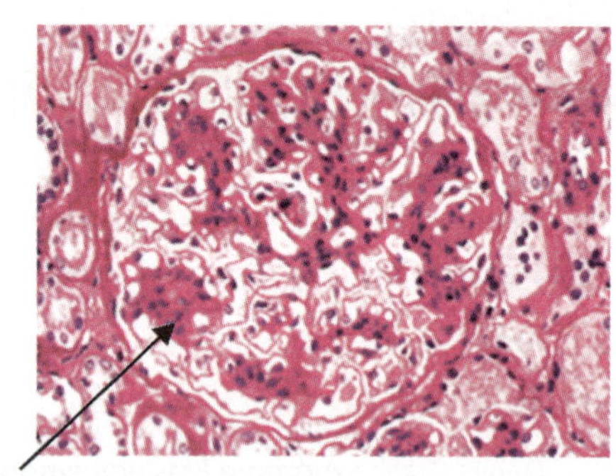

IgA Nephropathy showing mesangial deposits

Morphology

Light microscopy	Immunofluorescence microscopy	Electron microscopy
• **Mesangioproliferative glomerulonephritis:** mesangial widening and endocapillary proliferation[Q] • **Focal proliferative glomerulonephritis**	• **Mesangial deposition of IgA+ C3 and properdin, IgG, IgM+/-**[Q] • Early complement components are absent	Electron-dense deposits in mesangium[Q]

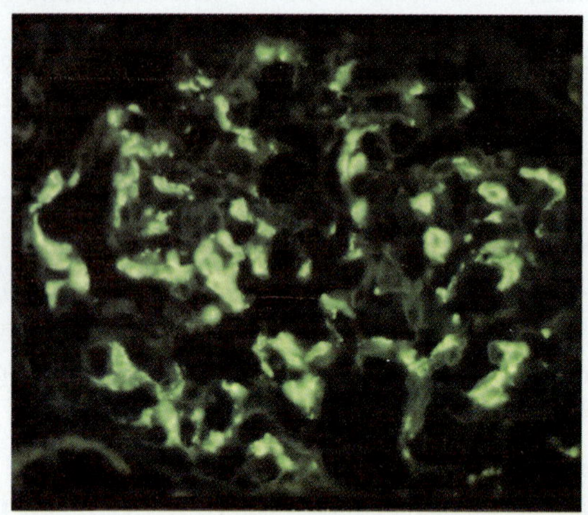

Immunofluorescence showing mesangial deposition of IgA

Clinical Course

- Two most common presentations of IgA nephropathy are:
  - Recurrent episodes of **macroscopic hematuria** 1–2 days following an **upper respiratory infection** often accompanied by **proteinuria** or
  - Persistent asymptomatic microscopic hematuria.
- **Nephrotic syndrome, however, is uncommon**
- **15–40% cases progress to ESRD in 20 years.**[Q]
- **15% recurs in patients who undergo transplantation**[Q]

High Yield Facts

- **Collapsing type** of FSGS has **worst prognosis**
- **Types II and III MPGN** are associated with complement factor H deficiency, presence of C3 nephritic factor, partial lipodystrophy (type II MPGN) or complement receptor deficiency (type III MPGN)
- Kidney changes in **AIDS** patient include **Collapsing variant of FSGS, MPGN, DPGN, IgA nephropathy (Mesangioproliferative glomerulonephritis), MCD and MGN**
- **Most specific histological lesion in diabetic nephropathy** (see chapter 18 Endocrine system) is Nodular glomerulosclerosis or **Kimmelstiel-Wilson lesions**
- **Most common** pathological lesion in diabetes nephropathy is **diffuse GBM thickening>diffuse glomerulosclerosis**

Hereditary Nephritis

Diseases with **mutations in collagen genes** that manifest primarily with **glomerular injury.**

Includes: Alport syndrome **and** Thin basement membrane lesion **(MC cause of benign familial hematuria)**[Q]

Alport Syndrome

- *Triad of:*
  - **Hematuria, sensorineural deafness, Eye disorders**: lens dislocation, posterior cataracts, and corneal dystrophy[Q]
- *Inheritance:*
  - **X-linked dominant**[Q] (85%, **MC** mode of inheritance) > Autosomal
- *Pathogenesis:* Mutations in subunits of collagen → Defective GBM synthesis
  - **COL4A5 (X-linked)**[Q], **COL4A3/4 (Autosomal)**[Q]
- *Morphology:*
  - **Light microscopy:** Mesangial proliferation, Capillary wall thickening,
    - **Foam cells**[Q]: Lipid containing tubular or interstitial cells
  - Immunofluorescence microscopy, **Absence of staining with COL4A5**[Q] (Not diagnostic)
  - **Electron microscopy**
    - **GBM: Irregular foci of thickening alternating with thinning**[Q]
    - Pronounced splitting and lamination of the **lamina densa:** distinctive **basket-weave appearance (diagnostic feature of Alport syndrome)**[Q].

THIN BASEMENT MEMBRANE LESION (BENIGN FAMILIAL HEMATURIA)

- **Inheritance:** Autosomal inheritance with **defective collagen 4 α3/4 (COL4A3/4)**[Q]
- **Morphology** on Light microscopy: Diffuse thinning of the GBM to widths between **150 and 225 nm**[Q] (compared with 300 to 400 nm in healthy adults)
- **Prognosis**: Excellent

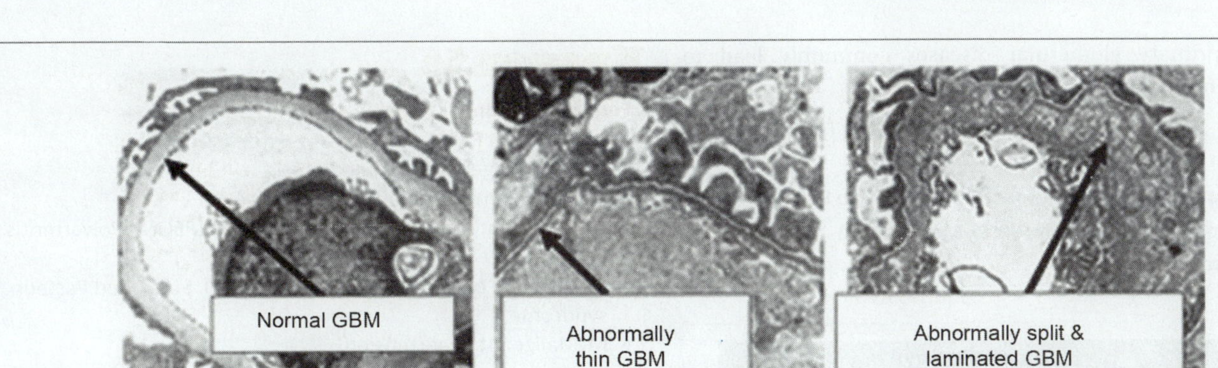

Alports' Syndrome (GBM showing splitting and lamination) arrow

TWO SPECIAL CONDITIONS NEED MENTION

Diabetic Nephropathy

This is nodular glomerulosclerosis (Kimmelstiel-Wilson lesion) of diabetes mellitus.

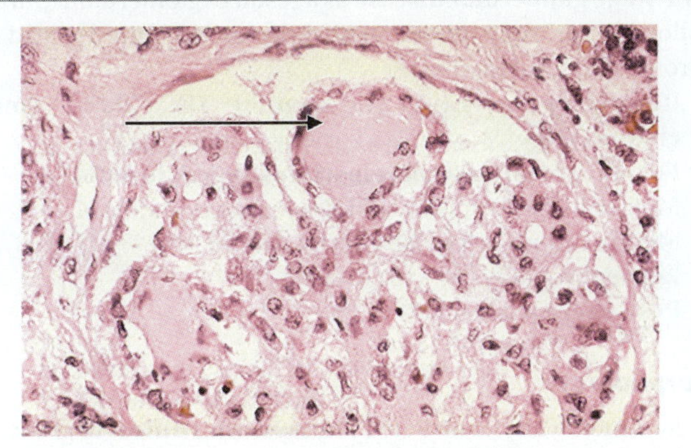

SLE Kidney

Classification of Lupus Nephritis (International Society of Nephrology)

- **Class I** : **Minimal Mesangial**[Q]
- **Class II** : **Mesangial Proliferative**
- **Class III** : **Focal** Lupus Nephritis[Q]
- **Class IV** : **Diffuse** Lupus Nephritis[Q]
- **Class V** : **Membranous** Lupus Nephritis[Q]
- **Class VI** : **Advanced** Sclerotic Lupus Nephritis

In lupus there is a full house pattern. They are all IgG, IgA, IgM. Alternative and classical cascade are involved

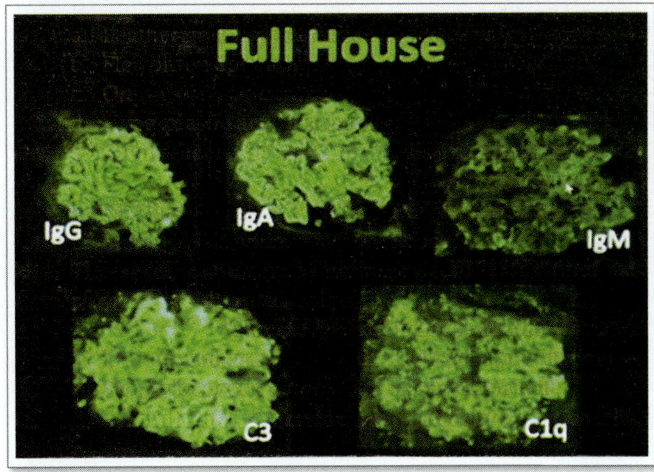

CHRONIC GLOMERULONEPHRITIS

It is end-stage glomerular disease as a result of glomerulone-phritis.

Following primary glomerular diseases commonly lead to chronic glomerulonephritis:

- **Rapidly progressive (Crescentic) GN (90%) (most common)**[Q]
- **Focal segmental glomerulosclerosis (50% to 80%)**
- Membranoproliferative GN (50%), Membranous, IgA nephropathy, **Post-streptococcal**

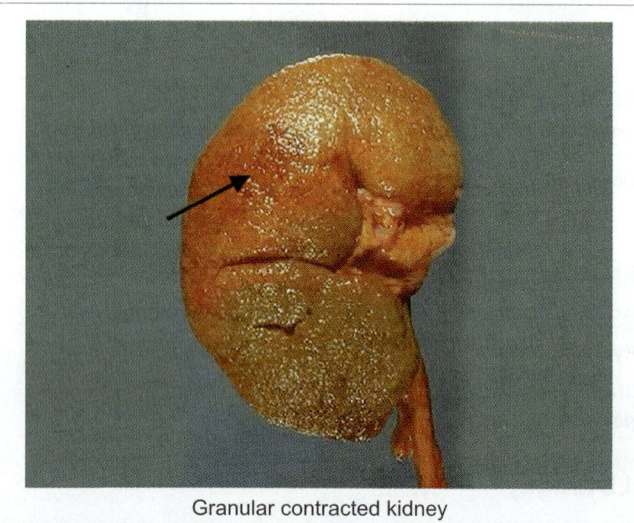
Granular contracted kidney

Morphology

- **Symmetrically contracted kidneys**[Q] with **diffusely granular cortical surfaces**
- On section, the **cortex is thinned,**[Q] and there is an increase in peripelvic fat.
- Replacement of glomeruli by **blue-staining collagen (Masson trichrome stain)**[Q]
- **Tubular atrophy**, irregular **interstitial fibrosis**, and **mononuclear leukocytic infiltration** of the interstitium.

Causes of Granular Contracted Kidney

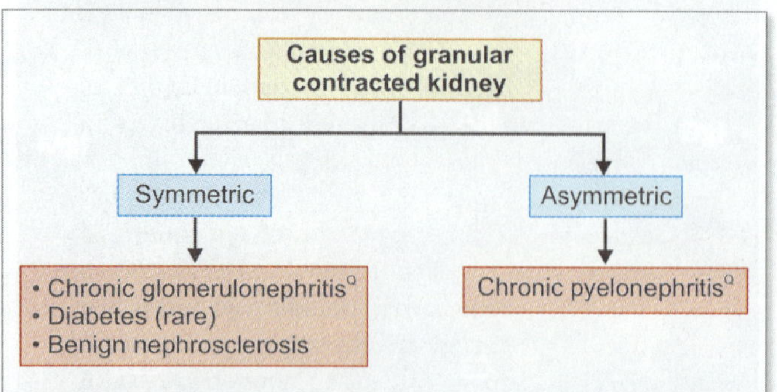

Flea-bitten kidney is seen in "World Health PSM"
- **W**orld - Wegener's granulomatosis
- **H**ealth - Henoch Schonlein purpura
- **P**-Post-streptococcal Glomerulonephritis (PSGN). Polyarteritis nodosa
- **S**-Sub acute bacterial endocarditis (SABE), SLE, Good Pasteur syndrome
- **M**-Malignant hypertension

THIN BASEMENT MEMBRANE LESION (BENIGN FAMILIAL HEMATURIA)

Inheritance: Autosomal inheritance with **defective collagen 4 α3/4 (COL4A3/4)**[Q]

Morphology on Light microscopy: Diffuse thinning of the GBM to widths between **150 and 225 nm**[Q] (compared with 300 to 400 nm in healthy adults)

Prognosis: Excellent

CHRONIC GLOMERULONEPHRITIS

End-stage glomerular disease as a result of glomerulonephritis. Following primary glomerular diseases commonly lead to chronic glomerulonephritis:

- **Rapidly progressive (Crescentic) GN (90%) (most common)**Q
- **Focal segmental glomerulosclerosis (50% to 80%)**
- Membranoproliferative GN (50%)
- Membranous (30% to 50%)
- IgA nephropathy (30% to 50%)
- **Post-streptococcal (1% to 2%)**

Morphology

- **Symmetrically contracted kidneys**[Q] with **diffusely granular cortical surfaces**
- On section, the **cortex is thinned,**[Q] and there is an increase in peri-pelvic fat.
- Replacement of glomeruli by **blue-staining collagen (Masson trichrome stain)**[Q]
- **Tubular atrophy**, irregular **interstitial fibrosis**, and **mononuclear leukocytic infiltration** of the interstitium.

Causes of Granular Contracted Kidney

Symmetric	Asymmetric
Chronic Glomerulonephritis[Q]	**Chronic Pyelonephritis**[Q]
Diabetes (rare)	
Benign Nephrosclerosiss	

ACUTE KIDNEY INJURY (AKI)/ACUTE RENAL FAILURE (ARF)

Causes of Acute Kidney Injury

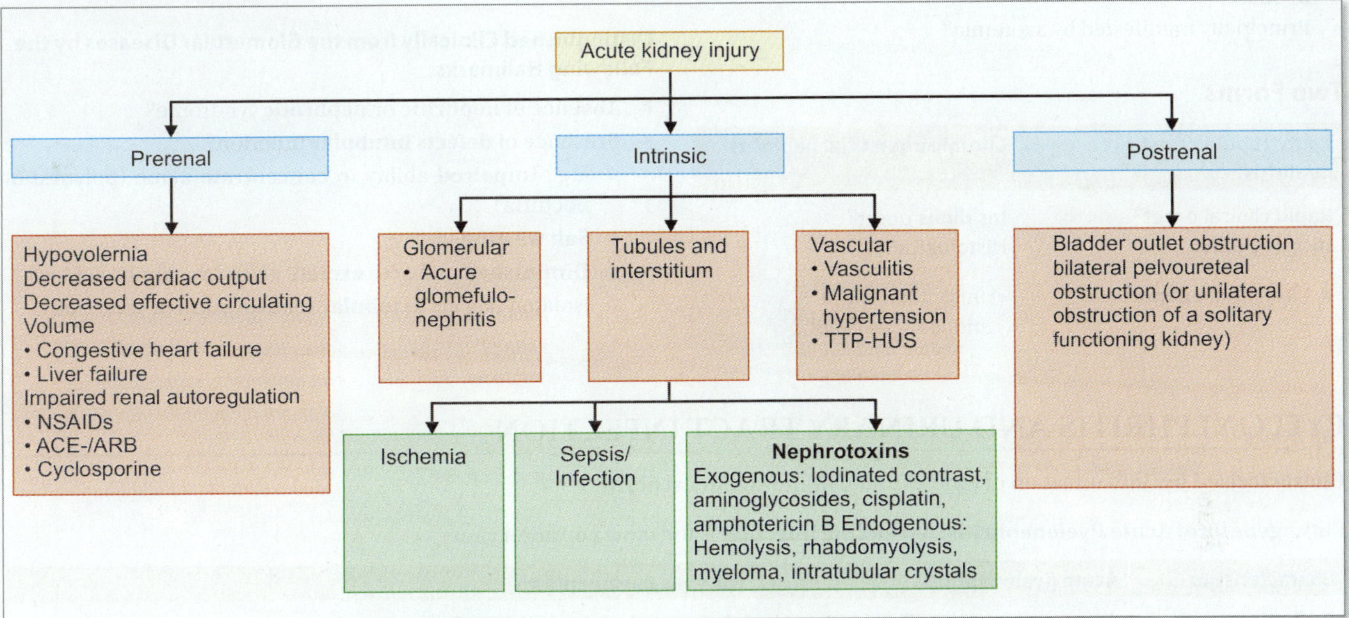

Definition: AKI is defined as any of the following:

- **Increase in Serum Cr by 0.3 mg/dl within 48 hours; or**
- **Increase in Serum Cr to 1.5 times baseline within the prior 7 days; or**
- **Urine volume <0.5 mL/kg/hr for 6 hours**

Acute Tubular Injury/Necrosis (ATN)

- **Structural tubular injury**[Q] due to renal hypoperfusion.
- **Ischemic and toxic ATN** account for 90% of cases of **acute intrinsic renal failure.**

Laboratory Findings in Acute Renal Failure

Index	Prerenal Azotemia	Oliguric Acute Renal Failure
BUN/P_{Cr} ratio[Q]	>20:1[Q]	10-15:1
Urine sodium (U_{Na}), meq/L[Q]	<20[Q]	>40
Urine osmolality (mosmol/L)	>500	<350
Fractional excretion of sodium	<1%[Q]	>2%
Urine/plasma creatinine (U_{Cr}/P_{Cr})	>40	<20

New Biomarkers of Acute Kidney Injury

Biomarker	Comments
N-Acetyl--(D) glucosaminidase (NAG)[Q]	Proximal tubule lysosomal enzyme
Retinol-binding protein	Early marker of tubular dysfunction
Cystatin C[Q]	Elevated urinary levels reflect tubular dysfunction; high levels may predict poorer outcome
Kidney injury molecule-1 (KIM-1)[Q]	Elevated urinary levels highly sensitive and specific for AKI
Clusterin	Elevated kidney and urinary levels are very sensitive for AKI
Neutrophil gelatinase associated lipocalin (NGAL)[Q]	Early indicator of AKI following cardiopulmo- nary bypass
Interleukin-18 (IL-18)	Elevated urinary level is an early marker of AKI and independent predictor of mortality in critically ill patients
Liver fatty acid–binding protein (L-FABP)	A biomarker in CKD and diabetic nephropathy
Sodium/hydrogen exchanger isoform (NHE3)	Urinary levels found to discriminate between prerenal azotemia and AKI in ICU patients
Exosomalfetuin-A	Acute phase protein synthesized in the liver; High Urinary levels in ICU patients with AKI

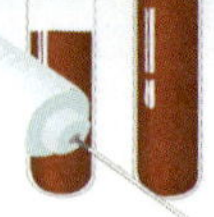

TUBULOINTERSTITIAL NEPHRITIS

Characterized by

- Inflammatory injuries to tubules and interstitium[Q] Insidious in onset
- Principally manifested by azotemia[Q]

Two Forms

Acute tubulointerstitial nephritis	Chronic interstitial nephritis
Rapid clinical onset[Q] **Histologically:** • **Interstitial edema**[Q]	**Insidious** onset[Q] **Histologically:** • Infiltration with mononuclear WBCs

• Neutrophillic infiltration in interstitium and tubules[Q]	• Prominent interstitial fibrosis
• **Tubular injury**	• **Tubular atrophy**[Q]

Distinguished Clinically from the Glomerular Diseases by the Following Hallmarks:

- **Absence** of **nephritic or nephrotic** syndrome[Q]
- **Presence** of **defects intubular function**[Q]
  - E.g.: **Impaired** ability to **concentrate urine** (polyuria or nocturia)
  - **Salt wasting**
  - **Diminished** ability to **excrete acids** (metabolic acidosis)
  - Isolated defects in **tubular reabsorption** or secretion

PYELONEPHRITIS AND URINARY TRACT INFECTION

Characterized by: Inflammation of tubules, interstitium, and renal pelvis

Pathogenesis of Acute Pyelonephritis: Ascending infection is the **most common** cause.

Characteristics	Acute pyelonephritis	Chronic pyelonephritis
Definition	Acute **suppurative inflammation** of the kidney	Chronic **tubulointerstitial inflammation** and **scarring** involve the calyces and pelvis
Etiology	Ascending urinary tract infection MC: **E. coli (MC)**[Q], *Proteus, Klebsiella, and Enterobacter*	Bacterial infection plays a dominant role; 2 forms: • **Reflux nephropathy**[Q]: Urinary infection on congenital **vesicoureteral reflux** • **Chronic obstructive pyelonephritis**[Q]
Morphology: Gross	• Discrete focal abscesses • Large wedge like areas	• Coarse, discrete, **Corticomedullary scars**[Q] (Hallmark) overlying dilated, blunted, or deformed calyces • **Flattening of the papillae**[Q]
Light Microscopy	• **Patchy interstitial suppurative inflammation (hallmark)** • Intratubular aggregates of neutrophils • **Neutrophilic tubulitis**[Q] • **Tubular necrosis**[Q]	• Involves **tubules and interstitium** • **Thyroidization of tubules**[Q]: Dilated tubules filled with casts resembling thyroid colloid • Chronic interstitial inflammation and fibrosis • Vessels demonstrate **obliterative intimal sclerosis** • **Hyaline arteriolo sclerosis**[Q] • **Periglomerular fibrosis**[Q] • **Secondary FSGS**[Q] may be seen.

Complications	• **Papillary Necrosis**
	   ▪ Major Causes
	     ♦ Analgesic nephropathy (Most common)[Q]
	     ♦ Sickle cell nephropathy
	     ♦ Diabetes with urinary tract infection
	 • **Pyonephrosis**[Q]
	 • **Perinephric abscess**[Q]
		• **Xanthogranulomatous pyelonephritis:**
		   ▪ A rare form of **chronic pyelonephritis**[Q]
		   ▪ Often associated with **Proteus infections**[Q] and obstruction
		   ▪ M.C age group: **5th -6th decade**[Q]
		   ▪ **Females** are most commonly affected
		   ▪ Associated features: **Large staghorn calculi**[Q] and **hydronephrosis**[Q]
		   ▪ Gross morphology: **large, yellowish orange** nodules that may be grossly confused with renal cell carcinoma.
		   ▪ **Microscopy:** Accumulation of **foamy (lipid laden) macrophages (Xanthoma cells)**[Q] with **plasma cells, lymphocytes.**

- **Most important factor in pyelonephritis: Vesicoureteral reflux**[Q]
- In the absence of vesicoureteral reflux, infection usually remains localized in the bladder
- An emerging **viral pathogen** causing **pyelonephritis** in **kidney transplantation** is Polyomavirus (> 6 months post-transplant)
- **Analgesic nephropathy is a high risk for development of transitional cell Carcinoma kidney**

Pyelonephritis can occur in following steps

- **Colonization**[Q] of the distal urethra and introitus (in the female) by coliform bacteria
- **Retrograde spread**[Q] from the **urethra to the bladder**
- Further spread from **bladder to kidneys** by the following mechanisms:
  - **Urinary tract obstruction** and **stasis** of urine[Q]
  - **Vesicoureteral reflux**[Q]-Incompetence of the vesicoureteral valve that allows bacteria to ascend the ureter into the renal pelvis.
  - Open ducts at the tips of the papillae (**intrarenal reflux**)[Q]

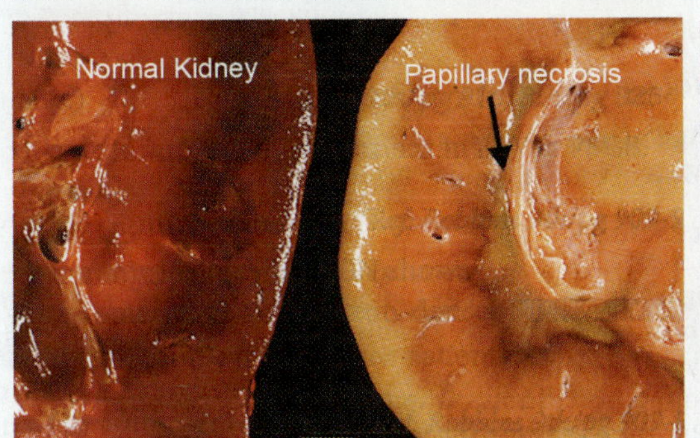

Papillary necrosis

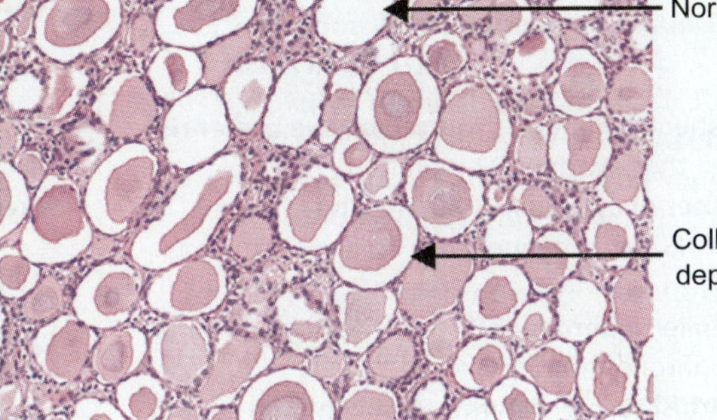

Thyroidization of tubules

INHERITED CYSTIC KIDNEY DISEASES

Disease		Gene	Protein	Renal Abnormality	Extrarenal Abnormality
Autosomal dominant polycystic kidney disease[Q]	AD AD	*PKD1* PKD2	Polycystin-1 Polycystin-2	Cortical and medullary cysts	**Cerebral aneurysms;**[Q] **liver and spleen cysts**[Q]
Autosomal recessive polycystic kidney disease[Q]	AR	*PKHD1*	Fibrocystin (polyductin)	Distal tubule and collecting duct cysts	**Hepatic fibrosis;**[Q] **Caroli's disease**[Q]
Nephronophthisis I (juvenile/adolescent)	**AR**	*NPHP1*	Nephrocystin	Small fibrotic kidneys; medullary cysts	**Retinitis pigmentosa**
Nephronophthisis II (infantile)	AR	*NPHP2 (INVS)*	Inversin	**Large kidneys;**[Q] widespread cysts	**Situs inversus**[Q]
Nephronophthisis III (juvenile/adolescent)	AR	*NPHP3*	Nephrocystin-3	Small fibrotic kidneys; medullary cysts	**Retinitis pigmentosa;** hepatic fibrosis
Medullary cystic kidney disease	**AD**	*MCKD1 /2*	Uromodulin	Small fibrotic kidneys; medullary cysts	**Hyperuricemia and gout**[Q]
Tuberous sclerosis	**AD**	*TSC1/2*	Hamartin/ Tuberin	**Renal cysts;**[Q] **angiomyolipomas;**[Q] **Renal cell carcinoma**[Q]	**Facial angiofibromas;**[Q] **CNS hamartomas**[Q]
Von Hippel-Lindau disease	AD	*VHL*	pVHL	**Renal cysts;**[Q] **Renal cell carcinoma**[Q]	**Retinal angiomas;**[Q] **CNS hemangioblastomas;**[Q] **pheochromocytomas**[Q]

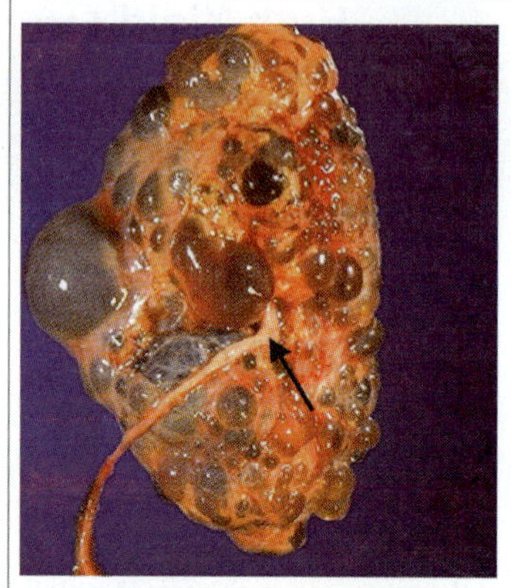

Autosomal dominant polycystic kidney disease showing distorted outline

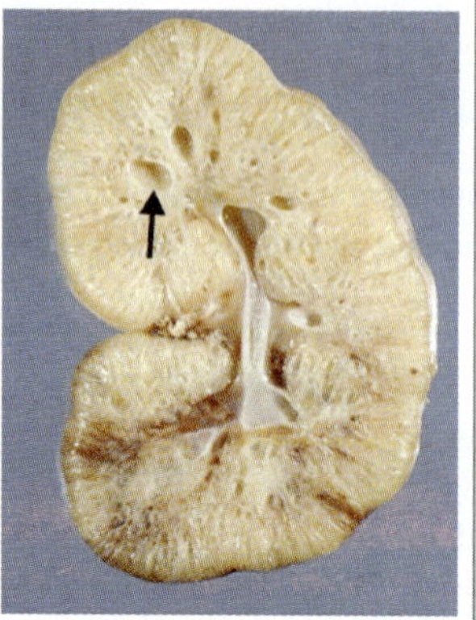

Autosomal recessive polycystic kidney disease showing smooth outline

High Yield Facts

- In ADPKD, patients with **PKD1 mutation have higher risk of ESRD**[Q] than those with PKD2 mutation
- **Extra-renal sites of cysts** in ADPKD are: **Liver (most common)**[Q]> CNS (berry aneurysm) > Spleen > Pancreas > Lung
- **Familial juvenile Nephronophthisis** is the most common variant of Nephronophthisis
- **Nephronophthisis** complex is the **most common genetic cause of ESRD in children**[Q]

Acquired (Dialysis-Associated) Cystic Disease

- Cystic degeneration in ESRD after prolonged dialysis.
- Increased risk of renal cell carcinoma

RENAL TUMORS

Benign Neoplasms

- **Renal Papillary Adenoma**
  - Small, discrete adenomas
  - Arises from the **renal tubular epithelium**[Q]
- **Angiomyolipoma**
  - **Benign neoplasm**[Q] consisting of vessels, smooth muscle, and fat
  - Originates from **perivascular epithelioid**[Q] cells.
- **Oncocytoma**
  - Epithelial neoplasm composed of **large eosinophilic cells**[Q] having small, round, **benign-appearing nuclei** that have large nucleoli.
  - Arise from the intercalated cells of collecting ducts
  - E/M: **eosinophilic cells** have **numerous mitochondria**.[Q]

Malignant Tumors

Renal Cell Carcinoma (RCC)

- **Age group**: most commonly in 6th and 7th decade[Q]
- **Male: Female ratio = 2:1.**[Q]

Risk Factors

• **Cigarette smoking (most important)**[Q] • **Obesity (particularly in women)**[Q] • Hypertension[Q] • Unopposed estrogen therapy • Exposure to asbestos • **Petroleum products**[Q] • Heavy metals.	There is also an **increased risk** in patients with: • **End-stage renal disease**[Q] • **Chronic kidney disease**[Q] • **Acquired cystic disease**[Q] • **Tuberous sclerosis.**[Q]

Classification of RCC

- **Sporadic**: Most common type
- **Hereditary forms:** Autosomal dominant, Young age affected

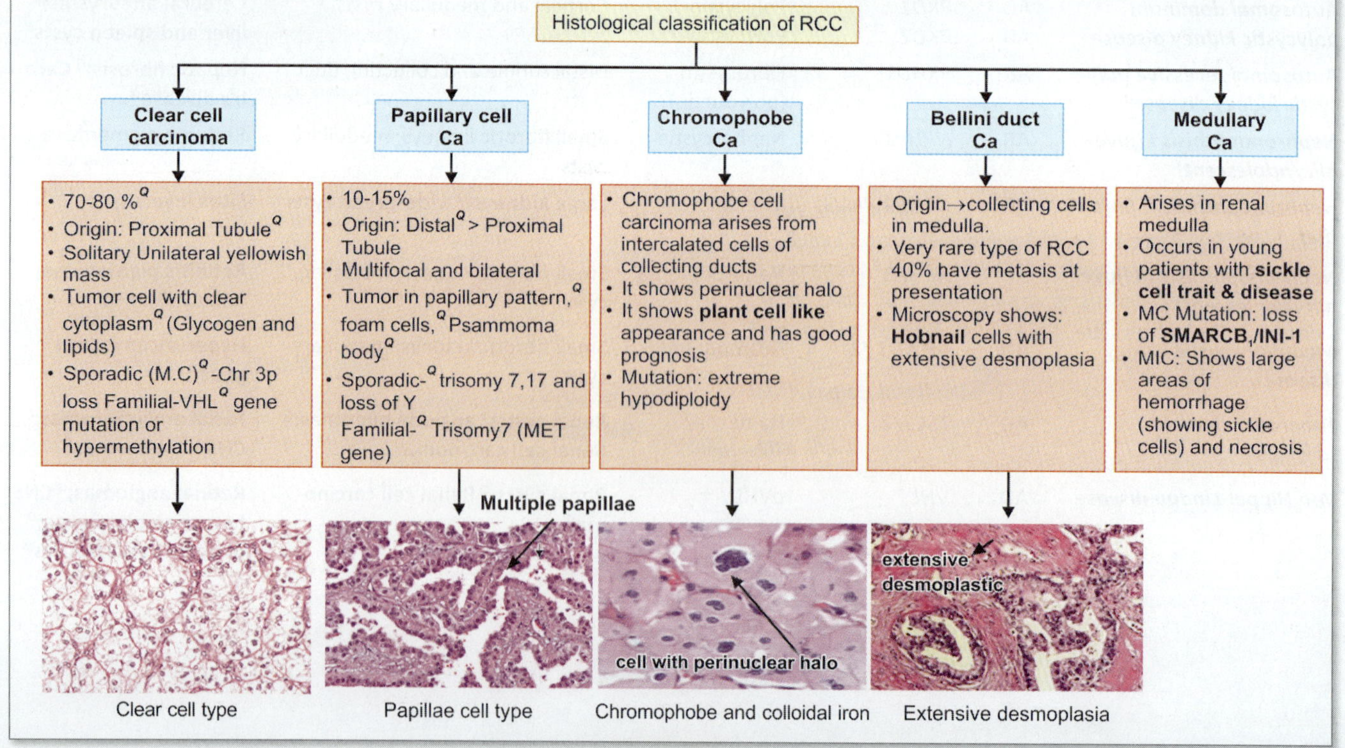

Clear cell type

Papillae cell type

Chromophobe and colloidal iron

Extensive desmoplasia

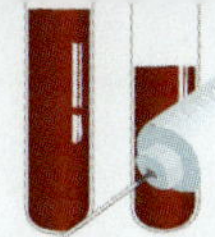

Latest Update

4 Types of Familial Variants
- **Von-Hippel-Lindau (VHL) syndrome:** AD
  - Sporadic and familial forms of clear cell carcinoma
- **Hereditary leiomyomatosis** and **renal cell cancer syndrome:** AD
  - Caused by mutations of the FH gene which expresses fumarate hydratase
- Characterized by cutaneous and uterine leiomyomata and an aggressive type of papillary carcinoma with increased tendency for metastatic spread.
- **Hereditary papillary carcinoma:** AD
  - Mutation in MET proto-oncogene papillary cell Ca
- **Birt-Hogg-Dubé syndrome:** AD
  - Mutations in BHD gene, which expresses folliculin.
  - Constellation of skin (fibrofolliculomas, trichodiscomas, and acrochordons), pulmonary (cysts or blebs), and renal tumors

Clinical Features

- Costovertebral pain, palpable mass, hematuria **(Most reliable sign)**[Q]

Metastasis

Most common locations of metastasis are: **lungs (50%)**[Q] **and bones (33%)**[Q]

Latest Update

Xp11 translocation
- Rare and seen in young Patients
- Tumor cells with clear cytoplasm and papillary structure
- Translocation of TFE3 on Chr Xp11.2

Paraneoplastic Feature of RCC

- Hypertension **(most common)**[Q]
- Polycythemia, Hypercalcemia
- **Hepatic dysfunction (Stauffer's syndrome)**[Q]
- **Feminization or masculinization**[Q]
- **Cushing syndrome (Rare)**[Q], Eosinophilia, Leukemoid reactions, Amyloidosis.

Urothelial Carcinoma of the Renal Pelvis

- **Originate from the urothelium of the renal pelvis**[Q]
- Range from **Benign papillomas to invasive urothelial (transitional cell) carcinomas.**[Q]
- Multiple lesions involving the pelvis, ureters, and bladder.
- Often associated with bladder urothelial tumor.
- Increased incidence with **Lynch syndrome** and **analgesic nephropathy.**[Q]
- Infiltration of the wall of the pelvis and calyces indicative of **poor prognosis.**[Q]

DISEASES OF URINARY BLADDER

MALACOPLAKIA

- A vesical **inflammatory reaction**[Q] is characterized macroscopically by soft, yellow, slightly raised **mucosal plaques** 3 to 4 cm in diameter
- It is a granulomatous disease with **defective intracellular lysosomal digestion** of bacteria in histiocytes. It is mostly caused by **E. coli.**[Q]

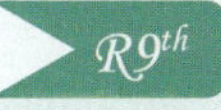

Von Hansemann histiocytes

Michaelis-Guttman bodies

Malakoplakia microscopy

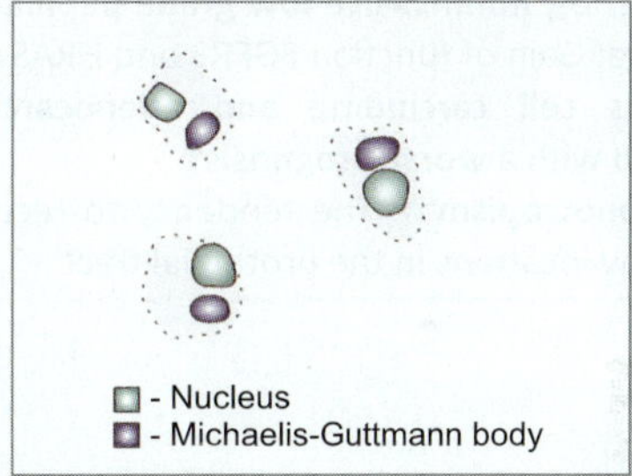

Microscopy

- Infiltration with **large, foamy macrophages**[Q] with a **Michaelis-Gutmann bodies**[Q] with multinucleate giant cells and lymphocytes.
- Laminated mineralized concretions resulting from deposition of calcium in enlarged lysosomes, typically present within the macrophages are called Michaelis Gutmann bodies. These histiocytes have pink-cytoplasm called as-**von Hansemann histiocytes**

BLADDER CARCINOMA

- ***Epidemiology:*** More common in men than in women, common age group affected: 50–80 years old
- ***Types:***
  - Epithelial tumors include **Urothelial or transitional cell type (most common)**[Q], Squamous[Q] and Glandular[Q]
- ***Precursor lesions:***
  - **Noninvasive** papillary tumors, **Flat noninvasive** urothelial carcinoma[Q]

- ***Risk factors:***
  - ○ **_Cigarette smoking_: Most important**[Q]
  - ○ **_Industrial exposure to arylamines_**[Q] like 2-naphthylamine, Benzidine, Acrolein
  - ○ **_Schistosoma haematobium_**[Q] infections (**Squamous Carcinoma** > Transitional Cell Ca)
  - ○ Long-term **analgesic use (Phenacetin)**[Q]
  - ○ Long-term exposure to **cyclophosphamide,** Exposure of bladder to **irradiation. Urolithiasis (predisposes to Squamous Cell Ca)**
- **_Genetic alterations:_**
  - ○ Monosomy 9 or del 9p or 9q (most common)
- Clinical feature:
  - ○ **_Painless hematuria_, Frequency, urgency, and dysuria** may be present
- **_Prognosis:_**
  - ○ Depends on the **histologic grade**[Q] of the papillary tumor and the **stage** at diagnosis.
  - ○ Involvement of **muscularis mucosa (detrusor muscle)**[Q] is associated with **worst prognosis**

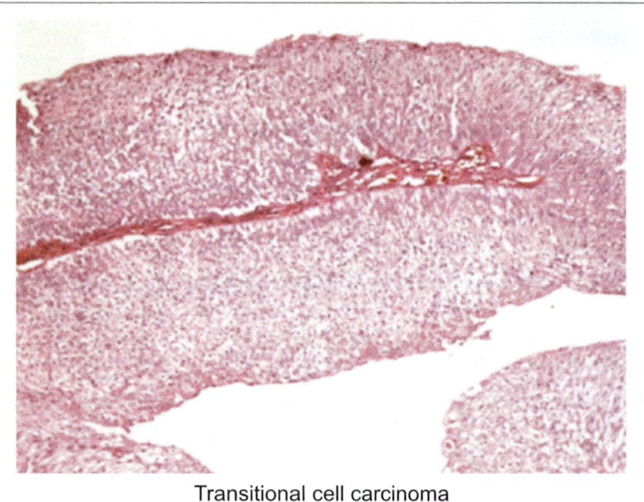
Transitional cell carcinoma

High Yield Facts

- **Noninvasive high grade urothelial carcinoma:** Loss of TP53 and RB genes, **noninvasive low grade papillary** urothelial Carcinoma: Gain of function FGFR3 and HRAS mutations
- **Squamous cell carcinoma and adenocarcinoma**[Q] are associated with a **worse prognosis**[Q]
- **"Polychronotropism"**[Q]: The tendency to recur over time and in new locations in the urothelial tract

High Yield Facts

Assessment of Glomerular Filtration Rate (GFR)
- **Direct measurement: By Inulin clearance**[Q] (Inulin is filtered at the glomerulus but neither reabsorbed nor secreted throughout the tubule)
- **Serum Creatinine:** Used as a surrogate to estimate GFR. It is the most widely used marker for GFR. Commonly used formulae used to calculate GFR from serum creatinine are:
  - **Cockcroft-Gault**[Q]
  - **Schwartz Formula**[Q]
- **Creatinine clearance**[Q]: An approximation of GFR; **CrCl = $(U_{vol} \times U_{Cr})/(P_{Cr} \times T_{min})$.**
- **Cystatin C**[Q]: **More sensitive marker** of **early GFR decline** than plasma creatinine

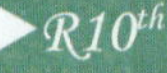 *R10ᵗʰ* **Latest** Update

C3 Glomerulopathy
Encompasses the following:
1. Dense-deposit disease (formerly known as type II MPGN) where dense glomerular intramembranous deposits are present in the glomerular capillary loops, which stain for C3 only by IF.
2. C3GN, a proliferative GN resembling MPGN type I without Ig deposits.
3. Rare diseases such as familial MPGN type III and complement factor H–related protein 5 abnormality–associated familial GN cases
   - **Immunofluorescence Characteristics:** C3 shows double-linear appearance of the glomerular capillary wall and a ring appearance around the mesangial deposits (mesangial rings)
   - IgG deposition should not be present
   - Type II MPGN is now classified under C3 glomerulopathy

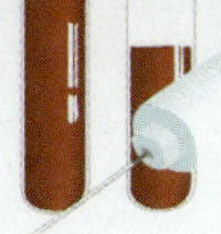

NEXT Pattern Questions

Q's

1. A 26-year-old patient presented with proteinuria, hematuria. PAS stain of renal biopsy demonstrates characteristic histological findings. Which of the following cannot be a possible etiology?

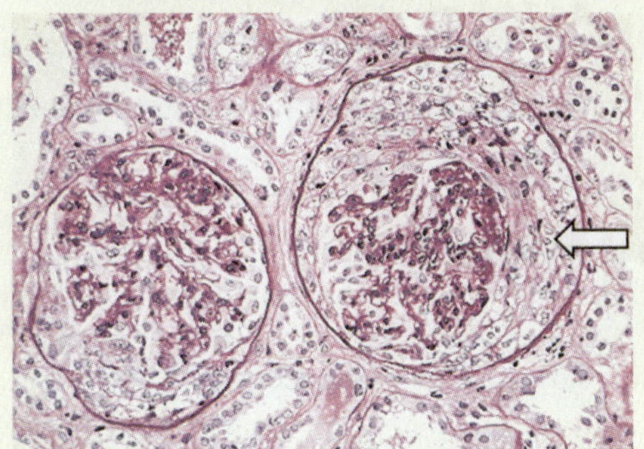

a. Good pasture syndrome b. Wegener's granulomatosis
c. IgA nephropathy d. Polyarteritis nodosa

Ans. (d) Polyarteritis nodosa

- With the history of nephritic syndrome and the image is suggestive of Crescent's, this is a case of RPGN. Now in the classification of RPGN, PAN is not a cause.

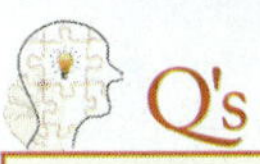

Q's

2. A 60-year-old male with complaints of hematuria, severe hypertension and mild facial puffiness with occasional hemoptysis. The DIF picture of the patient is given below. Which of the following is not true about the given condition?

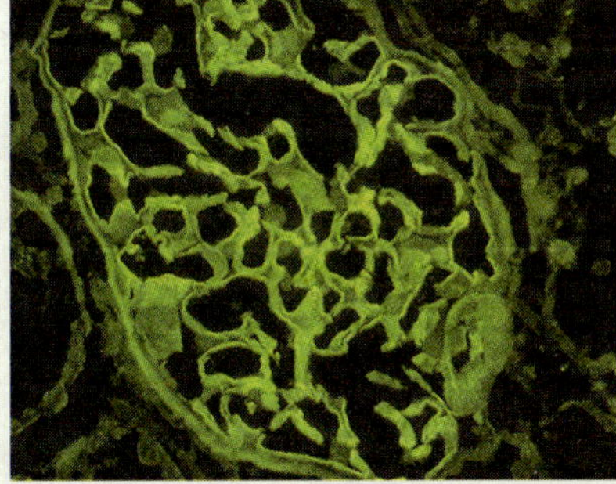

a. Antibody to alpha 3 chain of type 4 collagen part of non-collagenous domain is responsible
b. Strong association with HLA DR B1
c. Crescents are seen in >50% of the glomeruli
d. Dense depositions below podocytes are seen in electron microscopy

Ans. (d) Dense depositions below podocytes are seen in electron microscopy

- This is a case of nephritic syndrome and the DIF shows linear deposits, so it's a case of Good Pasteur syndrome. Since, it involves Anti GBM antibodies, so option D which is indicative of immune complex is false statement.

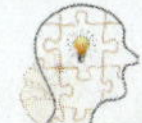

Q's

3. A patient presented with pus in urine. Urine culture was done which was negative. After a sudden onset renal failure the patient died. On autopsy the following finding was seen in kidney. What is the most likely diagnosis?

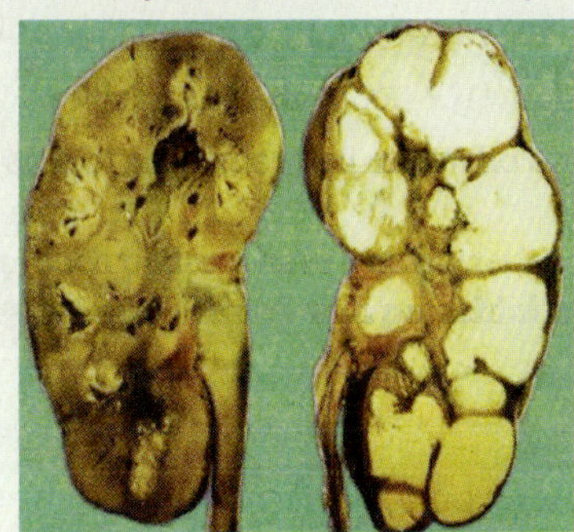

a. TB kidney b. Infected renal cysts
c. Renal cell carcinoma d. Renal stones

Ans. (a) TB kidney

- With the history of sterile pyuria, uremia and white cheesy caseous deposits in the kidney, this is a case of TB kidney.

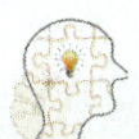

Q's

4. A 2-year-old child presented with purpuric skin lesions, abdominal pain, intestinal bleeding and arthralgia. Immunofluorescence study demonstrated IgA depostion as shown below. What is your diagnosis?

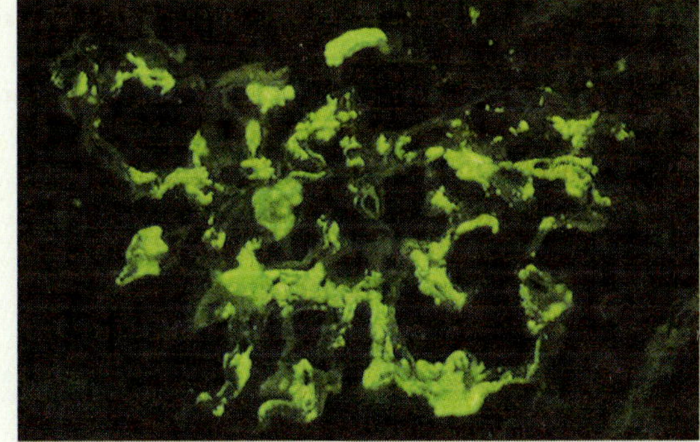

a. FSGS
b. Minimal change disease
c. Diabetic neuropathy
d. Henoch-Schönlein purpura

Ans. (d) Henoch-Schönlein purpura

- The history of this 2-year-old child is suggestive of Henoch schonlein purpura, and with an IgA deposition in the mesangium the biopsy is suggestive of IgA nephropathy.

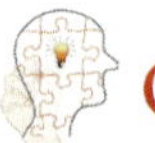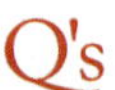

Q's

5. A 50-year-old male presented with blurring of vision. Urine examination showed proteinuria. Histopathology picture of kidney given below. What is not true about the finding in the associated condition?

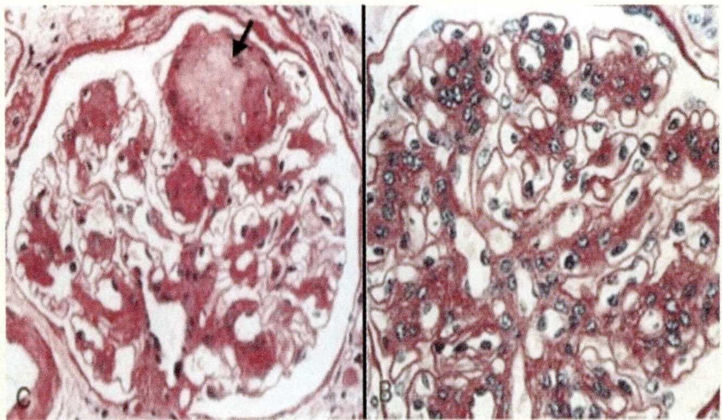

   a. Diffuse increase in mesangial matrix
   b. Sclerotic mesangial nodules
   c. GBM thinning and permeable
   d. Hyaline arteriosclerosis

Ans. (c) GBM thinning and permeable
   - The history of nephrotic syndrome and blurring of vision. Notice the first image shows Kimmelstiel-Wilson nodule suggestive of Diabetic nephropathy. The histology shows GBM thickening and more permeability.

Image-Based Questions

1. A 5-year-old male presented with mild hematuria, pedal edema and frothy urine. BP 110/70 mm Hg. Subsequently he was treated with steroid but he did not improve. The renal biopsy was carried out. The electron microscopy finding has been shown. What is your diagnosis?

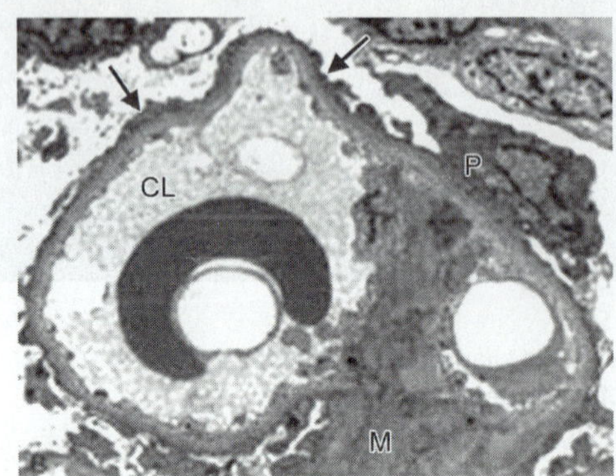

   a. Minimal Change disease   b. FSGS
   c. MPGN   d. PSGN

2. A 55-year-old diabetic male found to have microalbuminuria. Identify the lesion shown in renal biopsy of this patient.

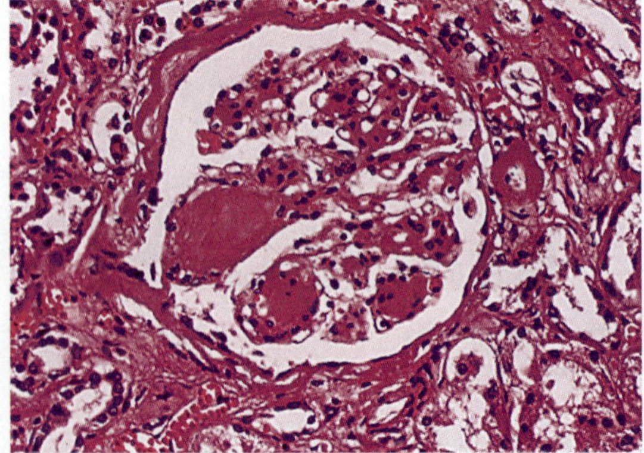

   a. Amyloidosis
   b. Kimmelstiel- wilson lesion
   c. Wire loop lesions
   d. Crescentric glomerulonephritis

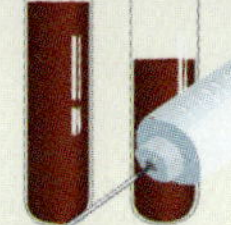

3. The morphological finding of kidney shown in the figure is associated with which of the following conditions?

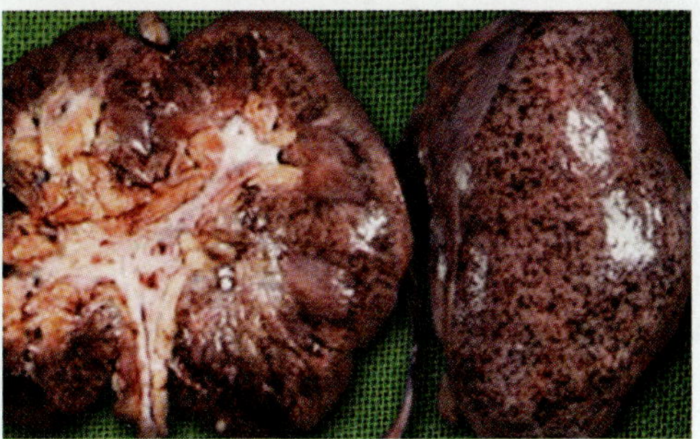

a. Chronic glomerulonephritis
b. Renal amyloidosis
c. Malignant hypertension
d. Acute pyelonephritis

4. Identify the kidney disease?

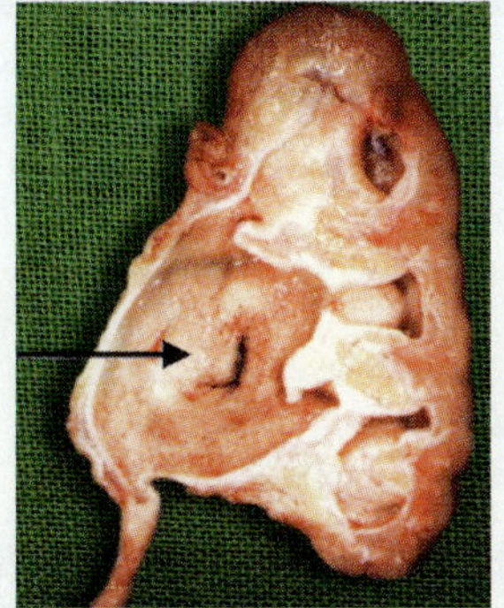

a. Polycystic disease   b. Hydronephrosis
c. Pyelonephritis   d. Chronic pyelonephritis

5. Which of the following conditions usually leads to the finding given below:

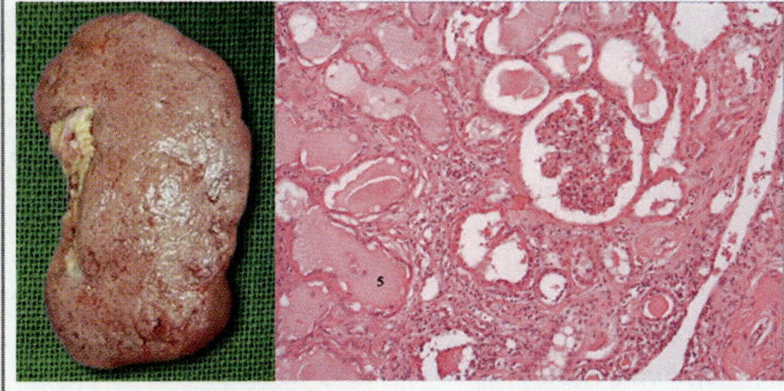

a. Benign hypertension   b. Malignant hypertension
c. Chronic pyelonephritis   d. Acute pyelonephritis

6. Most common histology of this gross lesion is:

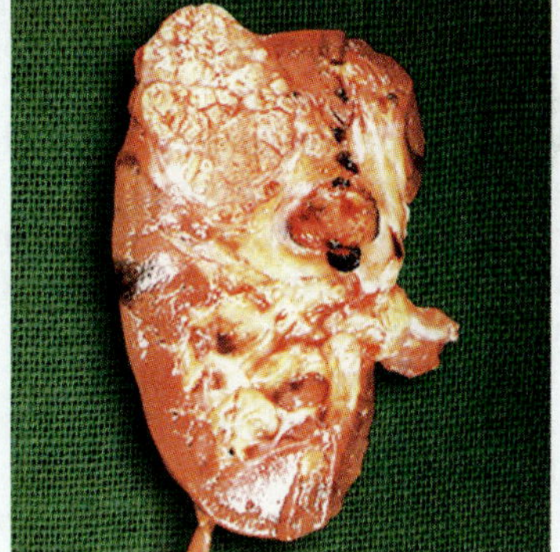

a. Clear cell type   b. Papillary Cell Ca
c. Belini duct Ca   d. Anaplastic Ca

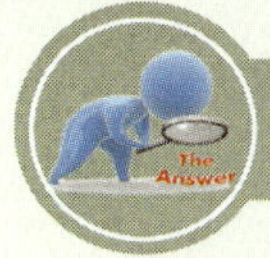

Answers of Image-Based Questions

1. **Ans. (a) Minimal Change disease**
   - History given here is that of nephrotic syndrome and electron microscopy shows flattening of foot processes of podocytes, a feature of minimal change disease.

2. **Ans. (b) Kimmelstiel-Wilson lesion**
   - In this case kidney biopsy from a patient suffering from diabetic nephropathy shows Nodular glomerulosclerosis suggested by diffuse increase in mesangial matrix and characteristic acellular PAS-positive nodules.

3. **Ans. (c) Malignant hypertension**
   - The given kidney gross shows small, pinpoint **petechial hemorrhages** may appear on the cortical surface from rupture of arterioles or glomerular capillaries, giving the kidney a peculiar "flea-bitten" appearance. The kidney size varies depending on the duration and severity of the hypertensive disease.

4. **Ans. (b) Hydronephrosis**
   - Marked dilation of the pelvis and calyces and thinning of the renal parenchyma.

5. **Ans. (c) Chronic pyelonephritis**
   - Gross surface is irregularly scarred. Microscopically shows changes involve predominantly tubules and interstitium. The tubules show atrophy in some areas and hypertrophy or dilation in others. Dilated tubules with flattened epithelium may be filled with casts resembling thyroid colloid (thyroidization)

6. **Ans. (a) Clear cell type**
   - The given gross shows Renal cell Carcinoma, the most common histology of which is clear cell type.

Answers of Image-Based Questions

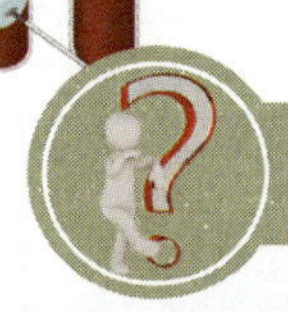

Multiple Choice Questions

STRUCTURE & FUNCTION

1. Maltese cross appearance in urinary sediment seen in which of the following disease other than nephrotic syndrome? *(AIIMS Nov 2019)*
 a. Felty syndrome
 b. Fanconi Syndrome
 c. Fabry disease
 d. Friedrich's ataxia

2. Dysmorphic RBC's in urine is/are seen in?
 (PGI May 18)
 a. Glomerulonephritis
 b. Renal vascular injury
 c. Renal stone
 d. Pyelonephritis
 e. Interstitial nephritis

3. Which of the following dyads are correctly matched regarding urinary casts and associated condition?
 a. Hyaline casts- may be normally present in healthy person *(PGI Nov 2017)*
 b. Muddy brown casts-acute tubular necrosis
 c. WBC cast - pyelonephritis
 d. Epithelial cast – acute glomerulonephritis
 e. Myogolobin cast - Rhabdomyolysis

4. Urinary cast better seen on microscope by?
 a. Centrifuge the urine first *(PGI May 2017)*
 b. Use immunofluorescence light
 c. See at edge of cover slip
 d. Increasing the light intensity
 e. Acidifying it first

5. A post renal transplant patient presented with complains of chronic renal failure. As a part of investigative workup, the patient urine microscopy suggested the following finding, identify the structure marked by arrow? *(Recent Question 2016-17)*

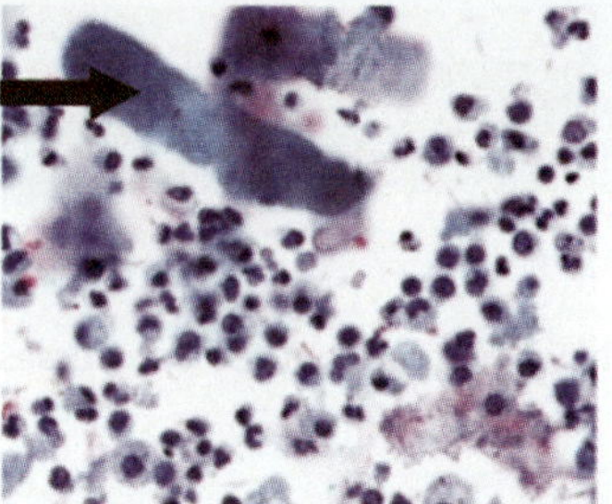

 a. Decoy cell
 b. Tubular epithelial cell
 c. Charcot leyden crystal
 d. Hyaline casts

6. Which one of the following tests is best for measuring glomerular function? *(Recent Question 2016-17)*
 a. Blood urea
 b. Serum creatinine
 c. Creatinine clearance rate
 d. Ultrasound of kidney

7. Match list I with list II and select the correct answer using the code given below the lists:
 (Recent Question 2016-17)

List I (Urine exam)	List II (Disease)
A. Red cell casts	1. Nephrotic syndrome
B. Microscopic haematuria	2. Chronic renal failure
C. Proteinuria	3. Polycystic kidney disease
D. Broad cell casts	4. Glomerulonephritis

Code:

	A	B	C	D
a.	A/4	B/3	C/1	D/2
b.	A/3	B/2	C/1	D/4
c.	A/2	B/3	C/4	D/1
d.	A/4	B/1	C/2	D/3

8. Identify the crystal in the urine analysis:
 (AIIMS Nov 2015)

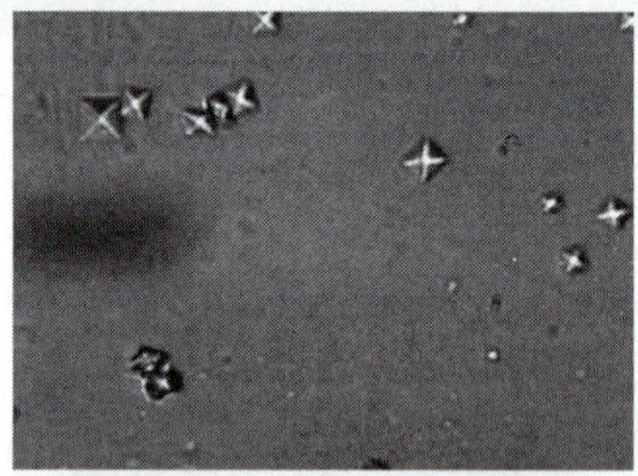

 a. Oxalate
 b. Uric acid
 c. Phospahates
 d. Cysteine

9. Identify the arrow marked structure in Urine routine microscopy? *(AP PGMEE 2015)*

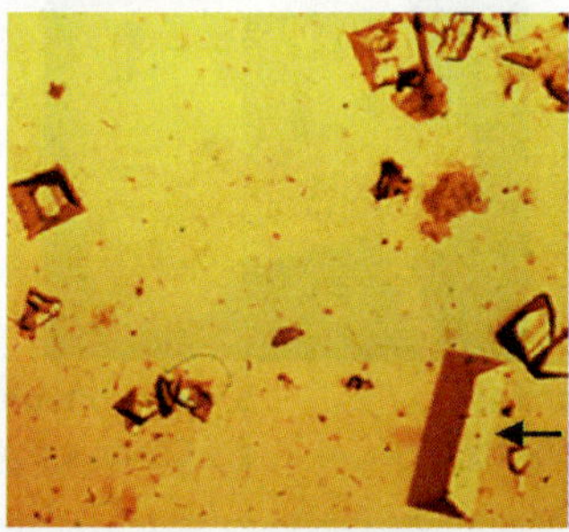

 a. Uric acid
 b. Ca oxalate
 c. Struvite
 d. Cysteine

10. Which of the following dyads are correct:
 a. WBC cast- Acute pyelonephritis *(PGI May 2015)*
 b. Broad cast-CRF
 c. Eosinophilic cast-interstitial nephritis
 d. RBC cast- Glomerulonephritis
 e. Broad cast : chronic pyelonephritis

11. Normal level of serum uric acid in males is:
 (Recent Question 2015)
 a. 3.1-7 mg/dl
 b. 2.5-5.6 mg/dl
 c. 1.5-3.3 mmol/L
 d. 1.8-4.4 mmol/L

12. The protein in glomerular basement membrane responsible for charge dependent filtration is:
 (Recent Question 2015, DPG 10)
 a. Albumin
 b. Collagen type IV
 c. Proteoglycan
 d. Fibronectin

13. Cast seen in Acute Glomerulonephritis is: *(WB PG 2015)*
 a. Hyaline cast
 b. Granular cast
 c. RBC cast
 d. WBC cast

14. What is the minimum number of red blood cells per microliter of urine required for diagnosis of hematuria?
 a. 3
 b. 5 *(APPGMEE 14)*
 c. 8
 d. 10

15. Urine analysis of a patient with hematuria and hypercalciuria is most likely to reveal?
- a. Isomorphic RBCs *(AIIMS Nov 11)*
- b. RBC casts
- c. Nephrotic range proteinuria
- d. Eosinophiluria

16. On kidney biopsy, PAS positive structures are:
- a. Glomerular basement membrane *(PGI Nov 10)*
- b. Tubule
- c. Neutrophils
- d. Interstitium
- e. Mesangial matrix

PSGN

17. Examine the renal histopathology slide. What is the probable diagnosis? *(JIPMER Nov 2019)*
- a. Membranoproliferative GN
- b. Rapidly proliferative GN
- c. PSGN
- d. Diabetic nephropathy

18. Not seen in post streptococcal glomerulonephritis (PSGN)? *(PGI May 2016)*
- a. Nephrotic range proteinuria
- b. Neutrophilic infiltration of tubules
- c. Subepithelial deposits
- d. Linear deposits along glomerular basement membrane

19. Post streptococcal glomerulonephritis presents with
- a. Asymptomatic hematuria *(Recent Question 2015)*
- b. Renal failure
- c. Massive anasarca
- d. Massive renomegaly

20. Most common renal lesions in HIV
- a. MPGN *(Recent Question 2015)*
- b. RPGN
- c. FSGS
- d. Membranous nephropathy

21. Which is seen in Electron microscopy in PSGN?
- a. Epithelial humps *(Recent Question 2015)*
- b. Spike and dome appearance
- c. Mesangeal deposits
- d. Subendothelial deposits

22. All are true about poststreptococcal glomerulonephritis except - *(Recent Question 2014)*
- a. Crescent formation
- b. Subepithelial deposits
- c. Granular deposits of IgG
- d. Deposition of IgA

23. The pathogenesis of acute proliferative glomerulonephritis -
- a. Cytotoxic T-cell mediated *(Recent Question 2014)*
- b. Immune complex mediated
- c. Antibody mediated
- d. Cell-mediated (Type IV hypersensitivity)

24. In Poststreptococcal glomerulonephritis:
- a. C3 decreases, ASO increases *(WBPG 2014)*
- b. C3 increases, ASO increases
- c. C3 decreases, ASO decreases
- d. C3 increases, ASO decreases

25. Poststreptococcal reactive arthritis is differentiated from Acute Rheumatic Fever by all except:
- a. Small joint involvement and often symmetric
- b. Caused by nongroupA hemolyticstreptococci
- c. Non-responsiveness to salicylate
- d. Shorter incubation period *(WB PG 2011)*

RPGN

26. A 50-year-old male presented with hematuria. Investigations revealed normal glucose levels, proteinuria and creatinine of 9 mg%. Electron microscopic image is shown below. What other investigations could help in the diagnosis?

(Recent Pattern Question 2020)

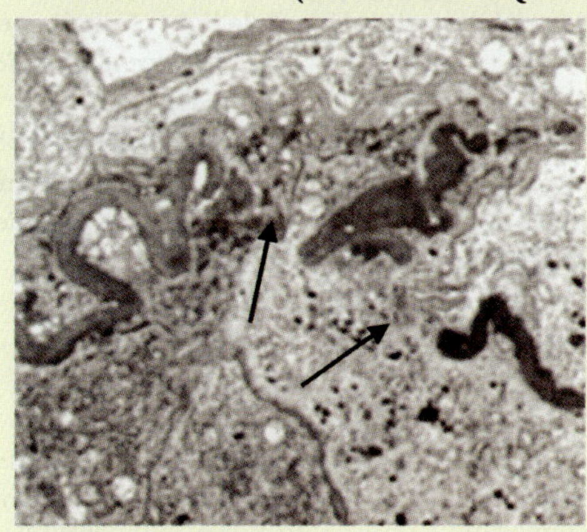

- a. ANA
- b. HIV serology
- c. Electrophoresis
- d. Anti GBM antibodies

27. Examine the gross kidney image. What is the diagnosis?
- a. Granular contracted kidney *(JIPMER Nov 2019)*
- b. Flea bitten kidney
- c. Spongy kidney
- d. Hemorrhagic kidney

28. Which of the following is correctly matched in RPGN?
- a. Type 1 IgA nephropathy *(JIPMER 18)*
- b. Type 2 Anti-GBM antibody
- c. Type 2- Wegener's granulomatosis
- d. Type 2- SLE nephritis

29. A patient presented with hemoptysis and hematuria. On renal biopsy, it show crescentic glomerulonephritis. Immunofluorescence microscopy shows linear IgG and C3 deposits. Which of the following is the most appropriate diagnosis? *(PGI May 18)*
- a. Thin basement disease
- b. Good pasture syndrome
- c. Wegener granulomatosis
- d. PSGN
- e. Minimal change disease

30. Rapid advanced renal parameters is clinically termed as Rapidly progressive glomerulonephritis. What exactly is the finding on microscopy?

(Recent Question 2016-17)
- a. Membrane thickening
- b. Segmental sclerosi
- c. Crescents
- d. Mesangial expansion

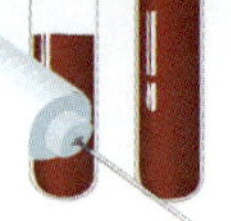

31. **Type I RPGN is seen in** *(Recent Question 2015)*
   a. SLE
   b. IgA nephropathy
   c. Henoch schonlein purpura
   d. Good pasture syndrome

32. **False regarding nephritic syndrome**
   (Recent Question 2015)
   a. Generalize edema   b. Proteinuria <3.5 g/day
   c. Hypoalbuminemia   d. Hypertension

33. **True regarding igA Nephropathy:** *(Recent Question 2015)*
   a. Usually in children < 10 years
   b. Microscopic hematuria is the most common presentation
   c. Recurrent gross hematuria following respiratory infection
   d. Decreased serum IgA

34. **Mesangial deposits of Lambda light chain is seen in**
   (Recent Question 2015)
   a. Amyloidosis   b. FSGS
   c. MPGN   d. Membranous nephropathy

35. **Most common cause of primary nephrotic syndrome in adult** *(Recent Question 2015)*
   a. Membranous nephropathy
   b. Minimal change disease
   c. Membranoproliferative glomerulonephritis
   d. Focal segmental glomerulosclerosis

36. **All of the following causes RPGN Except?**
   (Recent Question 2015)
   a. Wegeners   b. Polyarteritis nodosa
   c. HSP   d. Microscopic polyangitis

37. **Good pasture's syndrome is characterized by-**
   a. Necrotisting hemorrhagic interstitial pneumonitis
   b. Emphysema   *(Recent Question 2014)*
   c. Patchy consolidation
   d. Pulmonary edema

38. **Characteristic feature of Goodpasture's syndrome**
   (APPGMEE 14)
   a. Lumpy-bumpy deposits on immunofluorescence
   b. Serum antibodies against alpha 3 NC1 domain of collagen – IV
   c. Serum antibodies against alpha 1 NCI domain of collagen III
   d. Anti DNAse antibodies positive

39. **Feature of Goodpasture syndrome is/are:**
   (PGI May 2013)
   a. Antibody to α-chain of Type IV collagen (COL-4A)
   b. Basement membrane involvement
   c. Pulmonary hemorrhage
   d. Crescent formation
   e. Subendothelial deposits

OTHER GLOMERULONEPHRITIS

40. **Wire loop lesion seen in lupus nephritis is due to:**
   (JIPMER Nov 2019)
   a. Capillary wall thickening
   b. Basement membrane thickening
   c. Subepithelial deposits
   d. Sclerosis of mesangium

41. **Immunoflorescence staining pattern from a kidney biopsy from a 35yr old patient presenting with proteinuria has been shown below. What is the most probable cause?** *(AIIMS Nov 18)*

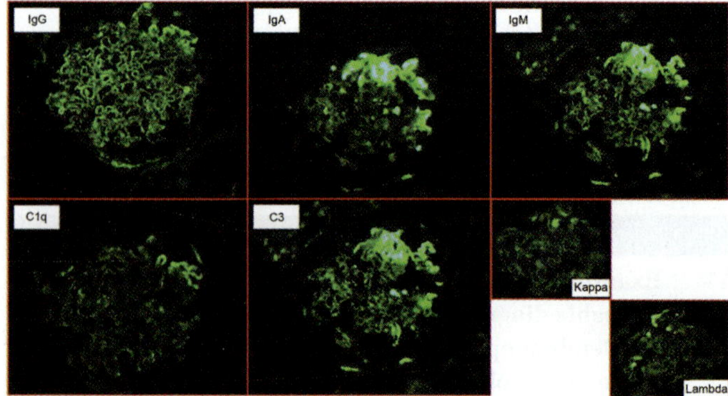

   a. FSGS
   b. PSGN
   c. Lupus nephritis
   d. Good pasteurs syndrome

42. **True about membranoproliferative glomerulonephritis is?** *(AIIMS May 2017)*
   a. Low C4 level
   b. Double basement membrane appearance on light microscopy
   c. Dense deposit along basement membrane on electron microscopy
   d. Mesangial hypocellularity
   e. GBM thickening

43. **Which of the following disease has deafness as well as hematuria?** *(JIPMER 2016)*
   a. Alport Syndrome
   b. Good pasture syndrome
   c. IgA nephropathy
   d. Cryoglobinemia

44. **A 4 years old child presents with rash on lower limbs, arthritis, and abdominal pain. Urine examination reveals microscopic hematuria. The most likely diagnosis is:**
   a. Thrombaesthenia   *(Recent Question 2016-17)*
   b. Idiopathic thrombocytopenic purpura
   c. Systemic lupus erythematosus
   d. Henoch Schonlein purpura

45. **In thin basement membrane disease the defect is in**
   (Recent Question 2015)
   a. Alpha-1 and alpha-2 chains of collagen type IV
   b. Alpha-3 and alpha -4 chains of collagen type IV
   c. Alpha-5 chain of collagen type IV
   d. Alpha-7 chain of collagen type IV

46. **Deposits in MPGN are** *(Recent Question 2015)*
   a. Subepithelial   b. Subendothelial
   c. Intramembranous   d. All of the above

47. **Tram track appearance of glomerular capillary wall is seen in** *(Recent Question 2015)*
   a. Membranoproliferative glomerulosclerosis
   b. Focal segmentral glomerulosclerosis
   c. IgA nephropathy
   d. Good pasture syndrome

48. Subepithelial humps are characteristic of
(Recent Question 2015)
a. Rapidly progressive glomerulobephritis
b. Focal segmental glomerulonephritis
c. Acute proliferative glomerulonephritis
d. Membranoproliferative glomerulonephritis

49. All the following are true regarding IgA nephropathy except *(Recent Question 2015)*
a. Can present as persistent microscopic hematuria
b. IgA 1 deposition in the mesangium
c. ACE inhibitors can be used
d. Decreased serum IgA level

50. Subendothelial deposits in glomerulus are seen in which of the following glomerulonephropathies?
a. MPGN *(Recent Question 2015)*
b. PSGN
c. Minimal change disease
d. FSGS

51. In renal biopsy of a 14-year-old boy with nephritic syndrome, glomeruli are showing proliferation of mesangial cells with GBM thickening and mesangial cell interposition. What is the most likely diagnosis in this case? *(APPGMEE 2015)*
a. Membranous nephropathy
b. Diffuse proliferative glomerulonephritis
c. Focal segmental glomerulosclerosis
d. Mesangiocapillary glomerulonepthritis

52. Dysmorphic RBC with ARF is seen in?
a. Glomerular disease *(Recent Question 2013)*
b. Renal carcinoma
c. Proximal tubule disease
d. Distal tubule disease

53. Mutation in COL4A5 chain the diagnosis:
a. Alport's syndrome *(AIIMS May 2013)*
b. Good pasture's syndrome
c. Hereditary Non-polyposis Colon Cancer
d. XerodermaPigmentosum

54. Mesangial cells of IgA Nephropathy overexpresses:
a. CD51 *(JIPMER 2012)*
b. CD61
c. CD71
d. CD81

55. Rapidly progressive glomerulonephritis is characterised by *(JIPMER 11)*
a. Crescents
b. Splitting of basement membrane
c. Neutrophil infilteration of the mesangium
d. Glomerulosclerosis

56. In which of the following are linear IgA deposits in mesangium noted: *(MH 11)*
a. Henoch Schonlein purpura
b. Malaria
c. Good Pasture's syndrome
d. Wegener's granulomatosis

57. Foot process effacement is seen on EM in:
a. Minimal change disease *(PGI Nov 10)*
b. Focal segmental GN
c. IgA nephropathy
d. Mesangial proliferative GN

58. Increased levels of C₃NeF are associated with?
(DNB Dec 10)
a. Type I MPGN	b. Type II MPGN
c. FSGS	d. Berger Disease

59. Membranous Lupus Nephritis is:
(Recent Question 2014)
a. Class II	b. Class III
c. Class IV	d. Class V

NEPHROTIC SYNDROME

60. True statement about minimal change disease
(Recent Question 2015)
a. Effacement of foot process on light microscopy
b. Severe hypoalbuminemia
c. Non selective proteinuria
d. Cyclosporine is the first line of treatment

61. Most common nephropathy in world is?
(Recent Question 2015)
a. IgA nephropathy	b. FSGS
c. Minimal Change ds	d. Adult PSGN

62. Most common cause of nephrotic syndrome in children- *(Recent Question 2015, 2014)*
a. Membranous GN
b. Minimal change disease
c. PSGN
d. RPGN

63. True about light microscopy in minimal change disease is: *(Recent Question 2014)*
a. Loss of foot process seen	b. Anti GBM Abs seen
c. IgA deposits seen	d. No change seen

64. A child presented with frothy urine, massive proteinuria and edema. Urine examination revealed RBC nil, WBC nil, nocasts, no crystal. No prior episode of similar presentation. What is your diagnosis? *(AIIMS May 2014)*
a. Minimal change disease
b. IgA nephropathy
c. Membranous glomerulonephritis
d. MPGN

65. Patients with minimal change disease are at risk of?
a. Spontaneous bacterial peritonitis *(PGI May 2014)*
b. Sepsis
c. DVT
d. Atherosclerosis
e. Renal Ca

66. Mutation in NPHS1 gene causes which disease?
a. Alport syndrome *(APPGMEE 14)*
b. Congenital Finnish type nephrotic syndrome
c. Focal segmental glomerulosclerosis
d. Nail patella syndrome

67. In which one of the primary Glomerulonephritides the glomeruli are normal by light microscopy but shows loss of foot processes of the visceral epithelial cells and no deposits by electron microscopy *(APPGMEE 14)*
a. Poststreptococcal glomerulonephritis
b. Membranoproliferative glomerulonephritis type
c. IgA nephropathy
d. Minimal change disease

68. Which of the following statement is true about Congenital nephrotic syndrome caused by Nephrin protein mutation: *(PGI May 2013)*

a. Cause steroid resistant nephrotic syndrome
b. Nephrin is a key component of the slit diaphragm
c. Coded by NPHS-1 gene
d. Symptom occur only after 1st month of age
e. Autosomal dominant pattern

69. A 7-year-old girl is brought with complaints of generalized swelling of the body. Urinary examination reveals grade 3 proteinuria and the presence of hyaline and fatty casts. She has no history of hematuria. Which of the following statements about her condition is true? *(AIIMS May 11)*

a. No IgG deposits or C3 deposition on renal biopsy
b. Her C3 level will be low
c. IgA nephropathy is the likely diagnosis
d. Alport's syndrome is the likely diagnosis

70. The most common gene defect in idiopathic steroid resistant nephrotic syndrome - *(AIIMS Nov 11, May 07, Nov 06, DNB Dec 09)*

a. ACE
b. NPHS 2
c. HOX II
d. PAX

71. Hypercoagulation in nephrotic syndrome is caused by-

a. Loss of antithrombin III *(AI 10)*
b. Decreased fibrinogen
c. Decreased metabolism of Vitamin K
d. Increase in protein C

72. Edema in nephrotic syndrome is due to -

a. Sodium and water retention *(AIIMS Nov 10)*
b. Increased venous pressure
c. Hypoalbuminemia
d. Hyperlipidemia

73. True about fibronectin nephropathy are all except:

a. Autosomal recessive inheritance *(AIIMS Nov 10)*
b. Glomerular enlargement with PAS+ trichrome+ mesangial deposit
c. Glomerulus do not consistently stain for Ig and complement
d. Ultrastructural feature is presence of large electron dense mesangialorsubendothelial deposit

MGN

74. A 60-year-old male with complaints for frothy urine and facial puffiness. The DIF and electron microscopic picture of the patient is given below. Diagnosis is?

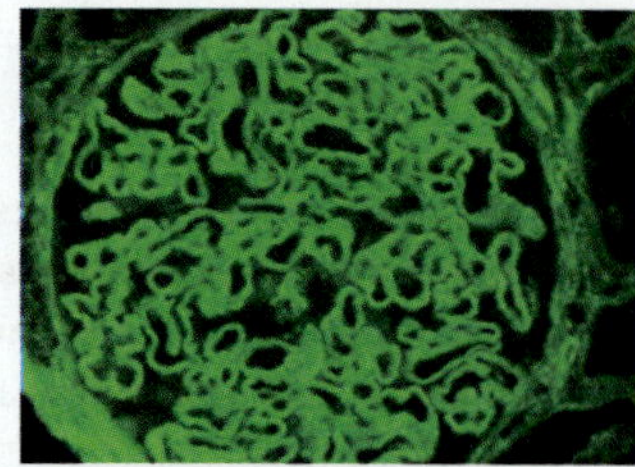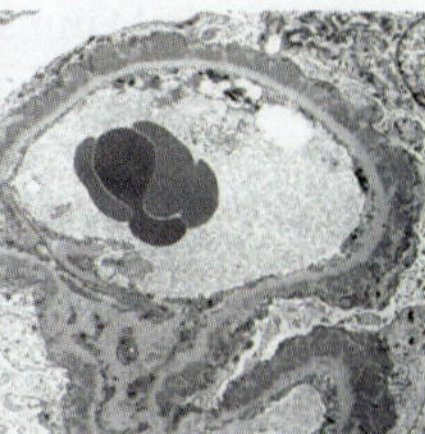

a. Membranoproliferative nephritis *(AIIMS May 2017)*
b. Membranous glomerulopathy
c. Minimal change disease
d. FSGS

75. Given below is the immunofluorescence image of kidney biopsy. Identify the condition?

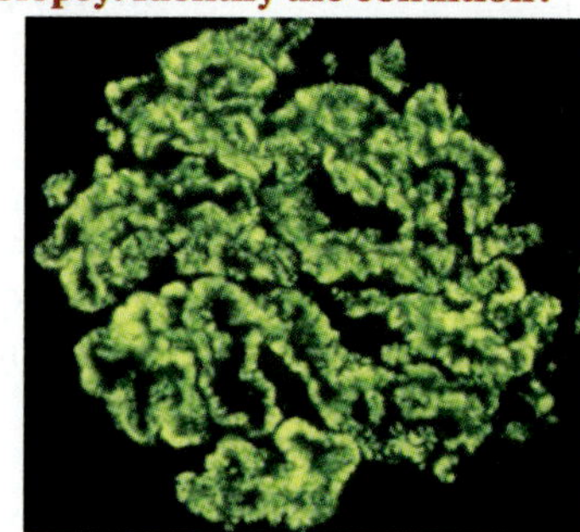

a. Good pasteurs syndrome *(Recent Question 2016-17)*
b. Membranous glomerulonephropathy
c. Berger's disease
d. Ig A nephropathy

76. Of all the types of lupus nephritis, the worst outcome is seen in? *(Recent Question 2016-17)*

a. Minimal mesangial
b. Diffuse nephritis
c. Focal segment nephritis
d. Membranous nephritis

77. A 45-year-old man presents with hematuria. Renal biopsy demonstrates a focal necrotizing glomerulitis with crescent formation. The patient gives history of intermittent hemoptysis and intermittent chest pain of moderate intensity. A previous chest X-ray had demonstrated multiple opacities, some of which were cavitated. The patient also has chronic cold like nasal symptoms. What is the most probable diagnosis?

a. Aspergillosis *(Recent Question 2016-17)*
b. Polyarteritis nodosa
c. Renal carcinoma metastatic to lung
d. Wegner's granulomatosis

78. Most common nephropathy associated with malignancy is? *(AIIMS May 2015)*

a. Membranous
b. MCD
c. IgA
d. FSGS

79. All the following are true regarding minimal change disease except *(Recent Question 2015)*

a. Most common cause of nephrotic syndrome in children
b. Massive proteinuria
c. Hematuria
d. Good response to steroids

80. Subendothelial deposits are seen in

a. Membranous nephropathy *(Recent Question 2015)*
b. MPGN type I
c. MPGN type II
d. IgA nephropathy

81. Which component of HBV causes glomerulonephritis- *(AIIMS May 2011)*

a. HbeAg
b. HBcAg
c. HBsAg
d. Anti HBs Ag antibody

FSGS

82. Collapsing variant of FSGS is seen in *(Recent Question 2015)*

a. NSAIDs
b. Heroin abuse
c. HIV
d. CMV

83. False statement in collapsing glomerulopathy:
(AP 2012)
a. It is a morphologic variant of FSGS (focal segmental glomerulosclerosis)
b. Microscopically retraction and /or collapse of the entire glomerular tuft is seen
c. There is no proliferation or hypertrophy of glomerular visceral epithelial cells
d. It may be idiopathic or HIV associated nephropathy

84. HIV infection causes - *(Recent Question 2014)*
a. Membranous glomerulonephritis
b. IgA glomerulopathy
c. Collapsing glonerulonephritis
d. RPGN

85. A person with radiologically confirmed reflux nephropathy develops nephrotic range proteinuria. Which of the following would be the most likely histological finding in the patient? *(AIIMS Nov 11)*
a. Focal segmental glomerulosclerosis
b. Nodular glomerulosclerosis
c. Membranous glomerulopathy
d. Proliferative glomerulonephritis with crescents

86. In glomerulus subendothelial deposits are seen in-
a. Good pasture syndrome *(Recent Question 2014)*
b. IgA nephropathy
c. MPGN type I   d. MPGN type II

87. Renal biopsy of a 14-year-old boy with nephritic syndrome shows proliferation of mesangial cells with Glomerular basement membrane thickening and mesangial cell interposition. What is the most likely diagnosis?
(APPGMEE 14)
a. Diffuse proliferative Glomerulonephritis
b. Mesangiocapillary Glomerulonephritis
c. Membranous nephropathy
d. Hemolytic Uremic syndrome

88. Type I membrano proliferative Glomerulonephritis is commonly associated with all EXCEPT
a. SLE *(APPGMEE 14)*
b. Persistant hepatitis C infections
c. Partial lipodystrophy
d. Neoplastic diseases

DIABETIC NEPHROPATHY

89. A 50-year-old male presented with blurring of vision. Urine examination showed proteinuria. Fundus examination showed dot and blot haemorrhages, microaneurysm and cotton wool spots. Histopathology pic of kidney given below. Your diagnosis? *(AIIMS May 2017)*

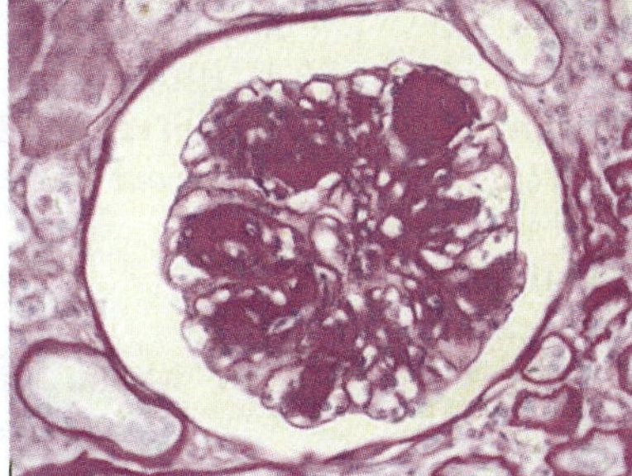

a. Kimmelstiel Wilson nodules
b. Crescents
c. Amyloid
d. Segmental sclerosis

90. Nodular glomerulosclerosis is seen in
a. Diabetes mellitus *(Recent Question 2015)*
b. Malignant hypertension
c. Amyloidosis
d. Multiple myeloma

91. Kimmelstiel-Wilson lesion is characteristic of-
(Recent Question 13 , 2014, AI 98, MH 2016)
a. HIV nephropathy
b. Diabetic nephropathy
c. Amyloidosis
d. Malignant hypertension

92. Characteristic type of nephropathy in DM is-
(DNB June 11, COMED 09)
a. Focal   b. Diffuse
c. Nodular   d. Crescent

PYELONEPHRITIS & PAPILLARY NECROSIS

93. A patient presented with with pus in urine. Urine culture was done which was negative. After a sudden onset renal failure the patient died. On autopsy the following finding was seen in kidney. What is the most likely diagnosis? *(JIPMER 2017)*

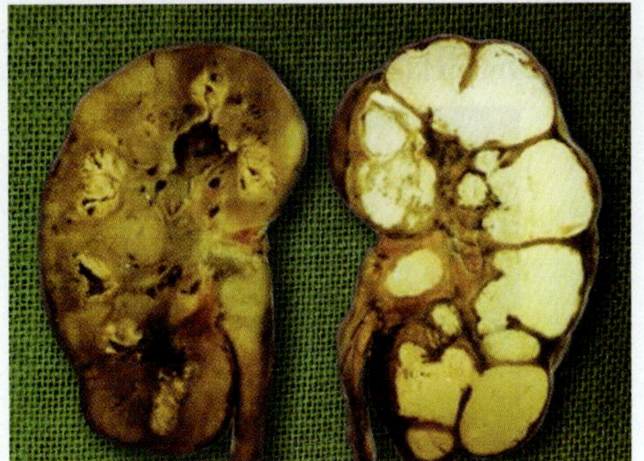

a. TB kidney   b. Infected renal cysts
c. Renal cell carcinoma   d. Renal stones

94. Characteristic feature of benign nephrosclerosis
a. Leather grain appearance *(Recent Question 2015)*
b. Flea bitten appearance
c. Onion skin appearance
d. Hyperplastic arteriosclerosis

95. Papillary necrosis is seen in all the following except
(Recent Question 2015)
a. NSAIDs   b. Diabetes mellitus
c. Sickle cell anemia   d. Shock

96. The most common infectious agent associated with chronic pyelonephritis is –
(Recent Question 2014, AIIMS May 2003)
a. Proteus vulgaris   b. Klebsiella pneumonia
c. Staphylococcus aureus   d. Escherichia coli

97. ENaC mutation is seen in: *(Recent Question 2015)*
a. Liddle syndrome   b. Gordon syndrome
c. Bartter syndrome   d. Gitelman syndrome

98. Least likely cause of renal papillary necrosis
a. Sickle cell disease *(APPGMEE 14)*
b. Analgesic nephropathy
c. Posterior urethral valves
d. Diabetes with UTI

99. **Acquired cystic diseases rather than inherited cause a 12- to 18-fold increased risk of renal cell carcinoma, which develops in 7% of dialyzed patients observed for 10 years. All of the following are seen in adult Polycystic kidney disease except?** *(PGI Nov 2016)*
   a. Large Kidney
   b. Small kidney
   c. Multilobulated on USG
   d. Cysts in liver and brain
   e. 10% progresses to ESRD

100. **Regarding adult polycystic kidney disease, which one of the following statements is not correct?**
   (Recent Question 2016-17)
   a. Inherited as autosomal dominant with 100% penetrance
   b. Often associated with hepatic cysts
   c. Associated with increased incidence of subarachnoid haemorrhage
   d. Renal cell carcinoma is a frequent association

101. **Hepatic fibrosis is found in** *(Recent Question 2016)*
   a. Medullary cystic kidney   b. ADPCKD
   c. ARPCKD   d. Nephrophthosis

102. **Chromosome a/w ADPKD** *(Recent Question 2016)*
   a. 14 and 16   b. 14 and 13
   c. 16 & 4   d. 12 & 16

103. **Gross section of kidney depicts what?** *(APPGMEE 2015)*

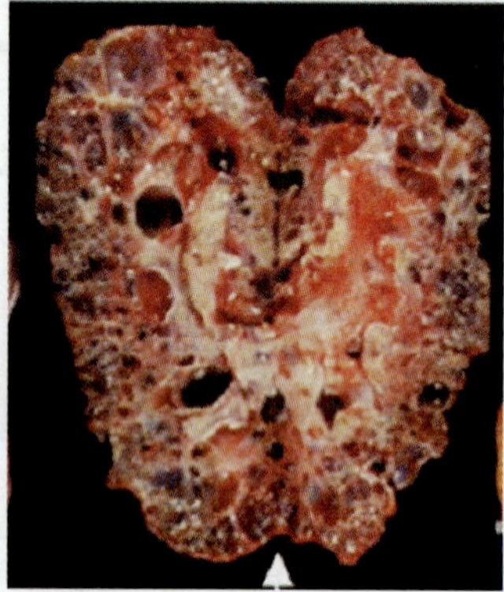

   a. RCC
   b. Medullary sponge kidney
   c. Hydatid cyst
   d. Polycystic kidney disease

104. **Balkan nephropathy is caused by?** *(APPGMEE 2015)*
   a. Fungal toxins   b. Lead
   c. Calcineurin inhibitors   d. Aristocholic acid

105. **True about Adult polycystic kidney disease:**
   (PGI May 12)
   a. Autosomal dominant pattern of inheritance
   b. 80% develop Nephrolithiasis
   c. Caused by mutation in two genes
   d. Somatic mutation can also occur
   e. Loss of heterozygosity may occur

106. **Which of the following statements about Xanthogranu-lomatous pyelonephritis is not true -** *(AI 11, 09)*
   a. Foam cells are seen
   b. Associated with tuberculosis
   c. Yellow nodules are seen
   d. Giant cells may be seen

VASCULAR DISEASES

107. **What is your diagnosis in the figure given below?**
   (Recent Question 2016-17)

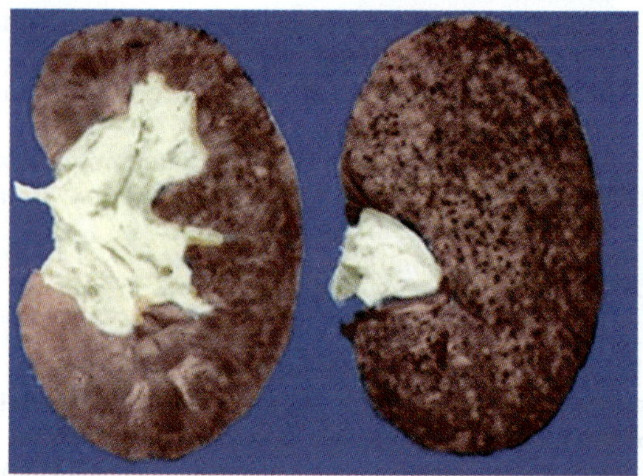

   a. Flea bitten kidney in malignant hypertension
   b. Amylodosis
   c. Ch. Glomerulonephritis
   d. Glomerulosclerosis

108. **A 40-year-old hypertensive male was admitted to the hospital with sudden onset of headache and altered sensorium. On Examination his Blood Pressure was observed to be 220/110mm Hg and the patient died four later. What is likely pathological finding in his kidneys -**
   a. Small kidney with granular surface   *(AI 12)*
   b. Small kidney with petechial hemorrhages
   c. Large kidney with waxy appearance
   d. Large kidney with granular surface

RENAL TUMORS

109. **Sickle cell anemia leads to which variety of Renal cell ca?** *(JIPMER 2017)*
   a. Medullary   b. Papillary
   c. Chromophobic   d. Belini duct Ca

110. **Loss of y chromosome is seen in in which Renal cell Ca?** *(JIPMER 2017)*
   a. Papillary   b. Chromophobe
   c. Chromophillic   d. Belini duct Ca

111. **MC tumors of kidney in children?** *(PGI Nov 2016)*
   a. Wilms tumor   b. Neuroblastoma
   c. PCKD   d. Angioliposarcoma
   e. Malignant rhabdoid tumor

112. **Chromosomal mutation in low grade transitional cell cancer of bladder is?** *(JIPMER 2016)*
   a. P53   b. Rb gene
   c. FGFR3   d. HRAS

113. **Most common histological type of renal cell cancer?**
   a. Clear cell ca   *(Recent Question 2016-17)*
   b. Clear cell sarcoma
   c. Metaplastic nephroma
   d. Xp translocation ca

114. **Hobnail pattern is seen in which type of renal carcinoma** *(Recent Question 2015)*
   a. Clear cell carcinoma
   b. Papillary carcinoma
   c. Chromophobe cell cancer
   d. Collecting duct carcinoma

115. **Multiple chromosomal losses are associated with the following type of renal cancer** *(Recent Question 2015)*
   a. Clear cell carcinoma
   b. Papillary carcinoma
   c. Chromophobe cell cancer
   d. Collecting duct carcinoma

116. **Most common histological variant of renal cell carcinoma is:**
   a. Papillary carcinoma *(Recent Question 2015)*
   b. Clear cell carcinoma
   c. Chromophobe renal carcinoma
   d. Collecting duct carcinoma

117. **Most common cystic disease of kidney is?**
   (Recent Question 2015)
   a. X linked recessive polycystic kidney disease
   b. X linked dominant polycystic kidney disease
   c. Autosomal recessive polycystic kidney disease
   d. Autosomal dominant polycystic kidney disease

118. **Most common gene associated with renal cell carcinoma is?** *(Recent Question 2015)*
   a. WT-1 b. BRCA-1
   c. VHL d. PATCH

119. **Clear cell variety of Renal cell carcinoma is related to gene located on chromosome:** *(Recent Question 2014)*
   a. 3 b. X
   c. 22 d. 20

120. **1 month post renal transplant a patient developed fever. Which of the following is the most likely organism responsible?** *(AIIMS May 2014)*
   a. Polyoma virus/ BK virus
   b. Hepatitis C virus
   c. Varicella virus
   d. HHV-6

121. **An emerging viral pathogen causing pyelonephritis in kidney allografts** *(Recent Question 2015)*
   a. Polyoma virus b. Marburg virus
   c. Ebola virus d. JC virus

122. **Histopathology showing large cells with plant like appearance with perinuclear halo is seen in which type of renal cell carcinoma?** *(PGI Nov 12)*
   a. Oncocytoma
   b. Papillary cell carcinoma
   c. Transitional cell Carcinoma
   d. Chromophobe RCC
   e. Clear cell carcinoma

123. **Clear cells are seen in:** *(PGI May 2011)*
   a. Rhabdomyosarcoma
   b. Adrenal cell carcinoma
   c. Renal cell Carcinoma
   d. Hodgkin's lymphoma
   e. NHL

124. **Chromophobe variant of renal cell carcinoma is associated with -** *(AI 10)*
   a. VHL gene mutations
   b. Trisomy 7 and 17
   c. 3 p deletions
   d. Monosomy of l and Y

125. **An emerging organism responsible for causing Pyelonephritis in Renal Allografts is?** *(DNB Dec 10)*
   a. Polyoma virus
   b. Herpes virus
   c. Hepatitis B virus
   d. Rota virus

126. **Findings of multiple myeloma in kidney are all except-** *(DPG 10)*
   a. Tubular casts b. Amyloidosis
   c. Wire loop lesions d. Renal tubular necrosis

DISEASES OF URINARY BLADDER

127. **Most common type of bladder cancer**
   a. Squamous cell carcinoma *(Recent Question 2015)*
   b. Urothelial cell carcinoma
   c. Adenocarcinoma
   d. Carcinoid

128. **Michaelis Gutmann bodies are seen in -**
   (Recent Question 2014, 2013/ AIIMS May 07/ DNB Dec 09)
   a. Xanthogranulomatous pyelonephritis
   b. Malakoplakia
   c. Nail patella syndrome
   d. Chronic Pyelonephritis

129. **90% of bladder cancer arise from-**
   a. Squamous cells *(Recent Question 2014)*
   b. Glandular cells
   c. Transitional cells
   d. Smooth muscle cells

130. **All are carcinogenic for bladder except?**
   a. Benzidine *(Recent Question 2014)*
   b. Isopropyl alcohol
   c. Acrolein
   d. Phenacetin

Answers with Explanations

1. Ans. (c) Fabry disease

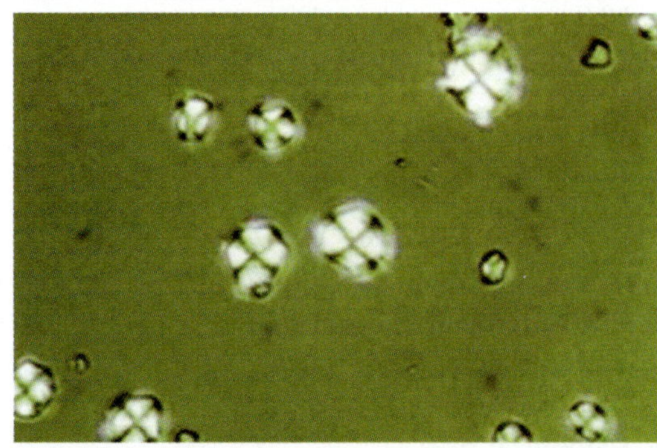

Round particles producing birefringent Maltese crosses under polarized light are commonly seen in the urinary sediment of patients with a nephrotic syndrome. The appearance of the Maltese crosses is due to the birefringence of lipid droplets, which consist mainly of cholesterol esters. These may also be seen in Fabry disease.

2. Ans. (a) Glomerulonephritis

3. Ans. (a, b, c, e) a. Hyaline casts- may be normally present in healthy person; b. Muddy brown casts- acute tubular necrosis; c. WBC cast - pyelonephritis; e. Myogolobin cast - Rhabdomyolysis

4. Ans. (a, b) a. Centrifuge the urine first; b. Use immunofluorescence light

5. Ans. (d) Hyaline casts

The given figure shows urine cytology in samples obtained during clinical rejection showing **numerous renal tubular cells, lymphocytes, and macrophages along with few Hyaline casts (as shown in the arrow).**

6. Ans. (c) Creatinine clearance rate

7. Ans. (a) A/4 B/3 C/1 D/2

8. Ans. (a) Oxalate *(Ref: Henry 22nd/457)*

9. Ans. (c) Struvite *(Ref: Henry 22nd/457)*

10. Ans. (a, b. d); a. WBC cast-Acute pyelonephritis b. Broad cast-CRF d. RBC cast-Glomerulonephritis

(Ref: Henry 22nd/457)

11. Ans. (a) 3.1-7 mg/dl *(Ref: Harrison 18th/pg Appendix)*

Normal levels of Uric acid

Females	0.15–0.33 mmol/L	2.5–5.6 mg/dL
Males	0.18–0.41 mmol/L	3.1–7.0 mg/dL

12. Ans. (c) Proteoglycan *(Ref: Robbins 9th/pg 900; 8th/pg 908)*

Glomerular basement membrane (GBM) contains Poly-anionic proteoglycans (negatively charged) (mostly heparan sulfate) and hence repels negatively charged proteins.

13. Ans. (c) RBC cast

(Ref: Henry's 22nd/ 466-469) Refer to Annexure

Cast seen in Acute Glomerulonephritis is RBC cast, which is pathognomonic

14. Ans. (b) 5 *(Ref: Henry's 22nd/ 457-458)*

Normal findings in analysis of urine sediment
- **Red blood cells:** 0–2/high-power field
- **White blood cells:** 0–2/high-power field
- **Bacteria:** None
- **Casts:** None except hyaline casts
- **Epithelial cells:** None

15. Ans. (a) Isomorphic RBCs *(Ref: Henry's 22nd/ 457-458)*

- **Hematuria:** Presence of >3 RBCs/hpf of urine
- Hematuria can be isomorphic (morphologically normal RBCs) or dysmorphic(RBCs with cellular protrusions or fragmentation)
- Hematuria due to nephrolithiasis lead to isomorphic RBCs with glomerulonephritis lead to dysmorphic RBCs.

Etiology of Hematuria

Isomorphic RBCs		Dysmorphic RBCs
Upper Tract	**Lower Tract**	**Renal disease:**
• Urolithiasis • Pyelonephritis • Renal cell cancer • Transitional cell Ca • Urinary obstruction • Benign hematuria	• Bacterial cystitis (UTI) • Benign prostatic hyperplasia • Strenuous exercise ("marathon runner's hematuria") • Transitional cell carcinoma • Spurious hematuria (e.g. menses) • Instrumentation • Benign hematuria	• Glomerulonephritis • Lupus nephritis • IgA nephropathy (Berger's disease) • Thin glomerular basement membrane disease • Hereditary nephritis (Alport's syndrome)

16. **Ans. (a, b, e); a. Glomerular basement membrane; b. Tubule; e. Mesangial matrix**

   (Ref: Rosai 10th/pg 1102-1104)

   PAS positive structures are GBM, tubule & mesangial matrix

17. **Ans. (c) PSGN** *(Ref: Robbins 9th/pg 909)*

18. **Ans. (a) Nephrotic range proteinuria b. Neutrophilic infiltration of tubules, d. Linear deposits along glomerular basement membrane**

   (Ref: Robbins 9th/ 909-12)

19. **Ans. (b) Renal failure**

   (Ref: Robbins 9th/pg 909; 8th/pg 917

20. **Ans. (c) FSGS** *(Ref: Robbins 9th/pg 918; 8th/pg 926*

   Most common renal involvement in HIV is FSGS.

21. **Ans. (a) Epithelial humps** *(Ref: Robbins 9th/pg 909-912)*

   Electron microscopy is PSGN shows
   Discrete, amorphous, electron-dense **SUBEPITHELIAL deposits ("Humps")**[Q]

22. **Ans. (d) Deposition of IgA** *(Ref: Robbins 9th/pg 909-912)*

23. **Ans. (b) Immune complex mediated**

   (Ref: R 9th/pg 909-912)

24. **Ans. (a) C3 decreases & ASO increases**

   (Ref: Robbins 9th/pg 909-912; 8th/pg 917-919)

25. **Ans. (b) Caused by non groupA hemolytic streptococci**

   (Ref: Robbins 9th/pg 909-912; 8th/pg 917-919)

   Both Post-streptococcal reactive arthritis and Acute Rheumatic fever are **caused by non-group A hemolytic streptococci**

26. **Ans. (d) Anti GBM antibodies** *(Ref: R 9th ed pg 912)*

   EM image show rupture of GBM. With a history to proteinuria and hypertension and high creatinine, RPGN can be an important differential.

27. **Ans. (b) Flea bitten kidney** *(Ref: Rob[bi]ns 9th/pg 912)*

28. **Ans. (d) Type 2- SLE nephritis**

29. **Ans. (b) Good Pasture syndrome**

30. **Ans. (c) Crescents** *(Ref: Robbins 9th ed. Pg. 912,)*

31. **Ans. (d) Good pasture syndrome**

   (Ref: Robbins 9th/pg 912)

32. **Ans. (a, c) a. Generalize edema, c. Hypoalbuminemia**

   (Ref: Robbins 9th/pg 909)

   Acute nephritic syndromes classically present with hypertension, hematuria, red blood cell casts, pyuria, and mild to moderate proteinuria.

33. **Ans. (c) Recurrent gross hematuria following respiratory infection**

   (Ref: Robbins 9th/pg 909; 8th/pg 917)

   IgA nephropathy is characterized by: **Recurrent hematuria** and presence of **IgA deposits in the mesangium**

34. **Ans. (a) Amyloidosis**

   (Ref: Robbins 9th/pg 261; 8th/pg 254; Harrison 18th/pg 947)

   Kidney involvement in Amyloidosis
   - **Deposition of monoclonal Ig or** λ (or kappa) light chains in the GBM
   - Distinctive **nodular glomerular lesions** resulting from the deposition of *non-fibrillar* light chains.
   - Glomeruli show **PAS-positive mesangial nodules, lobular accentuation & mild mesangial hypercellularity.**

35. **Ans. (d) Focal segmental glomerulosclerosis**

   (Ref: Robbins 9th/pg 912; 8th/pg 920)

   - **Most common cause** of **nephrotic** syndrome in **children** is **Minimal change disease**
   - Most common cause of nephrotic syndrome in **adults: FSGS**> MGN

36. **Ans. (b) Polyarteritis nodosa**

   (Ref: Robbins 9th/pg 912)

37. **Ans. (a) Necrotisting hemorrhagic interstitial pneumonitis**

   (Ref: Robbins 9th/pg 912-913; 8th/pg 920-921)

38. **Ans. (b) Serum antibodies against alpha 3 NC1 domain of collagen – IV** *(Ref: Robbins 9th/pg 912-913*

   Goodpasture syndrome
   - **It is type 1 RPGN & a type II hypersensitivity reaction.**
   - **It is characterized by s**erum antibodies against alpha 3 NC1 domain of collagen – IV.
   - This shows l**inear GBM fluorescence, while all other Glomerulonephritis, which are type 3 Hypersensitivity reactions show granular immune deposits.**

39. **Ans. (a, b, c, d); a. Antibody to** α**-chain of Type IV collagen (COL-4A); b. Basement membrane involvement; c. Pulmonary hemorrhage; d. Crescent formation**

   (Ref: Robbins 9th/pg 912-913; 8th/pg 920-921)

40. **Ans. (a) Capillary wall thickening** *(Ref: R 9th pg 222)*

41. Ans. (c) Lupus nephritis

Here, the typical "full-house" pattern with intense (+++) granular staining for IgA, IgG, IgM, kappa & lambda & C1 and C3 in a diffuse mesangiocapillary pattern can be seen which is suggestive of SLE.

Good Pasteur will show linear IgG and C3 dposits in basement membrane.

PSGN will show granular depotis of IgG & C3 and sometimes IgM in the mesangium and in sometimes GBM

FSGS will show IgM & C3 in sclerotic area or mesangium

42. Ans. (a, b, c) a. Low C4 level; b. Double basement membrane appearance on light microscopy; c. Dense deposit along basement membrane on electron microscopy

43. Ans. (a) Alport syndrome

44. Ans. (d) Henoch Schonlein purpura *(Ref: R 9/909-912)*

The clinical history is suggestive of nephritic syndrome with arthritis and purpura which is a triad of Henoch Schonlein purpura

45. Ans. (b) Alpha-3 and alpha -4 chains of collagen type IV

(Ref: Robbins 9th/pg 925; 8th/pg 932)

Thin basement membrane disease (TBMD)

- It is characterized by persistent or recurrent hematuria, but is not typically associated with proteinuria, hypertension, or loss of renal function or extrarenal disease.
- Genetic defects in *COL(IV) α3/COL(IV) α4* loci of type IV collagen
- Autosomal dominant or recessive inheritance
- GBM shows diffuse thinning compared to normal values for the patient's age in otherwise normal biopsies

46. Ans. (d) All of the above *(Ref: Robbins 9th/pg 920)*

- In MPGN type I, **Subendothelial**[Q]electron-dense deposits are most commonly seen
- **Mesangial/ subepithelial**[Q]deposits may also be present
- In MPGN type II, intramembranous deposits seen

47. Ans. (a) Membranoproliferative glomerulosclerosis

(Ref: Robbins 9th/pg 920; 8th/pg 928)

48. Ans. (c) Acute proliferative glomerulonephritis

(Ref: Robbins 9th/pg 910; 8th/pg 920)

49. Ans. (d) Decreased serum IgA level *(Ref: R 9th/pg 923)*

Serum IgA level is increased in IgA nephropathy

50. Ans. (a) MPGN *(Ref: Robbins 9th/pg 920; 8th/pg 928)*

51. Ans. (d) Mesangiocapillary glomerulonepthritis

(Ref: Robbins 9th/pg 920; 8th/pg 928)

Renal biopsy of a young male with nephritic syndrome showing mesangial cell proliferation with Glomerular basement membrane thickening and mesangial cell interposition is typical biopsy finding of **Mesangiocapillary Glomerulonephritis, also called MPGN**

52. Ans. (a) Glomerular disease

(Ref: Henry's 22nd/ 457-458)

Dysmorphic RBCs with ARF is seen in Glomerular disease, while isomorphic RBCs are seen in non-glomerular bleeds;

53. Ans. (a) Alport's syndrome

(Ref: Robbins 9th/pg 924-925; 8th/pg 931-932)

54. Ans. (c) CD71 *(Ref: Robbins 9th/pg 923-924)*

55. Ans. (a) Crescents *(Ref: Robbins 9th/pg 912-913)*

56. Ans. (a) Henoch Schonlein purpura

(Ref: Robbins 9th/pg 923-924)

57. Ans. (a, b, c, d); a. Minimal change disease; b. Focal segmental GN; c. IgA nephropathy; d. Mesangial proliferative GN

(Ref: Robbins 9th/pg 917-918; 8th/pg 924-926)

Foot process effacement is seen on EM in:

Minimal change disease, Focal segmental GN, IgA nephropathy, Mesangial proliferative GN

58. Ans. (b) Type II MPGN *(Ref: Robbins 9th/pg 920-921)*

Increased levels of C_3NeF are associated with **Type II MPGN.**

59. Ans. (d) Class V *(Ref: Robbins 9th/pg 222-224)*

Renal involvement in SLE:

Class I: Minimal Mesangial Lupus Nephritis[Q]

Class II: Mesangial Proliferative Lupus Nephritis

Class III: Focal Lupus Nephritis[Q]

Class IV: Diffuse Lupus Nephritis[Q]

Class V: Membranous Lupus Nephritis[Q]

Class VI: Advanced Sclerotic Lupus Nephritis

- **50%** patients of SLE have clinically significant **renal involvement**[Q]
- **Class I Lupus Nephritis Class I Lupus Nephritis is least common**[Q] **& class IV is the most common pattern**[Q]

"Wire loop lesions"[Q] characteristically seen in **Class IV Lupus Nephritis**[Q] is due to **sub-endothelial** immune complex deposits, on **light microscopy**- Also seen in **Class III/V Lupus nephritis**[Q]

60. Ans. (b) Severe hypoalbuminemia *(Ref: R 9th/pg 914)*

a. False	Effacement of foot process is seen on electron microscopy, while light microscopy is normal in minimal change disease
b. True	**Severe hypoalbuminemia is a feature of nephrotic syndrome due to minimal change disease**
c. False	c. Selective proteinuria
d. False	d. Cyclosporine is the first line of treatment

61.   **Ans. (a)   IgA nephropathy** *(Ref: Robbins 9th/pg 914)*

Most common nephropathy in world isIgA nephropathy

62.   **Ans. (b)   Minimal change disease** *(Ref: R 9th/pg 917-918)*

63.   **Ans. (d)   No change seen** *(Ref: Robbins 9th/pg 917-918)*

On light microscopy
Glomeruli appear normal[Q] minimal change disease

64.   **Ans. (a)   Minimal change disease** *(Ref: R 9th/pg 917-918)*

The child in this question presents with **first episode of massive proteinuria, frothy urine suggestive of lipiduria** and edema. Urine microscopy finding is not significant. This is suggestive of **nephrotic syndrome**, for which, the **most common cause in children is Minimal change disease.**

65.   **Ans. (a, b, c, d); a. Spontaneous bacterial peritonitis; b. Sepsis; c. DVT; d. Atherosclerosis**

(Ref: R 9th/pg 917-918)

Patients with minimal change disease are at risk of Spontaneous bacterial peritonitis, Sepsis, DVT and Atherosclerosis

Complications of Nephrotic syndrome:

Infection[Q]	• Staphylococcal and Pneumococcal infection. Eg Spontaneous bacterial peritonitis, Sepsis • Due to **loss of immunoglobulins[Q]** in the urine
Thrombotic & thromboembolic complications	• Due to loss of endogenous anticoagulants **(Antithrombin-III, protein C, protein S)[Q]** in urine • **Hypercoagulable state →Renal vein thrombosis / Deep vein thrombosis (**DVT) • Particularly in **membranous nephropathy[Q]**
Atherosclerosis	• Due to hyperlipidemia
Loss of other low molecular wt proteins	• **Transferrin** leads to **Iron deficiency anemia** • **Ceruloplasmin**leads to **copper deficiency anemia** • **Cholecalciferol binding protein** leads to**Vit D deficiency** • **Thyroglobulin binding protein** leads to **hypothyroidism**

66.   **Ans. (b)   Congenital Finnish type nephrotic syndrome**

(Ref: Nelson 19 thedpg 1803)

Mutation in NPHS1 gene causes Congenital Finnish type nephrotic syndrome

67.   **Ans. (d)   Minimal change disease** *(Ref: R 9th/pg 917-918)*

68.   **Ans. (a, b, c);   a. Cause steroid resistant nephrotic syndrome; b. Nephrin is a key component of the slit diaphragm; c. Coded by NPHS-1 gene**

(Ref: Nelson 19th/pg 1802)

• Congenital nephrotic syndrome Finnish type is a type of steroid resistant nephrotic syndrome

• It is caused by NPHS-1 gene mutation, which codes for Nephrin protein, a key component of the slit diaphragm

69.   **Ans. (a)   No IgG deposits or C3 deposition on renal biopsy**

(Ref: Robbins 9th/pg 917-918)

In the given scenario, a 7 year old girl presents with generalized swelling, massive proteinuria, but no hematuria and presence of hyaline and fatty casts. Therefore, she is suffering from Nephrotic Syndrome, the commonest cause of which is **Minimal change disease, in which there is no IgG or C3 deposition** on renal biopsy.

70.   **Ans. (b)   NPHS 2** *(Ref: Nelson 19thed/pg1802)*

Most common gene defect in idiopathic steroid resistant nephrotic syndrome NPHS 2 which codes for podocin;

71.   **Ans. (a)   Loss of antithrombin III**

(Ref: Robbins 9th/pg 914; 8th/pg 922)

72.   **Ans. (c)   Hypoalbuminemia** *(Ref: Harrison 19th ed/pg 253)*

73.   **Ans. (a)   Autosomal recessive inheritance**

(Ref: Rosai 10th/pg 1153)

Fibronectin glomerulopathy

Definition	Characterized by massive fibronectin deposition in the glomeruli.
Genetic basis	Caused by **mutations of FN1 gene on chromosome 2q34**
Inheritance	Hereditary **autosomal dominant** *(option A)* disease; **Both sexes** are equally affected
Clinical features	**Proteinuria** (nephrotic range), **microscopic hematuria** and slow **deterioration of renal function** over a period of several years.
Light microscopy	• **Glomeruli appear enlarged & lobulated** with minimal degree of hypercellularity • Most characteristic feature: **marked enlargement of mesangium & subendothelial** *(option D)* **space** due to **deposition of a homogeneous PAS +ve, Congo red –ve** *(option B)* **material**
Electron microscopy	**Dense granular appearance of the deposit in mesangium or subendothelium**
Immunohisto-chemical studies	• **Strong positivity for fibronectin** in the areas corresponding to the deposits. • Scanty immunoglobulins and complement factors may occasionally be seen, inconsistently.*(option C)*
Prognosis	**Poor prognosis**
Recurrence after renal transplant	The disease has been reported to **recur after renal transplantation.**

74. Ans. (b) **Membranous glomerulopathy**

(Ref: Robbins 9th ed p 915, 920)

The given image shows Membranous glomerulopathy with Diffuse capillary wall thickening in EM image and granular (IgG and C3 deposits) in immunofluorescence.

75. Ans (b) **Membranous glomerulonephropathy**

(Ref: Robbins 9th/pg 231-234; 8th/pg 221-229)

- Whenever you get an immunofluorescence image in a kidney biopsy, you must try to see if the deposits look granular (lumpy bumpy) or linear.
- If its linear the answer will be Good Pasteur's syndrome (Anti GBM antibody ds)
- If it is granular, it can be any other immune complex disease.

Among the given options, the only immune complex deposition disease is Membranous nephropathy.

76. Ans. (d) **Membranous nephritis**

77. Ans. (d) **Wegner's granulomatosis**

78. Ans. (a) **Membranous**

(Ref: Robbins 9th/pg 915; 8th/pg 922)

Most common nephropathy associated with malignancy is **Membranous in adults & minimal change in children**

79. Ans. (c) **Hematuria** *(Ref: Robbins 9th/pg 917; 8th/pg 924)*

80. Ans. (b) **MPGN type I**

(Ref: Robbins 9th/pg 920; 8th/pg 928)

81. Ans. (c) **HBsAg** *(Ref: Robbins 9th/pg 914; 8th/pg 922)*

- HBsAg causes Glomerulonephritis with Nephrotic syndrome
- HBsAg, immunoglobulin, and C3 deposition has been found in the glomerular basement membrane.

82. Ans. (c) **HIV** *(Ref: Robbins 9th/pg 920; 8th/pg 928;*

Collapsing variant of FSGS is seen in HIV

83. Ans. (c) **There is noproliferation or hypertrophy of glomerular visceral epithelial cells**

(Ref: Robbins 9th/pg 920; 8th/pg 928)

HIV-ASSOCIATED NEPHROPATHY (HIVAN) is characterized by collapse of entire glomerular tuft along with proliferation and hypertrophy of glomerular visceral epithelial cells[Q]

84. Ans. (c) **Collapsing glonerulonephritis**

(Ref: Robbins 9th/pg 920)

85. Ans. (a) **Focal segmental glomerulosclerosis**

(Ref: Robbins 9th/pg 918-919; 8th/pg 926-927)

Nephrotic syndrome in a patient with **reflux nephropathy** is caused by **Focal segmental glomerulosclerosis**, as a component of the adaptive response to loss of renal tissue

86. Ans. (c) **MPGN type I** *(Ref: Robbins 9th/pg 920-921)*

87. Ans. (b) **Mesangiocapillary Glomerulonephritis**

(Ref: Robbins 9th/pg 920-921; 8th/pg 928-929)

88. Ans. (c) **Partial lipodystrophy**

(Ref: Robbins 9th/pg 920-921; 8th/pg 928-929)

Types II & III MPGN are associated with complement factor H deficiency, presence of C_3 nephritic factor, partial lipodystrophy (type II MPGN) or complement receptor deficiency (type III MPGN)

89. Ans. (a) **Kimmelstiel Wilson nodules**

(Ref: Robbins 9th ed p 1118)

Diabetic Nephropathy:

The renal lesions include mainly: Glomerular lesions:
- Basement membrane thickening and increased mesangial matrix in patients
- Diffuse glomerulosclerosis
  - Increase in mesangial matrix associated with PAS+ basement membrane thickening, eventually obliterates mesangial cells, found in most individuals with disease of **more than 10 years duration**
- **Nodular glomerulosclerosis**
  - Intercapillary glomerulosclerosis or Kimmelstiel-Wilson diseas

90. Ans. (a) **Diabetes mellitus** *(Ref: Robbins 9th/pg 1118)*

Most specific histological lesion in diabetic nephropathy (see chapter 18 Endocrine system) is Nodular glomerulo-sclerosis or **Kimmelsteil -Wilson lesions**

91. Ans (b) **Diabetic nephropathy** *(Ref: R 9th/pg 1118-1119)*

92. Ans. (c) **Nodular** *(Ref: Robbins 9th/pg 1118-1119)*

93. Ans. (a) **TB kidney**

The clinical history is suggestive of sterile pyuria. The gross morphology shows greyish white are caseating necrotic material which is formed in patches, predominantly in the cortical areas involving the while circumference of the kidney. Hence, the first possibility is renal TB.

94. Ans. (a) **Leather grain appearance** *(Ref: R 9th/pg 938)*

95. Ans. (d) **Shock** *(Ref: Robbins 9th/pg 939; 8th/pg 930)*

Major Causes of Papillary Necrosis
i. Analgesic nephropathy (Most common)[Q]
ii. Sickle cell nephropathy
iii. Diabetes with urinary tract infection

96. Ans. (d) **Escherichia coli** *(Ref: Robbins 9th/pg 933-934)*

The most common infectious agent associated with chronic pyelonephritis is *Escherichia coli*

97. **Ans. (a)** **Liddle syndrome** *(Ref: Harrison 18th/Ch 285)*

98. **Ans. (c)** **Posterior urethral valves**

(Ref: Robbins 9th/pg 932)

99. **Ans. (b)** **Small kidney** *(Ref: Robbins 9/945)*

100. **Ans. (d)** **Renal cell carcinoma is a frequent association**

(Ref: Robbins 9/949-952)

101. **Ans. (c, d);** **c. ARPCKD, d. Nephrophthosis**

(Ref: Robbins 9th/pg 945; 8th/pg 956; Refer to pretext

102. **Ans. (c)** **16 & 4** *(Ref: Robbins 9th/pg 945; 8th/pg 956)*

PKD1 gene is located on chromosome 16p13.3, that encodes a large integral membrane protein named *polycystin-1*
PKD2 gene, located on chromosome 4q21, encodes *polycystin-2 that* accounts for most of the remaining cases of polycystic disease.

103. **Ans. (d)** **Polycystic kidney disease** *(Ref: R 9th/pg 945)*

104. **Ans. (d)** **Aristocholic acid** *(Ref: Robbins 9th/pg 929)*

Aristolochic Nephropathy or Balkans Nephropathy:

- **Chronic tubulointerstitial nephritis** caused by **aristolochic acid**, a supplement found in some herbal remedies in Europe in **Balkan region**
- Associated with **urothelial atypia**, occasionally culminating in tumors of renal pelvis & urethra.
- **Drug forms covalent adducts** with DNA and causes renal failure and interstitial fibrosis associated with a relative paucity of infiltrating leukocytes.
- **Increased incidence of carcinoma** in the kidney and urinary tract.

105. **Ans. (a, c, d, e); a. Autosomal dominant pattern of inheritance; c. Caused by mutation in two genes; d. Somatic mutation can also occur; e. Loss of heterozygosity may occur**

(Ref: Robbins 9th/pg 945-947 Harrison 18th/pg Chapter 284)

- Over **90%** of cases are inherited as an **autosomal dominant** trait, remainder due to spontaneous mutations. *(option A)*
- Mutations in the **PKD-1** gene on chromosome 16 (ADPKD-1) account for **85% of cases**, and mutations in the **PKD-2 gene on chromosome 4 (ADPKD-2)** account for the remainder. *(option C)*
- Direct mutation analysis of isolated cysts suggests that there is **loss of heterozygosity (option E)**, whereby **a somatic mutation in the normal allele (option D)** of a small number of tubular epithelial cells leads **to unregulated clonal proliferation of cells** that ultimately form the cyst lining.
- **Nephrolithiasis** is seen in **20%** of patients with ADPKD *(option B, false)*

106. **Ans. (b)** **Associated with tuberculosis** *(Ref: R 9th/pg 934)*

Xanthogranulomatous pyelonephritis is associated with proteus infections and not TB

107. **Ans. (a)** **Flea bitten kidney in malignant hypertension**

(Ref: Robbins 9th/pg 939; 8th/pg 950-951)

Small, pinpoint petechial hemorrhages appear on the cortical surface from rupture of arterioles or glomerular capillaries, giving the kidney a peculiar **"flea-bitten" appearance**.

108. **Ans. (b)** **Small kidney with petechial hemorrhages**

(Ref: Robbins 9th/pg 939; 8th/pg 950-951)

This is a case of a middle aged man who died of malignant hypertension
Kidneys in such patients have a characteristic flea-bitten appearance i.e. **Small kidney with petechial hemorrhages.**

109. **Ans. (a)** **Medullary**

110. **Ans. (b)** **Chromophobe**

111. **Ans. (a)** **Wilms' tumor**

(Ref: Nelson 20th ed/ pg 2466-68)

Wilms' tumor (WT), also known as nephroblastoma, is the most common primary malignant renal tumor of childhood; It is the second most common malignant abdominal tumor in childhood. The most common sites of metastases are the lungs, regional lymph nodes, and liver.

112. **Ans. (c)** **FGFR3** *(Ref: Robbins 9th/968)*

- **Noninvasive high-grade urothelial carcinoma** is associated with loss of the TP53 and RB tumor suppressor genes while **Noninvasive low-grade papillary urothelial carcinoma** is associated with gain of function FGFR3 and HRAS mutations.

113. **Ans (a)** **Clear cell ca**

114. **Ans. (d)** **Collecting duct carcinoma** *(Ref: R 9th/pg 953)*

115. **Ans. (c)** **Chromophobe cell cancer** *(Ref: R 9th/pg 953)*

116. **Ans. (b)** **Clear cell carcinoma**

(Ref: Robbins 9th/pg 953)

117. **Ans. (d)** **Autosomal dominant polycystic kidney**

(Ref: Robbins 9th/pg 953; 8th/pg 964)

118. **Ans. (c)** **VHL** *(Ref: Robbins 9th/pg 953; 8th/pg 964)*

119. **Ans. (a)** **3**

(Ref: Robbins 9th/pg953-955; 8th/pg 964-966)

Clear cell variety of Renal cell carcinoma is related to gene located on chromosome 3

120. Ans. (b) Hepatitis C virus (*Ref: Harrison 18th/Chapter 282*)

Most Common Opportunistic Infections in Renal Transplant Recipients

Peri-transplant (<1 month)	Early (1–6 months)	Late (>6 months)
• Wound infections • Herpesvirus • Oral candidiasis • Urinary tract infection	• *Pneumocystis carinii* • Cytomegalovirus • *Legionella Listeria* • Hepatitis B • Hepatitis C	• *Aspergillus Nocardia* • BK virus (polyoma) • Herpes zoster • Hepatitis B • Hepatitis C

121. Ans. (a) Polyoma virus

(*Ref: Robbins 9th/pg 953; 8th/pg 964*)

122. Ans. (a, d); a. Oncocytoma; d. Chromophobe RCC

(*Ref: Rosai 10th/pg 1183-1193*)

Histological distinction of Chromophobe RCC from Oncocytoma can be difficult;

123. Ans. (c) Renal cell Carcinoma (*Ref: R 9th/pg 953-955*)

124. Ans. (d) Monosomy of 1 and Y (*Ref: R 9th/pg 953-955*)

125. Ans. (a) Polyoma virus (*Ref: Harrison 18th/Chapter 282*)

An **emerging organism** responsible for causing **Pyelonephritis in Renal Allografts is Polyoma virus**

126. Ans. (c) Wire loop lesions (*Ref: Robbins 9th/pg 222-224*)

- Wire loop lesions are seen in Lupus nephritis
- Features of kidney involvement in Multiple myeloma are: Tubular casts, Amyloidosis & Renal tubular necrosis

Kidney involvement in Multiple myeloma:
- **Amyloidosis**, monoclonal light chain
- **Nodular glomerular lesions** due to deposition of *non-fibrillar* light chains (PAS +ve).

127. Ans. (b) Urothelial cell carcinoma

(*Ref: Robbins 9th/pg 964; 8th/pg 974*)

128. Ans. (b) Malakoplakia

(*Ref: Robbins 9th/pg 963; 8th/pg 975*)

- **Michaelis-Gutmann bodies**[Q] are Laminated mineralized concretions seen in malakoplakia

129. Ans. (c) Transitional cells (*Ref: Robbins 9th/pg 964-966*)

130. Ans. (b) Isopropyl alcohol (*Ref: Robbins 9th/pg 964-966*)

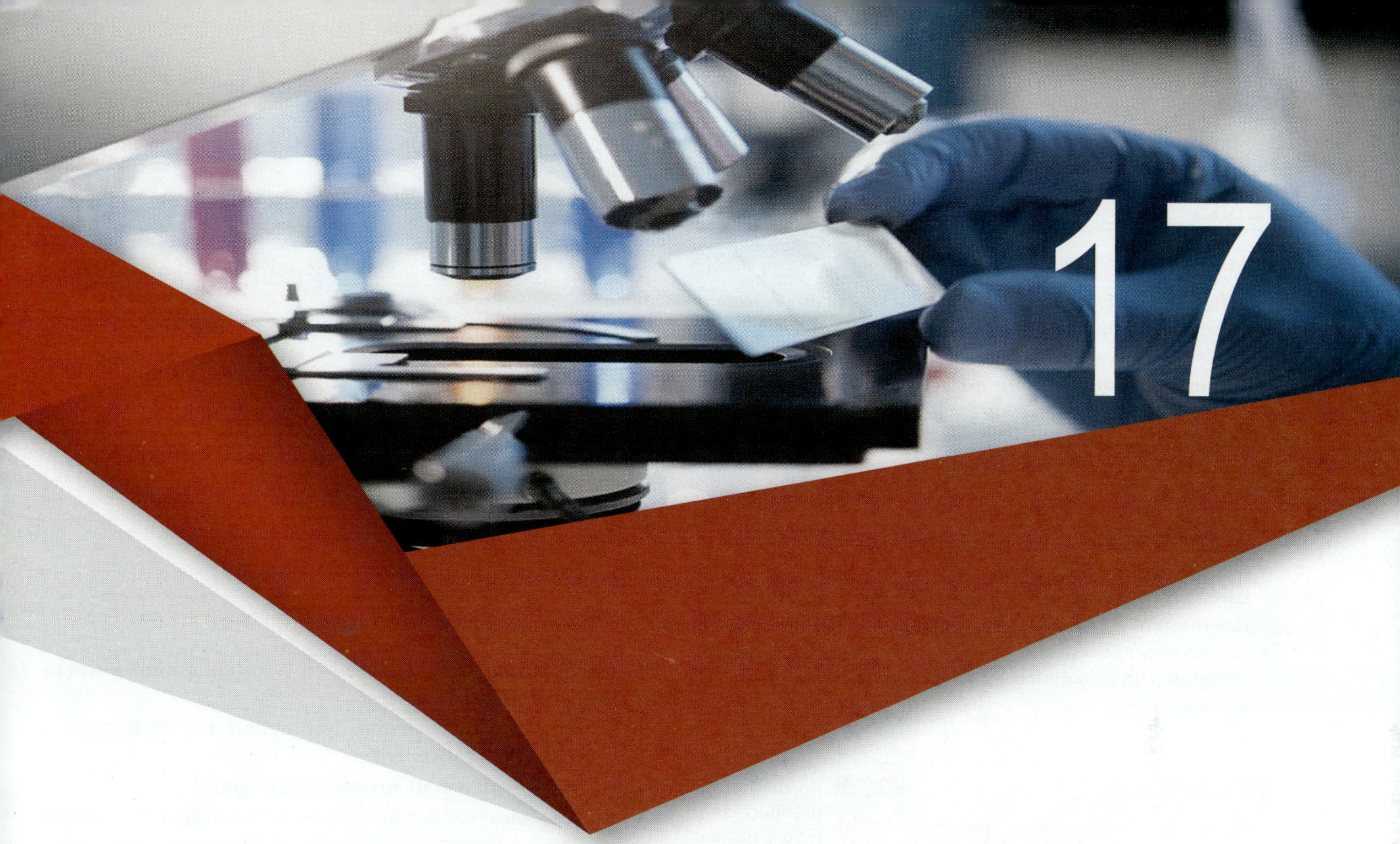

17

Male and Female Genitourinary Tract

Key Points

- » Most common testicular neoplasms in men over the age of 60 years-testicular lymphoma
- » Most common malignant paratesticular tumors are rhabdomyosarcomas in children
- » Yolk sac tumor most common testicular tumor in infants and children up to 3 years of age
- » HPVs are involved in the pathogenesis of cervical, vaginal, and vulvar cancers.
- » Most common tumor to develop in cryptorchid testis is seminoma
- » Primary adenocarcinoma of the fallopian tubes is rare and is usually serous papillary type
- » Superficial inguinal pouch is the most common site of ectopic testis

Key Recent Updates

- » ITGCN is now renamed as GCNIS i.e. germ cell neoplasm in situ
- » SOX, 2 is associated with embryonal carcinoma.

MALE GENITAL TRACT

PENIS

Inflammation

- **Balanoposthitis:**[Q] Nonspecific infection of glans & prepuce, mostly caused by **Candida, anaerobes & Gardenella.**[Q]
- Persistence of such infections leads to inflammatory scarring is a **common cause of phimosis.**[Q]

Tumors of Penis

Benign Tumors

Peyronie Disease	Condyloma Acuminatum
• **Characterized by fibrous bands involving corpus cavernosum** • **Results in penile curvature and pain during intercourse.**[Q]	• Caused by **HPV** types **6 & 11**[Q] • **Koilocytosis**[Q] **is characteristic** of HPV infection • **Recurs but rarely progresses to invasive cancer**

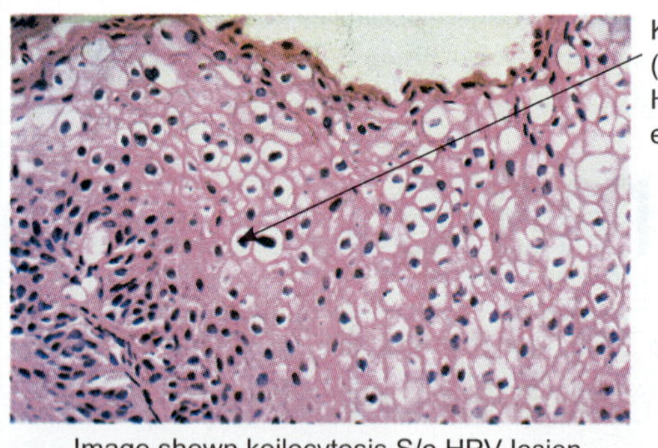

Image shown koilocytosis S/o HPV lesion

Carcinoma in situ: Precancerous Lesions

- Cytological changes of malignancy **confined to epithelium**
- 2 distinct lesions of CIS: **Bowen disease**[Q] **& bowenoid papulosis**

	Bowen's disease	Bowenoid papulosis
Age	**Older** than age 35 years[Q]	**Younger age**[Q]
No. of lesions	**Solitary** lesion[Q]	**Multiple lesions**[Q]
Prognosis	Transforms into **infiltrating squamous cell carcinoma**[Q] in 10%	**Never**[Q] develops into **invasive carcinoma** & in many cases regresses spontaneously.

Malignant Tumors: Squamous Cell Carcinoma

- **Risk factors:** HPV16 (Most common), HPV 18, Cigarette smoking
- Risk is **reduced by circumcision**; therefore it is *rare in* **Jews and Muslims**.

- **Occurs on the glans or shaft of the penis as an ulcerated infiltrative lesion**[Q]
- **Spread to inguinal nodes**[Q] and infrequently to distant sites.[Q]

- Most frequent penile neoplasm is condyloma acuminatum > carcinoma
- Both bowen disease and bowenoid papulosis are associated with HPV
- Verrucous carcinoma (also known as Giant condyloma or Buschke-Lowenstein tumor) refers to exophytic well-differentiated variant of squamous cell carcinoma, which is locally invasive, but rarely metastasize.

TESTIS AND EPIDIDYMIS

Cryptorchidism

- **Complete or partial failure of the intra-abdominal testes to descend into the scrotal sac**[Q]
- **Associated with testicular dysfunction and an increased risk of testicular cancer.**[Q]
- Grossly, testis is **small, brown and atrophic.**[Q]
- Microscopically: Atrophic tubules with thickened basement membrane, leydig cells are spared and appear predominant
- Higher **risk for testicular cancer:** from foci of **intratubular germ cell neoplasia within atrophic tubules**.
- Orchiopexy **reduces the risk of sterility and cancer.**[Q]

High Yield Facts

- Testicular atrophy occasionally occurs as a primary failure of **genetic origin**, such as in **Klinefelter's syndrome**[Q]
- **Ectopic testes** are the deviation of **testes** from normal path of descent.
- Ectopic testis is **fully developed** with **normal spermatogenesis**[Q] whereas undescended testis lacks spermatogenesis
- **Superficial inguinal pouch is the most common site of ectopic testis**[Q]
- **Most common tumor** to develop in cryptorchid testis is **seminoma**[Q]
- **Most common cause of non-specific inflammation of testis in:**
- A sexually active young patient (< 35 **years**) -*Chlamydia trachomatis* and *Neisseria gonorrhea*[Q]
- Men **older** than 35 **years** - *E. coli and pseudomonas.*[Q]

Inflammation

- More common in the **epididymis** than in the testis.
- **Gonorrhea & tuberculosis almost invariably arise in epididymis,** *whereas* **syphilis affects the testis**[Q] first.

Testicular Tumors

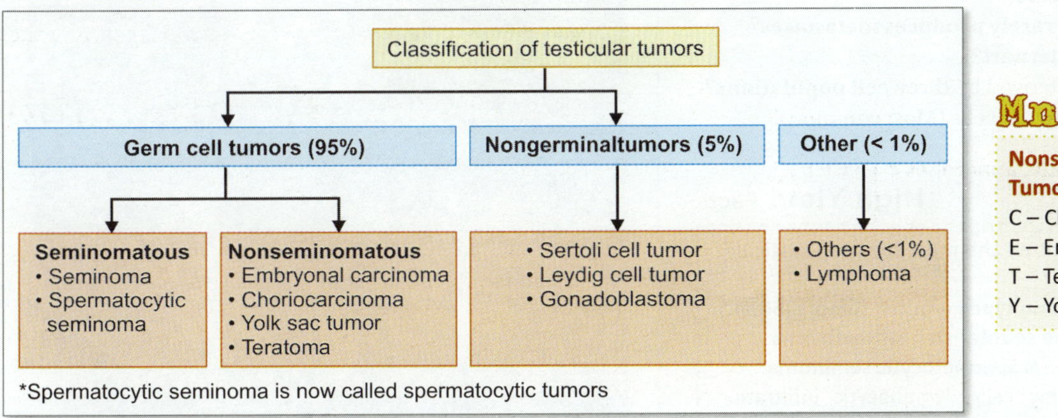

Mnemonic

Nonseminomatous Germ Cell Tumors

C – Choriocarcinoma
E – Embryonal Carcinoma
T – Teratoma
Y – Yolk Sac Tumors

Testicular Germ Cell Tumors

Most originate from a precursor lesion called **intratubular germ cell neoplasia (ITGCN)** except **spermatocyte seminoma; teratoma and Yolk Sac tumor in child.**[Q]

Predisposing Factors for Germ Cell Tumors are

- **Environmental Factors**: Increased risk by in uteroexposures to **pesticides and nonsteroidal estrogens.**[Q]
- **Testicular dysgenesis syndrome (TDS):** cryptorchidism, hypospadias, and poor sperm quality.
- **Cryptorchidism**
- **Klinefelter syndrome**: increased risk (50 times) of **mediastinal (not testicular) germ cell tumors**[Q]
- **Genetic Factors**:
  - **Strong familial predisposition** associated with the development of testicular germ cell tumors.
  - Isochromosome of short arm of chromosome **12, i(12p)**
  - Familial germ cell tumor risk: ligand for the receptor tyrosine kinase **KIT and BAK**

POINTS TO REMEMBER

Special Features of Testicular Germ Cell Tumors

- **Lymphatic spread**[Q] is common to all forms of testicular tumors
- Retroperitoneal para-aortic nodes are **the first to be involved.**[Q]
- Hematogenous spread Lung > Liver > Brain > Bones
- **Extragonadal site of germ cell tumors**[Q] include **mediastinum, retroperitoneum and pineal gland**[Q]
- Biopsy is associated with risk of tumor spillage, so contra-indicated
- The histology of metastases may differ from that of the testicular lesion.

Seminomatous Germ Cell Tumors

Seminoma

Clinical features: Peak incidence in **third decade, almost never occur in infants.**[Q]

Morphology:

- Sheets of **Monomorphic cells**[Q]
- **Sheets divided into poorly demarcated lobules by septa of fibrous tissue**

- **Septa show lymphocytic infiltration (T lymphocytes)**[Q]
- Classic **seminoma cell** - large and round to polyhedral and has a distinct cell membrane;
- **Clear or watery-appearing cytoplasm; Cytoplasm contains glycogen**[Q].

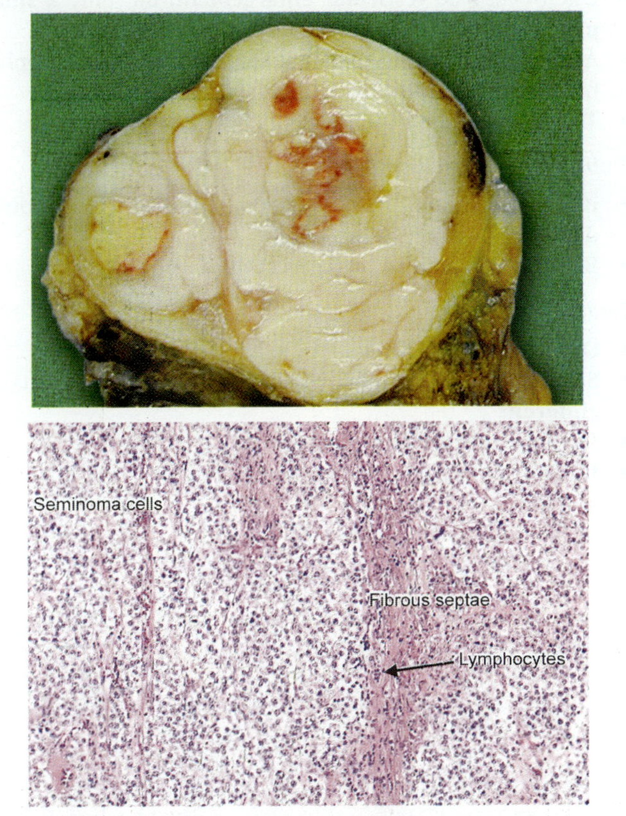

Tumor markers: **PLAP** (Placental alkaline phosphatase)[Q] **GGT** (Gamma glutamyl transpeptidase)[Q], hCG (15% cases)

Genetics: Seminomas contain isochromosome **12p and express OCT3/4 and NANOG.**[Q]

Spermatocytic Tumor

- It is **distinctive tumor both clinically** and **radiologically** as compared to seminoma[Q]

- **Do not arise from** an **intratubular germ cell neoplasia**[Q]
- Age of involvement >**65 years**[Q]
- **Slow growing tumor** that **rarely produces metastases**[Q]
- There is **no ovarian counterpart**[Q]
- Histologically, it is characterized by **three cell populations**[Q]- small cells, medium cells, giant cells (Most common).
- **Prognosis is excellent**[Q]

High Yield Facts

- Germ cell tumors constitute **the most common testicular tumor of men**[Q]
- **Seminoma: most common type germ cell tumors (50%).**[Q]
- **Dysgerminoma –Female counter part of seminoma**
- Spireme *chromatin is seen in* **Spermatocytic seminoma**[Q]
- Sheets of monomorphic cells, lymphocytic infiltration (T lymphocytes) is characteristic feature of seminoma

Nonseminomatous Germ Cell Tumors

Choriocarcinomas

- **Most aggressive** testicular tumor;[Q].
- Often cause **no testicular enlargement,** but only **a small palpable nodule**[Q]
- A mixture of malignant cytotrophoblasts and syncytiotrophoblasts seen
- **Tumor marker is hCG**

Embryonal cell carcinomas

- Present as sheets of undifferentiated cells; focal glandular differentiation may be present
- **Elevated AFP and hCG is seen in this tumor**[Q]

Teratomas

- Occur at any age from infancy to adult life.
- **Second most common testicular tumor in infants & children**[Q]
- **Derived from all three germ layers**[Q]
- **In children**, differentiated mature teratomas are considered **benign**[Q]
- In **post-pubertal males**, all teratomas are regarded as **malignant.**[Q]

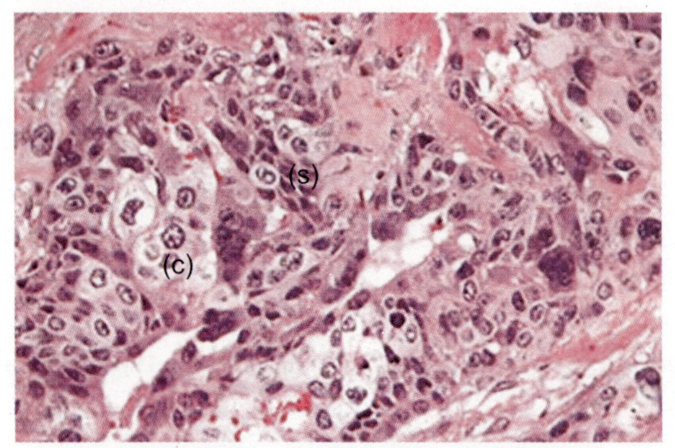

Choriocarcinoma: syncytiotrophoblasts (s) are multinucleated and have a dark staining cytoplasm. The cytotrophoblasts (c) are mononuclear and have a pale staining cytoplasm

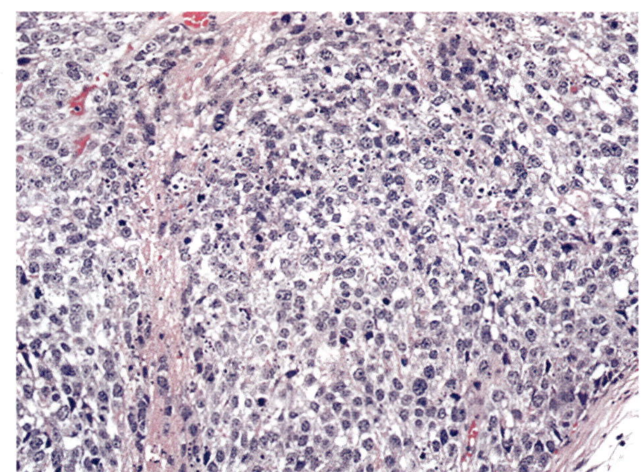

Embryonal cell ca: Characterized by large highly pleomorphic tumor cells

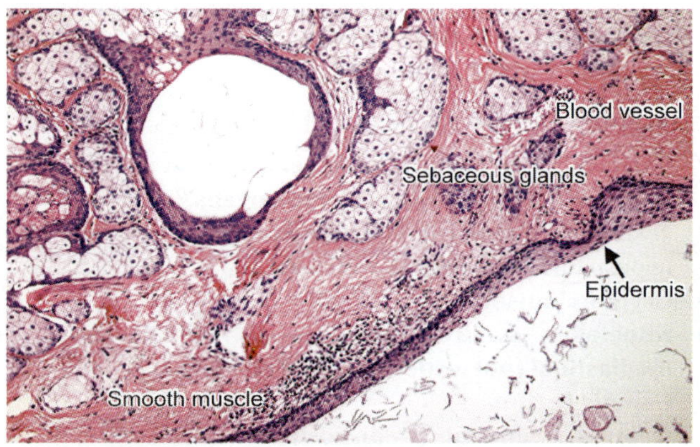

Teratoma: with >1 germ layers

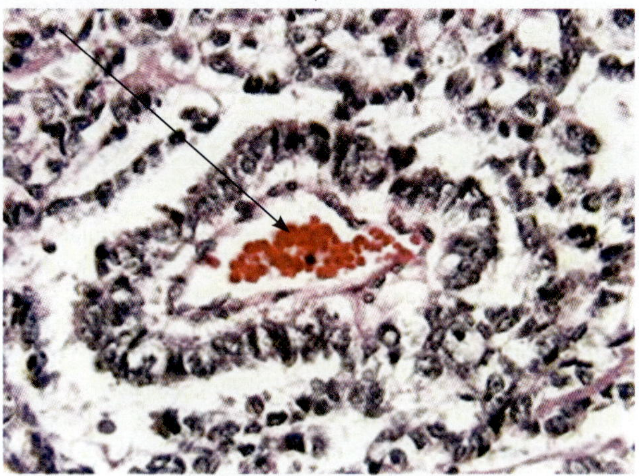

Mic: Shows Schiller-Duval body S/o YST

Yolk sac tumor (YST) or endodermal sinus tumor

- **Most common testicular tumor in infants and children up to 3 years of age.**[Q]
- **Schiller-Duval bodies or glomeruloid structures** (resembling endodermal sinuses).[Q]
- These have **excellent prognosis.**[Q]
- **Tumor marker–AFP**[Q]

- *YST*- **Most common testicular tumor in infants and children up to 3 years of age.**
- **Mixed Tumors:** About 60% of testicular tumors are composed of more than one of the "pure" patterns
- **Common mixtures include:** Teratoma, embryonal carcinoma, and yolk sac tumor
- **Teratocarcinoma**- embryonal carcinoma with teratoma.
- **Teratoma with malignant transformation**- malignant non–germ cell tumors arising in teratomas, like Squamous/cell carcinoma
- Secondary tumors are **chemoresistant**[Q]

Tumors of Sex Cord-Gonadal Stroma

Sertoli cell tumors: Androblastoma[Q]	Leydig cell tumors	Leydig cell tumor
• **Hormonally silent**[Q] • Present as a **testicular mass most commonly.**[Q] • Most are **benign**	• **Elaborate hormones**: androgens or androgens and estrogens • Most common presentation **is testicular swelling**[Q]. • Gynecomastia may be the **first symptom**[Q] • Cytoplasm: **Lipid droplets, vacuoles, or lipofuscin pigment** • Characteristic: **rod-shaped crystalloids of Reinke**[Q] • Most are **benign**[Q]	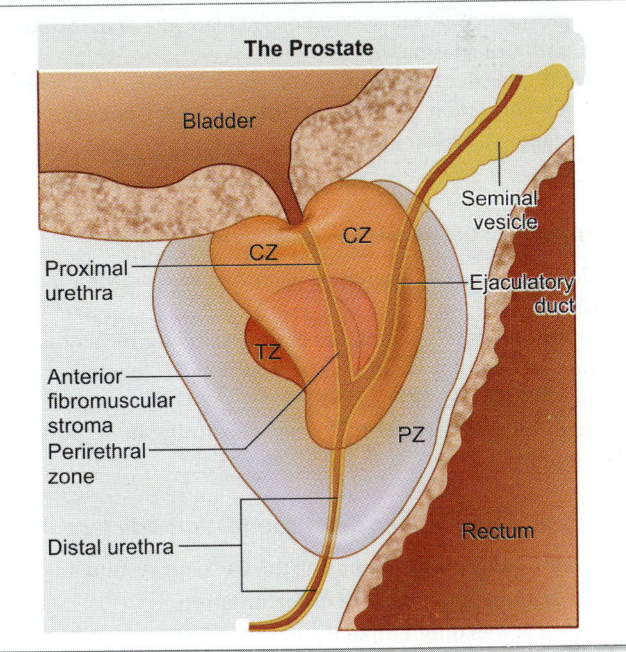Image showing crystals of Reinke

Gonadoblastoma

- Contains a **mixture of germ cells and gonadal stromal elements.**
- Almost always arise in gonads with **some form of testicular dysgenesis**
- **Hallmark oncogene:** TSPY gene

Testicular Lymphoma

- **Most common testicular neoplasms in men over the age of 60 years.**[Q]
- **Diffuse large B-cell lymphoma > Burkitt lymphoma > EBV-positive extranodal NK/T cell lymphoma**[Q]
- Prognosis is **extremely poor**; have a higher propensity for **central nervous system involvement**[Q]

High Yield Facts

- **Varicocele** results from **dilatation of testicular veins in pampiniform plexus.**[Q] **(left > right side)**
- **Varicocele** is associated with oligospermia (<20 million spermatozoa/mL of semen) and **is cause of infertility.**[Q]
- **Spermatocele is c**ystic enlargement of **efferent ducts or rete testis**[Q] with numerous spermatocytes present
- Most common **benign** paratesticular tumor is **adenomatoid tumor.**[Q]
- Most common **malignant** paratesticular tumors are **rhabdomyosarcomas in children**[Q]
- Most common **malignant** paratesticular tumors are **liposarcomas in adults.**[Q]

PROSTATE

- Prostate is a **combined tubuloalveolar organ,**[Q] weighing about 20 g in a normal adult;
- **Benign glands are two layered (basal cells and columnar cells), while in cancer single layered cells seen**[Q]

Nodular Hyperplasia—Benign Prostatic Hyperplasia (BPH)

- **The most common benign prostatic disease** in men older than age 50 years.
- It **mostly** originates from **transitional zone of prostate (carcinoma mostly arises from peripheral zone).**[Q]
- **Nodular hyperplasia is not considered to be a premalignant lesion.**[Q]
- **Median lobe hypertrophy**—nodular enlargement may project up into **floor of urethra as a hemispherical mass.**[Q]

- The **main androgen** in the prostate, is **dihydrotestosterone (DHT).**
- **5α-reductase** converts testosterone into the more potent **dihydrotestosterone**
- Both glands and stroma can become hyperplastic. Stromal or epithelial predominant hyperplasia may occur.
- Medium or large glands with 2 benign cell layers (secretory and basal) showing some architectural complexity including papillary infoldings.

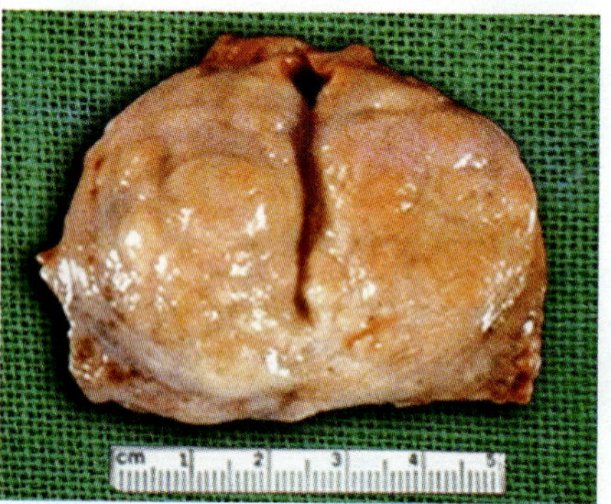

Gross showing nodular hyperplasia

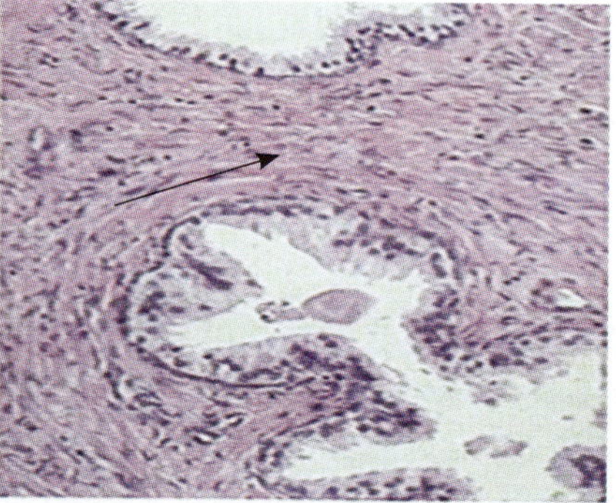

Microscopy showing normal gland stroma

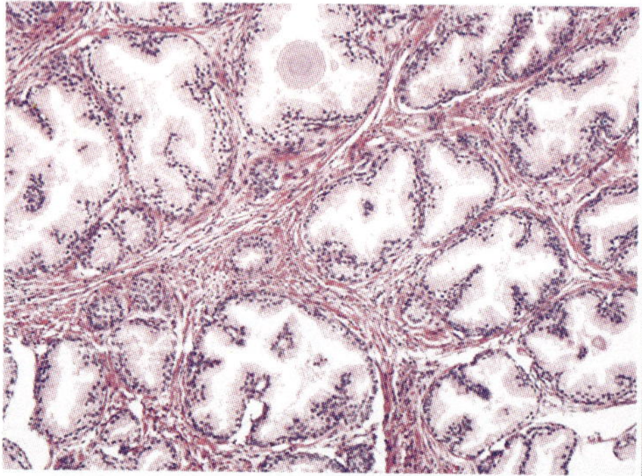

Microscopy showing glands (All are lined by two layer of cells) and stroma S/O BPH

High Yield Facts

- Chronic abacterial prostatitis is the **most common form** of prostatitis.[R9th] MC association is **Chlamydia or associated with Ureaplasma** [R9th]
- MC cause of Granulomatous prostatitis is intravesical administration of BCG (used for treatment of superficial bladder carcinoma).

Tumors of Prostate

- **Adenocarcinoma of prostate** *is most common form of cancer in men.*[Q]
- Most of the prostatic carcinomas are **acinar adenocarcinoma**[Q]
- Characterized by small glands that appear **"back to back"** without intervening stroma
- Most arise in peripheral zone, **classically in a posterior location.**[Q]

Grade and Stage are the Best Prognostic Predictors

- Prostate cancer is **graded** using the **Gleason system**
- **Five grades** on the **basis of differentiation.**[Q]
- Grade I is well differentiated and Grade 5 shows no glandular differentiation. Grade 2, 3 and 4 are in-between.

- **Primary grade is assigned to dominant pattern** and secondary grade to sub-dominant pattern.
- Combined Gleason score is derived by addition of these two grades
- **Staging of prostatic cancer is also important in the selection of the appropriate form of therapy**[Q]

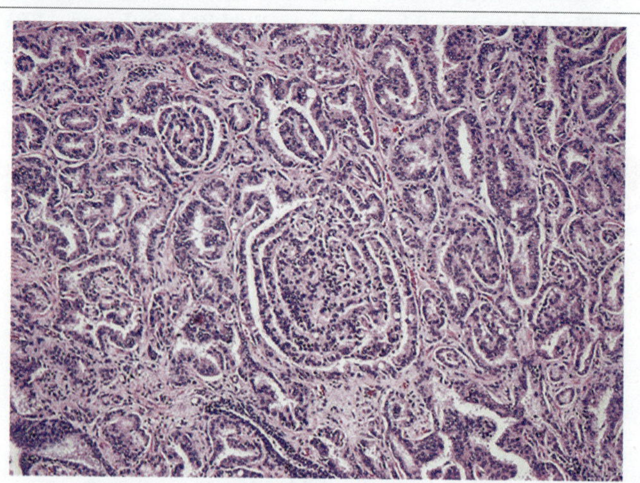

Characteristic morphologic features of prostatic adenocarcinoma (10x)

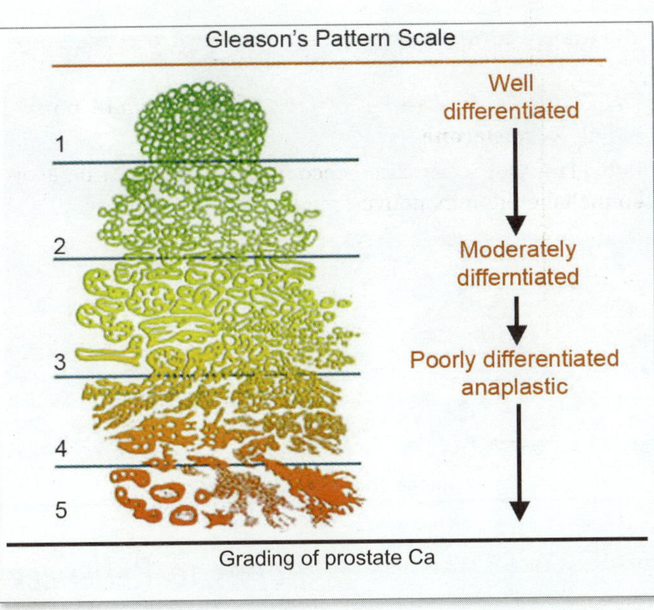

High Yield Facts

Prostatic Cancer
- Local extension **most commonly** involves periprostatic tissue, seminal vesicles, and the base of the urinary bladder
- **Fascia of Denonvilliers** prevents the backward extension of the tumor.[Q]
- Metastases spread via **lymphatics** to the obturator nodes[Q] and eventually to the para-aortic nodes.
- **Hematogenous spread** occurs chiefly to **bones (osteoblastic secondaries) most commonly to lumbar spine**
- **Most common epigenetic alteration** in prostate cancer is hypermethylation of the **glutathione S-transferase (GSTP1) gene**, which down-regulates GSTP1 expression[Q]

Genes that increase risk in prostatic carcinoma
- Germline mutations BRCA2: 20-fold increased risk
- Germline mutation in **HOXB13**: Homeobox gene that regulates prostatic development

FEMALE GENITAL TRACT

INFECTIONS OF FEMALE GENITAL TRACT

- *Neisseria gonorrhoeae* and *Chlamydia* **infections, are major causes of female infertility**[Q]
- *Trichomonas vaginalis*- **strawberry cervix.**[Q]
- *Gardnerella vaginalis*-**bacterial vaginosis**[Q]**: Causes green-gray, malodorous (fishy) vaginal discharge**[Q], Premature Labor

VULVA

Non-neoplastic Epithelial Disorders: Leukoplakia

Definition: White plaques on the vulva are **clinically** referred to as leukoplakia. It can be caused by:
- Inflammatory dermatoses (e.g., psoriasis, chronic dermatitis)
- Lichen sclerosus and squamous cell hyperplasia
- Neoplasias, such as vulvar intraepithelial neoplasia (VIN), Paget disease, and invasive carcinoma

Cysts of Vulva

Benign Exophytic Lesions

- **Fibroepithelial polyps, or skin tags**[Q]
- **Squamous papillomas**[Q]

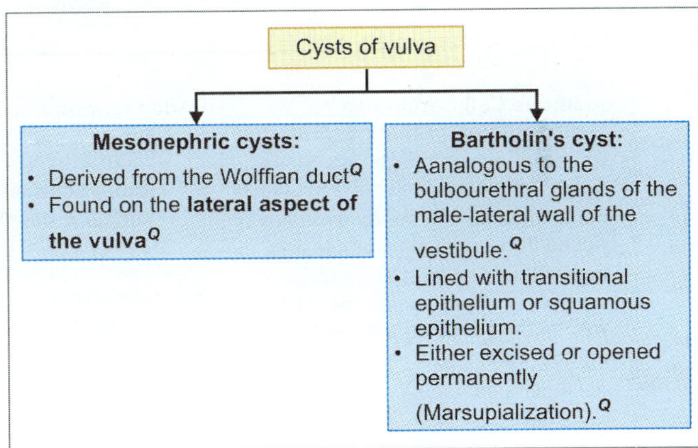

Squamous Neoplastic Lesions

Vulvar Squamous Cell Carcinomas are Divided into Two Groups

	Basaloid & Warty Carcinomas	Keratinizing Squamous Cell Carcinomas
Epidemiology	Less common[Q]	More common[Q]
Age affected	Younger ages[Q]	Older women[Q]
HPV association	High risk HPVs (type 16)[Q]	Unrelated to HPV (70% of cases)[Q]
Precursor lesions	Classic VIN (vulvar intraepithelial Neoplasia)	Long-standing lichen Sclerosis/ squamous cell hyperplasia[Q] Differentiated VIN or VIN simplex.[Q]

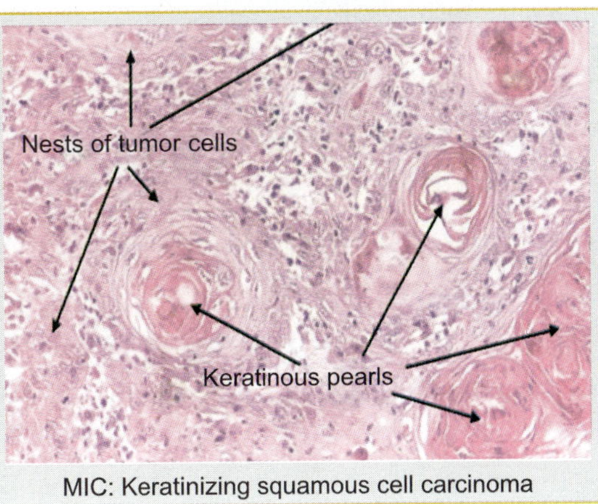

MIC: Keratinizing squamous cell carcinoma

Glandular Neoplastic Lesions

Papillary Hidradenoma

- Tubular ducts lined by a **layer of nonciliated columnar cells**[Q] with a layer of flattened "**myoepithelial cells**" underlying the epithelium

Extramammary Paget's Disease

- **Involved**: Epidermal apocrine gland-bearing areas, esp. **vulva, scrotum & perianal areas**
- **Gross:** Pruritic, erythematous, crusted, dry raised lesions
- **Microscopy:** Single or small clusters of large cells; Faintly basophilic or **vacuolated cells (Paget's cells),** Large nuclei and prominent nucleoli, Amorphous, granular cytoplasm
- **Stains used:** Stain positively with **PAS or mucicarmine stains.**[Q]
- **Immunohistochemistry:** CEA, S100, Melan-A, CAM 5.2, EMA, CK 7, GCDFP-15[Q]
- **D/D:** Malignant melanoma (malignant cells **melanin stain or S100** immunoperoxidase stain)

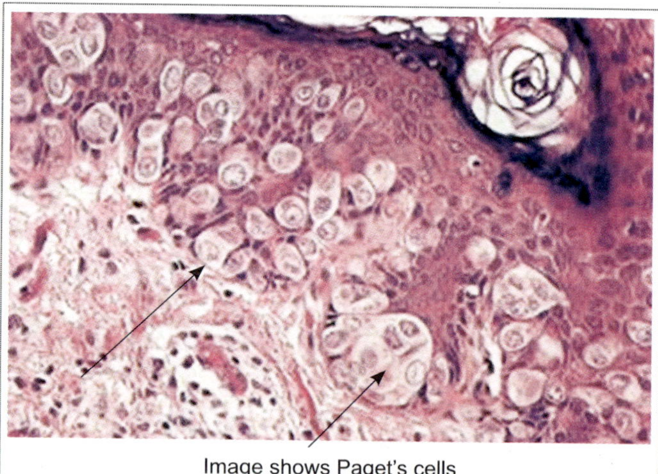

Image shows Paget's cells

- **Extramammary Paget's disease** is usually seen in **isolation** & associated with an underlying malignancy in **12%**[Q]
- **Mammary Paget's disease** is **almost always** associated with an underlying malignancy of the breast

VAGINA

Malignancies of Vagina		
Squamous Cell Carcinoma • **Most common primary carcinomas** • **Association with high risk HPVs**[Q] • The greatest risk factor is a **previous carcinoma of the cervix or vulva**[Q] • Arises from a premalignant lesion, **vaginal intraepithelial neoplasia**[Q] • Located in upper vagina (**posterior wall at the junction with the ectocervix**)[Q]	**Adenocarcinoma** • Rare • DES (**diethylstilbestrol**) causes **vaginal adenosis**[Q] and **clear cell** adenoca in daughters who were exposed in utero. • Located on the **anterior wall of the vagina,** usually in the **upper third.**[Q] • **Clear cell carcinoma**-composed of vacuolated, **glycogen-containing cells**[Q]	**Embryonalrhabdomyosarcoma or (sarcoma botryoides) ERMS** • Infants and children 5 years. • **Gross-grape like clusters** • **Microscopically** • **Tennis racket cells**-the tumor cells are small with small protrusions of cytoplasm from one end • **Cambium layer**-tumor cells are crowded beneath the vaginal epithelium

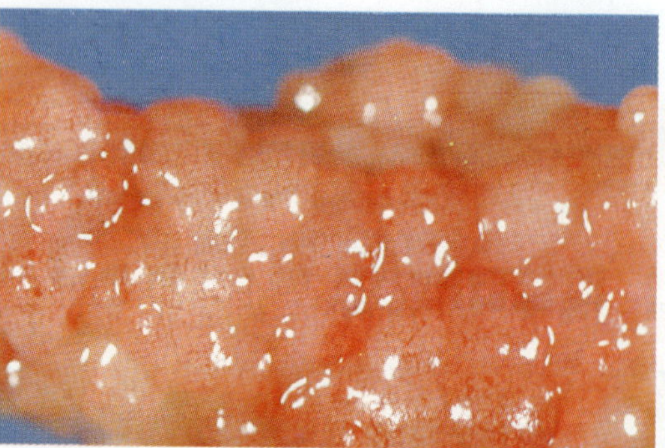

Gross: Grape like clusters S/O ERMS

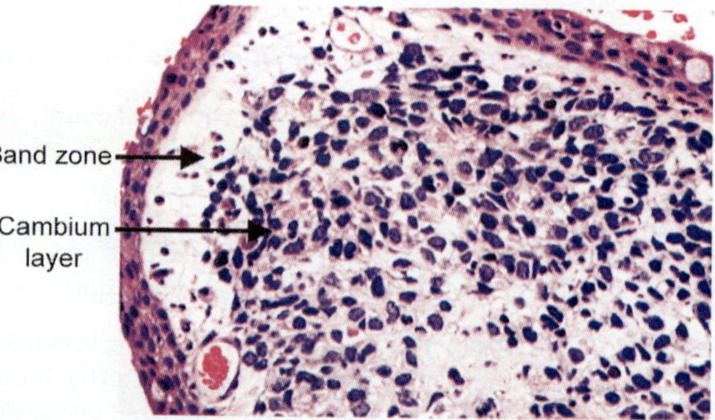

Mic: shows cambuim layer S/O ERMS

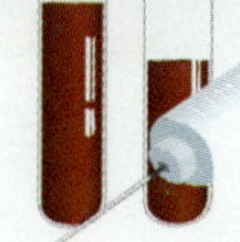

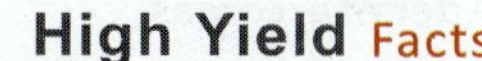

High Yield Facts

- **Gartner duct cysts** derived from **Wolffian (mesonephric) duct nests,** are found along **lateral walls of vagina**[Q]
- HSVs cause painful genital ulcerations[Q]
- HPVs are involved in the pathogenesis of cervical, vaginal, and vulvar cancers.[Q]
- Squamous cell carcinoma is the most common histologic type of vulvar cancer[Q]
- Most common malignant tumor to involve the vagina is carcinoma spreading from the cervix[Q]
- **Most common** primary **malignant tumor of vagina-squamous cell carcinoma**
- **Most common vaginal malignancy in infants: embryonal rhabdomyosarcoma (sarcoma botryoides).**[Q]
- Lesions in the lower **2/3ʳᵈ of the vagina metastasize** to the **inguinal nodes**[Q]
- Lesions in the **upper vagina** tend to spread to **regional iliac nodes**[Q]
- **Vaginal adenosis** is presence of metaplastic cervical or endometrial epithelium within the vaginal wall, derived **from persistent Müllerian epithelium islets in postembryonic life.**[Q]
- **Benign tumors** of the vagina include **stromal tumors (stromal polyps), leiomyomas, and hemangiomas**

CERVIX

Intraepithelial and Invasive Squamous Neoplasia

- CIN can be divided into three grades; CIN I, CIN II and CIN III

Cervical Dysplasia	CIN	Besthesda system	HPV type	Morphology
Mild	CIN I	Low grade SIL (L-SIL)	6,11	Koilocytic atypia, flat condyloma
Moderate, severe, carcinoma in situ	CIN II & CIN III	High grade SIL (H-SIL)	16,18	Progressive cellular atypia, loss of maturation

- Most common cancer subtype in cervix is squamous cell carcinoma (80% cases) > Adenocarcinoma (15%)

POINTS TO REMEMBER

Natural history of squamous intraepithelial lesions with approximate 2-year follow-up			
Lesion	Regress	Persist	Progress
LSIL	60[Q]	30	10 % to HSIL
HSIL	30	60[Q]	10% TO CARCINOMA

High Yield Facts

- **Koilocytic atypia** -The nuclear changes of LSIL, often accompanied by **cytoplasmic "halos."** These "halos" consist of perinuclear vacuoles, a cytopathic change created by **HPV-encoded protein called E5**[Q] that localizes to the membranes of the **endoplasmic reticulum.**[Q]
- Diagnosis of SIL is based on identification of **nuclear atypia**.
- **HPVs infect immature basal cells of the squamous** epithelium in areas of epithelial breaks**, or immature metaplastic squamous cells** present at the squamocolumnar junction[Q]
- **The ability of HPV** to act as a carcinogen depends on the viral proteins **E6 and E7**
- **High risk HPV types for cervical carcinoma:** 16, 18, 31, 33, 35, 39, 45, 51, 52, 56, 58, 59, 68 and others
- **Low risk HPV types for cervical carcinoma**: 6, 11, 42, 44 (associated with condyloma)
- **Nabothian cysts:** Obstruction of *mucous gland* ducts *in endocervix* results in small mucous (Nabothian) cysts.

UTERUS

- Endometrium and myometrium are relatively resistant to infections.

Endometrial Hyperplasia

- Increase in the number of glands relative to the stroma.
- It is divided into non-atypical and atypical hyperplasia based on nuclear atypia.[Q]
- Atypical hyperplasia is associated with an increased risk of endometrial carcinoma.[Q]

Malignant Tumors of Endometrium & Myometrium

Tumors of Endometrium

- Endometrial carcinoma is the most common invasive cancer of the female genital tract.
- Most of the endometrial carcinomas are **adenocarcinomas.**
- If there are areas of **benign** squamous differentiation within Endometrial Ca, they are called **adenoacanthomas.**

- If there are areas of **malignant** squamous differentiation, they are called **adenosquamous Endometrial Ca**
- **Endometrial carcinoma are divided into type 1 and type 2 tumors** *R9ᵗʰ*
- All tumors in type II endometrial tumors category are classified **as grade 3 irrespective of histologic pattern**

	Type 1	Type 2
Morphology	Endometrioid	Serous, Mixed Mullerian Tumor, Clear Cell
Genes	**PTEN** & (Most common), KRAS, FGF2	P 53, Aneuploidy
Prognosis	Indolent	Aggressive

Tumors of the Endometrium with Stromal Differentiation

Malignant Mixed Müllerian Tumors (Carcinosarcomas)

- Endometrial adenocarcinomas with a malignant mesenchymal component

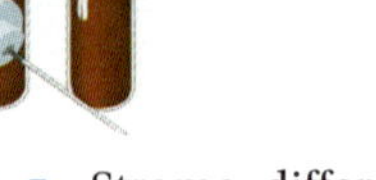

- Stroma differentiates into malignant mesodermal components, including muscle, cartilage
- Resemble endometrial Ca genetically & have **poor outcomes** with current therapies.

Adenosarcomas

Malignant appearing stroma, with **benign but abnormally shaped endometrial glands**.

Stromal Tumors

May be benign stromal nodules or endometrial stromal sarcomas.

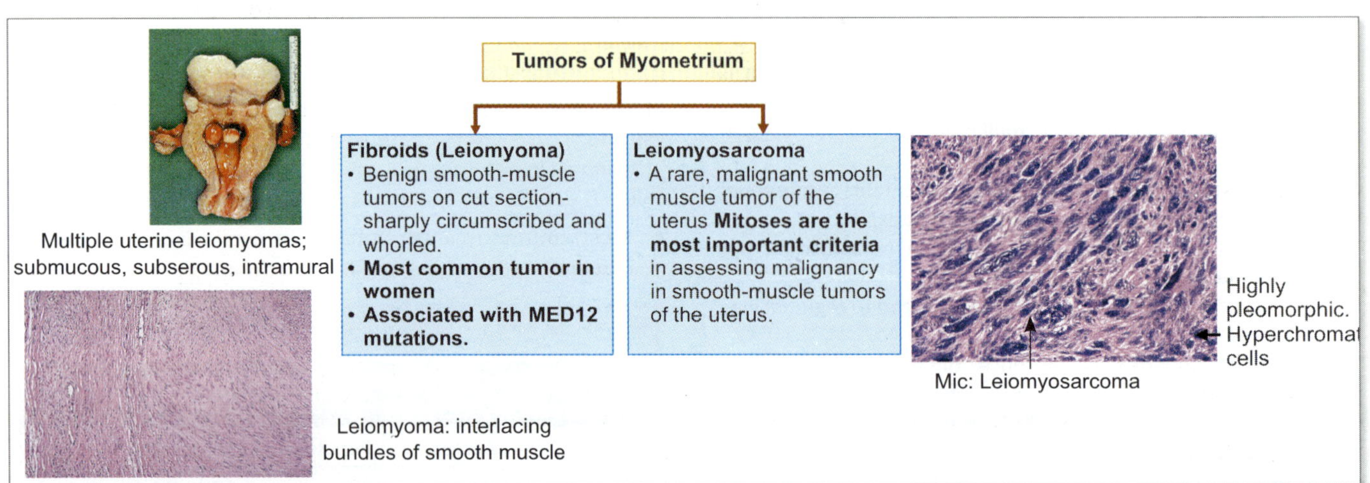

FALLOPIAN TUBES

- **Most common disorders infections followed by ectopic (tubal) pregnancy and endometriosis.**
- **Suppurative salpingitis Gonococcus–Most common (>most common primary lesion sparatubal cysts[Q]**
- **Hydatids of Morgagni paratubal cysts[QQ]**
- **Adenomatoid tumors[Q]**
- Primary adenocarcinoma of the fallopian tubes is rare and is usually **serous papillary type[Q]**

OVARIES

Cysts

- **Follicular cysts:** These are benign cysts of the ovary.
- **Chocolate cysts:** These refer to cystic areas of endometriosis that include hemorrhages and blood clots.
- Polycystic ovarian disease (PCOD)

Polycystic Ovarian Disease (Stein-Leventhal Syndrome)

Characterized by	Endocrine abnormalities	Abnormalities in ovary
• Hyperandrogenism • Menstrual abnormalities • Polycystic ovaries • Chronic anovulation • Decreased fertility[Q]	• **Excess androgens (androstenedione)Q** • **Increased estrogen levels[Q]** • Increased LH & decreased FSH levels • **High LH/FSH ratio** • Increased GnRH levels	• Enlarged with thick capsules • Hyperplastic ovarian stroma • Numerous follicular cysts lined by a hyperplastic theca interna.

Ovarian Tumors

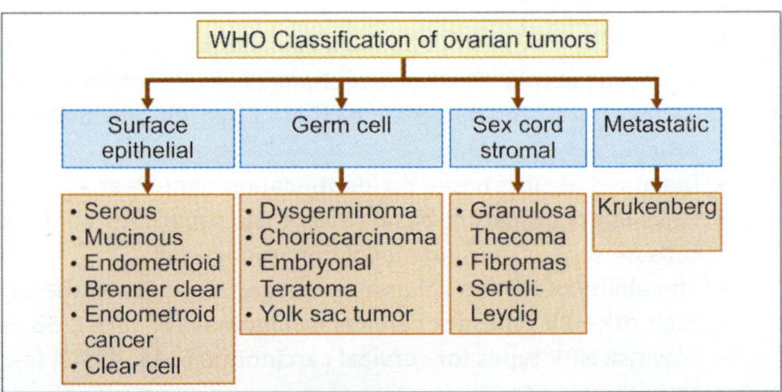

Surface Epithelial Tumors

- Derived from the surface coelomic epithelium, which embryonically gives rise to the Mullerian epithelium.
- Epithelial ovarian tumors are classified into benign, borderline or malignant
- Benign tumors are composed of **well-differentiated epithelial cells with minimal proliferation.[Q]**
- Borderline tumors show increased cell proliferation, but **lack stromal invasion.[Q]**
- Malignant tumors show increased epithelial atypia and are defined by the **presence of stromal invasion.[Q]**
- About 80% of all ovarian epithelial tumors are benign and occur in young women[Q]

Serous Ovarian Tumors

- **Associated Mutation BRCA1 and BRCA2, p53–High grade, KRAS, BRAF-low grade**
  - Most common malignant ovarian tumors; account for approximately 40% of all cancers of ovary

- ○ Composed of ciliated columnar serous epithelial cells, similar to **the lining cells of the fallopian tubes.**[Q]
- ○ They commonly involve the **surface of ovary, bilaterally**
- ○ **Concentric calcifications (psammoma bodies) seen**

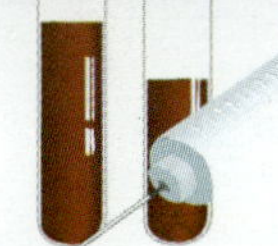

Serous Tumor

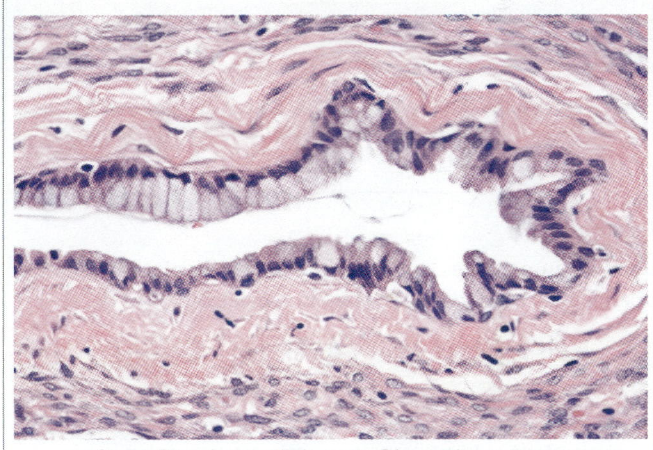

Multilocular serous cystadenoma with smooth inner surface with only solitary papillae

Microscopy showing multiple papillae

Microscopy Showing Psammoma body

Mucinous Ovarian Tumors

- **KRAS Consistent → mutation associated**
  - ○ Account for 20% to 25% of all ovarian neoplasms; **Most common- gastric or intestinal type differentiation**.
  - ○ Grossly unilateral, **more cysts and no surface involvement.**
  - ○ Tend to **produce larger cystic masses**
  - ○ **Mutation of the KRAS proto-oncogene is a consistently seen in mucinous tumors of ovary** ℛ9ᵗʰ

Brenner Tumor (Transitional Cell)

- 10% of ovarian tumors
- Unilateral
- Benign
- Contain Neoplastic epithelial cells resembling urothelium

Gross Showing multiple cysts S/o mucinous tumor

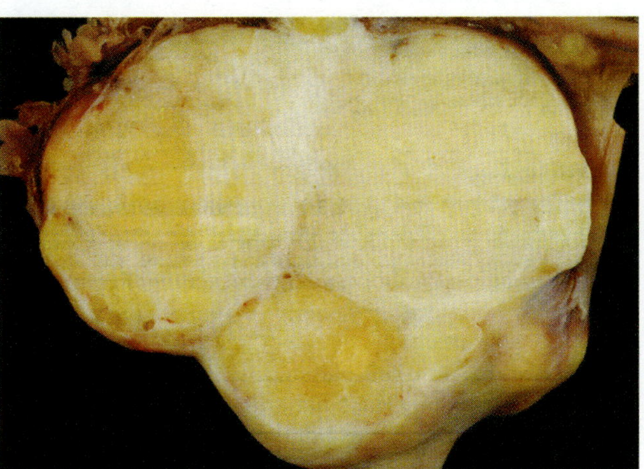

Gross: Solid yellow white tumor S/o Brenners tumor

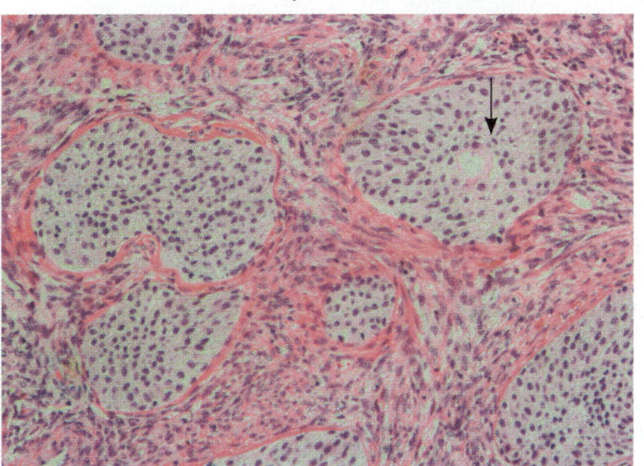

Nests of transistional epithelium in between stroma

Brenners tumor

Endometrioid Ovarian Tumors

- **20% endometriosis**
- 10% to 15% of all ovarian cancers;[Q] 15% to 20% of cases coexist with endometriosis[Q]
- Distinguished by the presence of tubular glands resembling benign or malignant endometrium.[Q]
- Molecular studies-striking similarities to endometrial endometrioid carcinoma; PI3K/AKT pathway signaling and mutations in mismatch **DNA repair genes** and **CTNNB1 (β-catenin).**[Q]

Germ Cell Tumors

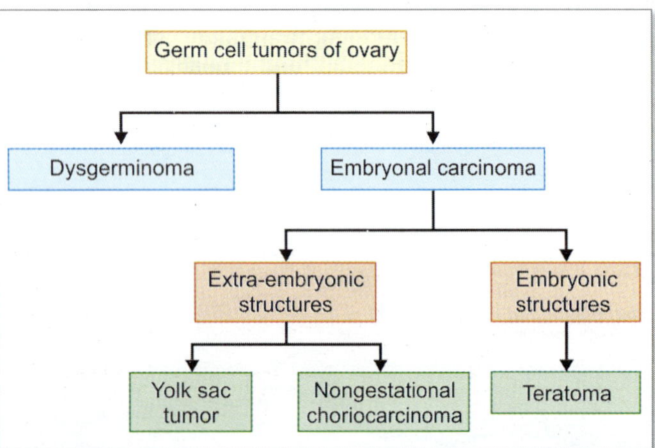

Teratomas

Divided into three categories: mature (benign), immature (malignant), monodermal or highly specialized

Mature (Benign) Teratomas	Immature Malignant Teratomas
• Most benign teratomas are **cystic (dermoid cysts)** • Arise from ectodermal differentiation of totipotential cells.[Q] • Arise from an ovum **after the first meiotic division**[Q] **Morphology:** • Unilocular cysts[Q] containing hair & cheesy sebaceous material with **tooth structures & areas of calcification.**[Q] • **Rokitansky protuberance**[Q] -The inner lining of cyst contains white shiny masses projecting from the wall toward the center of the cysts. Hair, other dermal appendages, bone and teeth are present, they usually arise from this protuberance	• Resembles **fetus or embryo tissues** rather than adult. • Seen chiefly in **prepubertal adolescents & young women**, the mean age being 18 years. • Microscopy: Immature neuroepithelium & cartilage; • Risk of extraovarian spread is dependent on **histologic grade of tumor** • Most recurrences **develop in the first 2 years**

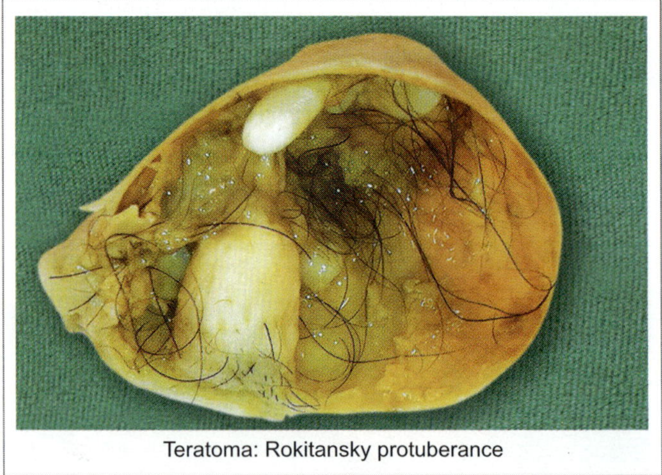

Teratoma: Rokitansky protuberance

Dysgerminoma

Characteristics: Ovarian counterpart of the **seminoma** of the testis; usually **unilateral** (80% to 90%) and **solid**

Genetics: Express **OCT-3, OCT4, and NANOG.** Onethird have activating mutations in the **KIT gene**

Morphology: Sheets or cords of cells separated by scant fibrous stroma, infiltrated with mature **lymphocytes**[Q] & occasional granulomas

Hormones elaborated: Most of these tumors have **no endocrine function (few produced hCG)**

- Tumor marker- **LDH, PLAP**
- All dysgerminomas are **malignant**

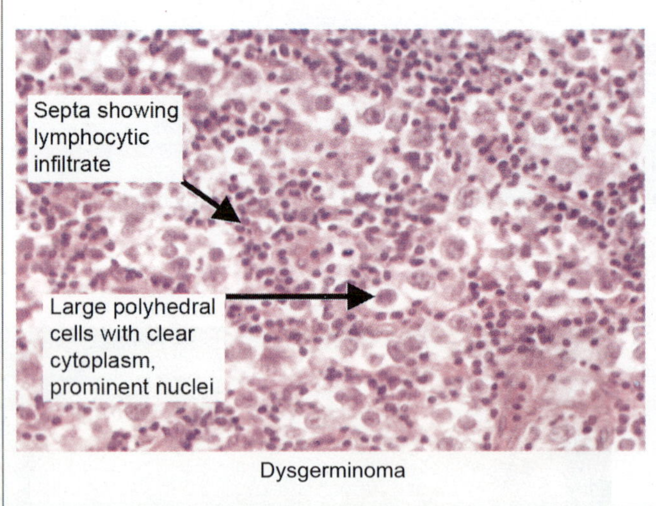

Dysgerminoma

Endodermal Sinus (Yolk Sac) Tumor

- **Second most common malignant tumor** of germ cell origin; usually **unilateral**
- Derived from differentiation of malignant germ cells **toward extraembryonic yolk sac structure.**
- Histology - Glomerulus-like structure composed of a central blood vessel enveloped by germ cells within a space lined by germ cells (**Schiller-Duval body**).

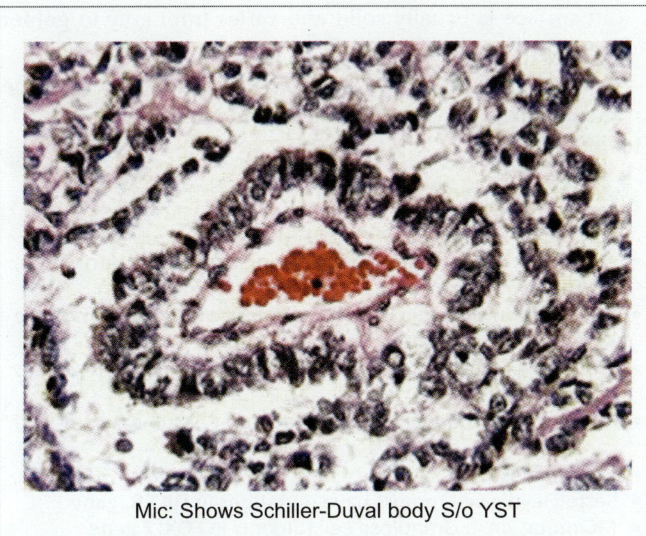

Mic: Shows Schiller-Duval body S/o YST

- Intracellular and extracellular **hyaline droplets** - **composed of a-fetoprotein and a1-antitrypsin.**
- Tumor Marker- **AFP**

Choriocarcinoma

- Most common of **placental origin**, is e.g. of **extra-embryonic differentiation of malignant germ cells.**
- Pure **ovarian** choriocarcinomas are rare – exist in combination with other germ cell tumors
- Elaborate high levels of **chorionic gonadotropins**[Q]
- Most common site of metastasis - **lung.**[Q]

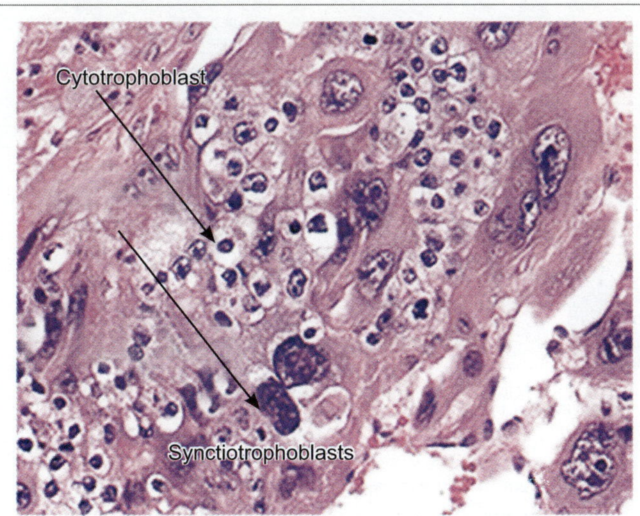

Mic: Admixed synctiotrophoblasts & cytotrophoblasts S/O Choriocarcinoma

Sex-Cord Stromal Tumors

Granulosa Cell Tumor

- **Most common** malignant tumor in this category;[Q] usually **unilateral** (80% to 90%) and solid cystic

- Hormonally active tumors have a **yellow coloration** due to intracellular lipids.
- Composed of cells that *stain positively with inhibin.*[Q]

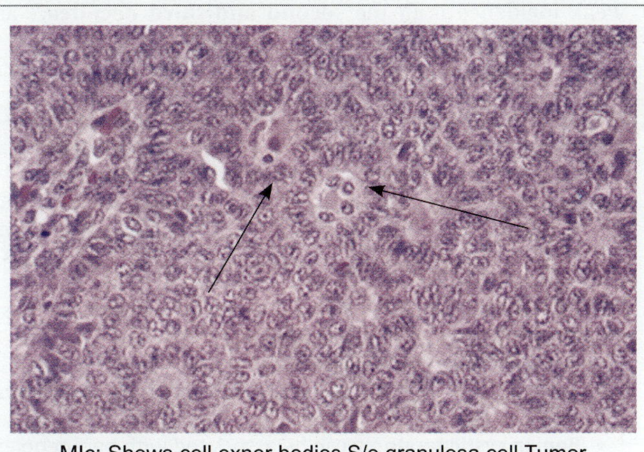

Mic: Shows cell exner bodies S/o granulosa cell Tumor

- Cells have coffee bean nuclei with grooves
- **Call Exner bodies**[Q] (small follicle like structure with eosinophilic material) are characteristic features
- **Clinical features depend upon the estrogenic activity of the tumor**[Q]
- Behavior of the **endometrium closely resembles that of metropathia hemorrhagica**[Q]
- Tumor cells may secrete estrogens → **precocious sexual development in girls/ ↑endometrial hyperplasia & Ca**
- Less commonly granulosa cell tumors **can secrete androgens** and produce masculinization.
- **Metastases 1st involve opposite ovary**[Q] followed by lumbar region, mesentery, liver and mediastinum.
- Tumor marker-Inhibin
- **FOXL2 gene** mutation (97% cases of Adult granulosa cell tumor)

High Yield Facts

Findings	Tumors
Call exner bodies	Granulosa cell tumor[Q]
Reinke's crystal[Q]	Hilus cell tumor/Leyding cell tumor
Signet ring cell[Q]	Krukenberg tumor
Hobnail cells	Clear cell carcinoma
Psammoma bodies	Papillary serous cystadenoma of ovary
Schiller duval body	Endodermal sinus (Yolk sac) tumour

Thecomas

- Are composed of **spindle-shaped cells with vacuolated cytoplasm.**
- Vacuolated because of *steroid hormone (estrogen) production,* which can be stained with an **Oil Red O stain.**

Sertoli-Leydig Tumors (Androblastomas)

- **Functional**[Q] tumors, which commonly produce **masculinization** due to secretion of androgens
- Peak incidence is in the **second and third decades;**[Q] are usually **unilateral;**[Q]

- Cut surface is usually solid and varies from gray to **golden brown**[Q] in appearance
- **Heterologous elements, such as mucinous glands, bone, and cartilage, may be present in some tumors**[Q]

High Yield Facts

- Patients with PCOD have risk of endometrial hyperplasia carcinoma due to *excess estrogen production*
- **Pseudomyxoma peritonei** results from spread of **mucinous tumor in appendix** & is marked by mucinous ascites, cystic epithelial implants on peritoneal surfaces, adhesions & frequent involvement of ovaries[Q]
- In contrast to choriocarcinomas arising in placental tissue, those arising in the ovary are generally unresponsive to chemotherapy and are often fatal.[Q]
- **Most common germ cell tumor in females is benign cystic teratoma**[Q]
- **Benign cystic teratoma** can be associated with paraneoplastic syndromes like **inflammatory limbic encephalitis.**

- About 1% of the dermoids undergo malignant transformation, **most commonly to squamous cell carcinoma**[Q]
- **Most common specialized/ monodermal teratoma** are struma ovarii and carcinoid
- Metastatic intestinal carcinoid **involving the ovaries is always bilateral.**[Q]
- **Stromal carcinoid is** a combination of struma ovarii and carcinoid in the same ovary.
- Gonadoblastoma have coexistent dysgerminoma in 50% cases
- Sertoli leydig cell tumors have mutations in **DICER, gene**
- MC mutation in Granulosa cell tumor is in **FOXL2 gene**

Metastatic Tumors of Ovary

- **Most common** occur from **tumors of Mullerian origin**: Uterus, fallopian tube, contralateral ovary, or pelvic peritoneum.
- **Most common extramullerian primaries are breast & GIT including colon, stomach, biliary tract, and pancreas.**[Q]

Krukenberg Tumor

- Refers to a **metastatic bilateral ovarian** malignancy whose primary site is **GIT or breast.**[Q]
- Composed of **mucin-producing, signet-ring cancer cells, most often of gastric origin.**[Q]
- Ca colon, appendix, breast (**especially invasive lobular carcinoma**), pancreas and gall bladder are other **primary sites.**

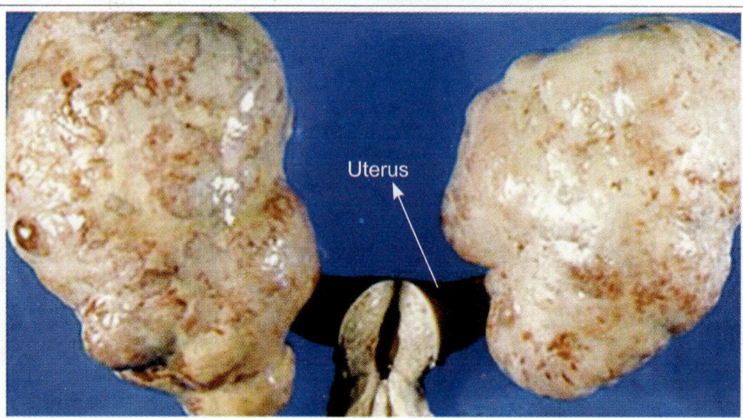

Gross B/L enlarged ovaries

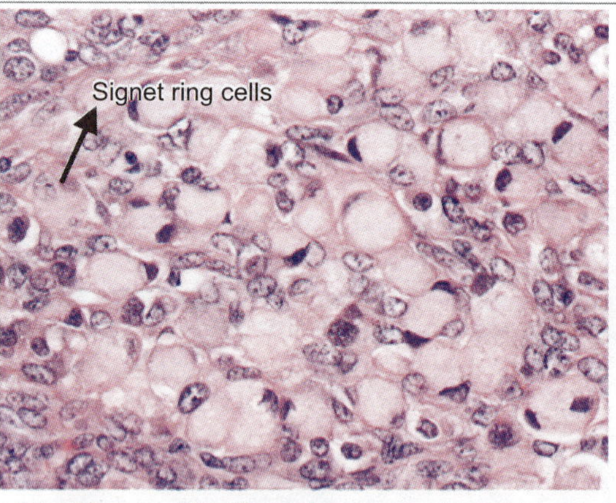

Mic: Shows cells with nucleus pushed to periphery S/O signet ring cell

IMPORTANT ADDITIONAL INFORMATION TO REMEMBER IN GENITAL SYSTEM

SEMEN ANALYSIS

In 2010 the World Health Organization (WHO) updated its reference values for the Semen Analysis

Cut-off reference values for semen characteristics as published in consecutive WHO manuals

The most common reasons for laboratory **semen analysis** in humans are

- As part of a couple's infertility investigation
- After a vasectomy to verify that the procedure was successful.
- Testing human donors for sperm donation,

Semen characteristics	WHO 2010
Volume (mL)	≥ 1.5
Sperm count (10^4/mL)	≥ 15
Total sperm count (10^6)	≥ 39
Total motility (%)	≥ 40
Progressive motility	≥ 32%
Vitality (%)	≥ 58
Morphology (%)	≥ 4
Leukocyte count (10^4/mL)	< 1.0

Prerequisites for Analysis

Liquefaction: Process when the gel formed by proteins from the seminal vesicles is broken up and the semen becomes more liquid. In the NICE guidelines, a liquefaction time < **60 minutes** -normal ranges. Semen analysis should be done **after liquefaction with through mixing**

Fructose Level

WHO specifies a normal level of 13 μmol per sample. Absence of fructose may indicate a problem with the seminal vesicles

Normal Values

PH

- Acidic ejaculate-one or both of the seminal vesicles are blocked.
- Basic ejaculate-infection

Motility

- **Grade a**: Sperm with progressive motility-swim fast in a straight line.
- **Grade b**: (non-linear motility): These also move forward but in a curved motion
- **Grade c**: These have **non-progressive motility**-they move their tails only.
- **Grade d**: These are immotile

Morphology

- A *motile sperm organelle morphology examination* (MSOME) is a particular morphologic investigation which increases light microscope's resolution 6000x times to assess sperm morphology

Vitality

- Number of live sperms is called viable
- A viable sperm will have intact cell membrane and won't take up **eosin Y dye**

Nomenclature Related to Sperm Quality

- *Aspermia:*
  - No semen (no or retrograde ejaculation)
- *Asthenozoospermia:*
  - Percentage of progressively motile (PR) spermatozoa **below** the lower reference limit
- *Azoospermia:*
  - **No spermatozoa** in the ejaculate
- *Cryptozoospermia:*
  - Spermatozoa absent from fresh preparation but **observed** in a **centrifuged** pellet
- *Necrozoospermia:*
  - Low percentage of live, and high percentage of immotile, spermatozoa in the ejaculate
- *Oligozoospermia:*
  - Total **number** (or concentration, depending on outcome reported) of spermatozoa below the lower reference limits

- *Teratozoospermia:*
  - Percentage of **morphologically normal** spermatozoa **below** the lower reference limit.

PAP SMEAR

Specimen Adequacy

Minimum Squamous Cellularity Criteria

- Conventional smear-8000 to 12000 well-preserved, well-visualised squamous cells.
- Liquid based prep-min 5000.

Endocervical Zone Component

- Atleast 10 well-preserved endocervical or squamous meta-plastic cells, singly or in clusters.

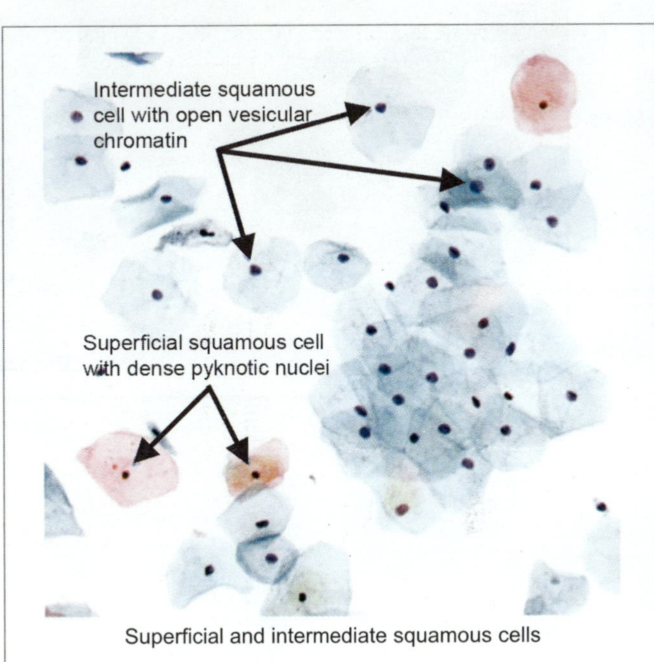

Superficial and intermediate squamous cells

Morphology

- Superficial cells display the most maturity, having been affected by estrogen
- Intermediate cells display mild maturation, having been affected by progesterone
- Parabasal cells are the least mature cells having not been affected by estrogen or progesterone
- **MATURATION INDEX (MI)** is a ratio obtained through performing a random count of three major cell types (parabasal cells, intermediate cells and superficial cells) that are shed from the squamous epithelium
- The cell count is expressed as a percentage that reads as follows:
- MI = % parabasal cells/% intermediate cells/% superficial cells.

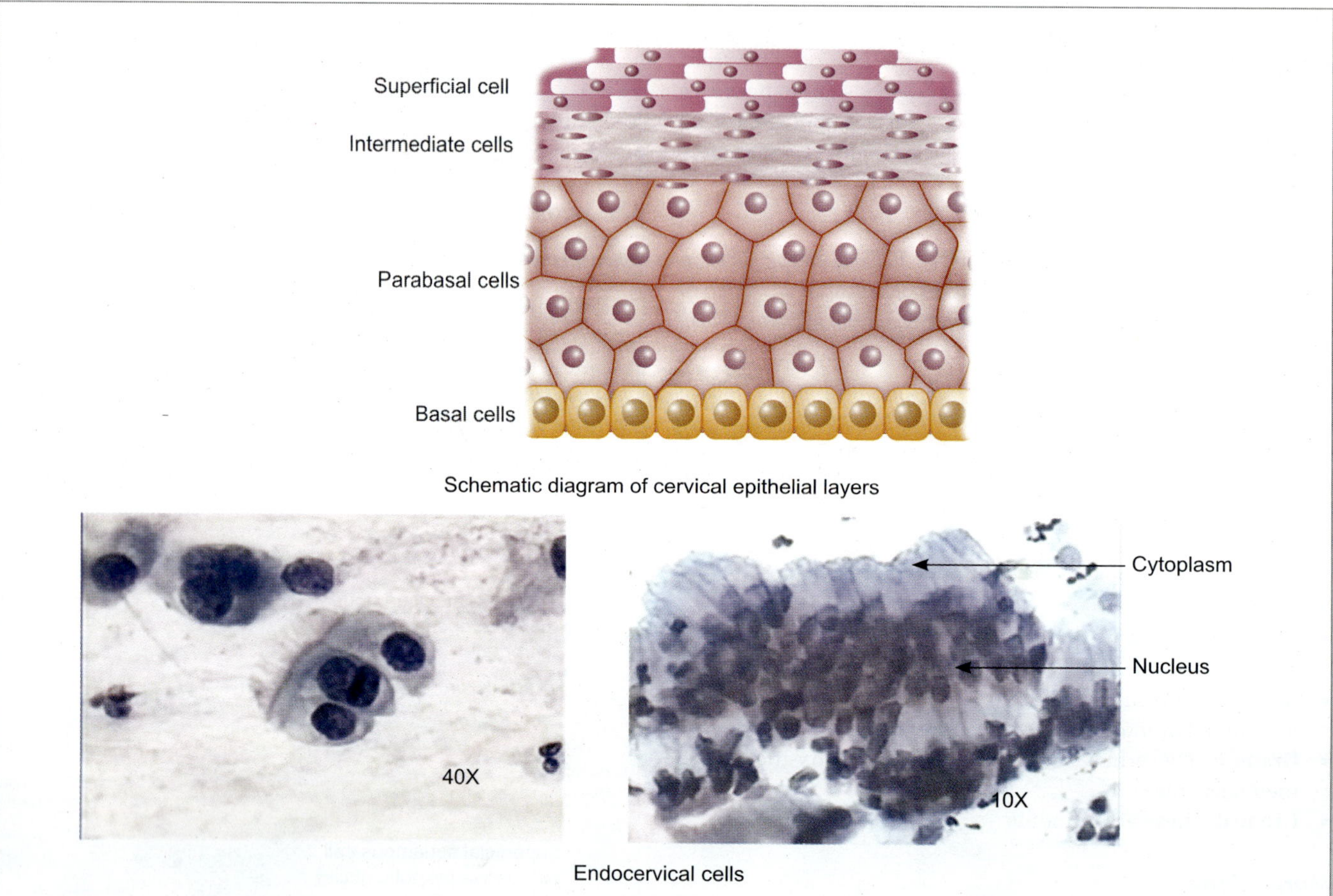

Schematic diagram of cervical epithelial layers

Endocervical cells

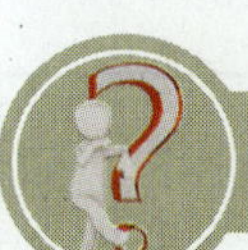

Few Images of Pap Smear

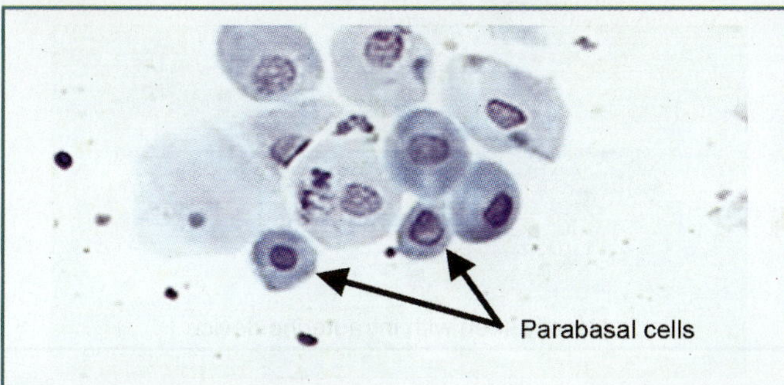

Bacterial Vaginosis

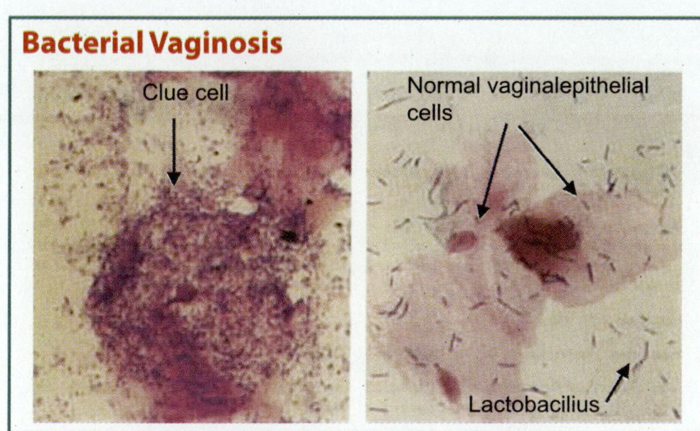

Squamous Cell Carcinoma, Pap

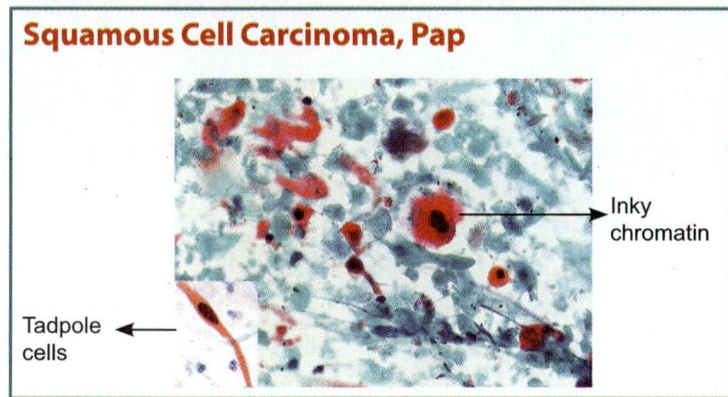

Herpes Simplex

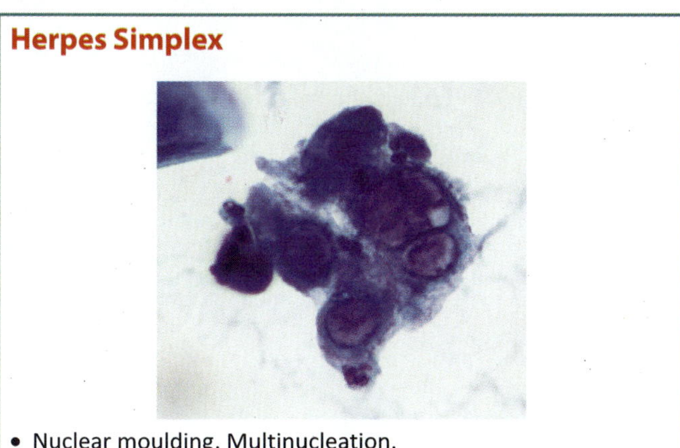

- Nuclear moulding, Multinucleation.
- Ground glass chromatin with prominent nuclear membrane

Human Papilloma Virus

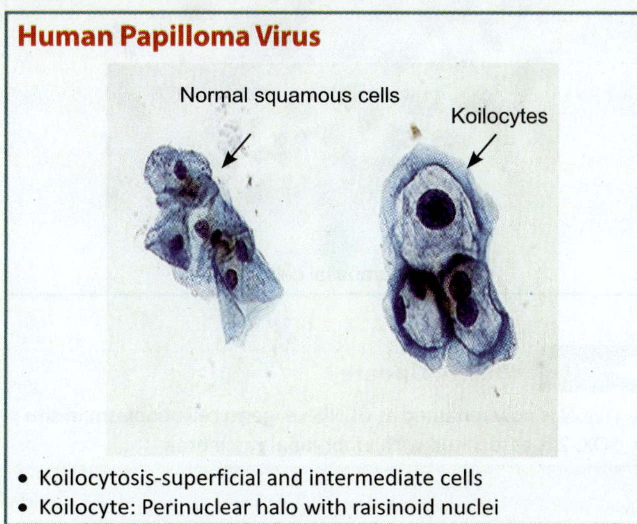

- Koilocytosis-superficial and intermediate cells
- Koilocyte: Perinuclear halo with raisinoid nuclei

Trichomonas

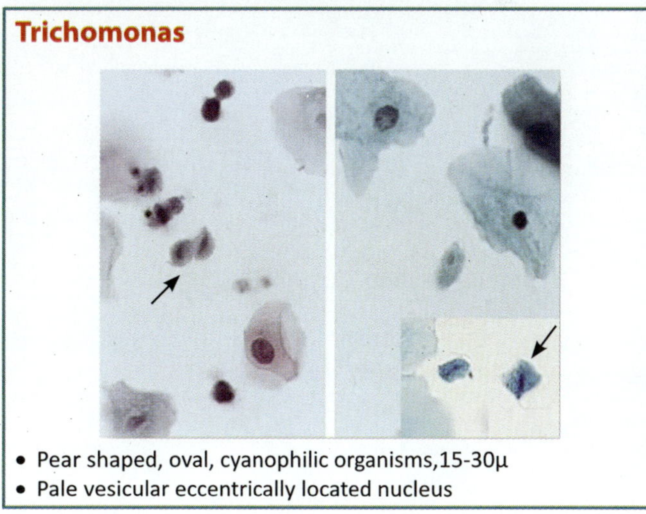

- Pear shaped, oval, cyanophilic organisms,15-30μ
- Pale vesicular eccentrically located nucleus

Candida

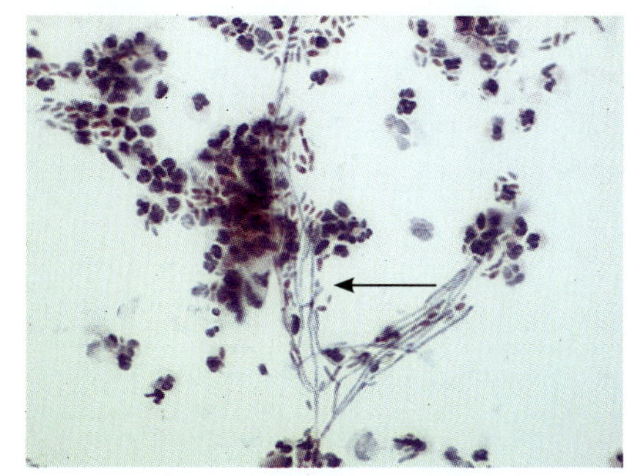

- Double contoured pale pink hyphae and pseudohyphae
- Pseudohyphae appear septate
- Spores are eosinophilic

Menopause

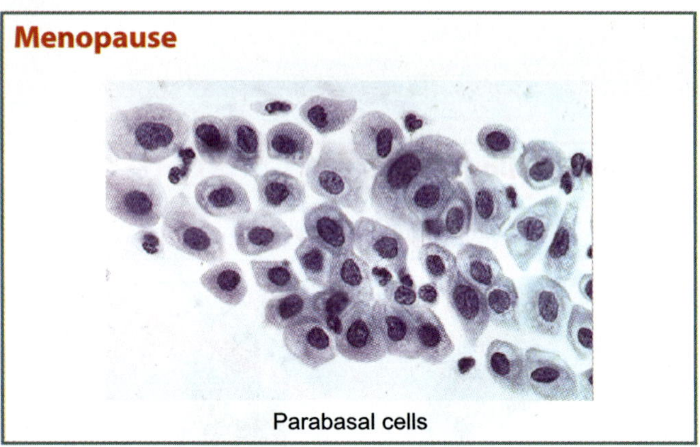

Parabasal cells

Actinomyces

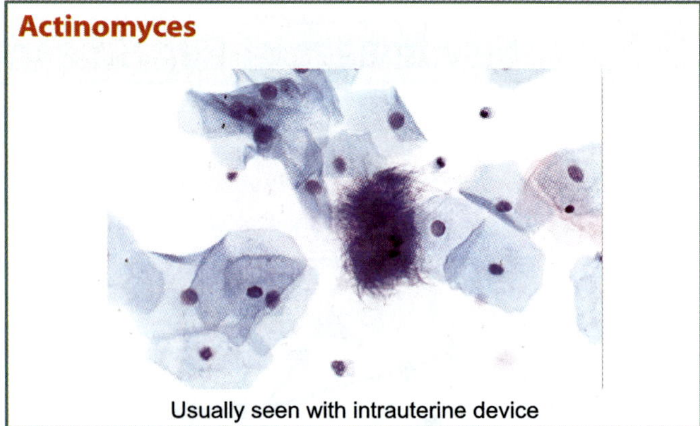

Usually seen with intrauterine device

- ITGCN is now renamed as GCNIS i.e. germ cell neoplasm in situ
- SOX, 2 is associated with embryonal carcinoma

Few Images of Pap Smear

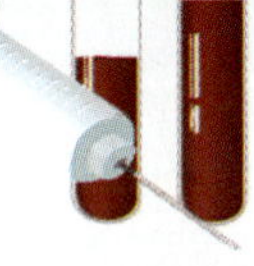

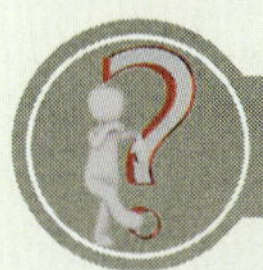

Image-Based Questions

1. A 32-year-female complained of menorrhagia. On pap smear, identify the cells marked in circle

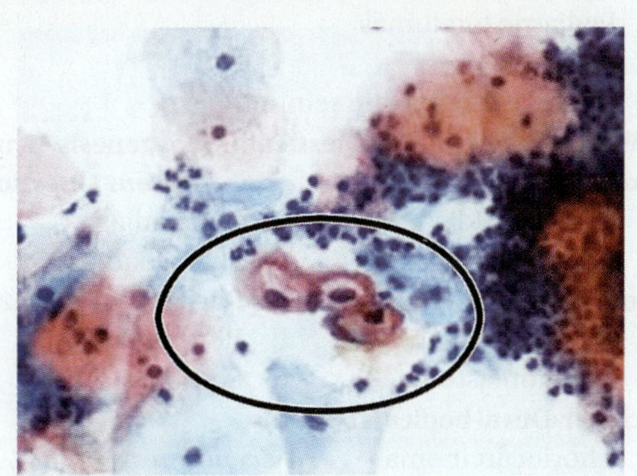

a. Koilocytes   b. Normal squamous cells
c. Candida   d. CMV

2. A 55-year-old female presented with Pruritic, erythematous, crusted, dry raised lesions over vulva. Diagnosis?

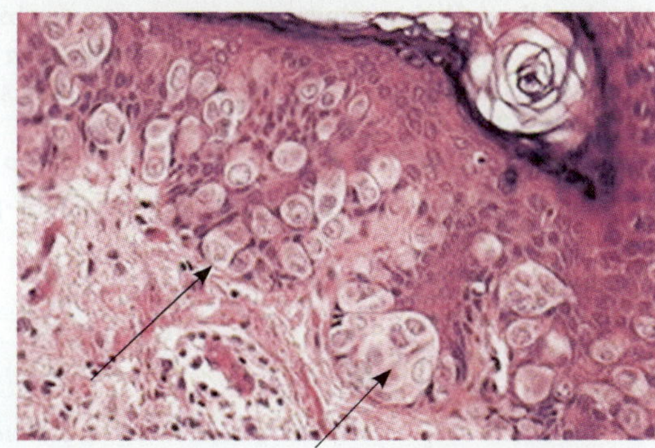

a. Paget's disease   b. Carcinoma vulva
c. CIS   d. Leukoplakia

3. A 25-year-old pregnant female has hcg levels which are markedly high. On USG, size of uterus exceeds the gestational age. Diagnosis:

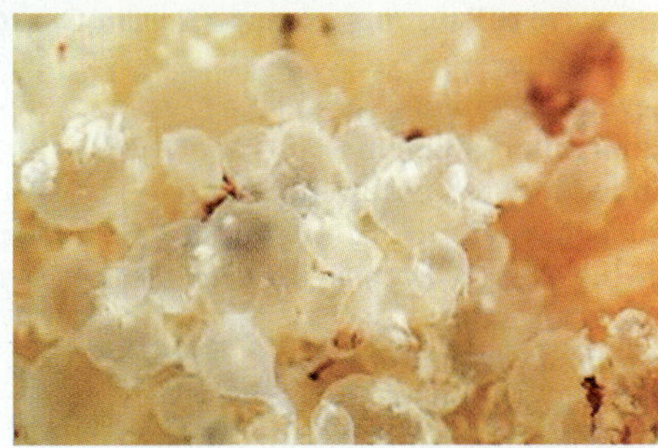

a. Choriocarcinoma   b. Hydatidiform mole
c. Normal pregnancy   d. PSTT

4. Identify the molecular subtype of breast cancer:

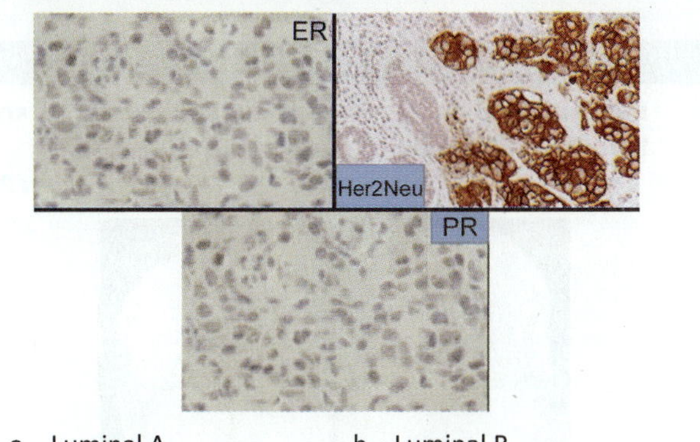

a. Luminal A   b. Luminal B
c. Her2 Neu positive   d. Triple negative

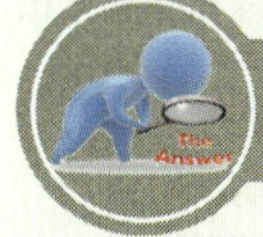

Answers of Image-Based Questions

1. Ans. (a) Koilocytes
- A **Koilocyte** is a squamous epithelial cell that has undergone a number of structural changes, which occur as a result of infection of the cell by human papillomavirus
- Koilocytes may have the following cellular changes:
  - Nuclear enlargement (two to three times normal size)
  - Irregularity of the nuclear membrane contour
  - A darker than normal staining pattern in the nucleus, known as Hyperchromasia
  - A clear area around the nucleus, known as a perinuclear halo.

2. Ans. (a) Paget's disease
- Here we see Single and small clusters of large cells; **vacuolated cells (Paget's cells),** Large nuclei and prominent nucleoli, Amorphous, granular cytoplasm

3. Ans. (b) Hydatidiform mole
- Complete hydatidiform mole, consisting of numerous swollen (hydropic) villi.

4. Ans. (c) Her2neu +
- ER, PR are nuclear stains whereas Her2neu is cytoplasmic and membranous stain. So here we see cytoplasmic and membranous positivity, hence Her2neu + cancer.

Multiple Choice Questions

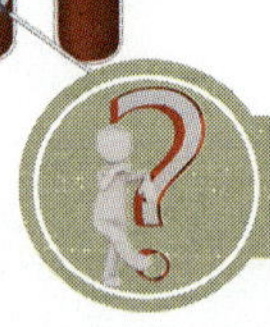

MALE GENITAL SYSTEM

PENIS

1. **Which of the following does not progress to carcinoma?**
(Recent Question 2016)
- a. Bowen's disease
- b. Bowenoid papulosis
- c. Leukoplakia
- d. Erythroplakia

2. **Corbus disease is:** *(AP 2013)*
- a. Dense fibrosis of dermis and buck fascia of penile corpus
- b. Balanitis circumscriptaplasmacellularis
- c. Gangrenous balanitis
- d. Erythroplasia of queyrat

3. **Verrucous carcinoma is-**
(Recent Question 2014, Kerala 2K)
- a. Extremely well differentiated squamous cell carcinoma
- b. Poorly differentiated squamous cell Ca
- c. Example of condyloma
- d. An example of adenocarcinoma

TESTIS

4. **Post surgery image of a tumor in scrotum is shown below. What could be your possible diagnosis?**
(Recent exam 2018)

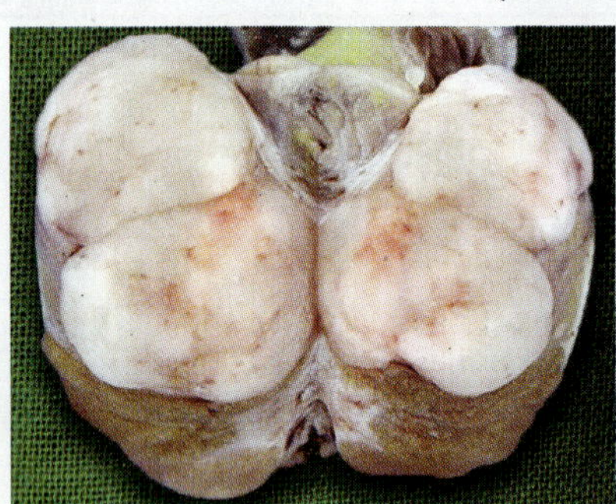

- a. Teratoma
- b. Seminoma
- c. Yolk sac tumor
- d. Lymphoma

5. **A surgeon suspecting testicular carcinoma in a patient asks the intern to send the sample for histopathology, what is the fluid in which the intern should send the sample to the pathologist?** *(AIIMS May 16)*
- a. Bouvin solution
- b. 10% formalin
- c. 95 % ethanol
- d. Alcohol

6. **All are true about seminomas except:**
(Recent Question 2015)
- a. Most common type of germ cell tumor
- b. Anaplastic seminomas is associated with a worse prognosis
- c. Almost never occur in infants
- d. Spermatocytic seminoma is slow growing with good prognosis

7. **Intratubular germ cell neoplasia is implicated as a cause for the following testicular tumor?**
- a. Pediatric yolk sac tumors *(Recent Question 2015)*
- b. Pediatric teratomas
- c. Seminomas
- d. Adult spermatocytic seminomas

8. **All the following are testicular dysgenesis syndromes except:** *(Recent Question 2015)*
- a. Cryptorchidism
- b. Epispadias
- c. Poor sperm quality
- d. Hypospadias

9. **Not seen in children** *(Recent Question 2014-15)*
- a. Neuroblastoma
- b. Retinoblastoma
- c. Hepatoblastoma
- d. Seminoma

10. **Schiller-Duval bodies is seen in:**
- a. Choriocarcinoma *(Recent Question 2014, DNB 11)*
- b. Embryonal cell Ca
- c. Endodermal sinus tumour
- d. Immature teratoma

11. **Alkaline phosphatase is a tumor marker of which tumor-** *(Recent Question 2014)*
- a. Seminoma
- b. Embryonal carcinoma
- c. Yolk sac tumor
- d. Embryonal sinus tumor

12. **All are germ cell tumors except-** *(Recent Question 2014)*
- a. Seminoma
- b. Leydig cell tumor
- c. Embryonal carcinoma
- d. Endodermal sinus tumor

13. **Microscopic feature of seminoma include all of the following except** *(Recent Question 2013, AP PGMEE 14)*
- a. Gland formation
- b. Lymphocytic infiltration
- c. Monomorphic cells
- d. Destruction of seminiferous tubules

14. **True about serum AFP level:** *(PGI May 2013)*
- a. Raised in testicular tumor
- b. Raised in 70% cases of HCC
- c. Correlation between tumor recurrence after surgery in HCC
- d. Correlation with HCC size
- e. Upper limit of normal in the serum is 200 ng/ml

15. **Commonest histological type of carcinoma testis is -**
(DNB 2012)
- a. Teratoma
- b. Yolk sac tumour
- c. Seminoma
- d. Chorio carcinoma

16. **AFP is elevated in:** *(PGI May 2011)*
- a. HCC
- b. Hepatoblastoma
- c. Infant hemangioendothelioma
- d. Amebic liver abscess
- e. Embryonic sarcoma

17. **Tumour marker for Endodermal Sinus Tumour**
- a. PLAP
- b. hCG *(JIPMER 11)*
- c. Alfa feto protein
- d. Cytokeratin

18. **A glomerulus-like structure composed of central blood vessel enveloped by germ cells within a space lined by germ cells, is seen in -** *(Karnataka 11)*
   a. Sertoli-Leydig cell tumor
   b. Granulosa cell tumor
   c. Endodermal sinus tumor
   d. Sex cord tumor with annular tubules

PROSTATE

19. **NKX3-1 immunohistochemical used for diagnosis of:** *(JIPMER Nov 2019)*
   a. Colorectal carcinoma
   b. Pancreatic carcinoma
   c. Prostate
   d. Renal cell carcinoma

20. **Gleason's grading system is for -** *(Recent Question 2014-15)*
   a. Carcinoma testis
   b. Carcinoma colon
   c. Carcinoma thyroid
   d. Carcinoma prostate

21. **Which of the following is not a variant of Prostate specific antigen (PSA)?** *(Recent Question 2014)*
   a. PSA density'
   b. PSA velocity
   c. PSA Nodularity
   d. Ratio of free and bound PSA in the serum

SEMEN ANALYSIS

22. **According to the 2010 WHO criteria what are the characteristics of normal semen analysis** *(AIIMS May 2015)*
   a. Volume 1.5 ml, count 15 million, morphology 4% progressive motility 32%
   b. Volume 2.0 ml, count 20 million, morphology 4% progressive motility 32%
   c. Volume 1.5 ml, count 20 million, morphology 4% progressive motility 32%
   d. Volume 2.0 ml, count 15 million, morphology 40% progressive motility 32%

23. **Semen analysis is to be done?** *(Recent Question 2014)*
   a. As early as possible in semisolid state
   b. After 15-30 minutes irrespective of liquefaction
   c. After 30-60 minutes irrespective of liquefaction
   d. After liquefaction with thorough mixing

24. **Teratozoospermia refers to?** *(Recent Question 2013)*
   a. Absence of semen
   b. Absence of sperm
   c. All dead sperms in ejaculate
   d. Morphologically defective sperms

FEMALE GENITAL SYSTEM

VULVA

25. **Extramammary paget's is seen in?** *(Recent exam 2018)*
   a. Uterus
   b. Vulva
   c. Vagina
   d. Ovary

26. **Predisposing factor for Carcinoma Vulva is all except:** *(Recent Question 2015)*
   a. Smoking
   b. Human papilloma virus (HPV) infection
   c. Fibroepithelial polyps
   d. Leukoplakia

VAGINA

27. **A grape like, polypoid, bulky mass protruding through vagina in a 4 yr old girl is characteristic of** *(MH PG 2014)*
   a. Fibrosarcoma
   b. Sarcoma botryoides
   c. Leiomyosarcoma
   d. Inflammatory polyp

28. **Sarcoma botryoides is a type of?** *(Recent Question 2015)*
   a. Rhabdomyosarcoma
   b. Lymphangioma
   c. Leimyoma
   d. Rhabdomyoma

CERVIX

29. **Identify the PAP Smear given below?** *(AIIMS May 16)*

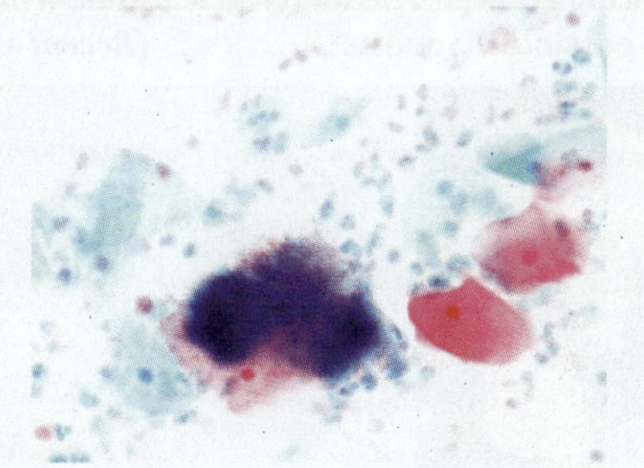

   a. Trichomonas
   b. Chlamydia
   c. Actinomycetes
   d. Herpes simplex type 2

30. **Findings of Cervical PAP smear taken during the late menstrual peri- od from a 45 year old lady suffering with a ovarian tumor is shown below. Which ovarian tumor is she most likely suffering from?** *(AIIMS May 16)*

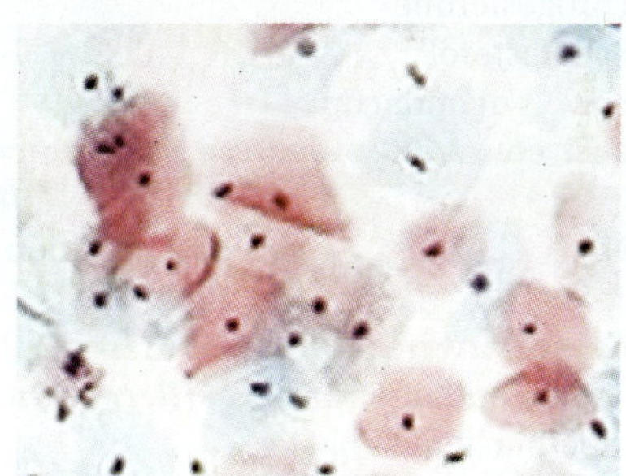

   a. Dysgerminoma
   b. Granulosa cell tumor
   c. Mucinous cyst adeno Ca
   d. Serous cyst adeo ca

31. **Which of the following marker favours diagnosis of preinvasive & invasive cervical cancer:** *(PGI May 16)*
   a. Ki67
   b. Oncoprotein E6
   c. p16INK4, cyclin E, and Ki-67
   d. Oncoprotein E8

CERVIX

32. **Most common cause of Cervical neoplasia is?** *(Recent Question 2015)*
   a. HPV-6
   b. HPV-11
   c. HPV-16
   d. HHV

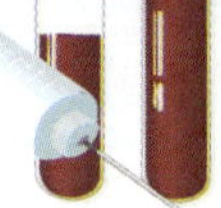

33. Risk factor of CA cervix *(Recent Question 2014-15)*
a. Smoking
b. Sex at 25 yrs
c. Decreased parity
d. Single sexual partner

34. 100/0/0 maturation index denotes
a. Atrophic smear *(Recent Question 2015)*
b. Pregnancy
c. Reproductive age female
d. None

UTERUS

35. Hysterectomy from a 35-year-old female showed the following gross and histological features. What could be your possible diagnosis? *(Recent exam 2018)*

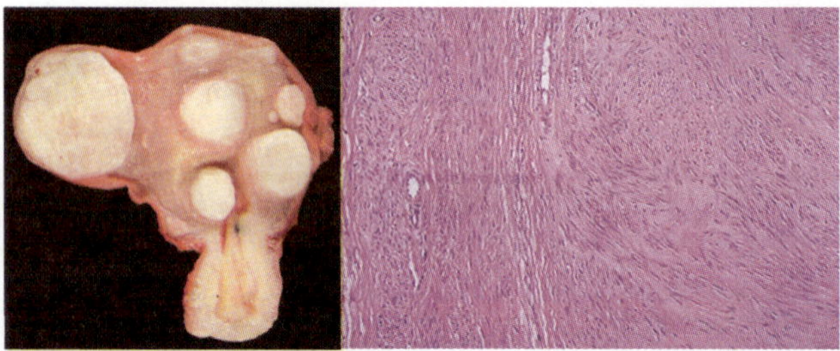

a. Carcinoma endometrium
b. Leiomyoma
c. Malignant mixed Müllerian tumor
d. Leiomyosarcoma

36. Endometriotic lesion histology represents it's?
a. High estrogen *(AIIMS May 2017)*
b. High progesterone
c. High cholesterol
d. High levels of prolactin

37. Gene most commonly involved in Endometrial carcinoma *(JIPMER 2016)*
a. PTEN
b. Braf mutation
c. RAS
d. REL

38. Swiss cheese pattern endometrium is seen in
a. Carcinoma endometrium *(Recent Question 2015)*
b. Metropathia hemorrhagica
c. Hydatidiform mole
d. Halban's disease

39. Endometrial Carcinoma risk in? *(Recent Question 2014)*
a. Sertoli Leydig cell
b. Immature teratoma
c. Gonadoblastoma
d. Granulosa theca cell tumor

40. Complete mole can be differentiated from partial mole by: *(Recent Question 2014, PGI May 12)*
a. P57
b. P53
c. P16inkga
d. P63
e. PED

41. True about Complete *(classic)* moles A/E
a. 90% have a 46, XX karyotype *(Recent Question 2014)*
b. Androgenesis
c. Duplication of the genetic material of one sperm
d. Arise from the fertilization of a single egg by two sperm

OVARY

42. A 35-year-old female with adnexal mass, CA 125 normal, LDH raised and CA 19.9 was normal. Gross and histopathology has been given below. What is your diagnosis? *(AIIMS Nov 16)*

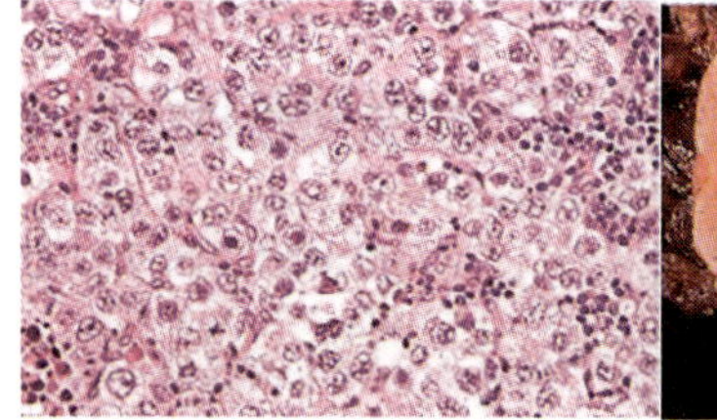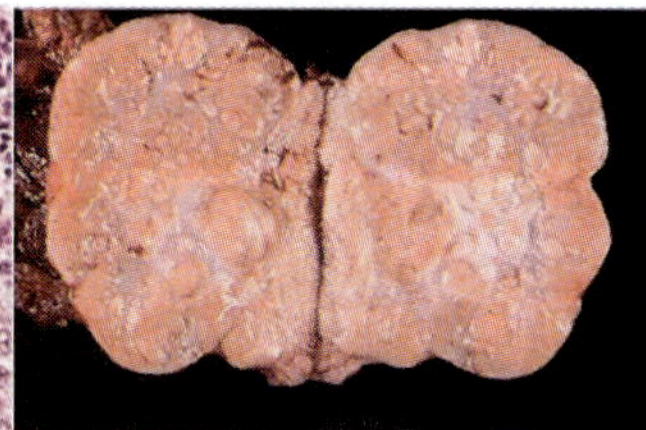

a. Choriocarcinoma
b. Dysgerminoma
c. Teratoma
d. Papillary serous cystadenoma

43. A 25 female patient presented with complains of feeling of mass per abdomen. On examination, a mass was found on left adnexal lesion with multiple solid cytic areas. The patient was operated and the mass was removed, which has been shown below. What is the true statement regarding the condition? *(AIIMS Nov 2016)*

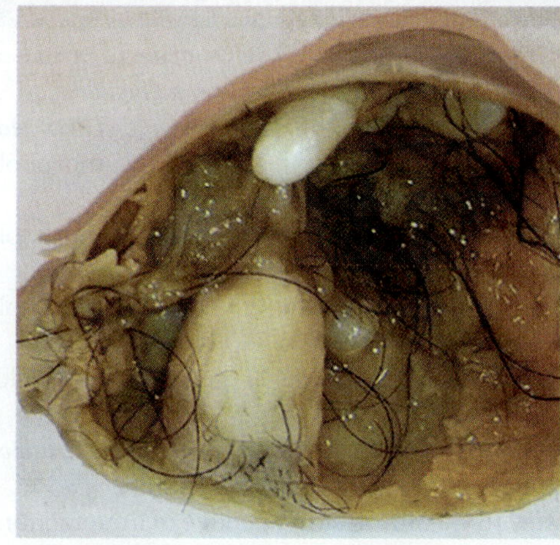

a. Specimen shows multiple solid cystic areas suggestive of dermoid cyst.
b. Specimen shows cystic areas suggestive of serous cyst adenoma
c. Specimen shows Choriocarcinoma
d. Specimen shows Dysgerminoma

44. Call exner bodies are seen in: *(Recent Question 2016-17)*
a. Dysgerminoma
b. Granulosa cell tumor
c. Thecoma
d. Arrhenoblastoma

45. BA lady with abdominal mass was investigated. On surgery, she was found to have b/l ovarian masses with smooth surface. On microscopy they revealed mucin secreting cells with signet ring shapes. What is your diagnosis? *(AIIMS May 2015)*
a. Dysgerminoma
b. Krukenberg tumour
c. Primary Adenocarcinoma of the ovaries
d. Dermoid cyst

46. **One of the following is a germ cell tumor of ovary:**
(MH PGMEE 2016, AP 2015)
a. Granulosa cell tumor
b. Mucinous cystadenoma
c. Brenner tumor
d. Benign cystic teratoma

47. **Fibroma belongs to** *(Recent Question 2014-15)*
a. Germ cell tumor
b. Sex cord stromal tumor
c. Surface epithelial stromal tumors
d. Metastatic tumors from non ovarian primary

48. **Which hormone is increased in PCOS?**
(Recent Question 2015)
a. LH b. FSH
c. Inhibin d. Estrogen

49. **Which of these tumors is unique to pregnancy?**
a. Luteoma *(Recent Question 2015)*
b. Serous cystadenoma
c. Mucinous cystadenoma
d. Teratoma

50. **Most common ovarian tumor** *(Recent Question 2013)*
a. Serous cystadenoma
b. Choriocarcinoma
c. Teratoma
d. Fibroma

51. **Rokitanski protruberences are seen in -**
a. Mucinous carcinoma *(Recent Question 2013)*
b. Teratoma
c. Epidermal cystoids adenoma
d. Papillary carcinoma

52. **Marker for ovarian carcinoma in serum is -**
(Recent Question 2013)
a. CA-125
b. Fibronectin
c. Acid Phosphatase
d. PSA

53. **True about CA-125:** *(PGI May 2013)*
a. Glycoprotein
b. It is a specific marker
c. Increased in colon carcinoma
d. Normal range in pre menopausal females is 200 U/ml
e. May be elevated in Pelvic inflammatory disease

54. **CA 125 is used for?** *(DNB Aug 12)*
a. Follow up of ovarian cancer
b. Diagnosis of pancreatic cancer
c. Diagnosis of stomach cancer
d. Diagnosis of ovarian cancer

55. **A 20-year-old female is diagnosed with granulosa cell tumor of the ovary. Which of the following biomarkers would be most useful for follow-up of patient'?**
a. CA 19-9 *(AIIMS 10, 11)*
b. CA 50
c. Inhibin
d. Neuron-specific-enolase

56. **Which one of the following is not true regarding chorio-carcinoma?** *(DNB 11)*
a. Aggressive malignancy
b. Raised HCG levels
c. Common below 20 yearsofage
d. Gonadal type is chemosensitive

Answers with Explanations

1.   Ans. (b) Bowenoid papulosis *(Ref: Robbins 9th/pg 970-71)*

Bowen disease	Bowenoid papulosis
Transforms into **infiltrating squamous cell carcinoma**[Q] in 10%	**Never**[Q] develops into **invasive carcinoma** & in many cases regresses spontaneously.

2.   Ans. (c) Gangrenous balanitis

(Ref:www.pathologyoutlines.com/topic/penscrotumgan-gren ousbalanitis.html)

- Corbus disease is rapidly progressing necrotizing inflammatory disease due to anaerobes in glans penis (Gangrenous balanitis)

3.   Ans. (a) Extremely well differentiated squamous cell carcinoma *(Ref: Robbins 9th/pg 971; 8th/pg 984)*

Verrucous carcinoma [also known as **Giant condyloma** or Buschke-Lowenstein tumor]
- **Exophytic well-differentiated variant of squamous cell carcinoma**[Q]
- **Locally invasive, but rarely metastasize.**[Q]
- **It** invades the underlying tissue **along a broad fronts**

4.   Ans. (b) Seminoma

(Ref: Robbins 9th ed p 976)

Seminomas produce bulky masses, sometimes ten times the size of the normal testis. The typical seminoma has a homogeneous, gray-white, lobulated cut surface, usually devoid of hemorrhage or necrosis. Generally the tunica albuginea is not penetrated, but occasionally extension to the epididymis, spermatic cord, or scrotal sac occurs.

Uniform cells divided into poorly demarcated lobules by deli-cate fibrous septa containing a lymphocytic infiltrate. The classic seminoma cell is large and round to polyhedral and has a distinct cell membrane; clear or watery-appearing cytoplasm; and a large, central nucleus with one or two prominent nucleoli.

5.   Ans. (b) 10% formalin

(Ref: Complete review of pathology 2nd ed / Annexure 4. http://www.adasp.org/Surveys/Question-about-Bouins-fixative-for-testis-biopsy.html)

This is a tricky Question !
When you first see the term analysis for sperm, the answer is bouin's fluid. But what the examiner wants to know is whether you know that for histological diagnosis, the fixative is 10% formalin

Remember: Bouins fluid should be used for testicular anlysis in cases of infertility or even CIS(carcinoma in situ) as Formalin induces marked shrinkage → difficulty in germ cell and CIS recognition.

But once you have known case of testicular carcinoma, then you need to make correct diagnosis on the basis of morphology, also preserve antigens for IHC and do molecular tests, which comes best when you fix the tissue in 10% buffered neutral formalin

6.   Ans. (b) Anaplastic seminomas is associated with a worse prognosis

(Ref: Genitourinary Pathology: A Volume in the Series: pg 610)

The term anaplastic seminoma is used when seminoma shows pleomorphism, robust mitotic activity and scant lymphocytic infiltrate. Anaplastic semioma has **same** prognosis as classical seminoma.

7.   Ans. (c) Seminomas *(Ref: Robbins 9th/pg 977; 8th/pg 989)*

Testicular germ cell tumour originate from a precursor lesion called **intratubular germ cell neoplasia (ITGCN)** except **spermatocyte seminoma**; pediatric **teratoma and Yolk Sac tumor**

8.   Ans. (b) Epispadias *(Ref: Robbins 9th/pg 975; 8th/pg 988)*

Testicular dysgenesis syndrome (TDS): cryptorchidism, hypospadias, and poor sperm quality

9.   Ans. (d) Seminoma *(Ref: Robbins 9th/pg 977; 8th/pg 989)*

10.   Ans. (c) Endodermal sinus tumour *(Ref: R 9th/pg 977)*

Yolk sac tumor or endodermal sinus tumor is the most common **testicular tumor in infants and children <3 yrs of age.** It has good prognosis

11.   Ans. (a) Seminoma *(Ref: R 9th/pg 975-76; 8th/pg 988-89)*

Seminoma

Most common type of germ cell tumors (50%).[Q]
Tumor markers:
PLAP (Placental alkaline phosphatase).[Q] **GGT** (Gamma glutamyl transpeptidase)[Q], hCG (15%)

12.   Ans. (b) Leydig cell tumor *(Ref: Robbins 9th/pg 975)*

13.   Ans. (a) Gland formation

(Ref: Robbins 9th/pg 976; 8th/pg 988-89)

14. **Ans. (a, b, c, d); a. Raised in testicular tumor; b. Raised in 70% cases of HCC; c. Correlation between tumor recurrence after surgery in HCC; d. Correlation with HCC size**

(Ref: Walker's Pediatric Gastrointestinal Disease 5th ed; volume 2 :914, Pediatric Hematology and Oncology, 18:11-26, 2001)

Increased AFP levels are seen in

- Omphalocele
- Hepatocellular carcinoma/hepatoma
- Hepatoblastoma
- Neural tube defects: ↑ α-fetoprotein in amniotic fluid and maternal serum
- **Non-seminomatous germ cell tumors (option A)**
  - Yolk sac tumor
  - Immature teratoma (rarely)
- Ataxia telangiectasia:
- Serum AFP has significant correlation with the size of tumour.
- Its concentration in adult serum is less than 20 ng/ml.- **option E is false**

15. **Ans. (c) Seminoma**

(Ref: Robbins 9th/pg 975; 8th/pg 988-89)

16. **Ans. (a, b, c, d); a. HCC; b. Hepatoblastoma; c. Infant hemangioendothelioma; d. Amebic liver abscess**

(Ref: Walker's Pediatric Gastrointestinal Disease 5th ed; volume 2 :914)

Infantile hemangioendothelioma - most common hepatic vascular tumor in infants < 6 months of age; same cases can be associated with raised AFP

Elevated AFP levels are commonly found in acute liver disorders like Fulminant acute hepatitis, Liver cirrhosis and few cases of Liver abscess (pyogenic, amebic)

Embryonal sarcoma of liver is not associated with raised AFP

17. **Ans. (c) Alfa feto protein** *(Ref: Robbins 9th/pg 979-80)*

Tumour Markers For Testicular Tumors	
Oncofetal substances	**Cellular Enzymes**
• **α-FP:** (Increases in **YST**)[Q] ▪ Produced by **trophoblastic cells**[Q] ▪ **Increases** in **Yolk sac tumour, embryonal carcinoma and terato carcinoma. (YET)**[Q] ▪ **Doesn't increase** in **pure choriocarcinoma**[Q] ▪ Metabolic **half life: 5-7 days**[Q]	• LDH: ▪ Not a specific tumour marker ▪ Most useful as a marker for **"bulk' disease** ▪ Raised serum LDH has poor prognosis • **PLAP** (Placental alkaline phosphatase): ▪ Elevated in **seminoma**[Q] • **GGT** (Gamma glutamyl transpeptidase): ▪ Marker of **seminoma testis**[Q] ▪ Marker for **"bulk"** disease

18. **Ans. (c) Endodermal sinus tumor**

(Ref: Robbins 9th/pg 977)

Yolk sac tumor or endodermal sinus tumor show Schiller-Duval bodies or glomeruloid structures

19. **Ans. (c) Prostate**

20. **Ans. (d) Carcinoma prostate** *(Ref: Robbins 9th/pg 982)*

21. **Ans. (c) PSA Nodularity** *(Ref: Robbins 9th/pg 982)*

Six variants in PSA Value

- **Age specific reference range**

Age	Cut off
40-49 years	0 to 2.5 ng/ml
50-59 years	0 to 3.5 ng/ml
60-69 years	0 to 4.5 ng/ml
70-79 years	0 to 6.5 ng/ml

Raising the PSA threshold in older men improves specificity

- **PSA velocity:**
  - Rate of change of PSA with time.
  - **According to BLSA study PSA Velocity Of more than 0.75 ng/ml/Year shows increased of prostate cancer.**
- **Free versus total PSA**
  - Free PSA (not bound to other proteins)/ total amount of PSA (free plus bound)
  - Lower proportion of free PSA-more aggressive cancer.
- **PSA density:**
  - It is the ratio of serum PSA value and volume of prostate (PSA/volume prostate)
  - Upper normal limit is 0.15.
  - Butter discrimnator between benign and malignant cancer than PSA
- **Ratio of free and bound PSA in the serum:**
  - It is calculated as Free PSA/Total PSA x 100
  - **Free PSA less than 10% indicates high risk of carcinoma.**
- **Pro-PSA.**
  - Pro-PSA refers to several different inactive precursors of PSA.
  - Pro-PSA is more strongly associated with prostate cancer

22. **Ans. (a) Volume 1.5 ml, count 15 million, morphology 4% progressive motility 32%**

(Ref: Who 2010 Manual Sperm Analysis)

In 2010 the World Health Organization (WHO) updated its reference values for the Semen Analysis

Semen characteristics	WHO 2010
Volume (mL)	≥ 1.5
Sperm count (10^4/mL)	≥ 15
Total sperm count (10^6)	≥ 39
Total motility (%)	≥ 40
Progressive motility	≥ 32%

23. **Ans. (d) After liquefaction with thorough mixing**

(Ref: www.who.int/reproductivehealth/publications/ infertility)

Liquefaction	Process when the gel formed by proteins from the seminal vesicles is broken up and the semen becomes more liquid In the NICE guidelines, a liquefaction time **<60 minutes** -normal ranges Semen analysis should be done **after liquefaction with through mixing**

24. **Ans. (d)** **Morphologically defective sperms**

(Ref: www.who.int/reproductivehealth/publications/ infertility)

25. **Ans. (b)** **Vulva** *(Ref: Robbins 9th ed p 999)*

Extramammary Paget's is rare lesion of the vulva is similar in its manifestations to Paget disease of the breast. In the vulva, it presents as a pruritic, red, crusted, maplike area, usually on the labia majora. aget disease is a distinctive intraepithelial proliferation of malignant cells. Paget cells are larger than surrounding keratinocyte and are seen singly or in small clusters within the epidermis. The cells have pale cytoplasm containing mucopolysaccharide that stains with periodic acid–Schiff (PAS), Alcian blue, or mucicarmine stains. In addition, the cells express cytokeratin 7.

26. **Ans. (c)** **Fibroepithelial polyps** *(Ref: Robbins 9th/pg 997)*

Predisposing factors for ca vulva
- Cigarette use
- Human papillomavirus (HPV) infection
- Lichen sclerosus
- Premalignant lesions like leucoplakia
- Cervical cancer.
- Patients that are infected with HIV tend to be more susceptible to vulvar cancer as well.

Option C- **Fibroepithelial polyps are also known as skin tags- they are benign exophytic lesions of vulva**

27. **Ans (b)** **Sarcoma botryoides** *(Ref: Robbins 9th/pg 1001)*

28. **Ans. (a)** **Rhabdomyosarcoma** *(Ref: Robbins 9th/pg 1001)*

29. **Ans. (c)** **Actinomycetes**

(Ref: Textbook of Interpretation of PAP smear, refer to pretext for details)

The image given shows a wooly appearance; periphery containing swollen filaments with clubs of filament organism. This is suggestive of **Actinomycetes**.

30. **Ans. (b)** **Granulosa cell tumor**

(Ref: Textbook of Interpretation of PAP smear, refer to pretext for details)

In the given PAP smear, predominance of Mature cells (orange coloured cells compared to parabasal cells: blue coloured), might be due to estrogen secretion from Granulosa cell tumor.

31. **Ans. (a, b, c)** **a. Ki67 b. Oncoprotein E6 c. p16INK4, cyclin E, and Ki-67** *(Ref: http)*

32. **Ans. (c)** **HPV-16**

(Ref: https://aidsinfo.nih.gov/guidelines/html/)

At least 12 HPV types are considered oncogenic, including HPV16, 18, 31, 33, 35, 39, 45, 51, 52, 56, 58, and 59
- HPV16 alone, though, accounts for approximately 50% of cervical cancers in the general population and HPV18 for another 10% to 15%. The other oncogenic HPV types each individually account for fewer than 5% of tumors.
- HPV types 6 and 11 cause 90% of genital warts, but are not considered oncogenic

33. **Ans. (a)** **Smoking**

Risk factorsfor ca cervix are	• Early age at first intercourse[Q] • Multiple sexual partners[Q] • Increased parity[Q] • High-risk HPVs (most important factor)	• Cigarette smoking, use of OCPs • **Genital infections[Q]** • History of HSIL • **Certain HLA & viral subtypes[Q]**

34. **Ans (a)** **Atrophic smear** *(Ref: Dutta Gyne 4th ed:105)*

MI is a ratio obtained through performing a random count of three major cell types (parabasal cells, intermediate cells and superficial cells) that are shed from the squamous epithelium.

The cell count is expressed as a percentage that reads as follows: **MI = % parabasal cells/ % intermediate cells/ % superficial cells.**
- **Atrophic smear** -100/0/0 means majorly parabasal cells i.e. no progesterone or estrogen.

35. **Ans. (b)** **Leiomyoma** *(Ref: Robbins 9th ed p 1020)*

Leiomyomas are sharply circumscribed, discrete, round, firm, gray-white tumors varying in size from small, barely visible nodules to massive tumors that fill the pelvis. Except in rare instances, they are found within the myometrium of the corpus. Leiomyomas are typically composed of bundles of smooth muscle cells that resemble the uninvolved myometrium. Usually, the individual muscle cells are uniform in size and shape and have the characteristic oval nucleus and long, slender bipolar cytoplasmic processes. Mitotic figures are scarce.

36. **Ans. (a)** **High estrogen** *(Ref: R 9th/p 721)*

Increased estrogen production by endometriotic stromal cells, due in large part to high levels of the key steroidogenic enzyme aromatase, which is absent in normal endometrial stroma. Mutations in specific genes (PTEN and ARID1A) in endometriotic cysts.

37. **Ans. (a)** **PTEN** *(Ref: Robbins 9th/pg 1015)*

Type 1 endometrial ca is MC and PTEN is MC involved in it.

38. Ans. (b) Metropathia hemorrhagica

(Ref: Textbook of gynecology by Rao:65)

Metropathia hemorrhagica

Anovulatory DUB associated with endometrial hyperplasia with acyclical bleeding

Overgrowth of endometrial stroma and glands producing swiss cheee appearance

39. Ans. (d) Granulosa theca cell tumor *(Ref: R 9th/pg 1032)*

Granulosa cell tumor
- The **most common** malignant **Sex-Cord Stromal Tumors of ovary**
- The main **clinical features depend upon the oestrogenic activity of the tumour**[Q]
- The tumor cells may secrete estrogens and **cause precocious sexual development in girls** or increase the risk for **endometrial hyperplasia and carcinoma in women**.

40. Ans. (a) P57 *(Ref: Robbins 9th/pg 1039)*

Gestational trophoblastic diseases include: benign hydatidiform mole (partial and complete), invasive mole, placental site trophoblastic tumor and choriocarcinoma

Hydatidiform mole:

There are two types of benign, noninvasive moles—complete and partial Both partial and complete, are composed of *avascular, grape-like structures* that **do not invade the myometrium**

Complete (classic) moles	Partial moles
All the chorionic villi are abnormal and fetal parts are not found	Only some of the villi are abnormal and fetal parts may be seen.
46, XX diploid pattern	Triploid or a tetraploid karyotype
MORPHOLOGY	
The chorionic villi are enlarged, scalloped in shape with central cavitation **(cisterns)** **Extensive**[Q] trophoblast proliferation	Focal villi enlargement Focal trophoblast proliferation
Risk of choriocarcinoma-**2.5%** Risk of persistent or invasive mole- **15%**	Have an increased risk of persistent molar disease, but are **not associated with choriocarcinoma.**[Q]

Immunostaining for p57, which is a gene that is paternally imprinted (inactivated) helps in differentiating the two moles. Because the complete mole arises only from paternal chromosomes, **immunostaining for p57 will be negative.**

41. Ans. (d) Arise from the fertilization of a single egg by two sperm *(Ref: Robbins 9th/pg 1039)*

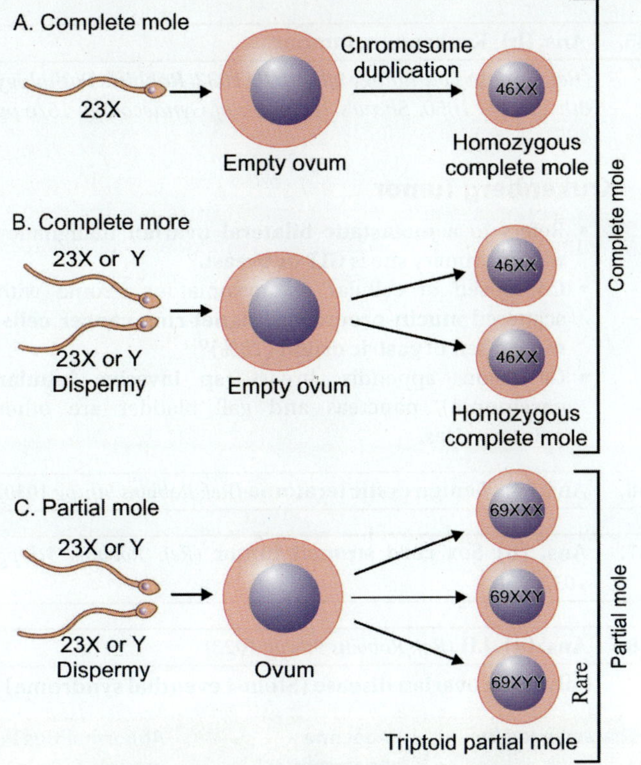

Figure: Origin of complete and partial hydatidiform moles.
A. Complete moles most commonly (90%) arise from fertilization of an empty ovum by a single sperm that undergoes duplication of its chromosomes–karyotype 46XX. **(a phenomenon called and rogenesis**[Q] **as it is derived from paternal chromosome).**
B. Less commonly,(10%) complete moles arise from dispermy in which two sperm fertilize an **empty ovum— karyotype**[Q] **46XX or 46XY karyotype.**
C. Partial moles arise from **two sperm fertilizing a single ovum.-OPTION D IS FALSE**

42. Ans. (b) Dysgerminoma

Here, you see, solid ovarian neoplasm with sheets of large polygonal cells separated by septa prominent nucleon. The septa is infiltrated by lymphocytes.

43. Ans. (a) Specimen shows multiple solid cystic areas suggestive of dermoid cyst.

(Ref: Robbins 9th/pg 1029)
- Dermoid cysts are the **commonest solid ovarian neoplasm found in young women**.

44. **Ans. (b)** **Granulosa cell tumor**

(Ref: Robbin's 9th/pg 1029)

45. **Ans. (b)** **Krukenberg tumour**

(Ref: Robbin's Pathology 9th Ed/Pg 1032; Robbin's Pathology 8th ED/PG 1050; Shaw's Textbook of Gynaecology 15/e pg 425)

Krukenberg Tumor

- Refers to a **metastatic bilateral ovarian** malignancy whose primary site is **GIT or breast.**[Q]
- Composed of cellular or myxomatous stroma with scattered **mucin-producing, signet-ring cancer cells, most often of gastric origin (70%)**[Q]
- Ca colon, appendix, breast (**sp invasive lobular carcinoma**), pancreas and gall bladder are other **primary sites.**

46. **Ans. (d)** **Benign cystic teratoma** *(Ref: Robbins 9th/pg 1030)*

47. **Ans. (b)** **Sex cord stromal tumor** *(Ref: Robbins 9th/pg 1032)*

48. **Ans. (a)** **LH** *(Ref: Robbins 9th/pg 1022)*

Polycystic ovarian disease (Stein-Leventhal syndrome)

Characterized by	Endocrine abnormalities	Abnormalities in ovary
• Hyperandrogenism • Menstrual abnormalities • Polycystic ovaries • Chronic anovulation • Decreased fertility[Q]	• **Excess androgens** (androstenedione)[Q] • **Increased estrogen levels**[Q] • Increased LH & decreased FSH levels • **High LH/FSH ratio** • Increased GnRH levels	• Enlarged with thick capsules • Hyperplastic ovarian stroma • Numerous follicular cysts lined by a hyperplastic theca interna.

49. **Ans. (a)** **Luteoma**

(Ref: Best Practice and Research Clinical Endocrinology and Metabolism (Elsevier Ltd.) 25:985–992)

A **luteoma** is a tumor that occurs in the ovaries during pregnancy.

It is associated with an increases of sex hormones, primarily progesterone and testosterone

Benign

Resolve themselves after delivery

50. **Ans. (a)** **Serous cystadenoma** *(Ref: Robbins 9th/pg 1023)*

- Most ovarian tumors are surface epithelial (65-70%)
- Serous cystadenoma is the most common surface epithelial tumor

51. **Ans. (b)** **Teratoma** *(Ref: R 9th/pg 1029; 8th/pg 1057-48)*

- *Mature (Benign) Teratomas*
- **Rokitansky protuberance**[Q]-The inner lining of cyst contains single or multiple white shiny masses projecting from the wall toward the center of the cysts. Hair, other dermal appendages, bone and teeth are present, they usually arise from this protuberance

52. **Ans. (a)** **CA-125**

(Ref: Robbins 9th/pg 1033; Am J Prev Med 13 (6): 444–6)

- CA125- is a glycoprotein
- Elevated levels in **epithelial ovarian cancers**
- CA-125 is the most frequently used biomarker for ovarian cancer detection

Elevated CA125- not a specific marker

- In other cancers, including **endometrial cancer, fallopian tube cancer, lung cancer, breast cancer and gastrointestinal cancer**.
- **Benign conditions**, such as endometriosis, PID, cirrhosis and diabetes mellitus

53. **Ans. (a, c, e); a. Glycoprotein; c. Increased in colon carcinoma; e. May be elevated in Pelvic inflammatory disease**

(Ref: Robbins 9th/pg 1033; 8th/pg 1052, Am J Prev Med 13 (6): 444–6)

54. **Ans. (a)** **Follow up of ovarian cancer**

(Ref: Robbins 9th/pg 1033; 8th/pg 1052, Am J Prev Med 13 (6): 444–6)

55. **Ans. (c)** **Inhibin** *(Ref: Robbins 9th/pg 1032)*

Elevated tissue and serum levels of **inhibin,**[Q] a product of granulosa cells, are associated with granulosa cell tumors

Option a- CA19-9- pancreatic cancer *(Ref: Eur J Surg Oncol. Apr 2007;33(3):266-70)*

Option D- NSE- Neuroblastoma

56. **Ans. (d)** **Gonadal type is chemosensitive**

(Ref: Robbins 9th/pg 1031)

- **In contrast to choriocarcinomas arising in placental tissue, those arising in the ovary are generally unresponsive to chemotherapy and are often fatal.**[Q]

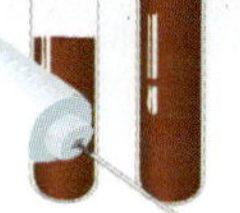

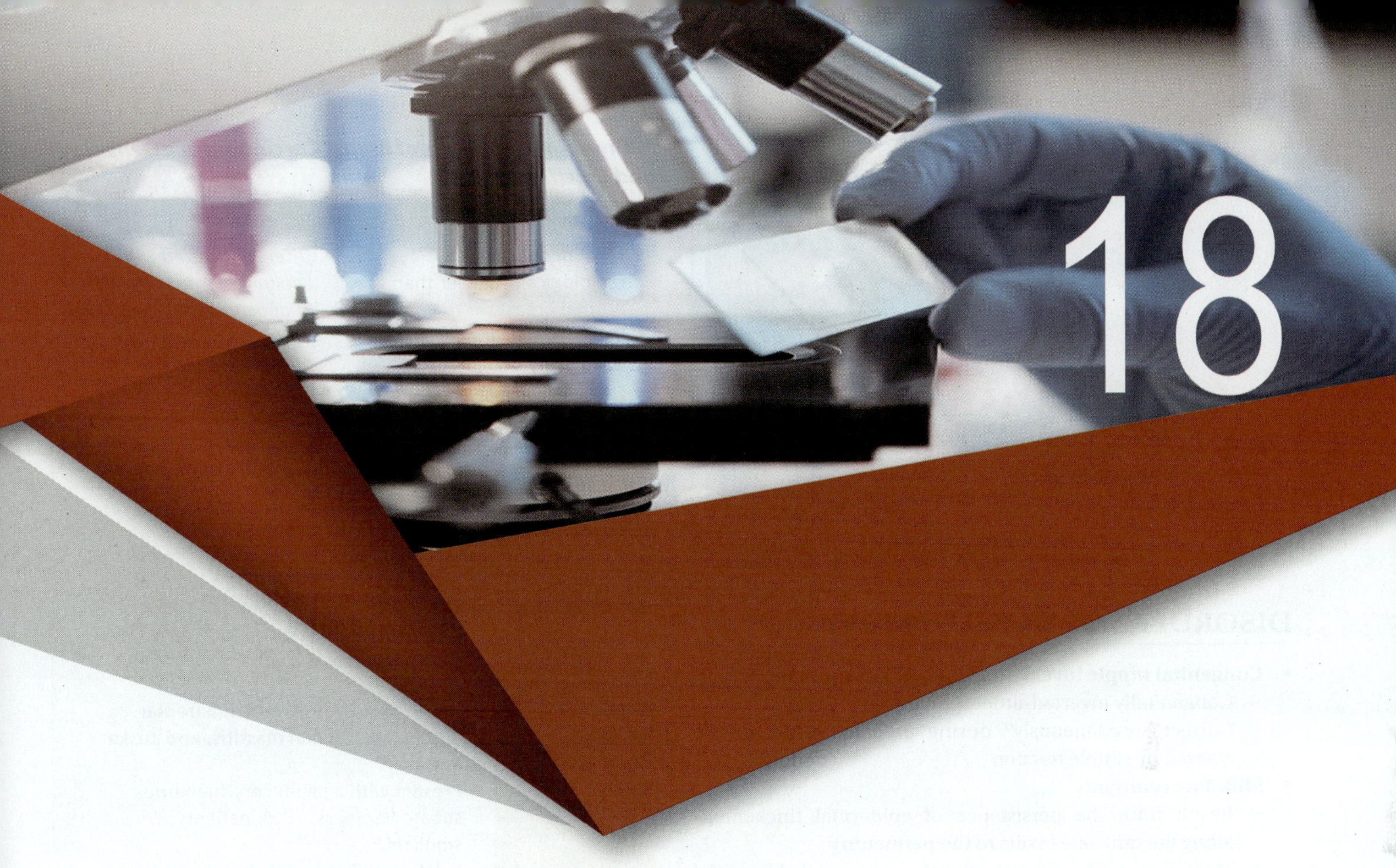

18

Breast

» Most common benign tumor of the female breast—fibroadenoma
» Most common malignant tumor of the female breast—ductal carcinoma
» Most common tumor of the female breast to be seen bilaterally—lobular carcinoma
» Extramammary Paget's disease is usually seen in isolation & associated with an underlying malignancy in 12%

» ITGCN is now renamed as GCNIS i.e. germ cell neoplasm in situ
» SOX, 2 is associated with embryonal carcinoma.

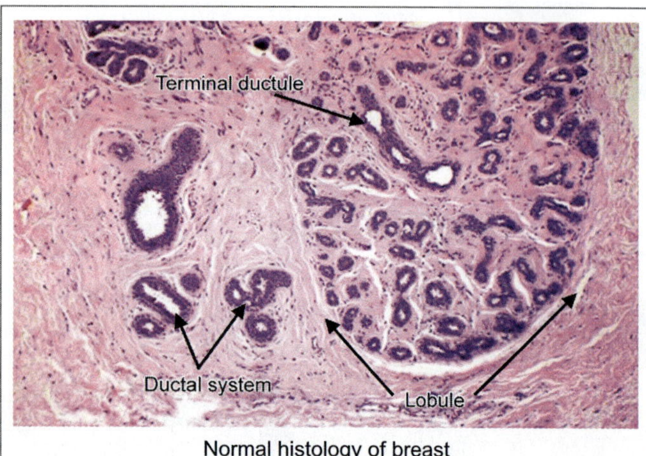

Normal histology of breast

DISORDERS OF DEVELOPMENT

- **Congenital nipple inversion**
  - Congenitally inverted-little significance
  - Correct spontaneously[Q] during pregnancy, or can be everted by simple traction
- **Milk-line remnants**
  - Result from the persistence of epidermal thickenings along the milk line (axilla to the perineum)
  - Most commonly come to attention as a result of painful premenstrual enlargements.
- **Accessory Axillary Breast Tissue**

Clinical Presentations of Breast Disease

- *Pain* (mastalgia or mastodynia) is **the most common**[Q] breast symptom.
- Discrete palpable masses are the **second most common** breast symptom.
- **Most common palpable lesions** are cysts, fibroadenomas, and invasive carcinomas
- Benign palpable masses are **most common in premenopausal women**[Q]
- Mass becomes palpable when size >2 cm
- Most common site of carcinomas-upper outer quadrant (50%)

Nipple discharge is a less common presenting symptom, but is of concern when it is spontaneous and unilateral.

Type of discharge	Cause
Milky discharges (*galactorrhea*)	• Elevated prolactin levels (e.g., by a pituitary adenoma), hypothyroidism, endocrine an ovulatory syndromes, OCP, tricyclic antidepressants, methyldopa, or phenothiazines • **Galactorrhea is not associated with malignancy.**[Q]
Bloody or serous discharges	• Solitary large duct papilloma, cysts, or carcinoma

Mammographic Signs of Breast Carcinoma are Densities and Calcifications

Densities	Calcifications
• Most neoplasms are radiologically denser than normal breast. • Rounded densities are **most commonly benign lesions** such as fibroadenomas or cysts	• *Often associated with benign lesions eg clusters of apocrine cysts, hyalinized fibroadenomas & sclerosing adenosis* • *Calcifications associated with malignancy are usually small, irregular, numerous, and clustered.*[Q]

Inflammatory Disorders

Account for less than 1% of breast symptoms.

Acute mastitis	• Occurs during the first month[Q] of breastfeeding; Most common cause is *Staphylococcus aureus*[Q]
Squamous metaplasia of lactiferous ducts	• Also known as **recurrent subareolar abscess, periductal mastitis, and Zuska disease.**[Q] • Present with a painful erythematous subareolar mass; >90% patients are **smokers.**[Q] • Relative **deficiency of vitamin A**[Q] associated with smoking or toxic substances in tobacco smoke alter the differentiation of the lactiferous ducts • **Keratinizing squamous epithelium**[Q] extending to an abnormal depth into orifices of nipple ducts.
Duct ectasia	• Occur in the fifth or sixth decade of life[Q], usually in multiparous women • Periareolar mass[Q] associated with thick, white nipple secretions & occasionally skin retraction • Not associated with cigarette smoking.[Q]
Fat necrosis	• Painless palpable mass, skin thickening or retraction, a mammographic density or calcifications. • About half of affected women have a history of breast trauma or prior surgery[Q] • Grossly-Ill-defined, firm, gray-white nodules containing small chalky-white foci[Q] • Microscopically- central areas of liquefactive fat necrosis with neutrophils and macrophages[Q]
Granulomatous mastitis	Can be a manifestation of systemic granulomatous diseases (e.g., granulomatosis with polyangiitis, sarcoidosis, TB, fungi) or of disorders that are localized to the breast (granulomatous lobular mastitis)[Q]

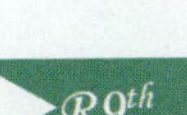

Latest Update

Lymphocytic Mastopathy (Sclerosing Lymphocytic Lobulitis)
- Presents with single or multiple hard palpable masses or mammographic densities [Q]
- Most common in women with **type 1 (insulin-dependent) diabetes** or **autoimmune thyroid disease**
- Granulomatous lobular mastitis is an uncommon disease that only occurs in parous women. [Q]-Caused by a hypersensitivity reaction to antigens expressed during lactation [Q]
- Cystic neutrophilic granulomatous mastitis is caused by Corynebacteria [Q]

Benign Epithelial Lesions

Non-proliferative breast changes (fibrocystic changes):

Cysts	Fibrosis	Adenosis
• Form by the dilation of lobules • **Bluedome cysts-** turbid, semi-translucent fluid of a brown or blue color in unopened cysts • Calcifications are common and may be detected by mammography	Cysts frequently rupture ↓ Release of secretory material into adjacent stroma ↓ Chronic inflammation & fibrous scarring lead to palpable firmness of the breast.	• Increase in number of acini per lobule • Acini - lined by columnar cells, • Benign or **show nuclear atypia ("flat epithelial atypia").**

High Yield Facts

- Flat epithelial atypia is **a clonal proliferation associated with deletions of chromosome 16q.** [Q]
- **Earliest recognizable precursor of low-grade breast cancers,** but does not convey an increased cancer risk

Proliferative Breast Disease without Atypia

Associated with a small increase in the risk of subsequent carcinoma in either breast[Q]

Epithelial Hyperplasia	• Defined by the **presence of more than two cell layers** [Q] • Normally, only myoepithelial cells & **single layer of luminal cells** are present
Sclerosing Adenosis	• Increased number of acini **compressed & distorted in central portion** of lesion but **dilated at the periphery;** Myoepithelial cells are usually prominent
Complex Sclerosing Lesion	• Have components of sclerosing adenosis, papillomas & epithelial hyperplasia. • One member of this group, the radial sclerosing lesion ("radial scar") • Radial scars are stellate lesions with a **central nidus of entrapped glands in a hyalinized stroma**
Papillomas	• Papillomas grows within a **dilated duct** • **Large duct papillomas** are situated in **lactiferous sinuses of the nipple (solitary with nipple discharge)** • **Small duct papillomas** are **multiple & located deeper within the ductal system** & usually present as **small palpable masses, or densities/ calcifications on mammogram**

Proliferative Breast Disease with Atypia

- Proliferative disease with atypia includes (ADH) and (ALH).
- Atypical hyperplasia is a clonal proliferation having some, but not all, of the histologic features that are required for the diagnosis of carcinoma in situ.

	Atypical ductal hyperplasia (ADH)	Atypical lobular hyperplasia (ALH)
Morphology	Histologic resemblance to ductal carcinoma in situ Monomorphic cells only partially fill involved ducts. [Q]	Resembles lobular carcinoma in situ Cells do not fill or distend **more than 50%**[Q] of the acini within a lobule
Mutation	Loss of 16q or gain of 17p[q]	Loss of E-cadherin[q]

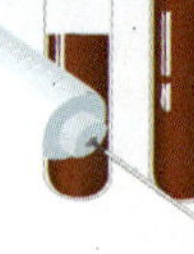

Epithelial Breast Lesions and the Risk of Developing Invasive Carcinoma

Pathological lesion	Relative Risk (Absolute Lifetime Risk)*
Nonproliferative Breast Changes (Fibrocystic changes)	1 (3%)[Q]
Proliferative Disease Without Atypia	1.5 to 2 (5%-7%)[Q]
Proliferative Disease with Atypia	4 to 5 (13%-17%)[Q]
Carcinoma in Situ	8 to 10 (25%-30%)[Q]

CARCINOMA OF THE BREAST

Based on the expression of estrogen receptor and HER2:

- Estrogen receptor (ER)-positive, HER2-negative (50% to 65% of tumors);[Q]
- HER2-positive (10% to 20% of tumors, which may either be ER-positive or ER-negative);[Q]
- ER-negative, HER2-negative (10% to 20% of tumors).[Q]

Etiology and Pathogenesis

- **Major risk factors** for the development of breast cancer are **genetic and hormonal**[Q]
- 12% of breast cancers occur due to inheritance of an identifiable susceptibility gene or genes.[Q]
- **Major risk factors for sporadic breast cancer are related to hormone exposure: gender, age at menarche and menopause, reproductive history, breastfeeding, and exogenous estrogens.**[Q]

Hereditary Breast Cancer

Gene (Location)	% of "Single Gene"	Risk by Age 70	Other Associated Cancers	Comments
BRCA1 **(17q)**[Q]	**52%** [Q]	40%- 90%	**Ovarian, male breast cancer** (but lower than BRCA2), prostate, pancreas, fallopian tube	**Poorly differentiated** and **triple negative**[Q] (basal-like)
BRCA2 **(13q)**[Q]	32%	30%-90%	**Ovarian, male breast cancer**, prostate, pancreas, stomach, melanoma, gallbladder, bile duct, pharynx	Bi-allelic germline Mutations; **Fanconi anemia**[Q]
TP53 **(17p)** Li-Fraumeni	3%	>90%[Q]	**Sarcoma, leukemia, brain tumors,** adrenocortical carcinoma	**MC sporadic breast Ca**[Q]
CHEK2 (22q)	5%	10%-20%	**Prostate, thyroid, kidney, colon**	**Increase risk for breast Ca after radiation exposure**[Q]

High Yield Facts

- BRCA1 and BRCA2 80- 90% of "single gene" familial breast cancers and 3% of all breast cancers
- BRCA1-associated breast cancers are poorly differentiated, have "medullary features" (a syncytial growth pattern with pushing margins and a lymphocytic infiltrate) and are triple negative (ER, PR,Her2neu negative)
- BRCA2-associated breast carcinomas also poorly differentiated, but are ER-positive
- Three other tumor suppressor genes—PTEN (Cowden syndrome), STK11 (Peutz-Jeghers syndrome), and ATM (ataxia telangiectasia)→<1% of all familial breast cancers.

CLASSIFICATION OF BREAST CARCINOMA

Noninvasive Carcinomas (Carinoma in situ)

Noninvasive carcinomas (carinoma in situ) may be located within the ducts (intraductal carcinoma) or within the lobules (lobular carcinoma in situ).

DCIS (Ductal Carcinoma in situ)

- Among the mammographically detected cancer, almost half are DCIS.[Q]

- DCIS most frequently presents as **mammographic calcifications**.[Q]

Histological types of DCIS (five types)

- Comedo carcinoma [Q]
- Cribriform [Q]
- Micropappilary[Q]
- Solid
- Papillary [Q]

Ductal carcinoma in situ (DCIS)

- Malignant clonal proliferation of epithelial cells limited to **ducts** by the **basement membrane**.
- **Myoepithelial cells are preserved**[Q] in involved ducts/lobules
- **Detected** by mammography as **calcifications**[Q]
- Divided into comedo and non-comedo- cribriform carcinoma, and intraductal papillary carcinoma
- **Comedocarcinoma-solid intraductal sheet of cells** with a central area of **necrosis**- undergoes calcification, can rarely present as **palpable mass**[Q]
- Associated with **erb B2/neu oncogene and poor prognosis.**
- Cribriform carcinoma: **round, duct like structures**[Q] within the solid intraductal sheet of epithelial cells
- Intraductal papillary carcinoma has a **papillary pattern.**[Q]

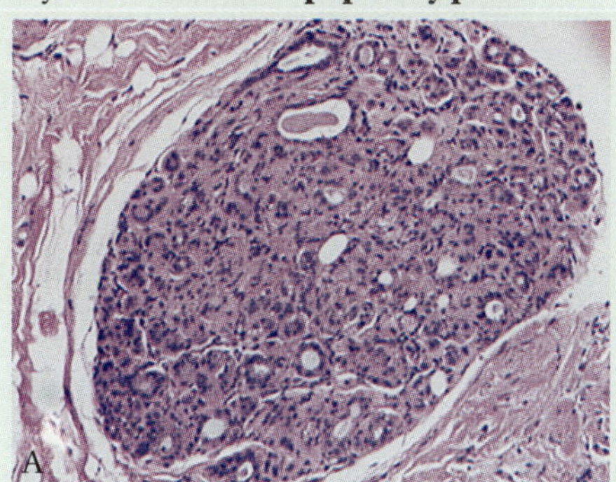

Lobular carcinoma in situ (LCIS)

- **Incidental biopsy finding**[Q]
- **Not associated with calcifications** or stromal reactions that produce mammographic densities
- **Bilateral in 20% to 40% of cases**
- LCIS is more common in **young women**,
- 80 - 90% of cases occurring before menopause.
- Cells **lack the cell adhesion protein E-cadherin**
- LCIS always expresses **ER and PR**

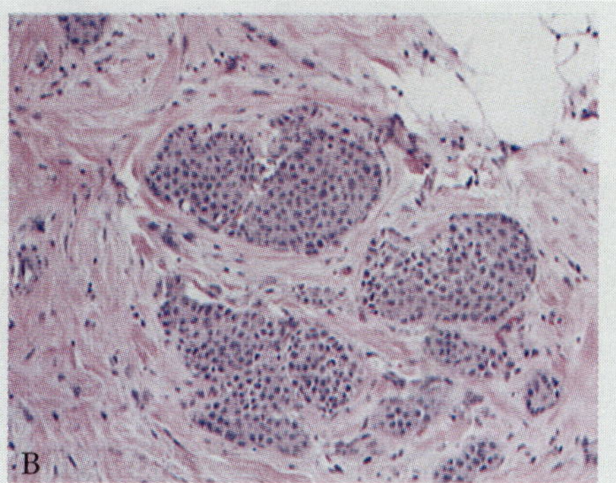

> **R 9th**   **Latest** Update
>
> **DCIS with microinvasion**
> - When there is an area of invasion through the basement membrane into stroma measuring no more than 0.1 cm. [Q]

INVASIVE (INFILTRATING) CARCINOMA

- Divided on the basis of molecular and morphologic characteristics

Molecular subtypes:

Molecular profiling of breast cancer is done on gene **profiling** [Q]

A. ER-positive, HER- negative (also termed "luminal" 60-70%):

- **Most common form**[Q] **of invasive breast cancer.**[Q]
- Essentially all are well differentiated carcinomas.
- Mucinous, papillary, cribriform, and lobular patterns may be present in this group[Q]

Based on proliferation rates, it is further divided into two subgroups.

ER-positive, HER2-negative, low proliferation (40% -55%) **Luminal A**	• **Most common form of invasive breast cancer.** [Q] • Majority of cancers in **older women and in men.** [Q] • MC type detected by mammographic screening and in women treated with menopausal hormone therapy [Q] • **Lowest incidence** of local **recurrence** & often **cured by surgery** [Q] • Respond well to hormonal treatment with long survival [Q] • **Metastasise late** but usually to bone.[Q]
ER-positive, HER2-negative, high proliferation (10%): **Luminal B**	• Most common type of carcinoma associated with **BRCA2 germline mutations**[Q]

B. HER2-positive (20% of cancers): 2nd MC subtype of invasive breast cancer

- **More common in young women and in non-white women.** [Q]
- **Majority of these carcinomas are poorly differentiated tumors** [Q]
- **No specific morphologic pattern associated with this cell type**
- **50% of apocrine**[Q] **Carcinomas and 40% of micropapillary carcinomas belong to this category.**[Q]
- **The associated DCIS is often extensive** [Q]
- >50% tumors **with germlineTP53 mutations** (Li-Fraumeni syndrome) develop carcinomas of this subtype
- Responds to trastuzumab (Herceptin),- humanized monoclonal antibody that specifically binds and inhibits HER2

C. ER-negative, HER2-negative tumors ("basal-like" triple negative Ca; 15%)-young premenopausal women as well as African American and Hispanic women

- The majority of carcinomas arising in women with BRCA1 mutations are of this type [Q]
- Almost all of these tumors are poorly differentiated.
- Spindle cell, squamous, and matrix producing patterns can also be seen. [Q]
- DCIS is generally very limited or not present. [Q]
- Cancers can metastasize when small in size, frequently to viscera and to the brain. [Q]
- Characterised by rapid growth, high proliferation-present as a palpable mass in the interval between mammographic screenings [Q]
- 30% completely respond to chemotherapy [Q]
- Local recurrence is common [Q]
- Express markers of typical myoepithelial cells (e.g. basal keratins, P-cadherin, p63 or laminin), progenitor cells or putative stem cells (cytokeratin 5 and 6) [Q]

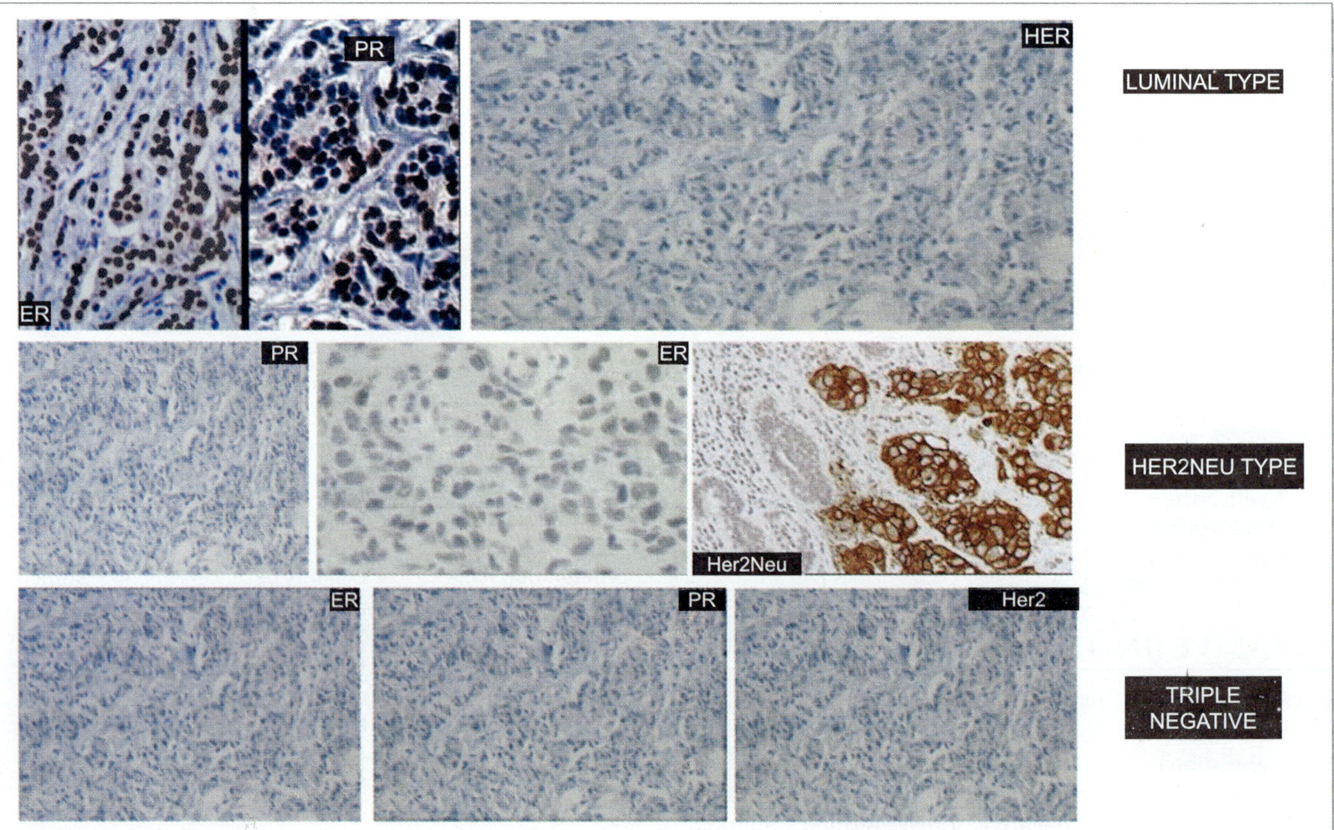

On the basis of morphology:

Invasive breast carcinoma 2 types: No- special type carcinoma (Intraductal) & Special carcinoma

Invasive Carcinoma, No Special Type (NST; Invasive Ductal Carcinoma) [Q]

- Majority of carcinomas (70 to 80%) belong to this subtype.
- **They MC present as a hard, irregular radiodense mass associated with a desmoplastic stromal reaction** [Q]
- On gross examination, most carcinomas are firm to" hard and have an irregular border.
- All types of invasive carcinoma are graded using **Modified Bloom Richardson Score.** [Q]
- Carcinomas are scored for **tubule formation, nuclear pleomorphism, and mitotic rate** [Q]
- The points added to divide carcinomas into grade I (well differentiated), grade II (moderately differentiated), and grade III (poorly differentiated) types.

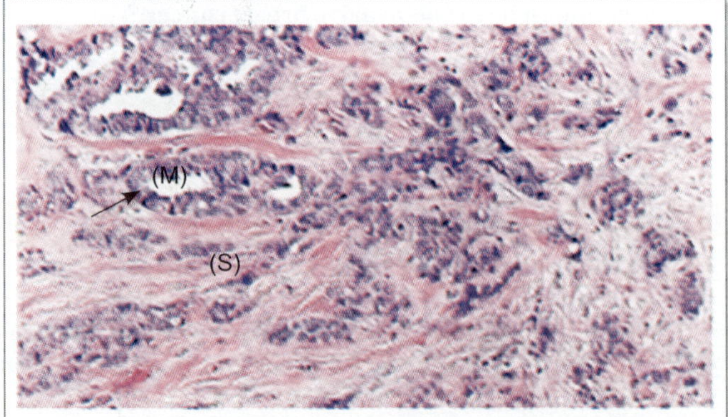

Inrasire ductal Ca: Malignant glands (M) inrading stroma (S)

Special -subtypes

• Lobular	• Cribriform	• Colloid
• Medullary	• Tubular	• Papillary
• Metaplastic	• Inflammatory carcinoma	• Micropapillary carcinoma
• Apocrine carcinoma		

Special histologic types of breast cancer often harbor unique genetic aberrations, sometimes have **distinct gene signatures**

1. Lobular carcinoma (invasive) of breast

- **Most cases show biallelic loss of expression of CDH1[Q] R9th, the gene that encodes E-cadherin.[Q]**
- **Loss of E-cadherin, lobular carcinomas are discohesive[Q] and fail to incite a desmoplastic response** [Q]
- **Seen bilaterally**
- **Most common type of breast carcinoma to present as an occult primary** [Q]
- **Characteristic patterns of metastatic spread:** involving the peritoneum and retroperitoneum, the leptomeninges (carcinomatous meningitis), the gastrointestinal tract, and the ovaries and uterus.[Q]
- **Histologic hallmark:** presence of discohesive infiltrating tumor cells as single cells in **single file pattern** [Q], **including signet-ring cells** [Q] **containing intracytoplasmic mucin droplets**[Q]
- Tubule formation is absent.
- Males and females with heterozygous germline mutations in CDH1 also have a greatly increased risk **of gastric signet ring cell carcinoma**[Q]

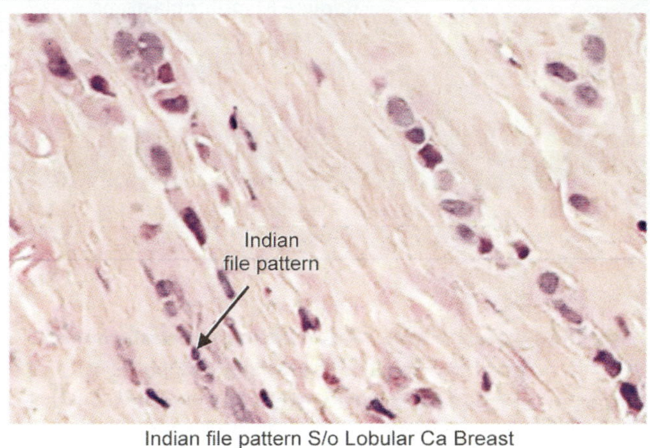

Indian file pattern S/o Lobular Ca Breast

2. Medullary Carcinoma

- Characterised by features that are characteristic of BRCA1-associated carcinomas.
- Comes under the category of **ER-negative, HER2-negative tumors**[Q]
- DCIS is **minimal or absent.**[Q]
- The tumor has a **soft, fleshy consistency and is well-circumscribed**
- Medullary carcinomas have **better prognosis** than do NST carcinomas[Q]

Characterized by

- Solid, syncytium-like sheets (occupying more than 75% of the tumor) of large cells with vesicular, pleomorphic nuclei, containing prominent nucleoli
- Frequent mitotic figures
- A moderate to marked lymphoplasmacytic infiltrate surrounding and within the tumor
- Pushing (non-infiltrative) border

R9th Latest Update

Current WHO classification system recommends grouping medullary carcinomas with similar carcinomas into one group termed "carcinomas with medullary features."[Q]

ER-negative, HER2-negative tumors
• Secretory carcinoma
• Spindle cell carcinoma
• Low-grade adenosquamous carcinoma
• Adenoid cystic carcinoma
• Medullary carcinoma

R9th Latest Update

Two special histologic types frequently overexpress HER2

Apocrine carcinoma	Micropapillary carcinoma
Resemble the cells that line sweat glands.	Shows a characteristic pattern of anchorage-independent growth. [Q] Although the cells are adherent to each other and express E-cadherin, they lack adhesion to the stroma [Q]

High Yield Facts

- *Special type carcinomas carry good prognosis but inflammatory carcinoma has poor prognosis*
- **Both lobular carcinoma of breast and signet ring carcinoma of GIT are characterized by the loss of E-cadherin** [Q]

PROGNOSTIC FACTORS

Major

- **Invasive carcinoma** has worse prognosis than in-situ carcinoma
- Distant **metastasis** indicates bad prognosis.

Lymph node status:

- ***Axillary lymph node*** *status: most important prognostic factor for invasive ca in the absence of distant metastases.*[Q]
- *Sentinel lymph node status: If negative for metastasis, it is unlikely that other more distant nodes will be involved and the patient can be spared the morbidity of a complete axillary dissection*[Q]

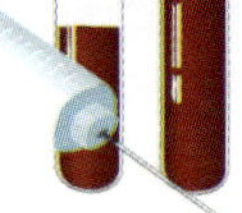

Lymphovascular invasion: strongly associated with the presence of lymph node metastases with poor prognostic factor

- **Tumor Size** <1 cm good prognosis, > 2 cm bad prognosis.
- **Local invasion** into skeletal muscle carries poor prognosis.
- **Inflammatory carcinoma** has poor prognosis

Minor

- **Molecular subtype**- explained above
- **Histological type:** Invasive ductal carcinoma (no special type; NST) carries poor prognosis.
- **Tubular, mucinous, lobular, papillary, adenoid cystic has better prognosis**
- **Metaplastic carcinoma or micro-papillary carcinoma have a poorer prognosis** [Q]
- Nottingham histological score (Scarff-Bloom-Ricahrdson **grade):** Grade 1 good prognosis, grade 3 poor
- **Estrogen and Progesterone receptor** positivity indicates **good response to anti-estrogen therapy.**
- **Strongly ER-positive cancers are less likely to respond to chemotherapy** [Q]
- **HER2/neu** overexpression: Poor prognosis
- High **proliferative rate** indicates worse prognosis
- **Aneuploidy** indicates bad prognosis

Male Breast Cancer

The incidence in breast cancer in men is only 1% of that in women

Risk Factors

- Increasing age [Q]
- First-degree relatives with breastcancer [Q]
- Exposure to exogenous estrogens or ionizing radiation [Q]
- Infertility [Q]
- Obesity [Q]
- Prior benign breast disease [Q]
- From 3% to 8% of cases areassociated with Klinefelter syndrome and decreased testicularfunction. [Q]
- From 4% to 14% of cases in males are attributed to germline BRCA2 mutations [Q]
- Male breast cancer is also observed in BRCA1 families, although not as frequently [Q]
- Most common histopathology- breast Carcinoma NSTQ
- ER positivity is more common [Q]
- Distant metastases to the lungs, brain, bone, and liver are common.
- Most cancers are treated locally with mastectomy and axillary node dissection

Stromal Tumors

Origin from intralobular carcinoma		Origin from interlobular carcinoma
Fibroadenoma: • Most common benign tumor of the female breast.[Q] • "Proliferative changes without atypia	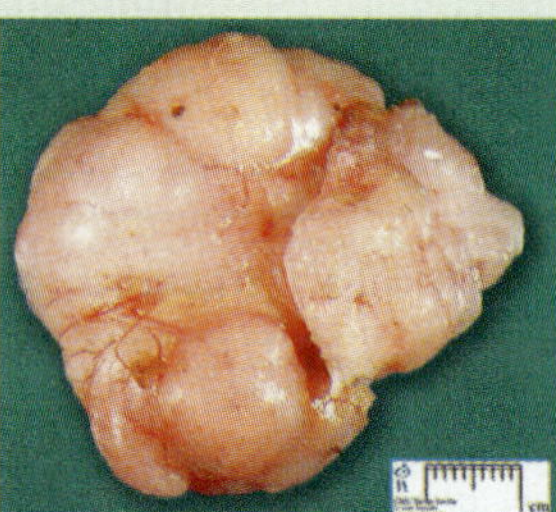 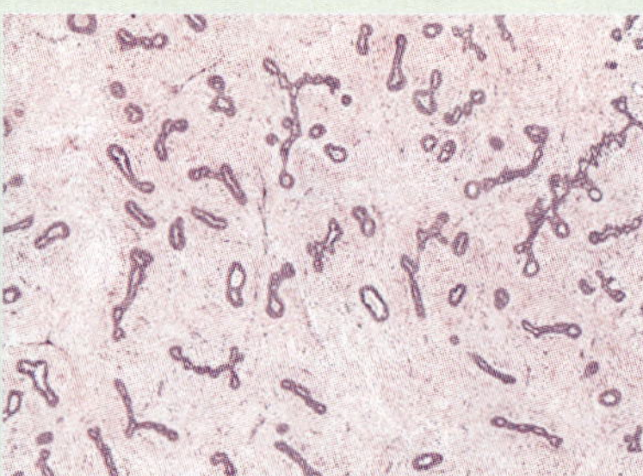	**Benign- Myofibroblastoma** only breast tumor that is equally common in males [Q]
Phyllodes Tumor/Cystosarcoma phyllodes: Gains in **chromosome 1q being the most frequent mutation** [Q] **Gross:** "leaf like due to stromal proliferations **Grade:** benign, intermediate and malignant	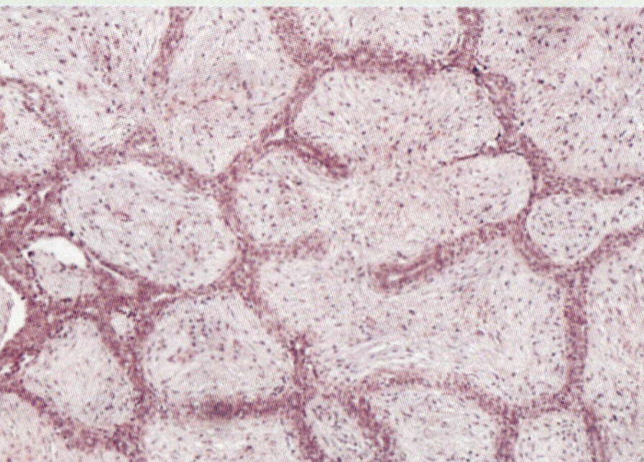	**Malignant:** • **Angiosarcoma: most common stromal malignancy** • Sporadic or associated with **radiation exposure or lymphedema.**[Q]

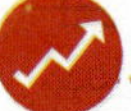

Complex fibroadenomas—fibroadenomas associated with cysts larger than 0.3 cm[Q], sclerosingadenosis[Q], epithelial calcifications[Q], or papillary apocrine change [Q]

NEXT Pattern Question

Q's

1. **24/f presented with painless left sided breast lump for last 2 months. Local examination revealed soft mobile, non tender mass. Excision biopsy was done and histopathological image is as shown below. What is your diagnosis?**

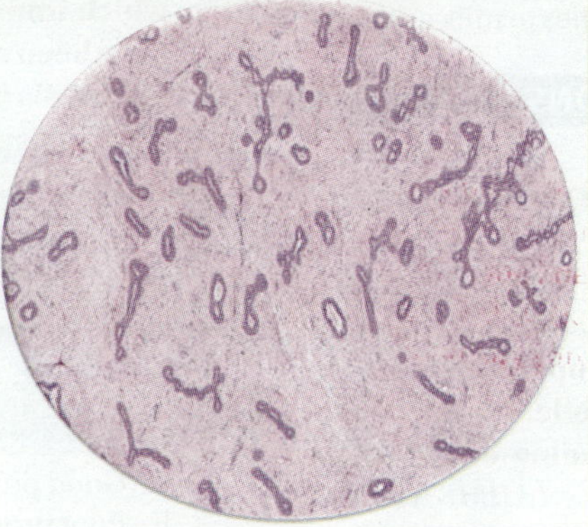

   a. Phyllodes tumor   b. Intraductal ca breast   c. Fibroadenoma   d. Ductal ca in situ

Ans. (c) Fibroadenoma
- Painless left sided breast lump which is soft mobile, non-tender mass looks like a benign lesion. The histopathology shows proliferation of pinkish stroma and ducts which have become distorted. This is suggestive of fibroadenoma.

Multiple Choice Questions

BREAST

INFLAMMATORY DISORDERS

1. **Granulomatous mastitis is caused by all except-**
(Recent Question 2014)

a. TB
b. Fungus
c. Staphylococcus
d. Antibodies to milk antigens

BENIGN EPITHELIAL LESIONS

2. **All are benign conditions except**

a. Fibroadenoma   *(Recent Question 2014-15)*
b. Cystosarcoma phyllodes
c. Pagets disease of nipple
d. Galactocele

3. **A 17/F underwent FNAC for a lump in the breast which was non-tender, firm and mobile. Which of the following features would suggest finding of a benign breast disease?**   *(AIIMS Nov 14)*

a. Dyscohesive ductal epithelial cells without cellular fragments
b. Tightly arranged ductal epithelial cells with bare nuclei
c. Stromal predominance with spindle cells
d. Polymorphism with single or arranged ductal epithelial cells

4. **Lesions affecting the terminal duct lobular unit (TDLU) in breast are all except -**   *(DPG 11)*

a. Nipple adenoma   b. Blunt duct adenosis
c. Intraductal papilloma   d. Fiboadenoma

CARCINOMA OF THE BREAST

5. **A 30-year-old female presented with 4 cm mass in the right breast. Biopsy showed densely packed cells with bland nuclei and mucin infiltrating the stroma. What is your diagnosis?**   *(Recent Pattern Question 2020)*

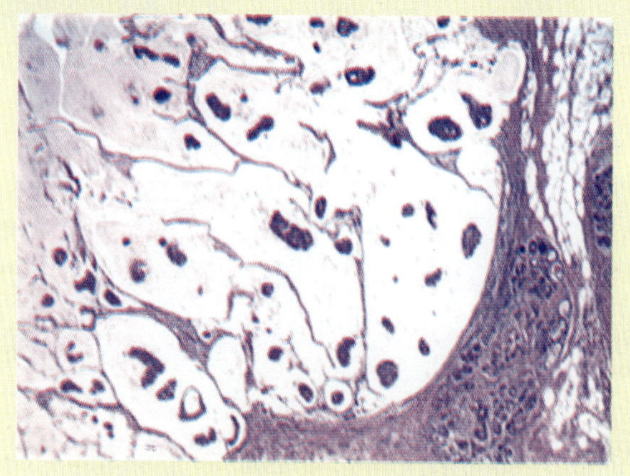

a. Invasive papillary carcinoma
b. Medullary carcinoma
c. Apocrine carcinoma
d. Colloid carcinoma

6. **Van Nuys prognostic indicator for DCIS does not include which of the following parameter?**
(Recent exam 2018)

a. DCIS size   b. Age of the patient
c. Type of DCIS   d. Excision margin

7. **The pictures below show breast biopsy specimen on which immu nohistochemical for ER,PR and Her2 neu have been done. Which of the following is true about the prognosis of the patient?**   *(AIIMS May 16)*

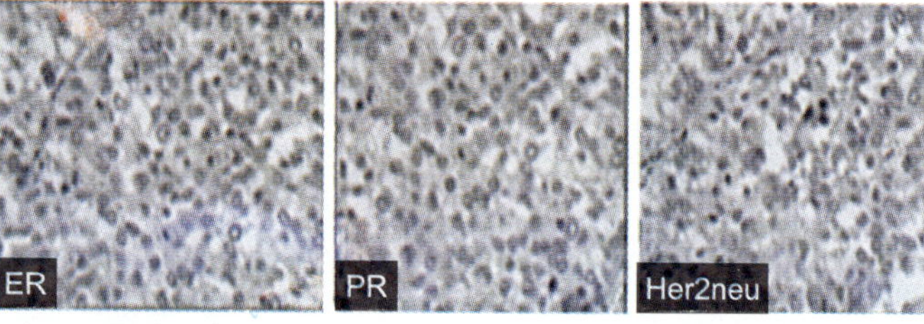

a. Good prognosis
b. Poor prognosis
c. Good prognosis with transtuzumab therapy can be given
d. Good prognosis without transtuzumab therapy should not be given

8. **Most important prognostic factor in Ca. Breast.**

a. Lymph Node status   *(JIPMER 16)*
b. Tumor Size
c. Progesterone receptor status
d. Stage

9. **Somatic mutation E17K in the PH domain of AKT-1 gene mutation is associated with?**
(Recent Question 2016)

a. Stomach   b. Breast
c. Ovary   d. Pancreas

10. **Cancer detected in one breast which to bl screened in contralateral breast**   *(Recent Question 2016)*

a. Lobular   b. Ductal
c. medullary   d. colloid

11. **Male breast cancer wrong statement-**

a. Brca2 seen in 6% cases   *(Recent Question 2016)*
b. Lobular carcinoma is common
c. DUCTAL carcimoma is most common subtype
d. Colloid carcinoma can be seen

12. **Cystosarcoma phylloides, true is?**   *(PGI Nov 2015)*

a. It has a spectrum of benign to malignant
b. Can be rarely seen in children
c. Always malignant
d. Always benign
e. Seen in elderly females

13. **Following is not true about the gene mutations leading to breast carcinoma**   *(Recent Question 2014-15)*

a. Most common mutation in inherited breast carcinoma is BRCA1
b. BRCA 1 mutation is present in most of the cases of breast carcinoma
c. Inherited breast carcinomas make about 3 % of the total cases
d. p53 mutation also increases chances of colon and brain cancer

14. **Breast CA with best prognosis** *(Recent Question 2015)*
    a. Mucinous
    b. Medullary
    c. Invasive ductal
    d. Lobular Ca

15. **All of the following are invasive carcinoma breast except-** *(Recent Question 2015)*
    a. Comedo carcinoma
    b. Colloid carcinoma
    c. Lobular carcinoma
    c. Medullary carcinoma

16. **The type of mammary ductal carcinoma in situ (DCIS) most likely to result in a palpable abnormality in the breast is:** *(Recent Question 2014)*
    a. Apocrine DCIS
    b. Neuroendocrine DCIS
    c. Well differentiated DCIS
    d. Comedo DCIS

17. **Molecular classification of breast cancer is based on?** *(AIIMS Nov 14)*
    a. Gene profiling
    b. ER, PR, and HER-2 neu
    c. histology
    d. Mutations

18. **The most common site for lymphagiosarcoma is:** *(AP PGMEE 14)*
    a. Liver
    b. Spleen
    c. Post mastectomy arm
    d. Retroperitoneum

19. **True about histology in infilterating lobular breast carcinoma:** *(JIPMER 11)*
    a. Single file pattern
    b. Pleomorphic cells in sheets
    c. Cribriform pattern
    d. Pin wheel pattern

20. **Modified Bloom Richardson criteria for CA breast includes:** *(PGI May 2010)*
    a. Desmoplasia
    b. Lymphovenous embolism
    c. Mitotic rate
    d. Tubule formation
    e. Nuclear polymorphism

21. **Breast Ca is not a/w:** *(PGI May 10)*
    a. BRCA I & BRCA 2
    b. Apocrine metaplasia
    c. Atypical ductal hyperplasia
    d. Fibroadenoma
    e. Moderate hyperplasia

22. **Most common carcinoma of breast is:** *(Recent Question 2016, MH PGMEE 2016, TN 97)*
    a. Ductal carcinoma
    b. Colloid carcinoma
    c. Lobular carcinoma
    d. Sarcoma phylloides

23. **Malignancy of the Breast is likely to be associated with** *(MH PGMEE 16, AI 94)*
    a. Sclerosing adenosis
    b. Atypical epithelial hyperplasia
    c. Cystic change
    d. Apocrine metaplasis

Answers with Explanations

1.   Ans. (c) Staphylococcus (*Ref: Robbins 9th/pg 1047*)

- **Granulomatous mastitis:** Can be a manifestation of systemic granulomatous diseases (e.g., granulomatosis with polyangiitis, sarcoidosis, TB, fungi) or of disorders that are localized to the breast (granulomatous lobular mastitis)[Q]

Granulomatous lobular mastitis- only occurs in parous women, caused by a **hypersensitivity reaction to antigens expressed during lactation**[Q]

2.   Ans. (c) Pagets disease of nipple

(*Ref: Robbins 9th/pg 1057*)

Option a and d are clearly benign
We get confused in option b and c
Now cystosarcoma phyllodes are usually benign but can be borderline or rarely malignant also
Mammary Pagets disease is always associated with an underlying carcinoma of the breast. Mammary Paget cells are malignant epithelial cells derived from underlying ductal adenocarcinoma of the breast that invade into the skin of nipple and areolar areas.

3.   Ans. (b) Tightly arranged ductal epithelial cells with bare nuclei

(*Ref: Gray Diagnostic Cytopathology 2nd ed: 279-80*)

- Option A- Dyscohesive ductal epithelial cells without cellular fragments- feature of ductal carcinoma
- Option B- **Tightly arranged ductal epithelial cells with bare nuclei- fibroadenoma (benign disease)**
- Option C- Stromal predominance with spindle cells- phyllodes tumor
- Option D- Polymorphism with single or arranged ductal epithelial cells- tubular carcinoma

4.   Ans. (a) Nipple adenoma (*Ref: Robbins 9th/pg 1044*)

Lesions arising from various parts of breast:

Normal	Lesions
Lobules and terminal ducts (Terminal Duct Lobular Unit or TDLU)	• Cyst, Adenosis, Multiple papillomatosis • Sclerosing adenomas • Hyperplasia, Atypical hyperplasia • Carcinoma
Large ducts	• Duct ectasia, Single intraductal papilloma • **Nipple adenoma**[Q], large duct adenoma • Squamous metaplasia of lactiferous ducts • Paget disease[Q]
Intralobular stroma	• Fibroadenoma (focal hyperplasia of stroma & epithelial component of TDLU) • Phyllodes tumor
Interlobular stroma	• Fat necrosis • Lipoma • Sarcoma

5.   Ans. (d) Colloid carcinoma (*Ref: Robbins 9th/pg 1057*)

6.   Ans. (c) Type of DCIS

(*Ref: Sterenberg diagnostic surgical pathology 5th ed p 312*)

The Van Nuys Prognostic Index (VNPI) classifies patients with DCIS to guide decisions on the best treatment option. The index uses patient age, tumour size, tumour growth patterns (histological grade) and the amount of healthy tissue surrounding the tumour after removal (resection margin width) to predict the risk of cancer returning.

7.   Ans. (b) Poor prognosis

(*Ref: Ref: Robbins 9th/pg 1064 Complete review of pathology 2nd ed/ pg 656*)

- The given image shows the breast tissue negatively stained for all three i.e ER, PR and Her2 neu.(called Triple negative); it signifies poor prognosis

8.   Ans. (a) Lymph Node status

(*Ref: Ref: Robbins 9th/pg 1064 Complete review of pathology 2nd ed/ pg 656*)

Axillary LN status is the most important prognostic indicator in breast ca

9.   Ans. (b) Breast

(*Ref: Atlasgeneticsoncology.org/Genes/AKT1*)

Hyper-activation of AKT1 has been found associated to several human cancers:
- Thyroid carcinoma
- Breast carcinoma
- Non-small cell lung carcinoma
- Gastric carcinoma

Now coming to question: Somatic mutation E17K occurs in the PH domain of AKT1 in 8% of human breast cancers. This mutation also occurs in 6% of colorectal cancers.

10.   Ans. (a) Lobular (*Ref: Robbins 9th/pg 1065; 8th/pg 1085*)

Lobular carcinomas are usually bilateral

11.   Ans. (b) Lobular carcinoma is common

(*Ref: Robbins 9th/pg 1054*)

From 4% to 14% of cases in males are attributed to germline BRCA2 mutations –OPTION A IS TRUE
Structure of the male breast does not have lobules and acini, lobular carcinoma cases are seen infrequently- OPTION B IS FALSE
Most common breast cancer in male is ductal carcimnoma NOS
Colloid carcinoma can be seen.

12. Ans. (a, b, e); a. it has a spectrum of benign to malignant; b. Can be rarely seen in children; e. Seen in elderly females *(Ref: Robbins 9th/pg 1051)*

It has a spectrum of benign to malignant- true

Phyllodes tumors occurs in a median age of fifth decade of life

Rare reports of phyllodes tumor in children have been described.

13. Ans. (b) BRCA 1 mutation is present in most of the cases of breast carcinoma

(Ref: Robbins 9th/pg 1054; 8th/pg 1077)

a. Most common gene involved in familial breast can-cer-BRCA1(52%) > BRCA1(32%)
b. **p53 mutation is present in most of the cases of breast carcinoma**
c. Inherited breast carcinomas make about 3 % of the total cases
d. p53 mutation increases risk of all cancers

14. Ans. (a) Mucinous *(Ref: Robbins 9th/pg 1064-65)*

- **Histological type:** Invasive ductal carcinoma (no special type; NST) carries poor prognosis.
- **Tubular, mucinous, lobular, papillary, adenoid cystic has better prognosis**
  - **Metaplastic carcinoma or micro-papillary carcinoma have a poorer prognosis[Q]**
  Remember mucinous > lobular

15. Ans. (a) Comedo carcinoma *(Ref: Robbins 9th/pg 1057)*

16. Ans. (d) Comedo DCIS *(Ref: 9th/pg 1057; 8th/pg 1080)*

Comedocarcinoma-solid intraductal sheet of cells with a central area of **necrosis**- undergoes calcification, can rarely present as **palpable mass[Q]**

17. Ans. (a) Gene profiling

(Ref: R 9th/pg 1061; 8th/pg 1080)

Molecular profiling of breast cancer is done on gene profiling[Q]
Gene profiling, measures relative quantities of mRNA for every gene, has 5 major patterns of gene expression.

18. Ans. (c) Post mastectomy arm *(Ref: Cancer 1948;1:64–81)*

- Lymphangiosarcoma is a misnomer because this malignancy seems to arise from blood vessels instead of lymphatic vessels.
- Most commonly, this tumor is a result of **lymphedema induced by radical mastectomy**
- **Stewart-Treves syndrome** is a rare, cutaneous angiosarcoma that develops in long-standing chronic lymphedema.

19. Ans. (a) Single file pattern *(Ref: R 9th/pg 1065; 8th/pg 1085)*

Lobular carcinoma (invasive) of breast-Histologic hallmark: presence of discohesive infiltrating tumor cells as single cells in single file pattern[Q], including signet-ring cells[Q] containing intracytoplasmic mucin droplets[Q]

20. Ans. (c, d, e); c. Mitotic rate; d. Tubule formation; e. Nuclear polymorphism *(Ref: Robbins 9th/pg 1064)*

- Invasive carcinoma are graded using **Modified Bloom Richardson Score.[Q]**
- Carcinomas are scored for **tubule formation, nuclear pleomorphism, and mitotic rate[Q]**
- The points added to divide carcinomas into grade I (well differentiated), grade II (moderately differentiated), and grade III (poorly differentiated) types.

21. Ans. (b, d); b. Apocrine metaplasia; d. Fibroadenoma
(Ref: Robbins 9th/pg 1051)

Apocrine metaplasia and fibroadenoma do not increase the risk of breast cancer.
All other 3 increase the risk of breast carcinoma.

Pathologic Lesion	Relative Risk (Absolute Life time Risk)
Nonproliferative Breast Changes (Fibrocystic changes) • Duct ectasia • Cysts, Adenosis, mild hyperplasia • Apocrine change • Fibrodenoma **without[Q]** complex features	1 (3%)[Q]
Proliferative Disease Without Atypia • Moderate or florid hyperplasia • Sclerosing adenosis • Papilloma • Complex sclerosing lesion (radial scar) • Fibroadenoma **with[Q]** complex features	1.5 to 2 (5% - 7%)[Q]
Proliferative Disease with Atypia • Atypical ductal hyperplasia (ADH) • Atypical lobular hyperplasia (ALH)	4 to 5 (13% - 17%)[Q]
Carcinoma in Situ • Lobular carcinoma in situ (LCIS) • Ductal carcinoma in situ (DCIS)	8 to 10 (20% - 30%)[Q]

22. Ans. (a) Ductal carcinoma *(Ref: Robbins 9th/pg 1057)*

- Almost all (>95%) of breast malignancies are adenocar-cinomas that first arise in the duct/lobular system as carcinoma in situ
- Distribution of invasive carcinoma, breast
- **Invasive Ductal Carcinoma**-70 to 80%
- **Invasive lobular Carcinoma**-10%
- **Mucinous**- 2%

23. Ans. (b) Atypical epithelial hyperplasia

(Ref: Robbins 9th/pg 1051)

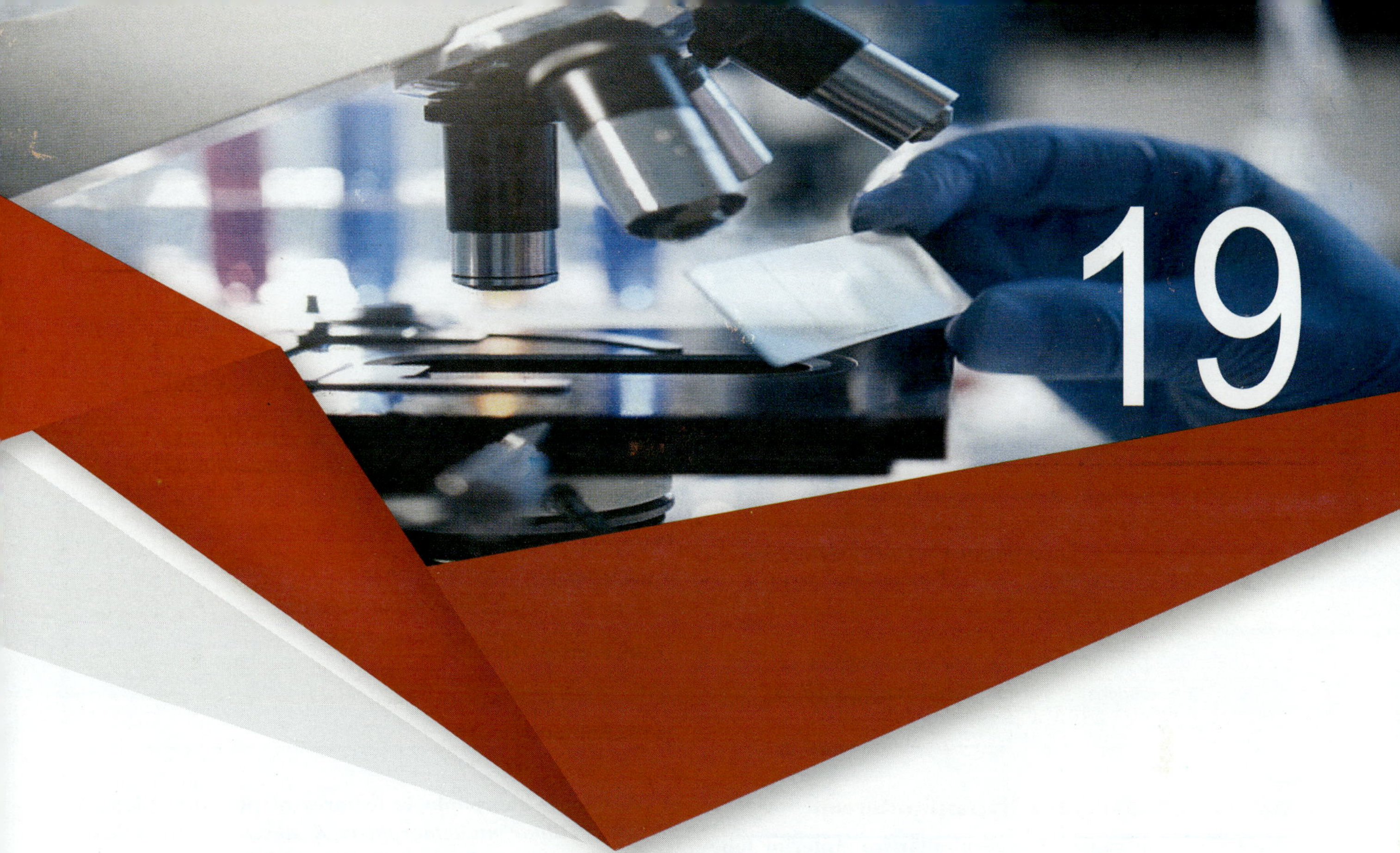

19

Endocrine System and its Disorders

Key Points

- Anterior lobe (adenohypophysis) consists of 80% of pituitary gland
- MC cause of hyperpituitarism is anterior lobe adenoma
- **Graves disease** is the most common cause of endogenous **hyperthyroidism & thyrotoxicosis**
- **Hürthle cell metaplasia or Oxyphil** change are a feature of **Hashimoto's Thyroiditis**
- Most common thyroid Cancer is **Papillary carcinoma**
- **Orphan Annie eye nuclei is a characteristic feature of papillary cell Ca thyroid**
- **Integrity of capsule** is most important in distinguishing **follicular adenomas from follicular Ca**
- **Most consistent** feature of **Diabetic nephropathy is diffuse thickening of basement membrane**
- **Earliest** manifestation of **Diabetic Nephropathy is Microalbuminuria**
- **Most common** cause of **primary adrenal insufficiency** in developed countries is **Autoimmune** adrenalitis while in India, it is **Tubercular adrenalitis** in **India**
- **Most common** subtype of congenital adrenal hyperplasia is caused by **deficiency of the enzyme 21-hydroxylase**
- **Primary hyperparathyroidism** is the most common manifestation of **Multiple Endocrine Neoplasia (MEN)-1**
- **Duodenum** is the **most common site of gastrinomas in individuals with MEN-1**

Key Recent Updates

- Most common mutation in papillary carcinoma, thyroid is **BRAF**
- Wet keratin is characteristic of craniopharyngioma.

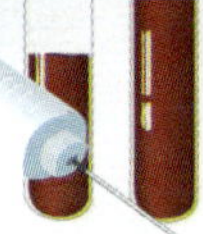

PITUITARY GLAND

Composed of two **morphologically** and **functionally distinct** components:

- **Anterior lobe (adenohypophysis): 80% of gland**[Q]
- **Posterior lobe (neurohypophysis):** 20% of the gland;

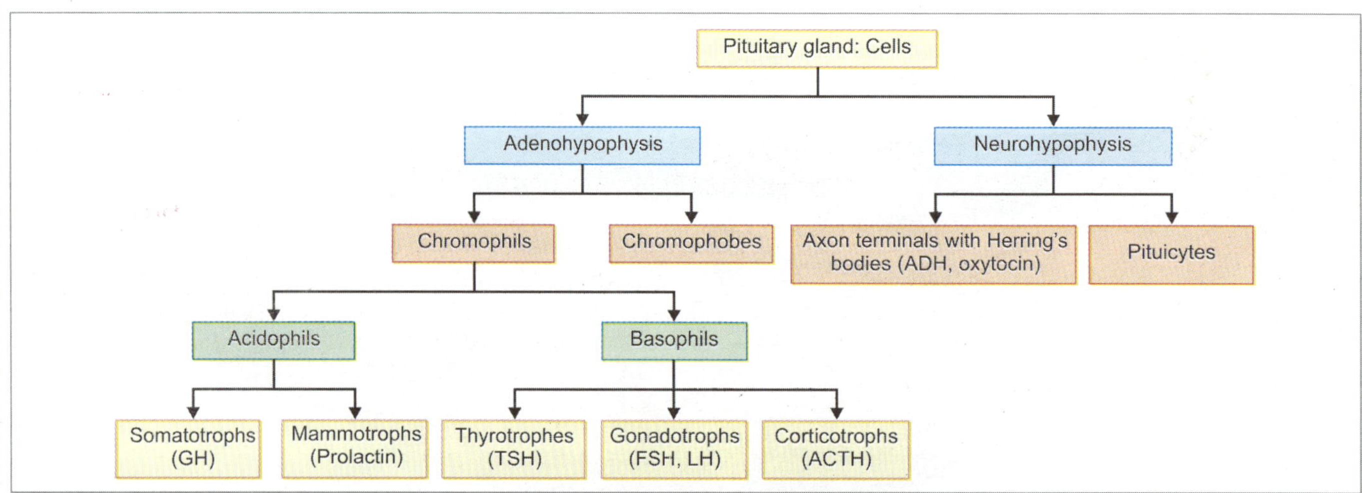

Pituitary Adenomas and Hyperpituitarism

- **Most Common cause of hyperpituitarism: Anterior lobe adenoma**[Q] > **Pituitary Carcinoma**[Q]
- GH and prolactin are the most common hormones secreted from Adenoma

Genetic Alterations in Pituitary Tumors

- Gain of function of: GNAS, PRKAR 1A, Cyclin D1, HRAS genes
- Loss of function of: MEN1, CDKN1B (p27), AIP, RB genes

Classification of Pituitary Adenomas

- Functional (i.e., associated with **hormone excess** and its clinical manifestations)
- **Non-functioning** (i.e., No hormone excess, **only mass effect**)
- **Microadenomas (<1 cm) (most common)**[Q]
- Macroadenomas (>1 cm)
- **Most common pituitary tumor** is **Adenoma**[Q]
- Most common cause of **hyperpituitarism** is **anterior lobe Microadenoma**[Q]
- Most common type of **microadenoma is Prolactinoma**[Q] > GH-adenoma

- **Distinctive morphologic features of pituitary Adenoma are:** *Cellular monomorphism & absence of a reticulin network staining*[Q]

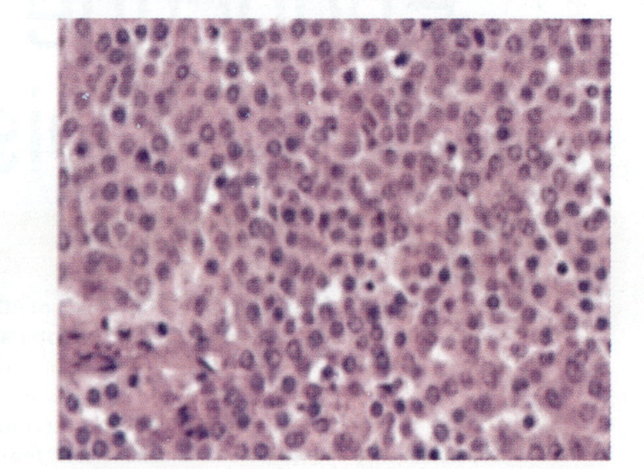

Two distinctive morphologic features **cellular monomorphism** and **absence of a reticulin network**

High Yield Facts

- Hormones secreted by posterior pituitary are: ADH (Vasopressin) & Oxytocin
- Crooke's hyaline change is seen in pituitary in Cushing syndrome. It is due to accumulation of cytokeratin intermediate filament

Posterior Pituitary Syndromes

- **Diabetes insipidus: ADH deficiency** → Excessive urination (polyuria) due to inability of kidney to reasorb water
- **Syndrome of inappropriate ADH (SIADH)**[Q]**: ADH excess** → resorption of excessive amounts of **free water**, resulting in **hyponatremia.**

HYPOTHALAMIC SUPRASELLAR TUMORS

- Result in **hyperfunction/ hypofunction** of the pituitary
- Most commonly **gliomas** and **craniopharyngiomas**

High Yield Facts

Craniopharyngiomas
3-4 cm, cause **mass effect**[Q] on optic chiasma or cranial nerves
Two distinct histologic variants: (Dystrophic calcification[Q] frequent in both)
- **Adamantinomatous** type: **(children)**[Q]: compact lamellar keratin formation
- **Papillary** type (adults)[Q]

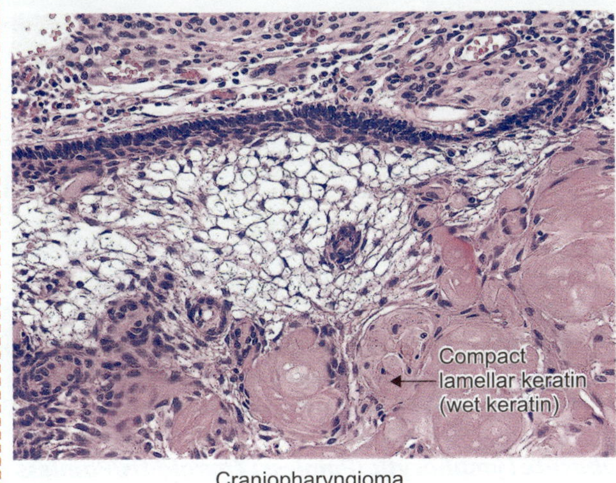

Craniopharyngioma

THYROID GLAND

Hyperthyroidism and Thyrotoxicosis

- **Thyrotoxicosis: A hypermetabolic state** caused by **elevated free T3 & T4**[Q]
- **Hyperthyroidism is hyperfunction of the thyroid gland**[Q]

High Yield Facts

- Thyroid **follicles** are lined by a **cuboidal to low columnar epithelium** filled with **PAS +ve thyroglobulin**
- **Hypothalamus** → TRH → **Thyrotrophs** (anterior pituitary)[Q] → TSH (thyrotropin)
- **Thyroid follicular epithelial cells** convert **thyroglobulin** into thyroxine **(T4)**[Q] & triiodothyronine **(T3)**[Q]
- **Parafollicular cells**, or C cells- synthesize and secrete the hormone **calcitonin**[Q]

Disorders Associated with Thyrotoxicosis

With Hyperthyroidism	Without Hyperthyroidism
Primary • **Graves disease**[Q] • **Toxic multinodular goiter**[Q] • **Toxic adenoma**[Q] • Iodine-induced hyperthyroidism • Neonatal thyrotoxicosis associated with maternal Graves disease *Secondary*: TSH-secreting pituitary adenoma	• Granulomatous (**de Quervain) thyroiditis**[Q] • **Subacute** lymphocytic thyroiditis (painless)[Q] • **Struma ovarii**: Ovarian teratoma with ectopic thyroid[Q] • Factitious thyrotoxicosis (exogenous thyroxine intake)

Grave's Disease

- *Most common:*
  - **Most common cause of endogenous hyperthyroidism**[Q]
  - **Most common cause of thyrotoxicosis**[Q]
- *Epidemiology:*
  - **Mean age: 20–40 yrs of age**[Q]**, Female: Male = 10:1**[Q]
- *Genetic basis:*
  - Polymorphisms in immune-function genes like **CTLA4 and PTPN22 and the HLA-DR3 allele**[Q]
- *Pathogenesis:*
  - **Autoimmune disorder** characterized by **autoantibodies against TSH receptor:**[Q]
  - **Thyroid-stimulating immunoglobulin (TSI)**[Q] (90% cases)
- *Clinical features (Triad):*
  - **Hyperthyroidism**[Q] with diffuse enlargement of the gland
  - **Infiltrative ophthalmopathy**[Q] with resultant exophthalmos
  - **Localized, infiltrative dermopathy**[Q] (pretibial myxedema)
- *Morphology:*
  - **Symmetrically enlarged**[Q] gland due to **diffuse hypertrophy and hyperplasia**[Q] of **thyroid follicular epithelial cells**[Q]

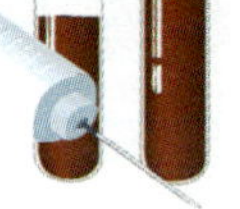

- *Laboratory findings:*
  - **Elevated** free **T4 and T3 levels** and **depressed TSH levels**[Q]

Hypothyroidism

Condition caused by a **structural or functional derangement**[Q] that **interferes** with **production of thyroid** hormone[Q]

- **Primary: Intrinsic abnormality**[Q] **in the thyroid**
- **Secondary: Pituitary** or **Hypothalamic disease**[Q]

High Yield Facts

- **Serum TSH**[Q] level is the **most useful single screening**[Q] test for hyperthyroidism
- **Low TSH** is confirmed with **measurement of free T4** (increased)
- **Radioactive iodine uptake:**
  - Diffusely increased uptake by the whole gland (Grave's disease)[Q]
  - Increased uptake in a solitary nodule: Toxic adenoma[Q]
  - Decreased uptake: Thyroiditis[Q]

Thyroiditis

Inflammation of the thyroid gland[Q]

Hashimoto's Thyroiditis

- *Definition:*
  - **Autoimmune destruction of thyroid gland** → **gradually progressive thyroid failure.**[Q]
- *Most common:*
  - **Cause of hypothyroidism in Iodine-sufficient areas of the world**[Q]
  - Clinically apparent cause of chronic thyroiditis
- *Epidemiology:*
  - Mean age: **45 - 65 years** of age; **Female: Male =10–20:1**[Q] **(Most Common in middle aged female)**[Q]
- *Pathogenesis:*
  - Breakdown in self tolerance to thyroid autoantigens
- *Etiology:*
  - **Autoimmune:** Defect in **regulatory T-cells (Tregs)**
  - **Genetic:** polymorphisms in **immune regulation-associated genes**
    - Cytotoxic T lymphocyte-associated antigen-4 **(CTLA4)**[Q]
    - Protein tyrosine phosphatase-22 **(PTPN22)**[Q]
- *Clinical Features:*
  - **P**ainless **enlargement** of the thyroid, usually associated with hypothyroidism
- *Increased risk for developing:*
  - **B-cell Non Hodgkins lymphoma**[Q]
  - **Autoimmune diseases:**
    - Endocrine (**type 1 diabetes, autoimmune adrenalitis**)[Q]
    - Non-endocrine (**SLE, myasthenia gravis, and Sjögren's syndrome**)[Q]

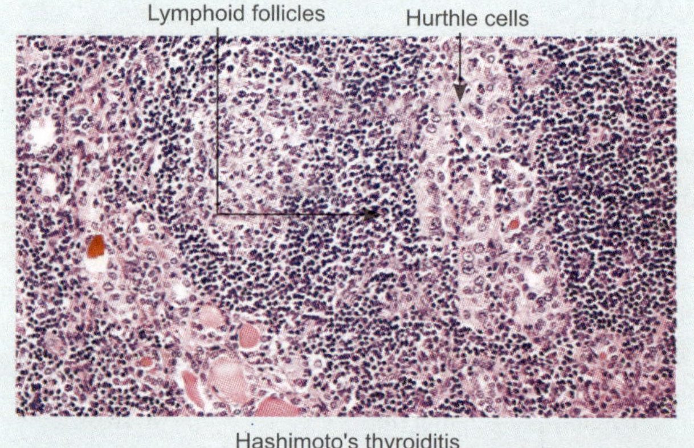

Hashimoto's thyroiditis

RECENT EXAM[Q]

Morphological changes in Thyroiditis
- **Infiltration** of the gland parenchyma by **small lymphocytes and plasma cells**[Q]
- Well-developed **germinal centers,** thyroid **follicles are atrophic**[Q]
- Hallmark: **Hürthle cell metaplasia or Oxyphil change** (cells with abundant eosinophilic, granular cytoplasm)
- **Intact capsule & fibrosis** confined to **gland**[Q]

Granulomatous Thyroiditis/De Quervain Thyroiditis

- *Epidemiology:*
  - Most common age group: **40 – 50 yrs**[Q]; **Female: Male = 4:1**[Q]
- *Etiology:*
  - Viral Infections: **Cox sackie virus**[Q]**, mumps**[Q]**, measles**[Q], Adenovirus
- *Clinical feature:*
  - **Thyroid pain**[Q] and goiter
- *Morphology:*
  - **Scattered follicles** disrupted & replaced by **neutrophils forming microabscesses**[Q]
  - **Multinucleate giant cells** enclose fragments of colloid[Q]

Subacute Lymphocytic (Painless) Thyroiditis/Painless Thyroiditis[Q]

- *Epidemiology*
  - Most common middle-aged adults ; F>M; **Self limiting**[Q];
- *Clinical feature*
  - Mild **hyperthyroidism** with **goitrous enlargement**[Q] of the gland
- *Morphology*
  - **Lymphocytic infiltration** with **large germinal centers**[Q]
  - **Patchy disruption** and **collapse**[Q] of thyroid follicles
  - Fibrosis and Hürthle cell metaplasia are **not prominent**[Q]

Riedel Thyroiditis

- *Characteristic:*
  - **Extensive fibrosis** involving **thyroid & contiguous neck structures**[Q]

- **Associated with:**
  - ○ Fibrosis in retroperitoneum[Q]
  - ○ Systemic autoimmune **IgG4-related disease** (fibrosis & tissue infiltration by plasma cells producing IgG4)[Q]

High Yield Facts

- In **hyperthyroidism**, there is **proximal muscle weakness**[Q]
- **Generalized lymphadenopathy** can occur in **Grave's disease**[Q]
- **Most common** type of thyroiditis is **Hashimoto's** thyroiditis[Q]
- **Hyperthyroidism may be seen initially in Hashimoto's** thyroiditis[Q]
- Most common type of thyroiditis **postpartum** is **subacute painless thyroiditis**[Q]
- **HLA DR3/5** are associated with **Hashimoto's** thyroiditis[Q]
- **HLA B5** is associated with **De** Quervain thyroiditis[Q]

Thyroid Carcinoma

Thyroid Ca	%	Genes Mc mutated	Route of Metastasis
Papillary	MC 85%	BRAF (MC), RET	Lymphatic
Follicular	5–15%	RAS/P13K 10% PAX/PPARG	Hematogenous
Medullary	<5%	RET	Regional : Lymphatic Distant : Hematogenous
Anaplastic	<5%	RAS, P53	Direct & hematogenous

Mc: Most common

Papillary Carcinoma

- **Epidemiology:**
  - ○ **Most common**[Q] form of thyroid cancer; most commonly seen at **20–40 yrs** of age
- **Morphology:**
  - ○ **Solitary or multifocal**[Q], Well **circumscribed** and **encapsulated**[Q]
  - ○ **Infiltrate adjacent parenchyma**[Q] along with areas of fibrosis and calcification
- **Variants of Papillary Ca:**
  - ○ *Follicular variant, Tall-cell variant, Diffuse sclerosing, Papillary Microcarcinoma*

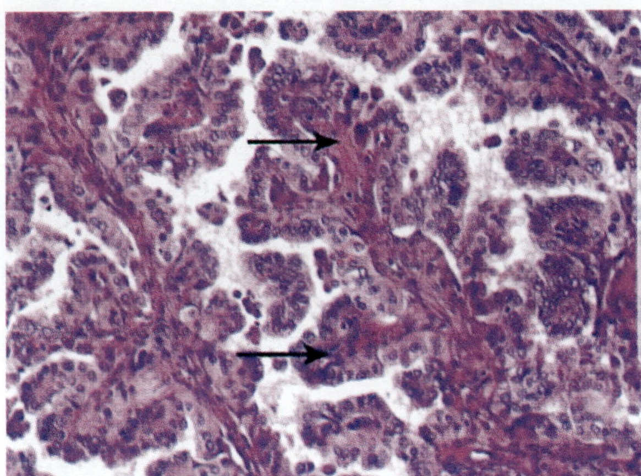

Papillary carcinoma, thyroid. A classical papillary carcinoma shows multiple finger like branching

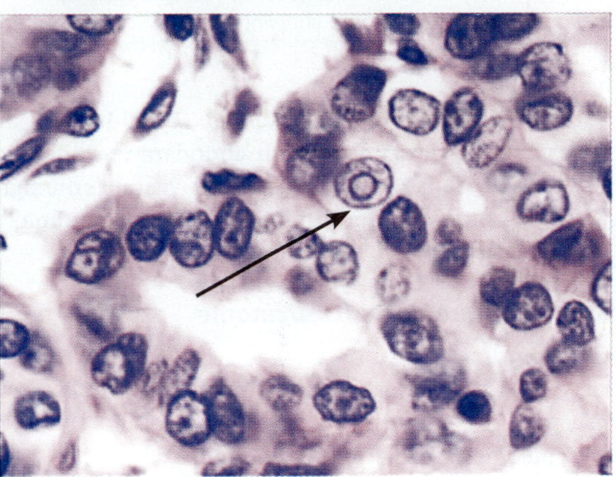

Orphan Annie Nuclie pseudoinclusions S/o papillary Ca

- **Microscopic hallmarks:**
  - ○ Branching papillae with a fibrovascular stalk covered by cuboidal epithelial cells
  - ○ **Nuclear features: Hallmark of diagnosis**
    - **Orphan Annie eye nuclei**[Q] (clear or empty appearing ground-glass appearance),
    - **"Pseudo-inclusions"**[Q] – invaginations in cytoplasm-appearance of **intranuclear**[Q] inclusions or **intranuclear grooves.**[Q]
  - ○ **Psammoma bodies**[Q] (Absent in follicular and medullary Ca)
  - ○ **Lymphatic invasion is common**[Q]

Mnemonic

Clinical criteria that point towards **neoplastic nature** of thyroid nodule (*"SoMe CRY"*)
- **S**olitary nodule[Q]
- **M**ale[Q]
- **C**old nodule on radioiodine uptake
- **R**adiation[Q] exposure history
- **Y**oung age[Q]

Follicular Carcinoma

- **Epidemiology:**
  - **2nd Most common**^{Q} primary thyroid cancer; MC in **mid to older** age, Female >**Males**^{Q}
  - More frequent in areas with **dietary iodine deficiency**^{Q}
- **Morphology:**
  - **Gross:** Single well circumscribed or widely infiltrative nodule
- **Clinical Course:**
  - **Slowly enlarging painless** nodules
  - Most frequently they are **cold nodule**
  - **Vascular (hematogenous) dissemination** to **bone, lungs, liver**^{Q}

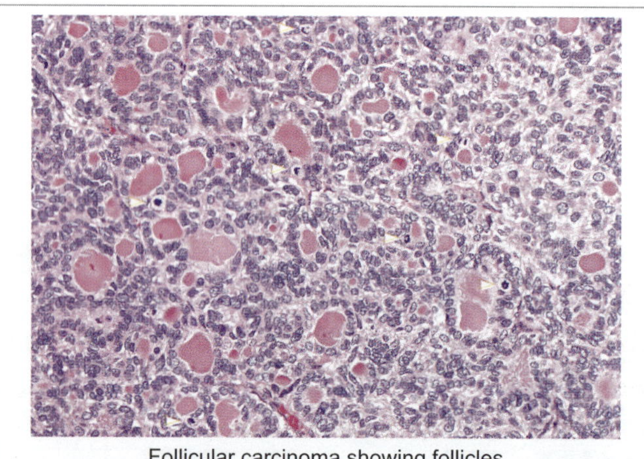
Follicular carcinoma showing follicles

  - Microscopically:
    - Small follicles containing colloid, **Hurthle cell or oncocytic variant**^{Q}: cells with abundant eosinophilic cytoplasm, **Capsular &/or vascular invasion** is the **sign of carcinoma** & **differentiates follicular adenoma**^{Q}, **Lymphatic spread is uncommon**^{Q}

Anaplastic (Undifferentiated) Carcinoma

- **Epidemiology**
  - Most common in **older persons**, (mean age of **65 years)**^{Q}
- **Microscopy**
  - Large, pleomorphic giant cells & spindle cells
- **Prognosis**
  - **Most aggressive** with a **mortality rate approaching 100%**^{Q}

Medullary Carcinoma

- **Definition:**
  - A Neuroendocrine neoplasm derived from the **parafollicular cells,**^{Q} **or C cells,** of thyroid
- **Inheritance:**
  - **70% sporadic (old age); 30% familial** (1st decade of life): **Autosomal dominant**
  - **As a part of MEN syndrome 2A or 2B**^{Q} or familial medullary thyroid carcinoma, or **FMTC**^{Q}
- **Clinical features:**
  - **Sporadic cases: Mass** in neck, dysphagia or hoarseness,
  - **Paraneoplastic syndromes: diarrhea**^{Q} (due to VIP), **Cushing syndrome**^{Q} (due to ACTH)

  - **Familial cases**: endocrine neoplasms in other organs (e.g., adrenal or parathyroid in MEN)
- **Gross Morphology:**
  - **Sporadic tumor** present as **Solitary nodule ("S for S")**
  - **Familial** cases- are **bilateral**^{Q} and **multicentric**^{Q}
- **Tumor Markers:**
  - **Calcitonin,** serotonin, ACTH, and vasoactive intestinal peptide (VIP)

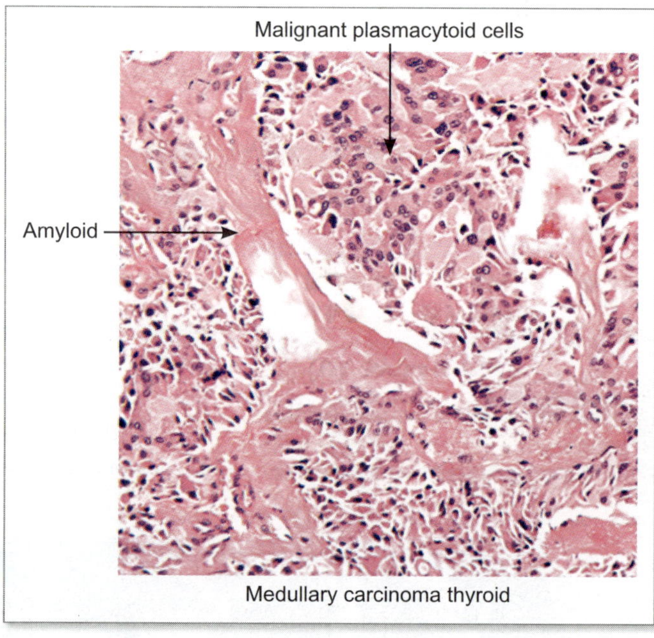

Medullary carcinoma thyroid

- **Microscopy:**
  - Polygonal **spindle-shaped cells** form nests, trabeculae and follicles
  - **Acellular amyloid deposits (A cal)**^{Q} are **characteristic** feature
  - **Electron microscopy:** membrane-bound **electron-dense granules**^{Q}
  - **Multicentric C-cell hyperplasia** in familial cases

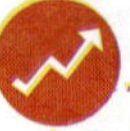

High Yield Facts

- **Integrity of capsule** is critical in distinguishing **follicular adenomas from follicular Ca**^{Q}
- **Follicular Carcinoma of Thyroid cannot be diagnosed by FNAC**^{Q}
- Most common thyroid Cancer is **Papillary carcinoma**
- Most common Thyroid Ca **post radiation exposure** is **Papillary CA**
- **Thyroid Carcinoma with best (excellent) prognosis: Papillary Ca thyroid**^{Q}
- **Thyroid Carcinoma with Worst prognosis: Anaplastic Carcinoma**^{Q}
- **Hypocalcemia**^{Q} is **not a prominent feature of Medullary Ca thyroid**, despite presence of raised calcitonin levels
- **Carcinoembryonic antigen (CEA)** is a useful biomarker in **calcitonin-negative Medullary Ca thyroid**

PARATHYROID GLANDS

The four parathyroid glands are composed of two cell types:

- **Chief cells:** Large amounts of **cytoplasmic glycogen (water clear appearance)**[Q]
- **Oxyphil cells: Acidophilic cytoplasm**, and are tightly packed with **mitochondria**

Hyperparathyroidism

Primary Hyperparathyroidism

Underlying Parathyroid lesions can be Adenoma (90%) > Primary hyperplasia > Parathyroid carcinoma

Lesion	Frequency	Morphology
Adenoma	**85% – 95%**[Q] (most common)	**Solitary lesions** with uniform, polygonal chief cells along with nests of oxyphil cells **(oxyphil adenomas)**
Primary hyperplasia	5%–10%	**Chief cell hyperplasia** with **water-clear cells involving all 4 glands**
Parathyroid carcinoma	~1%	Circumscribed lesion in a single gland **diagnosed by invasion** of **surrounding tissues** and **metastasis** as the only reliable criteria.

Molecular Defects

Sporadic adenomas:	Familial parathyroid adenomas:
• **Cyclin D1** overexpression • **MEN1 mutations on chr 11q**	• Multiple Endocrine Neoplasia (MEN syndrome-1 & 2) • **Familial hypocalciuric hypercalcemia:** (autosomal-dominant) • Loss-of-function mutations in **calcium-sensing receptor (CASR) gene**

Clinical Features

Skeletal abnormalities:

- **Osteoporosis:** Cortical bone more severely involved than medullary bone
- **Brown tumors:** Brown color-vascularity, hemorrhage & hemosiderin deposition
- **Osteitis fibrosa cystica (von Recklinghausen disease of bone)**

Metastatic Calcification

Nephrolithiasis, nephrocalcinosis, calcific deposits in stomach, lungs, myocardium, blood vessels.

Secondary Hyperparathyroidism

- *Definition:*
  - **Chronic hypocalcemia** leading to **compensatory over-activity** of the parathyroid glands.
- *Etiology:*
  - **Renal Failure (Most Common Cause)**[Q]
  - **Inadequate Dietary Intake of Calcium**
  - **Steatorrhea**[Q]
  - **Vitamin D Deficiency**[Q]
- *Clinical Features:*
  - Can cause **calciphylaxis**[Q] (**ischemic damage** to skin and other organs)
- *Morphology:*
  - Hyperplastic parathyroid glands with **chief cells (water-clear cells)**[Q]

Tertiary Hyperparathyroidism

Autonomous activity of gland with **hypercalcemia.**

> ## Pseudohypoparathyroidism
>
> **End-organ resistance** to the **actions of PTH**[Q].
> - Serum **PTH levels are normal or elevated**[Q]
> - Some cases have end-organ **resistance to TSH and FSH/LH and PTH**[Q]

Hypoparathyroidism

Etiology

- **Surgical removal of parathyroid: Most common cause**[Q]
- **Genetic causes of hypoparathyroidism**
  - **Autoimmune hypoparathyroidism:** mutations in AIRE gene (AIRE).
  - **Autosomal-dominant hypoparathyroidism**: mutations in CASR gene[Q]
  - **Familial isolated hypoparathyroidism (FIH)**
- **DiGeorge syndrome** : 22q11 deletion syndrome[Q]

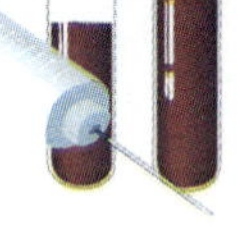

PANCREAS

Diabetes Mellitus

A Group of metabolic disorders sharing the common features of **hyperglycemia.**

Classification of Diabetes Mellitus

Type-1 diabetes (β-cell destruction causing absolute insulin deficiency).

Type-2 diabetes (combination of β-cell dysfunction and insulin resistance)

Genetic defects
- Maturity on set diabetes of the young (MODY).
  - **MODY-1** Hepatocyte nuclear factor 4α (HNF-4α)
  - **MODY-2** Glucokinase (GCK)
  - **MODY-3** Hepatocyte nuclear factor 1α (HNF-1α)
  - **MODY-4** Pancreatic and duodenal homebox-1 (PDX-1).
  - **MODY-5** Hepatocyte necrotic factor 1β (HNF-1β).
  - **MODY-6** Neurogenic differentiation factor 1β (Neuro D$_1$)
    - Neonatal diabetes: Activating mutations in KCNJ 11 and ABCC 8.
    - Maternally inherited diabetes and deafness (MIDD), Mitochondrial DNA mutations (m. 3243A → G)[Q]

Genetic defects in insulin action
- Type A insulin resistance
- Lipoatrophic diabetes (PPARG mutation)

Exocrine pancreatic defects
- Chronic pancreatitis
- Fibrocalculous pancreatopathy
- Neoplasia
- Cystic fibrosis, Hemochromatosis

Infections
- CMV
- Congenital rubella
- Coxsackie B

Endocrinopathies
- Acromegaly
- Cushing's syndrome
- Hyperthyroidism
- Pheochromocytoma
- Glucagonoma

Gestational diabetes mellitus
- **Drugs**
  - Glucocorticoids
  - Thyroid hormone
  - β-adrenergic agonists
  - Thiazides
  - Phenytoin

Genetic syndromes associated with diabetes
- Down's syndrome
- Klinefelter's syndrome
- Turner's syndrome
- Prader Willi syndrome

Diagnostic Criteria According to ADA and WHO

Diabetes

Presence of any 1 or more of the following:
- **Fasting** plasma glucose ≥126 mg/dL
- **Random** plasma glucose ≥200 mg/dL
- **2-hour plasma glucose ≥ 200 mg/dL** during oral glucose tolerance test **(OGTT)** with **75 g**
- Glycated hemoglobin **(HbA$_{1c}$)** level ≥ 6.5%

Impaired Glucose Tolerance (Pre-diabetes)

Presence of any 1 or more of the following:
- **Fasting** plasma glucose between **100 and 125 mg/dL (impaired fasting glucose)**
- **2-hour plasma glucose** between **140 and 199 mg/dL** following a **75-gm glucose OGTT**
- A glycated hemoglobin **(HbA$_{1c}$) level between 5.7% and 6.4%.**

Differences between Type 1 DM-(Insulin-dependent Diabetes Mellitus) and Type 2 DM (Non Insulin dependent Diabetes Mellitus)

Features	Type 1 Diabetes Mellitus	Type 2 Diabetes Mellitus
Onset	Childhood[Q] or adolescent	**Mostly adults[Q]**
Antibodies	Circulating **islet auto-antibodies[Q] (anti-insulin[Q]**, anti-GAD, anti-ICA 512)	**No auto-antibodies[Q]**
Complications	**Diabetic ketoacidosis[Q]** (DKA) in absence of insulin therapy	**Non-ketotic hyperosmolar coma > DKA.**
Genetics	1. Mostly linked to **MHC class I and II genes[Q]**. 2. **Polymorphism in CTLA4[Q]** and **PTPN 22[Q]** 3. Linked to insulin gene VNTR (variable number of tandem repeats)	1. No HLA-linkage[Q] 2. Related to diabetogenic and obesity related **candidates genes** (TCF7L2[Q], PPARG, FTO)
Pathogenesis	**Regulatory T-cell dysfunction[Q]** causing loss of self-tolerance to islet cell autoantigens.	1. **Insulin resistance[Q]** in peripheral tissue. 2. Failure of compensation by beta-cells. 3. Multiple obesity associated factors (non-esterified fatty acid, inflammatory cytokinesis)

Contd...

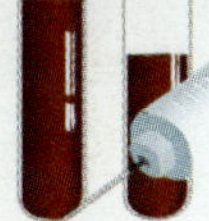

Features	Type 1 Diabetes Mellitus	Type 2 Diabetes Mellitus
Pathology	1. Insulitis[Q] (inflammatory infiltrates of T-cells and macrophages) 2. **Beta-cell depletion**[Q] 3. Islet atrophy	1. **No insulitis**[Q] 2. **Amyloid depostion**[Q] in islets 3. Islet cell hyperplasia (especially in non-diabetic newborns of diabetic mothers)
Diagnostic methods	Reduced insulin, C peptide ↓	↑ Insulin level, C peptide ↑

Pathological Changes in Diabetes

Changes in Pancreas

More common in type 1 than type 2 diabetes.

- **Reduction in the number and size of islets**
- **Leukocytic infiltrates** in the islets (insulitis) by T lymphocytes
- In type 2 diabetes → **amyloid deposition** within islets
- In **infants of diabetic mothers** → **Increase** in the number and size of islets

Diabetic Macrovascular Disease

- **Endothelial dysfunction** which predisposes to **atherosclerosis**
- **Hallmark: Accelerated atherosclerosis** of **aorta & large-medium-sized arteries**.[Q]
- **Hyaline arteriolosclerosis:** Amorphous hyaline thickening of arteriolar wall → Narrowing of lumen

Diabetic Microangiopathy

Nephropathy, Retinopathy, Neuropathy

- **Most consistent**[Q] morphologic feature of **Diabetes: Diffuse thickening of basement membrane in capillaries of skin, skeletal muscles, Retina, Glomeruli & renal medulla**

Diabetic Ocular Complications

- Diabetes-induced hyperglycemia can lead to **cataract**[Q]
- **Glaucoma** → damage to optic nerve[Q]
- **Retinal vasculopathy:**[Q] Can be non-proliferative or proliferative

Diabetic Neuropathy

- Can affect **central and peripheral nerves**[Q]
- **Distal symmetrical polyneuropathy**[Q] – most common pattern
- **Autonomic nervous system involvement**[Q]

Diabetic Nephropathy

Explained in chapter 16.

High Yield Facts

- **Most common type of MODY is MODY3**[Q]
- Myocardial infarction due to atherosclerosis is the most common cause of death in diabetics.[Q]
- Renal failure is second most common cause of death in DM[Q]
- **Dry Gangrene** of lower extremities is 100 times[Q] more common in diabetics
- Most profound histopathological changes of Diabetes are seen in Retina[Q]
- Fundamental lesion of Retinopathy is Neovascularization[Q]
- Earliest manifestation of Diabetic Nephropathy is **Micro-albuminuria**[Q]
- Risk of Nephropathy & ESRD is more in type 1 than type 2 Diabetes[Q]

Complications of Diabetes

- *Acute Metabolic Complications of Diabetes:*
  - Diabetic ketoacidosis (Type 1 > type 2 DM)
  - Hyperosmolar nonketotic hyperglycemia (Type 2 > type 1 DM)
  - **Hypoglycemia**[Q] **(most common acute complication)**
- *Chronic Complications of Diabetes: According to type of vessels involved*
  - **Macrovascular disease**: Large and medium sized
    - Accelerated atherosclerosis among diabetics
    - Increased risk of myocardial infarction
    - Stroke
    - Lower extremity ischemia
  - **Microvascular disease**: Small vessels
    - Retina- diabetic retinopathy, Macular edema
    - Kidneys- nephropathy
    - Peripheral nerves- neuropathy

Mechanisms of Chronic Complications in Diabetes

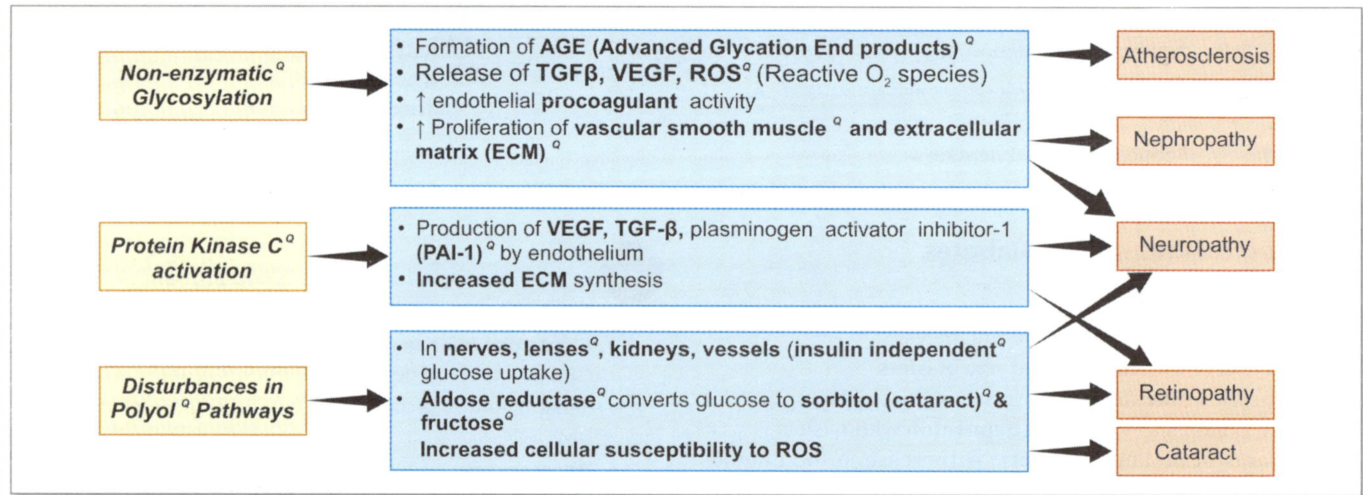

Pancreatic Neuroendocrine Tumors (Pannets)

- Tumors of the pancreatic islet cells ("islet cell tumors")
- 2% of all pancreatic neoplasms; may be single or multiple and benign or malignant
- May elaborate pancreatic hormones, or may be non-functional
- **Surest criteria for malignancy:** *metastases, vascular invasion & local infiltration.*[Q]
- 60%–90% of pancreatic endocrine neoplasms are malignant.

High Yield Facts

- **Most common pancreatic endocrine neoplasm is Insulinoma**
- *VIPoma causes WDHA syndrome* (watery diarrhoea, Hypokalemia and Achlorhydria)
- Deposition of amyloid in the extracellular tissue is a characteristic feature of many insulinomas
- **Diarrhea is** the most common presenting symptom of **gastrinoma**

R9th Latest Update

Mutations in PanNETs involve:

- MEN-1, PTEN, TSC2
- **A**lpha-**T**halassemia/mental **R**etardation syndrome, **X**-linked (**ATRX**)
- **D**eath-domain **a**ssociated protein (DAXX), which helps in telomere maintenance.

Functional Pancreatic Endocrine Neoplasms

- Insulinoma
- Zollinger-ellison's syndrome (Gastrinoma)
- Multiple endocrine neoplasia (MEN)

Insulinoma

Most common pancreatic endocrine neoplasm[Q], Deposition of **amyloid**[Q] is a characteristic feature, Focal or diffuse hyperplasia of the islets (nesidioblastosis)[Q]

Mnemonic

High Yield Facts

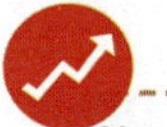

Nesidioblastosis

- Also called **congenital focal/diffuse beta-islet hyperplasia**.
- It is often associated with **hyperinsulinemic hypoglycemia**.
- It occurs due to increase in expression of growth factors **IGF2, IGF1Ra and TGFBR3 in islets**.
- It is associated with:
  - Beckwith-Weidman syndrome
  - Gastric bypass patients
  - Zollinger-Ellison syndrome

ADRENAL GLANDS

Paired organs lying above kidneys, which consists of: Cortex and Medulla

Adrenal cortex has 3 zones (from outermost to innermost—**G-F-R**)

Zones	Hormone Secreted
Zona Glomerulosa	Mineralocorticoids like Aldosterone
Zona Fasciculata	Glucocorticoids (principally cortisol)
Zona Reticularis	Sex steroids (estrogens and androgens)

Adrenal medulla is composed of **Chromaffin (Specialized neural crest/ neuroendocrine)**[Q] cells supported by **sustentacular**[Q] cells. **Chromaffin cells → Epinephrine & Norepinephrine**[Q]

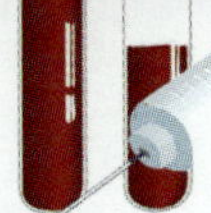

Adrenocortical Insufficiency

Caused by:

- **Primary adrenal disease (primary hypoadrenalism)** or
- Decreased stimulation of the adrenals due to a **ACTH deficiency (secondary hypoadrenalism)**

Adrenocortical Hyperfunction (Hyperadrenalism)

Includes:

Disease	Hormone over-produced
Cushing's syndrome	Cortisol
Hyperaldosteronism	Aldosterone[Q]
Adrenogenital or virilizing syndromes	Androgens[Q]

Hypercortisolism (Cushing's Syndrome)

Elevated glucocorticoid levels due to exogenous or endogenous causes. Homogeneous and paler cytoplasm of ACTH-producing cells due to intermediate keratin filaments in Pituitary is called: "**Crooke hyaline change**":

High Yield Facts

- **Most common** cause of **primary adrenal insufficiency** in developed countries: **Autoimmune** Adrenalitis[Q]
- Most common cause of primary adrenal insufficiency in **India: Tubercular Adrenalitis**[Q]
- Patients with **APS 1** develop antibody **against IL-17 & IL-22**
- **Hyperpigmentation** of skin in Addison's disease is caused by **POMC**[Q] → precursor of ACTH & MSH
- **Hypertension** is the most common manifestation of **primary hyperaldosteronism**[Q]
- **Plasma renin levels** distinguish **primary from secondary hyperaldosteronism**[Q]
- **Most common cause is of Cushing's syndrome is exogenous glucocorticoids ("iatrogenic")**[Q]
- **'Cushing disease'**[Q] refers to **ACTH producing pituitary Adenoma**
- Characteristic of **aldosterone-producing adenomas** is "**Spironolactone bodies**"[Q] (eosinophilic, laminated cytoplasmic inclusions), found after treatment with Spironolactone.

Adrenal Medulla Neoplasms

Let us first understand what is a Paraganglion System

Paraganglion System		
Definition: Neuroendocrine cells in **adrenal medulla & extraadrenal system** location[Q]		
Classification: (Based on their anatomic distribution)		
Parasympathetic	Branchiomeric	Close to the **major arteries & cranial nerves**; e.g. **carotid bodies**[Q]
	Intravagal	Distributed along the **vagus nerve**.[Q]
Sympathetic	Aorticosympathetic	Segmental ganglia distributed mainly along the abdominal aorta. e.g: **Organs of Zuckerkandl**[Q]

Neoplasms of Adrenal Medulla are of 2 types

- **Pheochromocytoma:** Neoplasms of **chromaffin cells that release catecholamines**
- **Neuroblastic tumors**: Neuroblastoma (Refer chapter 8)

Pheochromocytoma

Familial Syndromes Associated with Pheochromocytoma and extra-adrenal Paragangliomas

Syndrome	Gene	Associated Neoplasms
MEN-2A[Q]	*RET*[Q]	Medullary Thyroid Ca[Q] & Parathyroid hyperplasia[Q]
MEN-2B[Q]	*RET*[Q]	Medullary thyroid Ca[Q], Mucocutaneous Ganglioneuromas[Q]
NF1	*NF1*[Q]	Optic nerve glioma[Q]
Von Hippel-Lindau (VHL)	*VHL*[Q]	Renal cell Ca, Hemangioblastoma[Q], PanNET
Familial paraganglioma	*SDHD*	Paraganglioma

Diagnosis of Pheochromocytoma

- *Gross Morphology:*
  - **Small**, circumscribed lesions to **large hemorrhagic masses**
  - **Richly vascularized fibrous trabeculae** producing **lobular pattern**.
  - Incubation of **fresh tissue** with a **potassium dichromate** solution turns the tumor a **dark brown color (hence the name "chromaffin")**[Q].
- *Markers:*
  - **Chromogranin**[Q] and **Synaptophysin**[Q] in the chief cells
  - **S-100** in peripheral **sustentacular** cells[Q]
- *Definitive diagnosis of malignancy:*
  - Based on the **presence of metastases (vascular invasion)** & **not on histology.**
  - **Metastasis:** Involves regional **lymph nodes**[Q], **liver**[Q], **lung**[Q], **and bone**[Q]

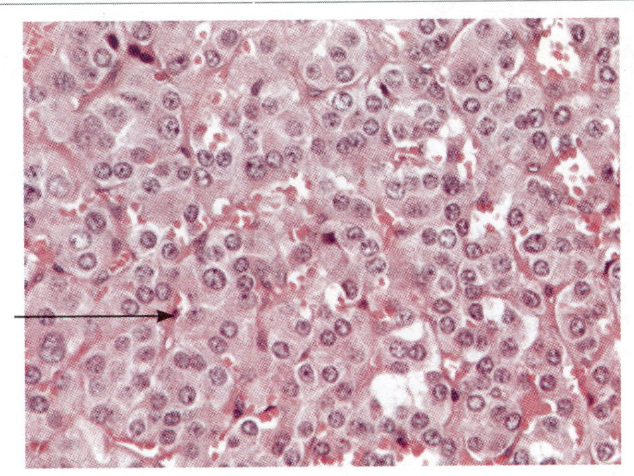

Zellballen pattern characterized by well defined nests of epithelioid cells & vascular fibrous stroma separating the nests of cells

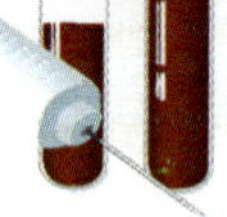

Microscopy

- Tumors made of **clusters of polygonal to spindle-shaped chromaffin cells** surrounded by **sustentacular cells**, creating **small nests (zellballen)**[Q], with rich vascularity.
- **"Salt and pepper"**[Q] nuclear chromatin: **characteristic** of neuroendocrine tumors.
- **Electron microscopy:** Membrane-bound, **electron-dense secretory**[Q] granules.

High Yield Facts

Adrenogenital Syndromes
- **Congenital adrenal hyperplasia (CAH):** Autosomal recessive inheritance[Q]
- **Most common subtype** is caused by deficiency of the enzyme 21-hydroxylase.[Q]
- **Bilateral hyperplasia of adrenal cortex due to excess ACTH is characteristic**[Q]

CAH with:	Female virilization	Male incomplete virilization
Hypertension	11 hydroxylase deficiency[Q]	17 hydroxylase deficiency[Q]
Salt crisis	21 hydroxylase deficiency[Q]	3 β hydroxy steroid dehydrogenase[Q]

MULTIPLE ENDOCRINE NEOPLASIA (MEN) SYNDROMES

- *Definition:*
  - **Genetically inherited diseases** resulting in **proliferative lesions (hyperplasia, adenomas, and carcinomas)** of multiple endocrine organs.
- *Characteristics:*
  - **Younger age** than sporadic tumors.
  - Involve multiple organs **synchronously (at same time)** or **metachronously (at different times)**
  - Tumors are often **multifocal**[Q], **more aggressive**[Q] and **recurrent**[Q]
  - **Preceded** by an asymptomatic stage of **endocrine hyperplasia.**[Q]

High Yield Facts

- **Primary hyperparathyroidism** is the most common manifestation of MEN-1.[Q]
- **Most frequent anterior pituitary tumor in MEN-1 is a prolactinoma.**[Q]
- **Most common thyroid Ca in MEN syndrome is Medullary Ca thyroid**
- **Duodenum**[Q] is the **most common site of gastrinomas** in individuals with **MEN-1.**
- **Medullary Thyroid Ca in MEN 2B is more aggressive**[Q] than in MEN 2A.
- **All individuals with RET mutation are advised prophylactic thyroidectomy.**

Multiple Endocrine Neoplasia (MEN) Syndromes

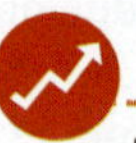

Mnemonic

MEN 1 (Wermer syndrome)	MEN 2A (Sipple syndrome)	MEN 2B
MEN1 (Chr 11q), encodes *Menin*	**RET on Chr 10q**	
3 "P" s **P**arathyroid Hyperplasia/Adenoma (MC) **P**ituitary : Hyperplasia/Adenoma **P**ancreas: Hyperplasia/Adenoma/NET Less common manifestations: *"CAP"* **C**arcinoid of Foregut **A**ngiofibroma/Lipoma **P**heochromocytoma	"HAPPY" **H**irschsprung disease **A**myloidosis Cutaneous lichen **P**heochromocytoma **P**arathyroid hyperplasia/Adenoma MTC (th**Y**roid Ca) • **N**euroblastoma • Wilms Tumor • Retinoblastoma	3 Ms Pheochromocytoma **M**TC **M**ucosal & gastrointestinal neuromas **M**arfanoid features

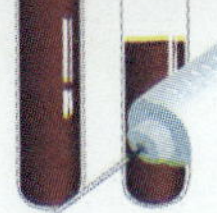

R10th Latest Update

- Mc mutation in papillary carcinoma now is BRAF
- Variants of papillary ca

Follicular variant	Nuclear features of papillary Ca, but follicular architecture More angioinvasive with less lymphatic metastasis
Tall-cell variant	More common in older individuals; Histopath: Tall columnar eosinophilic cells Higher vascular invasion, extra-thyroid extension & distant metastases is common
Diffuse sclerosing	More common on young and children; Extensive, diffuse fibrosis; abundant psammoma bodies, squamous metaplasia, extensive lymphocytes (resembles Hashimoto thyroiditis)-No BRAF mutation
Papillary Microcarcinoma	< 1 cm size; precursors of typical papillary carcinomas

NEXT Pattern Questions

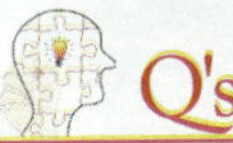

Q's

1. A 45-year-old patient presented with features of hypothyroidism from 2 to 3 years the histopathology is shown below. Based on histological features what is your diagnosis?

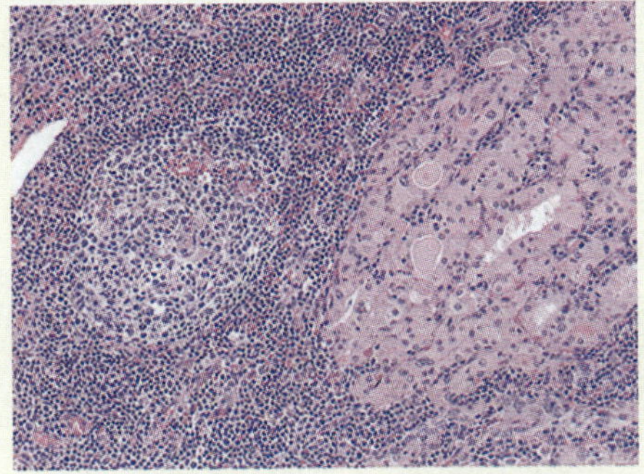

 a. Hashimoto's thyroiditis   b. Granulomatous thyroiditis
 c. Papillary carcinoma   d. Riders thyroiditis

Ans. (a) Hashimoto's thyroiditis

- Hypothyroidism history with lymphocytic infiltration in gland making germinal follicles. On the right side of the image you can see the oncocytes. This is suggestive of Hashimoto thyroiditis.

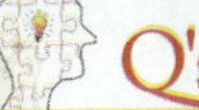

Q's

2. A 24-year-old patient presented with thyroid nodule, and ultrasound shows calcification. The histological features are shown in the diagram below, so what is your diagnosis?

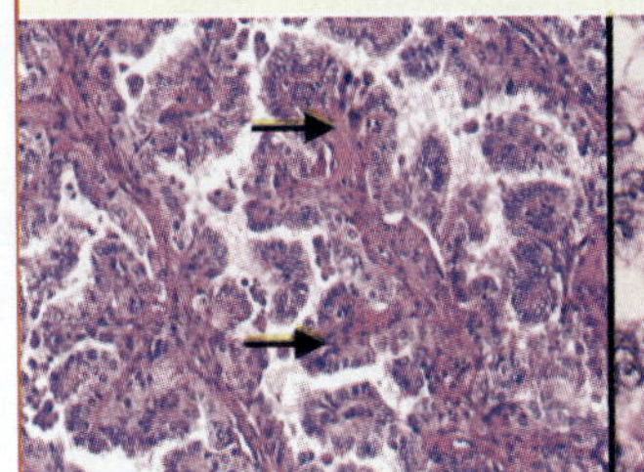

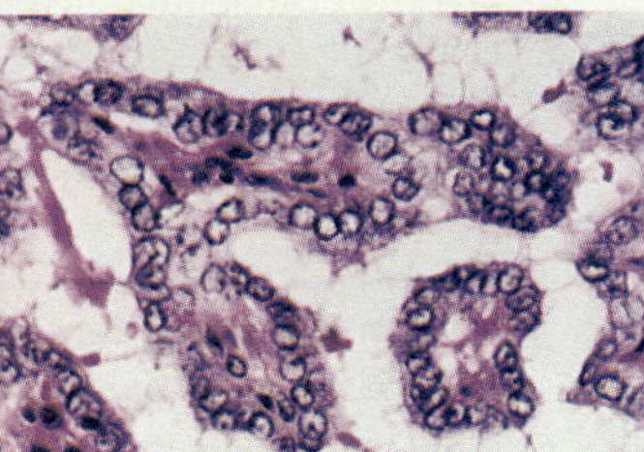

 a. Follicular carcinoma
 b. Medullary carcinoma
 c. Papillary carcinoma
 d. Anaplastic carcinoma

Ans. (c) Papillary carcinoma

- Thyroid nodule with calcification on a sonogram may be secondary to dystrophic calcification seen in papillary thyroid carcinoma. The histopath shows papillary pattern and annie-eye nuclei which is the hallmark of the same.

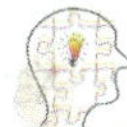

Q's

3. A patient presented with neck swelling. Cytology showed parafollicular cells along with clusters of plasmacytoid and scant amyloid. What investigation should be done to follow up the patient?

 a. Calcitonin   b. TSH level
 c. Anti TPO antibody   d. TRH

Ans. (a) Calcitonin

- Parafollicular cells along with clusters of plasmacytoid and scant amyloid is suggestive of medullary carcinoma thyroid gland. Serum calcitonin levels is used as a tumor marker in this case.

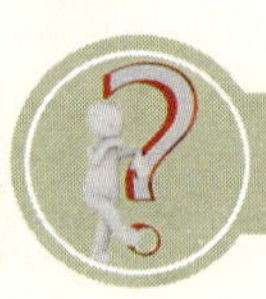

Image-Based Questions

1. A 25-year-old female presented with features of weight gain and loss of appetite and easy fatigue. On examination a swelling was noticed in anterior aspect of neck which moved with deglutination. Biopsy performed from neck revealed the following. What is your diagnosis?

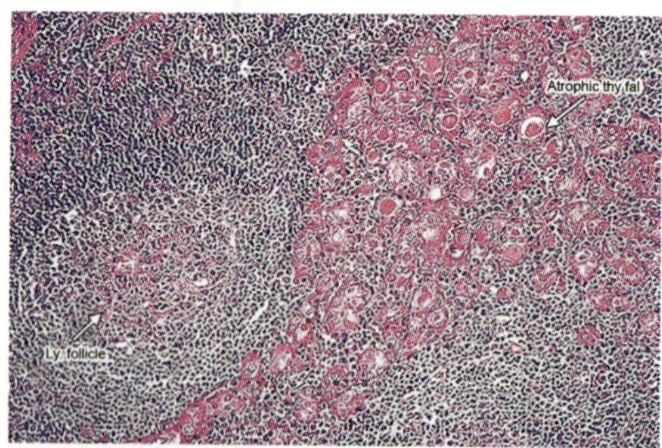

a. Reidel's thyroiditis
b. Hashimoto thyroiditis
c. Follicular carcinoma thyroid
d. Graves disease

2. A 24-year-old male presented with a swelling on anterior aspect of neck. On examination the swelling was firm and moved with deglutination. Biopsy from the lesion has been shown. What is the typical finding and diagnosis?

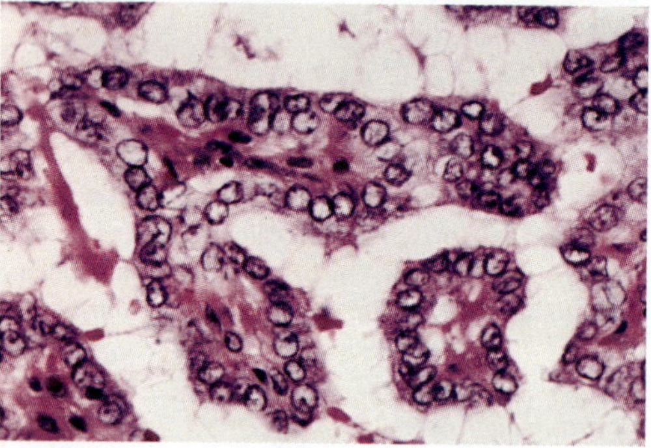

a. Orphan Annie eye nuclei; Follicular Ca thyroid
b. Orphan Annie eye nuclei; Papillary Ca thyroid
c. Hurthle cell change; Follicular Ca thyroid
d. Hurthle cell change; Papillary Ca thyroid

3. A 40-year-old male presented with a thyroid swelling and dysphagia. He gave history of on and off watery diarrhea. Biopsy of the lesion is shown. What is your diagnosis?

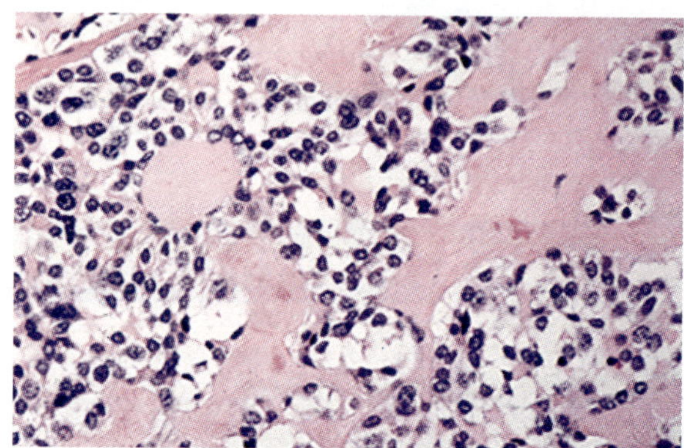

a. Follicular Ca thyroid
b. Papilllary Ca thyroid
c. Medullary Ca thyroid
d. Anaplastic cell Ca Thyroid

4. Biopsy from resected mass has been shown. What is the finding and diagnosis?

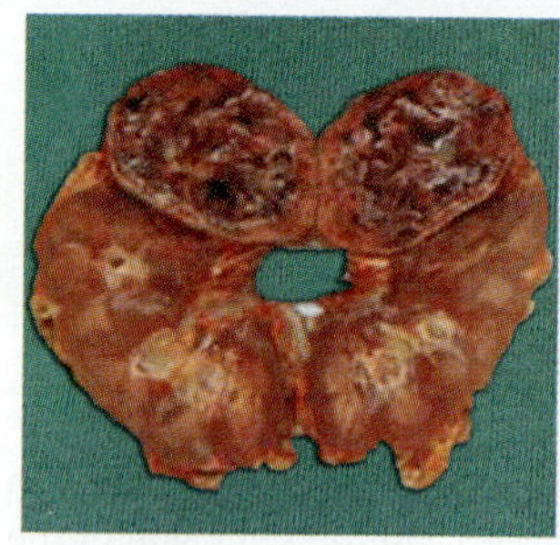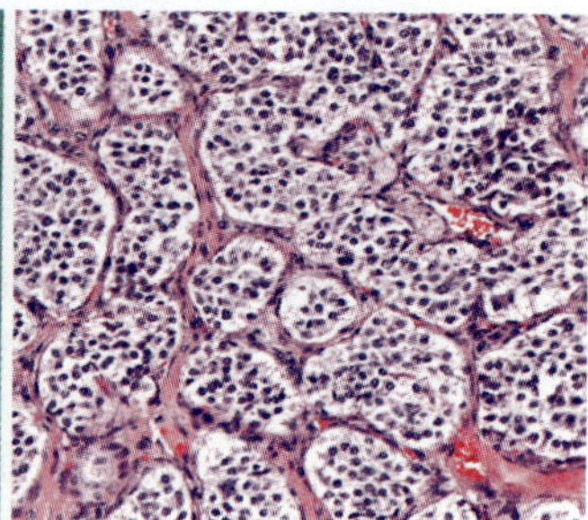

a. Zellballen in RCC
b. Zellballen in pheochrocytoma
c. Follicular Ca in renal metastasis
d. Homer Wright rosettes in neuroblastoma

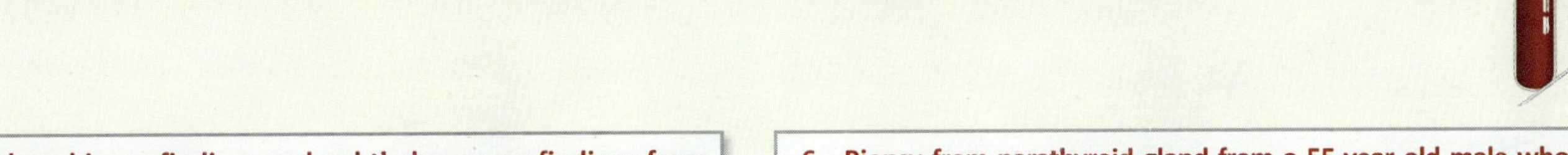

5. **Kidney biopsy findings and ophthalmoscopy findings from a patient of Type II diabetes of 25 years has been shown below. Identify the findings and pathology?**

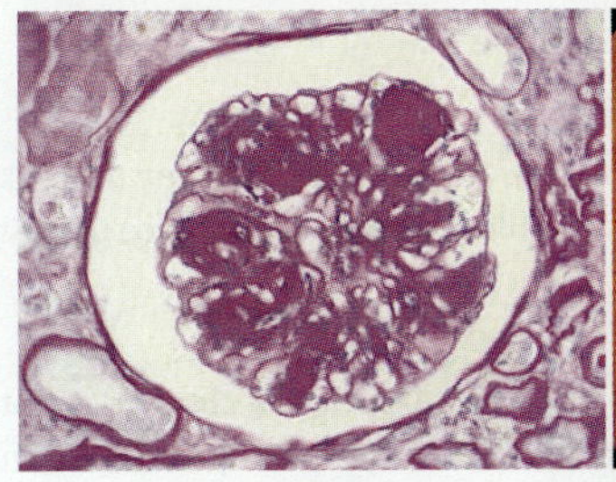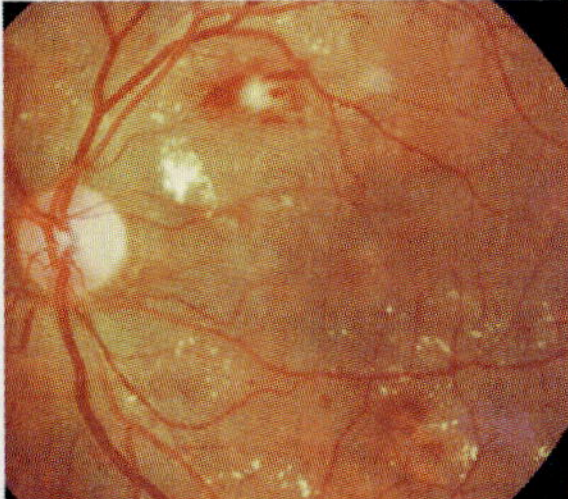

   a. Kimmelsteil Wilson lesion, diabetic non proliferative retinopathy due to macroangiopathy

   b. Diffuse glomerulosclerosis, diabetic proliferative retinopathy due to macroangiopathy

   c. Kimmelsteil Wilson lesion, diabetic non proliferative retinopathy due to microangiopathy

   d. Diffuse glomerulosclerosis, diabetic proliferative retinopathy due to microangiopathy

6. **Biopsy from parathyroid gland from a 55-year old male who presented to nephrology department of AIIMS has been shown below. He is a known case of chronic kidney disease with hypertension and type II diabetes. He has recently developed bone pain, lesions in skin and recurrent stones in kidney**

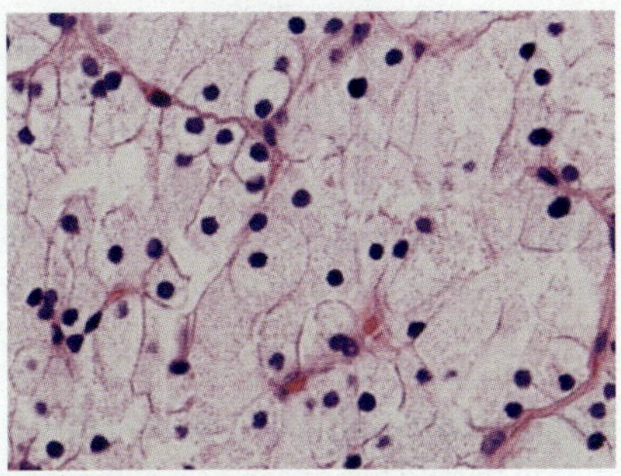

   a. Water clear cells in parathyroid hyperplasia

   b. Water clear cells in parathyroid Ca

   c. TB parathyroid

   d. Parathyroid Necrosis

7. **A 23-year-old female of Asian Indian origin was admitted to the orthopedic emergency department with pain in her left shoulder region, right knee, and left thigh following a trivial trauma. On physical examination of the patient, tenderness was found to be present in the left shoulder, right knee, and left thigh.On laboratory analysis, serum calcium level was 11.4 mg/dl (normal 8.4-10.7 mg/dl), serum alkaline phosphatase level was 780 IU/l (normal 50-240 IU/l), serum parathyroid hormone level was 456 pg/ ml (normal 7-53 pg/ml), vitamin D3 (1,25-dihydroxy cholecalciferol) was 32 pg/ml (normal 25-45 pg/ml). Biopsy done from the lesion has been shown below. What is your diagnosis?**

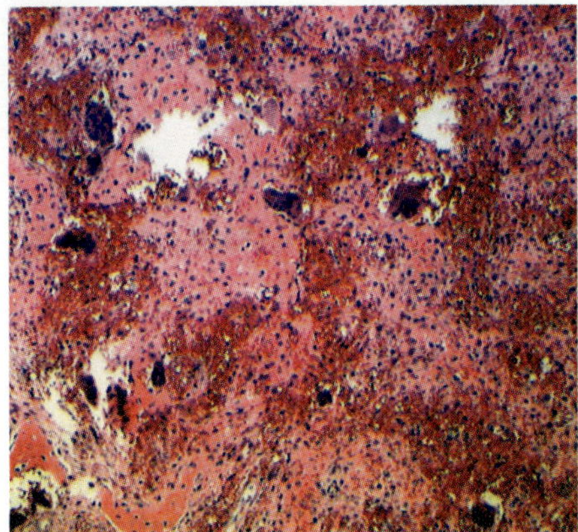

   a. Bone necrosis in secondary metastasis

   b. Bone fibrosis in tuberculosis

   c. Brown tumor in primary hyperparathyroidism

   d. Brown tumor in osteosarcoma

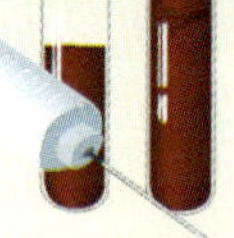
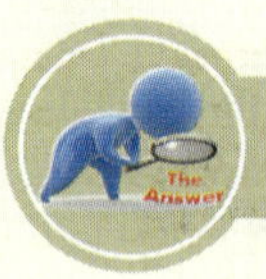

Answers of Image-Based Questions

1. Ans. (b) Hashimoto's thyroiditis
- The history given suggests a thyroid swelling. The given biopsy from the same shows thyroid parenchyma containing a dense lymphocytic infiltrate with **germinal centers**. Residual thyroid follicles are lined by deeply **eosinophilic Hürthle cells**. This suggests Hashimoto's thyroiditis.

2. Ans. (b) Orphan Annie eye nuclei; papillary Ca thyroid
- High power shows nuclei of papillary carcinoma cells contain finely dispersed chromatin, which imparts an **optically clear** or **empty** appearance, giving rise to the **ground glass** or **Orphan Annie eye nuclei**. In addition, invaginations of the cytoplasm may give the appearance of intranuclear inclusions ("pseudoinclusions") or intranuclear grooves. **The diagnosis of papillary carcinoma can be made based on these nuclear features,** even in the absence of papillary architecture.

3. Ans. (c) Medullary Ca thyroid
- Diarrhea in thyroid tumor can be a paraneoplastic syndromes due to VIP in a case of medullary Ca thyroid. Histology demonstrates abundant **deposition of amyloid**, visible here as homogeneous extracellular material, derived from calcitonin molecules secreted by the neoplastic cells.

4. Ans. (b) Zellballen in pheochrocytoma
- The tumor is enclosed within an attenuated cortex and demonstrates areas of hemorrhage. The histology of the same shows characteristic **nests of cells ("Zellballen")** with abundant cytoplasm

5. Ans. (c) Kimmelsteil Wilson lesion, Diabetic non proliferative retinopathy due to microangiopathy.
- Given kidney biospsy shows spherical, laminated, **nodules of matrix** at the **periphery of glomerulus** which are PAS-positive referred to as Nodular or Intercapillary Glomerulosclerosis or Kimmelstiel-Wilson disease. Remember retinopathy is a microangiopathy and not macroangiopathy.

6. Ans. (a) Water clear cells in parathyroid hyperplasia.
- The given histology shows abundant **optically clear cells** of variable size (hyperplasia and hypertrophy), with spherical clear vacuoles surrounded by thin eosinophilic material; basal nuclei, compact or alveolar patterns.

7. Ans. (c) Brown tumor in primary hyperparathyroidism
- Given histology shows brown **colour-vascularity, haemorrhage** & hemosiderin deposition in a case of primary hyperparathyroidism (Increased PTH hormaone levels, Calcium levels)

Multiple Choice Questions

PITUITARY

1. GNAS mutation is associated with malignancy of which cells? *(Recent Question 2016)*
   a. Lactotroph
   b. Somatotroph
   c. Thyrotroph
   d. None

2. Human chorionic thyrotropin is secreted from: *(Recent Question 2015)*
   a. Placenta
   b. Pituitary
   c. Hypothalamus
   d. Thyroid

3. Which of these organs are not affected in autoimmune polyglandular syndrome type 2? *(Recent Question 2015)*
   a. Parathyroid
   b. Thyroid
   c. Adrenal
   d. Pancreas

4. Proopiomelanocortin is not released from? *(Recent Question 2015)*
   a. Hypothalamus
   b. Liver
   c. Lung
   d. Adrenal gland

5. Posterior pituitary secretes- *(Recent Question 2014)*
   a. GH
   b. TSH
   c. ADH
   d. FSH

6. Findings of SIADH includes: *(PGI May 12)*
   a. ↑ Urine Na+
   b. ↑ S. Na+
   c. ↑ Urine osmolality
   d. ↑Serum osmolality
   e. Postural hypotension

7. A patient presents with Endocrinopathy, fibrous dysplasia of bone and hyperpigmentation. Diagnosis is?
   a. McCune Albright syndrome *(JIPMER 2011)*
   b. Addison's disease
   c. Alagille syndrome
   d. Lynch syndrome

THYROIDITIS

8. 25-year-old female presented with swelling in front of neck. TSH levels were elevated. Biopsy showed lymphocytic infiltration and Hurthle cells. Which of the following is the possible diagnosis?

(Recent Pattern Question 2020)

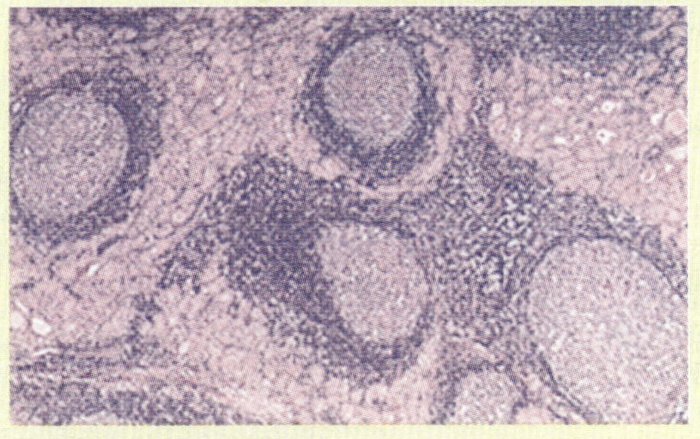

   a. Graves' disease
   b. Hashimoto's thyroiditis
   c. Medullary carcinoma thyroid
   d. Papillary carcinoma thyroid

9. Autoimmune thyroiditis is associated with all except- *(Recent Question 2014)*
   a. DM
   b. Myasthenia gravis
   c. SLE
   d. Psoriasis

10. Patients with Hashimoto's thyroiditis are at increased risk of developing: *(MH 10)*
   a. Papillary carcinoma
   b. Follicular carcinoma
   c. T-cell lymphoma
   d. B-cell Lymphoma

THYROID CARCINOMA

11. Patient came with swelling in midline of neck measuring 2 cm in size. Histopathological examination showed Orphan Annie-eye nuclei. What is the most likely diagnosis? *(Recent Pattern Question 2020)*
   a. Medullary carcinoma
   b. Papillary carcinoma thyroid
   c. Toxic nodular goiter
   d. Follicular thyroid carcinoma

12. Risk factors for solitary thyroid to be malignant? *(PGI Nov 2018)*
   a. Male sex
   b. Middle age
   c. Elderly age
   d. Iodine sufficiency

13. Papillary carcinoma of thyroid features?
   a. Haematological spread is early *(PGI Nov 2018)*
   b. Most commonly occurring thyroid carcinoma
   c. Capsular invasion is characteristic sign
   d. Shows worse prognosis than follicular type

14. 40-year-old female presented with neck swelling. Gross and histology is shown below. What is your diagnosis? *(Recent exam 2018)*

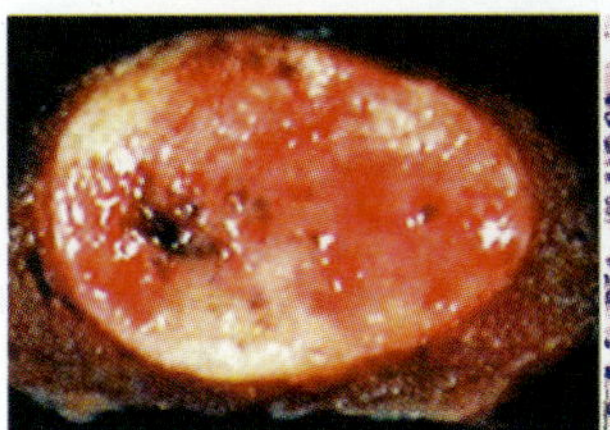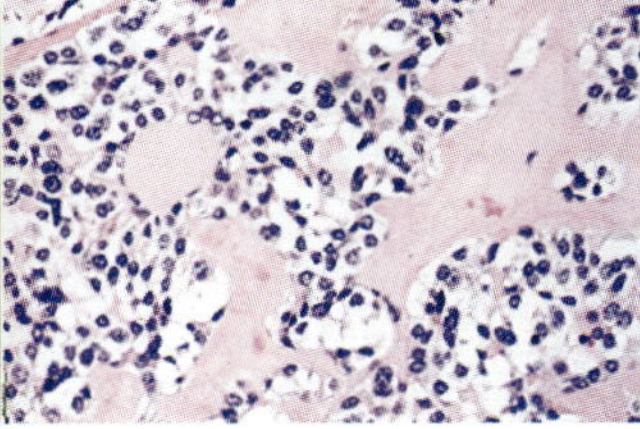

   a. Medullary carcinoma thyroid
   b. Hashimotos thyroiditis
   c. Anaplastic carcinoma
   d. Follicular carcinoma

15. A patient presented with neck swelling. Cytology showed showed parafollicular cells along with clusters of plasmacytoid and few spindle shaped cells. What investigation should be done to follow up the patient?
   a. Calcitonin
   b. TSH level *(JIPMER 2017)*
   c. Anti TPO antibody
   d. TRH

16. All the following condition can be diagnosed by FNAC except? *(AIIMS Nov 2016)*
   a. Follicular Ca thyroid
   b. Anaplastic Carcinoma
   c. Papillary carcinoma
   d. Medullary carcinoma

17. Lymphatic spread most commonly seen in which type of thyroid carcinoma? *(AIIMS May 2015)*
   a. Papillary
   b. Medullary
   c. Follicular
   d. Lymphoma

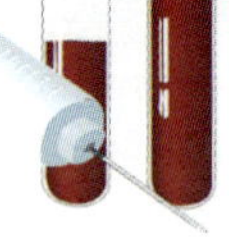

18. Which one of the following variants of papillary carcinoma thyroid occurs in younger individuals including children with lymphonodal metastases in almost all cases and morphologically simulates Hashimoto thyroiditis is: *(AP 2012)*
a. Tall-cell variant
b. Follicular variant
c. Diffuse sclerosing variant
d. Oncocyticvarient

19. Thyroglossal cyst is associated with which type of thyroid Ca? *(Recent Question 2015)*
a. Papillary
b. Medullary
c. Anaplastic
d. Lymphoma

20. About Reidel thyroiditis, which is true?
a. Extensive fibrosis involving thyroid *(PGI Nov 2015)*
b. Fibrosis in retroperitoneum
c. IgG4-related disease
d. Occurs in middle-aged women
e. Painful gland

21. Hematogenous route of metastasis is seen in which type of thyroid carcinoma? *(Recent Question 2016)*
a. Papillary
b. Medullary
c. Anaplastic
d. Follicular

22. Hurthle cell carcinoma is a variant of -
(Recent Question 2014)
a. Medullary carcinoma
b. Papillary carcinoma
c. Follicular carcinoma
d. Anaplastic carcinoma

23. Medullary ca of thyroid is associated with increase in:
(Recent Question 2014)
a. Calcitonin
b. Thyroglobulin
c. T3
d. T4

24. Which thyroid carcinoma has amyloid deposition:
(Recent Question 2014, MH 11)
a. Anaplastic
b. Follicular
c. Medullary
d. Papillary

25. True about Psammoma bodies are all except:
a. Seen in meningioma *(Recent Question 2013)*
b. Concentric whorled appearance
c. Dystrophic calcification
d. Seen in teratoma

26. Most common Thyroid ca post radiation exposure:
(Recent Question 2014)
a. Papillary CA
b. Medullary CA
c. Follicular CA
d. Anaplstic CA

27. Orphan annie-eye nuclei appearance is characteristic of *(Recent Question 2014, DNB Aug 12) (WB PG 2016)*
a. Papillary carcinoma thyroid
b. Carcinoma pituitary
c. Follicular ca thyroid
d. Medullary ca thyroid

28. Psammoma bodies can be seen in the following except?
a. Follicular carcinoma of thyroid *(AI 11)*
b. Papillary carcinoma of thyroid
c. Meningioma
d. Serous cytadenoma of ovary

29. Most common thyroid Cancer is - *(AP PGMEE 11, AI 00)*
a. Papillary carcinoma
b. Follicular carcinoma
c. Medullary carcinoma
d. Anaplastic carcinoma

PARATHYROID GLAND

30. Active form of Vit D? *(Recent Question 2015)*
a. $1,25\,(OH)_2\,Vit\,D_3$
b. $25\,OH\,Vit\,D_3$
c. $Vit\,D_3$
d. $Vit\,D_2$

31. The cut off for serum Calcium level below which it is called Hypocalcemia is: *(Recent Question 2015)*
a. 6 mg/dl
b. 7 mg/dl
c. 8 mg/dl
d. 9 mg/dl

32. Diagnostic feature of parathyroid carcinoma is-
(Recent Question 2014)
a. Cytology
b. Metastasis
c. Clinical features
d. All

33. Most common cause of primary hyperparathyroidism is: *(Recent Question 2014)*
a. Adenoma
b. Hyperplasia
c. Hypertrophy
d. Carcinoma

34. Gs-alpha mutation my lead to? *(Recent Question 2013)*
a. Mccune Albright syndrome
b. Pseudohypoparathyroidism
c. Pituitary adenomas
d. All of the above

35. Brown tumor of bone is seen in - *(AI 11)*
a. Hyperparathyroidism
b. Hypoparathyroidisrm
c. Hypo-thyroidism
d. Hyperthyroidism

PANCREAS

36. Whipple's triad is diagnostic of: *(AP PGMEE 2015)*
a. Gastrinoma
b. Insulinoma
c. somatostinoma
d. Glucogonoma

37. Which of these is the most common cause for insulin resistance? *(Recent Question 2015)*
a. Obesity
b. Post receptor defects
c. Liver dysfunction
d. Pancreatic dysfunction

38. Insulin resistance in liver disease is due to:
a. Decreased insulin release *(AIIMS May 2012)*
b. Steatosis
c. Hepatocyte dysfunction
d. Decreased 'C' peptide level

39. True about neuroendocrine tumors of pancreas is/are?
(PGI May 2011)
a. Insulinoma is most common neuroendocrine tumors of pancreas
b. VIPoma causes diarrhea
c. Diarrhea is most common symptom of gastrinoma
d. Somatostatinoma causes gall stone formation
e. Gastrinoma has high chance of malignancy

40. Nesidioblastoma is due to hyperplasia of-
a. Alpha cell
b. Beta cell *(PGI Dec 2011)*
c. Acinus
d. D cells

DIABETES

41. 70 M presented to AIIMS OPD with fatigue. Fasting sugar was 110 mg%, PP was 180 mg%, Hba1c was 6.1 %. What is your diagnosis? *(Recent Question 2016)*
a. Prediabetes
b. Stress induced
c. Normal
d. Diabetes

42. **For diagnosis of DM, fasting blood glucose level should be more than?** *(Recent Question 2014)*
    a. 126 mg/dl
    b. 140 mg/dl
    c. 100 mg/dl
    d. 200 mg/dl

43. **Which of the following drugs does not give rise to hyperglycemia?** *(Recent Question 2015)*
    a. Thiazides
    b. Phenytoin
    c. Chloroquine
    d. Prednisolone

44. **Which is the most common acute complication of diabetes?** *(Recent Question 2015)*
    a. Diabetic ketoacidosis
    b. Hyperosmolar nonketotic hyperglycemia
    c. Hypoglycemia
    d. Stroke

45. **Mechanisms responsible for chronic complications of Diabetes include all of the following except:** *(Recent Question 2015)*
    a. Non-enzymatic Glycosylation
    b. Protein Kinase C activation
    c. Disturbances in Polyol Pathways
    d. Chronic Inflammation

46. **Most commonly seen feature in kidney biopsy of a patient with Diabetic Nephropathy is:**
    a. Diffuse Mesangial Sclerosis   *(Recent Question 2014)*
    b. Diffuse glomerulosclerosis
    c. Nodular glomerulosclerosis
    d. Fibrin caps

47. **Which of the following is not an example of Diabetic Microangiopathy?** *(Recent Question 2014)*
    a. Nephropathy
    b. Stroke
    c. Retinopathy
    d. Neuropathy

48. **All of the following are ocular complications of Diabetes except:** *(Recent Question 2014)*
    a. Cataract
    b. Corneal opacity
    c. Proliferative Retinopathy
    d. Glaucoma

49. **Most common type of MODY is:** *(Recent Question 2013)*
    a. MODY 1
    b. MODY 2
    c. MODY 3
    d. MODY 4

50. **All of the following statement about Type 1 Diabetes are true except?** *(PGI Dec 11)*
    a. Family history is present in 90% cases
    b. Dependent on Insulin to prevent DKA
    c. Type of onset is usually predictable
    d. Autoimmune destruction of β-cells
    e. Often occurs in children

PHEOCHROMOCYTOMA

51. **True about pheochromocytoma:** *(PGI May 2019)*
    a. Before surgery alpha blockers are given
    b. Always forms part of MEN1 syndrome
    c. Mostly malignant
    d. Mostly familial
    e. Associated with von Hippel-Lindau disease

52. **All of the following are PNET Tumors except?** *(PGI Nov 2016)*
    a. Rhabdomyosarcoma
    b. Osteosarcoma
    c. Ewings Sa
    d. Medulloepithelioma
    e. Retinoblastoma

53. **Sustentacular cells of pheochromocytoma are positive for which of the following markers?** *(Recent Question 2016-17)*
    a. S-100
    b. Cytokeratin
    c. Vimentin
    d. Desmin

54. **Neuroendocrine tumors are positive for?** *(Recent Question 2016-17)*
    a. Synaptophysisn
    b. Langerin
    c. CD1 a
    d. CD 5a

55. **Zellballen pattern is found in histology of which of the following condition?** *(Recent Question 2016-17)*
    a. Neuroblastoma
    b. Paraganglioma
    c. Ewings Sarcoma
    d. RCC

56. **Carcinoid tumours commonly arise from:**
    a. G. cells in pancreas   *(Recent Question 2016-17)*
    b. Argentaffin cells of small intestine
    c. Pancreatic endocrine tumour
    d. Colon polyps

57. **Which of the following is paraganglioma:** *(Recent Question 2016-17)*
    a. Adrenal Pheochromocytoma
    b. Extra-adrenal Pheochromocytoma
    c. Carotid body tumour
    d. Carcinoid tumour
    e. Glomus tympanicum

58. **Pheochromocytomas has been associated with 'the rule of 10's. The following statements are true about Pheochromocytoma except?** *(Recent Question 2015)*
    a. 10% are bilateral
    b. 10% extra adrenal
    c. 10% inherited
    d. 10% malignant

59. **Pheochromocytoma is a tumour of** *(MH PG 2014)*
    a. Parathyroid
    b. Adrenal medulla
    c. Adrenal cortex
    d. Pituitary

60. **Which of the following are true about pheochromocytoma?** *(PGI May 2014)*
    a. Synthesizes epinephrine &norepinephrine
    b. Increased urinary 5HIAA
    c. Diagnosed by urinary catecholamine metabolites
    d. Tumor of adrenal cortex and sympathetic ganglion
    e. Tumor of adrenal medulla and sympathetic ganglion

61. **Tumor that follows rule of 10 is** *(Recent Question 2013, 2014)*
    a. Pheochromocytoma
    b. Oncocytoma
    c. Lymphoma
    d. Renal cell carcinoma

62. **Which of the following is most reliable feature of malignant transformation of pheochromocytoma –**
    a. Involvement of lymph nodes *(Recent Question 2013)*
    b. Capsular invasion
    c. Vascular invasion
    d. Pleomorphism

63. **Glomus Cells are found in -** *(Recent Question 2013)*
    a. Carotid body Tumour
    b. Thyroid carcinoma
    c. Livercarcinoma
    d. None

64. **Zellballen pattern is found in -** *(PGI Nov 11)*
    a. Pheochromocytoma
    b. Paraganglioma
    c. Acoustic neuroma
    d. Transitional renal cell carcinoma
    e. Schwannoma

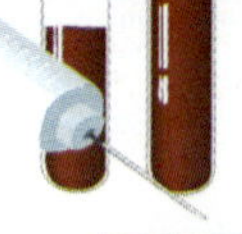

MEN

65. Most common site of gastrinoma in MEN 1 is:
(Recent Pattern Question 2020)
- a. Stomach
- b. Jejunum
- c. Duodenum
- d. Appendix

66. Which is found more in MEN2B than MEN2A?
- a. Medullary carcinoma thyroid *(PGI Nov 2018)*
- b. Hyperparathyroidism
- c. Pheochromocytoma
- d. Marfanoid features
- e. Mucosal neuromas

67. All are the features of MEN-1 except:?
- a. Pancreatic neuroendocrine tumour *(AIIMS Nov 2016)*
- b. Midgut carcinoid
- c. Posterior pituitary tumour
- d. Parathyroid adenoma

68. What is most probable diagnosis of a patient who has prolactinoma, parathyroid hyperplasia and family history of renal stones? *(Recent Question 2016-17)*
- a. MEN-I
- b. MEN-II
- c. NF1
- d. Li fraumeni syndrome

69. Which of the following is not associated with a mutation in RET gene? *(Recent Question 2015)*
- a. Leukemia
- b. MEN2A
- c. Hirschsprung's disease
- d. MEN1

70. Most common neuroendocrine tumor in MEN -1 is?
(Recent Question 2016)
- a. Insulinoma
- b. Gastrinoma
- c. Glucagonoma
- d. VIPoma

71. Which neuroendocrine tumor causes biliary sclerosis?
(Recent Question 2016)
- a. Somatostatinoma
- b. Gastrinoma
- c. Insulinoma
- d. Glucagonoma

72. Commonest thyroid tumor in MEN (multiple endocrine neoplasia) is: *(Recent Question 2014)*
- a. Follicular
- b. Papillary
- c. Anaplastic
- d. Medullary

73. Which of the following is not involved in MEN type IIA-
(Recent Question 2014)
- a. Parathyroid
- b. Adrenal
- c. Thyroid
- d. Pituitary

74. Wermer syndrome is - *(Recent Question 2014)*
- a. MEN 1
- b. MEN IIA
- c. MEN-IIB
- d. APS

75. MEN type I includes tumors of all except -
- a. Parathyroid *(Recent Question 2014)*
- b. Pituitary
- c. Pancreas
- d. Medullary carcinoma of thyroid

76. Which of the following is not true about medullary carcinoma of thyroid? *(MAHA 10)*
- a. Origin is from C cells of thyroid
- b. Component of MEN-1
- c. Multicentric in origin
- d. Amyloid deposition

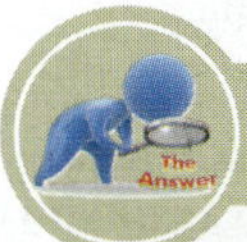

Answers with Explanations

1. Ans. (b) Somatotrophs *(Ref: Robbins 9th/pg)*

The mutation of guanine nucleotide-activating alpha subunit (GNAS) gene is the somatic mutation related to the McCune-Albright syndrome.

GNAS mutation is also detected in about 30% to 40% of sporadic growth hormone (GH) secreting tumors.

2. Ans. (a) Placenta *(Ref: Harrison's 18th/chapter 341)*

TSH secreted by placenta is called **Human chorionic thyrotropin.**

3. Ans. (c) Adrenal

(Ref: Robbins 9th/pg 1130; 8th/pg 1155-1156, Harrison 18th/chapter 318)

Autoimmune polyglandular syndrome

Disease	Gene	Characteristics
APS-1	AIRE (Chr 21q)	**A**utoimmune **P**oly **E**ndocrinopathy, **C**andidiasis, and **E**ctodermal **D**ystrophy[Q] **(APECED),** Hypoparathyroidism, rarely lymphomas
APS-2	HLA DR3, CTLA-4	Hypothyroidism, hyperthyroidism, premature ovarian failure, vitiligo, type 1 diabetes mellitus, pernicious anemia

4. Ans. (a) Hypothalamus

(Ref: Harrison 18th/chapter 339 Robbins 9th/pg1074; 8th/pg 1098)

- The **main source of POMC is pituitary gland**
- **Other sources of POMC are Adrenal, gut, reproductive tract, placenta, leukocytes, spleen, lung, liver, thyroid, heart, skin & brain**

5. Ans. (c) ADH *(Ref: Robbins 9th/pg1074; 8th/pg 1098)*

Posterior pituitary
Produces two hormones:
- Arginine vasopressin (AVP), also known as **antidiuretic hormone (ADH)**
- **Oxytocin**

6. Ans. (a) ↑ Urine Na+; (c) ↑ Urine osmolality

(Ref: Harrison 18th/chapter 100 Robbins 9th/pg 1081-1082; 8th/pg 1106)

In syndrome of inappropriate ADH (SIADH):[Q]
- **ADH excess** → resorption of excessive amounts of **free water**
- Excessive retention of water **expands extracellular & intracellular volume**, increases glomerular filtration

and atrial natriuretic hormone, suppresses plasma renin activity, and **increases urinary sodium excretion**.
- This **natriuresis reduces total body sodium**, resulting in **hyponatremia.**
- **Reduced serum osmolality** occur in the setting of an inappropriately **normal or increased urine osmolality**

7. Ans. (a) McCune Albright syndrome

(Ref: Robbins 9th/pg 1206-1207)

McCune-Albright syndrome

Genetics	It is due to **GNAS mutation→continuous activation of stimulatory G protein**
Patho-physiology	**Increased production of hormones** by glands regulated by the G protein system
Clinical features	Precocious puberty, Polyostotic fibrous dysplasia, unilateral Café au lait spots

8. Ans. (b) Hashimoto's thyroiditis

(Ref: Robbins 9th/pg 1086)

9. Ans. (d) Psoriasis *(Ref: Robbins 9th/pg 1086-1087)*

Patients with (autoimmune) Hashimoto thyroiditis are at increased risk for developing:

- **B-cell Non Hodgkins lymphoma**[Q]
- **Autoimmune diseases:**
  - Endocrine (**type 1 diabetes, autoimmune adrenalitis**)[Q]
  - Non-endocrine (**SLE, myasthenia gravis, and Sjögren syndrome**)

10. Ans. (d) B-cell Lymphoma

(Ref: Robbins 9th/pg 1086-1087)

11. Ans. (b) Papillary carcinoma thyroid *(Ref: R 9th pg 1086)*

12. Ans. (c, d); c. elderly age; d. Iodine sufficiency

13. Ans. (b) Most commonly occurring thyroid carcinoma

14. Ans. (a) Medullary carcinoma thyroid

(Ref: Robbins 9th ed p 1099)

Sporadic medullary thyroid carcinomas present as a solitary nodule. In contrast, bilaterality and multicentricity are common in familial cases. Larger lesions often contain areas of necrosis and hemorrhage and may extend through the capsule of the thyroid. The tumor tissue is firm, pale gray to tan, and infiltrative.

Microscopically, medullary carcinomas are composed of polygonal to spindle-shaped cells, which may form nests, tra-beculae, and even follicles. Small, more anaplastic cells are present in some tumors and may be the predominant cell type. Acellular amyloid deposits derived from calcitonin polypeptides are present in the stroma in many cases

15. Ans. (a) Calcitonin

Cytology showed showed parafollicular cells along with clusters of plasmacytoid and few spindle shaped cells are suggestive of medullary ca thyroid and so should be followed up by its tumor marker calcitonin.

16. Ans. (c) Papillary carcinoma *(Ref: R 9th ed. Pg. 631)*

The hallmark of all follicular adenomas is the presence of an intact, well-formed capsule encircling the tumor. **Careful evaluation of the integrity of the capsule is therefore critical in distinguishing follicular adenomas from follicular carcinomas**, which demonstrate capsular and/or vascular invasion. This can be demonstrated by biopsy of the gland and not FNAC which will demonstrate only the morphology of the tumor cells and not the entire gland histology

17. Ans. (a) Papillary *(Ref: Robbins 9th/pg 1097-1098)*

Thyroid carinoma type	Route of spread
Papillary	Lymphatic
Follicular	Hematogenous
Medullary	Regional lymphatic spread and hematogeneous *routes* to distant sites
Anaplastic	Direct

18. Ans. (c) Diffuse sclerosing variant

(Ref: Robbins 9th/pg 1097-1098)

Diffuse sclerosing variant of papillary carcinoma
- It occurs in younger individuals, including children.
- The tumor has a prominent papillary growth pattern intermixed with solid areas containing nests of squamous metaplasia.
- There is extensive, diffuse fibrosis throughout the thyroid gland, often associated with a prominent lymphocytic infiltrate, simulating Hashimoto thyroiditis.
- Lymph node metastases are present in almost all cases.
- Diffuse sclerosing variant carcinomas lack BRAF mutations, but RET/PTCtranslocations are found in approximately half the cases.

19. Ans. (a) Papillary *(Ref: Robbins 9th/pg 1097-1098)*

Papillary carcinoma accounts for 80% of cases of thyroglossal duct carcinomas, with the rest being squamous cell carcinoma

20. Ans. (a, b, c, d) a. Extensive fibrosis involving thyroid; b. Fibrosis in retroperitoneum; c. IgG4-related disease; d. Occurs in middle-aged women

(Ref: R 9th/pg 1097-1098)

Riedel Thyroiditis

It is a rare disorder that typically occurs in middle-aged women.

It presents with an insidious, painless goiter with local symptoms due to compression of the esophagus, trachea, neck veins, or recurrent laryngeal nerves.

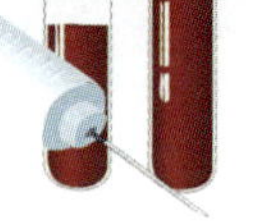

Dense fibrosis disrupts normal gland architecture and can extend outside the thyroid capsule.

Despite these extensive histologic changes, thyroid dysfunction is uncommon.

Fibrosis of retroperitoneum can also occur

Associated with Systemic autoimmune **IgG4-related disease** (fibrosis & tissue infiltration by plasma cells producing IgG4)

21.   Ans. (d) Follicular (*Ref: Robbins 9th/pg 1097-1098*)

22.   Ans. (c) Follicular carcinoma (*Ref: R 9th/pg 1097-1098*)

Hurthle cell or oncocytic variant of follicular carcinoma has characteristic cells with abundant eosinophilic cytoplasm.

Other variants of Papillary Ca are:

Follicular variant	Nuclear features of papillary Ca, but follicular architecture More angioinvasive with less lymphatic metastasis
Tall-cell variant	More common in older individuals; Histopath: Tallcolumnar eosinophilic cells Higher vascularinvasion, extra-thyroid extension and distantmetastases
Diffuse sclerosing	More common on young and children; Extensive, diffuse fibrosis;
Papillary Microcarcinoma	< 1 cm size; precursors of typical papillary carcinomas

23.   Ans. (a) Calcitonin (*Ref: Robbins 9th/pg 1099-1100*)

- **In Medullary Carcinoma Thyroid, serum Calcitonin is elevated.**
- **Elevated serum calcitonin** also provides a marker of **residual or recurrent** disease.
- All patients with **Medullary Carcinoma Thyroid** should also be tested for *RET* mutations, so that genetic counseling and testing of family members can be offered;

24.   Ans. (c) Medullary (*Ref: Robbins 9th/pg 1099-1100*)

Medullary carcinoma thyroid presents with **amyloid deposition of ACal type.**

25.   Ans. (d) Seen in teratoma (*Ref: Robbins 9th/pg 1096*)

Psammoma Bodies are

Lamellated, concentrically calcified structures formed by progressive acquisition of outer layers;

26.   Ans. (a) Papillary CA (*Ref: Robbins 9th/pg 1095-1097*)

Most common Thyroid Carcinoma post radiation exposure is **Papillary CA**

27.   Ans. (a) Papillary carcinoma thyroid

(*Ref: Robbins 9th/pg 1095-1097*)

28.   Ans. (a) Follicular carcinoma of thyroid

(*Ref: Robbins 9th/pg 1096; 8th/pg 38, 1122*)

29.   Ans. (a) Papillary carcinoma (*Ref: R 9th/pg 1095-1097*)

Most common thyroid Cancer is **Papillary carcinoma**

30.   Ans. (a) 1,25 (OH)2 Vit D3

(*Ref: Harrison 18th/chapter 352*)

Active form of Vit D is $1,25\,(OH)_2 Vit\ D_3$

31.   Ans. (c) 8 mg/dl (*Ref: Harrison 18th/Appendix*)

Normal Calcium level

Calcium	Serum	2.2–2.6 mmol/L	8.7–10.2 mg/dL
Calcium, ionized	Whole Blood	1.12–1.32 mmol/L	4.5–5.3 mg/dL

Hypocalcemia refers to total serum Ca< 8 mg/dl or ionized Ca< 1 mmol/L

32.   Ans. (b) Metastasis

(*Ref: Robbins 9th/pg 1104; 8th/pg 1129*)

Morphology in hyperparathyroidism

Parathyroid adenomas	**Solitary lesions** withuniform, polygonal chief cells along with nests of oxyphil cells **(oxyphil adenomas)**
Primary hyperplasia	**Chief cell hyperplasia** with abundant water-clear cells **("water-clear cell hyperplasia")** involving all 4 glands
Parathyroid Carcinomas	Circumscribed lesion in a single gland **diagnosed by invasion** of **surrounding tissues** and **metastasis** as the only **reliable criteria.**

33.   Ans. (a) Adenoma (*Ref: Robbins 9th/pg 1104*)

Most common cause of primary hyperparathyroidism is **Adenoma**

34.   Ans. (d) All of the above

(*Ref: Robbins 9th/pg 1077, 1101; 8th/pg 1101, 1127*)

GSα		
Loss of function	Gain of function	Gain or loss of function
• Pseudohypoparathyroidim type Ia • Pseudohypoparathyroidim type Ib	• Pituitary or thyroid adenomas • Leydig cell tumors • McCune-Albright syndrome	• Testotoxicosis with pseudo-hypoparathyroidism type Ia

Gi2α: Gain of function

- Pituitary adenomas
- Adrenal cortex and ovary tumors

35.   Ans. (a) Hyperparathyroidism (*Ref: R 9th/pg 1102*)

Skeletal Abnormalities in Hyperparathyroidism:

- Osteoporosis- cortical bone more severely involved than medullary bone
- Brown tumors: brown colour- due to increased vascularity, hemorrhage & hemosiderin deposition
- Osteitisfibrosacystica (von Recklinghausen disease of bone)

36. **Ans. (b)** **Insulinoma** *(Ref: Robbins 9th/pg 1121; 8th 1146)*

37. **Ans. (b)** **Post receptor defects**

(Ref: Robbins 9th/pg1111)

"Postreceptor" defects in insulin-regulated **phosphorylation/dephosphorylation** appear to play the predominant role in insulin resistance.

- PI-3-kinase signaling defect might reduce **translocation of GLUT4** to the plasma membrane.
- **Accumulation of lipid** within skeletal myocytes may **impair mitochondrial oxidative phosphorylation** and **reduce insulin-stimulated mitochondrial ATP production.**
- **Impaired fatty acid oxidation** and **lipid accumulation** within skeletal myocytes also may generate **reactive oxygen species** such as lipid peroxides.

38. **Ans. (c)** **Hepatocyte dysfunction**

(Ref: World J Hepatol. 2011 May 27; 3(5): 99–107)

Factors responsible for development of hepatogenous insulin resistance/diabetes:

- Hepatic parenchymal cell damage
- Portal-systemic shunting
- Hepatitis C virus

HCV genotype 3 can give rise to insulin resistance and non alcoholic fatty liver disease (NAFLD)

39. **Ans. (a, b, d, e); a. Insulinoma is most common neuroendocrine tumors of pancreas; b. VIPoma causes diarrhea; d. Somatostatinoma causes gall stone formation, e. Gastrinoma has high chance of malignancy** *(Ref: Harrison 18th/chapter 350)*

40. **Ans. (b)** **Beta cell**

(Ref: Robbins 9th/pg 1121; 8th/pg 1146)

- **Nesidioblastosis is** Focal or diffuse hyperplasia of the β-**cells**[Q] in pancreatic islets
- **Nesidioblastosis**can also be seen in:
  - Infant of diabetic mother[Q]
  - Beckwith-Wiedemann syndrome[Q]
  - Rare mutations in the β-**cell K+ channel protein or sulfonylurea receptor**

41. **Ans. (a)** **Prediabetes** *(Ref: Robbins 9th/pg 1106; 8th 1131)*

Diagnostic criteria according to ADA and WHO: Presence of any 1 or more of the following:

Criteria	Diabetes	Impaired glucose tolerance (pre-diabetes)
Fasting plasma glucose	≥126 mg/dL	between **100 and 125 mg/dL**
Random plasma glucose	≥200 mg/dL	–
2-hour plasma glucose during oral glucose tolerance test **(OGTT)** with 75 g	≥ 200 mg/dL	between **140 and 199 mg/dL**
Glycated hemoglobin **(HbA1C) level**	≥ 6.5%	between **5.7%** and **6.4%.**

42. **Ans. (a)** **126 mg/dl**

(Ref: Robbins 9th/pg 1106; 8th/pg 1131)

43. **Ans. (c)** **Chloroquine**

(Ref: Robbins 9th/pg 1107)

Important drugs that give rise to hyperglycemia are:

- Glucocorticoids[Q]
- Thyroid hormone
- β-adrenergic agonists[Q]
- Thiazides[Q]
- Phenytoin[Q]

44. **Ans. (c)** **Hypoglycemia**

(Ref: Robbins 9th/pg 1115-1116)

Acute Metabolic Complications of Diabetes:

- Diabetic ketoacidosis (Type 1 > type 2 DM)
- Hyperosmolar nonketotic hyperglycemia (Type 2 > type 1 DM)
- **Hypoglycemia**[Q] **(most common acute complication)**

45. **Ans. (d)** **Chronic Inflammation**

(Ref: Robbins 9th/pg1115-1116)

Mechanisms responsible for chronic complications of Diabetes are:

- Non-enzymatic Glycosylation
- Protein Kinase C activation
- Disturbances in Polyol Pathways

46. **Ans. (a)** **Diffuse Mesangial Sclerosis**

(Ref: Robbins 9th/pg1118-1119)

47. **Ans. (b)** **Stroke**

(Ref: Robbins 9th/pg1115-1116)

48. **Ans. (b)** **Corneal opacity**

(Ref: Robbins 9th/pg 1115-1116)

Diabetic Ocular Complications

- Diabetes-induced hyperglycemiacan lead to **cataract**[Q]
- **Glaucoma → damage to optic nerve**[Q]
- **Retinal vasculopathy:**[Q] **Can be non-proliferative or proliferative**

49. **Ans. (c)** **MODY 3**

(Ref: Robbins 9th/pg 1107; 8th/pg 1132)

Most common type of MODY is MODY3

Genetic defects of β-cell function:

Maturity-onset diabetes of the young (MODY)
- **MODY1:** Hepatocyte nuclear factor 4α **(HNF4A)**[Q]
- **MODY2:**Glucokinase **(GCK)**[Q]
- **MODY3:** Hepatocyte nuclear factor 1α **(HNF1A)**[Q]
- **MODY4:** Insulin promoter factor-1 **(IPF-1)**
- **Neonatal diabetes** (Mutations in **KCNJ11&ABCC8**)[Q]

50. **Ans. (a, c); a. Family history is present in 90% cases; c. Type of onset is usually predictable**

(Ref: Robbins 9th/pg 1106-1110; 8th/pg 1131-1134 Harrison 18th/chapter 344)

Discussing options about **Type 1 Diabetes**, one by one

a.	False as **Family history is present 10-20%cases**
b.	True as **insulin deficiency predisposes to DKA**
c.	False as the **rate of decline in beta cell mass varies widely** among individuals, with some patients progressing rapidly to clinical diabetes and others evolving more slowly. **Features of diabetes do not become evident until a majority of beta cells are destroyed (70–80%).**
d.	True as **circulating islet autoantibodies** (anti-insulin, anti-GAD, anti-ICA512) causes immune destruction of B cells
e.	True as **it usually involves normal wt children & young adults**

51. **Ans. (a) Before surgery alpha blockers are given; (c) Mostly malignant; (d) Mostly familial; (e) Associated with von Hippel-Lindau disease** *(Ref: R 9th pg 1135)*

Pheochromocytoma is often associated with MEN-2A, MEN-2B, NF1, Von Hippel-Lindau (VHL), Familial paraganglioma

52. **Ans. (c, d) c. Ewings Sa d. Medulloepithelioma**

(Ref: Robbins 9th/pg 1134-1136)

Primitive neuroectodermal tumors (PNETs) are a group of highly malignant tumors comThe following tumors are classified as peripheral primitive neuroectodermal tumors (pPNETs):

- Ewing sarcoma (osseus and extraosseous)
- Malignant peripheral primitive neuroectodermal tumors (pPNETs) or peripheral neuroepithelioma of bone and soft tissues
- Askin tumor (peripheral neuroepithelioma of the thoracopulmonary region)
- Other less common tumors (eg, neuroectodermal tumor, ectomesenchymoma, peripheral medulloepithelioma)

53. **Ans. (a) S-100** *(Ref: Robbins 9/1135)*

In pheochromocytoma: Immunoreactivity for neuroendocrine markers (chromogranin and synaptophysin) is seen in the chief cells, while the peripheral sustentacular cells stain with antibodies against S-100 which is a calcium-binding protein.

54. **Ans. (a) Synaptophysisn**

55. **Ans. (b) Paraganglioma** *(Ref: Robbins 9/1135)*

The histologic pattern in pheochromocytoma shows tumor cells composed of clusters of polygonal to spindle shaped chromaffin cells or chief cells that are surrounded by supporting sustentacular cells, creating small nests or alveoli called zellballen. These are supplied by a rich vascular network

56. **Ans. (b) Argentaffin cells of small intestine**

Carcinoid tumors arise from argentaffin cells of the crypts of Lieberkühn and are found from the distal duodenum to the ascending colon, areas embryologically derived from the midgut.

57. **Ans. (b, c, e) b. Extra-adrenal Pheochromocytoma c. Carotid body tumour e. Glomus tympanicum**

(Ref: Robbins 9th/ 741-42; Harrison 19th/ 2329-35; Davidson 22nd/ 781; CMDT 2016/ 1158; Danhert Radiology Review Manual 7th/401)

Pheochromocytomas and paragangliomas are catecholamine- producing tumors derived from the sympathetic or parasympathetic nervous system

58. **Ans. (c) 10% inherited**

(Ref: Robbins 9th/pg 1134-1135/8th 1159-1160)

59. **Ans. (b) Adrenal medulla (Ref: Robbins 9th/pg 1135)**

60. **Ans. (a, b, c, e); a. Synthesizes epinephrine & norepinephrine; b. Increased urinary 5HIAA; c. Diagnosed by urinary catecholamine metabolites; e. Tumor of adrenal medulla and sympathetic ganglion**

(Ref: Robbins 9th/pg 1134-1135; 8th/pg 1159-1160 Harrison 18th/chapter 343)

Biochemical tests for Pheochromocytoma:

- Pheochromocytomas synthesize & store catecholamines, which include **norepinephrine (noradrenaline), epinephrine (adrenaline), and dopamine.**
- Elevated plasma and urinary levels of **catecholamines** and the methylated metabolites, **metanephrines**, are the cornerstone for the diagnosis.
- Urinary tests for **vanillylmandelic acid (VMA), metanephrines (total or fractionated), and catecholamines** are widely available and are used commonly for initial testing.

61. **Ans. (a) Pheochromocytoma**

(Ref: R 9th/pg 1134-1135)

62. **Ans. (a) Involvement of lymph nodes**

(Ref: Robbins 9th/pg 1134-1135)

- **There is no histologic feature that reliably predicts clinical behavior.**
- **Therefore, the definitive diagnosis of malignancy in pheochromocytomas is based exclusively on the presence of metastases.**
- **Metastasis:** Involve regional **lymph nodes[Q], liver[Q], lung[Q], and bone[Q]**

63. **Ans. (a) Carotid body Tumour** *(Ref: Robbins 9th/pg 517)*

Glomus tumour (Carotid body tumor)

- Distinctive neoplasm which arises from **modified smooth muscle cells of the normal glomus body.**

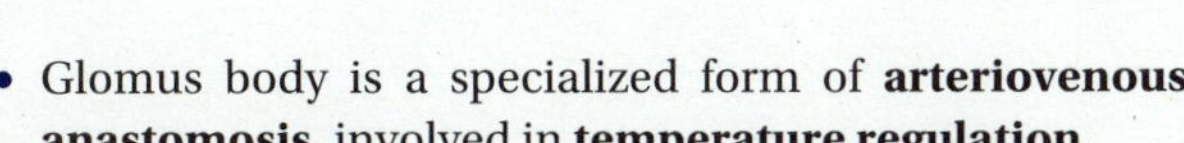

- Glomus body is a specialized form of **arteriovenous anastomosis**, involved in **temperature regulation**.
- There is a central coiled canal known as Suquet-Hoyer canal whichis lined by plump endothelial cells.

64.   Ans. (a, b);   a. Pheochromocytoma; b. Paraganglioma

(Ref: Robbins 9th/pg 1135; 8th/pg 1160)

Microscopic Feature of Pheochromocytoma

- Tumors made of **clusters of polygonal to spindle-shaped chromaffin cells** surrounded by **sustentacular cells**, creating **small nests (zellballen)**^{Q}, with rich vascularity.
- **"Salt and pepper"** nuclear chromatin: **characteristic** of neuroendocrine tumors.
- **Electron microscopy:** Membrane-bound, **electron-dense secretory**^{Q} granules.

Zellballen pattern is also found in Paraganglioma

65.   Ans. (c)   **Duodenum** *(Ref: Robbins 9th/pg 1136)*

66.   Ans. (d, e)   d. Marfanoid features; e. Mucosal neuromas

Multiple endocrine neoplasia type 2 (MEN 2) is classified into three subtypes: MEN 2A, FMTC (familial medullary thyroid carcinoma), and MEN 2B. All three subtypes involve high risk for development of medullary carcinoma of the thyroid (MTC); MEN 2A and MEN 2B have an increased risk for pheochromocytoma; MEN 2A has an increased risk for parathyroid adenoma or hyperplasia. Additional features in MEN 2B include mucosal neuromas of the lips and tongue, distinctive facies with enlarged lips, ganglioneuromatosis of the gastrointestinal tract, and a "marfanoid" habitus. MTC typically occurs in early childhood in MEN 2B, early adulthood in MEN 2A, and middle age in FMTC.

67.   Ans. (b)   **Midgut carcinoid** *(Ref: Robbins 9th ed. Pg. 1130)*

68.   Ans. (a)   **MENI** *(Ref: Robbins 9/1136)*

MEN-1, or Wermer syndrome, characterized by abnormalities involving the parathyroid (*Primary hyperparathyroidism resulting in renal stones*), pancreas, and pituitary glands (*prolactinoma*) ; thus the mnemonic device, the 3Ps.

69.   Ans. (d)   **MEN1** *(Ref: Robbins 9th/pg 1136/8th 1162)*

Multiple Endocrine Neoplasia (MEN) Syndromes; Refer to pretexts of this chapter

70.   Ans. (b)   **Gastrinoma** *(Ref: Robbins 9th/pg 1136/8th 1162)*

71.   Ans. (a)   **Somatostatinoma** *(Ref: Robbins 9th/pg 1136)*

Pancreatic endocrine tumors; Refer to pretexts

72.   Ans. (d)   **Medullary**

(Ref: Robbins 9th/pg 1136; 8th/pg 1162)

Commonest thyroid tumor in MEN is Medullary Carcinoma thyroid

73.   Ans. (d)   **Pituitary** *(Ref: Robbins 9th/pg 1136; 8th/pg 1162)*

74.   Ans. (a)   **MEN 1** *(Ref: Robbins 9th/pg 1136; 8th/pg 1162)*

Wermer syndrome is MEN 1

75.   Ans. (d)   **Medullary carcinoma of thyroid**

(Ref: Robbins 9th/pg 1136)

76.   Ans. (b)   **Component of MEN-1**

(Ref: Robbins 9th/pg 1099-1100, 1136; 8th/pg 1124-1125, 1162)

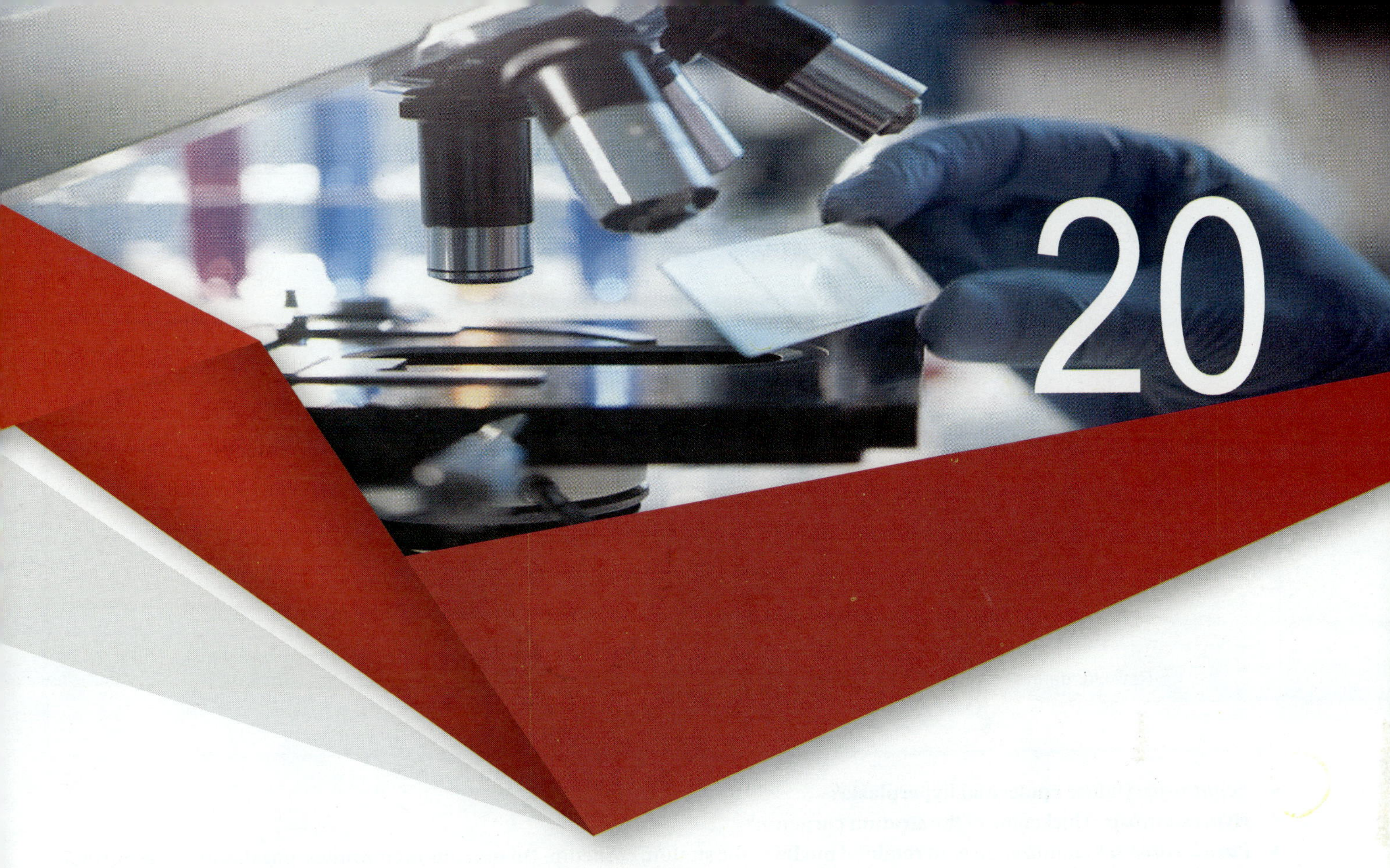

20

Skin and its Disorders

Key Points

- » **Erythema multiforme:** Characteristic clinical lesion-**target lesion**
- » **Auspitz sign:** Multiple, minute, bleeding points when the scale is lifted from the plaque
- » **Lichen planus: Hypergranulosis**
- » **Psoriasis: Stratum granulosum is thinned or absent**
- » *Pemphigus vulgaris:* **Suprabasal** acantholytic vesicle
- » **Verruca vulgaris** is the **most common type** of wart
- » Epithelioid granulomas are seen in **tuberculoid leprosy**
- » **Marjolin's ulcer:** SCC arising at site of chronic inflammation, presenting as **persistent ulceration**
- » **Mycosis fungoides:** Histologic hallmark - **Sézary-Lutzner cells**

Key Recent Updates

- » IgG antibodies to **desmoglein 1 & 3** are seen is **pemphigus vulgaris**
- » IgG autoantibodies to **hemidesmosomes** is seen in **Bullous pemphigoid.**

NORMAL SKIN HISTOLOGY

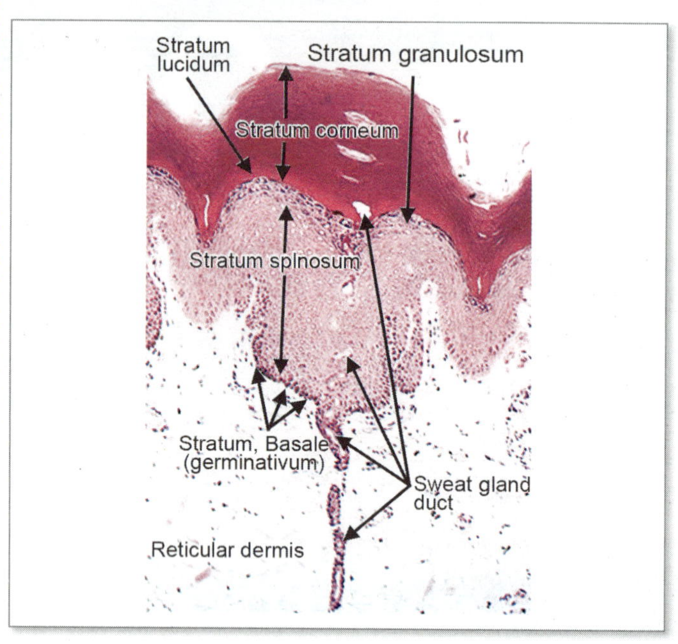

IMPORTANT DEFINITIONS

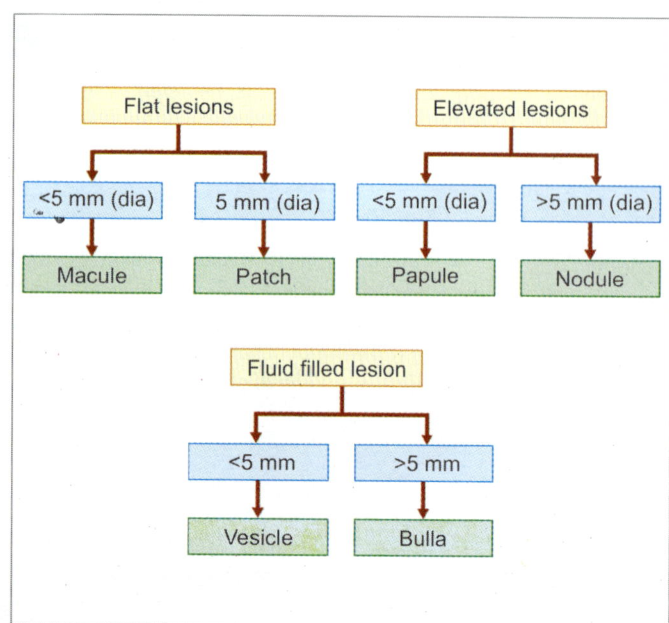

- *Acanthosis:* Diffuse **epidermal hyperplasia**[Q]
- *Hyperkeratosis:* Thickening of the **stratum corneum**[Q]
- *Parakeratosis:* Keratinization with **retained nuclei** in the stratum corneum. **On mucous membranes, parakeratosis is normal.**[Q]
- *Dyskeratosis:* Abnormal, **premature keratinization** within cells **below the stratum granulosum**[Q]
- *Spongiosis:* **Intercellular edema** of the epidermis[Q]
- *Acantholysis:* **Loss of intercellular connections**[Q]

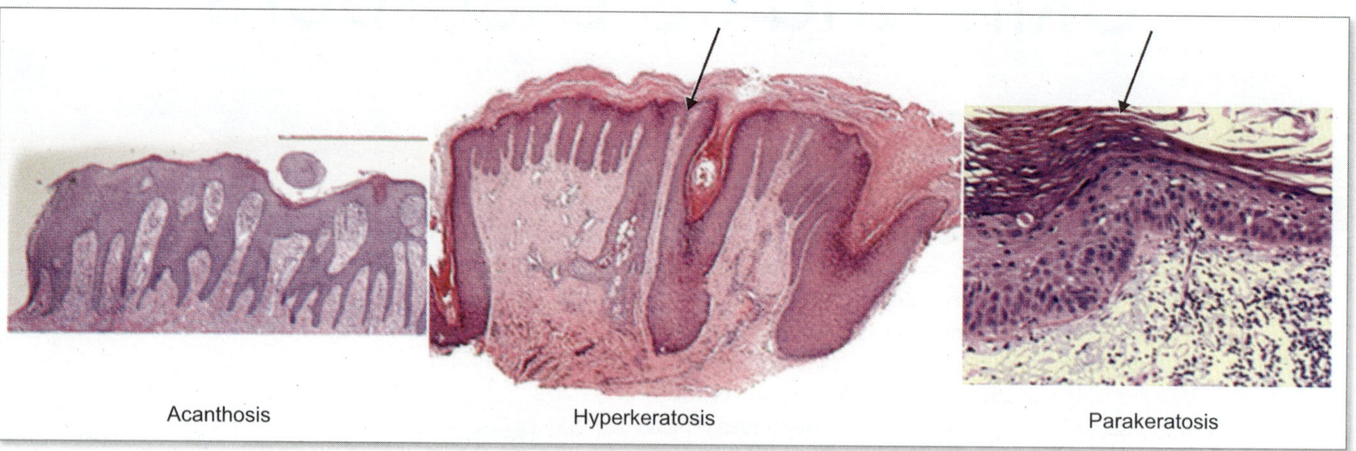

| Acanthosis | Hyperkeratosis | Parakeratosis |

ACUTE INFLAMMATORY DERMATOSES

Urticaria

- Localized **immediate hypersensitivity (type I) reaction**[Q]

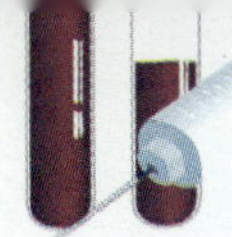

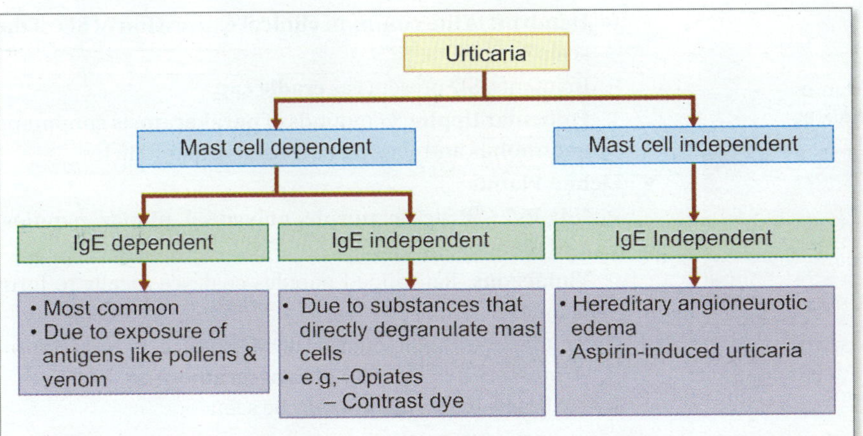

POINTS TO REMEMBER

- Hereditary Angioneurotic edema-deficiency of C1 inhibitor
- Angiedema-edema of both dermis and subcutaneous fat

ACUTE ECZEMATOUS DERMATITIS

- Eczematous dermatitis can be subdivided into the following categories:
  - **Allergic contact dermatitis, Atopic dermatitis, Drug-related eczematous dermatitis, Photoeczematous dermatitis, Primary irritant dermatitis.**[Q]
- Hallmark of acute eczema: spongiosis

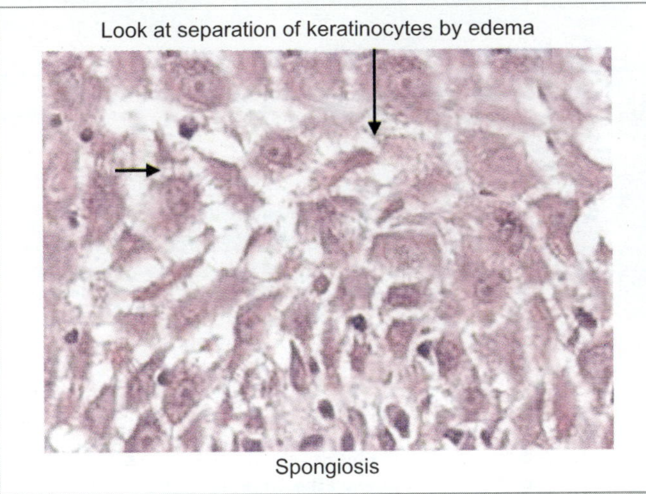

Look at separation of keratinocytes by edema

Spongiosis

ERYTHEMA MULTIFORME

- Characteristic clinical lesion-**target lesion**[Q]-shows central necrosis surrounded by a rim of perivenular inflammation[Q]

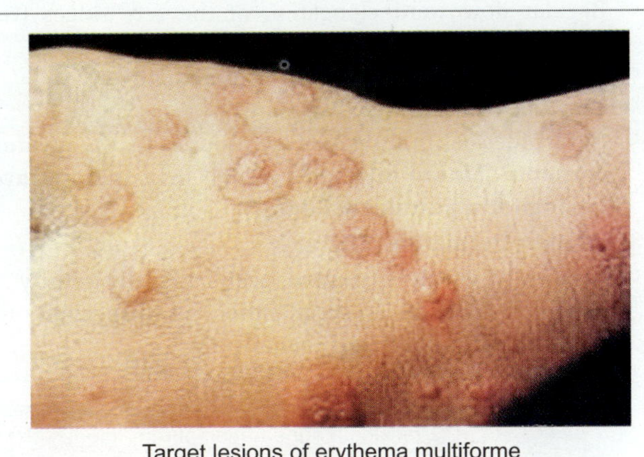

Target lesions of erythema multiforme

CHRONIC INFLAMMATORY DERMATOSES

- **Psoriasis**
  - Psoriasis is a **chronic inflammatory dermatosis**[Q] usually with **autoimmune basis**[Q]
  - **Most frequently - *skin of the elbows, knees, scalp, lumbosacral areas, intergluteal cleft, and glans penis.***[Q]
  - **Koebner's phenomenon**[Q] -lesions can be induced in susceptible individuals by local trauma.
  - Strong association with **HLA-C**, particularly with the **HLA-Cw*0602 allele**[Q]
  - **Auspitz sign**- multiple, minute, bleeding points when the scale is lifted from the plaque[Q]
  - ***Nail changes* occur in 30% of cases of psoriasis**[Q]

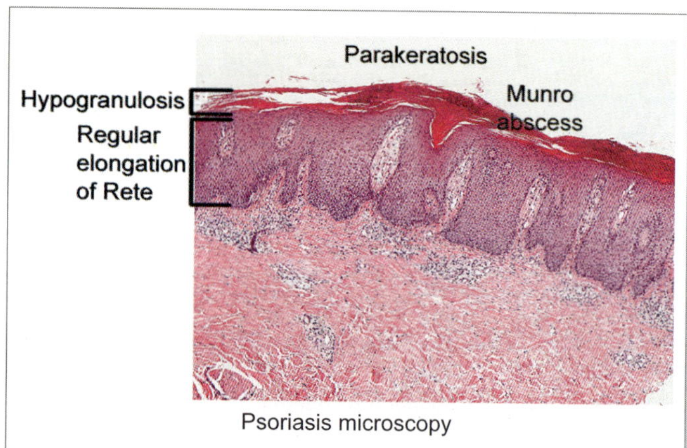

Psoriasis microscopy

- ○ Hyperkeratosis, parakeratosis, acanthosis
- ○ Regular downward elongation of the rete ridges (**test tubes in a rack**[Q])
- ○ **Stratum granulosum is thinned or absent**[Q]
- ○ Thinning of **suprapapillary plates**[Q]
- ○ Intraepidermal infiltrates of neutrophils in the **stratum corneum (Munro microabscesses)**[Q] & in **spinous layer (spongiform pustules of Kogoj)**[Q]
- ■ **Seborrheic Dermatitis (SD)**
  - ○ Classically involves regions with a high density of sebaceous glands, - scalp, forehead (especially the glabella), external auditory canal.

- ○ **Dandruff is the common clinical expression** of SD of the scalp[Q]
- ○ In infants, SD presents as **cradle cap**
- ○ **Follicular lipping**[Q] - mounds of **parakeratosis** containing neutrophils and serum at the ostia of hair follicles
- ■ **Lichen Planus**
  - ○ **"Six Ps"** : "**Pruritic, purple, polygonal, planar, papules, and plaques**"
  - ○ **Violaceous**, flat-topped papules coalesce focally to form plaques
  - ○ Papules are highlighted by white lines called **Wickham striae:**[Q] created by areas of **hypergranulosis**[Q]
  - ○ Koebner's phenomenon may be seen

Microscopy

- ■ Hyperkeratosis
- ■ **Hypergranulosis**[Q]
- ■ **Band of lymphocytes** are intimately associated with basal keratinocytes
  - ○ **Squamatization**[Q], degeneration, necrosis seen in basal keratinocytes
  - ○ **Colloid or Civatte bodies**[Q] -necrotic basal cells incorporated into the inflamed papillary dermis.

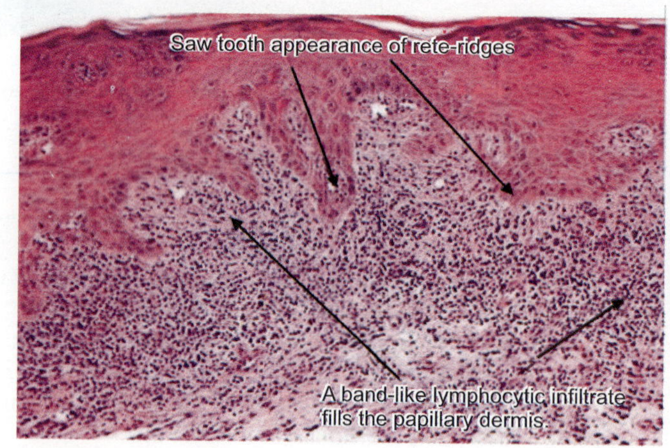

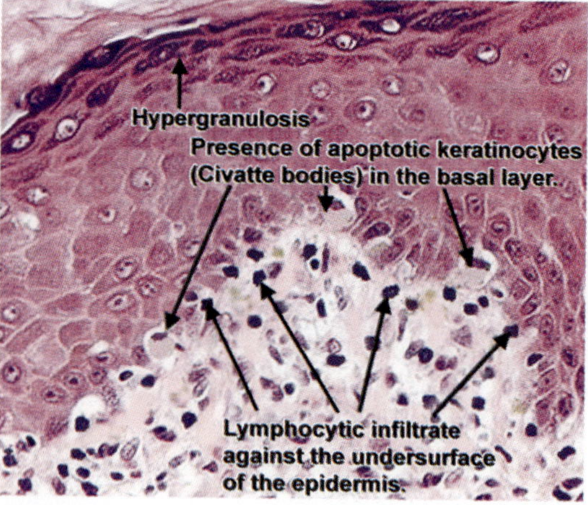

Lichen planus

Mnemonic

- • Pemphigu**S-S**uperficial separation[Q]- intraepidermal acantholysis[Q]-**flaccid bulla**[Q] which ruptures easily
- • Pemphigoi**D-D**eep separation at **d**ermo-epidermal junction[Q]- **tense bulla**[Q] that **does not** rupture easily

BLISTERING (BULLOUS) DISEASES

Caused **by autoantibodies**[Q] specific for epithelial or basement membrane proteins that lead to separation of keratinocytes (acantholysis)

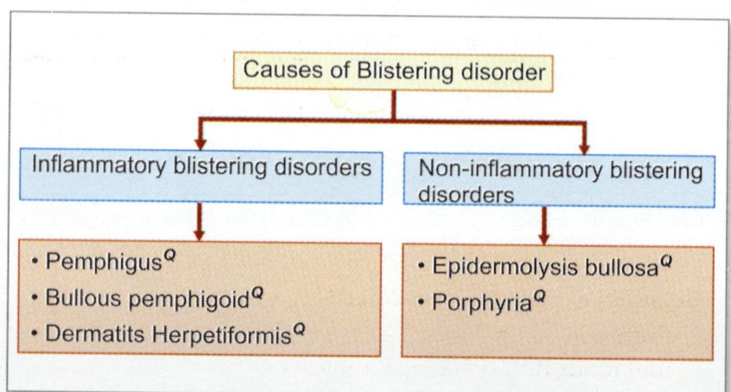

Skin biopsy and direct immunofluorescence (DIF) are crucial for diagnosis of immune-bullous diseases.[Q]

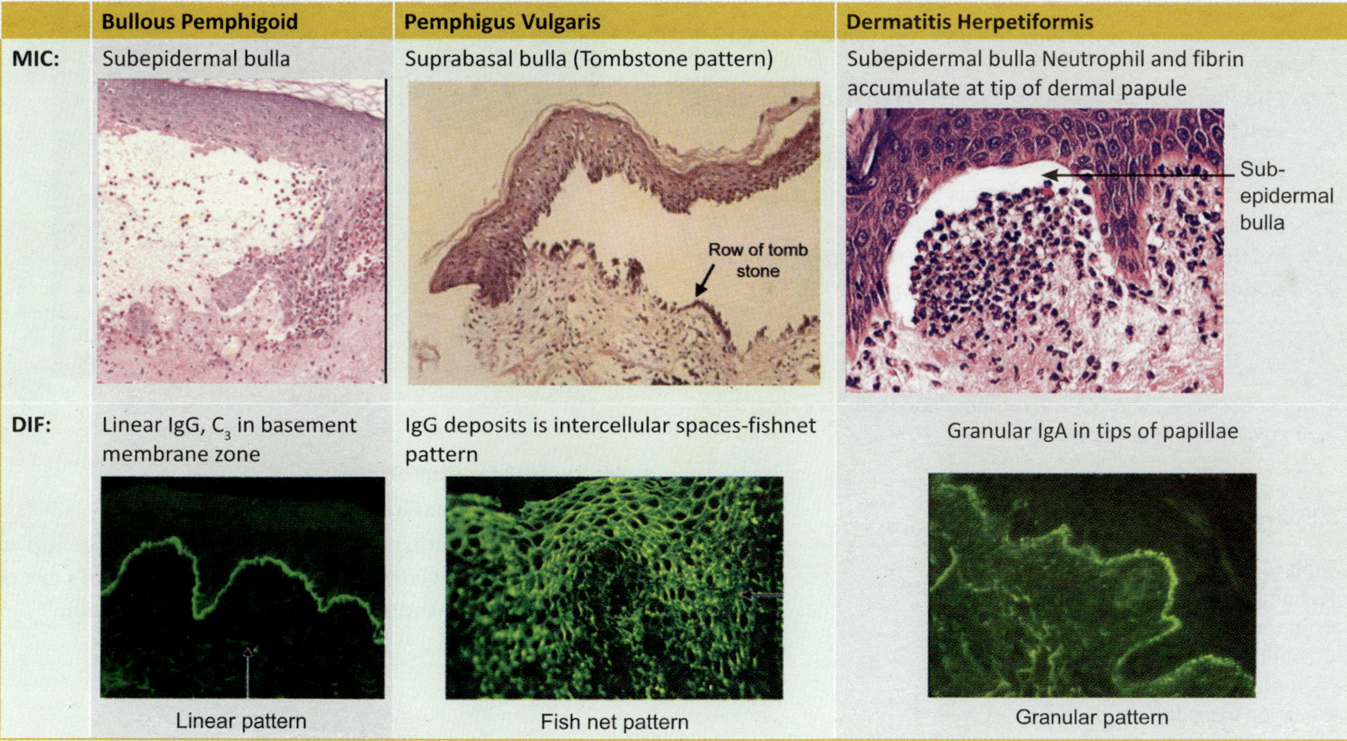

	Bullous Pemphigoid	Pemphigus Vulgaris	Dermatitis Herpetiformis
MIC:	Subepidermal bulla	Suprabasal bulla (Tombstone pattern)	Subepidermal bulla Neutrophil and fibrin accumulate at tip of dermal papule
DIF:	Linear IgG, C₃ in basement membrane zone	IgG deposits is intercellular spaces-fishnet pattern	Granular IgA in tips of papillae
	Linear pattern	Fish net pattern	Granular pattern

Other Bullous disorders

- **Pemphigoid gestations:** Spongiotic dermatitis and subepidermal bulla
- **Epidermolysis bullosa acquisita:** subepidermal bulla sparse inflammatory infiltrate
- **Pemphigus foliaceus:** subcorneal bulla

High Yield Facts

- **Pemphigus:** IgG autoantibodies to various **intercellular desmogleins. (Both desmoglein 1 & 3)**
- **Bullous Pemphigoid:** IgG autoAb to **hemidesmosome** proteins c. (Bullous Pemphigoid Antigen (BPAG) that attach epidermal cells to basement membrane)
- **Dermatitis Herpetiformis:** IgA auto-Ab to **fibrils** that bind epidermal BM & produces **subepidermal blisters.** Associated with **gluten-sensitive enteropathy** in most cases[Q]
- **Epidermolysis Bullosa: inherited defects in structural proteins that lend mechanical stability to the skin**[Q]

- **Dystrophic epidermolysis bullosa: inherited defects in collagen type 7**[Q]
- **Porphyria**: Vesicles are **subepidermal** in location and the adjacent dermis contains vessels with walls that are thickened by **glassy deposits of serum proteins, including immunoglobulins**[Q]
- **Seborrheic dermatitis is not a disease of the sebaceous glands**
- **Leiner disease**[Q] generalized seborrheic dermatitis in infants associated with diarrhea & failure to thrive

DISORDERS OF PIGMENTATION AND MELANOCYTES

- **Freckle (Ephelis): Most common**[Q] pigmented lesions of childhood in lightly pigmented individuals
- **Lentigo:** Essential histologic feature is linear (non-nested) melanocytic hyperplasia restricted to basal cell layer[Q]
- **Melanocytic Nevus (Pigmented Nevus, Mole)**
  - Common benign neoplasms, occur by acquired activating mutations RAS signaling pathway[Q]
  - Acquired **melanocytic nevi are the most common type and found in all individuals.**[Q]

- **Dysplastic Nevi:** Best regarded as **markers of melanoma risk** rather than premalignant lesions
  - They are characterized by architectural and cytologic atypia
  - Associated with **germline mutations in genes encoding cell cycle regulators (p16/INK4a, CDK4) and telomerase.**[Q]

- **Melanoma:** Highly aggressive malignancy linked to sun exposure;

- The two most important predisposing factors are inherited genes and sun exposure[Q]
- Shows striking **variations in color**, in contrast to benign nevus[Q]
- The borders of melanomas are **irregular and often notched**[Q]
- **Radial growth** describes the horizontal spread of melanoma within the epidermis and superficial dermis- **this is not associated with risk of metastasis.**[Q]
- **Vertical growth phase is signaled by the appearance of a nodule & correlates with metastatic potential.**[Q]

Points to Remember

- Acne, Rosacea, Panniculitis (Erythema nodosum) are disorders of epidermal appendages

Mnemonic

Mole: Signs of Trouble ABCDE
Asymmetry
Border irregular
Colour irregular
Diameter usually > 0.5 cm
Elevation irregular

High Yield Facts

- **Superficial spreading,- most common type of melanoma,**[Q] usually involving sun-exposed skin
- **Acral/mucosal lentiginous melanoma** - is **unrelated** to sun exposure.[Q]
- Melanoma is associated **with mutations** in **cell cycle regulators** (p16/INK4a, CDK4), growth factor receptors [e.g., **KIT], RAS, BRAF), and telomerase**[Q]
- **Marker- HMB-45 is very specific marker for melanocytes**[Q]
  - Few other familial syndromes, notably **CDKN2 A is a important risk factor of melanoma**

INFECTIONS

- *Verrucae (Warts):*
  - Caused by **human papilloma viruses**.
  - **Verruca vulgaris** is the **most common type**[Q] of wart.
  - **Condyloma acuminatum (venereal wart)** occurs on the penis, female genitalia, urethra, perianal areas, and rectum.
  - Diagnosis is based primarily on hyperplastic papillary architecture zones **of koilocytosis**[Q].

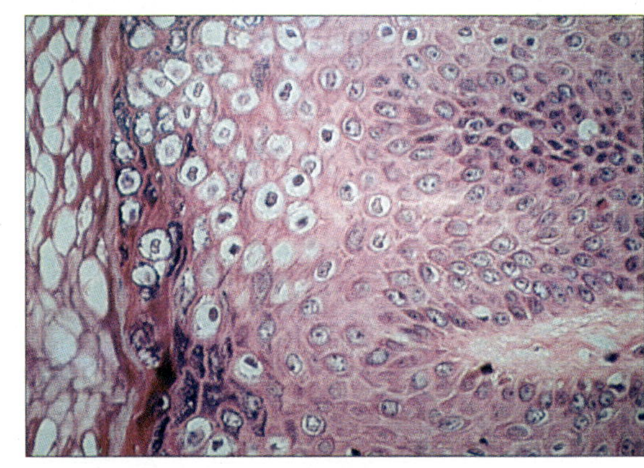

Verruca

- *Molluscum Contagiosum:*
  - Caused by a **poxvirus**.[Q]
  - **Diagnostic feature** is the **molluscum body**-large (up to 35 μm), homogeneous, cytoplasmic inclusion in cells of the **stratum granulosum and the stratum corneum**[Q]

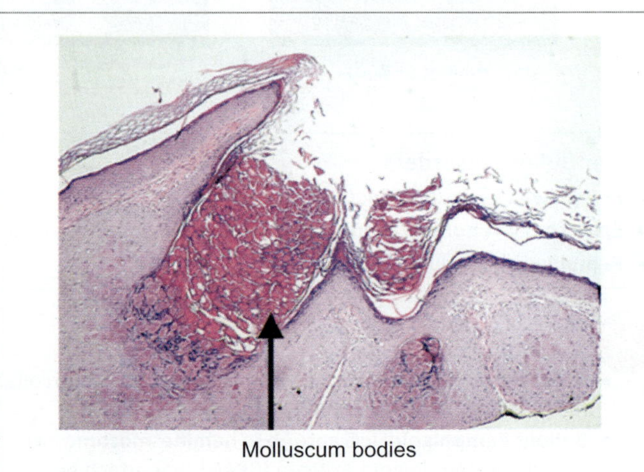

Molluscum bodies

- *Impetigo:*
  - **Common superficial bacterial infection** of skin caused by **Staphylococcus aureus**[Q]
- *Superficial Fungal Infections:*
  - Tinea capitis, Tinea barbae, Tinea corporis, **Tinea pedis (athlete's foot)** & Tinea versicolor[Q]
  - All of above are caused **by dermatophyte infections except Tinea versicolor which is caused by Malassezia furfur (a yeast, not a dermatophyte).**[Q]

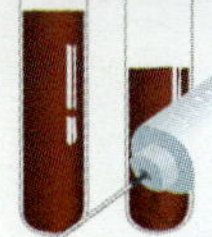

Clinical, Bacteriologic, Pathologic, and Immunologic Spectrum of Leprosy

Features	Tuberculoid (TT, BT) Leprosy	Lepromatous (LL) Leprosy
Skin lesions	**Sharply defined** macules or plaques with a tendency toward central clearing, **elevated borders**	**Symmetric, poorly marginated, multiple infiltrated nodules and plaques**[Q] or diffuse infiltration; **leonine facies and eyebrow alopecia**[Q]
Nerve lesions	Skin lesions **anesthetize early; nerve** near lesions sometimes **enlarged; nerve abscesses most common in BT**[Q]	**Hyperesthesia, a late** sign; nerve palsies variable; acral, distal, symmetric anesthesia common
Acid-fast bacilli (BI)	**0–1+**	**4–6+ GLOBI-** Macrophage cells laden with acid fast bacill[Q]
Lymphocytes	**2+**	0–1+
Macrophage differentiation	**Epithelioid**	**Foamy cells change the rule; Lepra cells**[Q] - large, mononuclear histiocytes (macrophages) with a foam like cytoplasm
Langhans' giant cells **Histopathology**[Q]	**1–3+**[Q] **Epithelioid granulomas** in the papillary dermis, specially **around neurovascular structures**[Q]	— **Diffuse infiltrate of foamy macrophages** is present in the dermis below a subepidermal zone of uninvolved papillary dermis (i.e., **grenz zone**).[Q]
Lepromin skin test	**+++**[Q]	—
Lymphocyte transformation test	**Generally positive**[Q]	1–2%
***M. leprae* PGL-1** antibodies	60%	**95%**[Q]

Image shows granuloma S/O Tuberculoid leprosy   Foamy cells S/O lepromatous leprosy
Acid-fast bacilli (BI): 0–1+   Acid-fast bacilli (BI): 4–6+ GLOBI- Macrophage cells laden with acid fast bacill[Q]

High Yield Facts

- **Globi:** Macrophage cells laden with acid fast bacill
- **Lepra cells**[Q]: Large, mononuclear histiocytes (macrophages) with a foam-like cytoplasm
- **Grenz zone**[Q] is seen in **lepromatous leprosy**
- **Epitheliod granulomas** are seen in **tuberculoid leprosy**

BENIGN EPITHELIAL TUMORS

- Derived from keratinizing stratified **squamous epithelium** of epidermis, hair follicles & **ductular epithelium** of cutaneous glands.
- Telltale sign of syndromes associated with **visceral malignancies**, such as **multiple trichilemmomas in Cowden's syndrome**[Q] or **multiple sebaceous neoplasms in Muir-Torre syndrome.**[Q]

SEBORRHEIC KERATOSES

- Middle-aged or older individuals
- Appear as part of a **paraneoplastic syndrome (Leser-Trélat sign)**[Q] possibly due to stimulation of keratinocytes by **TGF-alpha**[Q] produced by tumor cells, **most commonly carcinomas of the gastrointestinal tract.**[Q]
- **Sporadic** activating mutations in the **fibroblast growth factor receptor-3 (FGFR3)**[Q]
- Clinically: **coin-like, waxy plaques**.
- Inspection with a hand lens usually reveals small, **round, pore-like ostia impacted with keratin**[Q]
- Microscopy shows following **characteristic features:**
  - Hyperkeratosis
  - **Horn cysts**-keratin-filled cysts
  - **Invagination cysts**-invaginations of keratin into the main mass

ACANTHOSIS NIGRICANS

Thickened, hyperpigmented skin with a **"velvet-like"**[Q] texture, mostly seen in flexural areas

It is of two types

- In 80% of cases, associated with benign conditions like **obesity and diabetes.**[Q]
- In 20% cases, AN arises in association with cancers, **most commonly gastrointestinal adenocarcinomas**[Q]

FIBROEPITHELIAL POLYP, (ACROCHORDON, SQUAMOUS PAPILLOMA, SKIN TAG)

- **Most common cutaneous lesions**[Q]
- Occurs at **neck, trunk, face, and intertriginous areas**[Q]
- Become **more numerous or prominent during pregnancy**

ADNEXAL (APPENDAGE) TUMORS

- **Eccrine poroma:** Occurs predominantly on the palms and soles where sweat glands are numerous
- **Cylindroma:** Turban tumor (Microscopy shows zigzag puzzle pattern) see image below.
- **Brooke-Spiegler syndrome:** (associated with both trichoepithelioma and cylindroma)
- **Syringomas**
- **Sebaceous adenomas**-Can be associated with internal malignancy in **Muir-Torre syndrome**, a subset of hereditary non-polyposis colorectal carcinoma syndrome associated with germline deficits in **DNA mismatch repair**[Q] proteins.
- **Pilomatricomas**-shows **ghost cells**

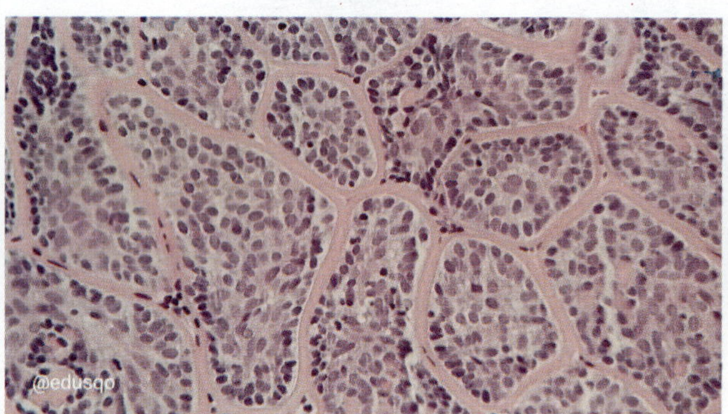

Cells arranged in zigzag puzzle separated by basement membrane like material diagnostic of cylindroma

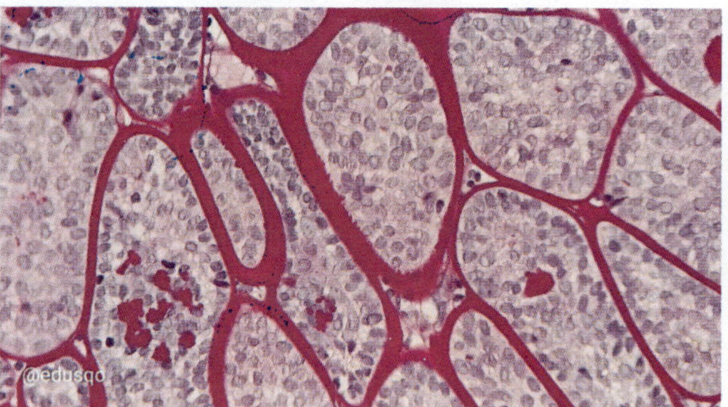

PAS+ basement membrane like material diagnostic of cylindroma

High Yield Facts

- Most appendage tumors are **benign.**[Q]
- Apocrine tumors are unusual in that **malignant forms seem to be more common**[Q] than benign.
- Sebaceous carcinoma arises from the **meibomian glands**[Q] of the eyelid and may follow an aggressive course.
- **Birt-Hogg-Dubé syndrome**-fibroepithelial polyps and tumors of perifollicular mesenchyme.[Q]

PREMALIGNANT AND MALIGNANT EPIDERMAL TUMORS

- **Carcinoma in Situ (Bowen's Disease)**
  - Occurs equally in **men and women**
  - Associated with HPV, Arsenic, solar radiation
  - **Morphology:** Full thickness dysplasia of the squamous epithelium.

High Yield Facts

Differential diagnosis of Bowen's disease include Bowenoid papulosis and Erythroplasia of Queyrat occurs primarily in men.

- **Bowenoid papulosis:**
  Histologically similar to squamous cell carcinoma in-situ. Features **favoring the diagnosis of bowenoid papulosis are:**
  - Presence of numerous mitotic figures in metaphase,
  - Basophilic inclusions in the granular layer
  - Koilocytes
- **Erythroplasia of Queyrat: Squamous cell carcinoma in situ** presenting on the **mucous membranes of the glans penis, vulva and oral mucosa^Q**

- **Actinic Keratosis**
  - **Sandpaper-like^Q** consistency, grossly.
  - Characterised by **cutaneous horns and pseudohorn cysts^Q.**
  - **Sites:** Sun-exposed sites (face, arms, dorsum of hands) are most frequently affected.
  - The lips may also develop similar lesions (termed **actinic cheilitis).**
  - Morphology
    - Hyperkeratosis, **parakeratosis^Q**
    - **Basal cell and squamous layer atypia** and **disorderly maturation^Q**
- **Squamous Cell Carcinoma (SCC):**
  - It is the **2nd most common tumor^Q** arising on sun-exposed sites in older people, exceeded only by basal cell Ca.
  - **M**ost important cause **DNA damage induced by exposure to UV light^Q**

Risk factors		
• Usually UV light / ionizing radiation	• Chronic ulcers	• **Necrobiosis lipoidica^Q**
• Actinic keratosis (precursor lesion)^Q	• **Epidermodysplasia verruciformis^Q**	• Osteomyelitis - draining sinuses
• Albinism (lack of pigmentation in skin)	• Tars/oils	• `PUVA treatment for psoriasis
• **Arsenic^Q**	• **Hidradenitis suppurativa^Q**	• **Xeroderma pigmentosa^Q:** disorder with diminished capacity for DNA repair after UV light exposure
• Burn scars	• Immunosuppression (post-transplant or HIV)	

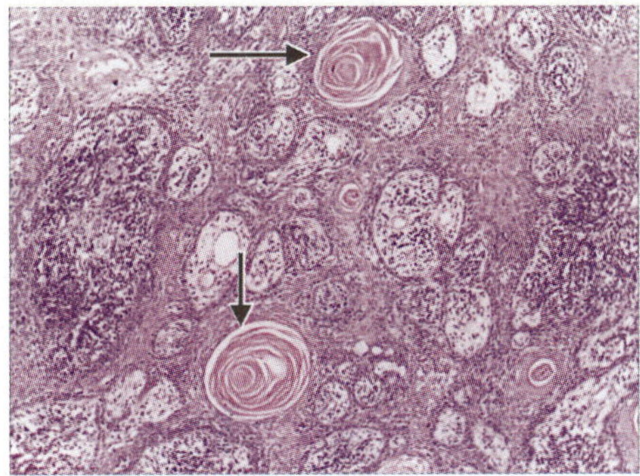

Mic: Keratin pearl and malignant squamous cells S/o SCC

- **Basal Cell Carcinoma-BCC**
  - Basal cell carcinoma is the **most common^Q** invasive cancer in humans
  - Locally invasive-**rarely metastasize.^{Q}**
  - **Most common mutations is—Sonic Hedgehog pathway**

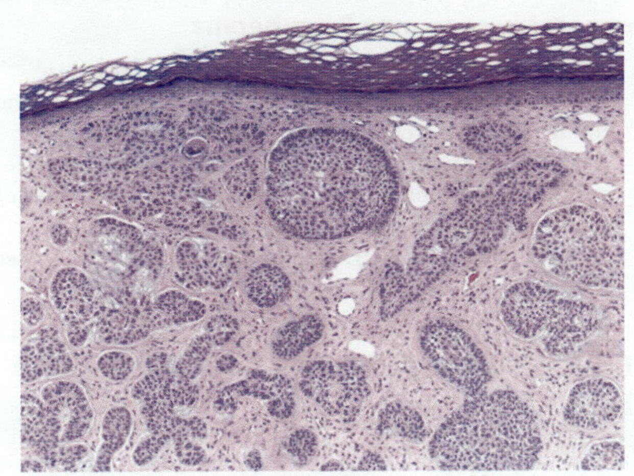

Peripheral palisading of nuclei S/O basal cell Ca

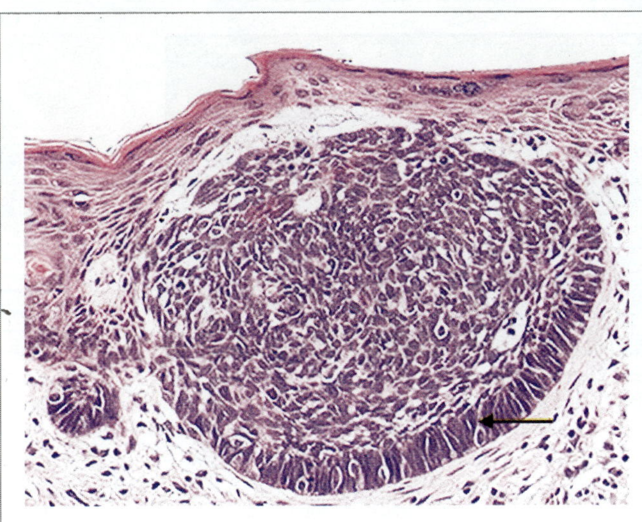

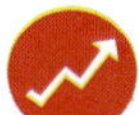

High Yield Facts

- **Cancers associated with sunlight exposure: BCC & SCC**
- HPVs cause autosomal recessive condition, **epidermodysplasia verruciformis,** which is marked by a **high susceptibility to cutaneous squamous cell carcinomas^Q**
- **Marjolins ulcer^Q:** SCC arising at site of chronic inflammation, presenting as **persistent ulceration^Q**
- **Rodent ulcer^Q- BCC (Due to local invasiveness of tumor)**
- Nevoid basal cell carcinoma syndrome (Gorlin syndrome)—autosomal dominant disorder; multiple basal cell Ca,^{Q} often before age 20, accompanied by other tumors (medulloblastomas^Q and ovarian fibromas^Q), odontogenic keratocysts^Q, pits of palms & soles.
- **Urticaria pigmentosa** is cutaneous form of mastocytosis

TUMORS OF THE DERMIS

Benign Fibrous Histiocytoma

- The **most common** form of fibrous histiocytoma is referred to as a **dermatofibroma**[Q]

Dermatofibrosarcoma Protuberans

- **Well-differentiated, primary fibrosarcoma of the skin**[Q]
- Deep extension from the dermis into subcutaneous fat, producing a characteristic **"honeycomb" pattern**[Q]
- The **molecular hallmark - balanced translocation between genes encoding collagen 1A1 (COL1A1) and the platelet-derived growth factor-β (PDGFB)**[Q]
- Characteristically has **storiform arrangement of fibroblasts (reminiscent of blades of a pinwheel)**[Q]

TUMORS OF CELLULAR MIGRANTS TO THE SKIN

In these lesions, progenitors arise elsewhere and then specifically home to the cutaneous microenvironment.

Mycosis Fungoides (Cutaneous T-Cell Lymphoma)

- **T-cell lymphoma** that presents in the skin and may evolve into generalized lymphoma
- Lesions involve truncal areas and include scaly, red-brown *patches*; raised, scaling *plaques* and fungating *nodules*
- **Histologic hallmark - Sézary-Lutzner cells**[Q], which form band-like aggregates within the superficial dermis
- These cells are **T-helper cells (CD4+)** have **hyperconvoluted or cerebriform contour**[Q]
- These invade the epidermis as single cells and small clusters (**Pautrier microabscesses**).[Q]
- Prognosis depends on **percentage** of body surface involved & **progression** from patch to plaque to nodule

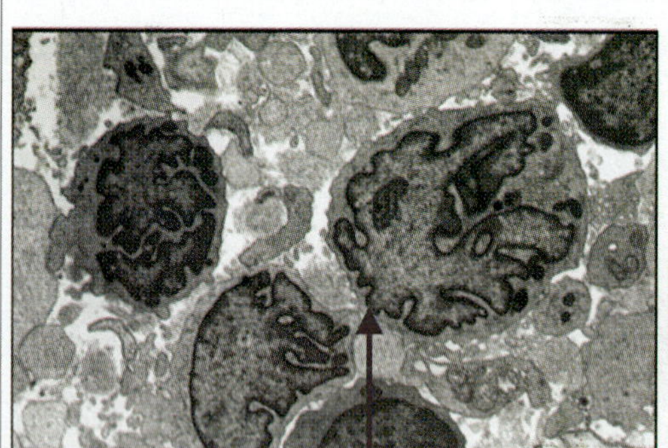
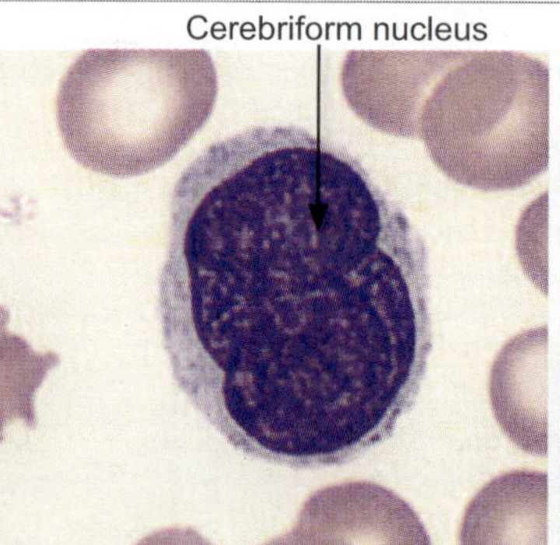

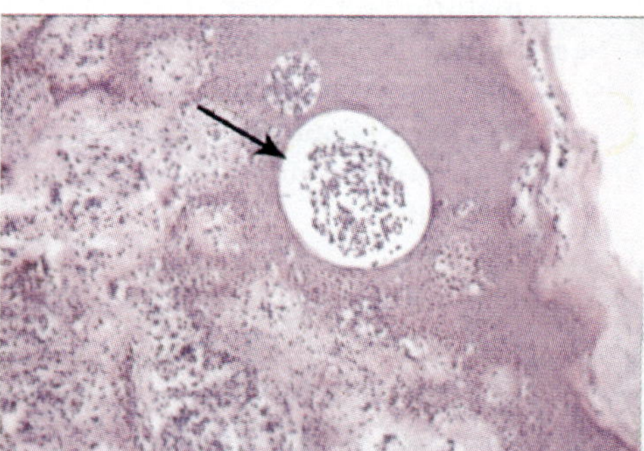

E.M Mycosis fungoides. Several T-lymphocytes with deeply indented and irregular ("cerebriform") nuclei

Sezary-Lutzner cell

Pautrier microabscess

Mastocytosis

- Characterized by increased numbers of mast cells in the skin and in other organs
- **Darier sign**-localized area of dermal edema and erythema (wheal) when lesional skin is rubbed[Q]
- **Dermatographism** - area of **dermal edema** due to **localized stroking** of normal skin with a pointed instrument[Q]
- Diagnosis of mast cells-metachromatic stains (**toluidine blue or Giemsa**)[Q]

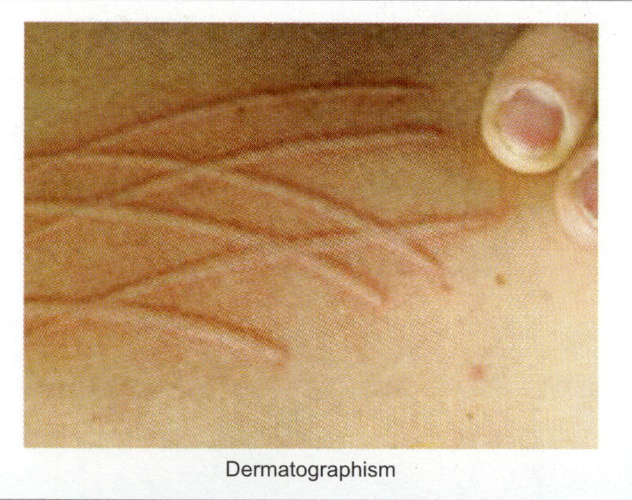

Dermatographism

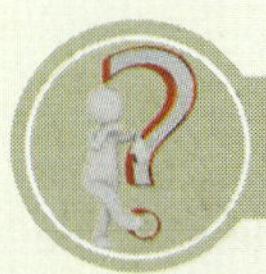

Image-Based Questions

1. **A 24-year-old male presents with following skin condition. Before doing biopsy, provisional diagnosis for the following condition is:**

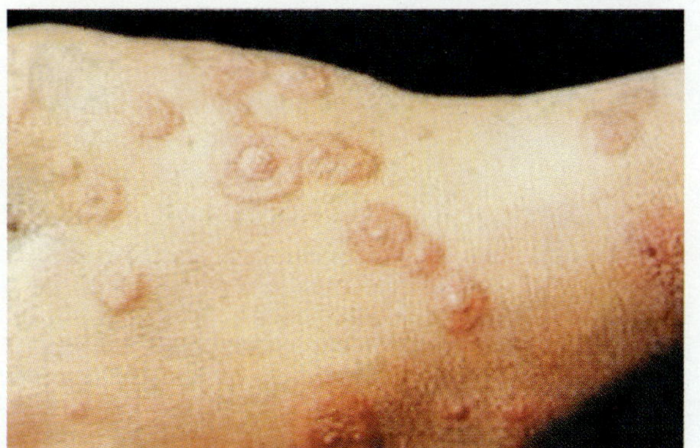

   a. Erythema multiforme
   b. Psoriasis
   c. Lichen planus
   d. Lichen striatus

2. **A 50-year-old female presents with blisters and erosions on the skin and mucous membranes, most commonly inside the mouth. Diagnosis:**

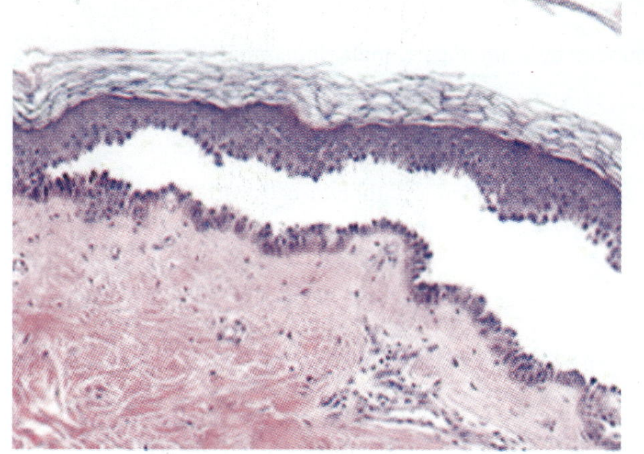

   a. Pemphigus vulgaris   b. Dermatitis herpetiformis
   c. Bullous pemphigoid   d. None

3. **A 50-year-old female presents with blisters and erosions on the skin and mucous membranes, most commonly inside the mouth. Direct immunofluorescence (DIF) on normal-appearing perilesional skin was done. It shows IgG within suprabasal intercellular spaces–fishnet pattern. Diagnosis:**

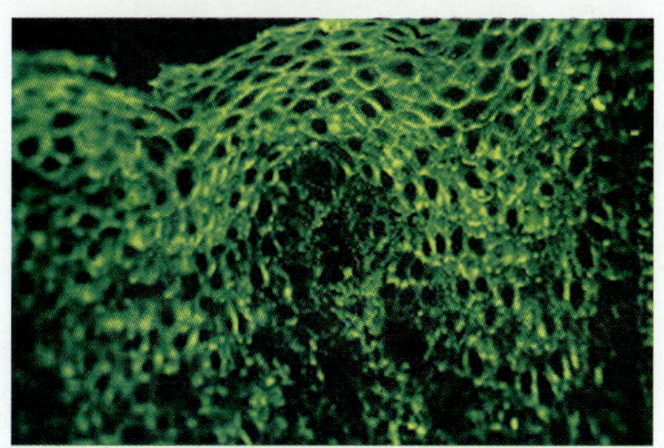

   a. Pemphigus vulgaris   b. Dermatitis herpetiformis
   c. Bullous pemphigoid   d. None

4. **A 60-year-old female presents with tense bullae on the flexural areas of the skin. Oral mucosa not involved. DIF shows Linear IgG, C3 in basement membrane zone. Diagnosis:**

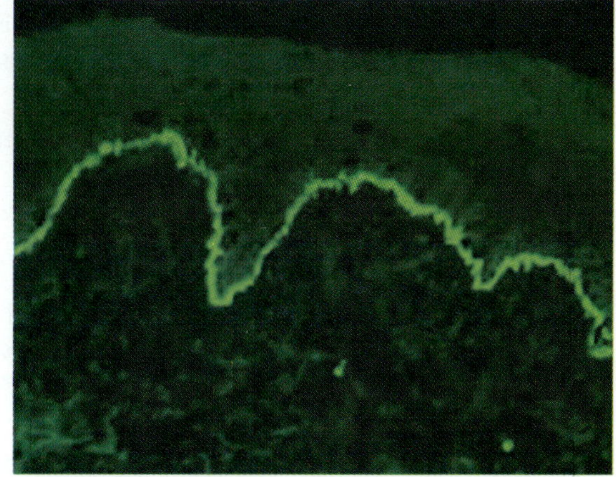

   a. Pemphigus vulgaris   b. Bullous pemphigoid
   c. Pemphigus vegetans   d. None

5. A 5-year-old child presents with Raised, firm, flesh colored nodules. On histopathological examination, following is seen. Diagnosis:

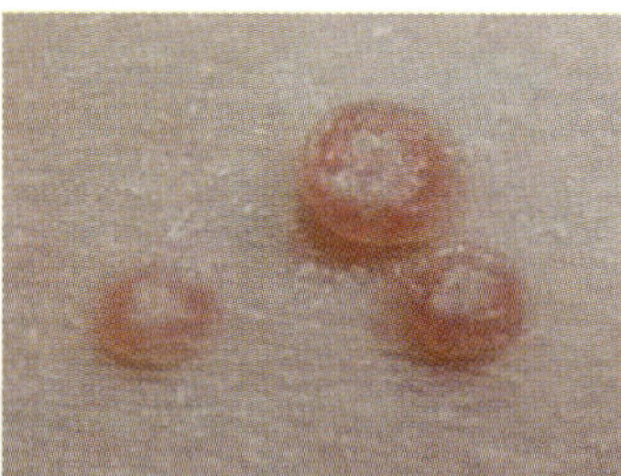

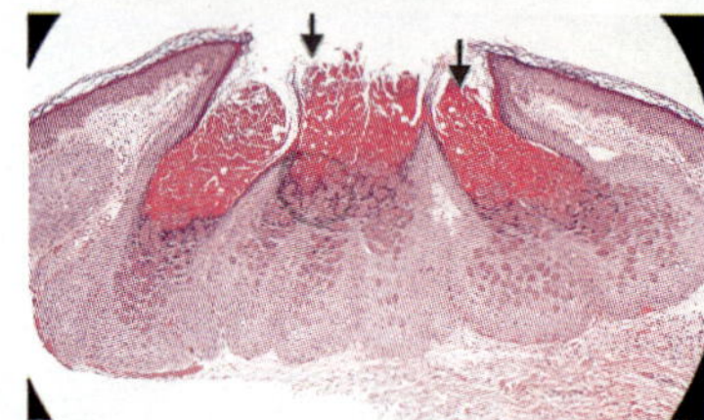

a. Myrmecia
b. Molluscum contagiosum
c. Herpes zoster
d. Herpes simplex

6. A 43-year-old smoker male, presents with growth in oral cavity. On examination, patient was diagnosed with well differentiated squamous cell carcinoma. Identify the structure marked with arrow.

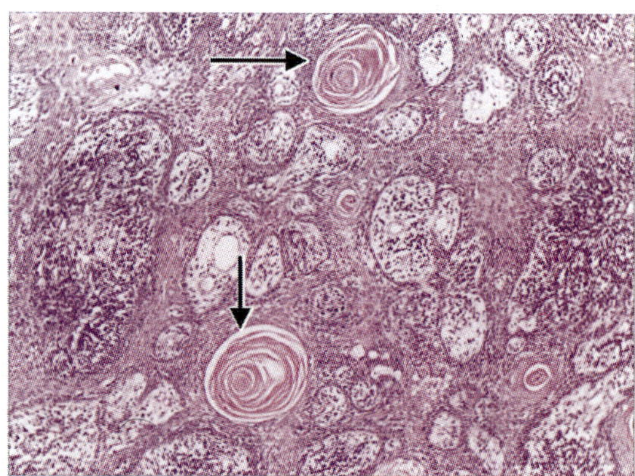

a. Keratin pearl
b. Koilocytes
c. Molluscum
d. None

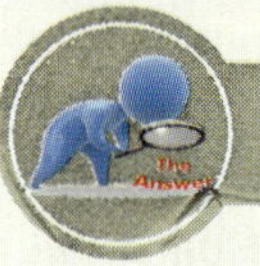

Answers of Image-Based Questions

1. **Ans. (a) Erythema multiforme**
   - Targetoid lesions are features of **Erythema multiforme**
   - Clinical **targetoid (target-like) lesion** shows central necrosis surrounded by a rim of perivenular inflammation

2. **Ans. (a) Pemphigus vulgaris**
   - Early lesions of pemphigus vulgaris show **suprabasal** epidermal acantholysis, clefting and blister formation
   - Basal cells are intact giving tombstone pattern
   - The blister cavity may contain inflammatory cells including eosinophils and rounded acantholytic cells with intensely eosinophilic cytoplasm and a perinuclear halo.

3. **Ans. (a) Pemphigus vulgaris**
   - DIF usually shows immunoglobulin G (IgG) deposited on the surface of the keratinocytes in and around lesions giving a fish net pattern. IgG1 and IgG4 are the most common subclasses.
   - Direct immunofluorescence (DIF) is usually done on normal-appearing perilesional skin

4. **Ans. (b) Bullous pemphigoid**
   - Linear IgG, C3 in basement membrane zone on DIF is a feature of Bullous pemphigoid

5. **Ans. (b) Molluscum Contagiosum**
   - Molluscum bodies are present (large cells with cytoplasmic, faintly granular eosinophilic inclusions that displace nuclei and contain viral particles) marked with arrow.

6. **Ans. (a) Keratin pearl**
   - Typical SCC has nests of squamous epithelial cells arising from the epidermis and extending into the dermis
   - We differentiated neoplastic cells in nests have pink cytoplasmic keratin.
   - Keratin pearl-a focus of central keratinization within concentric layers of abnormal squamous cells is a feature of well-differentiated SCC.

Multiple Choice Questions

OVERVIEW AND DEFINITIONS

1. Features of café au lait spots are all except: *(Recent Question 2015)*
a. Larger
b. Arise independent of sun exposure
c. Contain aggregated melanosomes
d. Most common pigmented lesions

2. Acanthosis means: *(AI 2014)*
a. Loss of intracellular connections
b. Abnormal premature keratinization
c. Diffuse epidermal hyperplasia
d. Thickening of stratum corneum

3. Spongiosis is seen in: *(Recent Question 2013)*
a. Acute eczema   b. Lichen Planus
c. Psoriasis   d. Pemphigus

4. True about Dyskeratosis congenita: *(PGI May 10)*
a. Pancytopenia   b. Nail dystrophy
c. Hyperkeratosis   d. X linked
e. Leukoplakia

INFLAMMATORY DERMATOSES

5. Munro microabscesses are seen in:
(WB PGMEE 16, MH 16)
a. Lichen planus
b. Mycosis fungoides
c. Psoriasis
d. Eczema

BLISTERING DISORDERS

6. A 20-year-old female presented with painful blister in skin and oral mucosa. Direct immunofluorescence picture of which is given below. Which of the following is not true regarding the same? *(AIIMS May 2017)*
a. Antibodies against hemidesmosomes
b. Antibodies against Desmoglein 1
c. Antibodies against Desmoglein 3
d. Basemene membrane deposition of IgG is the most common DIF picture in bullous lesions

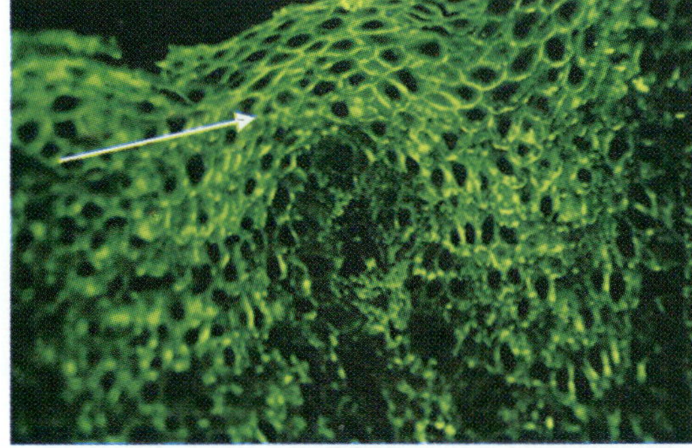

7. What is the diagnosis of the below histopathology image? *(AIIMS May 2017)*

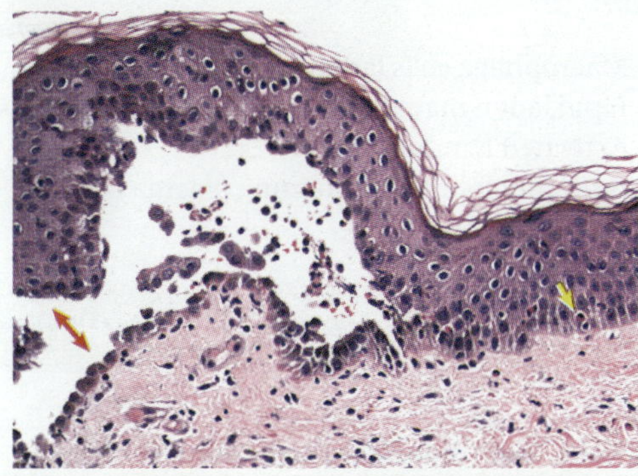

a. Pemphigus   b. Leismaniasis
c. Mycosis fungoides   d. Psoriasis

8. Fish net pattern seen in *(AIIMS Nov 16)*

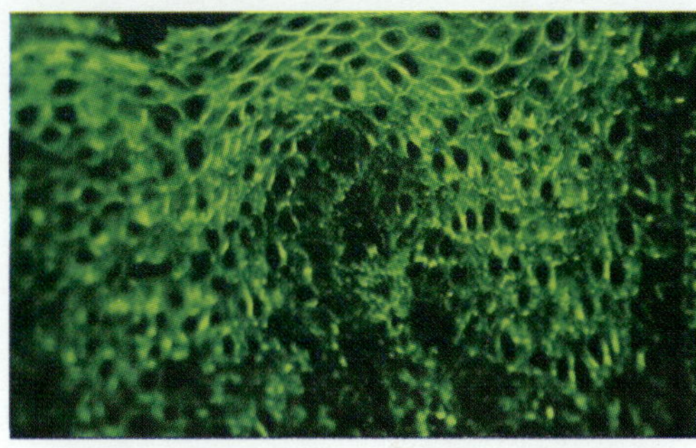

a. Pemphigus Vulgaris
b. Bullous pemphigoid
c. Behcet syndrome
d. All of above

9. Acantholysis means: *(Recent Question 2014)*
a. Diffuse epidermal hyperplasia
b. Loss of intercellular connections
c. Intercellular edema of the epidermis.
d. Abnormal keratinization

10. In congenital dystrophic variety of epidermolysis bullosa, mutation is seen in the gene coding for?
(AIIMS May 11)
a. Laminin 4
b. Collagen type VII
c. Alpha 6 integrin
d. Keratin 14 Infections

11. 'Row of tombstones' appearance is seen in:
(JIPMER 78, PGI 11)
a. Irritant dermatitis   b. Pemphigus
c. Pemphigoid   d. Herpes zoster

<table>
<tr><td colspan="2">INFECTIONS</td><td colspan="2">SKIN TUMORS</td></tr>
</table>

12. The "Lepra cells" are: *(Recent Question 2014)*
a. histologically
b. Histiocytes
c. Lymphocytes
d. Neutrophils Plasma cells

13. In lepromatous leprosy, globi consist of:
(Recent Question 2014)
a. Macrophage cells laden with acid fast bacill
b. Lipid laden macrophages and degenerated tissue
c. Activated lymphocytes
d. Immunoglobulin-containing plasma cells

14. Which of the following is a precancerous condition of the skin? *(MH PG 2014)*
a. Bowen disease
b. Seborrhoeic keratosis
c. Leprosy
d. Psoriasis

15. Mutation in malignant melanoma:
(Kerela 2016), (Recent Question 2015)
a. N-myc
b. CDKN2A
c. RbT
d. None

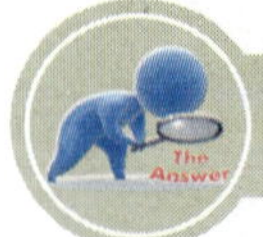

Answers with Explanations

1. Ans. (d) **Most common pigmented lesions**

(Ref: Robbins 9th/pg 1143)

Most common[Q] pigmented lesions- freckles
Other 3 options are features of café au lait spots

2. Ans. (c) **Diffuse epidermal hyperplasia**

(Ref: Robbin 9th/pg 1143)

Microscopic Lesions	Definition
Acanthosis	Diffuse **epidermal hyperplasia**[Q]
Hyperkeratosis	Thickening of the **stratum corneum**[Q]

3. Ans. (a) **Acute eczema** *(Ref: Robbins 9th/pg 1163; 1143)*

Microscopic Lesions	Definition
Spongiosis	**Intercellular edema** of the epidermis[Q]

4. Ans. (a, b, c, d, e); a. **Pancytopenia;** b. **Nail dystrophy;** c. **Hyperkeratosis;** d. **X linked;** e. **Leukoplakia**

(Ref: Table 41.4 Wintrobe's Clinical Hematology,12th Edition)

Dyskeratosis Congenita

- **Inherited Bone Marrow Failure Syndrome**
- Majority of patients present with pancytopenia
- Abnormal nails, reticular rash, leukoplakia
- X-linked recessive, autosomal dominant, and autosomal recessive inheritance patterns have been reported
- Patients exhibit a predisposition to bone marrow failure, malignancy, and pulmonary dysfunction.

5. Ans. (c) **Psoriasis** *(Ref: Robbins 9th/pg 1165; 8th/pg 1185)*

Psoriasis

- **Intraepidermal infiltrates of neutrophils**
  - In the **stratum corneum (Munro microabscesses)**[Q]
  - The **spinous layer (spongiform pustules of Kogoj)**[Q]

6. Ans. (a) **Antibodies against hemidesmosomes**

(Ref: Lever dermatopathology/ 10th 273)

Antibody targets for Pemphigus:

Diseases	Antigens
Pemphigus Vulgaris	
Mucosal	Desmoglein 3
Mucocutaneous	Desmoglein 3 &1
Pemphigus foliaceus	

The most common bullous lesion is bullous pemphigoid. – And the most common pattern of Immuno-fluorescence is Linear IgG deposit along basement membrane. **So, the best possible answer is A.**

7. Ans. (a) **Pemphigus**

(Ref: Robbins 9th/pg 1167)

Pemphigus Vulgaris

- Suprabasal blister formation
- Row of tombstone appearance

8. Ans. (a) **Pemphigus Vulgaris**

9. Ans. (b) **Loss of intercellular connections**

(Ref: Robbins 9th/pg 1165; 8th/pg 1168)

Acantholysis- Separation of keratinocytes- **Loss of intercellular connections**
Acanthosis- Diffuse epidermal hyperplasia
Spongiosis-Intercellular edema of the epidermis.

10. Ans. (b) **Collagen type VII**

(Ref: http://ghr.nlm.nih.gov/condition/dystrophic-epidermolysis-bullosa, J Med Genet. 2007 Mar; 44(3): 181–192.)

- Mutations in the COL7A1 gene seen in dystrophic epidermolysis bullosa
- COL7A1 mutations alter the structure or disrupt the production of **type VII collagen**, which impairs its ability to help connect the epidermis to the dermis.

11. **Ans. (b)** **Pemphigus**

(Ref: Robbins 9th/pg 1167)

Disease	Biopsy features	DIF
Pemphigus vulgaris	• Suprabasal acantholytic vesicle (tombstone pattern)[Q] • Mixed perivascular infiltrate with eosinophils[Q]	IgG within suprabasal intercellular spaces –fishnet pattern[Q]

12. **Ans. (b)** **Histiocytes**

(Ref: Sternberg's Diagnostic Surgical Pathology, 5th Edition. 862)

Lepra cells[Q] - large, mononuclear histiocytes (macrophages) with a foam like cytoplasm
Seen in lepromatous leprosy

13. **Ans. (a)** **Macrophage cells laden with acid fast bacill**

(Ref: Sternberg's Diagnostic Surgical Pathology, 5th Edition. 862)

GLOBI-Macrophage cells laden with acid fast bacill[Q]
Seen in lepromatous leprosy

14. **Ans. (a)** **Bowen disease**

(Ref: Clin Plast Surg. 1980 Jul;7(3):289-300.)

The most common precancerous skin lesions are actinic keratoses, Bowen's disease, and keratoacanthoma.
Actinic keratoses appear over the exposed areas of the body as the result of actinic radiation. Bowen's disease is most probably secondary to the effects of internal carcinogens. Keratoacanthomas are self-limited lesions that occasionally may transform into invasive squamous cell carcinoma.

15. **Ans. (b)** **CDKN2A** *(Ref: R 9th/pg 1148-50; 8th/pg 1172)*

Melanoma is associated with mutations in **cell cycle regulators** (p16/INK4a, CDK4), growth factor receptors [e.g., **KIT], RAS, BRAF**), and **telomerase**[Q]

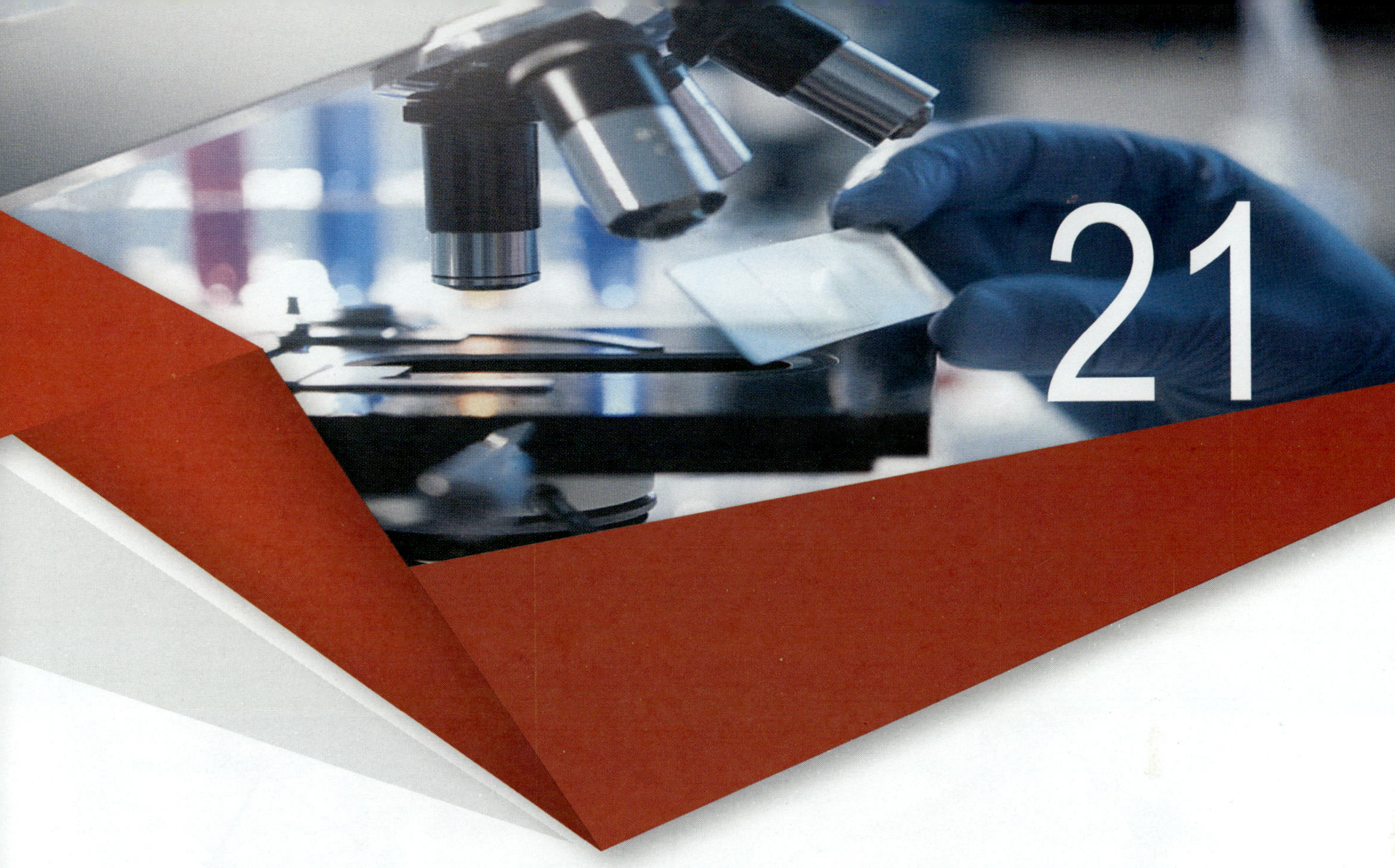

21

Central Nervous System and its Disorders

Key Points

- » Neural tube defects are most common CNS malformations
- » Most common type of intracranial aneurysm is Berry aneurysm
- » HIV Meningoencephalitis is characterized by microglial nodules
- » Most common intracranial tumors is metastasis
- » Most common primary tumor of CNS: Meningioma
- » Most common primary intracranial tumor of CNS: Glioma (astrocytoma)
- » Most common malignant tumor of CNS: Glioma (glioblastoma multiforme)
- » Most aggressive tumor in children: Medulloblastoma
- » Most common tumor in children: Pilocytic astrocytoma

Key Recent Updates

- » IDH_1 mutant glioblastomas have better prognosis
- » MC mutation in early onset familial Alzheimer's disease is PS_1.

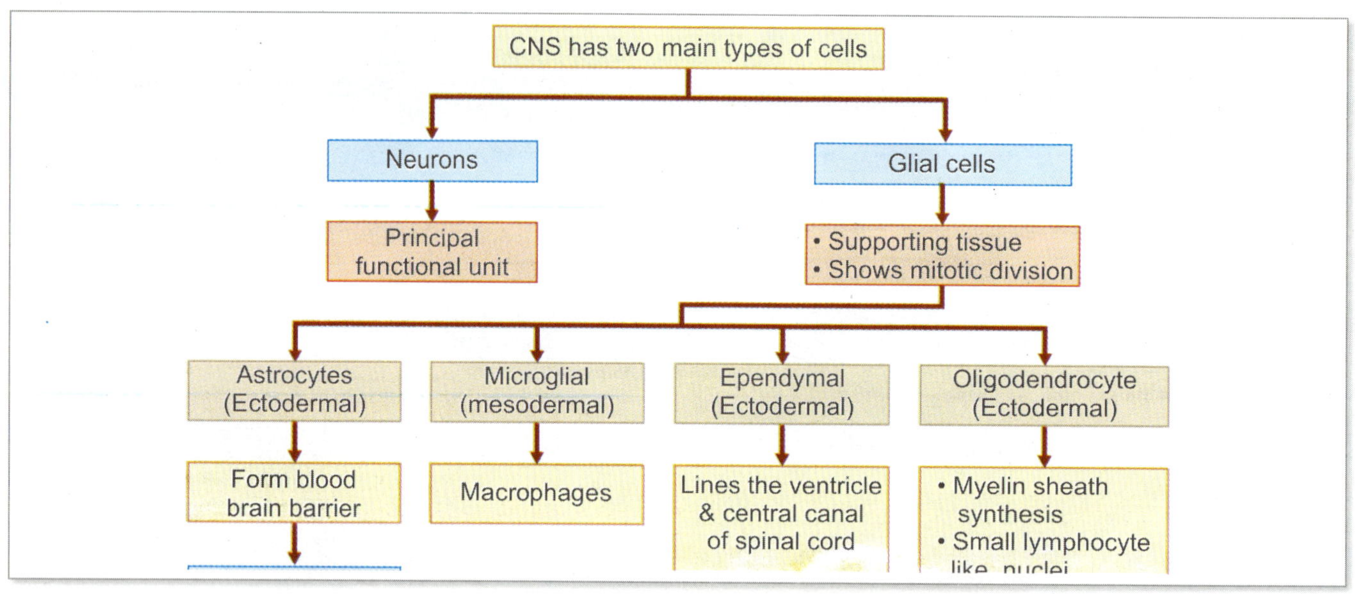

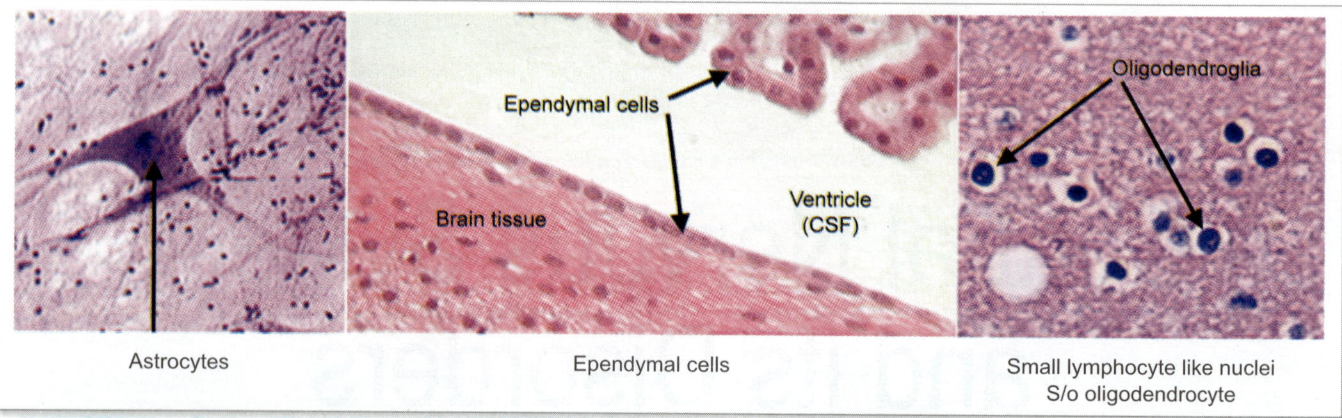

Astrocytes

Ependymal cells

Small lymphocyte like nuclei
S/o oligodendrocyte

CELLULAR PATHOLOGY OF THE CENTRAL NERVOUS SYSTEM

Neurons and glia of the CNS undergo a range of functional and morphologic **changes in the setting of injury.**

Reactions of Neurons to Injury

- The **characteristic** histologic feature is **cell loss**[Q] and **reactive gliosis**[Q]

Neuronal inclusions can be seen in

- **Viral infection**s
  - Intranuclear inclusions-Herpes infection (Cowdry body)[Q]
  - Cytoplasmic inclusions-Rabies (Negri body)[Q]
  - Both nucleus and cytoplasm-Cytomegalovirus infection.[Q]
- **Intracytoplasmic inclusions**[Q] in neurons,
  - Neurofibrillary tangles[Q] of Alzheimer's disease
  - Lewy bodies[Q] of Parkinson's disease
  - Lafora bodies[Q] in myoclonic epilepsy

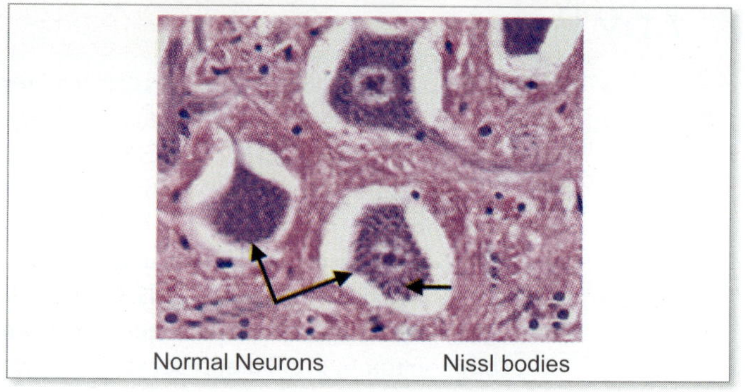

Normal Neurons   Nissl bodies

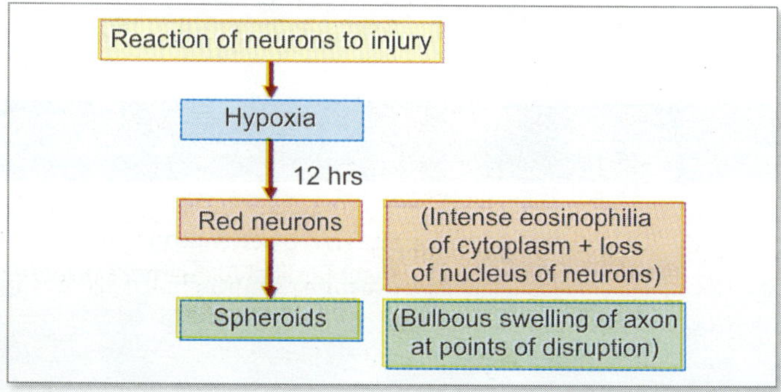

Reactions of Astrocytes to Injury

- **Gliosis**[Q] is the **most important histopathologic**[Q] indicator of **CNS injury** and is characterized by both **hypertrophy and hyperplasia of astrocytes.**

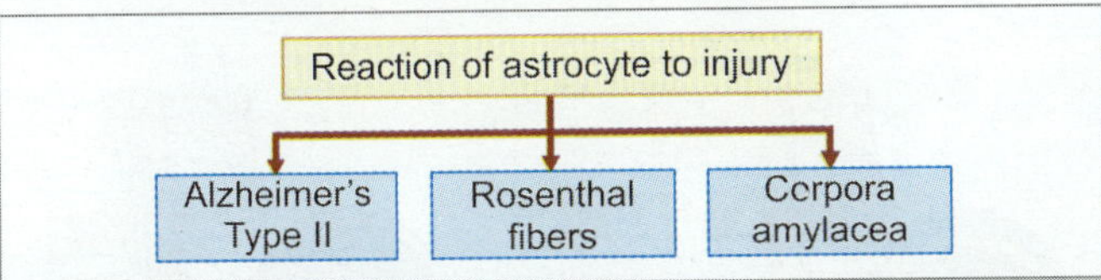

- **The Alzheimer type II astrocyte**[Q]:
  - Unrelated to Alzheimer's disease.[Q]
  - It is a gray matter cell with large nucleus with **intranuclear glycogen droplet**[Q]

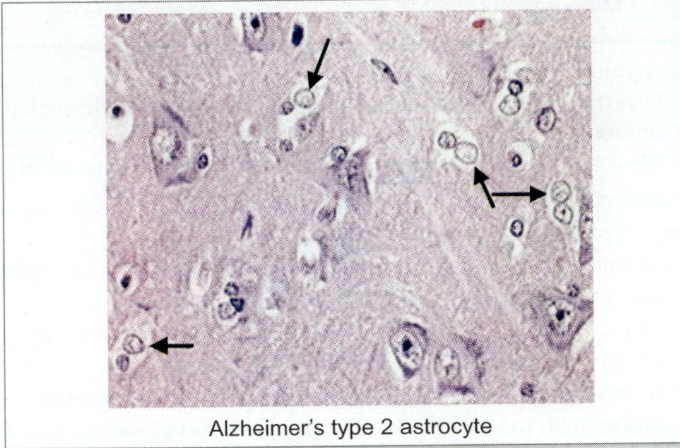

Alzheimer's type 2 astrocyte

  - Seen in **Long-standing hyperammonemia due to chronic liver disease, Wilson's disease, or hereditary metabolic disorders of the urea cycle.**[Q]
- **Rosenthal fibers:**

  - Brightly **eosinophilic structures / inclusions within cytoplasm of**[Q] astrocytic processes
  - Contain two **heat-shock proteins** (αB-crystallin and HSP27) as well as **ubiquitin**[Q]

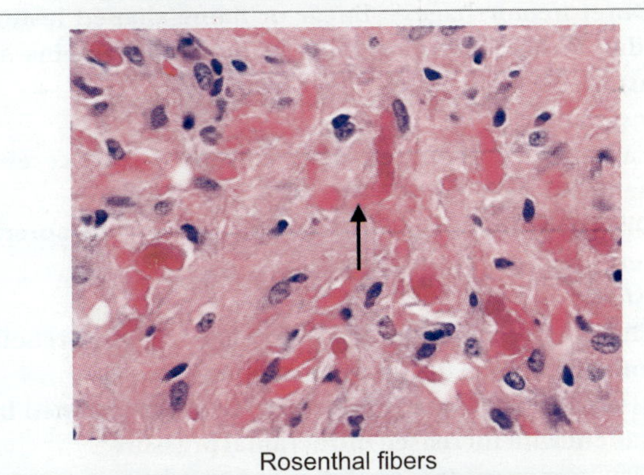

Rosenthal fibers

  - Seen in **Alexander's disease, pilocytic astrocytoma**[Q].
- **Corpora amylacea:**
  - **Periodic acid-Schiff (PAS)-positive**,[Q] concentrically **lamellated structures** and contains **glycosaminoglycan** polymers, as well as **heat-shock proteins** and **ubiquitin.**
  - Seen in **advancing age and are thought to represent a degenerative change in the Astrocyte.**[Q]

Reactions of Microglia to Injury

Microglia-Resident **macrophages** of the CNS[Q].
They respond to injury by[Q]
- Developing elongated nuclei (**rod cells**)[Q], as in **neurosyphilis**
- Forming **aggregates** around small foci of tissue necrosis → **microglial nodules**
- Forming **aggregates** around cell bodies of dying neurons → **neuronophagia**[Q].

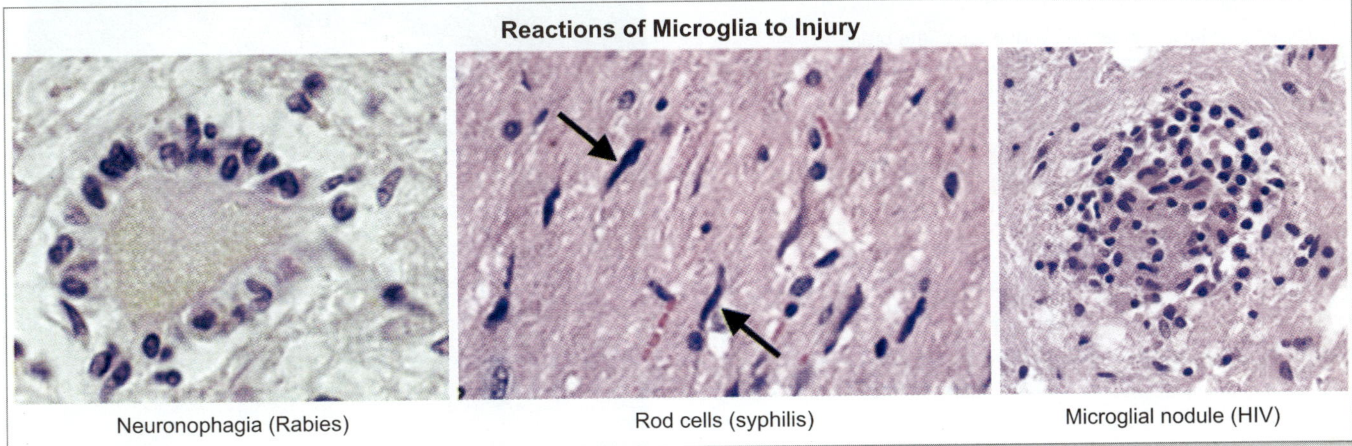

Reactions of Microglia to Injury

Neuronophagia (Rabies)

Rod cells (syphilis)

Microglial nodule (HIV)

Reactions of Other Glial Cells to Injury

- **Oligodendroglial nuclei** show viral inclusions in **progressive multifocal leukoencephalopathy**[Q]
- Ependymal cells-**ciliated columnar**[Q] epithelial cells **lining the ventricles**
- **Viral inclusions** in ependymal cells-**CMV**[Q]

CEREBRAL HERNIATION

- Most common cause of herniation is increased intracranial pressure.

Types of Herniation

- **Transtentorial:**
  - Occurs when the **medial aspect of the temporal lobe is compressed against the free margin of the tentorium**[Q]
  - **Duret hemorrhages**[Q] -linear or flame-shaped lesions[Q] -due to distortion or tearing of **penetrating veins and arteries**[Q] supplying the upper brainstem
- **Transfalcine:**
  - Caused by **asymmetric expansion of a cerebral hemisphere**[Q]
  - Displaces the cingulate gyrus-compresses the **anterior cerebral artery**[Q] and its branches.
- **Tonsillar:**
  - These are caused by displacement of the **cerebellar tonsils**[Q] through the **foramen magnum**[Q].
  - Also occur if a **lumbar puncture (LP) is performed in a patient with increased intracranial pressure**[Q].
  - May **compress the medulla and respiratory centers, causing death**[Q].

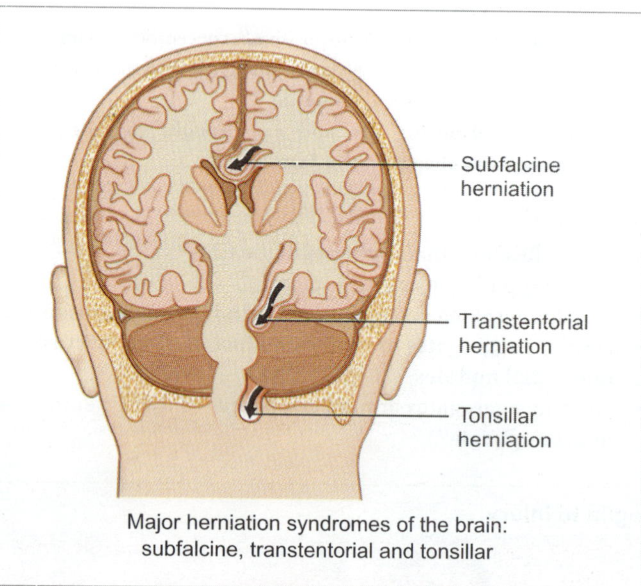

Major herniation syndromes of the brain: subfalcine, transtentorial and tonsillar

MALFORMATIONS AND DEVELOPMENTAL DISORDERS

NEURAL TUBE DEFECTS

- Neural tube defects are most common CNS malformations
- **Most common site** of neural tube defects is the **spinal cord.**[Q]

Types of Neural Tube Defects

Spinal dysraphism or spina bifida–can be of two types:
- **Spina bifida occulta**[Q] -can be **asymptomatic bony** defect
- **Spina bifida aperta**[Q] disorganized segment of spinal cord, associated with an overlying meningeal outpouching

Myelomeningocele–extension of **CNS tissue and meninges** through a defect in the vertebral column

Meningocele–applies when there is only a **meningeal extrusion**.

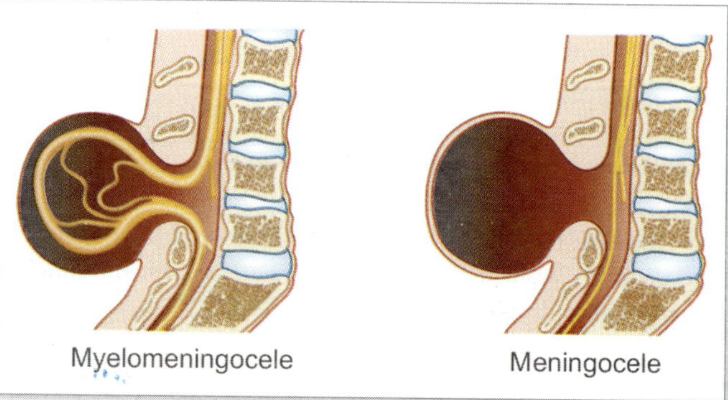

Myelomeningocele   Meningocele

Encephalocele
- Diverticulum of **malformed brain** tissue extending through a **defect in the cranium**.
- Most common in **posterior fossa**[Q] **cribriform plate in the anterior fossa**

Anencephaly
- Malformation of the anterior end of the neural tube, with absence of most of the brain and calvarium.
- Instead, there is a mass of disorganized glial tissue with vessels in this area called a **cerebrovasculosa**[Q]
- Neural tube defects are associated with ↑Alpha fetoprotein.
- Mutation in **DOUBLECORTIN (Dcx)** results in Lissencephaly in males and subcortical band heterotopia is females

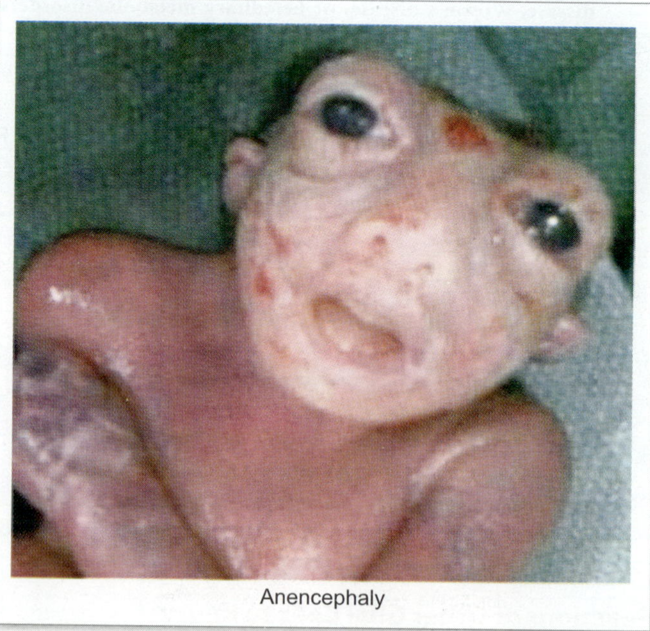

Anencephaly

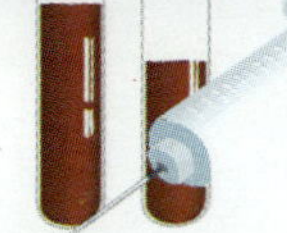

FOREBRAIN ANOMALIES

Lissencephaly	Polygyria	Holoprosencephaly	Arrhen-cephaly	Agenesis of the corpus callosum	Neuronal Heterotopia
↓ gyri	Small ↑gyri	Incomplete separation of cerebral hemispheres across midline	No olfactory nerves	• No white matter projections from one hemisphere to the other • **Bat wing anomaly**	Neurons in inappropriate locations along lines of migration
Lissencephaly	Polymicrogyria	Holoprosencephaly			

POSTERIOR FOSSA ANOMALIES

Developmental abnormalities of the brain include the **Arnold-Chiari malformation,** the **Dandy-Walker malformation**[Q]

- *Arnold Chiari:*
  - Small posterior fossa
  - Herniation of cerebellum & 4th ventricle into foramen magnum
  - Associated with hydrocephalus and lumbar myelomeningocele

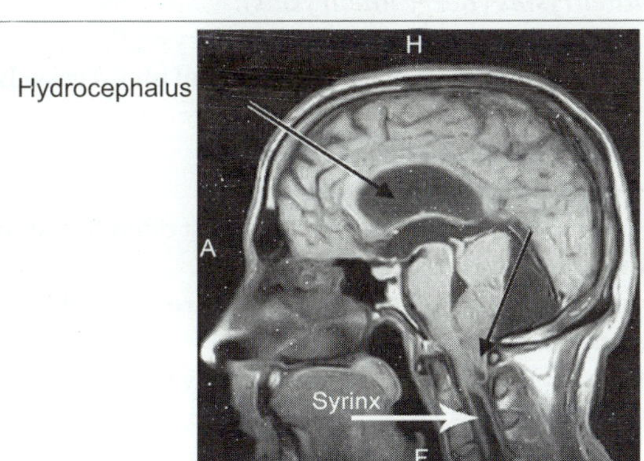

MRI Shows herniated cerebellum

- *Dandy Walker:*
  - Enlarged posterior fossa
  - Severe hypoplasia/Absence of cerebellar vermis
  - Cystic dilation of 4th ventricle hydrocephalus and agenesis of corpus callosum

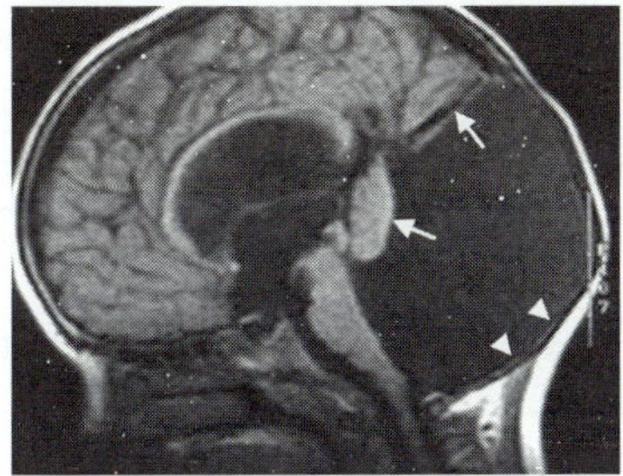
MRI Shows large posterior fossa and hypoplastic cerebellum

Mnemonic

Dandy-Walker syndrome: Components "Dandy Walker Syndrome":
- **D**ilated 4th ventricle
- **W**ater on the brain
- **S**mall vermis

High Yield Facts

- **Chiari type i malformation** is a less severe disorder in which low lying **cerebellar tonsils extend down into the vertebral canal.**[Q]
- Lucid interval is seen in epidural hemorrhage
- Worst headache is seen in SAH
- Self limited bleeding is SDH
- **Hypertension** MC causes **deep brain parenchymal hemorrhages**[Q]
- **Chronic hypertension** leads to development of *Charcot-Bouchard microaneurysms*[Q]
- **Cerebral amyloid angiopathy (CAA)**[Q] MC causes of **lobar hemorrhages**[Q].
- Cerebral amyloid angiopathy (AB$_{40}$)-MC cause of total hemorrhage

R9th Latest Update

- **Joubert syndrome:** Hypoplasia of the cerebellar vermis with elongation of the superior cerebellar peduncles and an altered shape of the brainstem; together these changes give rise to the **'molar tooth sign'**[Q] on imaging.
- Mutations affect genes that encode components of the **primary (non-motile) cilium.**[Q]

CEREBRAL HEMORRHAGE

It can be in epidural, subdural, subarachnoid, and intraparenchymal compartments

Site of Hemorrhage	Cause
• Epidural	• Rupture of dural arteries MC-middle meningeal artery
• Subdural	• Rupture of bridging veins
• Subarachnoid	• Rupture of Berry aneurysm in cerebral artery
• Ultra parenchymal	• Due to hypertension and cerebral amyloid angiopathy

Subarachnoid Hemorrhage (SAH)

- **MC cause is rupture of a saccular ("Berry") aneurysm in a cerebral artery.**[Q]
- **"Worst headache ever"**[Q]

High Yield Facts

Berry Aneurysm
- Developmental abnormalities[Q]
- Due to **the structural abnormality of the involved vessel (absence of smooth muscle and intimal elastic lamina.)**[Q]
- Called **congenital**[Q], although the aneurysm itself is **not present at birth**[Q] but develop over time
- Majority occur sporadically[Q],
- Increased incidence in autosomal dominant polycystic kidney disease, Ehlers-Danlos syndrome type IV, neurofibromatosis type 1 [NF1], and Marfan's syndrome, fibromuscular dysplasia of extracranial arteries,[Q] and coarctation of the aorta.[Q]
- 90% found **near major arterial branch**[Q] points in the **anterior circulation**[Q]
- The chance of rupture increases with age (**rupture is rare in childhood**[Q]).

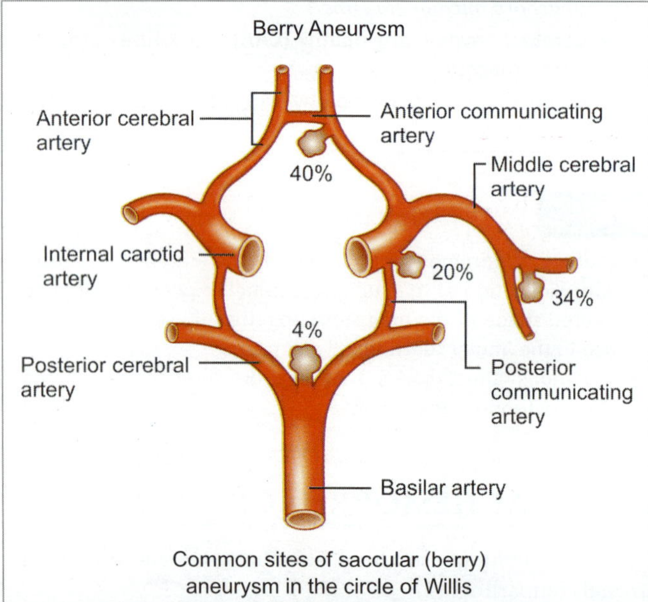

Common sites of saccular (berry) aneurysm in the circle of Willis

Intraparenchymal Hemorrhage

- **Ganglionic hemorrhages**[Q]: Hemorrhage in the *basal ganglia and thalamus*
- **Lobar hemorrhages.**[Q]: Hemorrhage is in the lobes of the *cerebral hemispheres*
- The two major causes: **Hypertension and cerebral amyloid angiopathy.**[Q]
- This deposition of Aβ40 weaken the vessel wall and lead to hemorrhage.
- The presence of either ε2 or ε4 **allele**[Q] increases the risk of repeat bleeding.

> **R9th** **Latest** Update
>
> - **Cerebral autosomal dominant arteriopathy with subcortical infarcts and leukoencephalopathy (CADASIL)**-autosomal dominant disorder caused by mutations in the **NOTCH3 gene.**[Q]
> - The disease is characterized clinically by recurrent strokes (usually infarcts, less often hemorrhages) and dementia.[Q]

INTRACRANIAL ANEURYSMS

- *Charcot-Bouchard aneurysms:*
  - Results from weakening of the wall of cerebral artery by **lipohyalinosis**[Q] (deposition of lipids and hyaline material) caused by **hypertension**[Q].
- *Saccular aneurysms (Berry aneurysms):*
  - **Most common type of intracranial aneurysm.**[Q]
  - Result of **congenital defects in the media of blood vessels**
  - Located at the **bifurcations of arteries**.
- *Atherosclerotic aneurysms:*
  - **Fusiform (spindle-shaped)**[Q] aneurysms
  - Located in *the* major cerebral vessels, most often found in the **anterior circulation**[Q]
  - They **rarely rupture**[Q], but may become **thrombosed.**[Q]
- *Mycotic (septic) aneurysms:*
  - Result from **septic emboli**[Q], most commonly from **subacute bacterial endocarditis**.[Q]
  - Causes **cerebral infarction**[Q], rather than subarachnoid **hemorrhage**[Q]

POINTS TO REMEMBER

- Hypertensive hemorrhage shows *a predilection for the distribution of the* **lenticulostriate arteries (branch of middle cerebral artery)** with small (**lacunar**) hemorrhages, or **large hemorrhages obliterating** *the* corpus striatum, including the **putamen and internal capsule**[Q].

CNS INFECTIONS

Meningitis

Inflammatory process of the leptomeninges and CSF within the subarachnoid space.

Causative Organisms of Meningitis[Q]

Type	Age group	Etiology
Acute Pyogenic Meningitis	Neonates	*Escherichia coli (India), group B streptococci (World)*
	Infants	*S.pnemoniae, Haemophilus influenzae*
	Adolescents & young adults	*S.pnemoniae, Neisseria meningitidis*
	Elderly	*Streptococcus pneumonia* *Listeria monocytogenes*
	Immunosuppressed individual	*Klebsiella or anaerobic organisms*
Chronic Meningitis		*Tuberculous, spirochetal or cryptococcal*
Aseptic meningitis		Viruses like enteroviruses

CSF Findings in CNS Infections

Parameters	Normal values	Bacterial Meningitis	Tuberculous Meningitis	Viral Meningitis
Pressure	50–180 mm water	Raised	Raised	Raised
Gross appearance	Clear and colorless	**Turbid**[Q]	**Clear (may clot)**[Q]	**Clear**[Q]
Protein	20–50 mg/dL	High	**Very High**[Q]	Slightly high
Glucose	40–70 mg/dL	**Very low**[Q]	Low	Normal
Chloride	110–125 mEq/L	Low	**Very low**[Q]	Normal
Cells	< 5/microlitre	Neutrophils 1,000–1,00,000 neutrophils/uL	Pleocytosis 100-1000 mononuclear/uL	**Lymphocytosis**[Q] 10-100 mononuclear/uL

Human Immunodeficiency Virus (HIV)

- **Directly** cause **meningoencephalitis,**[Q]
- **Indirectly**-increases the risk of **opportunistic infections**[Q] (toxoplasmosis, CMV) or EBV-positive CNS **lymphoma.**[Q]
- Meningoencephalitis-characterized by **microglial nodules**[Q] composed of **mononuclear cells, microglia, and scattered multinucleated giant cells,** usually found **near small blood vessels**[Q], which shows **prominent endothelial cells and perivascular foamy or pigment-laden macrophages**[Q]
- HIV-associated central nervous system (CNS) lymphoma is a **diffuse, large-cell non-Hodgkin's lymphoma**[Q] of **B-cell origin**[Q] that usually occurs in the brain (rarely in the spinal cord).
- It is a **late complication**[Q] of HIV infection.
- **Epstein-Barr virus (EBV)**[Q] is identified in almost **all cases**[Q].

Rabies Virus

- Rabies is **only communicable disease of man** that is **always fatal**[Q].
- Rabies is **dead end infection**[Q] caused by **enveloped, RNA (negative sense single stranded) virus**[Q].
- Most characteristic pathologic finding in CNS is the formation of **cytoplasmic inclusion bodies** called **Negri bodies**[Q].
- The **prominence of early brain stem dysfunction**[Q] distinguish it from other viral encephalitis.
- Diagnosis is made by **detection of rabies virus antigen** by **immunofluorescence**[Q].
- **Antemortem specimen**: **corneal smear**[Q], skin biopsy from neck or saliva.
- **Postmortem**: **Brain biopsy**[Q]
- **A definitive pathologic diagnosis of rabies can be based on the finding of negri bodies in the brain or spinal cord**[Q].

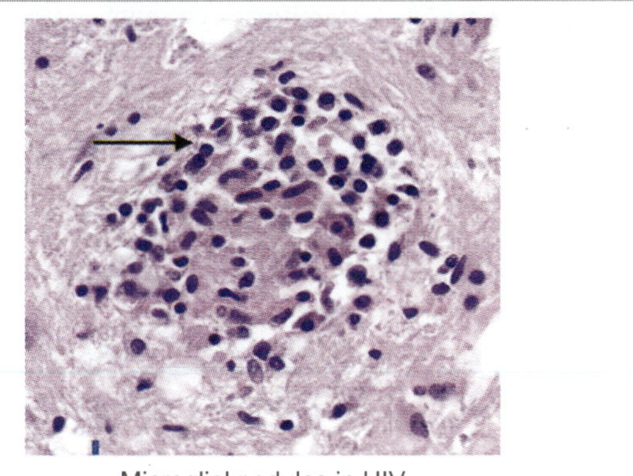

Microglial nodules in HIV

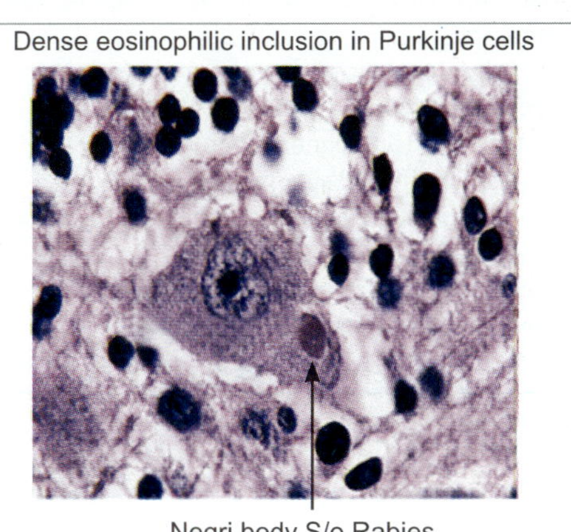

Dense eosinophilic inclusion in Purkinje cells

Negri body S/o Rabies

Negri bodies
- Composed of finely fibrillar matrix (**ribonuclear proteins** produced by the virus) and rabies virus particles
- Found **most abundantly in cerebellum (purkinje cells) & pyramidal neurons of hippocampus**. They are also seen in neurons of Ammon's horn, cerebral cortex, brainstem, hypothalamus, and dorsal spinal ganglia.

Neurosyphilis

- **Tertiary stage of syphilis**[Q], includes **syphilitic meningitis, paretic neurosvphilis, and tabes dorsalis**[Q]

Meningovascular Neurosyphilis	Paretic Neurosyphilis	Tabes Dorsalis
• **Obliterative endarteritis (Heubner arteritis)**[Q] • Perivascular infiltrates of lymphocytes and plasma cells[Q] • **Cerebral gummas (plasma cell-rich mass lesions)**[Q] can also occur.	• Occurs due to **invasion of the brain by T. pallidum.**[Q] • Characterized by **delusions of grandeur**[Q] that terminate in **severe dementia** (general paresis of the insane). • The lesions are characterized by **loss of neurons, proliferation of microglia (rod cells)**[Q], **gliosis, and iron deposits.**[Q]	• Result of **degeneration of the posterior columns of the spinal cord.**[Q] • Impaired joint position sensation, ataxia[Q] • Loss of pain sensation (leading to joint damage, i.e. Charcot joints)[Q] • *Argyll Robertson pupils* (pupils that react to accommodation but not to light).[Q]

CMV

- Enlarged cells (cytomegaly) with intranuclear and intracytoplasmic inclusions are seen with cytomegalovirus infection.[Q]
- Owl eyed inclusions seen in CMV[Q]

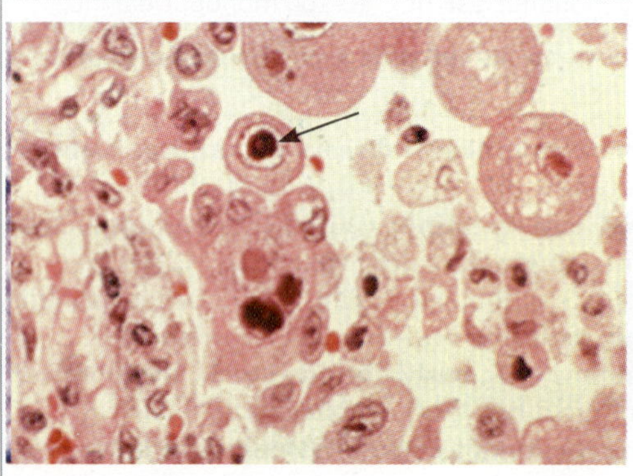

Features
- Cytomegaly
- Intranuclear inclusions (cowdry type)
- Cytoplasmic inclusions
- **S/o CMV**

- Vasculitis is characteristically absent in CNS involvement in AIDS
- Spinal cord involvement in AIDS leads to vacuolar myelopathy
- Herpes simplex virus produces Cowdry type A intranuclear inclusions[Q] in neurons and glial cells.[Q]
- Subacute sclerosing panencephalitis (SSPE)
  - Progressive clinical syndrome
  - Characterized by cognitive decline, spasticity of limbs, and seizures.
  - Occurs in children after an initial, early-age acute infection with measles.[Q]
- Babes nodules[Q] are seen in rabies encephalomyelitis

PROGRESSIVE MULTIFOCAL LEUKOENCEPHALOPATHY (PML)

- Demyelinating disease caused by the **JC polyomavirus**[Q], preferentially infects **oligodendrocytes**[Q].
- Occurs in **immunosuppressed individuals**[Q].
- The **pathognomonic feature** of PML is **"ground-glass" appearance of oligodendrocyte nuclei**[Q].

PRION DISEASES

- Prions are **abnormal forms of a cellular protein**[Q]
- Can be **sporadic, familial or transmitted.**[Q]

Humans[Q]	Animals[Q]
• Creutzfeldt-Jakob disease • Gerstmann-Sträussler-Scheinker syndrome • Fatal familial insomnia • Kuru	• Scrapie in sheep • Mink-transmissible encephalopathy • Chronic wasting • Disease of deer and elk • Bovine spongiform encephalopathy

- *Clinically:* Rapidly progressive dementia
- *Morphologically:* **Spongiform change**[Q] **without inflammation** hallmark of all prion diseases except **fatal familial insomnia,**[Q] which is characterized by neuronal loss and reactive gliosis .[Q]
- *Pathology:*
  - Normal PrP is a 30-kD cytoplasmic protein present in neurons.[Q]
  - Disease occurs when PrP undergoes a conformational change from its normal alpha-helix-containing isoform (PrPc) to an abnormal B-pleated sheet isoform, usually termed PrPsc.[Q]
  - PrP acquires resistance to digestion with proteases[Q]

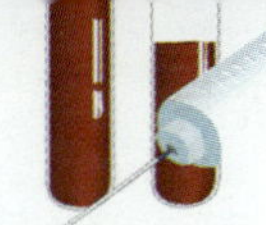

- ○ **Prion Diseases:** PrPsc, **independent of the means from which it originates**[Q], then facilitates, in a **cooperative fashion**[Q], the conversion of other PrPc molecules to PrPsc molecules.
  - ○ This transformation can occur sporadically or in familial fashion.
- ■ **Genetics: Mutations in the gene encoding PrPc (PRNP).**[Q]

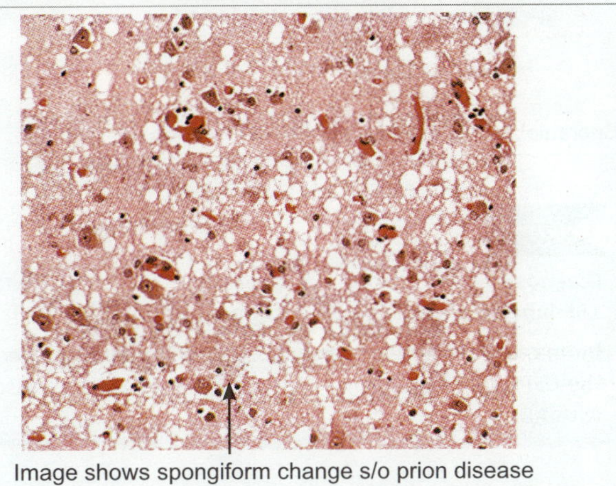

Image shows spongiform change s/o prion disease

- ■ **Diagnosis of Choice: Western blotting** of tissue extracts after partial digestion with proteinase K, **diagnostic.**[Q]

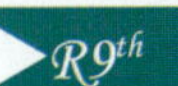

Latest Update

Prion Diseases
A polymorphic locus in **PRNP (codon 129 may be either Met or Val)**[Q] Homozygosity **increases risk of sporadic disease.**[Q]

Creutzfeldt-Jakob Disease (CJD)

- ■ **Most common** prion disease[Q]
- ■ Peak incidence in the **seventh decade**.[Q]
- ■ **Familial forms**-mutations in **PRNP**[Q]
- ■ Iatrogenic transmission-[Q]
  - ○ **Corneal, transplantation**[Q], Deep implantation of electrodes in the brain[Q], Administration of contaminated preparations of naturally derived human growth hormone[Q]
- ■ **Clinically- dementia, startle myoclonus**[Q]

Variant Creutzfeldt-Jakob Disease

- ■ **Young adults**[Q]
- ■ **No alterations in the PRNP gene** are present[Q]
- ■ Clinically-**behavioral disorders** prominently in the early stages[Q]
- ■ **Extensive cortical plaques surrounded by a "halo" of spongiform change**[Q]

NEURODEGENERATIVE DISEASES

- ■ Diseases that affect the gray matter of brain with **damage to the neurons**.[Q]
- ■ The **pathologic hallmark**[Q]-accumulation **of protein aggregates**[Q], hence the use of the term **"proteinopathy"**[Q].
- ■ The protein aggregates are recognized histologically as **inclusions-diagnostic hallmark**[Q] of the disease.
- ■ The protein aggregates typically are **resistant to degradation and are directly toxic to neuron**[Q]

Disease	Clinical pattern	Inclusions	Genetic causes
Alzheimer's Disease	Dementia	Aβ (plaques)[Q] Tau (tangles)[Q]	APP, PS1, PS2[Q]
Parkinson's disease (PD)	Hypokinetic movement disorder	**α-synuclein**[Q] Tau	**α-synuclein**[Q] LRRK2
Huntington's disease (HD)	Hyperkinetic movement disorder	Huntington[Q] (polyglutamine)	Htt
Amyotrophic lateral sclerosis (ALS)	Weakness with upper and lower motor neurons signs	SOD1[Q] TDP-43 FUS	SOD1 TDP-43, C9orf72 FUS

Alzheimer's Disease

- ■ **Most common cause** of **dementia in elderly**[Q] **(followed by vascular multi-infarct dementia)**[Q]
- ■ The **hallmark abnormality**[Q]-accumulation of two proteins (**Aβ and tau**) in specific brain regions
- ■ The etiology of AD is not well understood, Main risk factor-**age**[Q]
- ■ Grossly, **cortical atrophy (narrowed gyri and widened sulci)**[Q] is predominant in **frontal, temporal, and parietal** *lobes*
- ■ The **pathologic hallmark**[Q] are plaques and tangles.

High Yield Facts

- • Tangles are **not**[Q] specific to AD, being found in other diseases as well.
- • AD is associated with decrease in cerebral cortical level of acetylcholine. This degeneration occurs in **nucleus basalis of Meyernet**[Q]
- • Vascular amyloid in **cerebral amyloid angiopathy** is **Aβ40.**[Q]
- • **Medial temporal lobe, including hippocampus, entorhinal cortex and amygdala**[Q], are involved early in the course.
- • **Mutations in the gene for tau cause frontotemporal lobar degenerations**[Q] rather than AD
- • Beta-amyloid deposition is **necessary** but **not sufficient**[Q] for the development of Alzheimer's disease
- • **Hirano bodies**[Q] and Granulovacuolarde generation[Q] are other features seen in AD

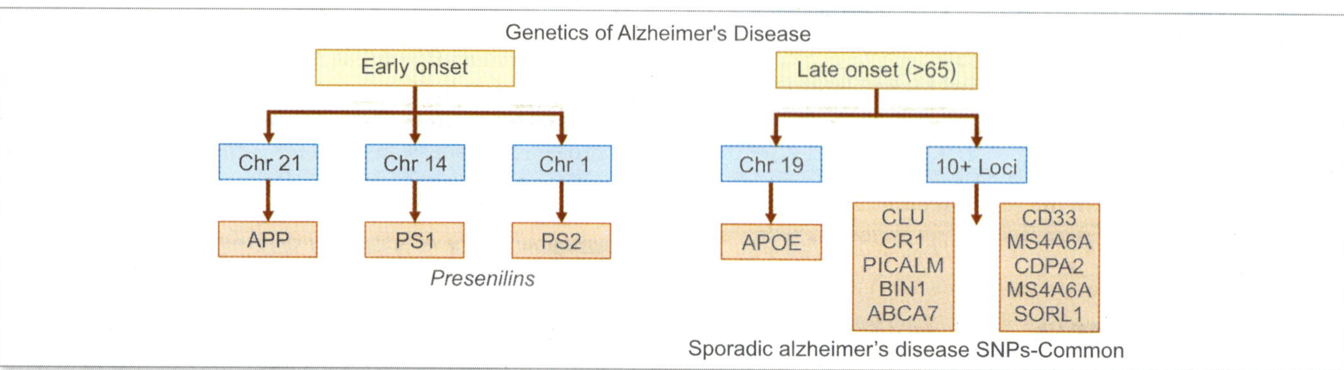

R⁹ᵗʰ Latest Update

1. Out of **APP**, **PSEN1** and **PSEN2** mutations in early-onset Alzheimer's disease occur in the order **PS1 > APP > PS2**.
2. Mutations in **PS-1** are the most common cause of early-age-of-onset **FAD**, representing perhaps 40–70% of all cases.
3. **ApoE4** remains the single most important biological marker associated with **AD** risk.

R⁹ᵗʰ Latest Update

Diagnosis: Demonstrate **Aβ deposition** in the brain through **18F-labeled amyloid binding compounds on PET scan.**[Q]

Biomarkers: Increased phosphorylated tau and reduced Aβ in the CSF[Q] provide evidence of neuronal degeneration associated with AD.

Plaques

- Deposits of aggregated **Aβ** peptides in the neuropil.
- Plaques are of two types diffuse and neuritic (senile).
- **Neuritic plaques** contain both **Aβ 40 and Aβ 42,**[Q] Diffuse **plaques** are predominantly made up of **Aβ 42.**[Q]
- **Diffuse plaques** —seen in brain of **trisomy 21**[Q] patients

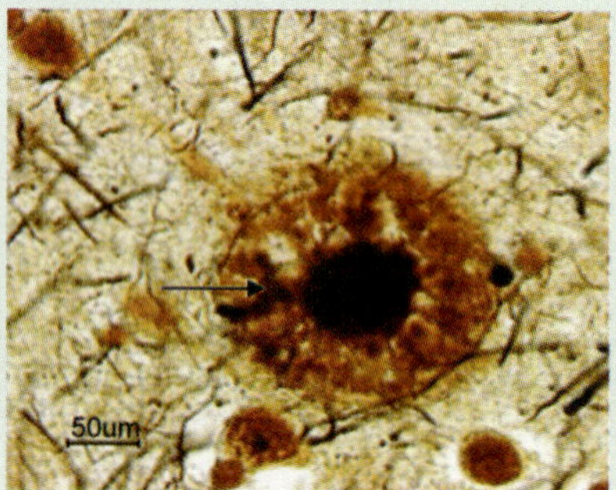

Plaques are aggregated Ab

Tangles

- Aggregates of the microtubule binding protein **tau**[Q].
- They are demonstrated by **silver (Bielschowsky) staining**[Q]
- They are commonly found in **cortical neurons,** especially in the **entorhinal cortex,** as well as in other sites such as **pyramidal cells of the hippocampus**[Q], the amygdala, the basal forebrain, and the raphe nuclei[Q]

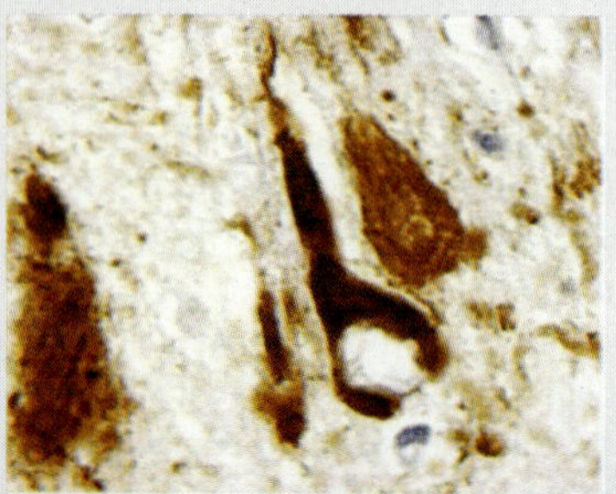

Neurofibrillary tangles are aggregates of tau protein

Lewy Body Disorders

- Lewy bodies are intracytoplasmic eosinophilic inclusions.
- Major component of the Lewy body is **alpha-synuclein**[Q], others being neurofilament antigens, parkin, and ubiquitin.
- The histologic features of Lewy body disorders depends on location of lewy bodies

Disease	Location	Symptoms
Classic Parkinson's disease	Nigrostriatal system[Q]	Extrapyramidal movement disorder
Lewy body dementia	Cerebral cortex[Q]	**Third most** common cause of dementia[Q]
Shy-Dragger syndrome	Sympathetic neurons in the spinal cord[Q]	Autonomic dysfunction

TUMORS

- **Most common tumor** of CNS- **metastasis**[Q]
- Most common **primary** tumor of CNS- **meningioma**[Q]
- Most common **primary intracranial tumor** of CNS- **glioma (astrocytoma)**[Q]
- Most common **malignant** tumor of CNS- glioma (**glioblastoma**)[Q]
- Most common **malignant** tumor in **children- medulloblastoma closely followed by pilocytic astrocytoma**[Q]
- Most common primary CNS tumor in children: **Pilocytic astrocytoma**.

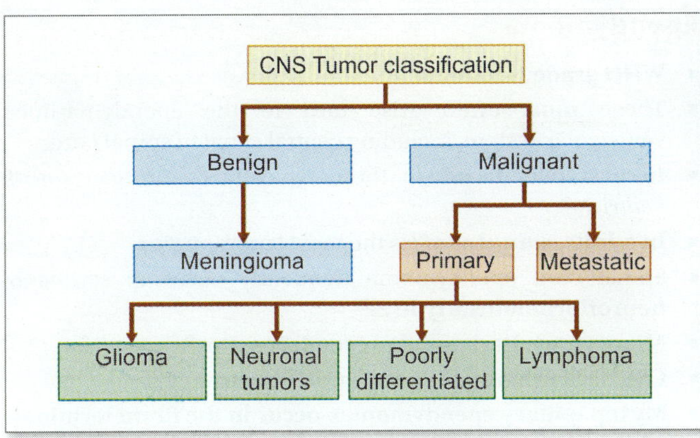

GLIOMAS

- These are **most common group of primary brain tumors.**
- These include **astrocytoma, oligodendroglioma and ependymoma.**

Astrocytoma

- **Most common primary malignant brain tumors in adults[Q].**
- The two major categories of astrocytic tumors are
  - **Localized astrocytomas*: Most common are the pilocytic astrocytomas.[Q]** (WHO grade I).
  - **Diffusely Infiltrating Astrocytomas:** Now classified as IDH wildtype and IDH mutant Gliblastoma

Localized Astrocytomas, Pilocytic Astrocytoma

- **WHO grade I[Q]**
- Occurs in **children and young[Q]**
- Located in the **cerebeilum but may also appear in the floor and walls of the third ventricle, the optic nerves.[Q]**
- Microscopically: Tumors are often biphasic, with both loose "microcystic" and fibrillary areas.[Q]
- Rosenthal fibers and eosinophilic granular bodies, are characteristic findings.[Q]

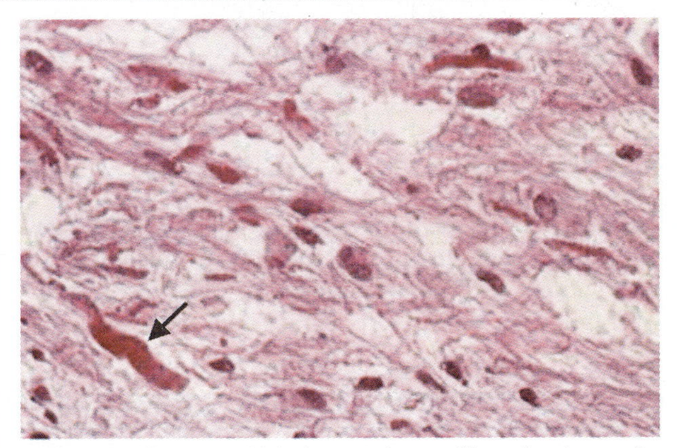

Rosenthal fibers are thick elongated worm-like or "corkscrew" eosinophilic (pink) bundle that is found on H&E staining of the brain

Diffusely Infiltrating Astrocytomas

- Range from diffuse astrocytoma (grade II) to anaplastic astrocytoma (grade III) to glioblastoma (grade IV).
- There **are no WHO grade** I infiltrating astrocytomas.

Glioblastoma (WHO Grade IV Astrocytoma)

- A **highly malignant** tumor characterized histologically by **serpentine areas of necrosis[Q]** surrounded by **peripheral palisading of tumor cells and vascular/endothelial cell proliferation.[Q]**
- The minimal criterion for **vascular/endothelial cell proliferation[Q]** is a double layer of endothelial cells.
- Massive endothelial proliferation can lead to formation of **glomeruloid body.[Q]**
- It frequently crosses midline (**"butterfly tumor"**).[Q]

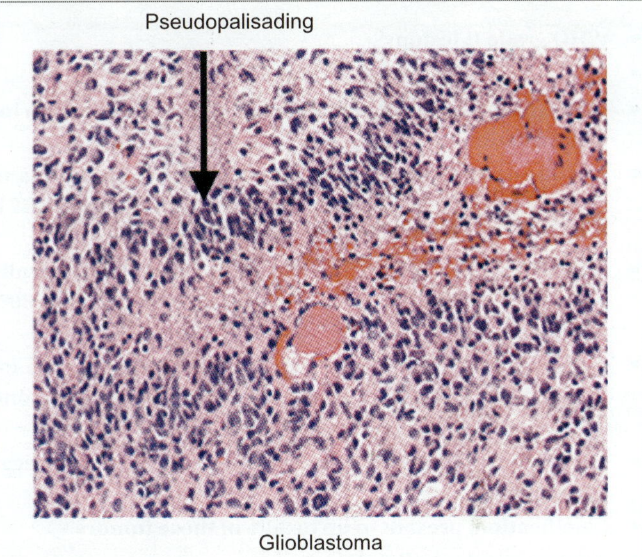

2016 WHO CNS Tumor Classification

	IDH-wildtype glioblastoma	IDH-mutant glioblastoma
Synonym	Primary glioblastoma	Secondary glioblastoma
Proportion of glioblastomas	~90%	~10%
Median age at diagnosis	~62 years	~44 years
Location	Supratentorial	Preferentially frontal
Necrosis	Extensive	Limited
Mutations	TERT (72%) EGFR (35%) PTEN (25%)	P53 (80%) ATRX (70%)
Prognosis	Bad	Good

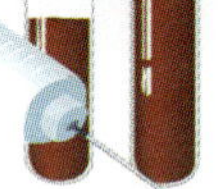

> **R10th** **Latest** Update
>
> **Molecular Genetics of malignant gliomas:**
> Genomically malignant gliomas are divided into four molecular subtypes: Classic, proneural, neural, and mesenchymal.[Q]
> - **Classic subtype-**majority of primary glioblastoma mutations of the PTEN, deletions of chromosome 10, amplification of the EGFR oncogene[Q]
> - **Proneural-**most common type associated with secondary glioblastoma[Q]; P53, and IDH, and IDH_2 mutations.
> - **Neural type-**neuronal markers, including NEFL, GABRA1, SYT1, and SLC12A5.[Q]
> - **Mesenchymal type** is characterized by deletions of the NF1 gene on chromosome 17 and TNF pathway genes, are highly expressed[Q]

Oligodendroglioma

- **WHO grade II lesions**[Q]
- Most common in the **fourth and fifth decades.**[Q]
- **Mostly in the cerebral hemispheres, with a predilection for white matter**[Q]
- **The most common genetic alterations are mutations of the isocitrate dehydrogenase genes (IDH1 and IDH2)-** present in up to **90% of oligodendrogliomas**[Q]
- **Deletions of portions of chromosomes 1p and 19q, typically occurring together as a co-deletion, are seen in up to 80% of cases.**[Q]
- Cytogenetic abnormalities have therapeutic significance for this type of tumor, as only tumors involving 19q or l p respond to chemotherapy
- **Microscopy:** Sheets of cells with clear halos (**"fried-egg"** appearance)[Q]
- **Calcification, present in up to 90% of these tumors.**[Q]
- **Perineuronal satellitosis.**[Q]

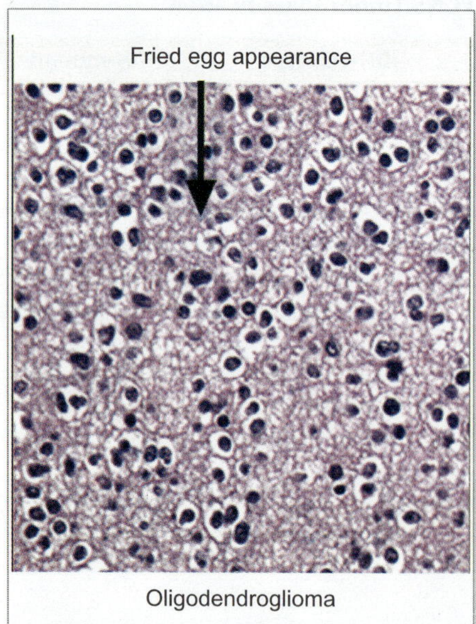

Oligodendroglioma

Ependymoma

- **WHO grade II lesions**[Q]
- These **most often** arise next to the ependyma-lined ventricular system, including central canal of spinal cord.
- **In first two decades-,** these typically occur *near fourth ventricle*[Q]
- **In adults,** *spinal cord*[Q] is the most common site.
- Spinal cord ependymoma frequently occur in setting of **neurofibromatosis type 2.**[Q]
- **Microscopy: Perivascular pseudorosettes**[Q]
- **CSF dissemination is a common occurrence**[Q]
- **Myxopapillary ependymomas-occur in the filum terminale of the spinal cord and contain papillary elements in a myxoid background, admixed with ependymoma-like cells.**[Q]

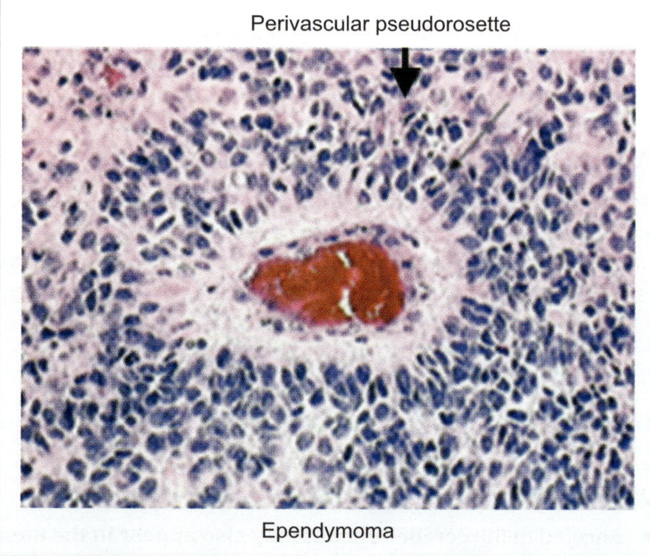

Ependymoma

NEURONAL TUMORS

- *Gangliogliomas:*
  - **Most common** of the neuronal tumors of the CNS
  - **Most commonly found in the temporal lobe.**[Q]
- *Dysembryoplastic neuroepithelial tumor:*
  - Low-grade (WHO Grade I) tumor of childhood that often presents as a seizure disorder
  - Well-differentiated **"floating neurons"**[Q] that sit in the pools of mucopolysaccharide-rich fluid of the myxoid background
- *Central neurocytoma:*
  - **WHO Grade II**, most commonly the lateral or third ventricle
  - **Neurocytic rosette**[Q] are characteristic feature

POORLY DIFFERENTIATED NEOPLASMS

- Medulloblastoma
- Atypical teratoid/rhabdoid tumor

High Yield Facts

- **Glial fibrillary acidic protein (GFAP):**
  - Intermediate filament expressed in astrocytes, ependymal cells and oligodendrocytes.[Q]
- **Few GFAP positive tumors[Q]**
  - Astrocytomas
  - Oligodendroglioma
  - Ependymoma
  - Medulloblastoma
  - Pituitary adenoma
  - Carcinoma of choroid plexuses
  - Hemangioblastoma

Medulloblastoma

- **WHO grade IV.[Q]**
- **Occurs predominantly in children and exclusively in the cerebellum[Q]**
- Largely undifferentiated tumor, appears as **Small round blue cell tumor[Q]**
- **Mitoses are abundant, and markers of cellular proliferation, such as Ki-67, are detected in a high percentage of the cells[Q]**
- **Homer-Wright rosettes[Q]**
- **Dissemination through the CSF** is a common complication-giving rise to **nodular masses** at some distance from the primary tumor called as "drop metastases."[Q]
- **Exquisitely radiosensitive[Q]**

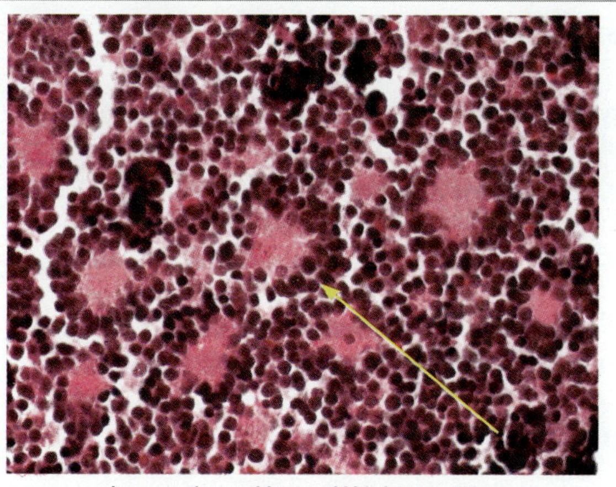

Image shows Homer-Wright rosettes

2016 CNS TUMOR CLASSIFICATION-MEDULLOBLASTOMA-Genetic profile predicts prognosis

Genetic profile	Prognosis
WNT-Activated	Best
SHH-activated TP53-mutant	High-risk tumor of infancy
SHH-activated, TP53-wildtype	Low-risk tumor of infancy
Non-WNT/non-SHH, group 3	• myc amplification • **WORST prognosis**
Non-WNT/non-SHH, group 4	Intermediate prognosis (17q alteration)

Atypical Teratoid/Rhabdoid Tumor

- **WHO grade IV**
- **Young children**
- Arise in **posterior fossa and supratentorial compartments[Q]**
- Highly **malignant tumor**
- Genetic alterations in **chromosome 22** (>90% of cases) are a **hallmark** of rhabdoid tumor[Q]
- MC mutation INI-1

PRIMARY CNS LYMPHOMA

- **Primary CNS lymphoma (PCNSL)** are uncommon tumors, accounting for only 1% of malignant CNS tumors
- **Most common** CNS neoplasm in HIV patient[Q]
- Predisposing factors include:
  - HIV/AIDS: approximately 2-6% of patients with HIV will develop PCNSL[Q], Prior EBV infection, Post transplantation, IgA deficiency, Wiskott-Aldrich syndrome
- The vast majority (>90%) of PCNSL are **B cell in origin[Q]**: **diffuse large B-cell lymphoma** is most common followed by high-grade, Burkitt-like B-cell lymphoma
- Malignant cells tend to accumulate around blood vessels.
- **Chemotherapy is highly effective[Q]**

MENINGIOMA

- Benign tumors of Adults; Most common primary brain tumor
- Attached to the dura,[Q] they commonly arise along the venous sinuses (parasagittal, sphenoid wings, and olfactory groove).
- Arise from meningothelial cells of the arachnoid[Q]
- Risk factors: Prior radiation therapy to the head and neck, typically decades earlier[Q]
- Meningiomas often express progesterone receptors and may grow more rapidly during pregnancy[Q]
- Most common cytogenetic abnormality is loss of region 12 on chromosome 22q[Q]
- Common lesion in the setting of **NF2[Q]**
- They may also grow en plaque, in which the tumor spreads in a sheet-like fashion along the surface of the dura-This form is commonly associated with hyperostotic reactive changes in the adjacent bone.[Q]

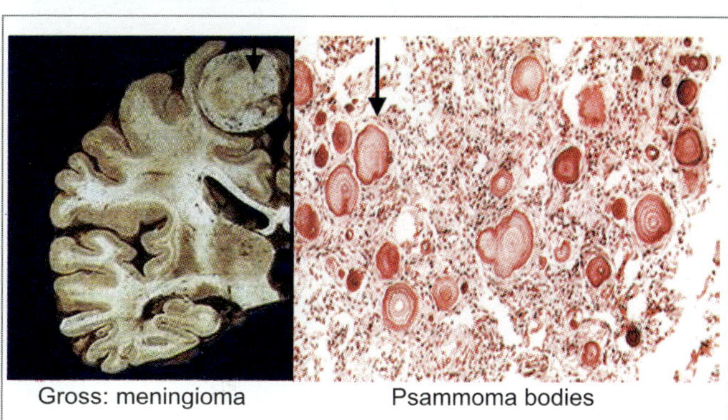

Gross: meningioma   Psammoma bodies

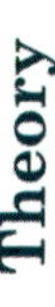

Mnemonic

Tumors with Calcifications-COM
- **C**raniopharyngioma-*suprasellar calcification.*[Q]
- **O**ligodendroglioma[Q]
- **M**eningioma

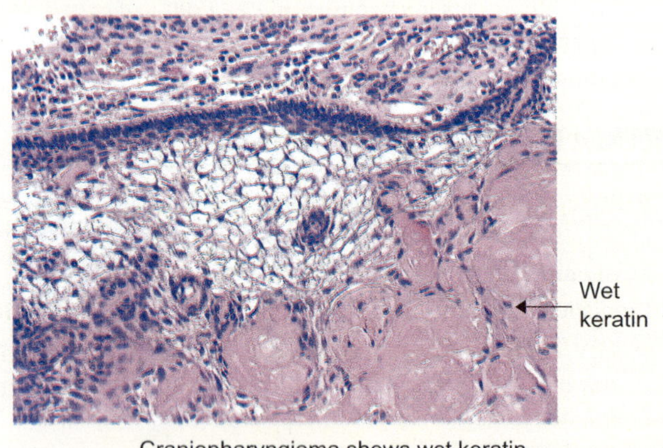

Craniopharyngioma shows wet keratin

Metastatic Tumors

These are **most common intracranial tumors**. Five most common sites of metastasis are, Lung, Breast, Skin (melanoma), Kidney, GIT

Site of Primary Tumor	Brain Metastases, %	Leptomeningeal Metastases, %	Spinal Cord Compression, %
Lung	40	24	18
Breast	19	41	24
Melanoma	10	12	4
Gastrointestinal tract	7	13	6
Genitourinary tract	10	12	4

NERVE SHEATH TUMORS

Peripheral Nerve Sheath Tumor

These include the three common types- schwannoma, neurofibroma, and malignant peripheral nerve sheath tumor (MPNST).[Q]

Features	Schwannomas	Neurofibromas		
General characteristics	• Benign tumors • **Arise directly from peripheral nerves.**[Q]	• Benign tumors • Heterogeneous in composition. • **The neoplastic Schwann cells admixed with perineurial like cells, fibroblasts, mast cells, and CD34+ spindle cells**[Q]		
Gross	**Well-circumscribed, encapsulated**	**Non-encapsulated** mass[Q]		
Morphology	• **Antoni A-** cellular areas • **Antoni B-** loose edematous areas • **Verocay bodies**[Q] foci of palisaded nuclei in cellular areas	**3 types of neurofibroma are there:**		
		Localized • **Low cellularity**[Q]	**Diffuse** • Diffusely **infiltrates** the dermis giving **plaque-like appearance**[Q] • **Pseudo-Meissner corpuscles or tactile-like bodies**	**Plexiform** • These tumors grow within and expand nerve fascicles. • **Bag of worms"**[Q] appearance • **CARROT SHAVINGS**
Genetics	Loss of NF2 gene product, **merlin**	**Loss of the NF1 gene product, neurofibromin**[Q]		
Malignant transformation	Extremely rare	Occur especially in plexiform neurofibroma[Q]		

Schwannoma

Plexiform neurofibroma

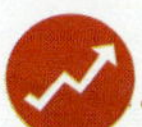

High Yield Facts

- **Most common tumor** of CNS- **metastasis**[Q]
- **Most common tumor** associated with **Brain Metastases-lung ca**[Q] **> breast > melanoma**
- **Most common tumor** associated with **Leptomeningeal Metastases**[Q] (also called carcinomatous meningitis, meningeal carcinomatosis) - **breast cancer**[Q] **> lung**
- **Choriocarcinoma** has high likelihood of metastasizing to brain whereas **prostatic carcinoma almost never grow in the brain.**[Q]
- **Acoustic neuroma**- Schwannoma that arises from the vestibulocochlear nerve (CN VIII). Located at the **cerebellopontine angle** or in the internal acoustic meatus

Malignant Peripheral Nerve Sheath Tumors (MPNST)

- *Origin:*
  - Sporadic- **de novo**[Q]
  - **NF1-associated tumors**[Q]- malignant transformation of a **(plexiform) neurofibroma.**[Q]

- *Morphology:*
  - Mitoses, necrosis, and nuclear anaplasia are common

High Yield Facts

- **Triton tumor**[Q] **-MPNST with focal areas that exhibit other lines of differentiation**, including glandular, cartilaginous, osseous, or rhabdomyoblastic morphology

Phakomatoses

Include **tuberous sclerosis, neurofibromatosis, von Hippel-Lindau disease, and Sturge-Weber syndrome.**

- **Tuberous sclerosis**: Explained in detail later
- **Von Hippel-Lindau** disease: Explained in detail later
- **Sturge-Weber syndrome** is a **non-familial**[Q] **congenital**[Q] disorder, display angiomas of the brain, leptomeninges, and ipsilateral face, which are called **port-wine stains (nevus flammeus)**[Q].

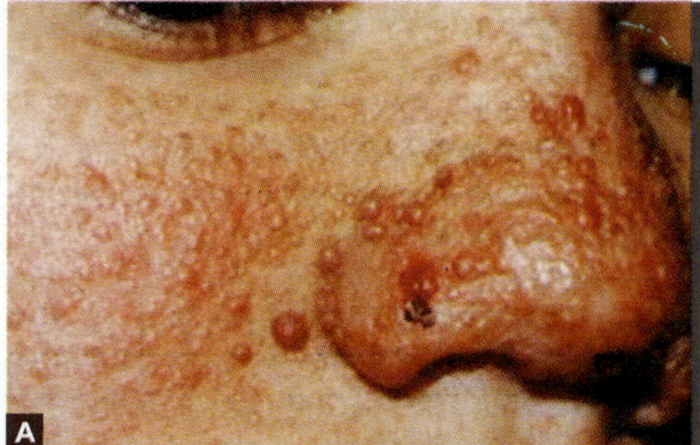

A

Adenoma sebaceum

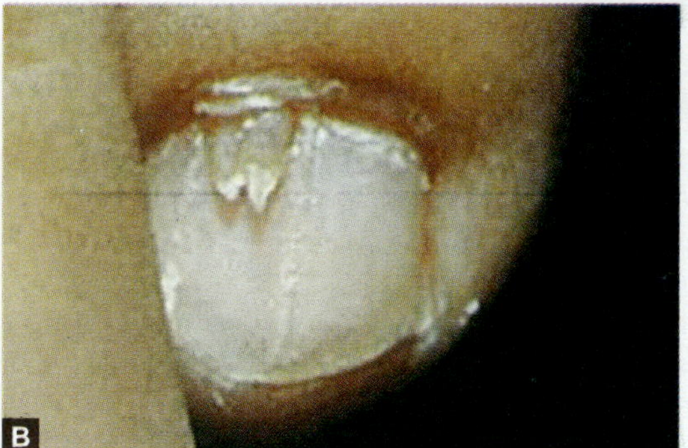

B

Subungual fibromas

FAMILIAL TUMOR SYNDROMES

Tuberous Sclerosis

- Autosomal dominant
- Mutations in **TSC I locus, which codes for hamartin**[Q], and the **TSC2 locus**, which codes for **tuberin.**[Q]
- These two proteins inhibit **mTOR**[Q] -plays a central role in the **regulation of cell growth**[Q].
- Clinical triad of angiofibromas ("adenoma sebaceum"), seizures, and mental retardation.[Q]
- Syndrome is associated with the development of **tumors**[Q] over **childhood and adolescence**[Q]

Systemic Changes

- *CNS:*
  - **Hamartomas**[Q] -
    - **Cortical tubers**[Q]—haphazardly arranged neurons-epileptogenic
    - **Subependymal nodules**[Q]—can protrude into ventricles (**candle drippings**)
  - **Neoplasm**[Q]
  - **Subependymal giant-cell astrocytomas**[Q]—**low**[Q] **grade** neoplasms, **develop from the hamartomatous (subependymal**[Q]**)** nodules in the same location
- *Kidney:* **Angiomyolipomas**[Q]
- *Retina:* **Glial hamartomas**[Q]
- **Lungs: Lymphangioleiomyomatosis**[Q]
- *Heart:* **Rhabdomyomas**[Q]
- *Skin:*
  - **Angiofibromas**[Q],
  - **Shagreen patches**[Q]- localized leathery thickenings
  - **Ash-leaf patches**[Q]- hypopigmented areas
  - **Subungual fibromas.**[Q]

Von Hippel-Lindau Disease

Autosomal dominant[Q], **gene on chromosome 3p25.3**[Q] **(tumor suppressor gene)**

- *CNS:* **Hemangioblastomas**[Q] (in 60–80% patients): **most common in the cerebellum and retina**[Q]
- *Kidney:* **Clear cell**[Q] Renal cell carcinomas (in 75% cases): **multifocal and bilateral**.[Q] Multiple benign cysts

- *Adrenal:* Pheochromocytomas (often **bilateral**[Q])
- *Pancreas:* **Cysts and serous cystadenomas**[Q] (most frequent lesions in pancreas)- seen in 77% cases. Neuroendocrine tumors occur in about 10-15 % of cases.[Q]
- *Miscellaneous:*
  - Extra adrenal paragangliomas
  - **Endolymphatic sac tumors**[Q] (11% of cases)
  - **Epididymal cysts**[Q] (often bilateral)- in 54% of men
  - Cystadenomas of the broad ligament ("**adnexal papillary tumor of probable mesonephric origin**")[Q] are highly specific

Mnemonic

Von Hippel-lindau: signs and symptoms (HIPPEL):

Hemanigoblastomas	**P**ort-wine stains
Increased renal cancer	**E**ye dysfunction
Pheochromocytoma	**L**iver, pancreas, kidney cysts

Neurofibromatosis (NF: Type 1 and 2)

Autosomal Dominant[Q] Inheritance

Mnemonic

NF1 (von Recklinghausen disease)	NF2
Mutations in Neurofibromin gene **(chr17q)**[Q]	Mutations in NF2/Merlin gene **(chr22q)**[Q]
"N-O S-P-A-C-E"	**"M-I-S-S M-E"**
• **N**-Neurofibroma[Q]	• **M**: Mutliple
• **O**-Optic glioma[Q]	• **I**: Inherited
• **S**-Scoliosis	• **S**: Schwannomas[Q]
• **P**-Positive family history	• **M**: Meningiomas
• **A**-Axillary freckling	• **E**: Ependymomas[Q]
• **C**-Café au lait spots[Q]	
• **E**-Eye (Lisch nodules)[Q]	

- NF1 patients have **increased risk** of **Meningioma**[Q], **Pheochromocytoma**[Q] and **Wilm's Tumor**[Q]
- Most common **tumor** in NF1 is **optic nerve glioma**[Q]
- **Most common Leukemia** in NF1 is **JMML**[Q] (Juvenile Myelomonocytic Leukemia)

Hereditary Syndromes Associated with Brain Tumors

Syndrome	Clinical Features	Mutation
Cowden syndrome	Dysplastic gangliogliocytoma of the cerebellum (**Lhermitte-Duclos disease**)	PTEN
Li-Fraumeni syndrome	**Medulloblastomas**	TP53
Turcot syndrome	Medulloblastoma or glioblastoma	**APC** or mismatch repair genes
Gorlin syndrome	Medulloblastoma	**PTCH gene**
Multiple endocrine neoplasia 1 (Werner's syndrome)	Pituitary adenoma, malignant schwannoma	**Menin** gene *MEN1* (11q13)

Mnemonic

Brain tumor spreading by CSF:
PGMEAL CSF

- **P**ineoblastoma
- **G**erminoma, Glioblastoma
- **M**edulloblastoma
- **E**pendymoma
- CNS **L**ymphoma
- **C**horoid plexuses carcinoma

R10[th] Latest Update

- Mutation of Rhabdoid tumor: **INI-1** mutation
- CNS tumors with mural nodules
  - Pilocytic astrocytoma
  - Pleomorphic xanthoastrocytoma
- CNS tumor with calcifications: Meningioma, oligodendroglioma, craniopharyngioma
- Genes in familiar Alzheimer's disease-PS_1 > APP > PS_2.

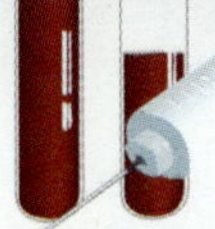

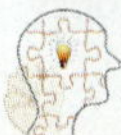

Q's

1. A 5-year-old patient presented with unconsciousness and projectile vomiting. MRI brain shows lesion in cerebellum and characteristic histological diagram is shown below. All of the following are true except:

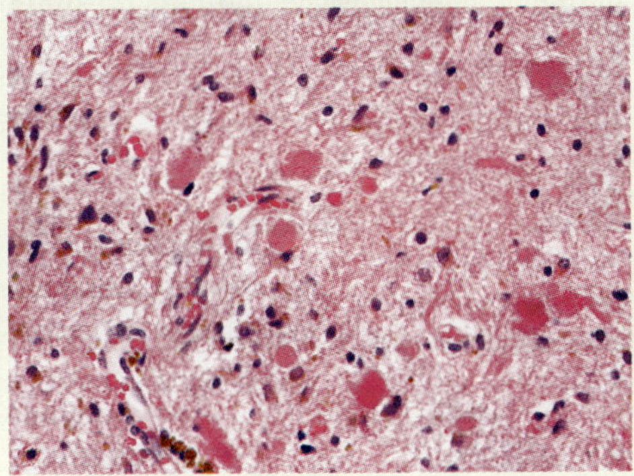

a. It can be solid and cystic
b. It is biphasic tumor shows microcystic and fibrillary area
c. Rosenthal fiber and eosinophilic granular bodies
d. Pseudopalisading necrosis is common

Ans. (d) Pseudopalisading necrosis is common

- Unconsciousness and projectile vomiting are suggestive of raised intracranial tension. Since the mass is in cerebellum, and biopsy shows the eosinophilic granular body and Rosenthal fibers, it is suggestive of Pilocytic astrocytoma. Pseudopalisading is a feature of Glioblastoma multiforme.

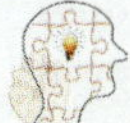

Q's

2. A patient presented with painless proptosis. Biopsy from the orbital mass showed the following image?

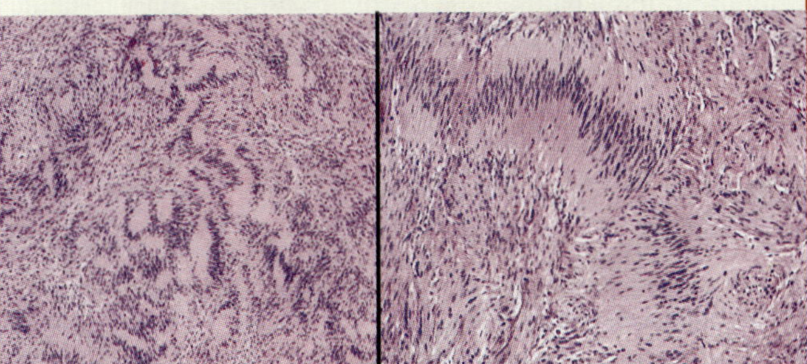

a. Neurofibroma
b. Rhabdomyoma
c. Leiomyoma
d. Schwannoma

Ans. (d) Schwannoma

- The image shows tumor cells arrange in palisading (Verocay body) and you can see the cellular areas Antoni A and acellular areas Antoni B. This is seen in Schwannoma.

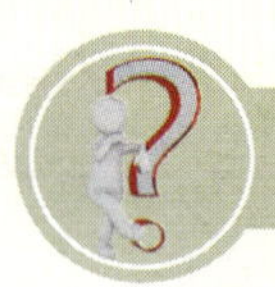

Image-Based Questions

1. A 10-year-old child with posterior fossa mass. On biopsy following features were seen. What are these dense eosinophilic fibers marked with arrow?

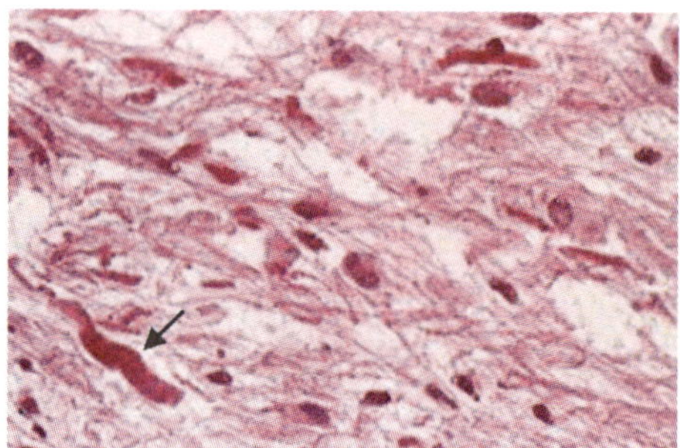

   a. Rosenthal fibers
   b. The Alzheimer type II astrocyte
   c. Corpora amylacea
   d. None

2. New born baby with lumbar mass. Diagnosis.

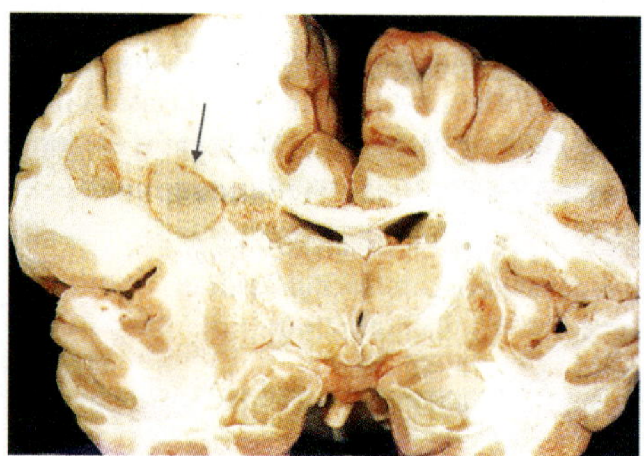

   a. Myelocele
   b. Lumbar meningomyelocele
   c. Spina bifida
   d. None

3. A 40-year-old male who died due to high fever. Autopsy finding?

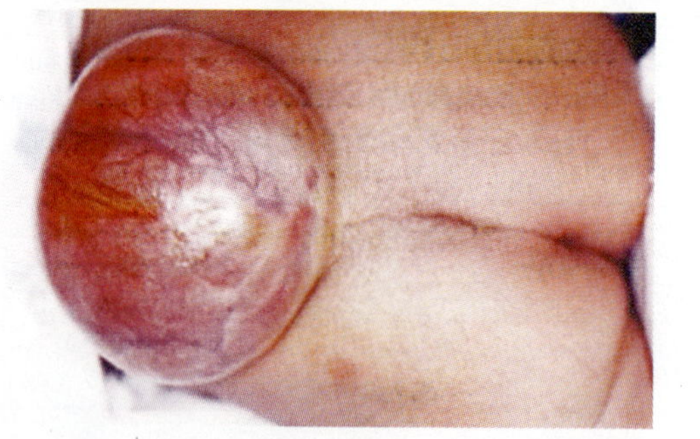

   a. Cerebral abscess
   b. Cerebral infarction
   c. Cerebral tumor
   d. None

4. Identify the lesion. Also mention the special stain and disease associated.

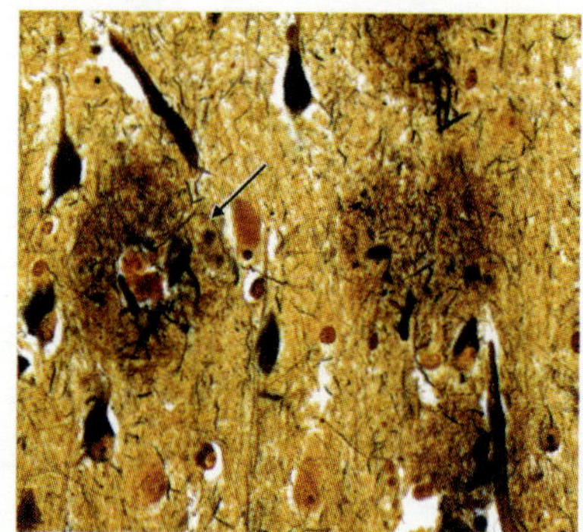

   a. Tangles
   b. Plaques
   c. Hirano bodies
   d. None

5. Identigy the Rosette and Diagnosis.

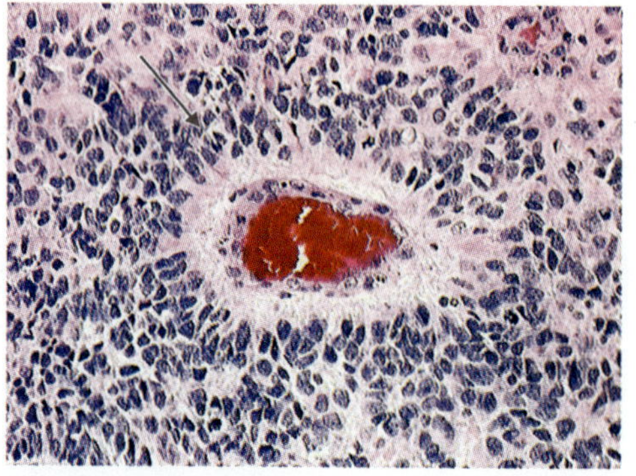

   a. Perivascular pseudorosette
   b. Homer-Wright rosette
   c. True rosette
   d. Flexner-Wintersteiner rosette

6. A 5-year-old child with posterior fossa mass. Biopsy from the mass shows the following rosettes.

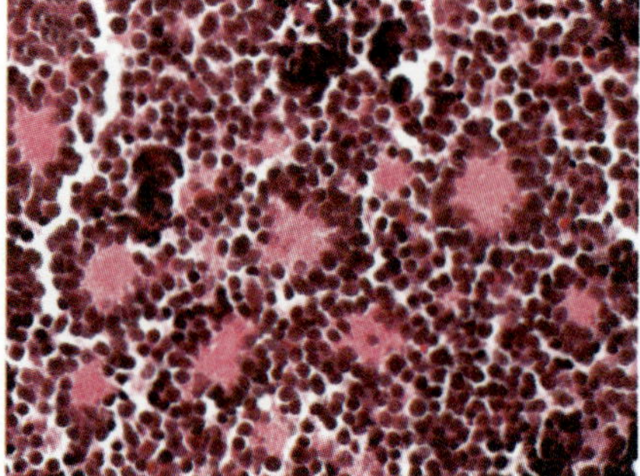

   a. Homer-Wright rosette
   b. Perivascular pseudorosette
   c. Flexner-Wintersteiner rosette
   d. None

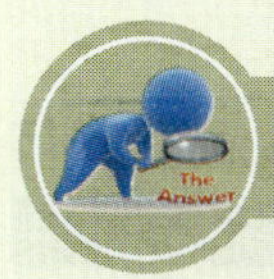

Answers of Image-Based Questions

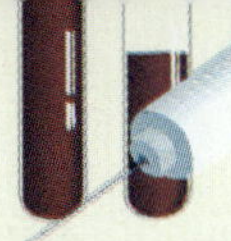

1. **Ans. (a) Rosenthal fibers**
   - Rosenthal fibers are eosinophilic, corkscrew fibers found in pilocytic astrocytoma, the most common primary brain tumor in children. They contain two heat-shock proteins (αB-crystallin and hsp27) as well as ubiquitin.
   - They are seen in Alexander disease and, pilocytic astrocytoma.

2. **Ans. (b) Lumbar meningomyelocele**
   - The lumbar region of a newborn baby with myelomeningocele. The skin is intact, and the placode-containing remnants of nervous tissue can be observed in the center of the lesion, which is filled with cerebrospinal fluid.

3. **Ans. (a) Cerebral Abscess**
   - Note well defined outline of cerebral abscess

4. **Ans. (b) Plaques**
   - Plaques (arrow) contain a central core of amyloid and a surrounding region of dystrophic neurites (Bielschowsky stain). These are seen in Alzheimer's disease.

5. **Ans. (a) Perivascular Pseudorosette**
   - In this pattern, a spoke-wheel arrangement of cells with tapered cellular processes radiates around a wall of a centrally placed vesse
   - Seen in ependymomas

6. **Ans. (a) Homer-Wright rosettes**
   - Type of pseudo rosette in which differentiated tumor cells surround the neuropil seen in neuroblastoma, medulloblastoma, pinealoblastoma

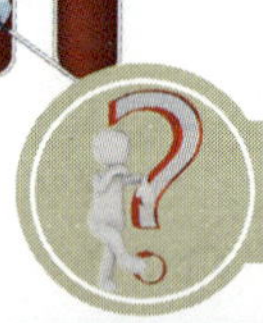

Multiple Choice Questions

CELLS OF CNS AND FUNCTIONS OF BRAIN CELLS

1. Most sensitive to hypoxia is: *(Recent Question 2016)*
a. Neuron
b. Liver cell
c. Stem cell
d. Muscle

2. Rosenthal fibres are: *(Recent Question 2015)*
a. Intranclear inclusions
b. Intracytoplasmic inclusions
c. Present extracellularly
d. Part of cell membrane

3. Rosenthal fibres in astrocytoma are composed of:
(Recent Question 2015)
a. Heat shock proteins   b. Fibrillar proteins
c. GFAP   d. Globulins

4. Phagocytosis in brain is caused by:
(Recent Question 2014, 2013, AIIMS Dec 94)
a. Astrocytes
b. Microglia
c. Oligodendrocytes
d. Ependymal cells

5. Which is a mesenchymal cell? *(Recent Question 2014)*
a. Microglia
b. Astrocytoma
c. Oligodendrocyte
d. Ependymal cells

6. The following cell types does not participate in repair after brain infarction: *(Recent Question 2014)*
a. Microglia   b. Astrocytes
c. Fibroblasts   d. Endothelium

7. Disease or infarction of neurological tissue causes it to be repaired by: *(AI 12)*
a. Fluid
b. Neuroglia
c. Proliferation of adjacent nerve cells
d. Blood vessel

8. Retraction ball is seen after injury to: *(PGI May 2011)*
a. Liver   b. Spleen
c. Brain   d. Kidney
e. Lungs

MALFORMATIONS AND DEVELOPMENTAL DISORDERS

9. Foix-Alajouanine disease of the spinal cord is a:
a. Arteriovenous malformation *(Recent Question 2016)*
b. Cavernous malformation
c. Capillary telangiectasia
d. Venous angioma

10. All of the following are the classical presentation of Craniovertebral junction anomalies except:
(AIIMS Nov 13)
a. Pyramidal signs   b. Low hairline
c. Short neck   d. Pupillary asymmetry

CNS INFECTIONS

11. A HIV pt presented with fever and neck rigidity and few days later the patient died even before any investigation could be performed. After autopsy the gross and histopathological image is given below. What is your diagnosis? *(AIIMS Nov 16)*

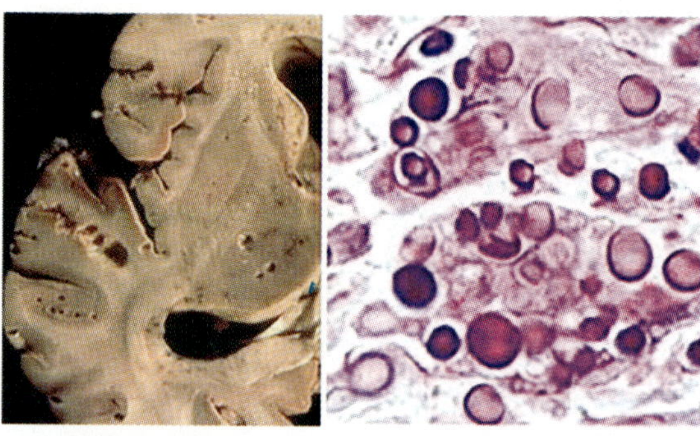

a. Cryptococcus
b. Toxoplasmosois
c. Herpes
d. Echinococcus multilocularis

12. In a patient suspected to be diagnosed with Rabies, a sample of corneal smear was taken. Which of the following investigations can be done from the specimen? *(JIPMER 16)*
a. RT PCR
b. Immunofluorescence test
c. Negri body visualization
d. Virus isolation

13. True about image below all except
(Recent Question 2016-17)

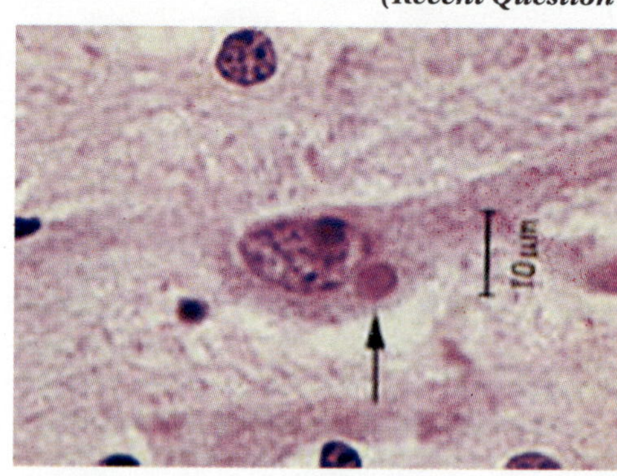

a. They are eosinophilic, sharply outlined bodies in nerve cells
b. These are Negri bodies seen in rabies
c. Consist of ribonuclear proteins produced by the virus
d. Consist of DNA

14. Hutchinson triad includes all except?
(Recent Question 2015)
a. Sabre skin   b. Eight nerve deafness
c. Upper incisor notch   d. Interstial keratitis

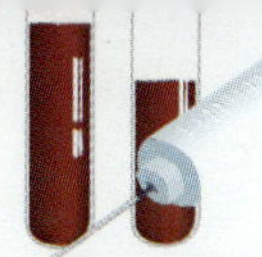

15. **Finding in histopathology of brain in rabies includes:**
    (PGI May 2015)
    a. Negri body
    b. Nodule
    c. Neuronophagia
    d. Vacuolar degenerative changes
    e. Inflammatory cell

16. **The appearance of cobweb formation in CSF indicates**
    (WB PGMEE 2016), (MH PG 2014)
    a. Pyogenic meningitis   b. Viral meningitis
    c. Tuberculous meningitis d. Fungal meningitis

17. **Owl eye inclusion bodies are seen in:**
    (Recent Question 2015)
    a. HSV   b. CMV
    c. EBV   d. Hepatitis B

18. **Progressive multifocal leucoencephalopathy spares:**
    a. White matter of cerebrum   *(Recent Question 2014)*
    b. White matter of parietal lobe
    c. White matter of periventricular area
    d. Spinal cord and optic nerve

19. **Perivascular lymphocytes & microglial nodules are seen in:**   *(Recent Question 2014)*
    a. Multiple sclerosis   b. HIV encephalitis
    c. CMV meningitis   d. Bacterial meningitis

20. **Which part of brain is not affected in HIV infection?**
    (JIPMER 2014)
    a. Hippocampus   b. Subcortical white matter
    c. Diencephalon   d. Brain stem

21. **Negri bodies are abundant in the following cells except?**   *(JIPMER 2014)*
    a. Subcortical white matter
    b. Purkinje cells
    c. Hippocampus
    d. Basal ganglia

22. **Negri bodies are seen in:**
    (WB PGMEE 2016, Recent Question 2013)
    a. Oligodendroglia   b. Neuron
    c. Microglia   d. Astrocytes

23. **In which stage of neurocysticercosis, there is no edema?**   *(AIIMS May 2012)*
    a. Vesicular   b. Vesicular colloidal
    c. Granular nodular   d. Nodular calcified

24. **Brain infarcts is/are seen in infection with:**
    (PGI May 2012, 2011)
    a. Toxoplasmosis   b. Rabies
    c. Cryptococcus   d. Aspergillosis
    e. TB

ANEURYSM

25. **Binswanger disease is a form of?** *(Recent Question 2016)*
    a. Hypertensive retinopathy
    b. Hypertensive nephropathy
    c. Hypertensive encephalopathy
    d. subcortical leukoencephalopathy

26. **Hypertensive hemorrhage is most commonly seen in?**
    (AIIMS May 2015)
    a. Basal ganglia   b. Thalamus
    c. Brain stem   d. Cerebrum

27. **Berry aneurysm-Defect lies in:**   *(AIIMS May 10)*
    a. Degeneration of internal elastic lamina
    b. Degeneration of medial muscle cell layer
    c. Deposition of mucoid material in media
    d. Low grade inflammation of vessel wall

PRION DISEASE

28. **What is the histological appearance of brain in Creutzfeldt-Jakob disease:**   *(Recent Question 2015)*
    a. Neuronophagia
    b. Spongiform change in brain
    c. Microabscesses
    d. Demyelination

29. **Spongiform degeneration of cerebral cortex occurs in**
    (Recent Question 2015)
    a. Creutzfeldt-Jakob disease
    b. Subacute sclerosing panencephalitis
    c. Fatal familial insomnia
    d. Cerebral toxoplasmosis

30. **Infectious protein with correct primary structure and wrong tertiary structure is?**   *(DNB Nov 12 Pattern)*
    a. Prion   b. Tau
    c. Huntington   d. Synuclein

NEURODEGENERATIVE DISEASE

31. **Which is the pathognomic feature of Alzheimer's disease?**   *(Recent exam 2018)*
    a. Lewy bodies
    b. Ballooned neurons
    c. Plaques and tangles
    d. Pick bodies

32. **Which of the following is/are features(s) of lewy body dementia:**   *(PGI May 16)*
    a. Plaque containing beta-amyloid peptide
    b. Deposition of α-synuclein protein
    c. Often resistant to standard treatment
    d. Common in elderly
    e. Risk of falling may present

33. **Features of Alzheimer's disease are all except?**
    a. Narrowing of ventricles   *(Recent Question 2016)*
    b. Hirano bodies
    c. amyloid
    d. neuritic plaques

34. **Knife-edge pattern of lobar atrophy of the brain is associated with which degenerative disease of the cerebral cortex:**   *(Recent Question 2015)*
    a. Alziemer's disease
    b. Frontotemporal dementias
    c. Pick's disease
    d. Progressive supranuclear palsy

35. **The nucleus involved in Alzheimer's disease is:**
    a. Basal nucleus of Meyernet   *(AIIMS 14)*
    b. Raphe nucleus
    c. Superior salivary nucleus
    d. Basal lobe of cerebellum

36. **In Alzheimer disease, pathology seen in brain is:**
a. Atrophy of parietal and temporal lobe *(AIIMS May 13)*
b. Atrophy of frontal and temporal lobe
c. Atrophy of occipital and temporal lobe
d. Atrophy of parietal and occipital lobe

TUMORS

37. **A 25-year-old male presented with swelling in the wrist joint. Histopathological examination showed spindle cells and Verocay bodies. What is the most likely diagnosis?** *(Recent Pattern Question 2020)*

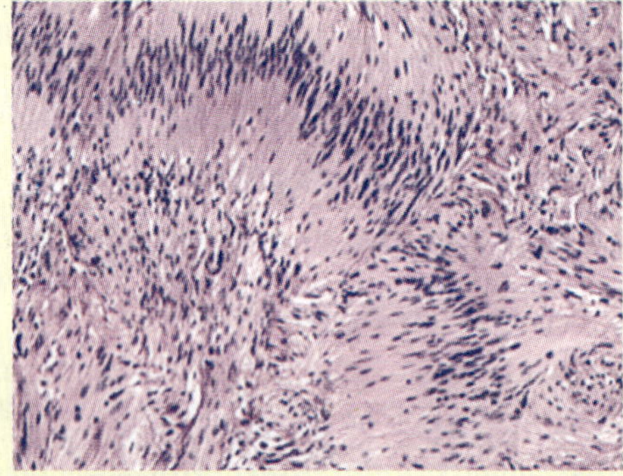

a. Neurofibroma
b. Schwannoma
c. Lipoma
d. Squamous cell carcinoma

38. **Which of the following condition is shown below?** *(AIIMS Nov 2019)*

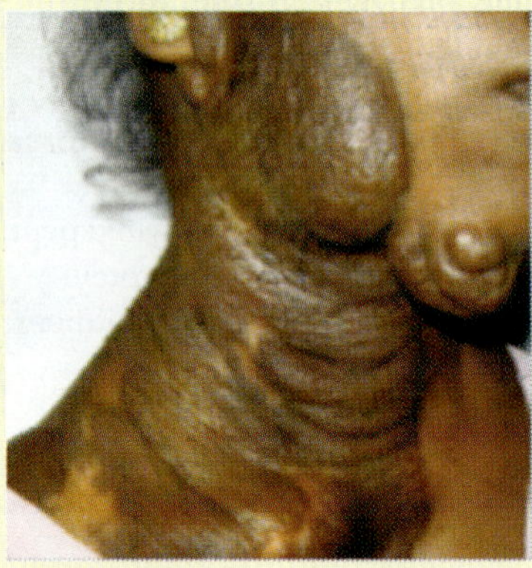

a. Plexiform neurofibroma
b. Von Hippel-Lindau syndrome
c. Marfan syndrome
d. Tuberous sclerosis

39. **A 15-year-old presents with a history of pain and swelling in the right thigh. Biopsy of the mass demonstrates osteosarcoma. His mother was diagnosed with breast cancer 1 year ago and his maternal grandmother died of breast cancer 10 years ago. The patient has three younger siblings. The siblings have an increased risk of developing which of the following cancers?** *(JIPMER Nov 2019)*

a. Wilms'
b. Neuroblastoma
c. Hepatoblastoma
d. Glioma

40. **A patient presented with painless proptosis. Biopsy from the orbital mass showed the following image?** *(AIIMS Nov 2017)*

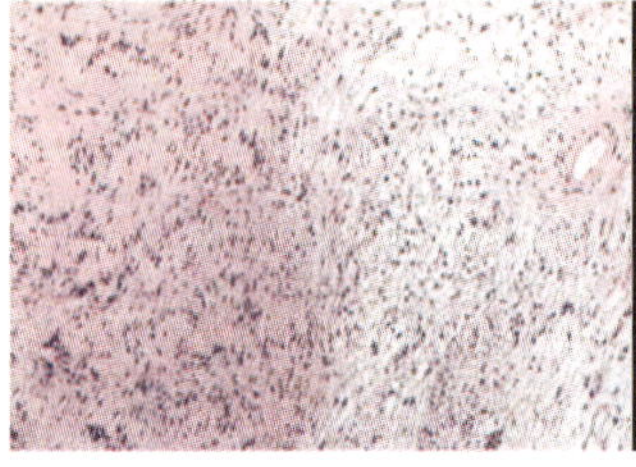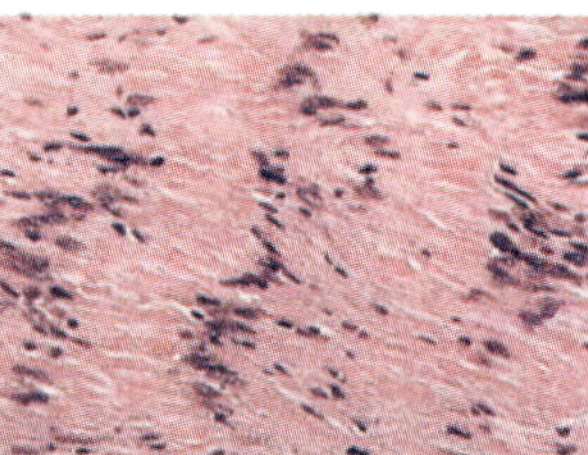

a. Neuofibroma
b. Rhabdomyoma
c. Leiomyoma
d. Schwannoma

41. **A 40-year-old lady is diagnosed to have brain tumor in frontal lobe. The lesion is characterized by focal necrosis surrounded by ring like enhancement** *(Recent Question 2016-17, JIPMER_May 2015)*
a. Glioblastoma multiforme
b. Oligodendroglioma
c. Ependymoma
d. Astrocytoma

42. **Homer Wright rossete is seen in:** *(Recent Question 2016)*
a. Neuroblastoma
b. Nephroblastoma
c. Ependymoma
d. Rhabdomyosarcoma

43. **Multiple schwannomas are seen with:**
a. NF1 *(Recent Question 2015)*
b. NF2
c. Noonan's syndrome
d. Tuberous sclerosis

44. **Perivascular pseudorosettes are classically seen in:**
a. Ependymoma *(Recent Question 2015)*
b. Oligodendroglioma
c. Astrocytoma
d. Medulloblastoma

45. **Most common cause of leptomeningeal metastasis is adenocarcinoma arising from:** *(Recent Question 2015)*
a. Breast
b. Thyroid
c. Bone
d. Liver

46. **In the following histopathology of schwannoma, the arrow marked lesion shows?** *(AIIMS Nov 2015)*

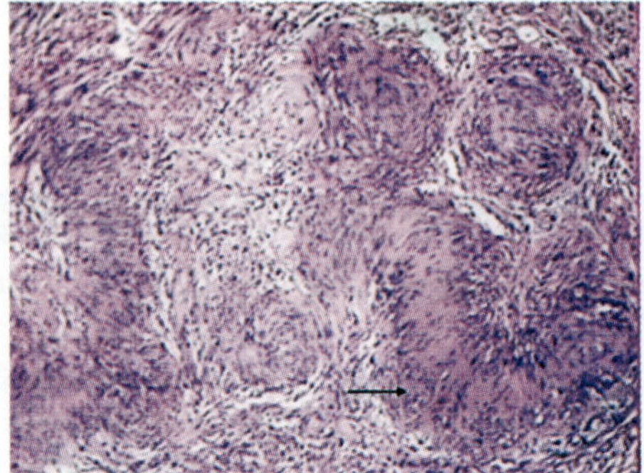

a. Antony A with verocay body
b. Rosettes
c. Antony B with verocay body
d. Pallisading

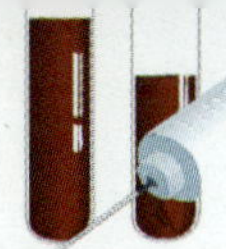

47. Flexner wintersteiner's rosettes are seen in: *(AP 2014)*
a. Hepatoblastoma
b. Neuroblastoma
c. Nephroblastoma
d. Retinoblastoma

48. True statement about metastases of malignant tumors of brain is: *(AP 2013)*
a. Drop metastases can occur in the spinal cord
b. Lymph node metastases in patients who have had brain surgery
c. Metastases through man made shunts
d. All of the above

49. Most common CNS tumor in NF1?
(Recent Question 2014)
a. Optic nerve glioma
b. Meningioma
c. Astrocytoma
d. Schamomma

50. Which of the following tumors is not derived from meninges: *(Recent Question 2014)*
a. Hemangioblastoma
b. Meningioma
c. Fibrous tumor
d. Hemangiopericytoma

51. Medulloblastoma most common metastasis is to:
(Recent Question 2014)
a. Lung
b. CNS
c. Liver
d. Bone

52. Most common CNS neoplasm in HIV patient:
a. Medulloblastoma
(Recent Question 2014)
b. Astrocytoma
c. Primary CNS lymphoma
d. Ependymoma

53. The commonest intracranial tumor is: *(AP PGMEE 14)*
a. Glioma
b. Pituitary tumor
c. Meningioma
d. Metastasis

54. Rosenthal fibres are seen in: *(Recent Question 2013)*
a. Pilocytic astrocytoma
b. Glioblastoma
c. Medulloblastoma
d. Ependymoma

55. Most common cerebellar tumor in children?
(MH 2016, Recent Question 2013)
a. Astrocytoma
b. Medulloblastoma
c. Ependymoma
d. PNET

56. Following is true about medullobastoma:
(Recent Question 2013)
a. It is seen mainly in over 50 age group
b. It is radiosensitive tumour
c. Only treatment is surgery
d. Seen in anterior cranial fossa

57. Receptor on neuronal membrane that induces development of glioma: *(AIIMS May 2013)*
a. CD-117
b. CD-133
c. CD-33
d. CD-45

58. Which of the following statement(s) is/are true about pilocytic astrocytoma: *(WB PGMEE 2016, PGI May 2013)*
a. Slow growing
b. Eosinophilic granular bodies
c. Most commonly involve cerebellum
d. Mostly cystic in nature
e. Mostly malignant
f. Negative GFAP

59. Most common site for medulloblastoma is:
(MH 2016, DNB 2012)
a. Cerebellum
b. Pituitary
c. Cerebrum
d. Basal ganglia

60. All of the following are neuronal tumors, except:
(AI 11)
a. Gangliocytoma
b. Gangliogliorna
c. Neurocytoma
d. Ependymoma

61. Most common site of glioblastoma multiforme is:
(DNB Pattern 11)
a. CP angle
b. Temporal lobe
c. Brain stem
d. Occipital lobe

62. True about meningioma: *(JIPMER 11)*
a. More common in men
b. 50% are malignant
c. 95 % cure rate following treatment
d. Arise from arachnoid layer

63. Which of the following brain tumors does not spread via CSF? *(DPG 11)*
a. Germ cell tumors
b. Medulloblastoma
c. CNS lymphoma
d. Craniopharyngioma

MISCELLANEOUS

64. Pseudolaminar necrosis is a feature of:
(Recent Question 2014-15)
a. Cerebral infarct
b. Renal infarct
c. Hepatic infarct
d. Cardiac infarct

65. Onion bulb appearance on nerve biopsy is seen in:
a. Amyloid neuropathy *(AIIMS Nov 11)*
b. Diabetic
c. CIDP
d. Leprous neuritis

FAMILIAL SYNDROMES

66. Koener's tumor are seen in? *(Recent Question 2015)*
a. Tuberous sclerosis
b. Neurofibromatosis
c. VHL
d. NF

67. True about turcot syndrome *(Recent Question 2015)*
a. Mutations in PTEN gene
b. CNS tumors
c. Non neoplastic polyps
d. Congenital hypertrophy of retinal pigment epithelium

68. About Neurofibromatosis are true, except:
(AIIMS May 14)
a. Autosomal recessive
b. Associated with cataract
c. Scoliosis
d. Multiple fibroma

69. Sturge-Weber syndrome is not associated with:
a. Seizures *(AIIMS 14)*
b. Hemiatrophy of cerebral cortex
c. Gyriform calcification in brain
d. Empty sella

Answers with Explanations

1. **Ans. (a) Neurons** *(Ref: Robbins 9th/pg 130; 8th/pg 129)*

- **Neurons** undergo irreversible damage after **3 to 4 minutes**[Q] of ischemia

2. **Ans. (b) Intracytoplasmic inclusions**
(Ref: Robbins 9th/pg 1253)

Rosenthal fibers-
- Brightly **eosinophilic structures/inclusions within cytoplasm of**[Q] astrocytic processes
- Contain two **heat-shock proteins (αB-crystallin and hsp27) as well as ubiquitin**[Q]
- Seen in **Alexander disease, pilocytic astrocytoma**[Q].

3. **Ans. (a) Heat shock proteins** *(Ref: Robbins 9th/pg 1253)*

4. **Ans. (b) Microglia** *(Ref: Robbins 9th/pg 1253; 8th/pg 1282)*

5. **Ans. (a) Microglia** *(Ref: Robbins 9th/pg 1253; 8th/pg 1282)*

- Microglial cells are mesodermal in origin.
- When the debris filled in the microglial cytoplasm is lipid- gitter cells
- **Option B, C and D**-All the other cells are derived from neuroectoderm

6. **Ans. (c) Fibroblasts** *(Ref: Robbins 9th/pg 1253; 8th/pg 1282)*

7. **Ans. (b) Neuroglia** *(Ref: Robbins 9th/pg 1253; 8th/pg 1282)*

8. **Ans. (c) Brain**

(Ref: Refer The Journal of Neuroscience. 24 (19): 4605—4613).

Axons are normally elastic, but when rapidly stretched as in diffuse axonal injury they become brittle, and the axonal cytoskeleton can be broken

Axonal transport continues up to the point of the break in the cytoskeleton, leading to a **buildup of transport products and local swelling at that point**

When it becomes large enough, swelling can tear the axon at the site of the break in the cytoskeleton, causing it to **draw back toward the cell body and form a bulb**

This bulb is called a **retraction ball,** the **hallmark of diffuse axonal injury**

9. **Ans. (a) Arteriovenous malformation**

(Ref: Toole's Cerebrovascular Disorders pg 351)

Foix-Alajouanine syndrome is an arteriovenous (AV) malformation of the spinal cord predominantly affecting the lower thoracic and/or lumbosacral levels

Foix-Alajouanine syndrome usually occurs in older patients (>50 years).

10. **Ans. (d) Pupillary asymmetry**

(Ref: William wilkins neurosurgery: 2732-35)

- Congenital anomalies included in craniovertebral anomalies–klippel fiel syndrome and down syndrome

In **Klippel-Feil syndrome,** head is cocked to one side with, **Low hairline posteriorly, Short neck,** Limited neck movement

11. **Ans. (a) Cryptococcus** *(Ref: Harrisons 19th/pg 2010)*

In Cryptococcal Meningitis:

- Hematoxylin and eosin stain shows **lightly basophilic cell wall surrounded by a clear zone**.
- Cryptococcus neoformans will stain with **Periodic acid– Schiff or silver methenamine**.
- **Mucicarmine stains the capsule**–shows clear zone containing car-minophilic material. Alcian blue also stains the capsule
- **Negative staining can be done by India ink stain**

12. **Ans. (b) Immunofluorescence test**

(Ref: http://www.cdc.gov/rabies/diagnosis/index.html)

Lab diagnosis of rabies
- RT-PCR: detecting the viral nucleic acid especially on **biological fluids** (saliva, cerebrospinal fluid, tears) and skin biopsy (ante mortem) and brain samples (post mortem)
- Serum and spinal fluid are **tested for antibodies to rabies virus**
- Skin biopsy specimens are examined for **rabies antigen in the cutaneous nerves at the base of hair follicles**
- Immunofluorescent antibody staining of the epithelial cells on **the corneal impression test (FAT)**

13. **Ans. (a, b, c, d) a. They are eosinophilic, sharply outlined bodies in nerve cells; b. These are Negri bodies seen in rabies; c. Consist of ribonuclear proteins produced by the virus d. Consist of DNA**

14. **Ans. (a) Sabre skin**

(Ref: Clinical Microbiology Reviews 12 (2): 187–209)

Hutchinson's triad-interstitial keratitis, Hutchinson incisors, and eighth nerve deafness

15. **Ans. (a, b, c, e); a. Negri body; b. Nodule; c. Neuronophagia; e. Inflammatory cell**

(Ref: Greenfield's Neuropathology, 8th ed/pg 1323)

Histopathologic evidence of rabies encephalomyelitis (inflammation) in brain tissue includes:
- Mononuclear infiltration
- Perivascular cuffing of lymphocytes or polymorphonuclear cells
- Neuronophagia
- Lymphocytic foci
- Babes nodules consisting of glial cells

16. **Ans. (c) Tuberculous meningitis**

(Ref: Robbins 9th/pg 1273 harshmohan 4th ed:857)

17. **Ans. (b)** **CMV** *(Ref: Robbins 9th/pg 1266)*

Enlarged cells **(cytomegaly)** with **intranuclear and intra-cytoplasmic inclusions** are seen with **cytomegalovirus infection.**[Q]

The intra nuclear inclusions appear like owl's eye inclusions in stained tissue sections

18. **Ans. (d)** **Spinal cord and optic nerve** *(Ref: R 9th/pg 1278)*

Progressive multifocal leukoencephalopathy (PML) typically spares the optic nerve and the spinal cord

19. **Ans. (b)** **HIV encephalitis** *(Ref: Robbins 9th/pg 1278)*

- HIV Meningoencephalitis-characterized by **microglial nodules**[Q] composed of **mononuclear cells, microglia, and scattered multinucleated giant cells.**

20. **Ans. (a)** **Hippocampus** *(Ref: R 9th/pg 1278; 8th/pg 1035)*

HIV encephalitis occurs especially in subcortical white matter, diencephalon and brainstem.

21. **Ans. (a)** **Subcortical white matter** *(Ref: R 9th/pg 1277)*

- Most characteristic pathologic finding in CNS in Rabies is the formation of **cytoplasmic inclusion bodies** called **Negri bodies**[Q] **(composed of finely fibrillar matrix and rabies virus particles)**
- They are most commonly seen in **cerebellum (purkinje cells) & pyramidal neurons of hippocampus**
- Basal ganglia involvement is common
- The **prominence of early brain stem dysfunction**[Q] distinguish it from other viral encephalitis.

22. **Ans. (b)** **Neuron**

(Ref: Robbins 9th/pg 1252)

Neuronal inclusions can be seen in

- **Viral infections**
- **Intranuclear inclusions**-herpes infection **(Cowdry body)**
- **Cytoplasmic inclusions**-rabies **(Negri body)**[Q]
- **Both nucleus & cytoplasm-CMV.**

23. **Ans. (d)** **Nodular calcified**

(Ref: AJNR 2001 22: 677-680)

4 main stages of NCC are:

1. **Vesicular:** viable parasite with intact membrane and therefore **no host reaction.**
2. **Colloidal vesicular:** As the membrane becomes leaky oedema surrounds the cyst. This is the **most symptomatic stage.**[Q]
3. **Granular nodular:** oedema decreases as the cyst retracts further; **enhancement persists.**
4. **Nodular calcified:** end-stage quiescent calcified cyst remnant; **no oedema.**[Q]

24. **Ans. (d, e); d. Aspergillosis; e. TB**

(Ref: Robbins 9th/pg 1280; The Brazilian Journal of Infectious Diseases 2004;8(2):175-17)

Brain infarcts is/are seen in infection with:

- **Aspergillus and mucor** have the tendency to invade blood vessels and cause thrombosis with cerebral infarction or vascular rupture with cerebral hemorrhage.

- Some infections, such as **cytomegalovirus, herpes zoster and tuberculosis** are known to produce vasculitis and infarction in the CNS.
- **HIV**

25. **Ans. (d)** **Subcortical leukoencephalopathy**

(Ref: International Neurology textbook pg 12)

Binswanger's disease (also known as **subcortical leukoencephalopathy**), also called *subcortical vascular dementia*, is a type of dementia caused by widespread, microscopic areas of damage to the deep layers of white matter in the brain

Hypertension and old age are risk factors.

26. **Ans. (a)** **Basal ganglia** *(Ref: Harrison 18th ed, chapter 370)*

Hypertensive hemorrhage is parenchymal and its most frequent sites of are the **basal ganglia, thalamus**, the cerebellum, the pons, and occasionally the subcortical white matter.

27. **Ans. (a, b); a. Degeneration of internal elastic lamina; b. Degeneration of medial muscle cell layer**

(Ref: Robbins 9th/pg 1270; 8th/pg 1297)

Berry aneurysm

- **Developmental abnormalities**[Q]
- Due to **the structural abnormality of the involved vessel (absence of smooth muscle and intimal elastic lamina.)**
- Please note : new edition of robbins has specifically mentioned degeneration of internal elastic lamina also.

28. **Ans. (b)** **Spongiform change in brain**
(Ref: Robbins 9th/pg 1281)

29. **Ans. (a)** **Creutzfeldt-Jakob disease** *(Ref: R 9th/pg 1281)*

30. **Ans. (a)** **Prion**

(Ref: http://www.rsc.org/chemistryworld/Issues/2005/October/prions, J G Safar, Proc. Nat. Acad. Sci. US, 2005, 102, 3501)

The primary structure of the human prion protein, both in its benign and pathogenic forms, consists of a linear chain of 253 amino acids.

The pathogenic form, designated PrP^{Sc}, where sc stands for scrapie (the earliest known prion disease which occurs in sheep), is **folded quite differently, even though its primary structure is essentially identical.**

31. **Ans. (c)** **Plaques and tangles** *(Ref: Robbins 9th ed p 1290)*

The major microscopic abnormalities of Alzheimer disease are neuritic (senile) plaques and neurofibrillary tangles.

32. **Ans. (b, c, d, e, f); b. Deposition of α-synuclein protein; c. Often resistant to standard treatment; d. Common in elderly; e. Risk of falling may present**

33. **Ans. (a)** **Narrowing of ventricles** *(Ref: Anderson 10th ed:2740; Robbins 9th/pg 1287-88; 8th/pg 1313)*

Compensatory ventricular enlargement due to extensive cortical atrophy is called hydrocephalus ex vacuo.

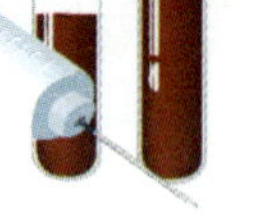

This is seen in **Alzheimer's and pick's disease.**
- The **pathologic hallmark**[Q] are plaques (both neuritic and senile) and tangles_Option d is true
- Vascular amyloid in **cerebral amyloid angiopathy** is **Aβ40**–Option c is true
- **Hirano bodies**[Q] and **Granulovacuolar degeneration**[Q] *are other features seen in AD.*–Option b is true

34.   Ans. (c) **Pick's disease** (**Ref: R** *9th/pg 1292; 8th/pg 1318*)

PICK'S disease
Asymmetric, atrophy of the frontal and temporal lobes
Sparing of the posterior two thirds of the superior temporal gyrus, parietal or occipital lobe
"Knife-edge" appearance- atrophy can be severe, reducing the gyri to a wafer-thin appearance
Pick cells- characteristic swelling of surviving neurons **(ballooning)**
Pick bodies- cytoplasmic, 3R tau containing bodies, stain strongly with silver methods

35.   Ans. (a) **Basal nucleus of Meyernet**

(*Ref: Harrison 18th ed: 3306, 17th pg 2541*)
AD is associated with decrease in cerebral cortical level of acetylcholine. This degeneration occurs in **nucleus basalis of Meyernet**[Q]

36.   Ans. (a) **Atrophy of parietal and temporal lobe**

(*Ref: Robbins 9th/pg 1290; 8th/pg 1313*)

Grossly, brain shows a variable degree of cortical atrophy marked by widening of the cerebral sulci that is most pronounced in the frontal, temporal, and parietal lobes.

37.   Ans. (b) **Schwannoma** (*Ref: R 9th pg 1317*)

38.   Ans. (a) **Plexiform neurofibroma** (*Ref: R 9th pg/1317*)

Plexiform neurofibromas represent an uncommon variant of NF-1 in which neurofibromas arise from multiple nerves as bulging and deforming masses involving also connective tissue and skin folds—hence the clinical description of lesions as "bags of worms".

39.   Ans. (d) **Glioma** (*Ref Robbins 9th/pg 1317*)

40.   Ans. (d) **Schwannoma**

Schwannomas often contain dense eosinophilic Antoni A areas(left) and loose, pale Antoni B areas (right), as well as hyalinized blood vessels (right). B, Antoni A area with the tumor cell nuclei aligned in palisading rows leaving anuclear zones and resulting in the formation of structures termed Verocay bodies

41.   Ans. (a) **Glioblastoma multiforme** (*Ref: Robbins 9th/pg 1307, Journal of Neuro-Oncology 108 (1): 11–27*)

When viewed with MRI, glioblastomas often appear as ring-enhancing lesions. The appearance is not specific, however, as other lesions such as abscess, metastasis, tumefactive multiple sclerosis, and other entities may have a similar appearance. But necrosis with ring enhancement Is a f/o Glioblastoma multiforme.
Oligodendroglioma usually shows calcifications.

42.   Ans. (a) **Neuroblastoma** (*Ref: Robbins 9th/pg 1306*)

Types of rosettes are given below:

Homer Wright rossete: Neuroblastoma, medulloblastoma	Perivascular pseudorosette: Ependymoma
Flexner wintersteiner rosette: Retinoblastoma	**True rosette:** Ependymoma

43.   Ans. (b) **NF2**

(*Ref: Robbins 9th/pg 1317*)

NF2 is **most commonly** characterized by **bilateral schwannomas of the vestibulocochlear nerves** (cranial nerve VIII) and **multiple meningiomas.**

44.   Ans. (a) **Ependymoma**

(*Ref: Robbins 9th/pg 1306*)

45.   Ans. (a) **Breast** (*Ref: Harrison 18th ed 3390, 17th ed: 2608*)

Site of Primary Tumor	Leptomeningeal Metastases, %
Lung	24
Breast	41[Q]
Melanoma	12
Gastrointestinal tract	13

46.   Ans. (a) **Antony A with verocay body** (*Ref: R 9th/ 1314*)

Morphology of schwannoma	Consists of: • **Antoni A:** cellular areas • **Antoni B:** loose edematous areas[Q] **Verocay bodies**[Q] (foci of palisaded nuclei) may be found in the more cellular areas.

47.   Ans. (d) **Retinoblastoma** (*Ref: Robbins 9th/pg 1306*)

48.   Ans. (d) **All of the above**

(*Ref: Robbins 9th/pg 1312; 8th/pg 1336*)

Dissemination through the CSF is a common complication-giving rise to **nodular masses** at some distance from the primary tumor called as **"drop metastases" is a feature of medulloblastoma**
Man made shunts provide a route for metastasis of malignant tumors
Lymphomatous metastases, on the other hand, tend to produce a more diffuse pial enhancement, as breast and prostate metastases.

49.   Ans. (a) **Optic nerve glioma** (*Ref: Robbins 9th/pg 1317*)
- **NF1-autosomal dominant disorders**
- Characterized by **neurofibromas of peripheral nerve, gliomas of the optic nerve, (Lisch nodules),** and cutaneous hyperpigmented macules (**café au lait spots).**
- **NF2** is **most commonly** characterized by **bilateral schwannomas of the vestibulocochlear nerves** (cranial nerve VIII) and **multiple meningiomas.**

50. Ans. (d) **Hemangiopericytoma**

(Ref: Robbins 9th/pg 1317, textbook of neuro-oncology :512)

Meningeal tumors

Meningothelial tumor	Meningioma
Mesenchymal non Meningothelial tumor	Hemigiopericytoma, meningeal solitary fibrous tumor

Hemangioblastomas are highly vascular neoplasms that occur as a mural nodule associated with a large fluid-filled cyst. It is associated with Von Hippel-Lindau Disease

51. Ans. (b) **CNS** *(Ref: Robbins 9th/pg 1312; 8th/pg 1336)*

52. Ans. (c) **Primary CNS lymphoma** *(Ref: R 9th/pg 1313)*

- **MC neoplasm in HIV**-central nervous system (CNS) lymphoma is a **diffuse, large-cell non-Hodgkin lymphoma**[Q] of **B-cell origin**[Q] that usually occurs in the brain (rarely in the spinal cord).
- It is a **late complication**[Q] of HIV infection.
  - **Epstein-Barr virus (EBV)**[Q] is identified in almost **all cases**[Q].

53. Ans. (d) **Metastasis** *(Ref: Robbins 9th/pg 1306)*

54. Ans. (a) **Pilocytic astrocytoma** *(Ref: Robbins 9th/pg 1307)*

55. Ans. (a) **Astrocytoma**

(Ref: Robbins 9th/pg 1306: See Ans 69)

- Most common pediatric brain tumor–Pilocytic astrocytoma
- Most aggressive pediatric brain tumor–Medulloblastoma

56. Ans. (b) **It is radiosensitive tumour** *(Ref: R 9th/pg 1312)*

Medulloblastoma is exquisitely radiosensitive[Q]**; Predominantly seen in children & exclusively in cerebellum**[Q]

57. Ans. (b) **CD-133**

(Ref: http://cdn.intechopen.com/pdfs/14462/InTec h-)
The most commonly used cell surface markers for glioma stem cells are CD133, CD15, and A2B5.
CD133 – on neuronal membrane that induces development of glioma.

58. Ans. (a, b, c, d); a. **Slow growing; b. Eosinophilic granular bodies; c. Most commonly involve cerebellum; d. Mostly cystic in nature** *(Ref: Robbins 9th/pg 1309)*

59. Ans. (a) **Cerebellum**

(Ref: Robbins 9th/pg 1312; 8th/pg 1336)

60. Ans. (d) **Ependymoma**

(Ref: Robbins 9th/pg 1306; 8th/pg 1330)

Gliomas	Neuronal tumors
Astrocytoma, oligodendroglioma and ependymoma	*Gangliogliomas Dysembryoplastic neuroepithelial tumor*

61. Ans. (b) **Temporal lobe** *(Ref: BRS neuroanatomy 4th ed: 87)*

Most common site of glioblastoma multiforme is temporal lobe, frontal lobe and basal ganglia

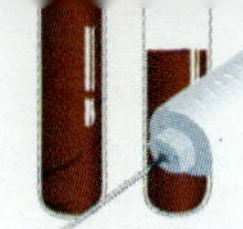

62. Ans. (d) **Arise from arachnoid layer** *(Ref: R 9th/pg 1314)*

Meningioma

- **Benign tumors of Adults**
- **Attached to the dura,**[Q] they commonly arise along the venous sinuses (parasagittal, sphenoid wings, and olfactory groove).
- **Arise from meningothelial cells of the arachnoid**[Q]

63. Ans. (d) **Craniopharyngioma** *(Ref: Robbins 9th/pg 1314)*

64. Ans. (a) **Cerebral infarct**

(Ref: AJNR Am J Neuroradiol. 2003 Apr;24(4):680-7)

Cortical pseudolaminar necrosis, also known as **laminar necrosis**, is the death of cells in the (cerebral) cortex of the brain in a band-like pattern, with a relative preservation of cells immediately adjacent to the meninges.
It is a feature of subacute cerebral infarction.

65. Ans. (c) **CIDP**

(Ref: Current therapy in neurological disease vol 1: 447, Fundamentals of Neurology: An Illustrated Guide :175, Harrison 18th ed:3475-3478)

Chronic inflammatory demyelinating polyneuropathy (CIDP) - immune-mediated inflammatory disorder of the peripheral nervous system.
Biopsy typically *reveals little inflammation and onion-bulb changes* (imbricated layers of **attenuated Schwann cell** processes surrounding an axon) that result from recurrent demyelination and remyelination
25% of patients with clinical features of **CIDP neuropathy** also have a monoclonal gammopathy of undetermined significance (MGUS).

66. Ans. (a) **Tuberous sclerosis** *(Ref: Robbins 9th/pg 516)*

Ungual fibromas or Koenen's tumors are angiofibromas which occur in the lateral nail groove, along the proximal nail fold or under the nail. They are seen in **Tuberous Sclerosis**

67. Ans. (b) **CNS tumors**

(Ref: Russell & Rubinstein's Pathology of Tumors of the Nervous System 7Ed, pg 997)

Turcot syndrome is characterised by:
- Intestinal polyposis
- CNS tumours: glioblastoma or medulloblastoma

68. Ans. (a) **Autosomal recessive** *(Ref: Robbins 9th/pg 1247)*

69. Ans. (d) **Empty sella** *(Ref: Robbins 9th/pg 516; 8th/pg 522)*

- **Sturge-Weber syndrome** is a **non-familial**[Q] **congenital**[Q] disorder
- There is intra cranial calcification in occipito parietal region- **serpentine/ rail road track**[Q] appearance
- **Associated with facial port wine nevi**[Q], ipsilateral venous angiomas in the cortical leptomeninges,
- **Mental retardation**[Q], **seizures**[Q], **hemiplegia, focal or diffuse atrophy**[Q] and skull radio-opacities.

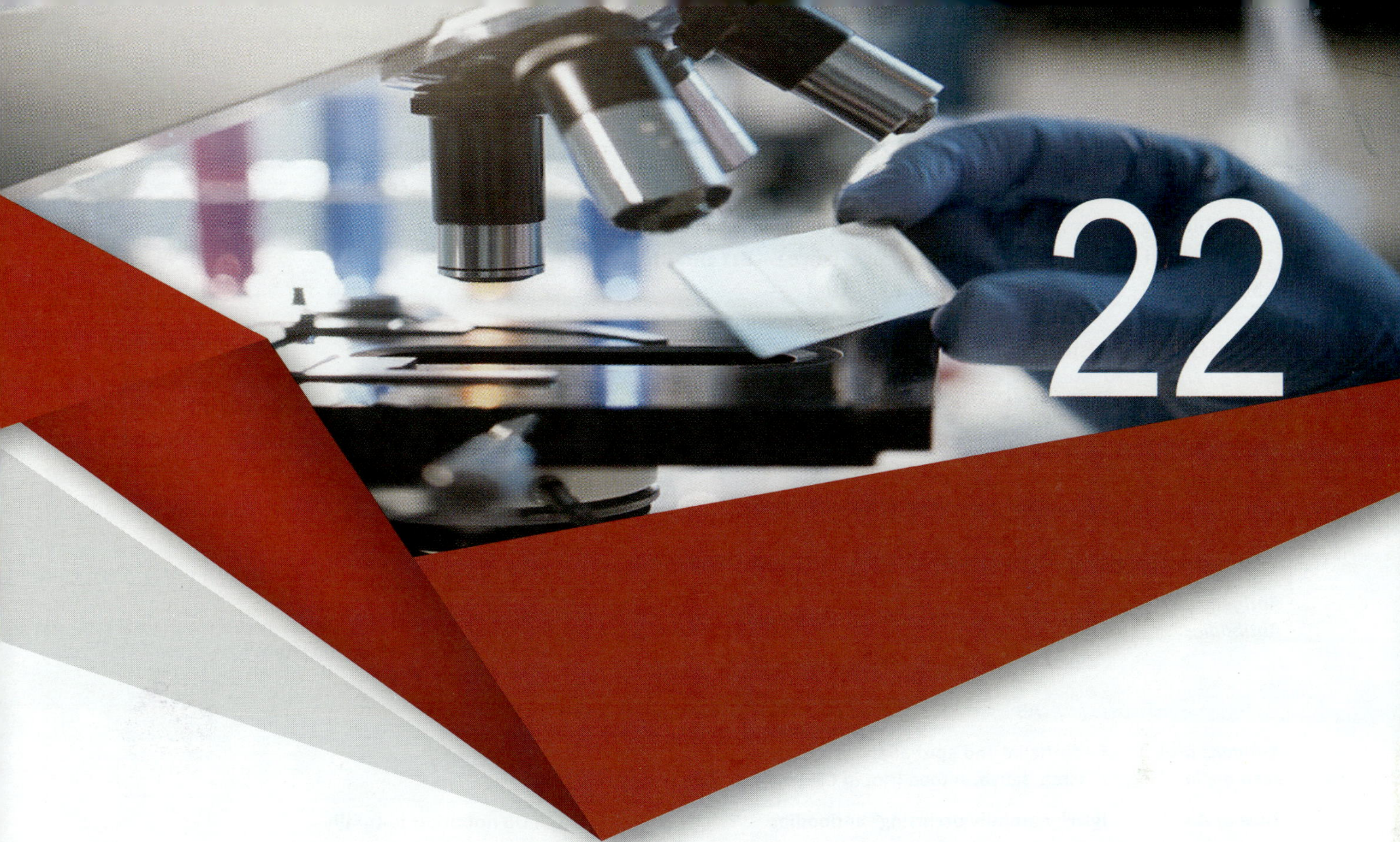

22

Blood Banking and Transfusion Medicine

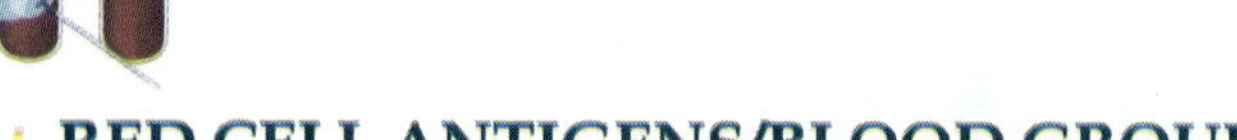

RED CELL ANTIGENS/BLOOD GROUPS

- A total of **30 blood group systems** have been described
- Each blood group system is a series of **red cell antigens**, determined by **genetic loci**
- **Major** blood group systems (of clinical importance): **ABO and Rh**
- **Minor** blood groups: e.g. **MNS, Duffy, Kell, Kidd**

The ABO and Rh Blood Group Systems

Properties	ABO system			Rh system
Blood groups	4 main blood groups: **A, B, AB and O**[Q]			Rh positive and negative
Genetic loci	On **chromosome 9**[Q]			On **chromosome 1**[Q]
Antigens and Antibodies	**Group**	**Antigen**	**Antibody**	• C, c, D, E, e Antigens[Q]
	O	H	Anti-A and Anti-B[Q]	• 'd' indicates the absence of D[Q]
	A	A	Anti-B[Q]	• Anti D Antibody: Most important[Q]
	B	B	Anti-A[Q]	
	AB	A and B	None[Q]	
Antigens also seen on/in	Endothelial and epithelial cells[Q] Plasma, saliva, semen (not in CSF)[Q]			No other cells[Q]
Type of Ab	IgM[Q]; naturally occurring[Q] antibodies			IgG[Q]; Do not occur naturally
Clinical importance	• Anti-A and anti-B Ab can cause **severe intravascular hemolysis after incompatible transfusion.**[Q] • ABO-**matching is required before transplantation**[Q] of solid organs			Rh -ve individuals **make anti-D Ab if:** • **Transfused with Rh +ve blood**[Q] or, • **Rh —ve pregnant women, is exposed to Rh +ve fetal RBCs**[Q] that have crossed the placenta.

Bombay Blood Group/Bombay Phenotype

- Absence of A, B, and H antigens on RBCs, and presence of **anti-A, anti-B, and anti-H** Antibodies
- Genetically: homozygous hh → cannot form the H precursor of A and B
- Clinical significance:
  ○ Their RBCs **type as group O**, but they **cannot receive blood group O** blood donation
  ○ Can only be safely transfused with other Bombay blood group which is rarely available

High Yield Facts

- The **Rh D antigen** is the **most immunogenic**[Q] RBC antigen **after A and B.**
- Immune **anti-K Ab (IgG) is the most common antibody**[Q] found outside the ABO and Rh systems.
- Antibodies to K1 (**Kell** group) can cause **severe hemolytic disease of the newborn.**[Q]
- Individuals **lacking Duffy antigens** are **immune to malaria**[Q] caused by *P. vivax* and *P. knowlesi*
- Erythroid-specific RBC antigens include: **Rh, Kell and MNS, not expressed in other tissues.**[Q]
- The **A, B and H antigens** are fully developed and reach **adult levels** by the age of **1 year.**[Q]
- Most red cell genes are expressed as **co-dominant**[Q] antigens (i.e. both genes expressed in heterozygote).
- Plasma **VWF and factor VIII levels are 25% lower in Gr. O**[Q] healthy individuals than other ABO groups.
- **Auto-anti-P Ab** ('Donath–Landsteiner antibody')[Q] is a potent **biphasic haemolysin**[Q] **(IgG)**[Q], responsible for **paroxysmal cold hemoglobinuria.**[Q]

BLOOD AND ITS COMPONENTS IN CLINICAL USE

Name	Description	Volume/Unit	Storage	Shelf Life	Indications	Special Remarks	Compatibility
Whole Blood	Donor blood plus anticoagulants	350 mL	2–6°C	35 days (CPDA) 42 days (SAGM)	• Acute blood loss with hypovolemia • Exchange transfusion	Per unit ↑ Hb by 1 gm/dL and Hct by 3–5%	ABO and Rh compatible with recipient
Packed RBCs	RBC concentrate (Hct 65-75%)^Q	350 mL	2–6°C	35 days (CPDA) 42 days (SAGM)	• Severe Anemia • Exchange transfusion	Same as above	Same as above
Random Donor Platelets (RDP)	Platelet Concentrate	50–70 mL	20–24°C in Platelet Agitator	5 days	Bleeding due to thrombocytopenia	Per unit ↑ platelet count by 10,000/uL	ABO compatible preferable
Single Donor Platelet (SDP)	Platelet concentrate from 1 donor by apharesis	200–300 mL	20–24°C in Platelet Agitator	5 days	Refractory/ severe thrombocytopenia	Per unit ↑ platelet by 30,000–50,000/uL	ABO and Rh compatible
Fresh Frozen Plasma (FFP)	Plasma from single donor frozen within 6 hrs of collection	200 mL	–30°C; thawed just before use	1 year	Hemophilia A/B, Liver disease, Warfarin overdose, DIC; TTP	Contains all coagulation factors and fibrinogen	ABO and Rh compatible
Cryoprecipitate (CP)	Precipitated proteins from FFP; Rich in Fibrinogen; f-VIII, XIII and vWF	10–20 mL	–30°C	1 year	vWD Hemophilia A Factor XIII def Fibrinogen def.	Each unit of factor VIII/kg plasma ↑ factor VIII by 2%	No compatibility testing required

DURATION TIMES FOR TRANSFUSION

Blood products	Start transfusion	Complete transfusion
Whole blood/PRBC	Within 30 minutes of removing from refrigerator	≤4 hours *Discard unit this period is exceeded*
Platelet concentrate	Immediately	Within 30 minutes
FFP	As soon as possible	Within 30 minutes
Cryoprecipitate	As soon as possible	Within 30 minutes

ADDITIVE SOLUTIONS USED FOR STORAGE OF BLOOD PRODUCTS

Name	Full form	Shelf life
ACD	Acid Citrate Dextrose	21 days
CPD	Citrate Phosphate Dextrose	21 days
CPD-A	Citrate Phosphate Dextrose with Adenine^Q	35 days
SAGM	Sodium Adenine Glucose Mannitol^Q (also contains CPD as anticoagulant)	42 days

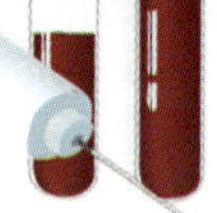

Action of Ingredients of Additive/Anticoagulant Solution

Ingredient	Action
Glucose	ATP generation by glycolysis[Q]
Adenine	Synthesis of ATP;[Q] Increases shelf life of RBCs to 42 days
Citrate	Prevents coagulation[Q] by chelating Calcium
Sodium di phosphate	Prevents fall in pH[Q]

ADVERSE EFFECTS OF BLOOD TRANSFUSION

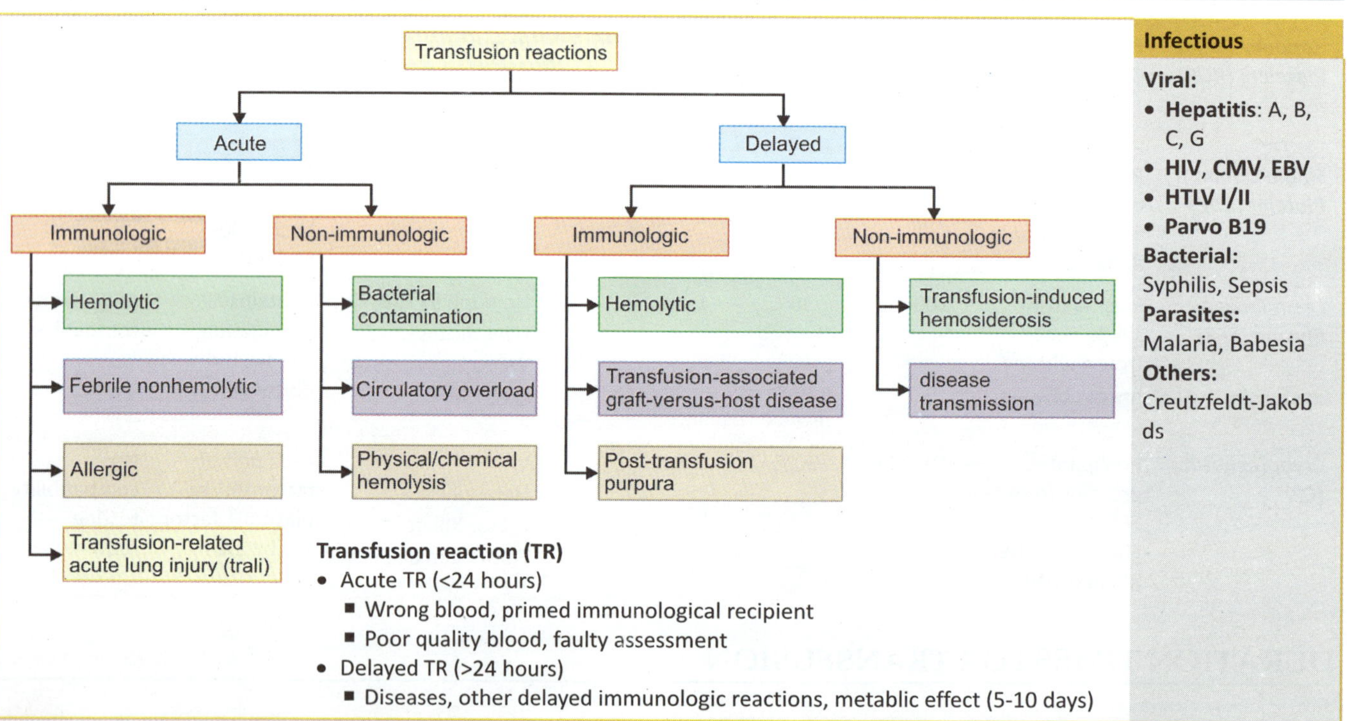

Transfusion reaction (TR)
- Acute TR (<24 hours)
  - Wrong blood, primed immunological recipient
  - Poor quality blood, faulty assessment
- Delayed TR (>24 hours)
  - Diseases, other delayed immunologic reactions, metablic effect (5-10 days)

High Yield Facts

- **Cryoprecipitate** is **not useful** in Hemophilia B.[Q]
- **FFP** is **relatively deficient in factor V and VIII.**[Q]
- To prevent hyperkalemia due to blood transfusion, it is **preferable to use blood <7 days old.**[Q]
- **TRALI** is caused by **Ab against patient's HLA type II and HNA (Human Neutrophilic Antigen),**[Q] in donor plasma; usually 1-4 hrs after starting transfusion
- **Hepatitis C** is the most common cause of **transfusion associated viral hepatitis**
- **Acute hemolytic transfusion reactions** are Type II Hypersensitivity reactions caused by **complement mediated hemolysis**
- **Most frequent transfusion reaction is FNHTR**
- **FNHTR** is caused by **antibodies against donor lymphocytes and HLA antigens**

Massive Transfusion

Definition	Replacement of ≥1 time the total blood volume, within 24 hours[Q] or Replacement of **more than 50% of the blood volume in 3 hours**[Q] in an adult
Complications	• **Metabolic Alkalosis >Acidosis**[Q] • **Hyperkalemia**[Q] → Ventricular arrhythmia or Cardiac Arrest; Hypokalemia (rare) • **Hypocalcemia**[Q] and/ or Citrate toxicity and Hypomagnesemia (rare) • Depletion of coagulation factors → Increased risk of **DIC** • Dilutional **thrombocytopenia** • Hypothermia

Transfusion Related Acute Lung Injury (TRALI)

Incidence	TRALI is reported by FDA as the most common cause of transfusion-associated fatality. Mortality rate, of TRALI at 5 to 10%.
Mechanism	• Antileukocyte antibodies in donor or patient plasma react with WBC complement system triggered to produce C3a and C5a tissue basophils and platelets release histamine and serotonin, lung capillary bed ■ Interstitial edema and fluid in alveolar air spaces, injury decreases gas exchange and hypoxia.
Clinical features	• Severe respiratory distress of sudden onset, caused by a syndrome of noncardiogenic pulmonary edema resembling the adult respiratory distress syndrome (ARDS). • Lung injury is generally transient with PO_2 levels returning to pretransfusion levels within 48–96 hours and CXR returning to normal within 96 hours.
Diagnosis	• Diagnosis of a TRALI reaction is based on the onset of acute lung injury (ALI) **within 6 hours of transfusion.** • Characterized by an acute onset of **hypoxemia (oxygen saturation <90% by pulse oximetry for a patient breathing room air or a PaO_2/FiO_2 ≤300 mm Hg),** bilateral infiltrates on frontal chest radiograph, and no evidence of circulatory overload.
Management	Management **involves supportive measures** for the pulmonary edema and hypoxia, including ventilatory support if required.

Transfusion Associated Graft versus Host Disease (TA-GVHD)

- Unlike transplant associated GVHD, TA-GVHD it is usually a fatal condition.
- Occurs in patients such as: – Immuno-deficient recipients of bone marrow transplants. – Immuno-competent patients transfused with blood from individuals with whom they have a compatible HLA tissue type, usually blood relatives particularly 1st degree. Signs and symptoms typically occur 10-12 days after transfusion and are characterized by: – Fever. – Skin rash and desquamation. – Diarrhoea. – Hepatitis. – Pancytopenia.
- **Management:** Treatment is supportive; there is no specific therapy.
- **Prevention:** Do not use 1st degree relatives as donors, unless gamma irradiation of cellular blood components is carried out to prevent the proliferation of transfused lymphocytes.

R10th **Latest** Update

Quality Control of Cryoprecipitate
(Ref: DGHS technical manual)

Parameter	Quality requirement
Volume	10–20 mL
Factor VIII	80-120 units
*von-Willebrand factor	40–70% of the original
*Factor XIII	20–30% of the original
Fibrinogen	150–250 mg
*Fibronectin	55 mg

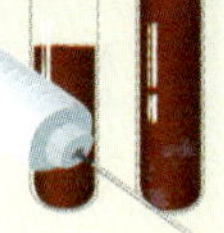

Image-Based Questions

1. Given below is blood group determination by slide method. What blood group does the results suggest?

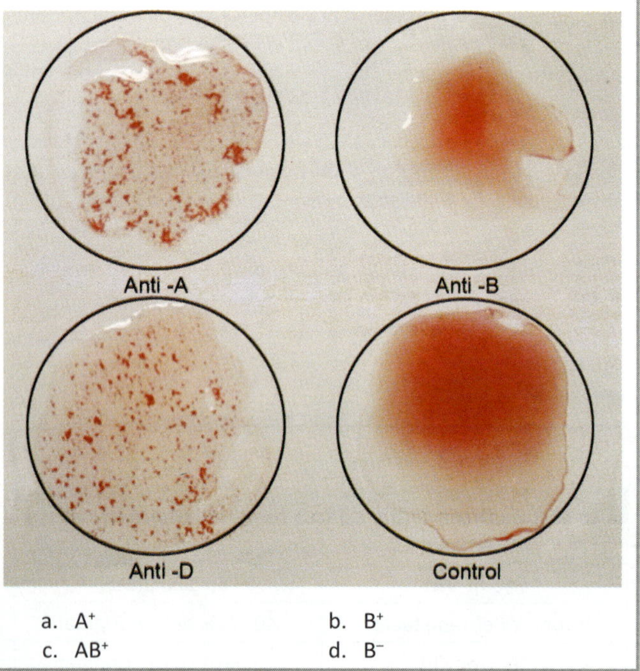

a. A⁺   b. B⁺
c. AB⁺   d. B⁻

2. Identify the instrument used in blood banking?

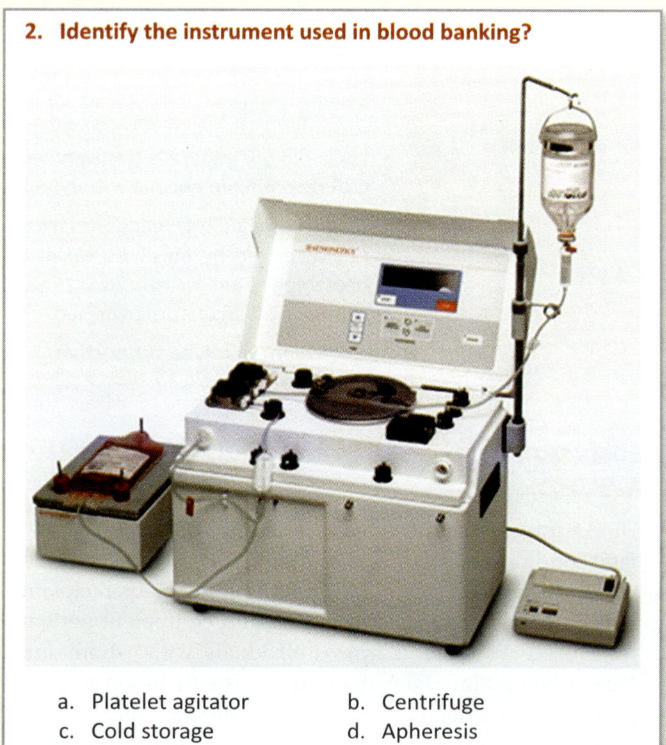

a. Platelet agitator   b. Centrifuge
c. Cold storage   d. Apheresis

3. The given product is used in the following indications?

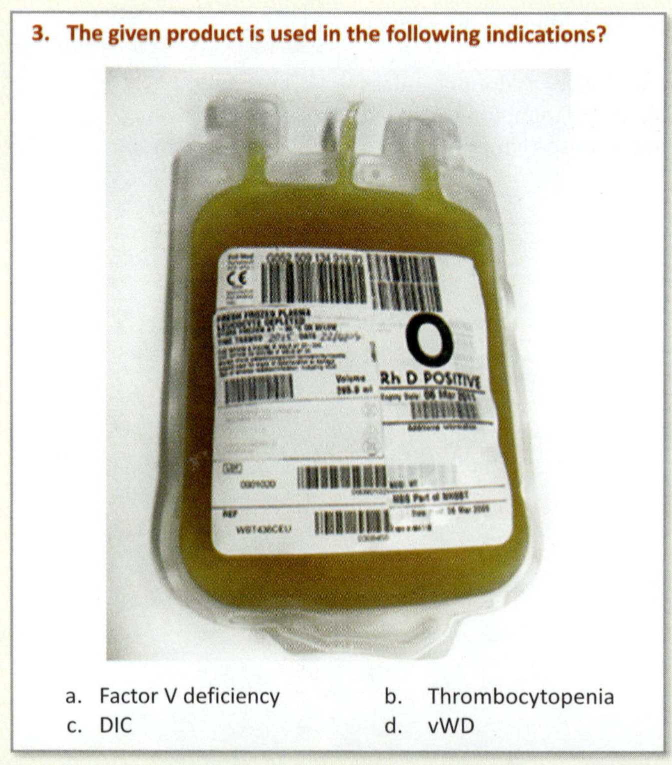

a. Factor V deficiency   b. Thrombocytopenia
c. DIC   d. vWD

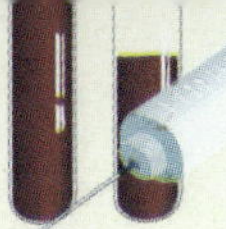

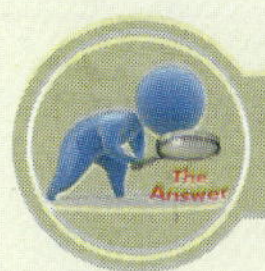

Answers of Image-Based Questions

1. **Ans. (a) A⁺**

   To determine the ABO type, red cells must be tested with anti-A and Anti-B and the serum/plasma tested with A and B red cells
   - **Forward grouping**-identifies the antigens on the red cells
   - **Reverse grouping**-identifies the presence of antibodies in the serum/plasma

ABO group	ABO Antisera (Forward)			ABO Cells (Reverse)			Rh D Antisera
	Anti-A	Anti-B	Anti-AB	A Cells	B Cells	O cells	Anti-D
A	+	0	+	0	+	0	
B	0	+	+	+	0	0	
AB	+	+	+	0	0	0	
O	0	0	0	+	+	+	

2. **Ans. (d) Apheresis**
   - The machine is used to separate out one particular component from donor's blood while returning the remainder back to the circulation. Mostly used to make single donor platelets (SDP)

3. **Ans. (c) DIC**
   - This is a bag of fresh frozen plasma (FFP) used to replace all coagulation factors in blood.

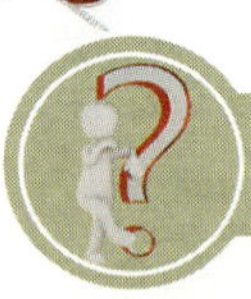

Multiple Choice Questions

1. **Why is CPDA better than ACD for storage of blood?**
   (Recent Pattern Question 2020)
   a. Improves oxygen transport
   b. More citrate ions
   c. It is less acidic
   d. Hypertonicity of blood

2. **Which of the following may show ABO incompatibility?**
   a. Cryoprecipitate   *(JIPMER Nov 2019)*
   b. Single donor platelets
   c. Platelets rich platelets
   d. FFP

3. **A patient comes with severe bleeding, 2 units PRBCs and 4 units of platelet concentrates have been collected from the blood bank. With only one IV access what will you do?**   *(AIIMS Nov 18)*
   a. Transfuse PRBC first and store Platelets at room temperature
   b. Transfuse PRBC first and store Platelets at 2-6°c
   c. Transfuse platelets first and store PRBC at 2-6°c
   d. Transfuse platelets first and store PRBC at room temp

4. **A trauma patient presents at emergency department. There is no time for cross matching. FFP of which blood group can be transfused safely?**   *(AIIMS Nov 18)*
   a. O RH D POSITIVE   b. O RH D NEGATIVE
   c. AB RH D POSITIVE   d. AB RH D NEGATIVE

5. **Which component is not stored in cold temperature?**
   a. RBC   *(PGI Nov 2018)*
   b. Whole blood
   c. Leucocyte removed RBC
   d. Platelet concentrate
   e. FFP

6. **Which of the following is true regarding blood transfusion of packed RBC?**   *(AIIMS May 18)*
   a. Started within 4 hours of receiving it from blood bank
   b. Completed within 4 hours of receiving from blood bank
   c. Wait till the patient is stable then transfuse, irrespective of any timing.
   d. Completed within 6 hours of receiving from blood bank.

7. **Storage temperature of RBC, Platelet, and Fresh Frozen Plasma (FFP) are?**   *(AIIMS May 18)*
   a. RBC 2-6 C, Platelet 20-22C, FFP -30 C
   b. RBC -30C, FFP 2-6 C, Platelet 20-22 C
   c. RBC 20-22 C, Platelet 2-6 C, FFP -30C
   d. RBC 20-22 C, FFP -30C, PLATELET 2-6 C

8. **Most immunogenic RBC blood group system?**
   (JIPMER 18)
   a. Kell   b. Duffy
   c. Kidd   d. K antigen

9. **Contraindication for platelet transfusion are all except?**
   a. Flavivirus infection   *(JIPMER 18)*
   b. Thrombotic thrombocytopenic purpura (TTP)
   c. Immune thrombocytopenic purpura (ITP)
   d. Heparin induced thrombocytopenia

10. **True about single donor platelet transfusion?**
    a. Equal to 6-8 RDP   *(JIPMER 18)*
    b. Stored in 2-6 degree
    c. 10 days shelf life
    d. Bedside leukodepletion done

11. **Which of the following is false regarding TRALI?**
    (Recent exam 2018)
    a. Due to release of mediators from the neutrophils in the lungs
    b. Occurs within 6 hours of transfusion
    c. Occurs more common when the donor is a multuiparous lady
    d. None

12. **A voluntary donor, underwent apheresis for platelet donation for the first time at a platelet count of 1.9 × 103/ mL. He started having tingling sensation (perioral) and numbness because?**   *(AIIMS Nov 2017)*
    a. His platelet count was low for donation
    b. It was his first donation
    c. Due to fluid depletion
    d. Due to citrate based anticoagulant

13. **Which of the following anticoagulant preservative can be used to store blood, so that it can be kept for 35 days?**
    a. Acid citrate dextrose (ACD)   *(AIIMS Nov 2017)*
    b. Citrate phosphate dextrose adenine (CADP-1)
    c. CPD Citrate phosphate dextrose
    d. CP2D citrate phosphate double dextrose

14. **What is the optimal use of ratio of RBC: FFP: PLATELETS in massive transfusion blood Products in severely Injured Trauma Patients?**   *(JIPMER 2016)*
    a. 1:1:1   b. 1:2:3
    c. 1:3:5   d. 2:1:4

15. **Which of the following blood components has the shortest shelf life?**   *(Recent Question 2016-17)*
    a. Red Blood Cells   b. Platelets
    c. Fresh frozen plasma   d. Cryoprecipitate

16. **Blood transfusion reaction can leads to:**
    a. Acute glomerulonephritis   *(PGI June 2016)*
    b. Myoglobinuria
    c. Hemoglobinuria
    d. Transfusion-related acute lung injury
    e. Acute renal tubular necrosis

17. **Packed RBC is stored at?**   *(AIIMS May 2016)*
    a. 2-6°C   b. -2 to -8°C
    c. -20°C   d. 20-24°C

18. **About Transfusion related lung injury what is not true?**
    a. Mortality < 10 % of cases   *(AIIMS Nov 2016)*
    b. Subsides within 2-3 weeks
    c. Supportive care is mainstay of treatment
    d. Steroids use is not well established.

19. **Which one of the following tests has the highest chance of detecting HIV infection in a blood donor during the window period?**   *(Recent Question 2016-17)*
    a. Demonstration of antibody to HIV by ELISA
    b. CD4 count
    c. P24 antigen detection
    d. Western blot test

20. Best blood product to be given in a patient of multiple clotting factor deficiency with active bleeding is? *(AIIMS May 2015)*
    a. Fresh frozen Plasma
    b. Whole blood
    c. Packed RBCs
    d. Cryoprecipitate

21. Which of the following is false about TRALI? *(AIIMS May 2015)*
    a. Develops within 24 hours
    b. Mostly seen after sepsis and cardiac surgeries
    c. It's a cause of non-cardiogenic pulmonary edema
    d. Plasma is more likely to cause it than whole blood

22. What is used in irradiation of blood products before transplant surgery? *(Recent Question 2016)*
    a. α Rays
    b. β Rays
    c. γ Rays
    d. X-Rays

23. Shelf life of γ irradiated packed RBCs is? *(Recent Question 2016)*
    a. 21 d
    b. 28 d
    c. 35 d
    d. 42 d

24. Chromosome of Rh gene is located on which chromosome? *(Recent Question 2016)*
    a. Chr 1
    b. Chr 3
    c. Chr 9
    d. Chr 19

25. ABO is located on which chromosome? *(Recent Question 2016)*
    a. Chr 1
    b. Chr 3
    c. Chr 6
    d. Chr 9

26. Bombay blood group contains? *(Recent Question 2016)*
    a. Anti H
    b. Anti A, Anti B, Anti H
    c. Anti A , Anti B
    d. H antibody

27. The major compatibility test before blood transfusion of cross matching of *(MH PG 2014)*
    a. Donor's red cells and Recipients serum
    b. Donor's serum and Recipients red cells
    c. Donor's serum and Recipients serum
    d. Donor's red cells and Recipients red cells

28. Spontaneous bleeding occurs when platelet count falls *(MH PG 2014)*
    a. 50,000/uL
    b. 40,000/uL
    c. 30,000/uL
    d. 20,000/uL

29. Life span of transfused platelets is? *(Recent Question 2016)*
    a. <24 hrs
    b. 1-3 days
    c. 3-5 days
    d. 7-14 days

30. Platelets in Single donor platelets is? *(Recent Question 2016)*
    a. 2×10^{11}
    b. 1×10^{11}
    c. 4×10^{11}
    d. 1×10^{12}

31. Shelf life is maximum for? *(Recent Question 2015)*
    a. Whole blood
    b. FFP
    c. Platelet concentrate
    d. PRBC

32. Indication of Cryoprecipitate? *(Recent Question 2015)*
    a. DIC
    b. vWD
    c. Hemophilia B
    d. Severe plasma loss

33. Which disease is transmitted by all the components of blood- *(Recent Question 2014)*
    a. Malaria
    b. Syphilis
    c. Toxoplasma
    d. H. pylori

34. Leuko-reduced blood products have lower WBCs than normal by what fold? *(Recent Question 2014)*
    a. 1 log reduction
    b. 2 log reduction
    c. 3 log reduction
    d. 4 log reduction

35. Cryoprecipitate is useful in- *(Recent Question 2014)*
    a. Hemophilia B
    b. Thrombasthenia
    c. Afibrinogenemia
    d. Warfarin reversal

36. Not true regarding fresh frozen plasma *(Recent Question 2013)*
    a. Supplies major coagulation factors
    b. ABO match required
    c. Should be used in replacement of factors in DIC
    d. To be used within 30 minutes of having trauma

37. Which of the following regarding Bombay blood group is false? *(AIIMS May 12)*
    a. Lack of H, A and B antigen on RBCs
    b. Lack of H, A and B substance in saliva
    c. Lack of antigens of several blood group systems
    d. H, A and B antibodies will always be present in serum

38. True about Blood transfusions? *(PGI June 12)*
    a. Antigen D determines Rh positivity
    b. Febrile reactions is due to HLA antigens
    c. Anti D is naturally occurring Ab
    d. Cryoprecipitate contains all coagulation factors
    e. FFP is rich in factor V and VIII

39. Rise in hemoglobin levels after one unit of whole blood transfusion is? *(DNB Aug 12 Pattern)*
    a. 0.55 g%
    b. 1 g%
    c. 1.5 g%
    d. 2 g%

40. In massive transfusion of blood, citrate toxicity is primarily due to? *(DNB Aug 12 Pattern)*
    a. Hemolysis
    b. Coagulopathy
    c. DIC
    d. Direct binding to calcium

41. Granulocyte transfusion is recommended when WBC count is below? *(DNB Aug 12 Pattern)*
    a. 2000/uL
    b. 1000/uL
    c. 500/uL
    d. 150/uL

42. Indication for fresh frozen plasma is/are: *(PGI Nov 2011)*
    a. Hypovolemia
    b. Nutritional supplement
    c. Coagulation factor deficiency
    d. Warfarin toxicity
    e. Hypoalbuminemia

43. ABO antigens are not found in - *(DNB June 10)*
    a. CSF
    b. Plasma
    c. Saliva
    d. Semen

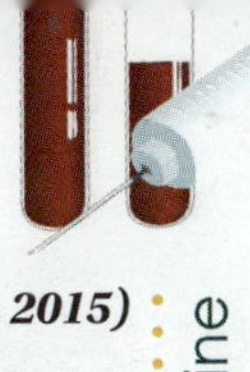

Answers with Explanations

1. **Ans. (a) Improves oxygen transport**
(*Ref: Wintrobe 12th ed/pg 677*)

2. **Ans. (d) FFP** (*Ref: Wintrobe 12th ed/pg 660*)

3. **Ans. (d) Transfuse platelets first and store PRBC at room temp**

The transfusion time of the PRBC is PRBC 100-150 mL/hour and platelets / plasma 150-300 mL/hour. So while the platelets are transfused, the PRBC are kept at room temperature as it can't be returned back to blood bank nor can be stored in ward refrigerator.

4. **Ans. (d) AB RH D NEGATIVE**

This question is based on antibodies in the plasma. As you know, AB blood group has both A & B antigen on RBC, but no antibodies. So, when plasma of AB blood group is given, there will be no antibodies to react with recipient's antigen, so is most preferred in this case without any cross-match done. The reason of choosing AB negative group is because small amount of RBC which might get contaminated while preparing FFP will not induce any alloimmunization in the receipient.

5. **Ans. (d) Platelet concentrate**

6. **Ans. (d) Completed within 4 hours of receiving from blood bank**

7. **Ans. (a) RBC 2-6 C, Platelet 20-22C, FFP -30 C**

8. **Ans. (a) Kell**

9. **Ans. (a) Flavivirus infection**

10. **Ans. (a) Equal to 6-8 RDP**

11. **Ans. (d) None**

12. **Ans. (d) Due to citrate based anticoagulant**

Citrate based anticoagulant may chelate the calcium causing hypocalcemia which may cause the tingling sensation (perioral) and numbness

13. **Ans. (b) Citrate phosphate dextrine adenine (CADP-1)**

14. **Ans. (a) 1:1:1**

(*Ref: ASH Education Book, December 4, 2010 vol. 2010 no. 1 465-469*)

Current data indicate that the early identification of coagulopathy and its treatment with RBCs, plasma, and platelets in a 1:1:1 unit ratio achieved with the use of fresh RBCs, thawed plasma, and platelets; limited use of crystalloids; and accompanied with rapid hemorrhage control may improve survival in the uncommon patient who presents with severe traumatic injury and life-threatening bleeding.

15. **Ans. (b) Platelets** (*Ref: Wintrobes 12th ed/pg 677*)

Shelf life for various components:
- Red Blood Cells- 35 to 42 days
- Platelets- 5-7 days (shortest)
- Fresh frozen plasma- 1 year
- Cryoprecipitate- 1 year

16. **Ans. (c, d, e) c. Hemoglobinuria d. Transfusion-related acute lung injury e. Acute renal tubular necrosis**

(*Ref: Robbins(SEA) 9th/665-66; Harrison 19th/138e5-6*)

17. **Ans. (a) 2-60C** (*Ref: Wintrobes 12th ed/pg 677*)

Storage temperature for various components:
- Red Blood Cells- 2-6 c
- Platelets- 22-24 c
- Fresh frozen plasma- -30c
- Cryoprecipitate- -30c

18. **Ans. (b) Subsides within 2-3 weeks**

(*Ref: Wintrobes 14th ed. pg. 575*)

Transfusion-related Acute Lung Injury (TRALI)

19. **Ans. (c) P24 antigen detection**

(*Ref: Centers for Disease Control and Prevention (CDC)*)

Based on the assumption that HIV RNA is first detected approximately ten days after exposure, window periods are as follows.
- First detection of HIV RNA: approximately ten days after exposure (7 to 21 days).
- First detection of p24: approximately 17 days after exposure (13 to 28 days).
- First detection of antibodies: approximately 22 days after exposure (18 to 34 days).
- Nucleic acid test (NAT) looks for HIV virus in the blood 7 to 28 days after infection.

Also Note

- Note that p24 is not used for HIV diagnosis, It is a test of immune status of a patient.
- Western blot is a specific test and not sensitive and so is not used for early diagnosis

20. **Ans. (a) Fresh Frozen Plasma**

(*Ref: Wintrobes 12thed/pg 677*)

FFP contains all coagulation factors and fibrinogen, so the choice when there is either multiple coagulation factor deficiency or unknown factor deficiency.

21. **Ans. (a) Develops within 24 hours**

(Ref: Wintrobes 12th ed/pg 699)

- **Transfusion related acute lung injury (TRALI)** is seen usually 1-4 hrs after starting transfusion.
- *In here, all the options look correct, but to choose the best option A is the best choice as the diagnosis of a TRALI reaction is based on the onset of acute lung injury (ALI) within 6 hours of transfusion.*

22. **Ans. (c) γ Rays** *(Ref: Wintrobes 12th ed/pg 699)*

Irradiation of Blood Products

Done to prevent Transfusion Associated Graft-Versus Host Disease (TA-GVHD) in immunocompromised host

Uses: The recommended dose for the irradiation is 2,500 cGy at the center of the irradiation field, with a minimum dose of 1,500 cGy at any point in the field.

Cellular blood products: whole blood, red blood cells, platelets, granulocytes

Who is at risk? Patients who are immunocompromised and patients receiving transfusion from a relative (directed donation) are at increased risk of TA-GVHD. TA-GVHD has also been reported rarely in patients with a 'normal' immune system.

Consequences: **Irradiation of red blood cells and whole blood** results in reduced post-transfusion red cell recovery and increases the rate of efflux of intracellular potassium. It has no clinically significant effect on red cell pH, glucose, 2,3 DPG levels or ATP. Packs irradiated within 14 days of collection **expire 28 days after collection**.

23. **Ans. (b) 28 d** *(Ref: Wintrobes 12th ed/pg 677)*

24. **Ans. (a) Chr1** *(Ref: Dacie/pg 486, 487)*

Genetic loci	ABO	Rh
Chromosome	9	1

25. **Ans. (d) Chr 9** *(Ref: Dacie/pg 486, 487)*

26. **Ans. (b) Anti A, Anti B, Anti H** *(Ref: Dacie/pg 487)*

Bombay phenotype is characterized by absence of A, B, and H antigens on RBCs, and presence of **anti-A, anti-B, and anti-H** Antibodies

27. **Ans. (a) Donor's red cells and Recipients serum**

(Ref: Dacie/pg 489)

Major compatibility test before blood transfusion requires cross-matching of donor's red cells which have the red cell Antigens with recipients serum having antibodies against those antigens

28. **Ans. (d) 20,000/uL** *(Ref: Wintrobes 12th ed/pg 660)*

In general, the risk of significant spontaneous hemorrhage increases gradually as the platelet count drops to $<50 \times 10^9$/L and is high at counts $<5 \times 10^9$/L. So among the options the best answer is 20,000/ul.

29. **Ans. (c) 3-5 days** *(Ref: Wintrobes 12th ed/pg 687)*

In healthy adults, the half-life of transfused platelets is 3 to 5 days. In thrombocytopenic patients, however, platelet survival is reduced.

30. **Ans. (d) 1×10^{12}** *(Ref: Wintrobes 12th ed/pg 677)*

- Single donor platelets contain at least 3×10^{11} platelets in approximately 300 mL of plasma
- Otherwise in platelets concentrates, there are 5.5×10^{10} platelets/unit

31. **Ans. (b) FFP** *(Ref: Wintrobes 12th ed/pg 677)*

32. **Ans. (b) vWD** *(Ref: Wintrobe's 12th ed/pg 695)*

Indications of cryoprecipitate are:

- vWD
- Hemophilia A (not Hemophilia B)
- Factor XIII deficiency
- Fibrinogen deficiency

33. **Ans. (a) Malaria**

(Ref: Wintrobe's 12th ed/pg 702-706)

*Singh et al. Asian J Transfus Sci. 2010 Jul; 4(2): 73–77,
** McCutcheon et al. PLoS One. 2011;6(8):e23169.

Transfusion transmitted infections are:

Viral	**Hepatitis**: A, B, C,G, **HIV, CMV, EBV, HTLV I/ II**, Parvo B19
Bacterial	Syphilis, Sepsis
Parasites	Malaria, Babesia
Others	Creutzfeldt-Jakob ds

- Most recognized infectious organisms, with the notable exception of non-lipid-enveloped viruses and prions, have been shown to be inactivated easily by plasma processing methods.
- **All clinically-relevant blood components transmit prion disease following a single blood transfusion**

Transmission of malaria by transfusion*

- Reported to occur mainly **from single-donor products: red cells, platelets or white cell concentrates** (because of contamination with residual red cells), **cryoprecipitate & frozen red cells** after thawing and washing.
- **Transmission from single-donor fresh-frozen plasma has not been reported**.
- Transmission from cryoprecipitate is rare and likely to reflect the preparation method and the degree to which the starting plasma is cell free.

So answer for this question should have been prion, but as **this is not given in options, Malaria is the best possible answer among options provided**

34. **Ans. (c) 3 log reduction**

(Ref: Wintrobe's 12th ed/pg 665-666)

- Leukoreduced blood products achieve 3 log reduction (10^{-3}) of WBC, thereby reducing the risk of FNHTR and CMV transmission.
- Risk of TRALI is not reduced by leukoreduction

35. Ans. (c) Afibrinogenemia

(Ref: Wintrobe's 12th ed/pg695)

Cryoprecipitate lacks Factor IX so is not useful in Hemophilia B

36. Ans. (d) To be used within 30 minutes of having trauma

(Ref: Wintrobe's 12th ed/pg 677)

37. Ans. (c) Lack of antigens of several blood group systems

(Ref: Dacie pg 487)

38. Ans. (a) Antigen D determines Rh positivity

(Ref: Wintrobe's 12th ed/pg 677-680, Rossi Principles of Transfusion Medicine 4th ed, pg 833-834)

Discussing options one by one

a.	True as presence of antigen D is Rh +ve while d (absence of D) denoted Rh -ve
b.	False as FNHTR is caused by **cytokines & pyrogens released from lymphocytes**
c.	False as Anti D is **IgG[Q] and do not occur naturally**
d.	False as it is rich in Fibrinogen; f-VIII, XIII & vWF only
e.	False as **FFP is relatively deficient in factor V & VIII.[Q]**

39. Ans. (b) 1 g% *(Ref: Wintrobe's 12th ed/pg 677)*

Hb increases by 1 gm/dl & Hct by 3–5% on transfusion of per unit PRBCs

40. Ans. (d) Direct binding to calcium

(Ref: W 12th ed/pg 701)

In **massive transfusion**, **large amount of citrate** present in blood bag **can chelate the calcium** causing hypocalcemia

41. Ans. (c) < 500/uL *(Ref: Wintrobe's 12th ed/pg 677)*

Indications for using granulocyte transfusion include:

- **Severe neutropenia**, defined as an absolute neutrophil count **< 0.5 x 10⁹ /L**
- A documented or presumed **severe bacterial or fungal infection**
- **No response of the infection** after 48 hours of appropriate antibiotic treatment
- Expected prolonged neutropenia
- Neutrophil recovery is expected and/or there is **anticipated therapy of curative potential planned**.

42. Ans. (c, d, e) c. Coagulation factor deficiency; d. Warfarin toxicity; e. Hypoalbuminemia

(Ref: Wintrobe's 12th ed/pg 677)

Indications of FFP are: Hemophilia A/B, Liver ds, Hypoalbuminemia, Warfarin overdose, DIC, TTP, Refractory vitamin K deficiency.

43. Ans. (a) CSF *(Ref: Wintrobe's 12th ed/pg 677)*

Antigens also seen on/in: **Endothelial & epithelial cells[Q] Plasma, saliva, semen (not in CSF)[Q]**

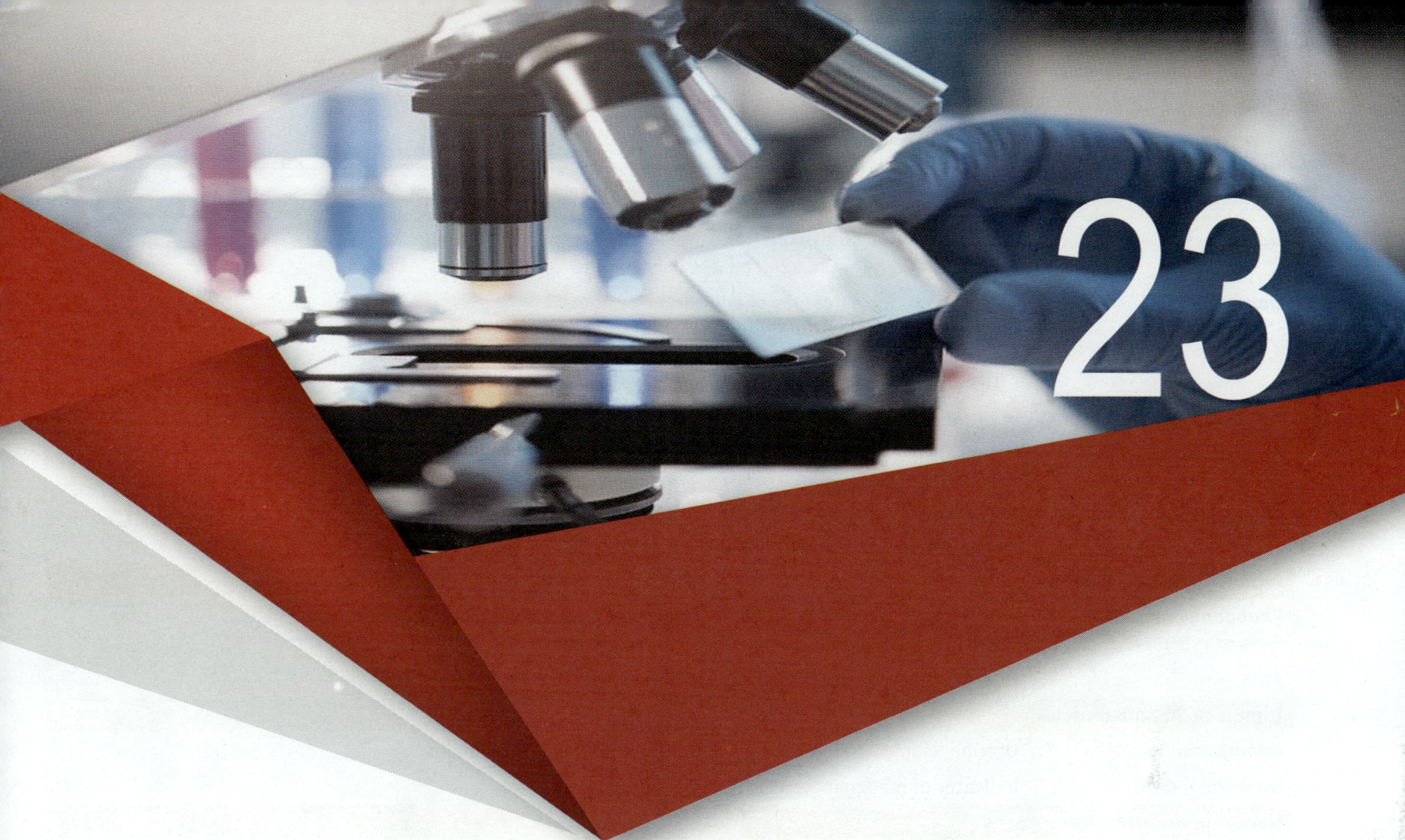

23

Tumors of Soft Tissue & Head & Neck

Key Points

- » **Lipoma is the most common soft tissue tumor**
- » **Most common sarcomas of adulthood is liposarcoma**
- » Most common site of Rhabdomyoma and Rhabdomyosarcoma is **head and neck**
- » **Prognosis of** Rhabdomyosarcoma **depends on histologic type & location of tumor influence survival**
- » **Embryonal variety is the most common Rhabdomyosarcoma**
- » **Most important indicator of malignancy in soft tissue tumor is mitotic index**
- » **t (X;18) is the cytogenetics seen in synovial cell sarcoma**
- » **Most common** salivary gland tumor (overall): Pleomorphic adenoma
- » Ameloblastoma is the **most common** odontogenic tumor
- » Retinoblastoma is the most common **primary malignant tumor of the eye** in children

Key Recent Updates

- » GIST & PNST are now included in soft tissue sarcoma.

SOFT TISSUE TUMORS

Fatty tumors	
Lipoma	• **Most common soft tissue tumor;**[Q] **Painless except angiolipoma**[Q] • Cytogenetics: Chr 6p, 12q and 13q involved
Liposarcoma	• **Most common sarcomas of adulthood**[Q] • **Most common: Proximal extremities & retroperitoneum**[Q] • **Morphology: Lipocytes** with supernumerary rings & giant rod chromosomes - 12q (*MDM2* oncogene) & **Lipoblasts** with scalloping of nucleus

Tumors & Tumor-like lesions of fibrous origin	
Fibromatoses	• **Superficial:** Palmar (**Dupuytren's contracture**), Plantar, Penile (**Peyronie disease**)[Q] • Deep: Desmoid tumors-Locally aggressive, Associated with Gardner's syndrome (APC)
Fibrosarcoma	• **Most common in extremities;**[Q] Aggressive, Recurs & Metastasizes • Herringbone pattern on Histology

Tumors of skeletal muscle	
Rhabdomyoma	• **Benign**; Most common in- **Head, Neck & heart**[Q]; Associated with Tuberous Sclerosis • Histology- Polygonal Rhabdomyoblast, **Spider cells**
RMS	Discussed below in detail

Tumors of Smooth muscles	
Leiomyoma	**Uterine** leiomyoma are the **most common Neoplasms in females**[Q]
Leiomyosarcoma	**Indicator of malignancy: Mitotic index**[Q]**>Atypia> Necrosis**

Tumors of uncertain histogenesis	
Synovial Cell Sarcoma	• **Only 10% intraarticular;**[Q] MC around knee • H/E: **Biphasic**[Q]- epithelial & mesenchymal (spindle cells) • Stains: Keratin, vimentin, S-100 & EMA; t(X;18) → poor prognosis[Q]

Lipoma

Herring bone pattern

RHABDOMYOSARCOMA (RMS)

- Malignant primitive mesenchymal tumor of skeletal muscle (**arises from pluripotent mucle cells**)
- **MC soft-tissue sarcoma of childhood & adolescence**[Q]
- **Most common—head/neck;**[Q] **2nd MC—genitourinary tract**
- **Diagnostic cell in all types is:**
  - **Rhabdomyoblast**- contains **eccentric eosinophilic granular cytoplasm**, rich in thick and thin filaments
  - **Tadpole or strap cells**[Q] - Elongated Rhabdomyoblasts that may contain cross-striations visible by light microscopy
- **Stains used- Desmin, MYOD1 & myogenin.**

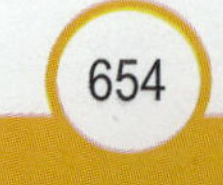

Classification: Histological sub-types include- Embryonal, Alveolar & Pleomorphic	
Embryonal RMS (Most common)[Q]	• Occurs in **children < 10 yrs** of age • **Chr 11p** involved • Histology: Consists of **primitive round & spindle cells** A submucosal zone of hypercellularity → **cambium layer[Q]**
Sarcoma botryoides	• A variant of **Embryonal RMS** • More common in **age < 5 yrs** • Arises from walls of hollow mucosal lined structures like vagina, bladder • **Grape-like clusters[Q]** seen • H/E: **Tennis racket cells[Q]** on light microscopy
Alveolar RMS (20%)	• Commonly arises in the deep musculature of the extremities • Cytogenetics: t(2;13) & t(1;13)
Pleomorphic RMS	• Rare; poor prognosis • Arise in the deep soft tissue of adults

Prognosis of RMS: Histologic type & location of tumor influence survival

• Best prognosis: Botryoid subtype
• Intermediate prognosis: Embryonal NOS
• Poor prognosis: pleomorphic and alveolar

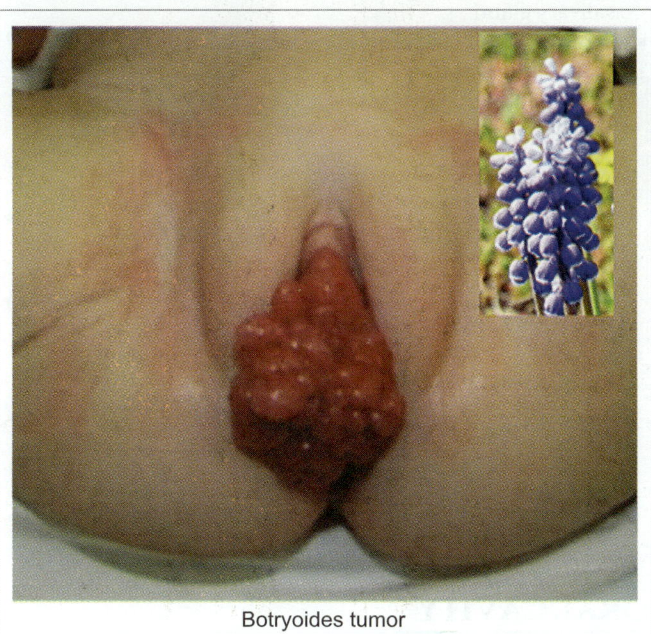

Botryoides tumor

Sarcomas in which Lymphatic Metastasis is seen -

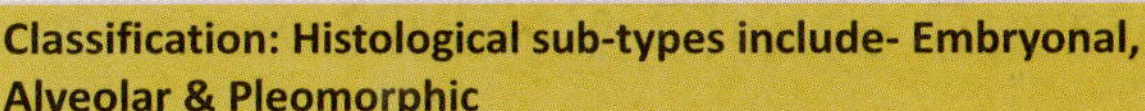

Mnemonic

RACE For MS

> **R : R**habdomyosarcoma
> **A : A**ngiosarcoma
> **C : C**lear cell sarcoma
> **E : E**pithelial cell sarcoma
> **For : F**ibrosarcoma
> **M : M**alignant fibrous histiocytoma
> **S : S**ynovial cell sarcoma

High Yield Facts

• **Most common** salivary gland tumor (overall): **Pleomorphic adenoma[Q]**
• **Most common benign** salivary gland tumor: Pleomorphic adenoma[Q]
• **Most common malignant** salivary gland tumor: Mucoepidermoid carcinoma[Q]
• Most common salivary gland tumor in **children**: Hemangioma[Q]
• Most common **malignant** salivary gland tumor in **children**: Mucoepidermoid carcinoma.[Q]
• **Salivary gland tumor with worst prognosis is Adenoid cystic carcinoma**
• **Salivary gland tumor being malignant is inversely proportional to size of the gland.[Q]**

SALIVARY GLAND TUMORS

Histological classification of common benign and malignant salivary gland tumors

Benign Tumors[Q]	Malignant Tumors[q]
• Pleomorphic adenoma • Warthin tumor's • Oncocytoma • Other adenoma (Basal cell adenoma)	• Mucoepidermoid carcinoma • Adenocarcinoma NOS • Acinic cell carcinoma • Adenoid cystic carcinoma

Benign Neoplasms

Pleomorphic Adenoma

■ Commonest neoplasm of salivary gland.
■ Most common salivary gland involved: **Parotid[Q]** > Submandibular > Minor salivary gland.
■ Shows both epithelial and mesenchymal differentiation. Thus known as **mixed tumor[Q]**
■ Carcinoma arising in pleomorphic adenoma is called carcinoma, e.g. pleomorphic adenoma.
■ The malignant component of Ca ex pleomorphic adenoma is most often **adenocarcinoma not otherwise specified**

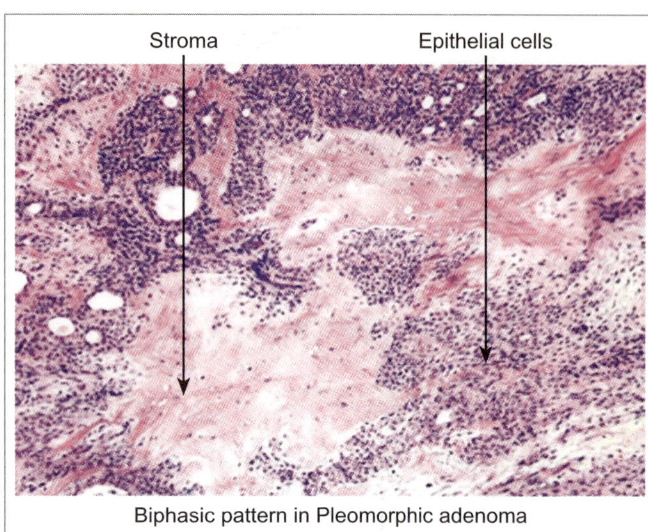

Biphasic pattern in Pleomorphic adenoma

Warthin's Tumor

- Also known as papillary **cystadenoma lymphomatosum**[Q]
- **Second most common** benign salivary gland tumor (after pleomorphic adenoma)[Q]
- Common tumor of parotid gland with double layer of epithelial cells resting on dense lymphoid stroma[Q]
- **Surface palisading of oncocytic** columnar cells are seen[Q]

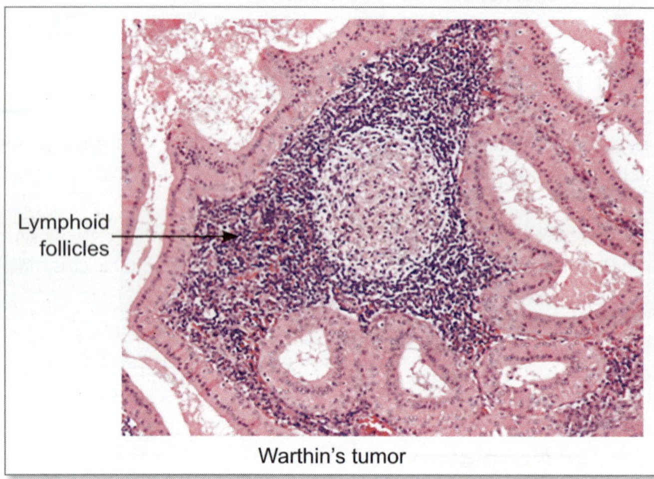

Warthin's tumor

Malignant Neoplasms

Mucoepidermoid Carcinoma

- **Most common** malignant salivary gland tumor[Q]
- Occur mainly in **parotids**
- **Most common radiation induced** neoplasm in salivary glands
- Consist of variable number of **squamous cell, mucus secreting cells and intermediate cells.**[Q]

Adenoid Cystic Carcinoma

- **Malignant tumor** most commonly seen in **minor salivary glands**

- Among major salivary glands, **parotid gland** is the **most common site**
- **Microscopically:** Cribriform arrangements of bland cells arranged around cystic spaces - these are not truly cystic and are thought to be filled with material produced by tumour cells.
- Unpredictable tumor with **perineural invasion.**

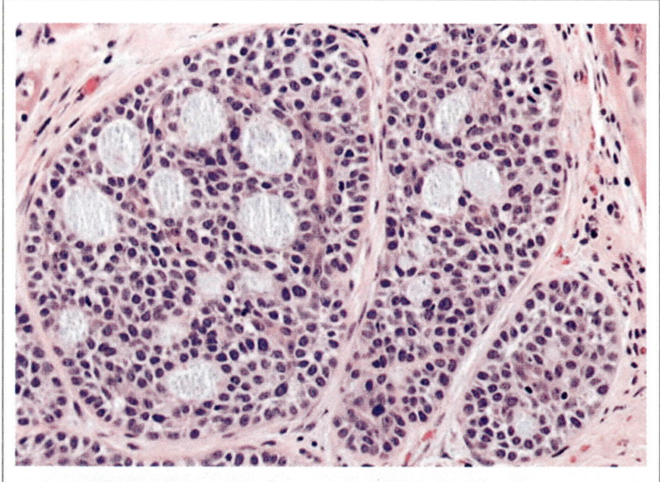

Acinic Cell Carcinoma

- Relatively **uncommon malignant tumor**
- **2nd childhood salivary gland** malignancy after mucoepidermoid carcinoma
- Most commonly arise in **parotid** > submandibular> minor salivary gland.
- Composed of cells resembling **normal serous acinar cells**[Q]

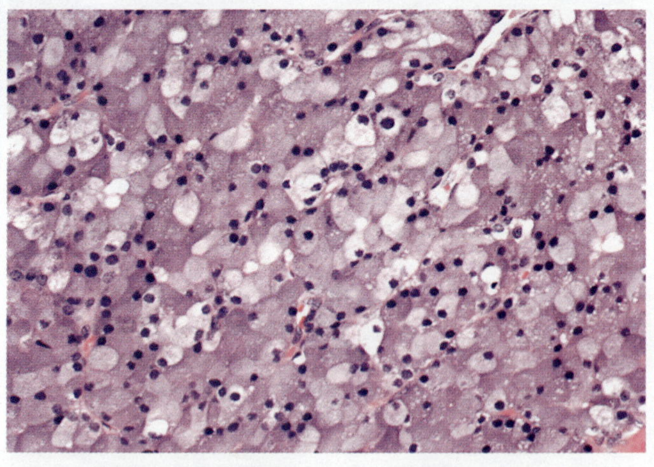

ORAL CAVITY

Ameloblastoma

- It is the **most common** odontogenic tumor[Q]
- Most commonly occur in 3-5 decade
- Most common site- **Posterior mandible (80%)**[Q]
- **Risk factors:** impacted teeth, dentigerous cyst
- It is benign but locally aggressive

Morphology of Ameloblastoma

- Columnar basal cells in palisading arrangement with vacuolated cytoplasm.
- Hyperchromatic nuclei **polarized away** from basement membrane.
- **Suprabasal cells** loosely textured and non-cohesive, resembling **stellate reticulum.**
- Treatment include wide surgical excision.
- Metastasizes rarely to lungs or CNS.
- Metastases associated with tumor of **long duration, multiple** surgical procedures, **radiation therapy.**

High Yield Facts

- **Precancerous Lesions of Oral Cavity are:** Leukoplakia (most common) & Erythroplakia
- **Most Common Malignancy of Oral Cavity** is Squamous Cell Carcinoma (classically linked to tobacco, HPV infection)

RETINOBLASTOMA

- Most common **primary malignant tumor of the eye** in children[Q]
- **Cell of origin is a neuronal progenitor.**[Q]

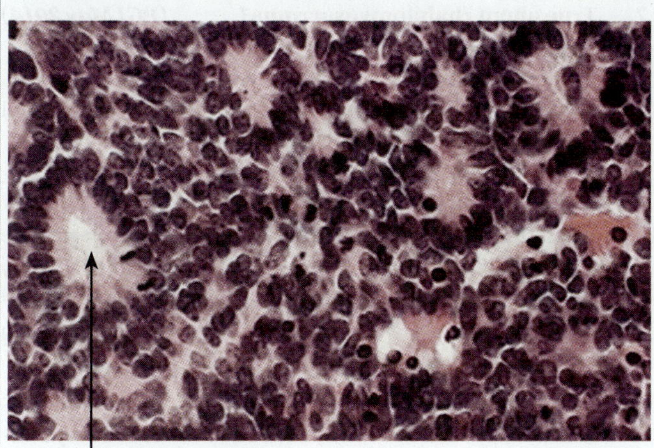

Rossette in Retinoblastoma

Genetics

- Caused by **loss of function mutation of the Retinoblastoma (Rb) gene**[Q]
- **Familial (40% cases; autosomal dominant):**
  - Carrying **germline mutation** in one copy of the gene (**first hit**).[Q]
  - **Spontaneous somatic mutation** in the second normal allele (**second hit**) → retinoblastoma[Q]
  - **Often bilateral** with increased risk of **developing osteosarcoma**[Q] and other **soft tissue sarcomas**.
- **Sporadic** cases (60%):
  - **Somatic mutation in both the alleles**.
  - Involves **only one eye and there is no increased risk of other cancer**[Q]

Morphology

- Small, round cells with **hyperchromatic nuclei.**[Q]
- **Flexner Wintersteiner rosettes**[Q] (a single layer of tumor cells aggregated around a central lumen)
- **Fleurettes**[Q] (a single layer of cells with **tapering cytoplasmic processes** that protrude into **the center of the rossette**)

Adverse Prognostic Factors

- **Extraocular extension**[Q], invasion along optic nerve[Q] and choroidal invasion.[Q]

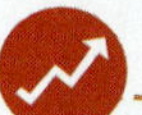

High Yield Facts

- Rb gene was the first tumor suppressor gene discovered
- **Trilateral retinoblastoma**: **Bilateral** retinoblastoma along with **pinealoblastoma**
- **Fleurettes** are seen in well differentiated tumors and **represent photoreceptor differentiation.**[Q]

> **R10th Latest Updates**
- GIST & peripheral nerve sheath tumors (PNST) are included in soft tissue sarcomas
- Undifferentiated-unclassified tumors is added & include pleomorphic sarcoma
- Round cell & mixed types of liposarcoma categories are removed

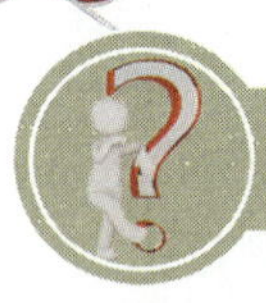

Multiple Choice Questions

1. **Which of the following translocation is seen in Myxoid liposarcoma?** *(Recent Pattern Question 2020)*
   a. t (11:22)
   b. t (14:18)
   c. t (x:18)
   d. t (12:16)

2. **Which of the following is not small round cell tumor?** *(AIIMS Nov 2019)*
   a. Neuroblastoma
   b. Retinoblastoma
   c. Hemangioblastoma
   d. Ewing sarcoma

3. **In alveolar variant of rhabdomyosarcoma, the resultant fusion protein is believed to function as:** *(JIPMER Nov 2019)*
   a. Activated growth factor receptor
   b. Chimeric transcription factor
   c. Constitutively active kinase
   d. Novel growth factor

4. **Sarcoma spreading by lymphatic spread is:** *(Recent Question 2016-17)*
   a. Alveolar RMS
   b. Embroynal RMS
   c. Liposarcoma
   d. Fibrosarcoma

5. **Spindle shaped cells is/are seen in which sarcoma:** *(PGI May 2015)*
   a. Osteosarcoma
   b. Chondromyosarcoma
   c. Embryonal rhabdomyosarcoma
   d. Leiomyosarcoma
   e. Fibrosarcoma

6. **Most common site of Rhabdomyosarcoma is:** *(Recent Question 2016)*
   a. Head and neck
   b. Trunk
   c. Urogenital
   d. Lungs

7. **Hyperglycemia is associated with:** *(Recent Question 2016)*
   a. Osteosarcoma
   b. Chondroblastoma
   c. Chondrosarcoma
   d. Osteoma

8. **Olliers disease also known as?** *(Recent Question 2016)*
   a. Osteosarcoma
   b. Enchondromatosis
   c. Multiple myeloma
   d. Enchondrosis

9. **Cambium layer is seen in:** *(Recent Question 2015)*
   a. Embryonal rhabdomyosarcoma
   b. Pleomorphic rhabdomyosarcoma
   c. Alveolar rhabdomyosarcoma
   d. Undifferentiated rhabdomyosarcoma

10. **Which of the following are primarily spindle cell tumor?** *(PGI Nov 2015)*
    a. Rhabdomyosarcoma
    b. Fibrosarcoma
    c. Leimyosarcoma
    d. Kaposi sarcoma

11. **Most common soft tissue tumor is:** *(Recent Question 2015)*
    a. Fibroma
    b. Lipoma
    c. Leiomyoma
    d. Rhabdomyoma

12. **Most common Sarcoma of adulthood is:** *(Recent Question 2015)*
    a. Liposarcoma
    b. Fibrosarcoma
    c. Rhabdomyosarcoma
    d. Leiomyosarcoma

13. **Most common site of Fibrosarcoma is:** *(Recent Question 2014)*
    a. Head and Neck
    b. Extremities
    c. Abdominal wall
    d. Joints

14. **Which of the following is associated with Tuberous Sclerosis:** *(Recent Question 2014)*
    a. Fibroma
    b. Lipoma
    c. Leiomyoma
    d. Rhabdomyoma

15. **Tadpole cells or comma shaped cells on histopathology are seen in:** *(Recent Question 2014)*
    a. Trichoepithelioma
    b. Spideroma
    c. Rhabdomyosarcoma
    d. Histiocytoma

16. **Most important indicator of malignancy in smooth muscle tumors is:** *(Recent Question 2014)*
    a. Mitotic index
    b. Atypia
    c. Necrosis
    d. Cellularity

17. **True about rhabdomyosacroma?** *(PGI May 2014)*
    a. Arise from pluripotent cells
    b. Tennis racket cells on light microscopy
    c. Sarcoma botryoides, is a variant of embryonal rhabdomyosarcoma
    d. Most common type is Embryonal
    e. Most common site is lower extremity

18. **Retinoblastomas arising in the context of germ-line mutations not only may be bilateral, but also may be associated with ______ (so called "trilateral" retinoblastoma)** *(AP PGMEE 14)*
    a. Medulloblastoma
    b. Pinealoblastoma
    c. Neuroblastoma
    d. Hemangioblastoma

19. **Immunohistochemical stain marker of Rhabdomyosarcoma** *(JIPMER 2014)*
    a. Desmin
    b. Vimentin
    c. Cytokeratin
    d. Neurofilamment

20. **Primitive Neuro Ectodermal Tumor of bones and soft tissues shows which of the following cytogenetic abnormalities?** *(PGI May 2013)*
    a. EWS-ETVI
    b. EWS-ERG
    c. EWS-FLI1
    d. EWS-ATFI
    e. EWS-WTl

21. **Bible Bump is a:** *(Recent Question 2016, 2013)*
    a. Synovial cyst
    b. Malformation
    c. Neurofibroma
    d. Myxomatous degeneration

22. **"Biphasic pattern" on histology is seen in which tumor:** *(DPG 10, MH 02)*
    a. Rhabdomyosarcoma
    b. Synovial cell sarcoma
    c. Osteosarcoma
    d. Neurofibroma

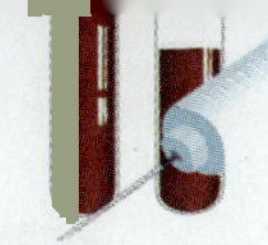

23. **Glomus tumor is seen in:** *(AIIMS Nov 10)*
    a. Retroperitoneum
    b. Soft tissue
    c. Distal portion of digits
    d. Proximal portion of digits

TUMORS OF ORAL CAVITY

24. **Most common cancer of oral cavity histologically is:**
    (Recent Question 2016-17)
    a. Squamous cell Ca
    b. Adeno ca
    c. Adenocystic Ca
    d. Odontogenic ca
    (Recent Question 2016-17)

25. **True about Dentigerous cyst:**
    a. Arises in relation to unerupted teeth
    b. It most commonly encroaches maxillary antrum
    c. Mandibular third molar is common site
    d. Common in mandible

26. **Most malignant salivary gland tumor is:**
    a. MucoepidermoidCa   *(Recent Question 2016)*
    b. Acinic cell carcinoma
    c. Adenoid cystic carcinoma
    d. Pleomorphic adenoma

27. **Cystic spaces lined by double layer of neoplastic epithelial cells resting on dense lymphoid tissue is a feature of:** *(AP PGMEE 2015)*
    a. Aneurismal bone cyst
    b. Dermoid cyst
    c. Warthin tumor
    d. Hashimoto's thyroiditis

28. **Warthins tumor true statement is:** *(PGI Nov 2015)*
    a. Sinuses are present
    b. Clefts are present
    c. Pallisading cells are seen
    d. Papillary CystadenomaLymphomatosum
    e. Arises from sublingual gland commonly

29. **Most common site of Ameloblastoma is:**
    a. Anterior Mandible   *(Recent Question 2014)*
    b. Posterior Mandible
    c. Maxilla
    d. Zygomatic bone

30. **The most common pre-malignant condition of oral carcinoma is:** *(Recent Question 2014)*
    a. Leukoplakia
    b. Erythroplakia
    c. Lichen planus
    d. Fibrosis

31. **Most common salivary gland tumor?**
    a. Mucoepidermoid carcinoma   *(Recent Question 2013)*
    b. Pleomorphic adenoma
    c. Warthims tumor
    d. Oncocytoma

32. **Pleomorphic adenoma has:** *(Recent Question 2013)*
    a. Columnar cells enclosing lymphoid stroma
    b. Exclusively myoepithelial cells
    c. Epithelial cells in chondroid matrix
    d. Nests of squamous cells and vacuolated cells containing mucin

33. **Which of the following head and neck tumor has worst prognosis?** *(MH 11, DNB June 08)*
    a. Adenoid cystic carcinoma
    b. Acinic cell carcinoma
    c. Cystadenolymphoma
    d. Mucoepidermoid carcinoma

34. **Most common type of salivary neoplasm:** *(PGI Nov 10)*
    a. Adenocysticcacinorna
    b. Mixed cell parotid neoplasm
    c. Epidermoid carcinoma
    d. Adenocarcinoma
    e. Adenolymphoma

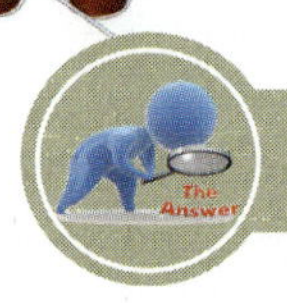

Answers with Explanations

1. Ans. (d) t (12:16) *(Ref: Robbins 9th/pg 1220)*

- Malignant tumor composed of primitive nonlipogenic mesenchymal cells, signet ring lipoblasts and prominent myxoid stroma with a highly characteristic branching vascular pattern. It shows Recurrent molecular alteration with either t(12;16)(q13;p11.2) *FUS-DDIT3* or very rarely (~2%) t(12;22)(q13;q12) *EWSR1-DDIT3* rearrangements

2. Ans. (c) Hemangioblastoma *(Ref: Robbins 9th/pg/1222)*

Diffuse round cell pattern is seen in: Ewing's sarcoma, Primitive neuroectodermal tumor (PNET), Merkel cell carcinoma, Embryonal rhabdomyosarcoma (ERMS), Small cell carcinoma, Lymphoma

Round cell pattern with rosettes

- Flexner's (also called Flexner – Winterstein, true rosettes) –e.g., Retinoblastoma, PNET
- Homer Wright rosette-center has no lumen, but abundant fibrillary material e.g., neuroblastoma.

3. Ans. (b) Chimeric transcription factor *(Ref: Robbins 9th/pg 1253)*

4. Ans. (d) Fibrosarcoma *(Ref: Robbins 9/730-740)*

5. Ans. (a, c, d, e); a. Osteosarcoma c. Embryonal rhabdomyosarcoma, d. Leiomyosarcoma, e. Fibrosarcoma *(Ref: Robbins 9th/pg 474)*

Differential diagnoses of spindle cell sarcomas:

- Fibrosarcoma
- Benign fibrous histiocytoma
- Embryonal rhabdomyosarcoma
- Leiomyosarcoma
- Synovial sarcoma: t(X;18) (p 11;q11) fusion of SYT-SSX.
- Malignant Peripheral Nerve Sheath Tumours (MPNST)
- **Vascular tumors:** hemangio-endothelioma, hemangio-pericytoma, angiosarcoma, lymphangiosarcoma, and Kaposi's sarcoma.

Note that osteosarcoma has osteoblasts which are plump cells and not typical spindle cells.

6. Ans. (a) Head and neck *(Ref: Robbins 9th/pg 1253)*

- **MC site of rhabdomyosarcoma is head/neck; genito-urinary tract**

7. Ans. (c) Chondrosarcoma

(Ref: Cancer 42:603-610, 1978; Hypoglycemia as Paraneoplastic syndrome in some tumors: Mesenchymal tumors, sarcomas, adrenal, hepatic, gastrointestinal, kidney, prostate, Cervix (small-cell carcinoma)

The first association of hyperglycemia was made by Glicksman and Rawson who noted a 25% incidence of "diabetes" in patients with sarcomas of bone. Marcove

and Francis found hyperglycemia in 85% of their chondrosarcoma patient. and Turner and Horne reported similar abnormalities associated with fibrosarcoma

8. Ans. (b) Enchondromatosis *(Ref: Robbins 9th/pg)*

Ollier disease is a rare, non inherited disease of unknown cause characterized by multiple enchondromas.

9. Ans. (a) Embryonal rhabdomyosarcoma

(Ref: Robbins 9th/pg 1253)

In **Sarcoma botryoides**, a variant of embryonal rhabdomyosarcoma, histology shows a **cambium layer** where the tumors abut the mucosa of an organ, they form a submucosal zone of hypercellularity.

10. Ans. (a, b, d) a. Rhabdomyosarcoma; b. Fibrosarcoma; d. Kaposi sarcoma *(Ref: Robbins 9th/pg 474)*

11. Ans. (b) Lipoma *(Ref: Robbins 9th/pg 1220; 8th/pg 1249)*

12. Ans. (a) Liposarcoma *(Ref: Robbins 9th/pg 1220)*

13. Ans. (b) Extremities

(Ref: Robbins 9th/pg 1221; 8th/pg 1250)

Fibrosarcoma

- It is **most common in extremities**
- It shows **Herringbone pattern** on histopathology
- It is **Aggressive, Recurs and Metastasizes**

14. Ans. (d) Rhabdomyoma

(Ref: Nelson Textbook of Pediatrics, 19th Edition, 2011; pg 2049)

Tuberous Sclerosis

It is inherited as an **autosomal dominant trait** with variable expression

Important **clinical manifestations of Tuberous Sclerosis** include:

Skin Lesions	CNS Lesions	Other Tumors
- **Facial angiofibroma** - Ungual/ periungual fibroma (non-traumatic) - **Ash-leaf macules** - **Shagreen patch** - Confetti skin lesions	- **Cortical tubers** - **Subependymal nodule** - **Subependymal giant cell astrocytoma**	- **Multiple retinal hamartomas** - **Cardiac rhabdomyoma** - **Renal angiomyolipoma**

15. Ans. (c) Rhabdomyosarcoma *(Ref: Robbins 9th/pg 1222)*

In Rhabdomyosarcoma, **diagnostic cell in all types is:**

- **Rhabdomyoblast** - contains **eccentric eosinophilic granular cytoplasm**, rich in thick and thin filaments

- **Tadpole or strap cells**[Q] - Elongated Rhabdomyoblasts that may contain cross-striations visible by light microscopy

16. Ans. (a) Mitotic index *(Ref: Robbins 9th/pg 1223)*

Indicator of malignancy in soft tissue tumors (Leiomyosarcoma): **Mitotic index**[Q] **>Atypia> Necrosis.**

17. Ans. (a,b,c,d) a. Arise from pluripotent cells; b. Tennis racket cellson light microscopy; c. Sarcoma botryoides, is a variant of embryonal rhabdomyosarcoma; d. Most common type is Embryonal. *(Ref: Robbins 9th/pg 1222)*

18. Ans. (b) Pinealoblastoma *(Ref: Robbins 9th/pg 1339)*

- "Trilateral" retinoblastoma refers to **bilateral Retinoblastomas pluspinealoblastoma,** occurring in individuals inheriting a germline mutation of one *RB* allele; it is associated with a dismal outcome
- **Retinoblastoma is the most common primary intraocular malignancy of children.**

19. Ans. (a) Desmin *(Ref: Robbins 9th/pg 1222; 8th/pg 1253)*

20. Ans. (a,b,c) a. EWS-ETVI; b. EWS-ERG; c. EWS-FLI1

(Ref: Robbins 9th/pg 1219; 8th/pg 1249)

Cytogenetics in Ewing's Sarcoma

- t(11;22) → fusion of EWS gene with FLI1 gene → **EWS-FLI1 (most common**, 90%)

21. Ans. (a) Synovial cyst

(Ref: Atlas of Soft tissue & bone pathology, 2015; pg 54)
- It is also known as a **'ganglion cyst', 'myxoid cyst', 'Gideon's Disease', 'Bible Cyst'** or **'Bible bump'**
- It is a non-neoplastic soft tissue lump that may occur in any joint, but most often occurs in the hands or feet.
- Caused by leakage of fluid from the joint into the surrounding tissue.

22. Ans. (b) Synovial cell sarcoma *(Ref: R 9th/pg 1220-1224)*

A **biphasic tumor** refers to neoplastic tissue which is characterized by **two different cellular elements.**

Biphasic tumors include

• **Spindle Cell Carcinoma**	• **Mesothelioma**
• Nasopharyngeal Carcinoma –	• **Pleomorphic adenoma**
• **Synovial Sarcoma (SC)**	• **Melanoma**
	• Malignant Mixed Mullerian tumor

An example of Triphasic tumor is Wilm's tumor

23. Ans. (c) Distal portion of digits *(Ref: Robbins 9th/pg 517)*

24. Ans. (a) Squamous cell Ca *(Ref: R 9/PG 732)*

25. Ans. (a) Arises in relation to unerupted teeth, (c) Mandibular third molar is common site, (d) Common in mandible

(Ref: Robbins 9th/ 734; Manipal Surgery 4th/292-93; Harshmohan 7th/511-12)
- **Dentigerous cyst** is defined as a cyst that originates around the crown of an *unerupted tooth* and is thought to be the result of fluid accumulation between the developing tooth and the dental follicle.
- Radiographically, these are unilocular lesions most often associated with **impacted third molar (wisdom)** teeth. Histologically, they are lined by a thin layer of stratified squamous epithelium. Often, there is a dense chronic inflammatory cell infiltrate in the connective tissue stroma.
- Complete removal of the lesion is curative.

26. Ans. (a) Mucoepidermoid Carcinoma

(Ref: R 9th/pg 757-758)

27. Ans. (c) Warthin's tumor *(Ref: Robbins 9th/pg 757-758)*

Histology of Warthin tumour:

- Cystic spaces are lined by a **double layer of neoplastic epithelial cells resting on** a **dense lymphoid stroma** sometimes bearing **germinal centers.**
- The **double layer of lining cells is distinctive**; the upper layer consists of palisading columnar cells while the lower layer is comprised of cuboidal to polygonal cells.

28. Ans. (b, c, d); b. Clefts are present; c. Pallisading cells are seen; d. Papillary Cystadenoma Lymphomatosum

(Ref: Robbins 9th/pg 757- 758)

29. Ans. (b) Posterior Mandible *(Ref: Robbins 9th/pg 735)*

30. Ans. (a) Leukoplakia *(Ref: Robbins 9th/pg 731)*

Precancerous lesions of oral cavity

- Leukoplakia (most common)
- Erythroplakia

Most common malignancy of oral cavity: squamous cell carcinoma (classicaly linked to tobacco, HPV infection)

31. Ans. (b) Pleomorphic adenoma

(Ref: Robbins 9th/pg 744)

32. Ans. (c) Epithelial cells in chondroid matrix

(Ref: Robbins 9th/pg 744)

33. Ans. (a) Adenoid cystic carcinoma

(Ref: R 9th/pg 744)

34. Ans. (b) Mixed cell parotid neoplasm

(Ref: R 9th/pg 744)

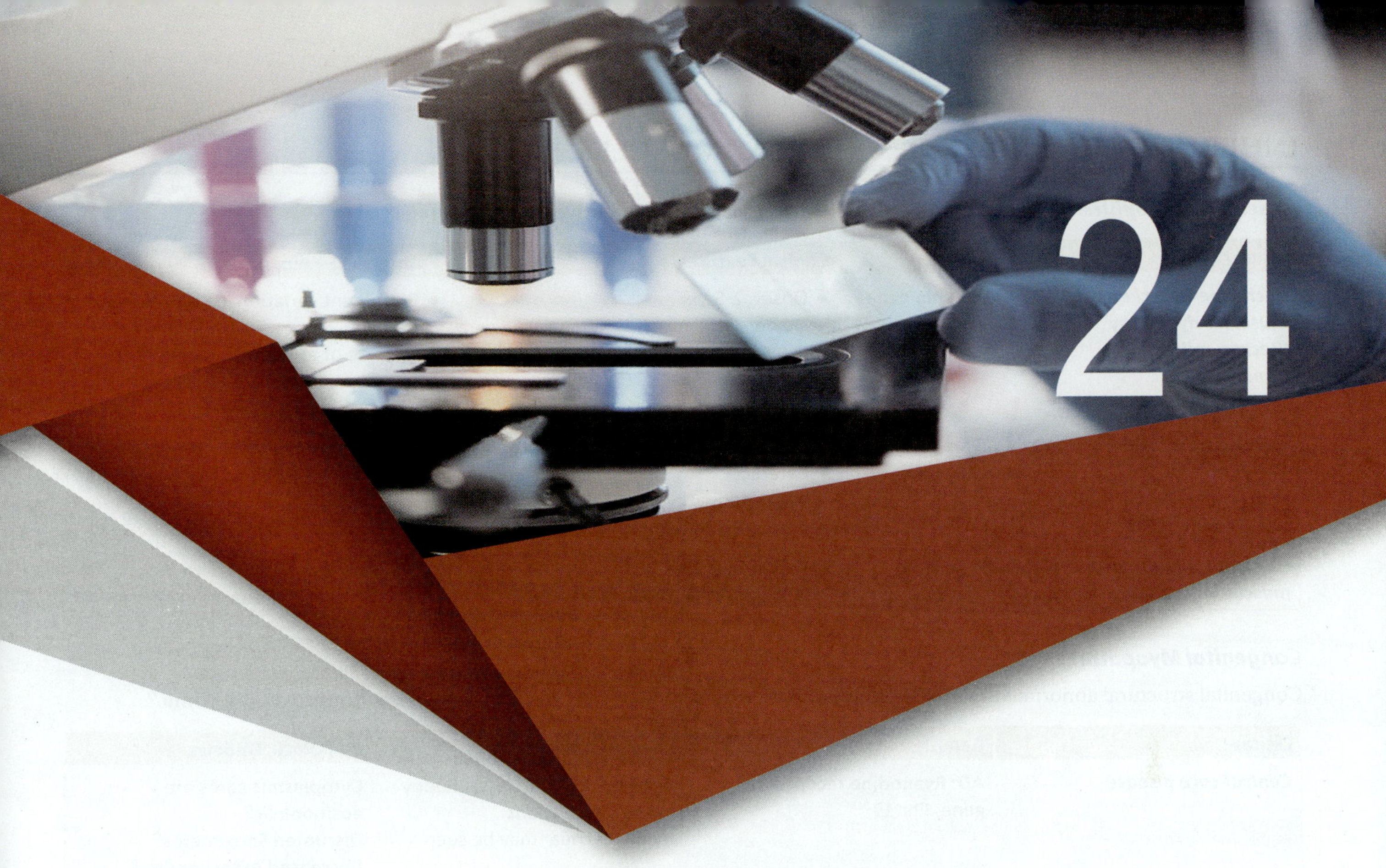

24

Diseases of Muscles

Key Points

- **Duchenne & Becker Muscular dystrophy** are X-linked recessive myotonic dystrophy
- **Central-core disease, Nemaline and Myotubular** (centronuclear) are congenital myopathies

Key Recent Updates

- Duchenne muscular dystrophy (DMD) is caused by mutations is DMD gene, largest gene is human body.

INHERITED DISORDERS OF SKELETAL MUSCLES

Muscular Dystrophies: Inherited disorders of skeletal muscle with **progressive muscle damage**[Q]

Disease	Genetics	Clinical Features	Pathologic Findings
Duchenne & Becker Muscular dystrophy (Becker: milder disease)	**XR**;[Q] **Dystrophin gene**[Q] on **Chr X**;[Q]	• Onset: 2-5 yrs • Gower sign • Pseudohypertrophy of calf muscles • **CPK level** ↑[Q]	• Prominent **variation in size**[Q] of muscle fibers • Mixture of **atrophic & regenerating myofibers**[Q] seen • **Fatty infiltration**[Q] (See fig 1)
Myotonic dystrophy	**AD**;[Q] CTG repeats in DMPK gene on Chr19	• Skeletal muscle weakness (myotonia) • Cataract • Endocrinopathy • Cardiomyopathy	• **Intrafusal fibers**[Q] of muscle spindle affected
Fascioscapulohumeral muscular dystrophy	**AD**; DUX4 gene on Chr 4	• **Facial muscle &** • **Shoulder** girdle muscle weakness	• **Dystrophic** myopathy with **inflammatory infiltrates** in muscle

Congenital Myopathies

Congenital structural abnormalities of skeletal muscles, that present in infancy and remains **static or improves over time**.[Q]

Disease	Genetics	Clinical Findings	Pathologic Findings
Central-core disease	**AD; Ryanodine receptor**-1[Q] gene; Chr 19	**Early-onset** weakness; "floppy infant"; **Malignant hyperthermia**[Q] may be seen	**Cytoplasmic cores are eosinophilic**[Q] **Disrupted Sarcomeres**[Q] **Decreased mitochondria**[Q]
Nemaline myopathy (See fig 2)	AD or AR; **NEM gene**	Hypotonia at birth; "floppy infant"	Aggregates of **sub-sarcolemmal spindle-shaped particles ('Nemaline rods')**[Q]
Myotubular (centronuclear) myopathy	XL, AD or AR myotubularin (*MTM1*) gene	Severe congenital hypotonia, "floppy infant"; poor prognosis	Abundance of **centrally located nuclei in type I fibers**[Q]

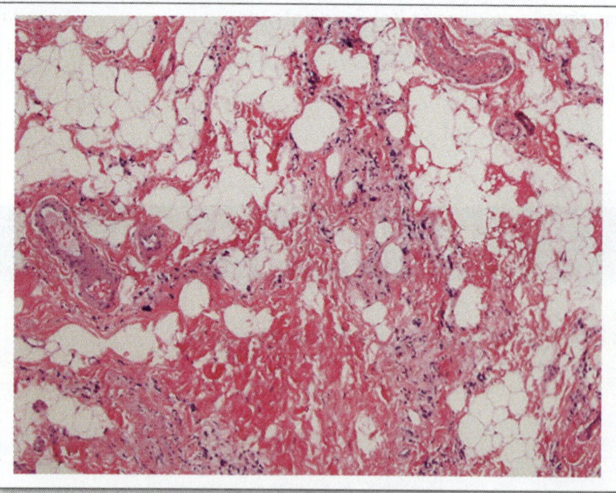

Fig. 1: End stage muscle with atrophic fibres and fibrofatty replacement (H&E) in Duchenne muscular dystrophy

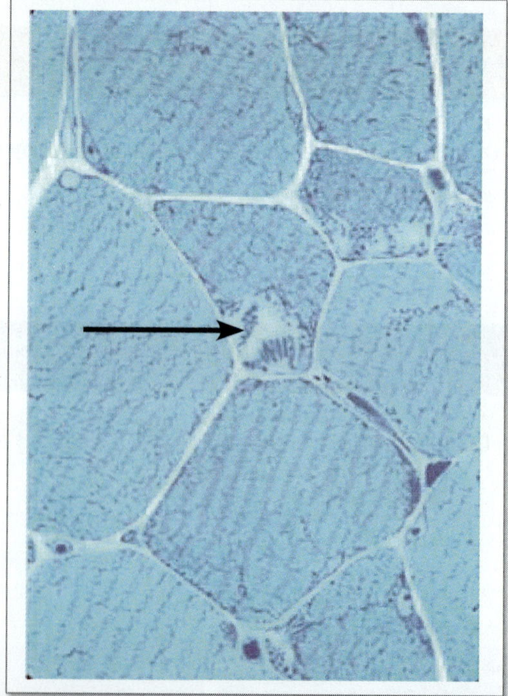

Fig. 2: Rod (nemaline) myopathy. A. Muscle fibers contain dark aggregates of rods (toluidine blue, 1000×)

INFLAMMATORY MYOPATHIES

- Disorders include polymyositis (PM), dermatomyositis (DM)
- **Features**
  - ○ Symmetric proximal muscle weakness
  - ○ Increased serum levels of muscle derived enzymes
  - ○ Nonsuppurative inflammation of skeletal muscle.

Polymyositis (PM)

- Primarily occurs in persons aged 40 to 60 years.
- Increased risk of malignant neoplasms (15%–20% of cases), particularly lung and bladder cancer, and non-Hodgkin malignant lymphomas.
- **Laboratory findings**
- Antibody findings
  - ○ Serum ANA increased in 30% to 60% of cases.
  - ○ Anti–transfer RNA synthetase (Jo-1) antibodies increased in 25% of cases.
- Muscle biopsies show necrotic and regenerating muscle and a lymphocytic and macrophage infiltrate.
- Muscle atrophy is not a prominent feature

Dermatomyositis (DM)

Cutaneous findings are key.
- Reddish-purple papules called Gottron patches are noted over the knuckles and proximal interphalangeal (PIP) joints in both hands

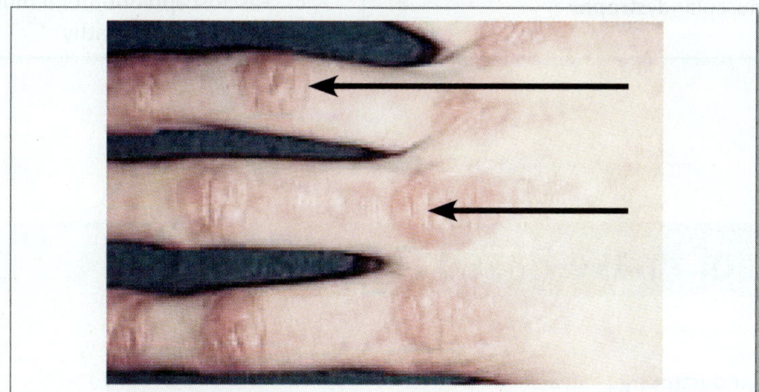

- Purple-red eyelid discoloration occurs (called heliotrope eyelids or "raccoon eyes".

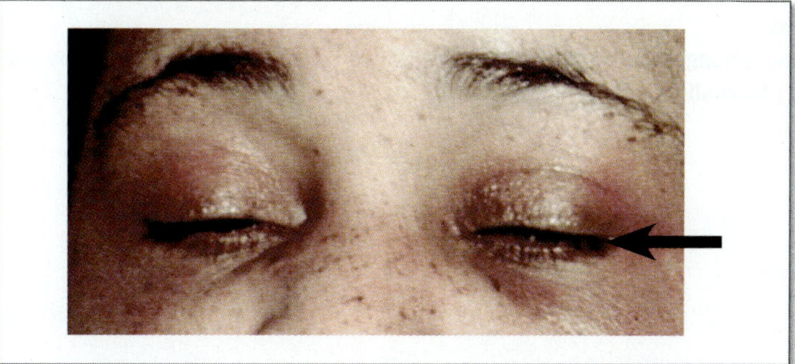

Laboratory Findings

- Similar to those described for Polymyositis (PM)
- Muscle biopsies show an inflammatory reaction (primarily lymphocytic).
  - ○ Unlike PM, atrophy of muscle fibers is a **prominent feature**.
  - ○ Damage to the capillaries in the muscle leads to ischemia and atrophy of the muscle fibers.

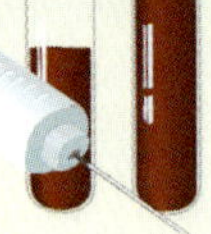
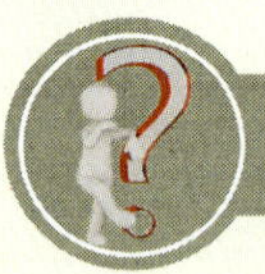

Image-Based Questions

1. **A 5-year-old male presented to AIIMS pediatrics OPD with a chief complaint of difficulty in climbing stairs and getting up from sitting position. There was history of maternal uncle having the same illness. On examination, there was pseudohypertrophy of calf muscle. Biopsy of the muscle was performed as shown below. What is your diagnosis?**

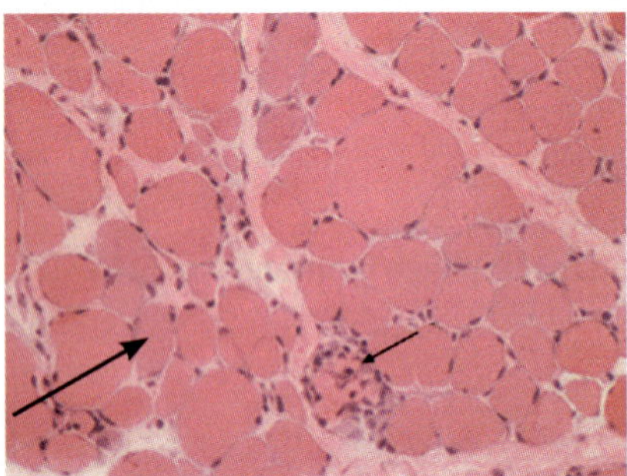

   a. Duchenne muscular dystrophy
   b. Myotonic dystrophy
   c. Fascioscapulohumeral muscular dystrophy
   d. Nemaline myopathy

2. **Electron microscopy of muscles was performed in infant who presented with hypotonia at birth. What is the most likely diagnosis?**

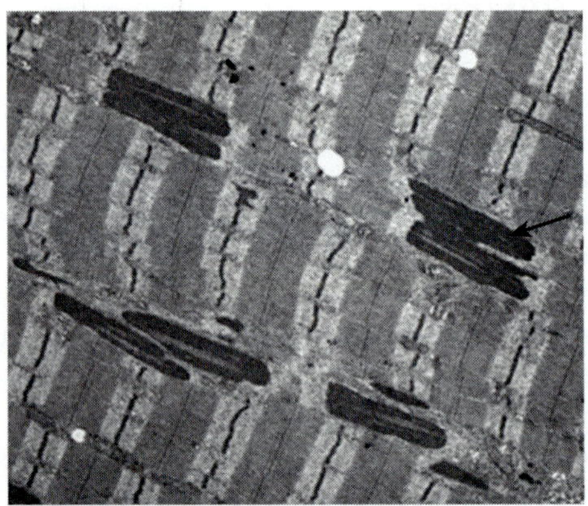

   a. Duchenne muscular dystrophy
   b. Myotonic dystrophy
   c. Fascioscapulohumeral muscular dystrophy
   d. Nemaline myopathy

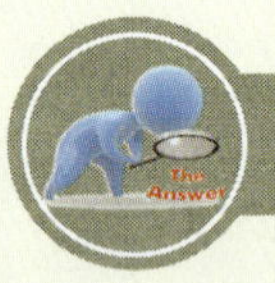

Answers of Image-Based Questions

1. **Ans. (a) Duchenne muscular dystrophy**
   - This is myopathy with X-linked inheritance suggested by same history in maternal uncle. On muscle biopsy prominent variation in size of muscle fibers can be seen.

2. **Ans. (d) Nemaline myopathy**
   - This is a congenital myopathy suggested by clinical features since birth. Electron microscopy shows aggregates of **subsarcolemmal spindle-shaped particles ('Nemaline rods')**

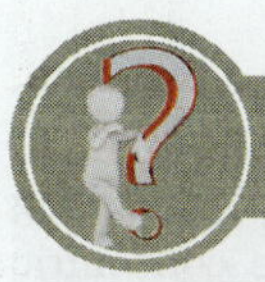

Multiple Choice Questions

BONE LESIONS

1. X-ray foot shows lytic lesion in the calcaneus, biopsy done from the lesion shows the following. What is your diagnosis? *(AIIMS Nov 18)*

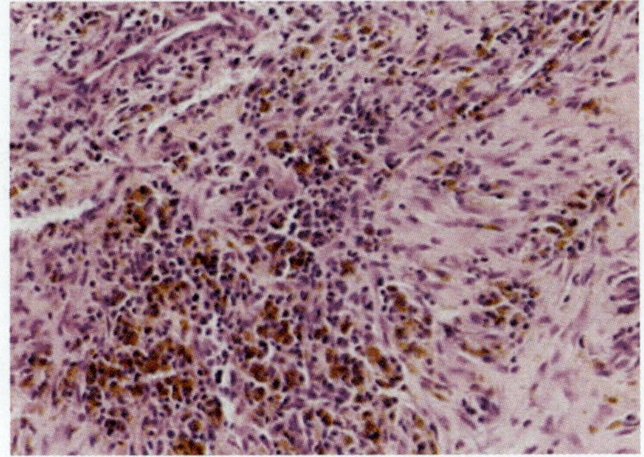

a. Pigmented villonodular synovitis.
b. Onchonosis
c. Osteomyelitis
d. Eumycosis

MUSCULAR DYSTROPHY AND MYOSITIS

2. Absence of dystrophin and presence of small muscle fibers are seen in: *(Recent Pattern Question 2020)*
a. Duchenne muscular dystrophy
b. Becker muscular dystrophy
c. Myotonic dystrophy
d. Dermatomyositis

3. Juvenile myoclonic epilepsy is due to mutation in: *(JIPMER Nov 2019)*

a. GABRA 1
b. CHRNA 2
c. COL4A1
d. FMRI

4. Parking lot inclusions are seen in:
a. Mitochondrial myopathy *(Recent Question 2015)*
b. Nemaline myopathy
c. Central myopathy
d. Lipid Myopathies

5. Perifascicular atrophy of muscle fibres is seen in- *(Recent Question 2014, 2013)*

a. Steroid myopathy
b. Dermatomyositis
c. Inclusion body myositis
d. Nemaline myopathy

6. Dystrophin is lacking in: *(Recent Question 2013, AIIMS May 93, 03)*
a. Polio
b. Duchenne's muscular dystrophy
c. Peroneal muscular atrophy
d. None of the above

7. Myasthenia gravis is associated with: *(Recent Question 2013)*

a. Thymoma
b. Thymic carcinoma
c. Thymic hyperplasia
d. Lymphoma

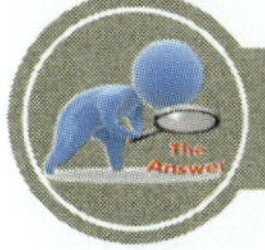

Answers with Explanations

1. **Ans. (a)** **Pigmented villonodular synovitis**

Definition: Rare neoplastic-like villonodular hyperplasia of synovium and tendon sheaths in young adults composed of mononuclear cells and multinuclear giant cells with hemosiderin deposition

- It Develops in synovial lining of joints, tendon sheaths and bursae, usually of knee (80%), ankle, hip, shoulder, elbow joint; nodular variant occurs in hands and wrists
- Almost always monoarticular
- Occasionally invades underlying bone - radiograph shows pressure erosions of the bones about the ankle, including the calcaneus, caused by large hyperdense, irregular soft-tissue mass. The bone erosions have well-defined, sclerotic margins.

Microscopic (Histologic) Description

- Hyperplastic synovium with papillary projections composed of foamy cells and hemosiderin containing macrophages

- Also large clefts, pseudoglandular or alveolar spaces lined by synovial cells, multinucleated (10 - 70 nuclei) giant cells, epithelioid cells

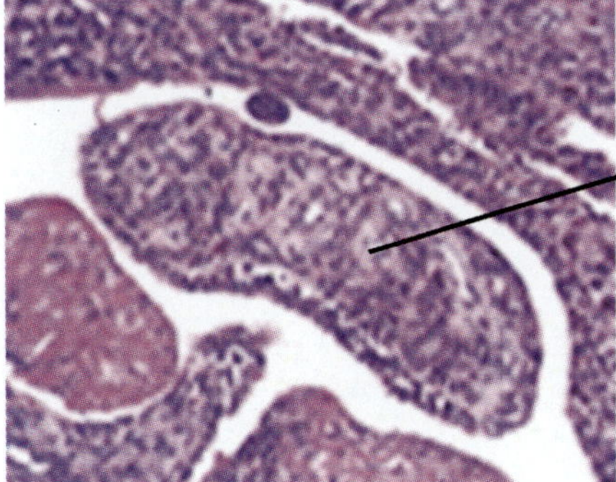

The papillary and villous structures show proliferation of polygonal cells in a background of fibroconnective tissue which is covered by synovial lining

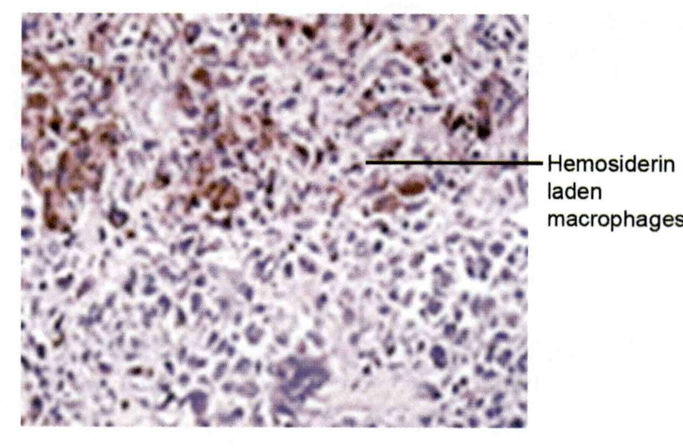

2. **Ans. (a)** **Duchenne muscular dystrophy**
(Ref: Robbins 9th/pg 1274)

3. **Ans. (a)** **GABRA 1** *(Ref: Robbins 9th/pg 1242)*

4. **Ans. (a)** **Mitochondrial myopathy** *(Ref: R 9th/pg 1274)*

In mitochondrial diseases, electron micrography showing morphologically abnormal mitochondria with concentric membranous rings ("phonograph records") & rhomboid paracrystalline inclusions ("parking lot" inclusions).

5. **Ans. (b)** **Dermatomyositis** *(Ref: Robbins 9th/pg 1238)*

6. **Ans. (b)** **Duchenne's muscular dystrophy**

(Ref: Robbins 9th/pg 1242-1243)

7. **Ans. (c)** **Thymic hyperplasia** *(Ref: Robbins 9th/pg 1236)*

- Thymic hyperplasia is found in 65% and thymoma in 15% of patients with myasthenia gravis.

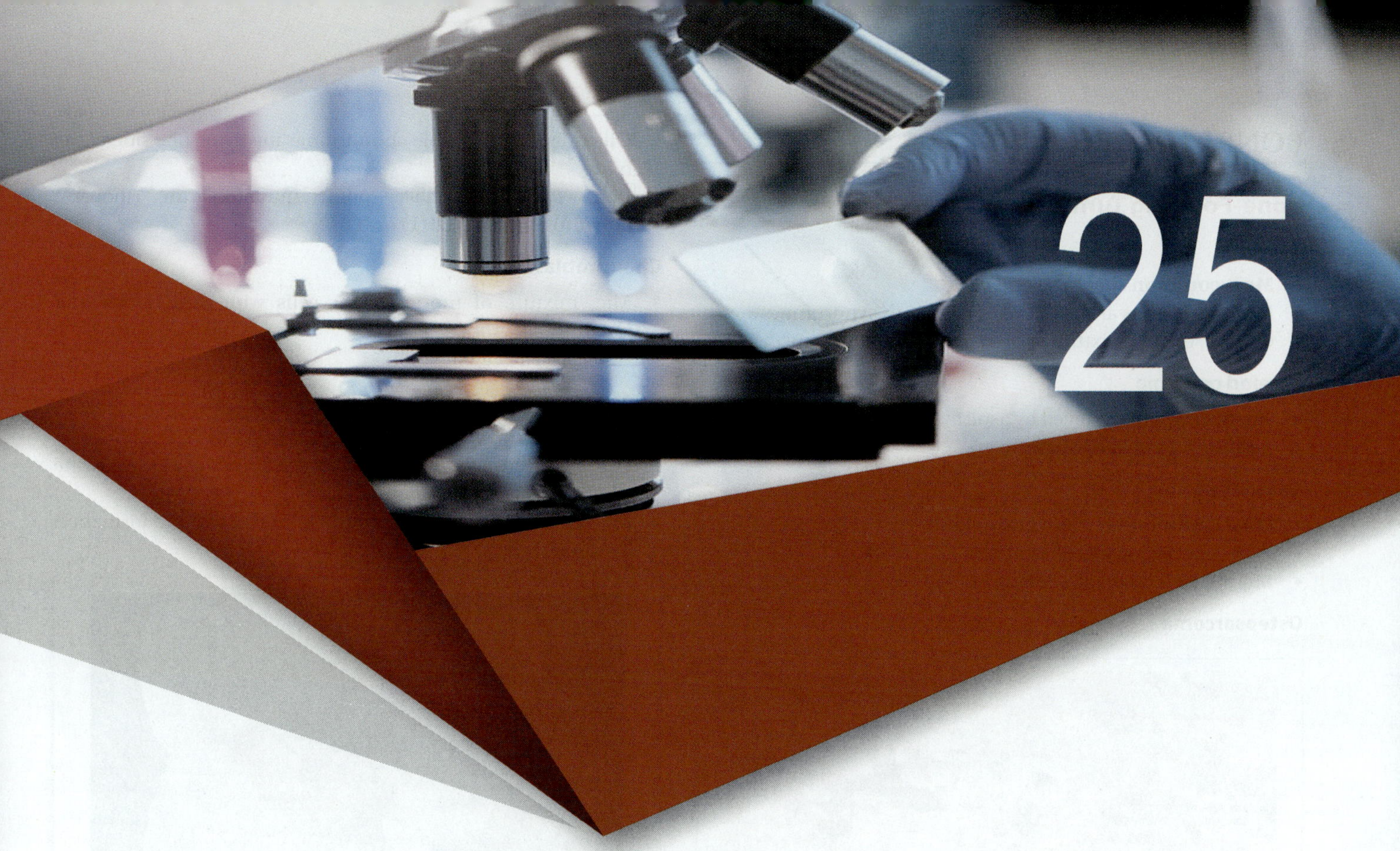

25

Tumors of Bone and Joints

» Most common mutation seen in osteosarcoma is germ line mutation in **retinoblastoma gene**
» **Ext** gene mutations are seen in osteochondroma
» **Giant cells** are seen in osteoclastoma, osteosarcoma, chondroblastoma, fibrous dysplasia, non ossifying fibrous and chondromyxoid fibroma

BONE TUMORS

Bone-Forming Tumors

Osteoma

- **Most common** site: head and neck
- Multiple lesions are a feature of Gardner's syndrome
- Composed of a mixture of woven and lamellar bone.

Osteiod osteoma

- Nocturnal pain- relieved by aspirin
- Less than 2 cm in diameter

Osteoblastoma

- **Most common** site: vertebral column
- Pain- not responsive to aspirin
- More than 2 cm in diameter

Osteosarcoma

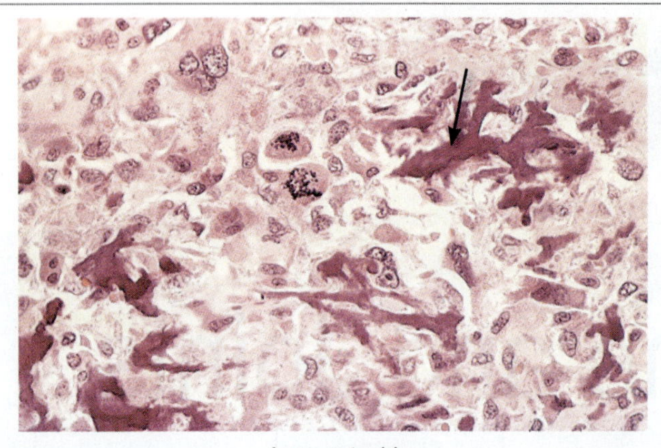

Lacy osteoid

- **Most common** site: metaphyseal region of the long bones of the extremities
- Shows osteiod (eosinophilic, glassy appearance) or bone produced directly by tumor cells without interposition of cartilage
- Metastatize via blood mainly to lungs
- **Most common** mutation: RB gene mutations (70%)

Cartilage-Forming Tumors

Osteochondroma

- **Most common** site: metaphysis near the growth plate of long bones
- **Most common** solitary tumor
- Multiple autosomal dominant disorder due to inactivity of EXT1 or EXT2 genes

Chondroma
Within Medulla: Enchondromas

On Bone surface: juxtacortical chondromas

- Maffucci syndrome: multiple chondromas associated with soft tissue spindle cell, Hemangiomas

- Ollier disease: multiple chondromas involving one side of the body
- Both syndromes have point mutations in isocitrate dehydrogenase I (IDH1) or IDH2

Chondroblastoma

- Mic: mixture of mononuclear cells with oval nuclei and longitudinal groove.
- Chicken wire calcification

Chondrosarcoma

- **Most common** site: pelvis, shoulder and ribs
- Gross: glistening white tumor image shows glistening white tumor S/o chondrosarcoma
- Mic: cartilaginous matrix and lack of direct bone formation by tumor cells

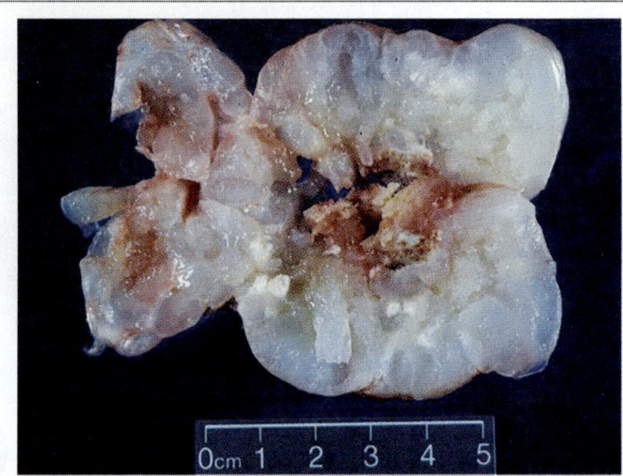

Glistening white tumor

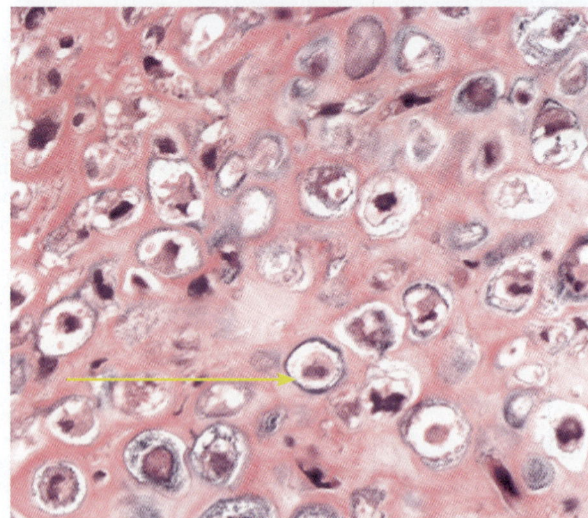

Chondrosarcoma showing malignant chondrocytes with moderate pleomorphism

Fibro-osseous Tumors

Fibrous Dysplasia

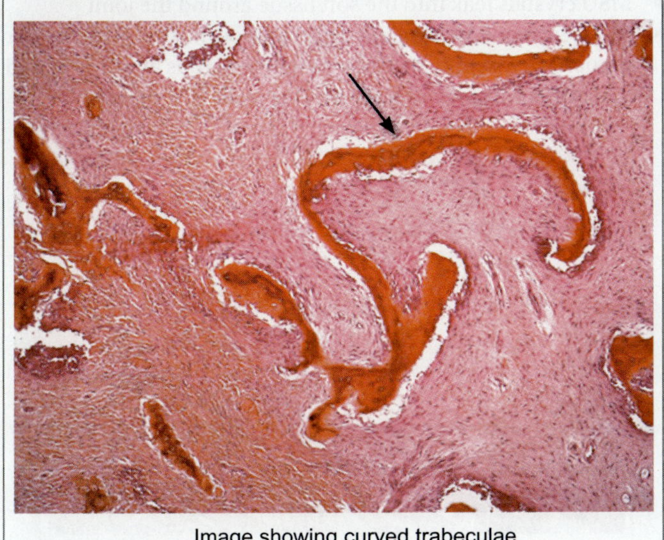

Image showing curved trabeculae

- **Most common** Mutation: GNAS gene
- Mic: curved trabeculae of woven bone (mimicking Chinese characters), surrounded by cellular fibroblastic proliferation

Miscellaneous Bone Tumors

Osteoclastoma/ Giant cell tumor

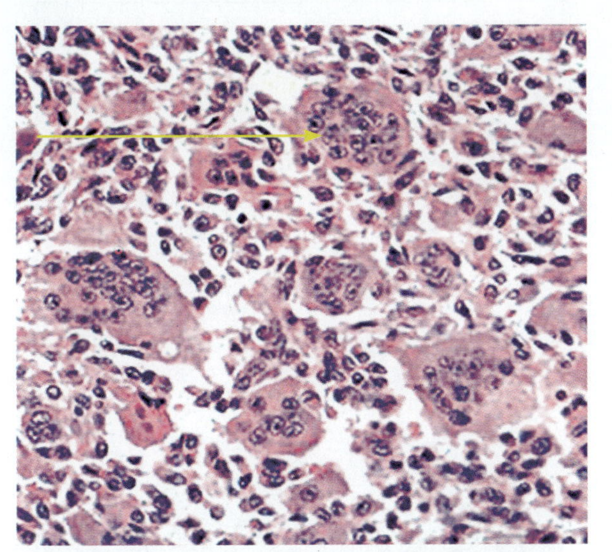

Osteoclastoma/Giant cell tumor showing giant cells in background of oval to spindle shaped mononuclear cells

- **Most common** site: epiphyses of long bones
- Benign but locally aggressive bone tumor
- Neoplastic component: mononuclear cells
- Mononuclear cells → RANK ligand → proliferation of non-neoplastic osteoclast-like cells.

Ewings tumor/ PNET

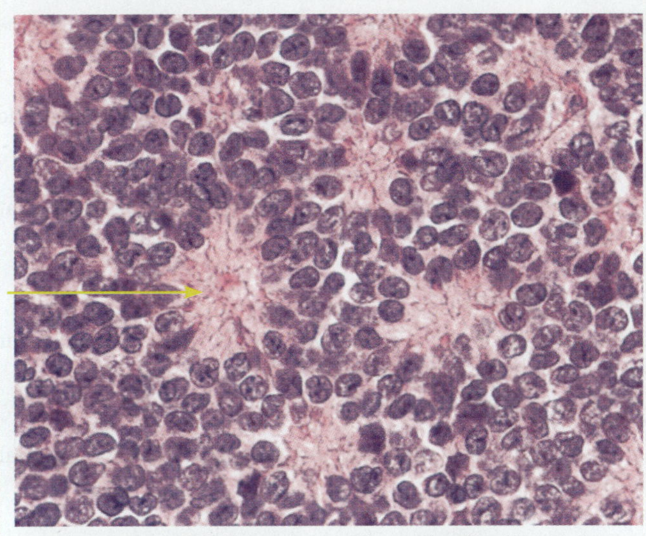

Ewings tumor/PNET showing small round cells with rosettes

- **Most common** Mutation: t(11;22)(q24;q12) in 95% cases or t(21;22)(q22;q12).
- **Most common** site: diaphyses of long bones
- Gross: characteristic periosteal reaction with deposition of bone in onion-skin pattern.
- Mic: uniform small, round cells with scant glycogen-rich cytoplasm
- Homer-Wright rosettes suggests neural differentiation (PNET)

JOINTS

Joint Disorders

Classification of Joint Disorders

Group I
- Noninflammatory
- Examples—osteoarthritis (OA), neuropathic joint

Group II
- Inflammatory
- Examples—rheumatoid arthritis (RA), gout

Group III
- Septic
- Examples—Lyme disease, disseminated gonococcemia

Group IV
- Hemorrhagic
- Examples—trauma, hemophilia A and B

Osteoarthritis (OA)

Definition—progressive degeneration of articular cartilage
- Targets weight-bearing joints

Joint findings

- Erosion and clefts in articular cartilage
- Reactive bone formation occurs at the joint margins (osteophytes)
- Subchondral cysts
- Bone eventually rubs on bone - This produces dense, sclerotic bone.
- No ankylosis (fusion) of the joint
- Joint mice- Refers to fragments of articular cartilage that break free into the joint space

Rheumatoid Arthritis (RA)

Definition—systemic disorder associated with chronic joint inflammation that most commonly affects peripheral joints

Clinical findings

Symmetric involvement of second/third metacarpophalangeal (MCP) and PIP joints

- Causes ulnar deviation, morning stiffness
- **Swan neck deformity**
  - Flexion of the DIP joint
  - Extension of the PIP joint
- **Boutonnière deformity**
  - Extension of the DIP joint
  - Flexion of the PIP joint

Laboratory findings

- Positive serum antinuclear antibody (ANA) test (30% of cases)
- Positive serum RF (70%–90% of cases)
- Normal to increased serum C3, decreased synovial C3
- Increased serum total protein
  - Due to increase in γ-globulins (IgG) in chronic inflammation
  - Polyclonal gammopathy on serum protein electrophoresis

Gouty Arthritis

Definition—Tissue deposition of monosodium urate (MSU) due to prolonged hyperuricemia

- Most commonly involve the first metatarsophalangeal joint (MTP; called podagra; joint in the foot with the most trauma)

Acute gout

Laboratory findings

- Hyperuricemia
  - Increased serum uric acid >7 mg/dL in men
  - Increased serum uric acid >6 mg/dL in women
- Absolute neutrophilic leukocytosis
- Joint aspiration is confirmatory. Shows Negatively birefringent MSU crystals

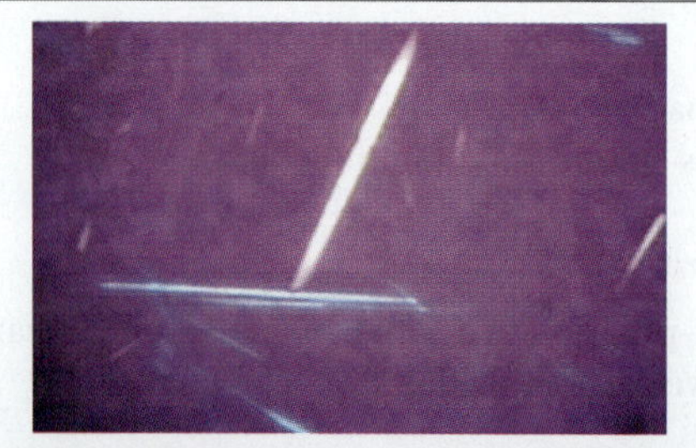

Showing Negatively Birefringent Crystals

Chronic gout

Distal joints are preferential sites.
UA crystals accumulate in the joint and produce a tophus.

- MSU crystals leak into the soft tissue around the joint
- MSU excites a brisk giant cell reaction in the periarticular tissue.-Microscopic sections reveal numerous multinucleated giant cells within which are MSU crystals that polarize.

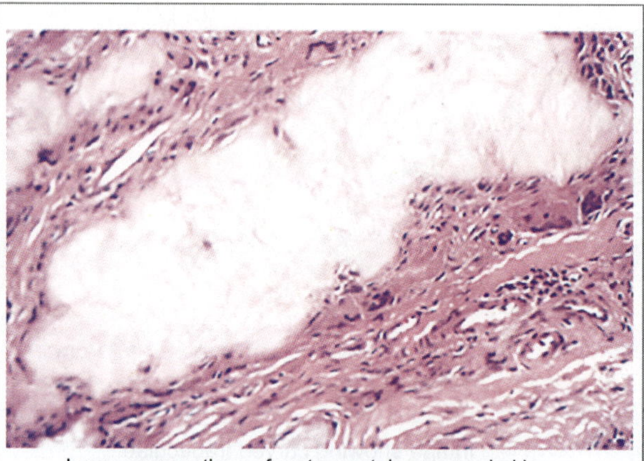

Large aggregations of urate crystals surrounded by an intense foreign body giant cell reaction

- Tophi destroy subjacent bone, causing erosive arthritis that breaks down bone and leaves overhanging edges (sometimes called rat bites)

Pseudogout -Calcium Pyrophosphate Dihydrate Deposition (CPPD) Disease

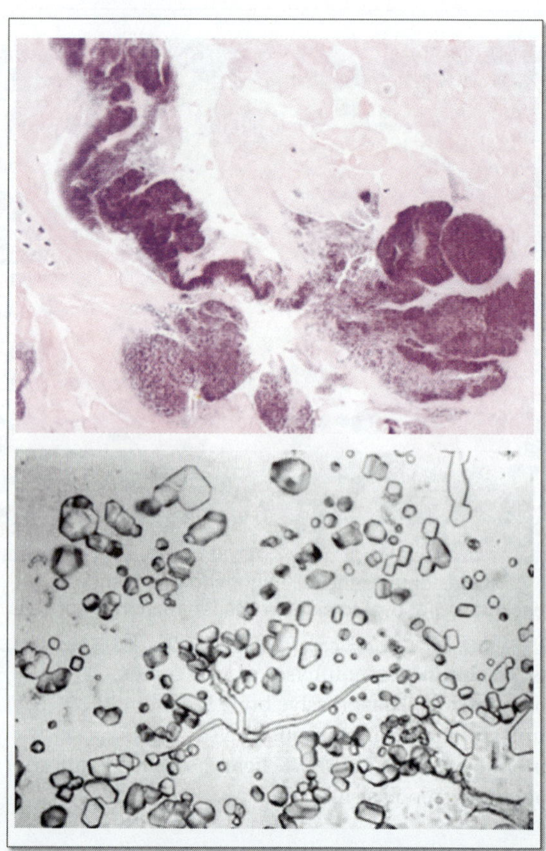

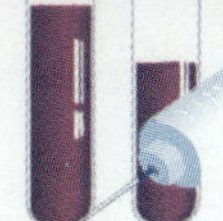

- Most common joint involved is the knee.
- Calcium pyrophosphate crystals deposit in articular cartilage
  - Crystals produce linear deposits in articular cartilage
  - It is called chondrocalcinosis when it deposits in articular cartilage.
- If the patient has acute pain, redness, swelling, and limitation of motion in the joint, the combination is called pseudogout.
- Crystals-rhomboid, positively birefringent
- The crystals form chalky, white friable deposits, which are seen histologically in hematoxylin and eosin stained preparations as oval blue-purple aggregates

Joint Tumors

Tenosynovial Giant Cell Tumor

- Develop in the synovial lining of joints, tendon sheaths, and bursae
- 2 types:
- Diffuse tumors-Also called as pigmented villonodular synovitis (MC site-knee)
- Localized type -also known as giant cell tumor of tendon (MC site-wrist) -it is the most common mesenchymal neoplasm of the hand
- Microscopically both show similar changes (Giant cells are more in local variant whereas hemosiderin laden macrophages are predominant in PVNS)

- Both variants show proliferating synoviocytes, macrophages, and may contain hemosiderin or foamy lipid. Scattered multinucleated giant cells and patchy fibrosis are commonly present.

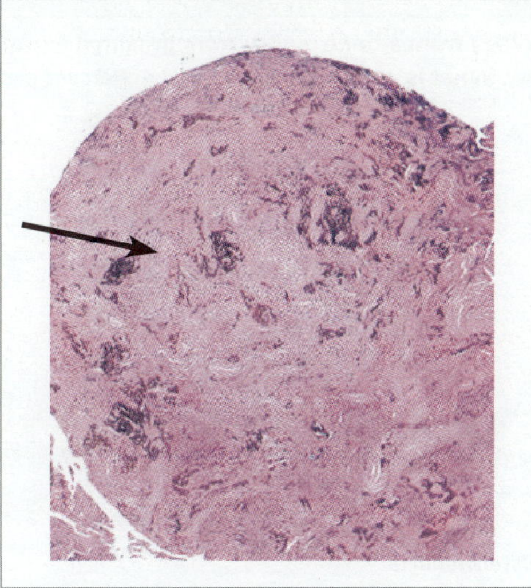

Showing Pigmented Macrophage and Proliferating Synoviocytes suggestive of Pigmented villonodular synovitis

NEXT Pattern Question

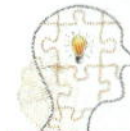

Q's

1. **30 Y/male presented painful enlarging mass in the wrist associated with tenderness. After CT amputation was done, cut section of femur is shown along with corresponding histopathological image. Identify type of tumor?**

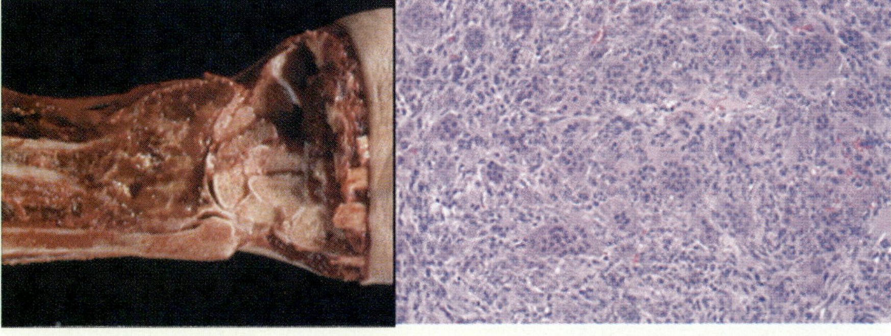

  a. Osteosarcoma   b. Aneurysmal bone cyst   c. Osteoclastoma   d. Pagets disease

Ans. (c) Osteoclastoma

- Painful enlarging mass with the lytic lesion in wrist joint. The histopath is suggestive of giant cells in with the mononuclear tumor cells, this is suggestive of Osteoclastoma.

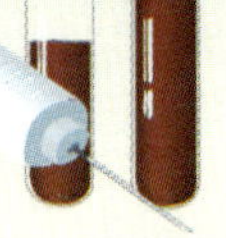

Image-Based Questions

1. Histology from a bone biopsy from proximal femur is given below. What is your diagnosis? *(Recent exam 2018)*

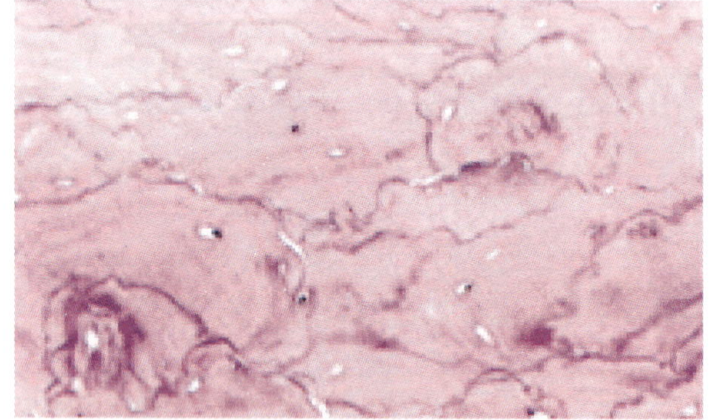

a. Osteomalacia
b. Paget's disease
c. Osteoporosis
d. Osteosclerosis

2. X-ray shows lytic lesion in calceneus in young adult. Biopsy shows following diagnosis:

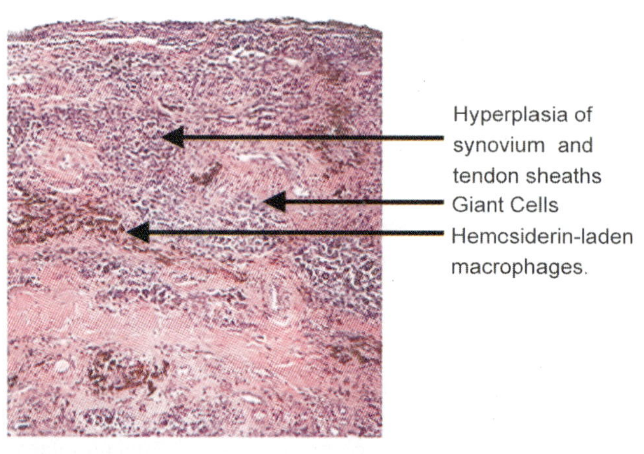

a. Pigmented villonodular synovitis
b. Ochronosis
c. Osteomylitis
d. Eumycosis

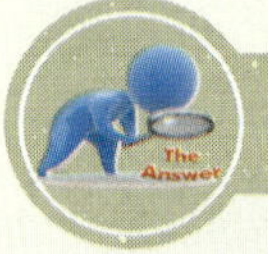

Answers of Image-Based Questions

1. Ans. (b) Paget's disease
Robbins 9th/pg 1190
- Paget disease shows remarkable histologic variation over time and from site to site. The hallmark is a mosaic pattern of lamellar bone, seen in the sclerotic phase. This jigsaw puzzle-like appearance is produced by unusually prominent cement lines, which join haphazardly oriented units of lamellar bone.

2. Ans. (a) Pigmented villonodular synovitis
Image shows hyperplasia of synomin along with hemosiderin laden macrophages and giant cells s/o Pigmented villonodular synovitis.

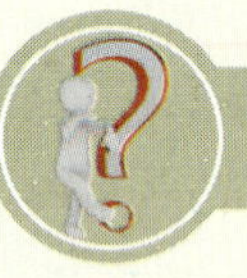

Multiple Choice Questions

1. All are true about Paget's disease of bone except: *(PGIMay2019)*

a. Initially woven pattern, but ultimately lamellar pattern
b. Mosaic pattern in final stage
c. Osteoclasts may have up to 100 nuclei
d. Fibrous connective tissue replaces bone marrow
e. Cortical thickening

2. A 25-year-old female presented with swelling around the knee joint. Biopsy showed giant cells interspersed with mononuclear cells. What is your diagnosis? *(Recent Pattern Question 2020)*

a. Rheumatoid arthritis
b. Osteosarcoma
c. Aneurysmal bone cyst
d. Giant cell tumor

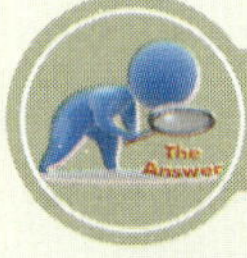

Answers with Explanations

1. Ans. (a) Initially woven pattern, but ultimately lamellar pattern *(Ref: Robbins 9th/pg 1190)*

2. Ans. (d) Giant cell tumor *(Ref: R9th pg 1187)*

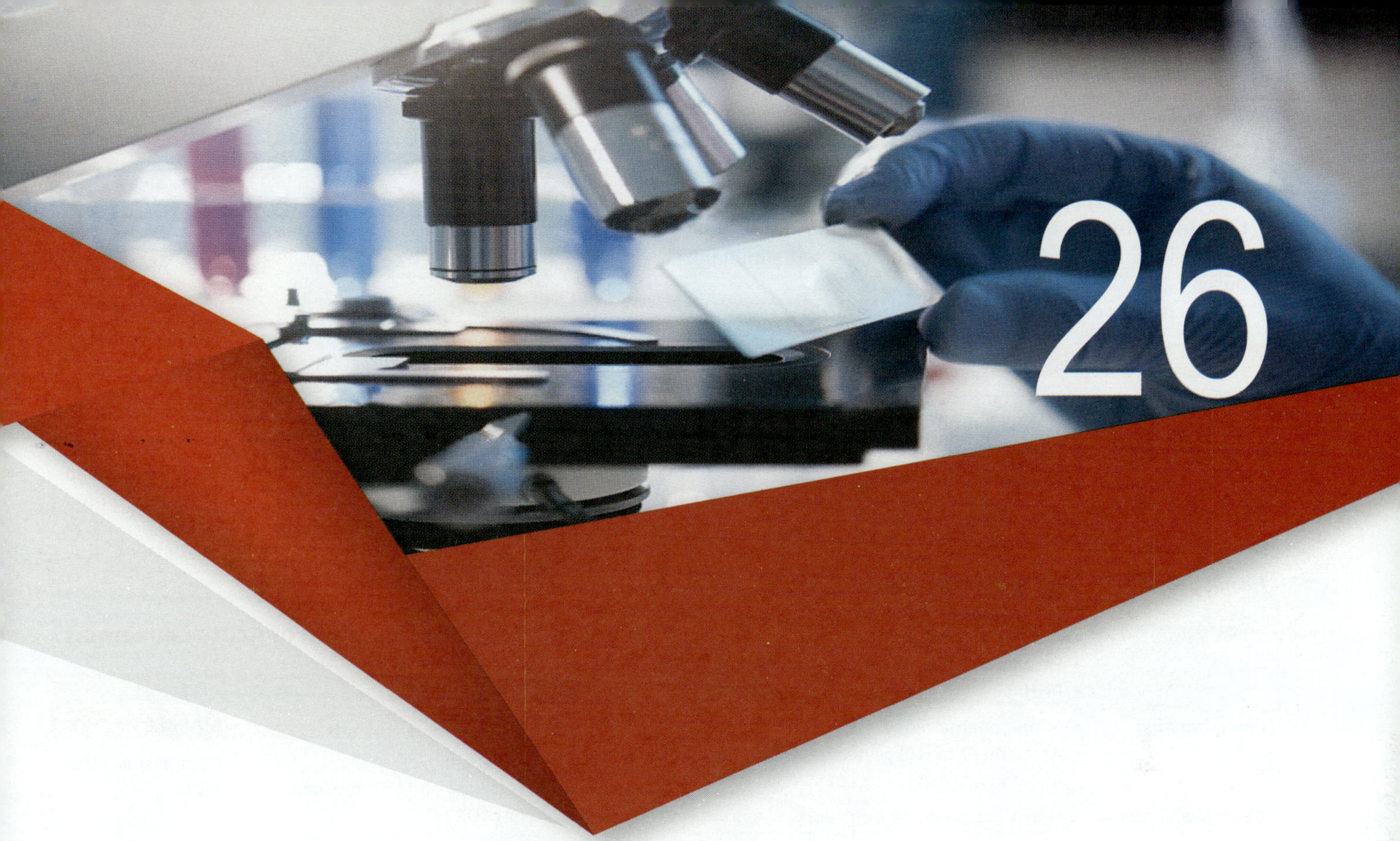

Recent Techniques in Pathology

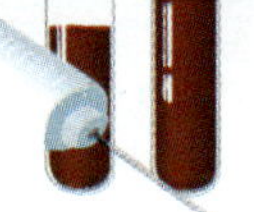

FLOW CYTOMETRY

- Flow cytometry provides rapid analysis of **multiple charac-teristics** of **single cells** made to **flow in a single** line.
- Expression of **several antigens** can be assessed simultane-ously
- The usefulness of FCM immunophenotyping are:

Field	Clinical Application
Immunology	• Histocompatibility cross-matching • Transplantation rejection • **HLA-B27 detection** • Immunodeficiency studies
Oncology	• **DNA content** and S phase of tumors • Measurement of **proliferation markers**
Hematology	• **Leukemia and lymphoma** • Anti-platelet antibodies • Anti-neutrophil antibodies • **Fetomaternal hemorrhage** quantification • **PNH**
Blood banking	• Immunohematology • Assessment of leukocyte contamination of blood products
Genetic disorders	• Leukocyte adhesion deficiency

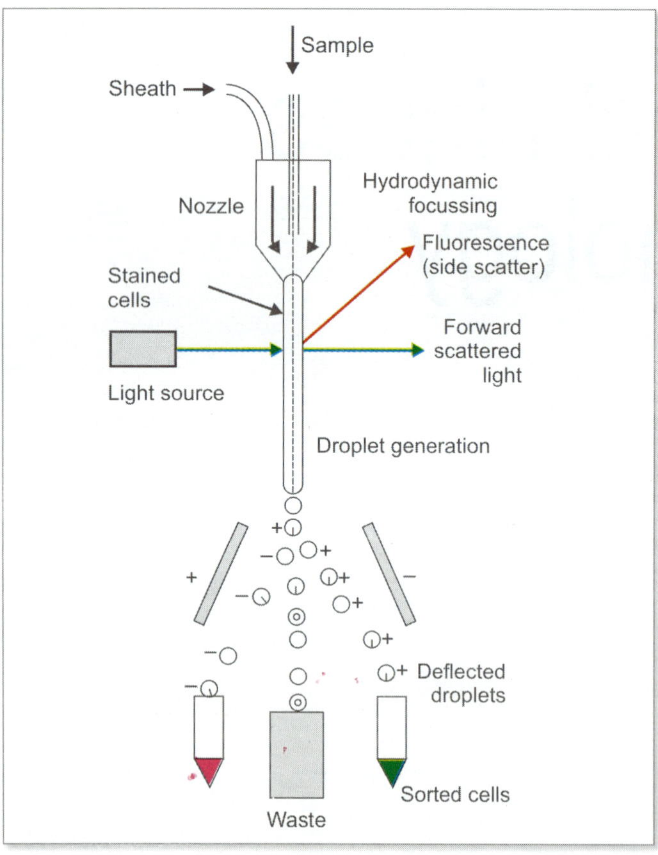

PANEL OF MARKERS FOR FLOW CYTOMETRY

Leukemia	ALL		AML
	B-Cell	**T-Cell**	
First-line	CD19, CD22, CD79a, CD20	CD7, CD2, cCD3	CD13, CD33, CD117, anti-MPO
	TdT, HLA-DR, CD34		
Second-line	cμ, SmIg	CD1a, CD5, CD4, CD8 anti-TCR	CD41, CD42, CD62p, antiglycophorin-A (CD235a), CD11c, CD64

Immunological Classification of Acute Leukemias

Lymphoblastic leukaemia/lymphomas (ALL)- (TdT +)			
B-ALL	**MARKERS**	**T-ALL**	**MARKERS**
B-cell precursor	CD19+ and/or cCD79a+ and/or cCD22+	*T-cell precursor*	Cytoplasmic CD3+, CD7+
Pro-B-ALL	No expression of other B-cell markers	*Pro-T-ALL*	No expression of other T-cell markers
Common-ALL	CD10+, cytoplasmic μ-)	*Pre-T-ALL*	CD2+ and/or CD5+
Pre-B-ALL	Cytoplasmic μ+	*Cortical T-ALL*	CD1a+
		Mature T-ALL	Membrane CD3+

Miscellaneous leukemia	Markers

Mixed phenotype acute leukemias (MPAL) (coexpression of myeloid and lymphoid markers)	**MYELOID COMPONENT:** anti-MPO/cytochemical MPO and/ or monocytic component
	LYMPHOID COMPONENT:
	• **B-lymphoid Differentiation:**
	  ▪ **Strong CD19** plus B-cell marker (CD10, CD22 or CD79)
	  ▪ **Weak/negative CD19** and strong expression of two of the specified B-cell markers.
	• **T-lymphoid Component-** CD3 whether cytoplasmic or membrane.

Myeloid antigen positive ALL	• Leukemia with aberrant markers
Lymphoid antigen positive AML	

Common Phenotypes of B-cell Lymphoproliferative Disorders

Diagnosis	CD5	CD10	CD19	CD20	CD23	CD79b	FMC-7	CD25	CD11c	CD103
SLL/CLL*	+	–	+	+(W)	++	–	–	–/+	+/–	–
Mantle cell lymphoma	+	–	+	+	–	+	+	–	–	–
Follicle center lymphoma	–	+	+	+	–/+	+/–	+/–	–	–	–
Marginal zone lymphoma	–	–	+	+	–	+/–	+/–	–/+	+	–
Hairy cell leukemia	–	–	+	+	–	+/–	+/–	+	++	++

*SLL/CLL small lymphocytic lymphoma/chronic lymphocytic leukemia: +, positive; –, negative; +/–, occasionally positive; w. weak; Red color indicates most important marker for the entity

HIGH PERFORMANCE LIQUID CHROMATOGRAPHY (HPLC)

- A technique for separating mixtures into their components in order to **analyze**, **identify**, and **purify** the mixture or components.

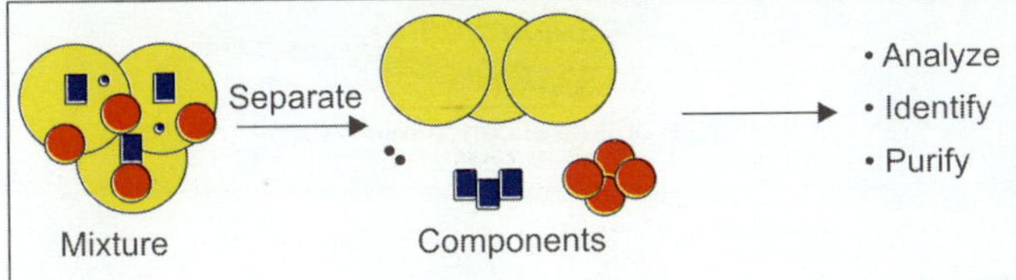

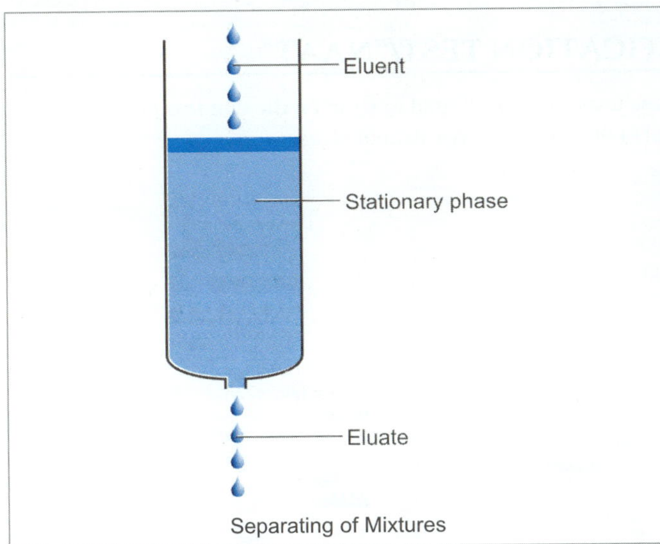

Separating of Mixtures

Important Terminologies used in HPLC

- **Retention time:** Time taken for analyte to pass through the system under set conditions.
- **Stationary Phase:** Fixed in place either in a column or on a planar surface, acts as a adsorbent (atoms that accumulate on the surface of the material)
- **Mobile Phase:** Carries the analyte through the stationary phase, acts as eluent **(solvent that carry the analyte in elution)**

- **Eluent:** Substance used as a solvent in elution
- **Eluate:** Solution of the solvent and the substance that was adsorbed to another

Applications

- Detection of hemoglobin abnormalities
- Toxicology
- Therapeutic and overdose drug monitoring
- HbA_1C levels in DM monitoring
- Protein analysis (Transferrin)
- Nucleic acid sequencing (as replacement to PCR in HLA typing)

High Yield Facts

- Normal Adult Hb %:
  - HbA: 96.5-97.5%
  - HbA_2: 2.5-3.5%
  - HbF: <1%
- **HbA_2>4%** suggests β-thalassemia trait
- **HbA_2>8%** suggests HbE
- HbA_2, HbE and LEPORE **co elute**.

Hb HPLC

Principle: Depends on the interchange of **charged groups** on resin with charged groups on the hemoglobin molecule. Each hemoglobin variant has a specific elution time, which should always be matched with controls

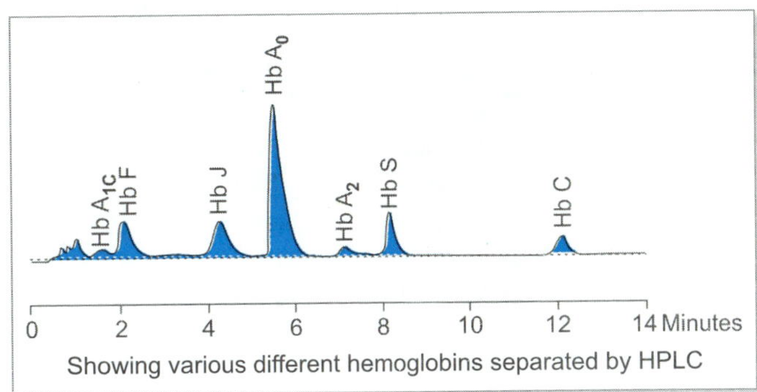

Showing various different hemoglobins separated by HPLC

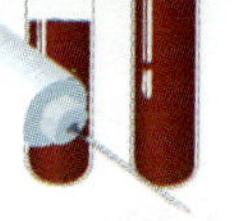

IMMUNOFLUORESCENCE

A technique that utilizes **fluorescent-labeled antibodies** to detect specific target antigens.

Types

- *Direct Immunofluorescence*
  - Uses **fluorescent-tagged antibodies** to bind directly to the target antigen.
  - DIF techniques can also be used to detect non-antibody targets in the skin, such as infectious organisms. In this case, a fluorophore-labeled primary antibody directed against the suspected antigen is used to detect the presence or absence of the organism
- *Indirect Immunofluorescence:* A primary, unlabeled antibody binds to the target, after which a fluorophore-labeled second antibody (directed against the Fc portion of the primary antibody) is used to detect the first antibody.

Purpose

To detect circulating autoantibodies

Fluorescence Detection

It is based on the use of fluorochromes that emit light when excited by light of a shorter wavelength.

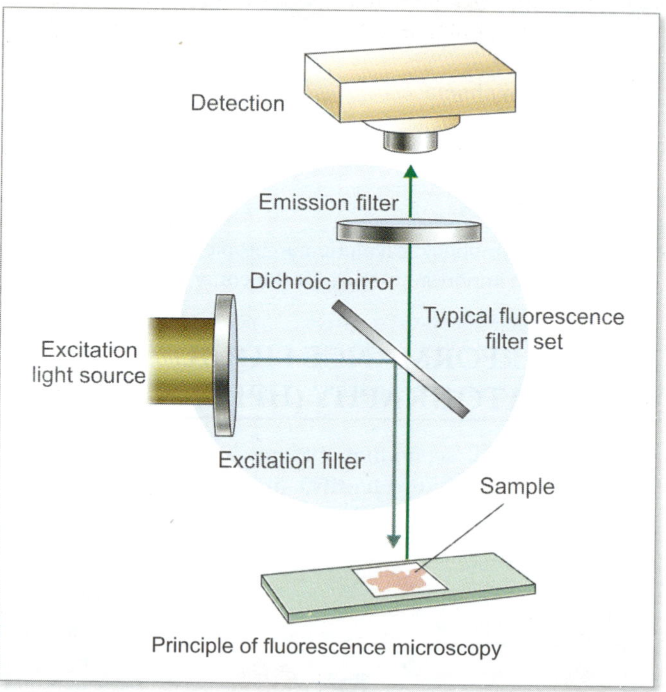

Principle of fluorescence microscopy

NUCLEIC ACID TEST/NUCLEIC ACID AMPLIFICATION TEST/"NAAT"

It is a molecular technique used to detect a **virus or a bacterium**. These tests were developed to **shorten the window period**. The term includes any test that directly detects the genetic material of the infecting organism or virus.

Polymerase Chain Reaction

- PCR was invented by **Kary Mullis** in 1983.
- He shared the **Nobel Prize** in chemistry with Michael Smith in 1993.

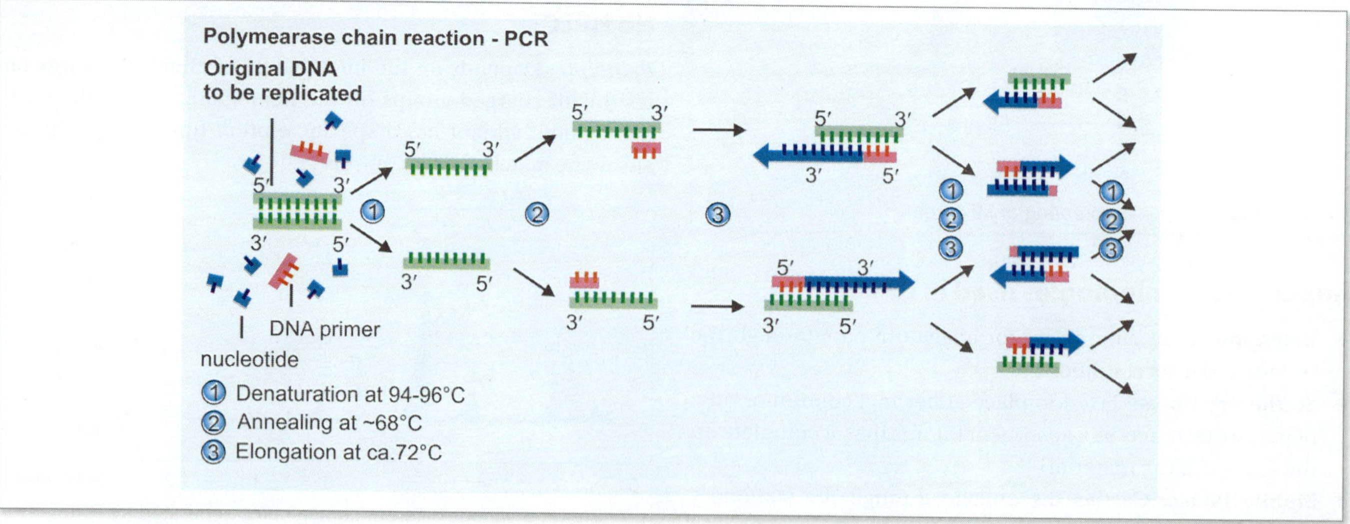

Principle

- **DNA polymerase** adds nucleotides to the 3` end designed **primer (oligonucleotide)** when it is **annealed** to target template DNA.
- Thus, if primer is annealed to a single-stranded template that contains a region complementary to the oligonucleotide, DNA polymerase can use the oligonucleotide as a primer and **elongate its 3′ end** to generate an extended region of **double stranded DNA**.

Types: 2 main Types

- **Real Time PCR:** Quantitative estimation of sample (viral load, DNA, RNA etc)
- **Reverse Transcriptase PCR:** Diagnosis of genetic disorders & semi-quantitatively calculation of specific expression level of particular RNA.

  Reaction Requires: Template DNA, target sequence, specific primers, mixture of dNTPs (Deoxynucleotides), and heat-stable *Taq* DNA polymerase (& **Mg^{2+}** for its activity).

  Taq Polymerase:
- Thermostable DNA polymerase named after the **thermophilic bacterium**
- DNA polymerase from *E. coli* originally used in PCR

FLUORESCENCE IN SITU HYBRIDIZATION (FISH)

- Cytogenetic technique that uses fluorescent probes binding to only **complementary sequences** of parts of the chromosome.
- Used to **detect and localize** the presence or absence of specific DNA sequences on chromosomes.
- FISH can also be used to detect and localize specific RNA targets (**mRNA, lncRNA and miRNA**) in cells, circulating tumor cells, and tissue samples. In this context, it can help define the **spatial-temporal patterns of gene expression** within cells and tissues.

---

1. Flow cytometry is used to detect? *(JIPMER 2017)*
   a. Antibody response
   b. To get differential leukocyte count
   c. **T lymphocytes types**
   d. To separate blood cells

Uses of FISH

Diagnostic	Research
Identification of specific chromosome abnormalities	Identification of new non-random abnormalities
The characterization of marker chromosomes	Gene mapping
Interphase FISH for specific abnormalities in cases of failed cytogenetics	Identification of regions of amplification or deletion by CGH
Monitoring disease progression	Identification of translocation breakpoints
Monitoring the success of bone marrow transplantation	Study of 3D chromosome organization in interphase nuclei

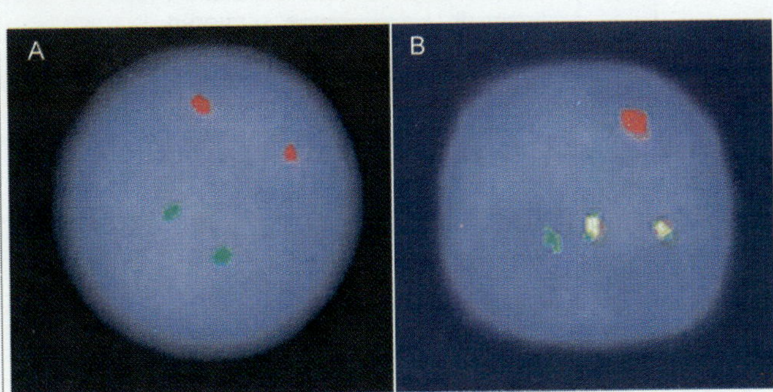

FISH with dual fusion probes on two separate nuclei to detect. (A) Normal nuclei (green and red separate) while (B) nuclei containing BCR/ABL double fusions indicated by green-red fusion (yellow) signals.

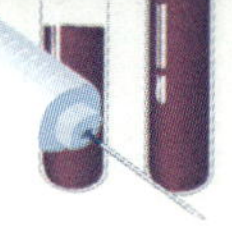
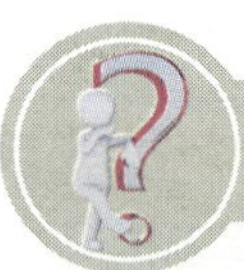

Image-Based Questions

1. Forward scatter in Flowcytometry indicates?

(AIIMS May 2015)

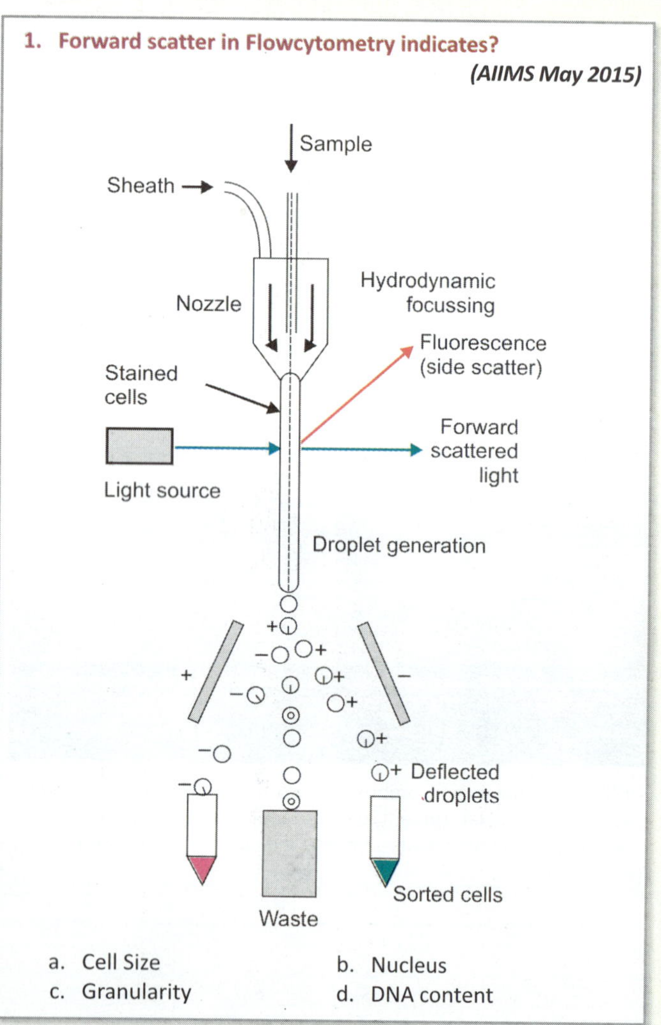

a. Cell Size
b. Nucleus
c. Granularity
d. DNA content

2. Identify the HPLC pattern: *(Recent Question 2016)*

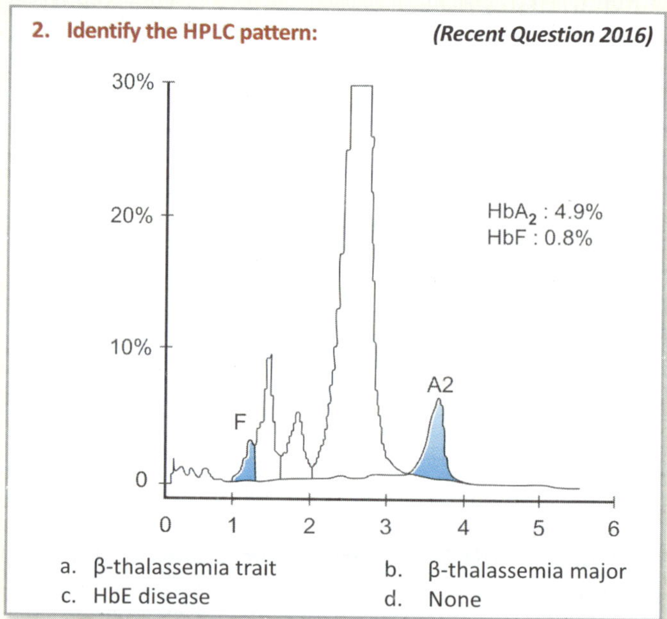

a. β-thalassemia trait
b. β-thalassemia major
c. HbE disease
d. None

3. The given technique is very important in the diagnostic field. Which of the following os an important component for viewing by this technique? *(AIIMS May 2015)*

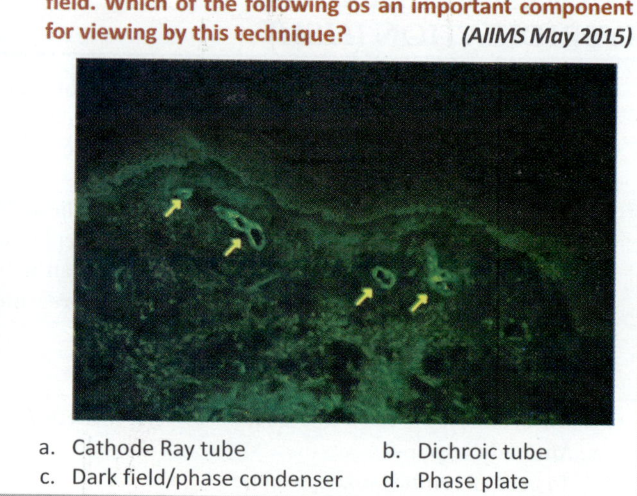

a. Cathode Ray tube
b. Dichroic tube
c. Dark field/phase condenser
d. Phase plate

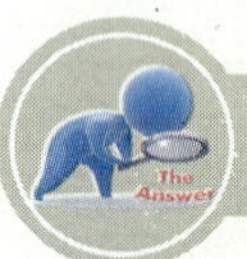

Answers of Image-Based Questions

1. Ans. (a) Cell Size

On flow cytometry
- Forward scatter-cell size
- Side scatter-granularity

2. Ans. (a) β-thalassemia trait-HbA2 >4%

3. Ans. (b) Dichroic tube

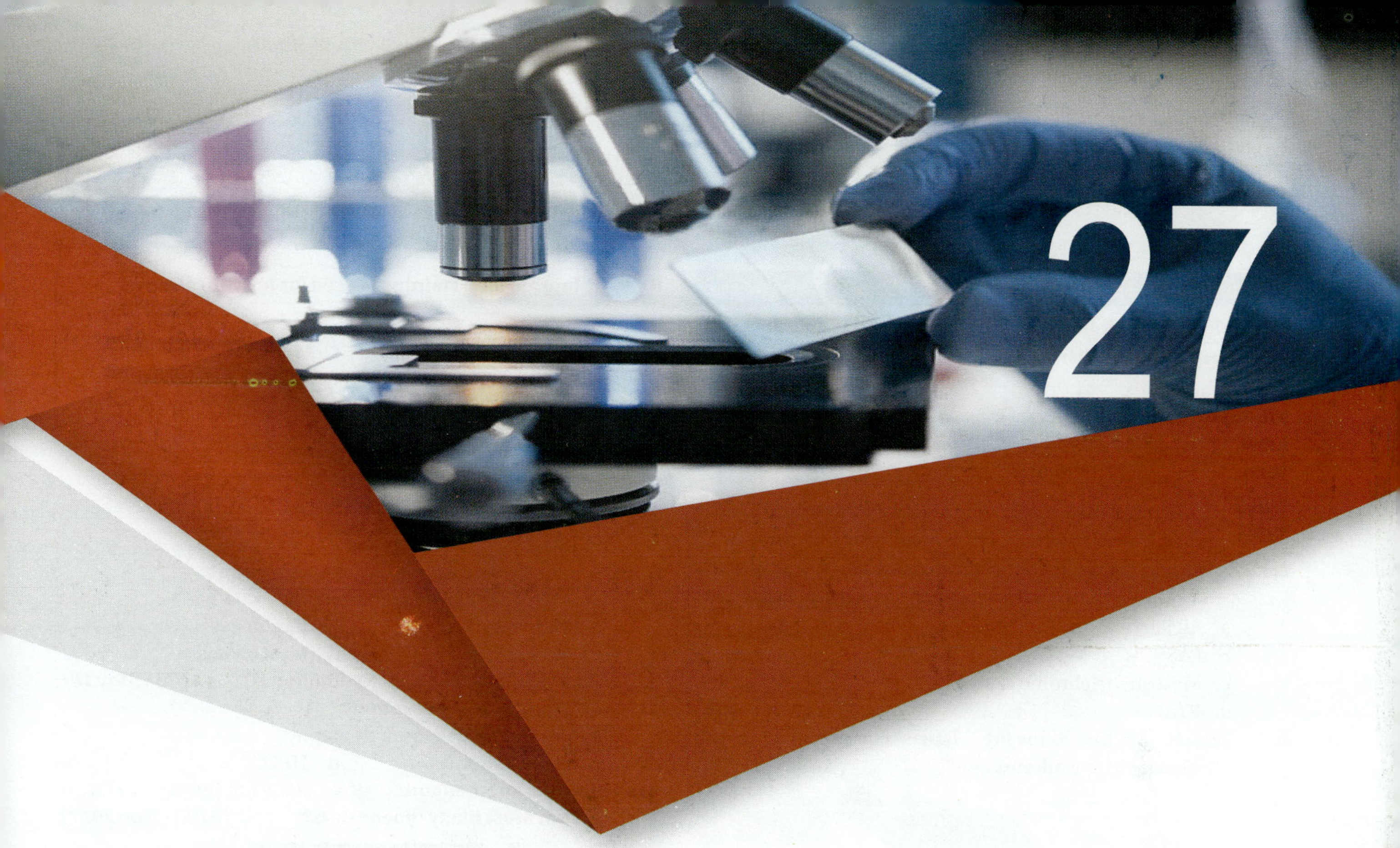

Stains and Fixatives

Multiple Choice Questions

STAINS & FIXATIVES

1. Match the following viral intracellular bodies with respect to the disease? *(AIIMS Nov 2019)*

Column A	Column B
a. HPV	1. Henderson-Paterson bodies
b. CMV	2. Decoy cells
c. Molluscum contagiosum	3. Owl eye inclusion
d. Polyomavirus	4. Koilocyte

2. Which of the following stain is used for Acidic mucin? *(AIIMS May 18)*

a. Alcian blue
b. PAS
c. Masson's trichrome stain
d. PTAH

3. Which of the following labels corresponds to the condenser of the microscope? *(AIIMS May 18)*

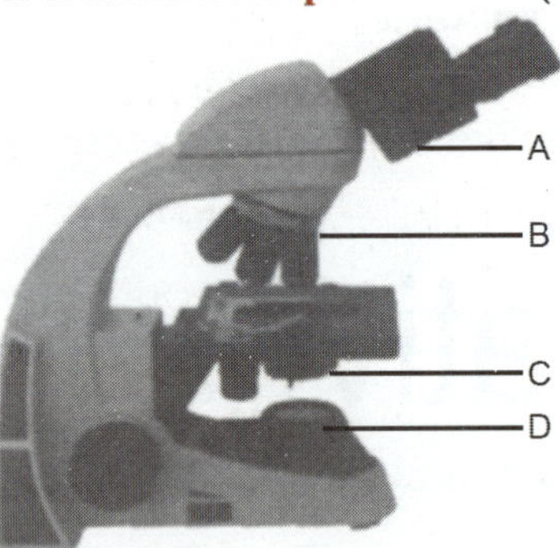

a. C
b. B
c. D
d. A

4. Which of the following are false about electron microscopy? *(PGI May 18)*

a. High resolving power
b. Can see both live and dead objects
c. Vacuum is required
d. Three-dimensional images can be obtained
e. Coloured images are seen

5. Microscopy which can be performed with minimum optical illumination? *(PGI May 18)*

a. Dark field
b. Phase contrast
c. Bright-field microscopy
d. Fluorescent microscopy
e. Inverted microscopy

6. Toluidine blue staining is used for identification of? *(AIIMS May 18)*

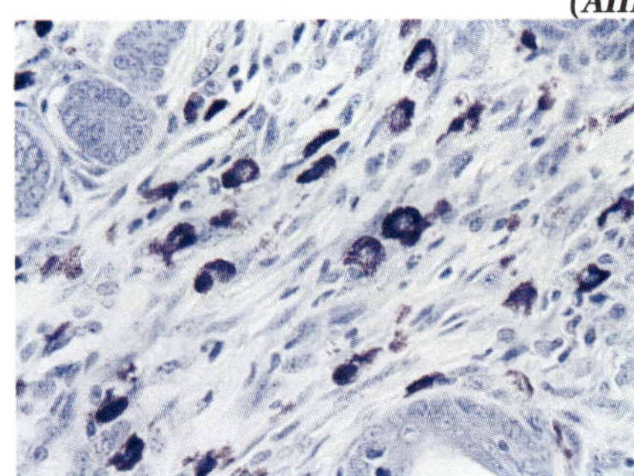

a. Mast cell   b. Fibroblast
c. Melanocyte   d. Macrophages

7. Best method for HbA1c estimation is? *(AIIMS May 18)*

a. Affinity chromatography
b. Ion exchange chromatography
c. Electrophoresis   d. HPLC

8. Gomori methenamine silver stain for fungus is shown below. Most likely diagnosis is? *(AIIMS Nov 2017)*

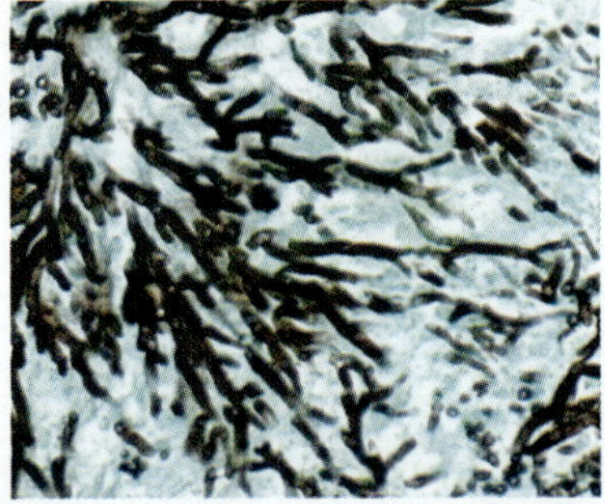

a. Acute angle branching with septate hyphae - Aspergillus
b. Right angle branching and aseptate hyphae- Mucor
c. Acute angle branching with septate hyphae - Mucor
d. Right angle branching and aseptate hyphae- Aspergillus

9. Identify the stain done on a section of liver shown below? *(AIIMS May 2017)*

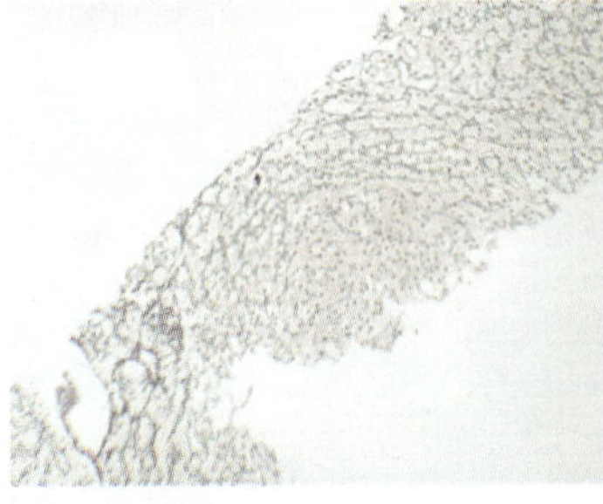

a. Sweets reticulin stain
b. Gremilus silver stain
c. Warthin starry silver stain
d. Steiner silver stain

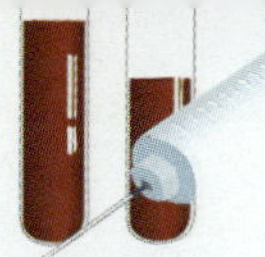

10. **For detection of carcinoma lip, stain used is?**
    a. Giemsa   *(AIIMS Nov 2016)*
    b. Crystal violet
    c. Toulidine blue
    d. Hematoxylin and eosin

11. **Given below is the histopathology of liver biopsy of hemochromatosis. Which of the following stain is used?**
                                                       (AIIMS Nov 2016)

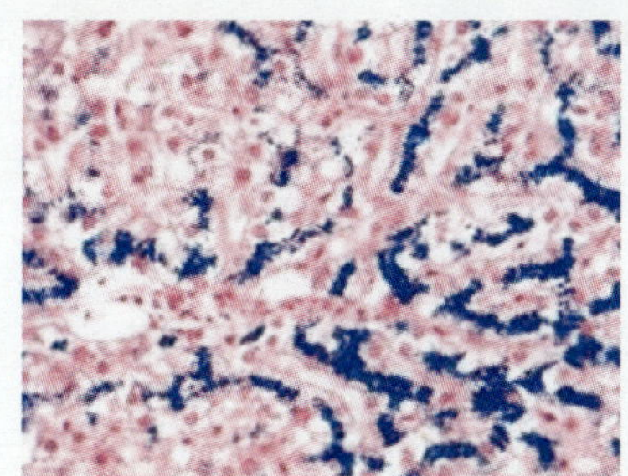

    a. Von kossa   b. Alcian blue
    c. Prussian blue   d. Crystal violet

12. **Which of the following is a correct match?**
    a. Perl stain -Iron   *(PGI Nov 2016)*
    b. Von Gieson-Collagen
    c. Mason Trichrome-elastin
    d. PAS-glycogen
    e. PAS- Acidic and neutral mucin

13. **Which of the following stain and the material stained by it is correct?**
                                                       (PGI Nov 2016)
    a. Perl stain-Iron
    b. Collagen- Von kossa
    c. Elastin-Von Geison
    d. Copper-modified rhodamine
    e. Oil red O - Glycogen

14. **Toluidine blue has been established as a diagnostic adjunct in detecting oral lesions related to invasive carcinomas, carcinoma in situ or early asymptomatic oral carcinomas Stain used for hemachromatosis**
                                                       (Recent Question 2016-17)
    a. Prussian blue stain   b. Von Kossa
    c. Sudan black   d. Methenamine silver

15. **Oil red O stain is used for?**   *(AIIMS May 2015)*
    a. Frozen specimen
    b. Glutaraldehyde fixed specimen
    c. Alcohol fixed specimen
    d. Formalin fixed specimen

16. **Which of the following cellular component gives purplish blue color with H & E reagent:**
                                                       (PGI May 2015)
    a. Reticulum   b. Elastin
    c. P-selectin   d. Collagen
    e. Heterochromatin

17. **Which of the following stain is used for staining of glycogen?**
                                                       (Recent Question 2016)
    a. PAS   b. Oli Red –O
    c. Sudan black   d. Von kossa

18. **Perl' stain is for:**   *(Recent Question 2015)*
    a. Iron   b. Copper
    c. Melanin   d. Glycogen

19. **Stain used for copper:**   *(Recent Question 2015)*
    a. Congo red   b. Prussian blue
    c. PAS   d. Rubeanic acid

20. **Tissues for electron microscopy are fixed in:**
                                                       (Recent Question 2015)
    a. Carnoy's fixative   b. 10% buffered formalin
    c. 4% gluteraldehyde   d. 50% glycerine

21. **Frozen section was introduced by:**
                                                       (Recent Question 2015)
    a. Virchow   b. Feulgen
    c. Morgagni   d. Cohnheim

22. **Stain for collagen:**   *(Recent Question 2015)*
    a. Von gieson   b. Von kossa
    c. Alizarin red   d. Rubeanic acid

23. **Stain for axons:**   *(Recent Question 2015)*
    a. Phosphotungstic acid-Hematoxylin (PTAH)
    b. Luxol fast blue
    c. Bileschowsky's silver
    d. Masson fontana

24. **Stain for hepatitis B surface antigen:**
    a. Fite-wade   *(Recent Question 2015)*
    b. Grocott's silver methanamine
    c. Shiata's orciein
    d. Grimelius

25. **Histopathological specimens are commonly preserved in:**
                                                       (Recent Question 2015)
    a. 10%formalin   b. 4% gluteraldehyde
    c. Rectified spirit   d. Saturated saline solution

26. **PTAH stain is used for staining:**
    a. Myelin   *(Recent Question 2015)*
    b. Axon
    c. Muscle and glial filamets
    d. Melanin

27. **Heart failure cells can be stained by:**
                                                       (Recent Question 2015)
    a. PAS   b. Prussian blue
    c. Congo red   d. Gram stain

28. **Gauge of commonly used FNAC needle is?**
                                                       (Recent Question 2015)
    a. 26-29   b. 22-26
    c. 18-22   d. 16-18

29. **Ocular basement membrane is stained by:**
                                                       (Recent Question 2015)
    a. Alcian blue   b. PAS
    c. Methylene blue   d. Geimsa stain

30. **Acid mucin is best demonstrated by the stain:**
    a. Alcian blue   *(Recent Question 2015)*
    b. Periodic Acid Schiff (PAS)
    c. Van Giesen
    d. Reticulin

31. **The fixative used in histopathology:**
                                                       (Recent Question 2014; AIIMS May 12)
    a. 10% buffered neutral formalin
    b. Bouins fixative
    c. Glutaraldehyde
    d. Ethyl alcohol

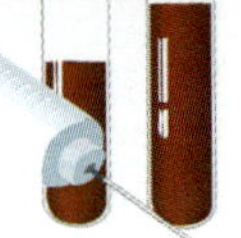

32. **Stain used for glycogen:** *(Recent Question 2014)*
   a. PAS
   b. Congo red
   c. Prussian blue
   d. Alician blue

33. **Which of the following statement is TRUE?**
   a. Gomori Methamine silver stain stains fungi green
   b. Gram +ve stains bacteria black *(AIIMS May 2014)*
   c. Gram –ve stains red
   d. Calcoflor stains red in colour

34. **Most common fixative used in electron microscopy:**
   (AIIMS May 2013, Nov 2012)
   a. Glutaraldehyde
   b. Formalin
   c. Picric acid
   d. Absolute alcohol

35. **Staining done for sebaceous cell carcinoma:**
   a. Oil Red O
   b. PAS *(AIIMS May 2013)*
   c. Methamine silver
   d. KOH

36. **Liver in hemochromatosis is stained by:**
   (Recent Question 2013)
   a. Masson Fontana
   b. Prussian blue
   c. Masson trichrome
   d. Congo red

37. **Stain used for melanin:** *(Recent Question 2013)*
   a. Masson Fontana
   b. Prussain blue
   c. Masson trichrome
   d. Congo red

38. **Which of the following is a negative stain:**
   (Recent Question 2013)
   α. Negrosin
   β. Fonatana
   χ. ZN stain
   δ. Albert stain

39. **The most common fixative used in pathology is?**
   a. Gluteraldehyde
   b. Alcohol *(AI 11)*
   c. Formaldehyde
   d. Picric acid

40. **Fixative used for histopathology is?** *(DNB Dec 11)*
   a. 10%formalin
   b. Normal saline
   c. Rectified spirit
   d. 100% alcohol

41. **Resolving power of a light microscope does not depend on?** *(AIIMS Nov 2016)*
   a. Power of eyepiece
   b. Wavelength of light used
   c. Power of the lens
   d. Thickness of the specimen

42. **The following image is taken from a Neubauer chamber after charging of fluid. If the dilution factor is 20, what is the total cell count per cu.mm?**
   (Recent Question 2016-17; AIIMS Nov 2016)

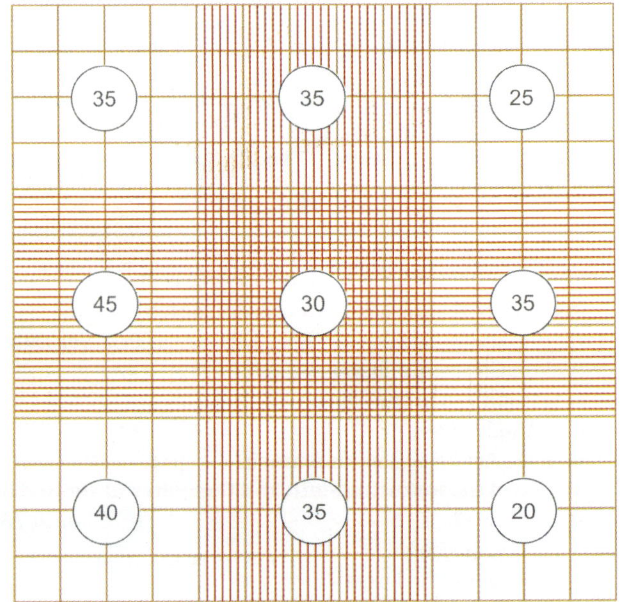

   a. 6000
   b. 3000
   c. 7000
   d. 1100

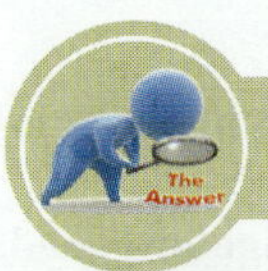

Answers with Explanations

1. Ans. (a) 4, (b) 3, (c) 1, (d) 2

Viral Inclusion Bodies

Intracyto-plasmic		Henderson-Peterson bodies (Molluscum Contagiosum)	
		Negri bodies (Rabies)	
		Guarnieri bodies (Smallpox)	
		Paschen bodies (Smallpox)	
		Bollinger bodies (Fowl pox)	
		Borrel bodies (Fowl pox)	
Intranuclear	Acidophilic	Cowdry type A	Varicella zoster virus
			Herpes simplex virus
			Yellow fever virus
		Cowdry type B	Polio virus
	Basophilic	Cowdry type B	Adeno virus
			Cytomegalo virus

2. Ans. (a) Alcian blue

3. Ans. (a) C

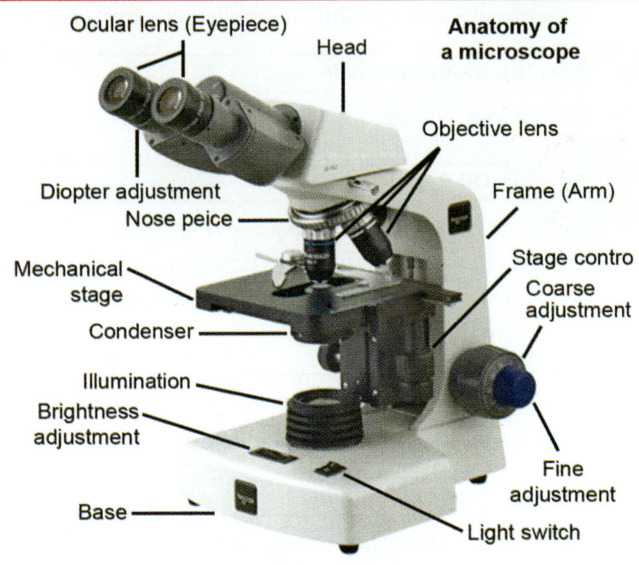

4. Ans. (b, e); b. Can see both live and dead objects; e. Coloured images are seen

5. Ans. (a) Dark field

Darkfield microscopy reduces the amount of light entering the lens system of a microscope in two ways. First, it blocks the center of the beam of light that would otherwise fill the objective lens. Second, only the light which is scattered by the specimen and enters the objective lens is seen

6. Ans. (a) Mast cell

Toluidine blue (also known as tolonium chloride) is an acidophilic metachromatic dye that selectively stains acidic tissue components (sulfates, carboxylates, and phosphate radicals), has an affinity for nucleic acids, and therefore binds to nuclear material of tissues with a high DNA and RNA content. Mast cell granules stain purple in color due to the presence of heparin and histamine.

7. Ans. (d) HPLC

Four basic types of methods are used most commonly to measure HbA1c: immunoassay, ion-exchange high-performance liquid chromatography (HPLC), boronate affinity HPLC, and enzymatic assays. The gold standard is HPLC method

8. Ans. (a) Acute angle branching with septate hyphae - Aspergillus

Mucor- Broad base with obtuse branching
Aspergillus- Acute branching, Septate hyphae with narrow base

9. Ans. (a) Sweets reticulin stain

(Ref: Bancroft histochemical techniques. p. 180)

Reticulin stain: Demonstrates reticular fibers and basement membrane material. Reticular fibers are thin, usually type III collagen, widespread in connective tissue throughout the body. Staining procedures are Gordon and Sweet's reticulin stain (mc) & Gomori reticulin stain

10. Ans. (c) Toulidine blue

(Ref: Early Diagnosis and Treatment of Cancer Series: Head and Neck Cancers, Wayne Koch Pg. 54)

- **Toluidine blue** stain is used as a marker to **differentiate lesions at high risk of progression** in order to improve early diagnosis of oropharyngeal carcinomas.
- Toluidine blue, an **acidophilic metachromatic dye** of **thiazine group** selectively stains acidic tissue components (sulfates, carboxylates and phosphate radicals), thus staining DNA and RNA.

11. Ans. (c) Prussian blue

(Ref: Bancroft's histological techniques, 7th ed)

12. Ans. (a) Perl stain -Iron, (d) PAS-glycogen

(Ref: Bancroft's histological techniques, 7th ed)

Note:
- **Verhoff-Von gieson** stain is for elastin fibres
- **Alcian blue** is for differentiating Acidic and neutral mucin
- **Masson trichrome** is for collagen

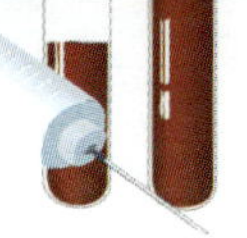

13. Ans. (a) **Perl stain-Iron,** (c) **Elastin-Von Geison,** (d) **Copper-modified rhodamine,** (e) **Oil red O - Glycogen**

(*Ref: Bancroft's histological techniques, 7th ed*)

14. Ans. (a) **Prussian blue stain**

(*Ref: Bancroft's histological techniques, 7th ed*)

15. Ans. (a) **Frozen specimen**

(*Ref: Bancroft's histological techniques, 7th ed*)

16. Ans. (a, e) **a. Reticulum; e. Heterochromatin**

(*Ref: Bancroft's histological techniques, 7th ed*)

H&E Stain (Hematoxylin and Eosin)

- Hematoxylin, a natural dye product, acts as a basic dye that stains blue or black.
- Nuclear heterochromatin stains blue and the cytoplasm of cells rich in ribonucleoprotein also stains blue.
- The cytoplasm of cells with minimal amounts of ribonucleoprotein tends to be lavender in color.
- The aniline dye, eosin, is an acid dye that stains cytoplasm, muscle, and connective tissues various shades of pink and orange.
- This difference in staining intensity is useful in differentiating one tissue from another.

17. Ans. (a) **PAS** (*Ref: Bancroft's staining 7th ed*)

18. Ans. (a) **Iron** (*Ref: Bancroft's staining 7th ed*)

19. Ans. (d) **Rubeanic acid** (*Ref: Bancroft's staining 7th ed*)

20. Ans. (c) **4% gluteraldehyde**

(*Ref: Bancroft's staining 7th ed*)

21. Ans. (d) **Cohnheim** (*Ref: Bancroft's staining 7th ed*)

22. Ans. (a) **Von gieson** (*Ref: Bancroft's staining 7th ed*)

23. Ans. (c) **Bileschowsky's silver**

(*Ref: Bancroft's staining 7th ed*)

24. Ans. (c) **Shiata'sorciein** (*Ref: Bancroft's staining 7th ed*)

25. Ans. (a) **10% formalin** (*Ref: Bancroft's staining 7th ed*)

26. Ans. (c) **Muscle and glial filamets**

(*Ref: Bancroft's staining 7th ed*)

27. Ans. (b) **Prussian blue** (*Ref: Bancroft's staining 7th ed*)

28. Ans. (b) **22-26**

(*Ref: Bancroft's histological techniques, 7th edition*)

- **FNAC** is **Fine-Needle Aspiration Cytology** or Needle aspiration biopsy.
- A needle attached to a syringe is used to **collect cells from lesions or masses** in various body organs by microcoring, often with the application of **negative pressure (suction) to increase yield.**

- FNAC can be performed **under palpation or imaging guidance** (USG or CT scan)
- For FNAC, **Fine needles of 23 to 27 gauge** are used; most commonly used is a **25-gauge needle.**
- Core needle biopsy (CNB) is increasingly replacing FNAC because of the **inability of FNAC to distinguish carcinoma in-situ from invasive carcinoma**

29. Ans. (b) **PAS** (*Ref: Bancroft's staining 7th ed*)

PAS is used to stain **carbohydrates (polysaccharides), neutral mucus (glycoproteins and glycolipids), tissue basement membrane, fungal cell wall.**

30. Ans. (a) **Alcian blue** (*Ref: Bancroft's staining 7th ed*)

31. Ans. (a) **10% buffered neutral formalin**

(*Ref: Bancroft's histological techniques, 7th edition*)

32. Ans. (a) **PAS**

(*Ref: Bancroft's histological techniques, 7th edition*)

33. Ans. (c) **Gram –ve stains red**

(*Ref: Bancroft's histological techniques, 7th edition*)

Discussing the options one by one:
A. False, as it stains fungi black, against a green background
B. False, as Gram +ve stains bacteria blue
C. True
D. False, as it stains Acanthamoeba white & not red

34. Ans. (a) **Glutaraldehyde**

(*Ref: Bancroft's histological techniques, 7th edition*)

35. Ans. (a) **Oil Red O**

(*Ref: Bancroft's histological techniques, 7th edition*)

Oil red O stain, Sudan III, Sudan IV & Sudan black are used to stain Fat, seen in sebaceous cell carcinoma

36. Ans. (b) **Prussian blue**

(*Ref: Bancroft's histological techniques, 7th edition*)

Iron accumulates in Liver in **hemochromatosis**

37. Ans. (a) **Masson Fontana**

(*Ref: Bancroft's histological techniques, 7th edition*)

38. Ans. (a) **Negrosin**

(*Ref: Bancroft's histological techniques, 7th edition*)

Examples of **negative stain** are:
- **Negrosin:** Stains bacteria, Cryptococcus, test for viability (sperms)
- **India Ink:** Stains Cryptococcus

39. Ans. (c) **Formaldehyde**

(*Ref: Bancroft's histological techniques, 7th edition*)

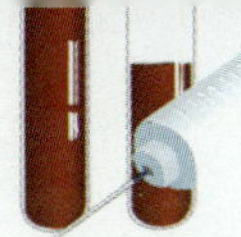

40. Ans. (a) 10% formalin

(Ref: Bancroft's histological techniques, 7th edition)

41. Ans. (d) Thickness of the specimen

(Ref: Laboratory Diagnosis of Infectious Diseases: Essentials of Diagnostic Pg. 130)

- **Resolving power:** It is defined as the **inverse of the distance or angular separation between two objects** which can be just resolved when viewed through the optical instrument.
- Resolving power of a microscope:
- For microscopes, the resolving power is the **inverse of the distance between two objects that can be just resolved**. This is given by the famous Abbe's criterion given by Ernst Abbe in 1873 as

$$\Delta d = \frac{\lambda}{2n \sin\theta}$$

$$\text{Resolving power} = \frac{\lambda}{\Delta d} = \frac{2n\sin\theta}{\lambda}$$

- Where n is the refractive index of the medium separating object and aperture. Note that to achieve high resolution $n \sin\theta$ must be large. **This is known as the Numerical aperture**.

Thus, for good resolution:
- **$\sin\theta$ must be large.**
- To achieve this, the objective lens is kept as close to the specimen as possible.
- A **higher refractive index (n)** medium must be used. Oil immersion microscopes use oil to increase the refractive index.
- **Decreasing the wavelength** by using X-rays and gamma rays. While these techniques are used to study inorganic crystals, biological samples are usually damaged by x-rays and hence are not used.

42. Ans. (a) 6000

(Ref: Text book of practical physiology GK Pal. Pg. 63)

Note the squares:

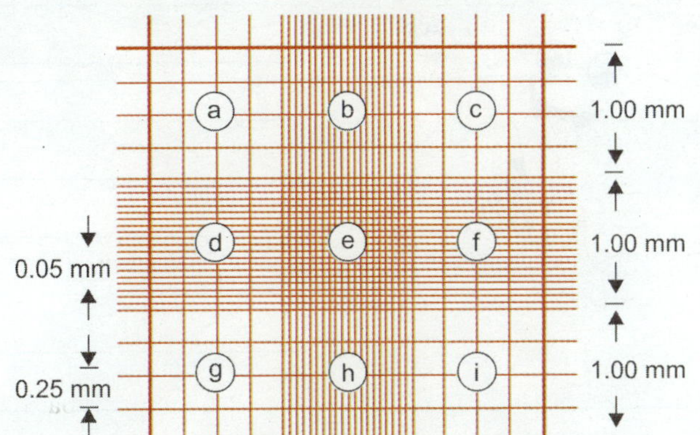

- Each of the squares (a to i) has a dimension of 1mm x1mm
- When you keep a cover slip over this chamber, the depth is 0.1mm
- So the total volume is 1X1X 0.1mm 3 = 0.1mm3 or ul Calculation:
- Concentration of cells = n/v xd
- Where (n = number of cells, V = volume, d = dilution)
- Coming back to the question: total number of cells in the 4 squares (a, c, g,i) = 35 + 25 + 40 + 20 = 120
- Volume of 4 squares= 4 × 0.1 = 0.4mm3
- So concentration = 120/0.4 × 20 = **6000/mm³ or uL**

Note